MW00454209

APPLIED CLINICAL PHARMACOKINETICS

NOTICE

Medicine is an ever-changing science. As new research and clinical experience broaden our knowledge, changes in treatment and drug therapy are required. The author and the publisher of this work have checked with sources believed to be reliable in their efforts to provide information that is complete and generally in accord with the standards accepted at the time of publication. However, in view of the possibility of human error or changes in medical sciences, neither the author nor the publisher nor any other party who has been involved in the preparation or publication of this work warrants that the information contained herein is in every respect accurate or complete, and they disclaim all responsibility for any errors or omissions or the results obtained from the use of such information contained in this work. Readers are encouraged to confirm the information contained herein with other sources. For example and in particular, readers are advised to check the product information sheet included in the package of each drug they plan to administer to be certain that the information contained in this book is accurate and that changes have not been made in the recommended dose or in the contraindications for administration. This recommendation is of particular importance in connection with new or infrequently used drugs.

APPLIED CLINICAL PHARMACOKINETICS

by

LARRY A. BAUER, PharmD
Associate Professor
Departments of Pharmacy and Laboratory Medicine
Schools of Pharmacy and Medicine
University of Washington
Seattle, Washington

McGRAW-HILL

Medical Publishing Division

New York Chicago San Francisco Lisbon London
Madrid Mexico City Milan New Delhi San Juan Seoul Singapore Sydney Toronto

McGraw-Hill

A Division of The ***McGraw-Hill*** *Companies*

APPLIED CLINICAL PHARMACOKINETICS

Copyright © 2001 by The McGraw-Hill Companies.
All rights reserved. Printed in the United States of America.
Except as permitted under the United States Copyright Act
of 1976, no part of this publication may be reproduced or
distributed in any form or by any means, or stored
in a data base or retrieval system, without the prior written
permission of the publisher.

1234567890 DOCDOC 0987654321

ISBN 0-8385-0388-8

This book was set in Times Roman by Rainbow Graphics.
The editors were Stephen Zollo and Karen G. Edmonson.
The index was prepared by Steven Shimer.
The production supervisor was Richard Ruzycka.
The text was designed by Joan O'Connor.
The illustration manager was Charissa Baker.
R. R. Donnelley and Sons was the printer and binder.

This book is printed on acid-free paper.

Library of Congress
Cataloging-in-Publication Data

Bauer, Larry A.
Applied clinical pharmacokinetics / by Larry A. Bauer.
p. ; cm.
Includes bibliographical references and index.
ISBN 0-8385-0388-8 (hardback)
1. Pharmacokinetics. I. Title.
[DNLM: 1. Pharmacokinetics. 2. Pharmaceutical Preparations—administration & dosage. QV 38 B344a 2001]
RM301.5 .B384 2001
615′.7—dc21

00-045078

I am most grateful to my family,
especially my wife (S.P.B.)
and daughters (L.A.B. & L.E.B.),
for allowing me the time
to fulfill a life-long dream.

—L.A.B.

P.S. Mom, I finally did it!

CONTENTS

PART IV ANTICONVULSANTS

PART V IMMUNOSUPPRESSANTS

PART VI OTHER DRUGS

ABOUT THE AUTHOR

Larry A. Bauer, Pharm.D. is an Associate Professor at the University of Washington School of Pharmacy and has been on the faculty since 1980. He also holds an adjunct appointment at the same rank in the Department of Laboratory Medicine, where he is a toxicology consultant. He received his Bachelor of Science in Pharmacy degree (1977) from the University of Washington and his Doctor of Pharmacy degree (1980) from the University of Kentucky. He also completed an ASHP-accredited hospital pharmacy residency (1980) specializing in clinical pharmacokinetics from A. B. Chandler Medical Center at the University of Kentucky under the preceptorship of Dr. Paul Parker. Dr. Bauer is a fellow of the American College of Clinical Pharmacology and the American College of Clinical Pharmacy.

Dr. Bauer's specialty area is clinical pharmacokinetics, and he teaches courses and offers clinical clerkships in this area. His research interests include the pharmacokinetics and pharmacodynamics of drug interactions, the effects of liver disease and age on drug metabolism, and computer modeling of population pharmacokinetics. He has over 135 published research papers and abstracts. Dr. Bauer is a member of several clinical pharmacology and clinical pharmacy professional organizations. He is a reviewer for several scientific publications, was Consulting Editor of *Clinical Pharmacy* (1981–1990) and Field Editor of *ASHP Signal* (1981–1983), and is currently on the editorial boards of *Clinical Pharmacology and Therapeutics* and *Antimicrobial Agents and Chemotherapy.* Also, he is a Regent of the American College of Clinical Pharmacology. Dr. Bauer has precepted three postdoctoral fellows in clinical pharmacokinetics who currently have faculty appointments in schools of pharmacy or positions in the pharmaceutical industry.

PREFACE

Being a practitioner for over 20 years, I have had an opportunity to see the development of therapeutic drug monitoring almost from its inception. What began in the late 1960s and early 1970s as a way to optimize cardiac glycoside and aminoglycoside antibiotic treatment for patients has, in the 21st century, blossomed into an integral part of patient care for many drugs. On any given day, our clinical laboratory at the University of Washington reports the results of over 200 patient drug concentration assays to clinicians.

The structure of this book is uniform for each chapter and is derived from my lectures in clinical pharmacokinetics. In each chapter, the introduction is a brief discussion of the clinical pharmacology and mechanism of action for the specific drug and is followed by a section that describes the therapeutic concentration range and anticipated adverse effects of the drug as well as a general monitoring scheme for the agent. Next, clinical monitoring parameters for therapeutic response and toxicity and basic clinical pharmacokinetic parameters for the compound are discussed. The sections that follow describe the effects of disease states and conditions on the pharmacokinetics and dosing of the drug, and the drug interactions that may occur with concurrent use of other agents. Each chapter concludes with a comprehensive presentation (with examples) of various methods of computing initial drug doses and of modifying drug therapy regimens using serum concentrations to adjust doses. All dosing methods in this text are ones that are published in peer-reviewed literature. In addition, they are techniques with which I have personal clinical experience and which have produced acceptable results in my practice and clinical clerkships. Finally, problems (with solutions) are included for each chapter so that the various dosing methods can be practiced. The problems are made up of brief clinical vignettes, which, given a brief background, request that initial doses be computed or that dosage regimens be modified using drug concentrations.

This text is meant to teach clinical pharmacokinetic and therapeutic drug-monitoring techniques to all clinical practitioners, regardless of professional background. Pharmacists, physicians, nurse practitioners, and physician assistants are among those who can benefit from the text. With the advent of the almost-universal Doctor of Pharmacy degree in colleges of pharmacy, this book can be used in a pharmaceutics, pharmacokinetics, therapeutics, or clinical pharmacy course sequence. It is also possible to use this textbook in a self-directed manner to self-teach or to review important concepts and techniques. Every effort was made to make the chapters "student-friendly." Abbreviations are held to an absolute minimum. When they are used, they are defined near the place where they are used. Rather than using appendices, important information is repeated in each drug section so that readers do not need to jump from section to section for critical data. Multiple dosage computation and adjustment techniques for each drug, ranging from the simplest to the sophisticated, are presented. The easiest pharmacokinetic equations that produce accurate results are used in each instance.

My strong belief is that clinical pharmacokinetics cannot be practiced in a vacuum. Individuals interested in using these dosing techniques for their patients must also be excellent clinical practitioners. Although it is true that "kinetics = dose," clinicians must be able to select the best drug therapy among many choices and appropriately monitor patients for therapeutic response, adverse drug effects, potential drug interactions, disease states and conditions that alter drug dosage, and so on. Thus, it is not acceptable to simply suggest a dose and walk away from the patient, satisfied that the job has been done. It is my sincere hope that this book will help clinicians increase their knowledge in the area of therapeutic drug monitoring and improve care to their patients.

Larry Bauer, PharmD

APPLIED CLINICAL PHARMACOKINETICS

Part I

BASIC CONCEPTS

1

CLINICAL PHARMACOKINETIC AND PHARMACODYNAMIC CONCEPTS

INTRODUCTION

Clinical pharmacokinetics is the discipline that applies pharmacokinetic concepts and principles to humans to design individualized dosage regimens that optimize the therapeutic response of a medication and minimize the chances of an adverse drug reaction. Pharmacokinetics is the study of the absorption, distribution, metabolism, and excretion of drugs.[1] When drugs are given extravascularly (e.g., orally, intramuscularly, or applied to the skin by a transdermal patch), *absorption* must take place for the drug molecules to reach the systemic circulation. To be absorbed, the drug molecules must pass through several physiologic barriers before reaching the vascular system. For example, when a medication is given orally, the drug dosage form must release drug molecules via dissolution, and the molecules must pass through the various layers of the gastrointestinal tract, where they enter capillaries. *Distribution* occurs when drug molecules that have entered the vascular system pass from the bloodstream into various tissues and organs, such as the muscle and heart. *Metabolism* is the chemical conversion of the drug molecule, usually by an enzymatically mediated reaction, into another chemical entity referred to as a *metabolite.* The metabolite may have the same or a different pharmacologic effect as that of the parent drug or may even cause toxic side effects. *Excretion* is the irreversible removal of drug from the body and commonly occurs through the kidney or biliary tract.

Pharmacodynamics is the relationship between drug concentration and pharmacologic response. It is extremely important for clinicians to realize that the change in drug effect is usually not proportional to the change in drug dose or concentration (Figure 1-1). For example, when a drug dose or concentration is increased from a baseline value, the increase in pharmacologic effect is greater when the initial dose or concentration is low, compared with the change in drug effect observed when the initial dose or concentration

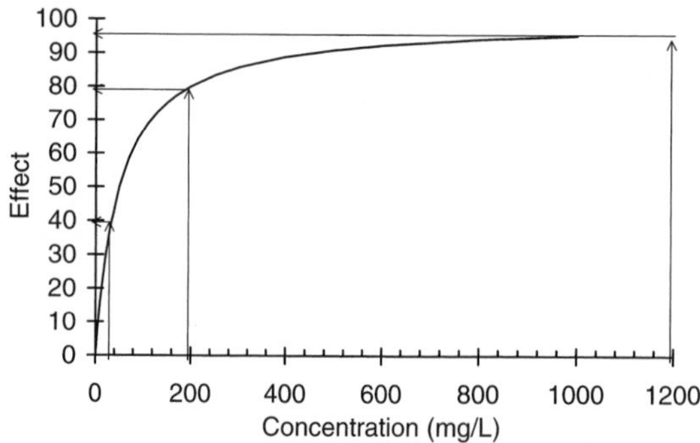

FIGURE 1-1 The relationship between drug concentration and response is usually a hyperbolic function: Effect = $(E_{max} \cdot C)/(EC_{50} + C)$, where E_{max} is the maximum effect and EC_{50} is the drug concentration where the drug effect equals $E_{max}/2$. After a dosage change is made and drug concentrations increase, the drug effect does not change proportionally. Furthermore, the increase in pharmacologic effect is greater when the initial concentration is low compared with the change in drug effect observed when the initial concentration is high. In this graph, the drug effect changes ~50% (from ~40 to 80 units) with a fivefold increase in concentrations at low levels (from ~40 to 200 mg/L) but only ~20% (from ~80 to 95 units) when a sixfold increase in concentrations is made at high concentrations (from ~200 to 1200 mg/L).

is high. Thus, the increase in pharmacologic effect that one observes in a patient as the dose is increased is subject to the law of diminishing returns and eventually reaches a maximum. Most drugs follow this pattern because their pharmacologic effect is produced by forming a complex with a drug receptor. After the drug-receptor complex is formed, the pharmacologic effect is expressed. Often, toxic side effects of drugs follow the same type of dose- or concentration-response relationship, although it is shifted to the right on the dose or concentration axis. In clinical situations, patients may need to tolerate some drug side effects to obtain the maximal pharmacologic effect of the agent.

LINEAR AND NONLINEAR PHARMACOKINETICS

When drugs are given on a constant basis, such as in continuous intravenous infusion or oral medication given every 12 hours, serum drug concentrations increase until the rate of drug administration equals the rate of drug metabolism and excretion. At that point, serum drug concentrations become constant during a continuous intravenous infusion or exhibit a repeating pattern over each dosage interval for medications given at a scheduled time (Figure 1-2). For example, if theophylline is given as a continuous infusion at a rate of 50 mg/h, theophylline serum concentrations increase until the removal of theophylline via hepatic metabolism and renal excretion is 50 mg/h. If cyclosporine 300 mg is given orally every 12 hours, cyclosporine blood concentrations will follow a repeating pattern over the dosage interval, increasing after a dose is given (owing to drug absorption from the gastrointestinal tract) and decreasing after absorption is complete. This repeating pattern continues, and eventually drug concentrations for each dosage interval become superimposable when the amount of cyclosporine absorbed into the body from the gastro-

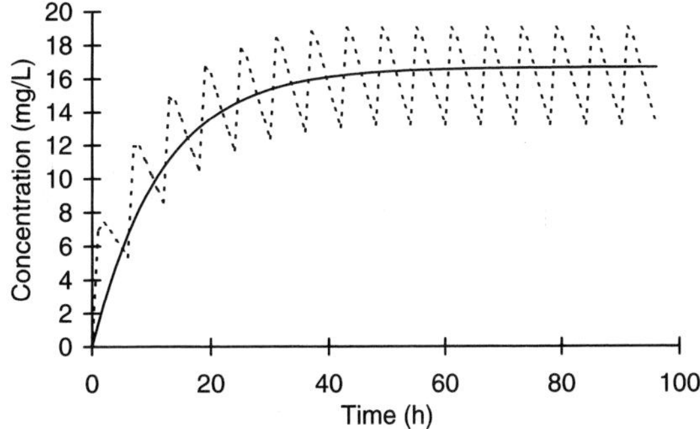

FIGURE 1-2 When medications are given on a continuous basis, serum concentrations increase until the rate of drug administration equals the elimination rate. In this case, the solid line shows serum concentrations in a patient receiving intravenous theophylline at a rate of 50 mg/h and oral theophylline 300 mg every 6 hours (*dashed line*). Because the oral dosing rate (dose/dosage interval = 300 mg/6 h = 50 mg/h) equals the intravenous infusion rate, the drug accumulation patterns are similar. For the intravenous infusion, serum concentrations increase in a smooth pattern until steady state is achieved. During oral dosing, the serum concentrations oscillate around the intravenous profile, increasing during drug absorption and decreasing after absorption is complete and elimination takes place.

intestinal tract equals the amount removed by hepatic metabolism over each dosage interval. Regardless of the mode of drug administration, when the rate of drug administration equals the rate of drug removal, the amount of drug contained in the body reaches a constant value. This equilibrium condition is known as *steady state* and is extremely important in clinical pharmacokinetics because steady-state serum or blood concentrations are usually used to assess patient response and compute new dosage regimens.

If a patient is administered several different doses until steady state is established and steady-state serum concentrations are obtained from the patient after each dosage level, it is possible to determine a pattern of drug accumulation (Figure 1-3). If a plot of steady-state concentration versus dose yields a straight line, the drug is said to follow *linear pharmacokinetics*. In this situation, steady-state serum concentrations increase or decrease proportionally according to dose. Therefore, if a patient has a steady-state drug concentration of 10 μg/mL at a dosage rate of 100 mg/h, the steady-state serum concentration will increase to 15 μg/mL if the dosage rate is increased to 150 mg/h (e.g., a 50% increase in dose yields a 50% increase in steady-state concentration).

Although most drugs follow linear pharmacokinetics, in some cases drug concentrations do not change proportionally with dose. When steady-state concentrations change in a disproportionate fashion after the dosage is altered, a plot of steady-state concentration versus dose is not a straight line, and the drug is said to follow *nonlinear pharmacokinetics*. When steady-state concentrations increase more than expected after a dosage increase, the most likely explanation is that the processes removing the drug from the body have become saturated. This phenomenon is known as *saturable* or *Michaelis-Menten pharmacokinetics*. Both phenytoin[2] and salicylic acid[3] follow Michaelis-Menten pharmacokinetics. When steady-state concentrations increase less than expected after a dosage increase, there are two typical explanations. Some drugs, such as valproic acid[4] and

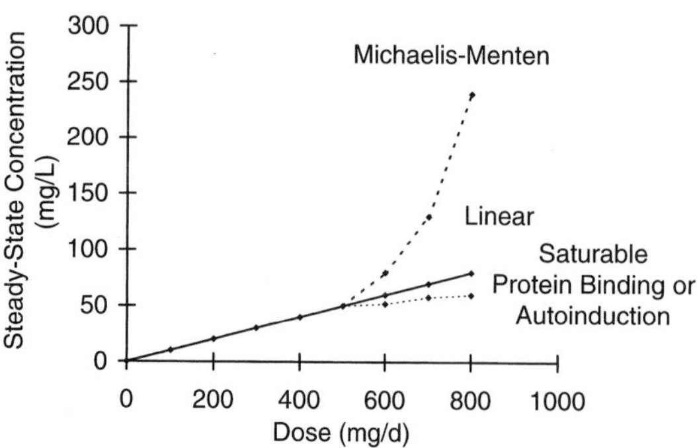

FIGURE 1-3 When doses are increased for most drugs, steady-state concentrations increase in a proportional fashion leading to linear pharmacokinetics (*solid line*). However, in some cases proportional increases in steady-state concentrations do not occur after a dosage increase. When steady-state concentrations increase more than expected after a dosage increase (*upper dashed line*), Michaelis-Menten pharmacokinetics may be taking place. If steady-state concentrations increase less than expected after a dosage increase (*lower dashed line*), saturable plasma protein binding or autoinduction are likely explanations.

disopyramide,[5] saturate plasma protein binding sites so that as the dosage is increased steady-state serum concentrations increase less than expected. Other drugs, such as carbamazepine,[6] increase their own rate of metabolism from the body as the dose is increased, so that steady-state serum concentrations increase less than anticipated. This process is known as *autoinduction* of drug metabolism. In either case, the relationship between steady-state concentration and dosage for drugs that follow nonlinear pharmacokinetics is fraught with significant intersubject variability. Drugs that exhibit nonlinear pharmacokinetics are often very difficult to dose correctly.

Steady-state serum concentration–dose plots for medications are determined in humans early during the drug development process. Because of this, by the time a new drug is available for general use it is usually known whether the drug follows linear or nonlinear pharmacokinetics, and it is not necessary to determine this relationship in individual patients. Thus, the clinician treating a patient knows whether to anticipate linear or nonlinear pharmacokinetics and can assume the appropriate situation when adjusting drug doses. Dealing with drugs that follow linear pharmacokinetics is more straightforward and relatively easy. If a patient has been taking a medication long enough for steady state to have been established and if a dosage adjustment is necessary because of lack of drug effect or the presence of drug toxicity, steady-state drug concentrations will change in proportion to dose for drugs that follow linear pharmacokinetics. For example, if a patient is taking procainamide 500 mg every 8 hours for the treatment of a cardiac arrhythmia but still has the arrhythmia, a clinician could obtain a steady-state procainamide serum concentration. If the procainamide concentration was too low (e.g., 4 μg/mL before the next dose), a dosage increase could help suppress the arrhythmia. Using linear pharmacokinetic principles, one could determine that a dosage increase to 750 mg every 8 hours would increase the steady-state procainamide serum concentration to 6 μg/mL (e.g., new steady-state concentration = [new dose/old dose] × old steady-state concentration; new steady-state concentration = [750 mg/500 mg] × 4 μg/mL = 6 μg/mL).

CLEARANCE

Clearance (Cl) is the most important pharmacokinetic parameter because it determines the maintenance dose (MD) that is required to obtain a given steady-state serum concentration (Css): MD = Css · Cl. If one knows the clearance of a drug and wants to achieve a certain steady-state serum concentration, it is easy to compute the required maintenance dose. Target steady-state concentrations are usually chosen from previous studies in patients that have determined minimum effective concentrations and maximum concentrations that produce the desired pharmacologic effect but avoid toxic side effects. This range of steady-state concentrations is known as the *therapeutic range* for the drug. The therapeutic range should be considered as an initial guideline for drug concentrations in a specific patient; drug dosage and steady-state concentrations should then be titrated and individualized based on therapeutic response. For example, the therapeutic range of theophylline is generally accepted as 10 to 20 μg/mL for the treatment of asthma, with concentrations of 8 to 12 μg/mL considered as a reasonable starting point. If it was known that the theophylline clearance for a patient was 3 L/h and the desired steady-state theophylline serum concentration was 10 μg/mL, the theophylline maintenance dose to achieve this concentration would be 30 mg/h (10 μg/mL = 10 mg/L; MD = Css · Cl; MD = 10 mg/L · 3 L/h = 30 mg/h).

The definition of *clearance* is the volume of serum or blood completely cleared of the drug per unit time. Thus, the dimension of clearance is volume per unit time, such as liters per hour (L/h) or milliliters per minute (mL/min). The liver is most often the organ responsible for drug metabolism, whereas in most cases the kidney is responsible for drug elimination. The gastrointestinal wall, lung, and kidney can also metabolize some drugs, and some medications are eliminated unchanged in the bile. Drug metabolism is characterized as Phase I reactions, which oxidize drug molecules, or Phase II reactions, which form glucuronide or sulfate esters with drug molecules. In either case, the resulting metabolite is more water-soluble than the parent drug and is more likely to be eliminated in the urine.

Most drug metabolism is catalyzed by enzymes contained in the microsomes of hepatocytes known as the cytochrome P-450 enzyme system. This family of enzymes is very important to understand because specific enzymes are responsible for the metabolism of each drug entity. Once it is known that a patient is deficient in one of the enzymes—usually because the clearance of a known drug substrate is very low, resulting in high steady-state serum concentrations for a low to moderate dose—it can be inferred that all drugs metabolized by that enzyme have a low clearance and that doses of other drugs that are substrates of the enzyme may be empirically reduced. If a metabolic drug interaction occurs between one medication and another known to be a substrate for a specific enzyme, it can be assumed that a drug interaction will occur between that drug and other substrates of the same enzyme. The enzymes are classified using a series of numbers and letters and indicate how closely related the enzymes are to each other using amino acid sequencing.

As an example of the classification scheme, the enzyme known as CYP3A4 is named because it is part of the cytochrome P-450 family (CYP); the major family group is "3," the subfamily group within the family is "A," and the specific, individual enzyme within the subfamily is "4." Thus, using this scheme, one can tell that CYP2C9 and CYP2E1 belong to the same family, and CYP2C9 and CYP2C19 belong to the same subfamily and are closely related but different enzymes. Table 1-1 lists the cytochrome P-450 enzymes

TABLE 1-1 Cytochrome P-450 Enzymes, Substrates, Inhibitors, and Inducers

CYTOCHROME P-450 ENZYME	SUBSTRATES	INHIBITORS	INDUCERS
CYP1A2	Acetaminophen Caffeine Desipramine Imipramine Nortriptyline Phenacetin Tacrine Theophylline *(R)*-Warfarin Zileuton	Allopurinol Cimetidine Ciprofloxacin Enoxacin Erythromycin Fluvoxamine Isoniazid	Charcoal-broiled meat Omeprazole Phenobarbital Primidone Rifampin Tobacco smoke
CYP2C9	Diclofenac Ibuprofen Imipramine Naproxen Phenytoin Piroxicam Ritonavir Tolbutamide Torsemide *(S)*-Warfarin	Amiodarone Cimetidine Cotrimoxazole Disulfiram Fluconazole Fluvastatin Fluvoxamine Isoniazid Itraconazole Ketoconazole Metronidazole Sulfinpyrazole Ticlopidine Zafirlukast	Barbiturates Carbamazepine Phenobarbital Phenytoin Primidone Rifampin
CYP2C19 PM: ~4% Caucasians ~20% Japanese and Chinese	Amitriptyline Desmethyldiazepam Diazepam Hexobarbital Imipramine *(S)*-Mephenytoin Omeprazole Propranolol *(R)*-Warfarin	Felbamate Fluoxetine Fluvoxamine Omeprazole Ticlopidine	
CYP2D6 PM: ~8% Caucasians ~1% Japanese and Chinese	Amitriptyline Chlorpromazine Clozapine Codeine Debrisoquin Desipramine Dextromethorphan Encainide Fentanyl Flecainide Fluoxetine Fluvoxamine Fluphenazine Haloperidol Hydrocodone	Amiodarone Chloroquine Cimetidine Fluoxetine Paroxetine Perphenazine Propafenone Propoxyphene Quinidine Ritonavir Sertraline Thioridazine	

TABLE 1-1 ***(continued)***

CYTOCHROME P-450 ENZYME	SUBSTRATES	INHIBITORS	INDUCERS
CYP2D6 *(continued)*	Imipramine Labetalol Maprotiline Methamphetamine Metoprolol Mexiletine Nortriptyline Oxycodone Paroxetine Perhexiline Perphenazine Propafenone Propranolol Risperidone Sertraline Sparteine Thoridazine Timolol Tramadol Trazodone Venlafaxine		
CYP2E1	Acetaminophen Chlorzoxazone Enflurane Ethanol Halothane Isoflurane Isoniazid	Disulfiram	Ethanol Isoniazid
CYP3A4	Alfentanil Alprazolam Amiodarone Amlodipine Astemizole Atorvastatin Bepridil Bromocriptine Carbamazepine Cerivastatin Cisapride Clarithromycin Cortisol Cyclosporine Delavirdine Dexamethasone Diazepam Diltiazem Disopyramide Doxorubicin Erythromycin	Clarithromycin Clotrimazole Danazole Delavirdine Diltiazem Erythromycin Fluconazole Fluvoxamine Grapefruit juice Indinavir Isoniazid Itraconazole Ketoconazole Metronidazole Mibefradil Miconazole Nefazodone Nelfinavir Norfloxacin Quinidine Ritonavir	Barbiturates Carbamazepine Phenobarbital Phenytoin Primidone Rifabutin Rifampin Troglitazone

TABLE 1-1 Cytochrome P-450 Enzymes, Substrates, Inhibitors, and Inducers *(continued)*

CYTOCHROME P-450 ENZYME	SUBSTRATES	INHIBITORS	INDUCERS
CYP3A4 *(continued)*	Ethinyl estradiol	Saquinavir	
	Etoposide	Troleandomycin	
	Felodipine	Verapamil	
	Fenofexadine	Zafirlukast	
	Fentanyl		
	Finasteride		
	Fluconazole		
	Hydrocortisone		
	Imipramine		
	Indinavir		
	Isradipine		
	Itraconazole		
	Ketoconazole		
	Lansoprazole		
	Lidocaine		
	Loratadine		
	Losartan		
	Lovastatin		
	Methylprednisolone		
	Mibefradil		
	Miconazole		
	Midazolam		
	Nefazodone		
	Nelfinavir		
	Nicardipine		
	Nifedipine		
	Nimodipine		
	Nisoldipine		
	Nitrendipine		
	Progesterone		
	Prednisolone		
	Quinidine		
	Quinine		
	Rifabutin		
	Ritonavir		
	Saquinavir		
	Sertraline		
	Simvastatin		
	Sufentanil		
	Tacrolimus		
	Teniposide		
	Terfenadine		
	Testosterone		
	Triazolam		
	Troleoandomycin		
	Verapamil		
	Vinblastine		
	Vincristine		
	Zolpidem		

PM = poor metabolizer.
From Hansten PD, Horn JR. Hansten and Horn's Drug Interactions Analysis and Management. Vancouver, WA: Applied Therapeutics, 1998:521.

responsible for most drug oxidative metabolism in humans, along with examples of known substrates, inhibitors, and inducers.[7] Also, some ethnic groups are deficient in certain enzyme families to a varying extent, and this information is included. Some drugs are transported by P-glycoprotein from the blood into the bile where the drug is eliminated by biliary secretion.

The kidney eliminates drugs by glomerular filtration and tubular secretion in the nephron. After drug molecules have entered the urine by either of these processes, the molecules may reenter the blood by means of a process known as *tubular reabsorption.* Glomerular filtration and usually tubular reabsorption are passive processes. *Tubular secretion* is an active process usually mediated by a transport molecule that facilitates the transfer of drug across the kidney tubule. Most drug tubular secretion takes place in the proximal tubule of the nephron, whereas tubular reabsorption usually takes place in the distal tubule of the nephron. Some drugs eliminated by the kidney are transported from the blood into the urine by P-glycoprotein.

The clearance for an organ such as the liver or kidney, which metabolizes or eliminates drugs, is determined by the blood flow to the organ and the ability of the organ to metabolize or eliminate the drug.[8] Liver blood flow (LBF) and renal blood flow (RBF) are each ~1 to 1.5 L/min in adults with normal cardiovascular function. The ability of an organ to remove or extract the drug from the blood or serum is usually measured by determining the extraction ratio (ER), which is the fraction of drug removed by the organ, and is computed by measuring the concentrations of the drug entering (C_{in}) and leaving (C_{out}) the organ: $ER = (C_{in} - C_{out})/C_{in}$. Liver or renal blood flow and the extraction ratio for a drug are rarely measured in patients. However, the extraction ratio is often determined during the drug development process, and knowledge of this parameter can be extremely useful in determining how the pharmacokinetics of a drug will change during a drug interaction or when a patient develops hepatic, renal, or cardiac failure.

The drug clearance for an organ is the product of the blood flow to the organ and the extraction ratio of the drug. Therefore, hepatic clearance (Cl_H) of a drug would be determined by taking the product of liver blood flow and the hepatic extraction ratio (ER_H) for the drug ($Cl_H = LBF \cdot ER_H$), and renal clearance (Cl_R) for a medication would be determined by multiplying renal blood flow and the renal extraction ratio for the agent ($Cl_R = RBF \cdot ER_R$). For example, verapamil has a hepatic extraction ratio of 90% ($ER_H = 0.90$). For patients with normal liver blood flow (LBF = 1.5 L/min), hepatic clearance would be expected to be 1.35 L/min ($Cl_H = LBF \cdot ER_H$, $Cl_H = 1.5\ L/min \cdot 0.90 = 1.35\ L/min$; Figure 1-4). The total clearance for a drug is the sum of the individual clearances for each organ that extracts the medication. For example, the total clearance for a drug that is metabolized by the liver and eliminated by the kidney is the sum of hepatic and renal clearance for the agent: $Cl = Cl_H + Cl_R$.

Hepatic Clearance

The physiologic determinants of hepatic clearance have been extensively studied.[8–10] Another way to think of hepatic clearance is to recognize that its value is a function of the intrinsic ability of the enzyme to metabolize a drug (intrinsic clearance); the fraction of drug present in the bloodstream that is not bound to cells or proteins, such as albumin, α_1-acid glycoprotein, or lipoproteins, but is present in the unbound, or "free," state (unbound fraction of drug); and liver blood flow. The *intrinsic clearance* (Cl'_{int}) is the inherent abil-

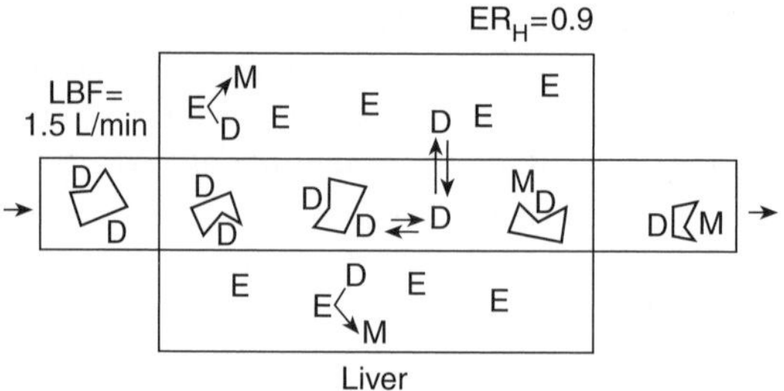

FIGURE 1-4 This schematic depicts the liver (*large box*) with the blood vessel supplying blood to it. When drug molecules (*D*) enter an organ (blood flows from left to right) that clears the drug, they may be bound to plasma proteins (*trapezoid shapes*) or exist in the unbound state. The unbound, or "free," drug molecules are in equilibrium with the bound drug in the blood and unbound drug in the tissue. Drug–protein complexes are usually too big to diffuse across biological membranes into tissues. Drug molecules that have entered hepatic tissue may encounter an enzyme (*E*) that metabolizes the drug. When this occurs, the drug is chemically converted to a metabolite (*M*), which can diffuse back into the blood and leave the liver along with drug molecules that were not metabolized. The clearance of drug is equal to the blood flow to the organ (*LBF*) times the extraction ratio (EH_H) for the organ.

ity of the enzyme to metabolize the drug and is the quotient of the Michaelis-Menten constants V_{max} (maximum rate of drug metabolism) and Km (drug concentration at which the metabolic rate is $V_{max}/2$; $Cl'_{int} = V_{max}/Km$) for the unbound drug. The unbound fraction of drug in the blood or serum (f_B) is the unbound drug concentration divided by the total (bound + unbound) drug concentration. The relationship among the three physiologic factors and hepatic drug clearance is:

$$Cl_H = \frac{LBF \cdot (f_B \cdot Cl'_{int})}{LBF + (f_B \cdot Cl'_{int})}$$

Fortunately, most drugs have a large hepatic extraction ratio ($ER_H \geq 0.7$) or a small hepatic extraction ratio ($ER_H \leq 0.3$), and the relationship is simplified in these situations. For drugs with a low hepatic extraction ratio, hepatic clearance is mainly a product of the free fraction of the drug in the blood or serum and intrinsic clearance: $Cl_H = f_B \cdot Cl'_{int}$. In this case, drug interactions that displace drug molecules bound to proteins increase the fraction of unbound drug in the blood ($\uparrow f_B$), and more unbound drug molecules are able to leave the vascular system (drug–protein complexes are far too big to exit the vascular system) and enter hepatocytes, where the additional unbound drug is metabolized and hepatic drug clearance increases. In addition, drug interactions that inhibit or induce the cytochrome P-450 enzyme system (decreasing or increasing Cl'_{int}, respectively) change the hepatic clearance of the medication accordingly. The hepatic clearance of drugs with low extraction ratios does not change much when liver blood flow decreases secondary to liver or cardiac disease. Examples of drugs with low hepatic extraction ratios are valproic acid, phenytoin, and warfarin.

For drugs with high hepatic extraction ratios, hepatic clearance is mainly a function of liver blood flow: Cl_H = LBF. The rate-limiting step for drug metabolism in this case is how much drug can be delivered to the liver, because the capacity to metabolize drug is very large. In this case, hepatic clearance is very sensitive to changes in liver blood flow because of congestive heart failure or liver disease. However, the hepatic clearance of drugs with high extraction ratios does not change much when protein-binding displacement or enzyme induction or inhibition occurs owing to drug interactions. Examples of drugs with high hepatic extraction ratios are lidocaine, morphine, and most tricyclic antidepressants.

Renal Clearance

The physiologic determinants of renal clearance are glomerular filtration rate (GFR), the free fraction of drug in the blood or serum (f_B), the clearance of drug via renal tubular secretion (Cl_{sec}), and the fraction of drug reabsorbed in the kidney (FR): $Cl_R = [(f_B \cdot GFR) + Cl_{sec}](1 - FR)$.[11,12] Average glomerular filtration rates in adults with normal renal function are 100 to 120 mL/min. Since tubular secretion is an active process, it has been described by an equation similar to that used to explain liver metabolism:

$$Cl_{sec} = [RBF \cdot (f_B Cl'_{sec})]/[RBF + (f_B Cl'_{sec})],$$

where Cl'_{sec} is the intrinsic clearance due to active tubular secretion. Thus, the entire equation is:

$$Cl_R = [(f_B \cdot GFR) + \frac{RBF \cdot (f_B Cl'_{sec})}{RBF + (f_B Cl'_{sec})}](1 - FR)$$

If the renal clearance of a drug is greater than glomerular filtration rate, it is likely that the drug was eliminated, in part, by active tubular secretion. The aminoglycoside antibiotics and vancomycin are eliminated primarily by glomerular filtration. Procainamide, ranitidine, and ciprofloxacin are eliminated by both glomerular filtration and active tubular secretion.

In some cases, glomerular filtration rate and renal tubular secretion function may be measured in patients with renal disease. However, for the purposes of drug dosing, glomerular filtration rate is approximated by measuring or estimating creatinine clearance for a patient. Creatinine is a by-product of muscle metabolism that is eliminated primarily by glomerular filtration.

VOLUME OF DISTRIBUTION

Volume of distribution (V) is an important pharmacokinetic parameter because it determines the loading dose (LD) required to achieve a particular steady-state drug concentration immediately after the dose is administered: $LD = Css \cdot V$ (Figure 1-5). However, the exact volume of distribution for a patient is rarely known because it is necessary to have administered a dose on a previous occasion to compute the volume of distribution. Thus, an average volume of distribution measured in other patients with similar demographics (e.g., age, weight, and gender) and medical conditions (e.g., renal failure, liver failure, and heart failure) is usually used to estimate a loading dose (Figure 1-6). Because of this, most patients do not actually attain steady state after a loading dose, but it is hoped that serum drug concentrations will be high enough that the patient will experience the pharmacologic effect of the drug.

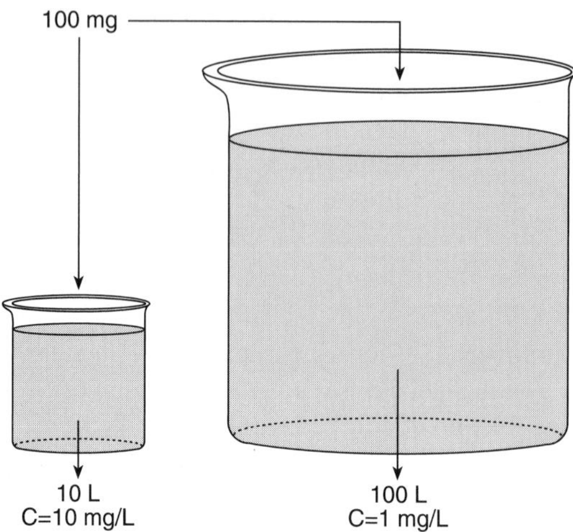

FIGURE 1-5 The volume of distribution (V) is a hypothetical volume that is the proportionality constant that relates the concentration of drug in the blood or serum (*C*) and the amount of drug in the body (A_B): $A_B = C \cdot V$. It can be thought of as a beaker of fluid representing the entire space that drug distributes into. In this case, one beaker, representing a patient with a small volume of distribution, contains 10 L, whereas the other beaker, representing a patient with a large volume of distribution, contains 100 L. If 100 mg of drug is given to each patient, the resulting concentration will be 10 mg/L in the patient with the smaller volume of distribution, but 1 mg/L in the patient with the larger volume of distribution. If the minimum concentration needed to exert the pharmacologic effect of the drug is 5 mg/L, one patient will receive a benefit from the drug, whereas the other will have a subtherapeutic concentration.

The volume of distribution is a hypothetical volume that relates drug serum concentrations to the amount of drug in the body. Thus, the dimension of volume of distribution is in volume units, such as liters or milliliters. At any given time after drug has been absorbed from extravascular sites and the serum and tissue drug concentrations are in equilibrium, the serum concentration for a drug (C) is equal to the quotient of the amount of drug in the body (A_B) and the volume of distribution: $C = A_B/V$. The volume of distribution can be very small if the drug is primarily contained in the blood (warfarin V = 5–7 L) or very large if the drug distributes widely in the body and is mostly bound to bodily tissues (digoxin V = 500 L).

The physiologic determinants of volume of distribution are the actual volume of blood (V_B) and size (measured as a volume) of the various tissues and organs of the body (V_T). Therefore, a larger person, such as a 160-kg football player, would be expected to have a larger volume of distribution for a drug than a smaller person, such as a 40-kg grandmother. How the drug binds in the blood or serum compared with the binding in tissues is also an important determinant of the volume of distribution for a drug. For example, warfarin has such a small volume of distribution because it is highly bound to serum albumin so that the free fraction of drug in the blood (f_B) is very small. Digoxin has a very large volume of distribution because it is very highly bound to tissues (primarily muscle), so that the free fraction of drug in the tissues (f_T; f_T = unbound drug concentration in the tis-

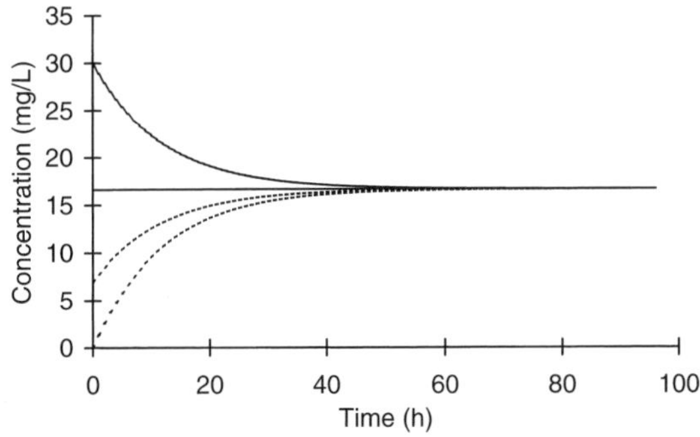

FIGURE 1-6 If the volume of distribution (V) is known for a patient, it is possible to administer a loading dose (LD) that will attain a specified steady-state drug concentration (Css): LD = Css · V. This example depicts the ideal loading dose given as an intravenous bolus dose followed by a continuous intravenous infusion (*solid line starting at 16 mg/L*) so that steady-state is achieved immediately and maintained. If a loading dose was not given and a continuous infusion started (*dashed line starting at 0 mg/L*), it would take time to reach steady-state concentrations, and the patient may not experience an effect from the drug until a minimum effect concentration is achieved. This situation would not be acceptable for many clinical situations in which a quick onset of action is needed. Since the volume of distribution is not known for a patient before a dose is given, clinicians use an average volume of distribution previously measured in patients with similar demographics and disease states to compute loading doses. When this is done, the patient's volume of distribution may be smaller than average and result in higher than expected concentrations (*solid line starting at 30 mg/L*) or larger than average and result in lower than expected concentrations (*dotted line starting at 7 mg/L*). In these cases, it still takes 3 to 5 half-lives to reach steady state, but therapeutic drug concentrations are achieved much sooner than by intravenous infusion only.

sue/total tissue drug concentration) is very small. The equation that relates all of these physiologic determinants to the volume of distribution is[13]:

$$V = V_B + \frac{f_B}{f_T} V_T$$

This equation can help clinicians understand why a drug has a large or small volume of distribution or why the volume of distribution might change under various circumstances. An example is how the volume of distribution changes when a plasma protein binding drug interaction occurs. If a drug that is highly bound to plasma proteins is given to a patient and a second drug that is also highly bound to the same protein is given concurrently, the second drug will compete for plasma protein binding sites and displace the first drug from the protein. In this case, the free fraction in the serum of the first drug will increase ($\uparrow f_B$), resulting in an increased volume of distribution: $\uparrow V = V_B + (\uparrow f_B/f_T)V_T$.

HALF-LIFE AND ELIMINATION RATE CONSTANT

When drugs that follow linear pharmacokinetics are given to humans, serum concentrations decline in a curvilinear fashion (Figure 1-7). When the same data are plotted on a semilogarithmic axis, serum concentrations decrease in a linear fashion after drug absorp-

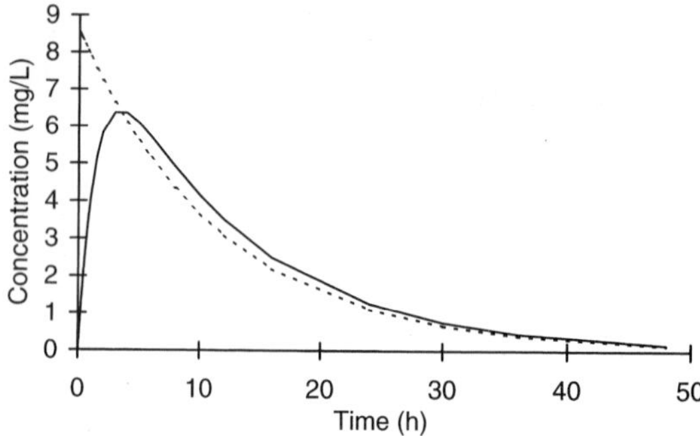

FIGURE 1-7 Serum concentration–time profile for a patient receiving 300 mg of theophylline orally (*solid line*) and by intravenous bolus (*dashed line*). If these data are plotted on rectilinear axes, serum concentrations decline in a curvilinear fashion in both cases. When the drug is given orally, serum concentrations initially increase while the drug is being absorbed and decline after drug absorption is complete.

tion and distribution phases are complete (Figure 1-8). This part of the curve is known as the *elimination phase.* The time that it takes for serum concentrations to decrease by half in the elimination phase is a constant and is called the *half-life* ($t_{1/2}$). The half-life describes how quickly drug serum concentrations decrease in a patient after a medication is administered, and the dimension of half-life is time (e.g., h, min, d).

Another common measurement used to denote how quickly drug serum concentrations decline in a patient is the elimination rate constant (k_e). The dimension for the elimination rate constant is reciprocal time (e.g., h^{-1}, min^{-1}, d^{-1}). If the amount of drug in the body is known, the elimination rate for the drug can be computed by taking the product of the elimination rate constant and the amount of drug in the body (A_B): elimination rate = $A_B \cdot k_e$. The half-life and elimination rate constant are related to each other by the following equation, so it is easy to compute one when the other is known: $t_{1/2}$ =

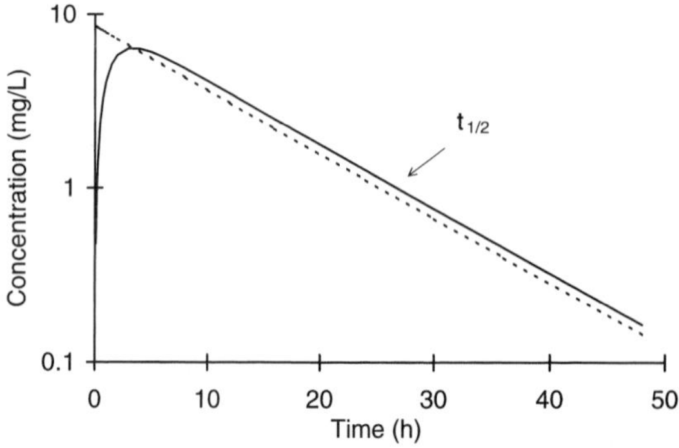

FIGURE 1-8 Serum concentration–time profile for a patient receiving 300 mg of theophylline orally (*solid line*) and by intravenous bolus (*dashed line*). If these data are plotted on semilogarithmic axes, serum concentrations decline in a straight line in both cases. When the drug is given orally, serum concentrations initially increase while the drug is being absorbed and decline after drug absorption is complete. This same data set is plotted in Figure 1-7 on rectilinear axes.

$0.693/k_e$. The elimination rate constant can also be measured graphically by computing the slope of the log concentration versus time graph during the elimination phase: using $\log_{10}$, $k_e/2.303 = (\log C_1 - \log C_2)/(t_1 - t_2)$; or, using natural logarithms (ln), $k_e = (\ln C_1 - \ln C_2)/(t_1 - t_2)$.

The half-life is important because it determines the time to steady state during the continuous dosing of a drug and the dosage interval. The approach to steady-state serum concentrations is an exponential function. If a drug is administered on a continuous basis for 3 half-lives, serum concentrations are ~90% of steady-state values; on a continuous basis for 5 half-lives, serum concentrations equal ~95% of steady-state values; or on a continuous basis for 7 half-lives, serum concentrations achieve ~99% of steady-state values (Figure 1-9). Generally, drug serum concentrations used for pharmacokinetic monitoring can be safely measured after 3 to 5 estimated half-lives because most drug assays have 5% to 10% measurement error. Note that the half-life of a drug in a patient is not usually known but is estimated using values previously measured during pharmacokinetic studies conducted in similar patients.

The dosage interval for a drug is also determined by the half-life of the medication. For example, if the therapeutic range of a drug is 10 to 20 mg/L, the ideal dosage interval would not let maximum serum concentrations exceed 20 mg/L or allow the minimum serum concentration to go below 10 mg/L (Figure 1-10). In this case, the dosage interval that would produce this steady-state concentration–time profile would be every half-life. After a dose is given, the maximum serum concentration would be 20 mg/L. In 1 half-life, the serum concentration would be 10 mg/L, and the next dose would be administered to the patient. At steady state, this serum concentration–time profile would be repeated after each dose. During drug development, it is very common to use the drug half-life as the initial dosage interval for the new drug compound until the pharmacodynamics of the agent can be determined.

The half-life and elimination rate constant are known as *dependent parameters* because their values depend on the clearance and volume of distribution of the agent: $t_{1/2} = (0.693 \cdot V)/Cl$, $k_e = Cl/V$. The half-life and elimination rate constant for a drug can change

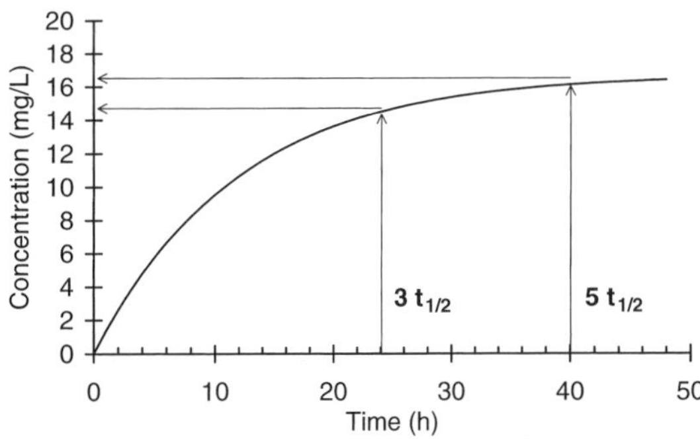

FIGURE 1-9 Serum concentration–time graph for a drug that has a half-life equal to 8 hours. The arrows indicate concentrations at 3 half-lives (24 h, ~90% of Css) and at 5 half-lives (40 h, ~95% of Css). Since most drug assays have 5% to 10% measurement error, serum concentrations obtained between 3 and 5 half-lives after dosing commenced can be considered to be at steady state for clinical purposes and used to adjust drug doses.

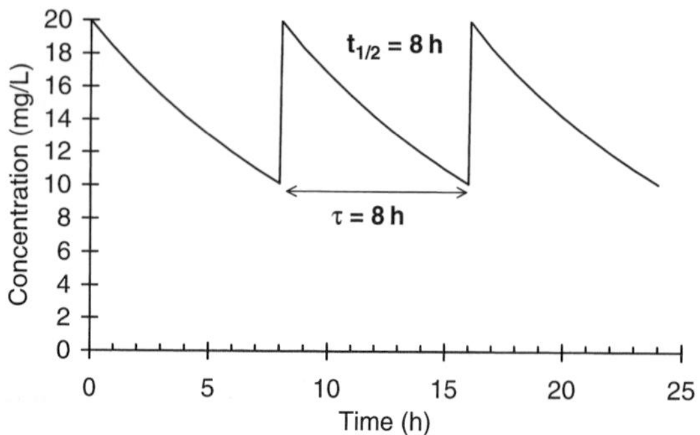

FIGURE 1-10 The dosage interval for a drug is determined by the half-life of the agent. In this case, the half-life of the drug is 8 hours, and the therapeutic range of the drug is 10 to 20 mg/L. To ensure that maximum serum concentrations never go above and minimum serum concentrations never go below the therapeutic range, it is necessary to give the drug every 8 hours (τ = dosage interval).

either because of a change in clearance or a change in the volume of distribution. Because the values for clearance and volume of distribution depend solely on physiologic parameters and can vary independently of each other, they are known as *independent parameters.*

MICHAELIS-MENTEN OR SATURABLE PHARMACOKINETICS

Drugs that are metabolized by the cytochrome P-450 enzymes and other enzyme systems may undergo Michaelis-Menten or saturable pharmacokinetics. This is the type of nonlinear pharmacokinetics that occurs when the number of drug molecules overwhelms or saturates the enzymes' ability to metabolize the drug.[2,3] When this occurs, steady-state drug serum concentrations increase in a disproportionate manner after a dosage increase (see Figure 1-3). In this case, the rate of drug removal is described by the classic Michaelis-Menten relationship that is used for all enzyme systems: rate of metabolism = $(V_{max} \cdot C)/(Km + C)$, where V_{max} is the maximum rate of metabolism, C is the substrate concentration, and Km is the substrate concentration where the rate of metabolism = $V_{max}/2$.

The clinical implication of Michaelis-Menten pharmacokinetics is that the clearance of a drug is not a constant as it is with linear pharmacokinetics, but it is concentration- or dose-dependent. As the dose or concentration increases, the clearance rate decreases as the enzyme approaches saturable conditions: $Cl = V_{max}/(Km + C)$. This is why concentrations increase disproportionately after a dosage increase. For example, phenytoin follows saturable pharmacokinetics with average Michaelis-Menten constants of V_{max} = 500 mg/d and Km = 4 mg/L. The therapeutic range of phenytoin is 10 to 20 mg/L. As the steady-state concentration of phenytoin increases from 10 mg/L to 20 mg/L, clearance decreases from 36 L/d to 21 L/d [$Cl = V_{max}/(Km + C)$; Cl = (500 mg/d)/(4 mg/L + 10 mg/L) = 36 L/d; Cl = (500 mg/d)/(4 mg/L + 20 mg/L) = 21 L/d]. Unfortunately, there is so much interpatient variability in Michaelis-Menten pharmacokinetic parameters for a drug (typically, V_{max} = 100 to 1000 mg/d and Km = 1 to 10 mg/L for phenytoin) that dosing drugs that follow saturable metabolism is extremely difficult.

The volume of distribution is unaffected by saturable metabolism and is still determined by the physiologic volume of blood (V_B) and tissues (V_T) as well as the unbound concentration of drug in the blood (f_B) and tissues (f_T): $V = V_B + (f_B/f_T)V_T$. Also, half-life ($t_{1/2}$) is still related to clearance and volume of distribution using the same equation as for linear pharmacokinetics: $t_{1/2} = (0.693 \cdot V)/Cl$. However, since clearance is dose- or concentration-dependent, half-life also changes with dosage or concentration changes. As doses or concentrations increase for a drug that follows Michaelis-Menten pharmacokinetics, clearance decreases and half-life becomes longer for the drug: $\uparrow t_{1/2} = (0.693 \cdot V)/\downarrow Cl$. The clinical implication of this finding is that the time to steady state (3 to 5 $t_{1/2}$) is longer as the dose or concentration is increased for a drug that follows saturable pharmacokinetics.

Under steady-state conditions, the rate of drug administration equals the rate of drug removal. Therefore, for a drug that is removed solely by metabolism via one enzyme system, the Michaelis-Menten equation can be used to compute the maintenance dose (MD) required to achieve a target steady-state serum concentration (Css):

$$MD = \frac{V_{max} \cdot Css}{Km + Css}$$

When the therapeutic range for a drug is far below the Km value for the enzymes that metabolize the drug. This equation simplifies to: $MD = (V_{max}/Km)$ Css or, since V_{max}/Km is a constant, $MD = Cl \cdot Css$. Therefore, when Km >> Css, drugs that are metabolized follow linear pharmacokinetics. When the therapeutic range for a drug is far above the Km value for the enzyme system that metabolizes the drug, the rate of metabolism becomes a constant equal to V_{max}. Under these conditions, only a fixed amount of drug is metabolized because the enzyme system is completely saturated and cannot increase its metabolic capacity. This situation is also known as *zero-order pharmacokinetics. First-order pharmacokinetics* is another name for linear pharmacokinetics.

Based on these facts, it can be seen that any drug that is metabolized by enzymes undergoes Michaelis-Menten pharmacokinetics. But the therapeutic ranges of most drugs are far below the Km for the enzymes that metabolize the agent. Because of this, most medications that are metabolized follow linear pharmacokinetics. However, even in these cases saturable drug metabolism can occur in drug overdose cases in which the drug concentration far exceeds the therapeutic range for the medication.

BIOAVAILABILITY

When a drug is administered extravascularly, the entire dose may not enter the systemic circulation. For example, an orally administered tablet may not completely dissolve so that part of the dose is eliminated in the stool, or a transdermal patch may not release the entire dose before it is removed from the skin. The fraction of the administered dose that is delivered to the systemic circulation is known as the *bioavailability* of the drug and dosage form. When medications are given orally, intramuscularly, subcutaneously, or by other extravascular routes, the drug must be absorbed across several biologic membranes before entering the vascular system. In these cases, drug serum concentrations rise while the drug is being absorbed into the bloodstream, reach a maximum concentration (C_{max}) when the rate of drug absorption equals the rate of drug elimination, and eventually decrease according to the half-life of the drug. The phase of the curve over which absorption takes place is known as the *absorption phase,* and the time that the maximum concentration occurs is called T_{max} (Figure 1-11).

If a medication is given orally, drug molecules must pass through several organs before entering the systemic circulation. During absorption from the gastrointestinal tract, the drug molecules encounter enzymes that may metabolize the agent (primarily CYP3A4 substrates, since ~90% of cytochrome P-450 contained in the gut wall is CYP3A4) or even pump the drug back into the lumen and prevent absorption from taking place (primarily P-glycoprotein substrates). After drug molecules are absorbed from the gastrointestinal tract, they enter the portal vein. The portal vein and hepatic artery together supply blood to the liver, and the sum of portal vein (~⅔ total LBF) and hepatic artery (~⅓ total LBF) blood flows make up liver blood flow, which is ~1 to 1.5 L/min. If the drug is hepatically metabolized, part of the drug may be metabolized by the liver even though most of the drug was absorbed from the gastrointestinal tract. Drugs that are substrates of CYP3A4 and CYP2D6 are particularly susceptible to presystemic metabolism by the liver. Blood leaving the liver by the hepatic vein enters the inferior vena cava and eventually is pumped through the lung by the right side of the heart before entering the left side of the heart and being pumped into the arterial system. To a lesser extent, some drugs are metabolized by the lung or irreversibly eliminated into expired air.

The loss of drug from these combined processes is known as *presystemic metabolism* or the *first-pass effect.* Since the entire oral dose that was absorbed must take this route before entering the systemic vascular system, large amounts of drug can be lost through these processes. For example, the oral bioavailability of both propranolol (a substrate of CYP2D6 and CYP2C19) and verapamil (a substrate of CYP3A4 and P-glycoprotein) is ~10%, even though the oral dosage forms for each agent releases 100% of the drug into the gastrointestinal tract.

For drugs that follow linear pharmacokinetics, bioavailability is measured by comparing serum concentrations achieved after extravascular and intravenous doses in the same individual. Rather than compare drug concentrations at each time point, a composite of

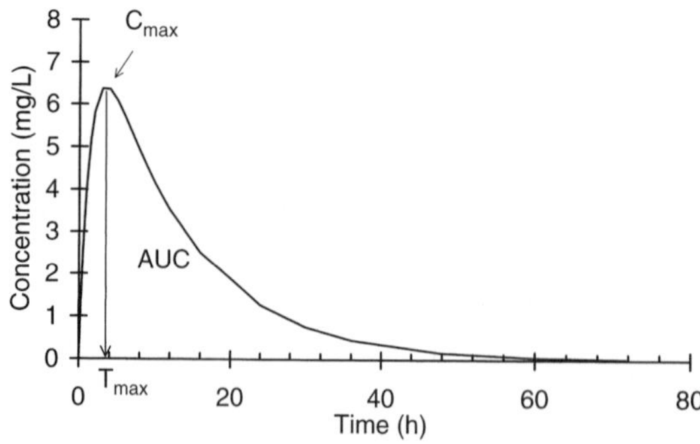

FIGURE 1-11 Area under the serum concentration–time curve (*AUC*), the maximum concentration (C_{max}), and the time that the maximum concentration occurs (T_{max}) are considered primary bioavailability parameters. When the AUC, C_{max}, and T_{max} are the same within statistical limits for two dosage forms of the same drug, the dosage forms are considered to be bioequivalent.

drug concentrations over time is derived by measuring the total area under the serum concentration–time curve (AUC) for each route of administration (see Figure 1-11). If the extravascular and intravenous doses are the same, the bioavailability of a drug can be calculated by taking the ratio of the AUCs for each route of administration. For example, if 10 mg of a drug were administered to a subject on two separate occasions by intravenous (IV) and oral (PO) routes of administration, the bioavailability (F) would be computed by dividing the AUC after oral administration (AUC_{PO}) by the AUC after intravenous administration (AUC_{IV}): $F = AUC_{PO}/AUC_{IV}$. If it is not possible to administer the same dose intravenously and extravascularly because poor absorption or presystemic metabolism yields serum concentrations that are too low to measure, the bioavailability calculation can be corrected to allow for different size doses for the different routes of administration: $F = (AUC_{PO}/AUC_{IV})(D_{IV}/D_{PO})$, where D_{IV} is the intravenous dose and D_{PO} is the oral dose.

Bioequivalence

When the patent expires for drug entities, generic drugs are manufactured, which are less expensive than brand name products. This is because the drug company manufacturing the generic drug does not have to prove that the drug is safe and effective, since those studies were done by the pharmaceutical company producing the brand name drug. Although generic drug products are not required to have the same absorption characteristics to be marketed by a pharmaceutical company, a desirable attribute of a generic drug dosage form is that it produces the same serum concentration–time profile as its brand name counterpart. When it meets this requirement, the generic drug product is said to be *bioequivalent* to the brand name drug. In theory, it should be possible to substitute a bioequivalent generic drug dosage form for a brand name product without a change in steady-state drug serum concentrations or therapeutic efficacy.

Bioequivalence is achieved when the serum concentration–time curve for the generic and brand name drug dosage forms are deemed indistinguishable from each other using statistical tests. Concentration–time curves are superimposable when the area under the total serum concentration–time curve, maximum concentration, and time that the maximum concentration occurs are identical within statistical limits. To achieve the Food and Drug Administration's (FDA) definition of oral bioequivalence and be awarded an "AB" rating in the FDA publication, *Approved Drug Products with Therapeutic Equivalence Evaluations* (also known as *The Orange Book*), the pharmaceutical company producing a generic drug product must administer single doses or multiple doses of the drug until steady state is achieved using both the generic and brand name drug dosage forms to a group of 18 to 24 humans and prove that the AUC (from time = 0 to infinity after a single dose, or over the dosage interval at steady state), C_{max}, and T_{max} values are statistically identical for the two dosage forms. The ratio of the area under the serum concentration–time curves for the generic ($AUC_{generic}$) and brand name (AUC_{brand}) drug dosage forms is known as the relative bioavailability ($F_{relative}$), since the reference AUC is derived from the brand name drug dosage form: $F_{relative} = AUC_{generic}/AUC_{brand}$. Many states allow the substitution of generic drugs for brand name drugs if the prescriber notes on the prescription order that generic substitution is acceptable and the generic drug dosage form has an AB rating.

PROBLEMS

1. Define the following terms:
   a. absorption
   b. distribution
   c. metabolism
   d. elimination
   e. steady state
   f. linear or first-order pharmacokinetics
   g. nonlinear pharmacokinetics
   h. saturable or Michaelis-Menten pharmacokinetics
   i. autoinduction
   j. therapeutic range
   k. zero-order pharmacokinetics
   l. bioavailability
   m. bioequivalent
   n. clearance
   o. volume of distribution
   p. half-life
   q. elimination rate constant

2. Two new antibiotics are marketed by a pharmaceutical manufacturer. Reading the package insert, you find the following information:

DOSE	CURACILLIN STEADY-STATE CONCENTRATIONS (mg/L)	BETTERMYCIN STEADY-STATE CONCENTRATIONS (mg/L)
0	0	0
100	15	25
250	37.5	62.5
500	75	190
1000	150	510

   What type of pharmacokinetics does each of these drugs follow?

3. A patient with liver failure and a patient with heart failure need to be treated with a new antiarrhythmic drug. You find a clinical research study that contains the following information for Stopabeat in patients similar to the ones you need to treat: normal subjects: clearance = 45 L/h, volume of distribution = 175 L; patients with liver failure: clearance = 15 L/h, volume of distribution = 300 L; patients with heart failure: clearance = 30 L/h, volume of distribution = 100 L. Recommend an intravenous loading dose and continuous intravenous infusion maintenance dose to achieve a steady-state concentration of 10 mg/L for your two patients based on these data, and estimate the time it will take to achieve steady-state conditions.

4. After the first dose of gentamicin is given to a patient with renal failure, the following serum concentrations are obtained:

TIME AFTER DOSAGE ADMINISTRATION (h)	CONCENTRATION (μg/mL)
1	7.7
24	5.6
48	4.0

Compute the half-life and the elimination rate constant for this patient.

5. Average values of Michaelis-Menten pharmacokinetic parameters for phenytoin in adults are V_{max} = 500 mg/d and Km = 4 mg/L. What are the expected average doses of phenytoin that would produce steady-state concentrations at the lower and upper limits of the therapeutic range (10 to 20 mg/L)?

6. A new immunosuppressant, Noreject, is being studied in the renal transplantation clinic where you work. Based on previous studies, the following area under the serum concentration–time curves (AUC) were measured after single doses of 10 mg in renal transplant recipients: intravenous bolus AUC = 1530 mg · h/L, oral capsule AUC = 1220 mg · h/L, oral liquid AUC = 1420 mg · h/L. What is the bioavailability of the oral capsule and oral liquid? What is the relative bioavailability of the oral capsule compared with the oral liquid?

ANSWERS TO PROBLEMS

1. The following are definitions of terms in question 1:
   - **a.** Passage of drug molecules through physiologic/biologic barriers before reaching the vascular system
   - **b.** Passage of drug molecules from the bloodstream into tissues and organs
   - **c.** Chemical conversion of a drug molecule into a metabolite
   - **d.** Irreversible removal of drug from the body
   - **e.** Rate of drug administration equals the rate of drug removal so that serum concentrations and amount of drug in the body are constant
   - **f.** Situation in which steady-state serum concentration or area under the serum concentration–time curve (AUC) changes proportionally with dosage changes
   - **g.** Situation in which steady-state serum concentration or area under the serum concentration–time curve (AUC) changes disproportionally with dosage changes
   - **h.** Type of nonlinear pharmacokinetics in which an increase in dose results in a disproportionally large increase in steady-state serum concentration or area under the serum concentration–time curve; results from overwhelming or "saturating" the enzymes' ability to metabolize the drug
   - **i.** Situation in which a drug increases its own rate of metabolism by inducing more drug-metabolizing enzyme to be produced
   - **j.** Minimum and maximum serum or blood concentrations that produce the desired pharmacologic effect without producing unwanted adverse effects
   - **k.** A constant amount of drug eliminated per unit time usually owing to complete saturation of the enzyme system responsible for the metabolism of the drug
   - **l.** Fraction of administered dose that is delivered to the systemic circulation

m. A dosage form of a drug that produces the same serum concentration–time profile as another dosage form of the same drug; usually measured by showing that the two dosage forms have the same area under the serum concentration–time curve, maximum serum concentration, and time that maximal serum concentration occurs values within statistical limits

n. Volume of serum or blood completely cleared of drug per unit of time

o. Proportionality constant that relates serum concentrations to amount of drug in the body

p. Time required for serum concentrations to decrease by half after absorption and distribution phases are complete

q. Terminal slope (using an ln C versus time plot) of the serum concentration–time curve after absorption and distribution phases are complete

2. A plot of steady-state concentration versus doses is a straight line for Curacillin, but a curved line for Bettermycin (see table for problem 2). Since this relationship is a straight line for Curacillin, it follows linear or first-order pharmacokinetics. Because the steady-state concentration versus dose plot is curved upward indicating disproportionally large increases in concentration after a dosage increase, Bettermycin follows nonlinear pharmacokinetics. The type of nonlinear pharmacokinetics is Michaelis-Menten or saturable pharmacokinetics.

3. The patient with liver failure would likely have pharmacokinetic parameters similar to the liver failure patients in the research study (Cl = 15 L/h, V = 300 L): LD = V · Css, LD = (300 L)(10 mg/L) = 3000 mg intravenous bolus; MD = Cl · Css, MD = (15 L/h)(10 mg/L) = 150 mg/h intravenous infusion. The half-life would be estimated using the clearance and volume of distribution: $t_{1/2}$ = (0.693 V)/Cl, $t_{1/2}$ = [(0.693)(300 L)]/(15 L/h) = 13.9 h. Steady state would be achieved in 3 to 5 $t_{1/2}$ of 42 to 70 h.

The patient with heart failure would likely have pharmacokinetic parameters similar to the heart failure patients in the research study (Cl = 30 L/h, V = 100 L): LD = V · Css, LD = (100 L)(10 mg/L) = 1000 mg intravenous bolus; MD = Cl · Css, MD = (30 L/h)(10 mg/L) = 300 mg/h intravenous infusion. The half-life would be estimated using the clearance and volume of distribution: $t_{1/2}$ = (0.693 V)/Cl, $t_{1/2}$ = [(0.693)(100 L)]/(30 L/h) = 2.3 h. Steady state would be achieved in 3 to 5 $t_{1/2}$ of 7 to 12 hours.

4. The serum concentration–time profile is plotted on semilogarithmic paper (see table for problem 4), and the best straight line is drawn through the points. Because all of the concentrations fall on the straight line, any two concentration–time pairs can be used to compute the elimination rate constant (k_e): k_e = (ln C_1 – ln C_2)/(t_1 – t_2), k_e = (ln 7.7 – ln 4)/(48 h – 1 h) = 0.0139 h^{-1}. The elimination rate constant can be used to calculate the half-life for the patient: $t_{1/2}$ = 0.693/k_e, $t_{1/2}$ = 0.693/0.0139 h^{-1} = 50 h.

5. Since phenytoin follows saturable pharmacokinetics, the Michaelis-Menten equation can be used for concentrations of 10 mg/L and 20 mg/L: MD = (V_{max} · Css)/(Km + Css); MD = [(500 mg/d)(10 mg/L)]/(4 mg/L + 10 mg/L) = 357 mg/d for Css = 10 mg/L; MD = [(500 mg/d)(20 mg/L)]/(4 mg/L + 20 mg/L) = 417 mg/d for Css = 20 mg/L.

6. The bioavailability of the capsule and liquid: $F = AUC_{PO}/AUC_{IV}$; capsule F = (1220 mg · h/L)/(1530 mg · h/L) = 0.80 or 80%; liquid F = (1420 mg · h/L)/(1530 mg · h/L) = 0.93 or 93%. The relative bioavailability: $F_{relative} = AUC_{CAPSULE}/AUC_{LIQUID}$; $F_{relative}$ = (1220 mg · h/L)/(1420 mg · h/L) = 0.86 or 86%.

REFERENCES

1. Shargel L, Yu ABC. Applied biopharmaceutics and pharmacokinetics. East Norwalk, CT: Appleton & Lange, 1999:30.
2. Ludden TM, Allen JP, Valutsky WA, et al. Individualization of phenytoin dosage regimens. Clin Pharmacol Ther 1977;21:287–293.
3. Levy G. Pharmacokinetics of salicylate elimination in man. J Pharm Sci 1965;54:959–967.
4. Bowdle TA, Patel IH, Levy RH, Wilensky AJ. Valproic acid dosage and plasma protein binding and clearance. Clin Pharmacol Ther 1980;28:486–492.
5. Lima JJ, Boudoulas H, Blanford M. Concentration-dependence of disopyramide binding to plasma protein and its influence on kinetics and dynamics. J Pharmacol Exp Ther 1981; 219:741–747.
6. Bertilsson L, Höjer B, Tybring G, Osterloh J, Rane A. Autoinduction of carbamazepine metabolism in children examined by a stable isotope technique. Clin Pharmacol Ther 1980;27:83–88.
7. Hansten PD, Horn JR. Hansten and Horn's Drug Interactions Analysis and Management. Vancouver, WA: Applied Therapeutics, 1998:521.
8. Rowland M, Benet LZ, Graham GG. Clearance concepts in pharmacokinetics. J Pharmacokinet Biopharm 1973;1:123–136.
9. Wilkinson GR, Shand DG. A physiological approach to hepatic drug clearance. Clin Pharmacol Ther 1975;18:377–390.
10. Nies AS, Shand DG, Wilkinson GR. Altered hepatic blood flow and drug disposition. Clin Pharmacokinet 1976;1:131–155.
11. Levy G. Effect of plasma protein binding on renal clearance of drugs. J Pharm Sci 1980; 69:482–491.
12. Øie S, Bennet LZ. Altered drug disposition in disease states. Annu Rep Med Chem 1980;15:277–296.
13. Gibaldi M, McNamara PJ. Apparent volumes of distribution and drug binding to plasma proteins and tissues. Eur J Clin Pharmacol 1978;13:373–378.

2

CLINICAL PHARMACOKINETIC EQUATIONS AND CALCULATIONS

INTRODUCTION

Clinical pharmacokinetic dosage calculations are conducted using the easiest possible equations and methods. This is because there are usually only a few (sometimes as little as one or two) drug serum concentrations on which to base the calculations. Drug serum concentrations are expensive (typically \$25 to \$75 each), and obtaining them can cause minor discomfort and trauma to the patient. This situation is much different from that found in pharmacokinetic research studies, in which 10 to 15 drug serum concentrations may be used to calculate pharmacokinetic parameters and more complex equations can be used to describe the pharmacokinetics of the drug. Since the goal of therapeutic drug monitoring in patients is to individualize the drug dose and serum concentrations to produce the desired pharmacologic effect and to avoid adverse effects, it may not be possible, or even necessary, to compute pharmacokinetic parameters for every patient or clinical situation.

ONE-COMPARTMENT MODEL EQUATIONS FOR LINEAR PHARMACOKINETICS

When medications are administered to humans, the body acts as if it is a series of compartments[1] (Figure 2-1). Often, the drug distributes from the blood into the tissues quickly, and a pseudoequilibrium of drug movement between blood and tissues is established rapidly. When this occurs, a one-compartment model can be used to describe the serum concentrations of a drug.[2,3] In some clinical situations, a one-compartment model can be used to compute doses for a drug even if drug distribution takes time to com-

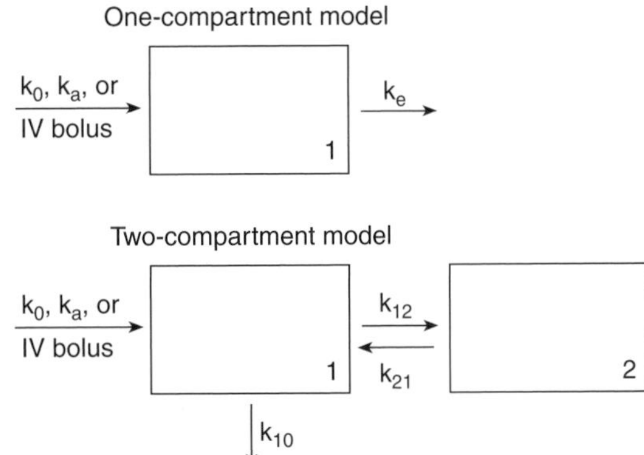

FIGURE 2-1 Using compartment models, the body can be represented as a series of discrete sections. The simplest model is the one-compartment model, which depicts the body as one large container in which drug distribution between blood and tissues occurs instantaneously. Drug is introduced into the compartment by infusion (k_0), absorption (k_a), or intravenous bolus; distributes immediately into a volume of distribution; and is removed from the body by metabolism and elimination via the elimination rate constant (k_e). The simplest multicompartment model is a two-compartment model, which represents the body as a central compartment into which drug is administered and as a peripheral compartment into which drug distributes. The central compartment (1) is composed of blood and tissues that equilibrate rapidly with blood. The peripheral compartment (2) represents tissues that equilibrate slowly with blood. Rate constants represent the transfer between compartments (k_{12}, k_{21}) and elimination from the body (k_{10}).

plete.[4,5] In this case, drug serum concentrations are not obtained in a patient until after the distribution phase is over.

Intravenous Bolus Equation

When a drug is given as an intravenous bolus and the drug distributes from the blood into the tissues quickly, the serum concentrations often decline in a straight line when plotted on semilogarithmic axes (Figure 2-2). In this instance, a one-compartment model intravenous bolus equation can be used: $C = (D/V)e^{-k_e t}$, where t is the time after the intravenous bolus was given (t = 0 at the time the dose was administered), C is the concentration at time = t, V is the volume of distribution, and k_e is the elimination rate constant. Most drugs given intravenously cannot be given as an actual intravenous bolus because of side effects related to rapid injection. A short infusion of 5 to 30 minutes can prevent these types of adverse effects, and if the intravenous infusion time is very short compared with the half-life of the drug so that a large amount of drug is not eliminated during the infusion time, intravenous bolus equations can still be used.

For example, a patient is given a theophylline loading dose of 400 mg intravenously over 20 minutes. Because the patient received theophylline during previous hospitalizations, it is known that the volume of distribution is 30 L, the elimination rate constant equals 0.116 h^{-1}, and the half-life ($t_{1/2}$) is 6 hours ($t_{1/2} = 0.693/k_e = 0.693/0.115 h^{-1} = 6$ h). To compute the expected theophylline concentration 4 hours after the dose was given, a one-compartment model intravenous bolus equation can be used: $C = (D/V)e^{-k_e t} = (400\ mg/30\ L)e^{-(0.115\ h^{-1})(4\ h)} = 8.4$ mg/L.

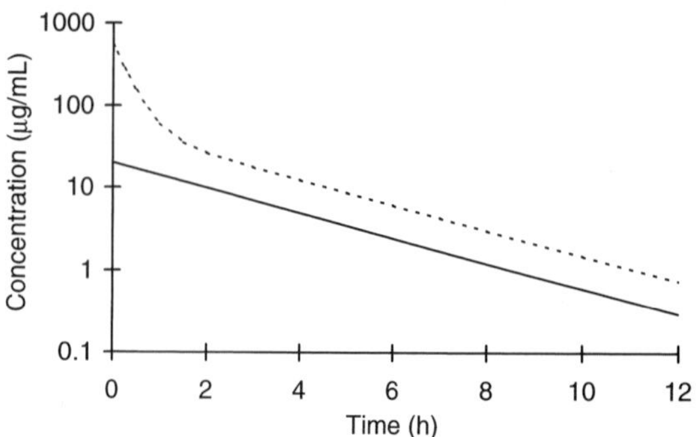

FIGURE 2-2 The *solid line* shows the serum concentration–time graph for a drug that follows one-compartment model pharmacokinetics after intravenous bolus administration. Drug distribution occurs instantaneously, and serum concentrations decline in a straight line on semilogarithmic axes. The *dashed line* represents the serum concentration–time plot for a drug that follows two-compartment model pharmacokinetics after an intravenous bolus is given. Immediately after the dose is given, serum concentrations decline rapidly. This portion of the curve is known as the distribution phase. During the distribution phase, drug is distributed between blood and tissues and is removed from the body via hepatic metabolism and renal elimination. Later, serum concentrations decline more slowly during the elimination phase. During the elimination phase, drug is primarily being removed from the body.

If drug distribution is not rapid, it is still possible to use a one-compartment model intravenous bolus equation if the duration of the distribution phase and infusion time is small compared with the half-life of the drug and only a small amount of drug is eliminated during the infusion and distribution phases.[6] The strategy in this situation is to infuse the medication and wait for the distribution phase to be over before obtaining serum concentrations in the patient. For instance, vancomycin must be infused slowly over 1 hour to avoid hypotension and red flushing around the head and neck areas. In addition, vancomycin distributes slowly to tissues with a 1/2- to 1-hour distribution phase. Because the half-life of vancomycin in patients with normal renal function is approximately 8 hours, a one-compartment model intravenous bolus equation can be used to compute concentrations in the postinfusion, postdistribution phase without a large amount of error. As an example of this approach, a patient is given an intravenous dose of 1000 mg vancomycin. Since the patient has received this drug before, the known volume of distribution is 50 L, the elimination rate constant is 0.077 h^{-1}, and the half-life is 9 h ($t_{1/2} = 0.693/k_e = 0.693/0.077\ h^{-1} = 9$ h). To calculate the expected vancomycin concentration 12 hours after the dose was given, a one-compartment model intravenous bolus equation can be used: $C = (D/V)e^{-k_e t} = (1000\ mg/50\ L)e^{-(0.077\ h^{-1})(12h)} = 7.9$ mg/L.

Pharmacokinetic parameters for patients can also be computed for use in the equations. If two or more serum concentrations are obtained after an intravenous bolus dose, the elimination rate constant, half-life, and volume of distribution can be calculated (Figure 2-3). For example, a patient was given an intravenous loading dose of 600 mg phenobarbital over a period of about 1 hour. One day and 4 days after the dose was administered phenobarbital serum concentrations were 12.6 mg/L and 7.5 mg/L, respectively. By plotting the serum concentration–time data on semilogarithmic axes, the time it takes for

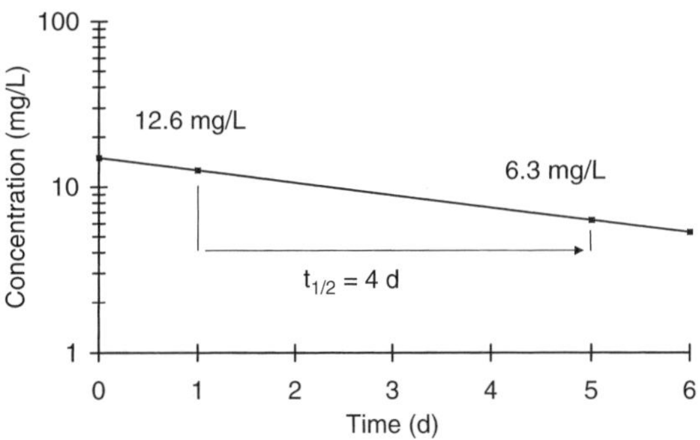

FIGURE 2-3 Phenobarbital concentrations are plotted on semilogarithmic axes, and a straight line is drawn connecting the concentrations. Half-life ($t_{1/2}$) is determined by measuring the time needed for serum concentrations to decline by half (i.e., from 12.6 mg/L to 6.3 mg/L) and is converted to the elimination rate constant ($k_e = 0.693/t_{1/2} = 0.693/4\ d = 0.173\ d^{-1}$). The concentration–time line can be extrapolated to the concentration axis to derive the concentration at time zero (C_0 = 15 mg/L) and used to compute the volume of distribution ($V = D/C_0$).

serum concentrations to decrease by half can be determined and is 4 days. The elimination rate constant can be computed using the following relationship: $k_e = 0.693/t_{1/2} = 0.693/4\ d = 0.173\ d^{-1}$. The concentration–time line can be extrapolated to the y-axis, where time = 0. Since this was the first dose of phenobarbital and the predose concentration was zero, the extrapolated concentration at time = 0 (C_0 = 15 mg/L in this case) can be used to calculate the volume of distribution (Figure 2-4): $V = D/C_0$ = 600 mg/(15 mg/L) = 40 L.

Alternatively, these parameters could be obtained by calculation without plotting the concentrations. The elimination rate constant can be computed using the following equation: $k_e = -(\ln C_1 - \ln C_2)/(t_1 - t_2)$, where t_1 and C_1 are the first time–concentration pair and t_2 and C_2 are the second time–concentration pair; $k_e = -$ [ln (12.6 mg/L) – ln (7.5 mg/L)]/(1 d – 4 d) = 0.173 d^{-1}. The elimination rate constant can be converted into the half-life using the following equation: $t_{1/2} = 0.693/k_e = 0.693/0.173\ d^{-1} = 4$ d. The volume of distribution can be calculated by dividing the dose by the serum concentration at time = 0. The serum concentration at time = 0 (C_0) can be computed using a variation of the intravenous bolus equation: $C_0 = C/e^{-k_e t}$, where t and C are a time–concentration pair that occur after the intravenous bolus dose. Either phenobarbital concentration can be used to compute C_0. In this case, the time–concentration pair on day 1 is used (time = 1 d, concentration = 12.6 mg/L): $C_0 = C/e^{-k_e t} = (12.6\ mg/L)/e^{-(0.173\ d^{-1})(1\ d)} = 15.0$ mg/L. The volume of distribution is then computed: $V = D/C_0$ = 600 mg/(15 mg/L) = 40 L.

Continuous and Intermittent Intravenous Infusion Equations

Some drugs are administered using a continuous intravenous infusion, and if the infusion is discontinued the serum concentration–time profile decreases in a straight line when graphed on a semilogarithmic axis (Figure 2-5). In this case, a one-compartment model intravenous infusion equation can be used to compute concentrations (C) while the infusion is running: $C = (k_0/Cl)(1 - e^{-k_e t}) = [k_0/(k_e V)](1 - e^{-k_e t})$, where k_0 is the drug in-

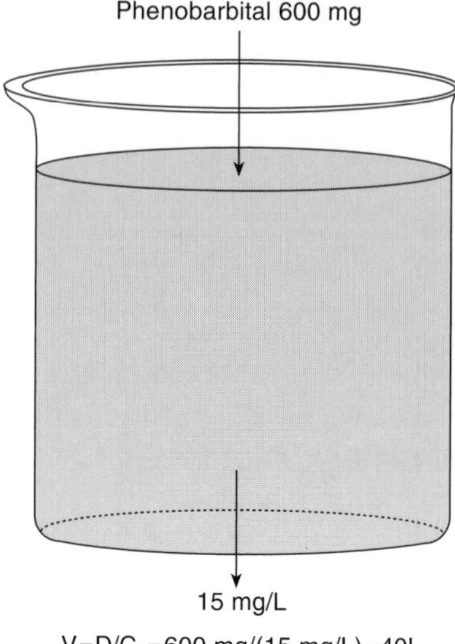

FIGURE 2-4 For a one-compartment model, the body can be thought of as a beaker containing fluid. If 600 mg of phenobarbital is added to a beaker of unknown volume and the resulting concentration is 15 mg/L, the volume can be computed by taking the quotient of the amount placed into the beaker and the concentration: $V = D/C_0 = 600$ mg/(15 mg/L) = 40 L. C_0 = concentration at time zero.

fusion rate (in amount per unit time, such as milligrams per hour [mg/h] or micrograms per minute [μg/min]), Cl is the drug clearance (since $Cl = k_eV$, this substitution was made in the second version of the equation), k_e is the elimination rate constant, and t is the time duration that the infusion has been running. If the infusion is allowed to continue until

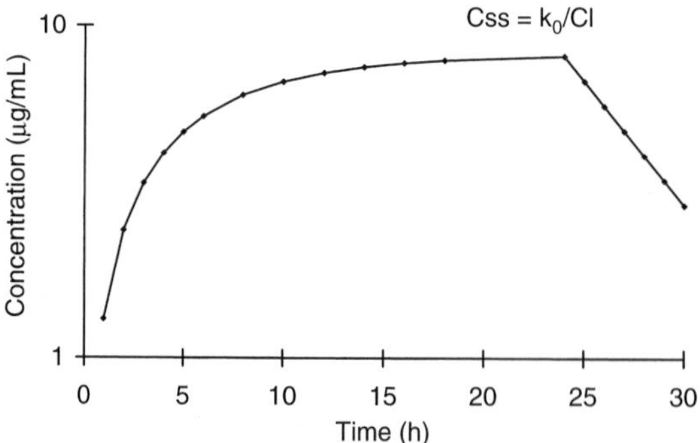

FIGURE 2-5 If a drug is given as a continuous intravenous infusion, serum concentrations increase until a steady-state concentration (*Css*) is achieved in 5 to 7 half-lives. The steady-state concentration is determined by the quotient of the infusion rate (k_0) and drug clearance (*Cl*): Css = k_0/Cl. When the infusion is discontinued, serum concentrations decline in a straight line if the graph is plotted on semilogarithmic axes. When using $\log_{10}$ graph paper, the elimination rate constant (k_e) can be computed using the following formula: Slope = $-k_e/2.303$.

steady-state is achieved, the steady-state concentration (Css) can be calculated easily: Css $= k_0/Cl = k_0/(k_eV)$.

If the infusion is stopped, postinfusion serum concentrations ($C_{postinfusion}$) can be computed by calculating the concentration when the infusion ended (C_{end}), using the appropriate equation in the preceding paragraph and the following equation: $C_{postinfusion} = C_{end}e^{-k_et_{postinfusion}}$, where k_e is the elimination rate constant and $t_{postinfusion}$ is the postinfusion time ($t_{postinfusion} = 0$ at end of infusion and increases from that point).

For example, a patient is administered 60 mg/h of theophylline. It is known from previous hospital admissions that the patient has the following pharmacokinetic parameters for theophylline: V = 40 L and $k_e = 0.139\ h^{-1}$. The serum concentration of theophylline in this patient after receiving the drug for 8 hours and at steady state can be calculated: $C = [k_0/(k_eV)]\ (1 - e^{-k_et}) = [(60\ mg/h)/(0.139\ h^{-1} \cdot 40\ L)](1 - e^{-(0.139\ h^{-1})(8\ h)}) = 7.2\ mg/L$; $Css = k_0/\ (k_eV) = (60\ mg/h)/(0.139\ h^{-1} \cdot 40\ L) = 10.8\ mg/L$. The theophylline serum concentration can be computed 6 hours after the infusion stopped in either circumstance. If the infusion ran for only 8 hours, the serum concentration 6 hours after the infusion stopped would be $C_{postinfusion} = C_{end}e^{-k_et_{postinfusion}} = (7.2\ mg/L)e^{-(0.139\ h^{-1})(6\ h)} = 3.1\ mg/L$. If the infusion ran until steady state was achieved, the serum concentration 6 hours after the infusion ended would be $C_{postinfusion} = C_{end}e^{-k_et_{postinfusion}} = (10.8\ mg/L)e^{-(0.139\ h^{-1})(6\ h)} = 4.7$ mg/L.

Even if serum concentrations exhibit a distribution phase after the drug infusion has ended, it is still possible to use one-compartment model intravenous infusion equations for the drug without a large amount of error.[4,5] The strategy used in this instance is to infuse the medication and wait for the distribution phase to be over before measuring serum drug concentrations in the patient. For example, gentamicin, tobramycin, and amikacin are usually infused over 30 minutes. When administered this way, these aminoglycoside antibiotics have distribution phases that last about 30 minutes. Using this strategy, aminoglycoside serum concentrations are obtained no sooner than 30 minutes after a 30-minute infusion to avoid the distribution phase. If aminoglycosides are infused over 1 hour, the distribution phase is very short and serum concentrations can be obtained immediately. For example, a patient is given an intravenous infusion of gentamicin 100 mg over 60 minutes. Because the patient received gentamicin before, it is known that the volume of distribution is 20 L, the elimination rate constant is $0.231\ h^{-1}$, and the half-life is 3 h ($t_{1/2} = 0.693/k_e = 0.693/0.231\ h^{-1} = 3\ h$). To compute the gentamicin concentration at the end of infusion, a one-compartment model intravenous infusion equation can be used: $C = [k_0/(k_eV)]\ (1 - e^{-k_et}) = [(100\ mg/1\ h)/(0.231\ h^{-1} \cdot 20\ L)](1 - e^{-(0.231\ h^{-1})(1\ h)}) = 4.5\ mg/L$.

Pharmacokinetic constants can also be calculated for use in the equations. If a steady-state concentration is obtained after a continuous intravenous infusion has been running uninterrupted for 3 to 5 half-lives, the drug clearance (Cl) can be calculated by rearranging the steady-state infusion formula: $Cl = k_0/Css$. For example, a patient receiving procainamide by intravenous infusion ($k_0 = 5$ mg/min) has a steady-state procainamide concentration measured as 8 mg/L. Procainamide clearance can be computed using the following expression: $Cl = k_0/Css = (5\ mg/min)/(8\ mg/L) = 0.625\ L/min$.

If the infusion did not run until steady state was achieved, pharmacokinetic parameters can still be computed from postinfusion concentrations. In the following example, a patient was given a single 120-mg dose of tobramycin as a 60-minute infusion, and concentrations at the end of infusion (6.2 mg/L) and 4 hours after the infusion ended (1.6 mg/L) were obtained. By plotting the serum concentration–time information on semilogarithmic axes, the half-life can be determined by measuring the time it takes for serum concentrations to decline by half (Figure 2-6), which equals 2 hours in this case. The elimination rate constant (k_e) can be calculated using the following formula: $k_e = 0.693/t_{1/2} = 0.693/2\ h = 0.347\ h^{-1}$. Alternatively, the elimination rate constant can be calculated without plotting the concentrations using the following equation: $k_e = -(\ln C_1 - \ln C_2)/(t_1 - t_2)$, where t_1 and C_1 are the first time–concentration pair and t_2 and C_2 are the second time–concentration pair; $k_e = -[\ln (6.2\ mg/L) - \ln (1.6\ mg/L)]/(1\ h - 5\ h) = 0.339\ h^{-1}$ (note the slight difference in k_e due to rounding errors). The elimination rate constant can be converted into the half-life using the following equation: $t_{1/2} = 0.693/k_e = 0.693/0.339\ h^{-1} = 2\ h$.

The volume of distribution can be computed using the following equation[4]:

$$V = \frac{k_0(1 - e^{-k_e t'})}{k_e[C_{max} - (C_{predose} e^{-k_e t'})]}$$

where k_0 is the infusion rate, k_e is the elimination rate constant, t' = infusion time, C_{max} is the maximum concentration at the end of infusion, and $C_{predose}$ is the predose concentration. In this example, the volume of distribution is:

$$V = \frac{(120\ mg/1\ h)(1 - e^{-(0.339\ h^{-1})(1\ h)})}{0.339\ h^{-1}[(6.2\ mg/L) - (0\ mg/L \cdot e^{-(0.339\ h^{-1})(1\ h)})]} = 16.4\ L$$

Extravascular Equation

When a drug is administered extravascularly (e.g., orally, intramuscularly, subcutaneously, or transdermally), absorption into the systemic vascular system must take place (Figure 2-7). If serum concentrations decrease in a straight line when plotted on semilogarithmic axes after drug absorption is complete, a one-compartment model extravascular equation can be used to describe the serum concentration–time curve: $C = \{(Fk_aD)/[V(k_a - k_e)]\}$

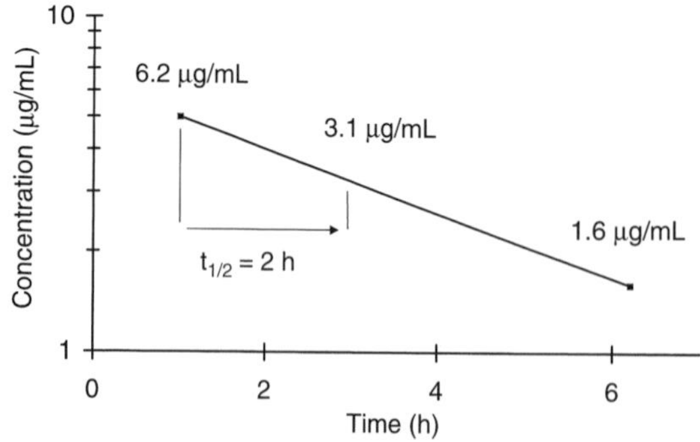

FIGURE 2-6 Tobramycin concentrations are plotted on semilogarithmic axes, and a straight line is drawn connecting the concentrations. Half-life ($t_{1/2}$) is determined by measuring the time needed for serum concentrations to decline by half (i.e., from 6.2 mg/L to 3.1 mg/L) and is converted to the elimination rate constant ($k_e = 0.693/t_{1/2} = 0.693/2\ h = 0.347\ h^{-1}$). Volume of distribution is computed using the equation given in the text.

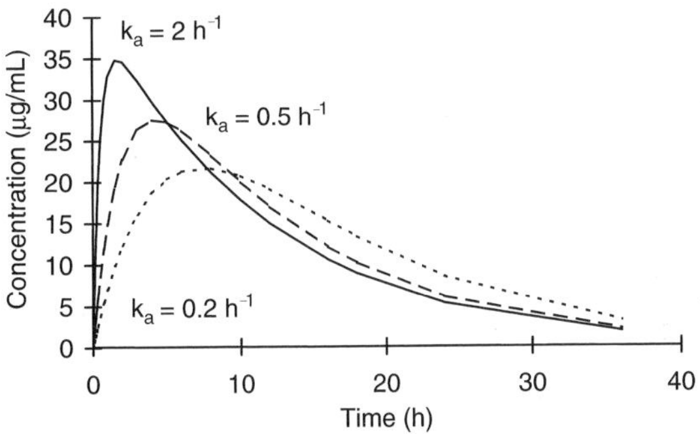

FIGURE 2-7 Serum concentration–time curves for extravascular drug administration for agents following one-compartment pharmacokinetics. The absorption rate constant (k_a) controls how quickly the drug enters the body. A large absorption rate constant allows drug to enter the body quickly, whereas a small elimination rate constant permits drug to enter the body more slowly. The *solid line* shows the concentration–time curve on semilogarithmic axes for an elimination rate constant of 2 h^{-1}. The *dashed* and *dotted lines* depict serum concentration–time plots for elimination rate constants of 0.5 h^{-1} and 0.2 h^{-1}, respectively.

$(e^{-k_e t} - e^{-k_a t})$, where t is the time after the extravascular dose was given (t = 0 at the time the dose was administered), C is the concentration at time = t, F is the bioavailability fraction, k_a is the absorption rate constant, D is the dose, V is the volume of distribution, and k_e is the elimination rate constant. The absorption rate constant describes how quickly drug is absorbed, with a large number indicating fast absorption and a small number indicating slow absorption (see Figure 2-7).

An example of the use of this equation would be a patient who is administered 500 mg of oral procainamide as a capsule. From prior clinic visits, it is known that procainamide in this patient has a half-life of 4 hours, an elimination rate constant of 0.173 h^{-1} ($k_e = 0.693/t_{1/2} = 0.693/4\ h = 0.173\ h^{-1}$), and a volume of distribution of 175 L. The capsule that is administered to the patient has an absorption rate constant of 2 h^{-1} and an oral bioavailability fraction of 0.85. The procainamide serum concentration 4 hours after a single dose would be:

$$C = \frac{Fk_aD}{V(k_a - k_e)}(e^{-k_e t} - e^{-k_a t})$$

$$C = \frac{(0.85)\,(2\ h^{-1})(500\ mg)}{(175\ L)\,(2\ h^{-1} - 0.173\ h^{-1})}(e^{-(0.173\ h^{-1})\,(4\ h)} - e^{-(2\ h^{-1})\,(4\ h)})$$

$$C = 1.3\ mg/L$$

If the serum concentration–time curve displays a distribution phase, it is still possible to use one-compartment model equations after an extravascular dose is administered. To do this, serum concentrations are obtained only in the postdistribution phase. Because the absorption rate constant is also hard to measure in patients, it is also desirable to avoid drawing drug serum concentrations during the absorption phase in clinical situations.

When only postabsorption, postdistribution serum concentrations are obtained for a drug that is administered extravascularly, the equation simplifies to $C = [(FD)/V]e^{-k_e t}$, where C is the concentration at any postabsorption, postdistribution time; F is the bioavailability fraction; D is the dose; V is the volume of distribution; k_e is the elimination rate constant; and t is any postabsorption, postdistribution time. This approach works very well when the extravascular dose is rapidly absorbed and not a sustained- or extended-release dosage form. An example would be a patient receiving 24 mEq of lithium ion as lithium carbonate capsules. From previous clinic visits, it is known that the patient has a volume of distribution of 60 L and an elimination rate constant of 0.058 h^{-1}. The bioavailability of the capsule is known to be 0.90. The serum lithium concentration 12 hours after a single dose would be $C = [(FD)/V]e^{-k_e t} = [(0.90 \cdot 24\ mEq)/60\ L]e^{-(0.058\ h^{-1})(12\ h)} = 0.18\ mEq/L$.

Pharmacokinetic constants can also be calculated and used in these equations. If two or more postabsorption, postdistribution serum concentrations are obtained after an extravascular dose, the volume of distribution, elimination rate constant, and half-life can be computed (Figure 2-8). For example, a patient is given an oral dose of valproic acid 750 mg as capsules. Six and 24 hours after the dose, the valproic acid serum concentrations are 51.9 mg/L and 21.3 mg/L, respectively. After graphing the serum concentration–time data on semilogarithmic axes, the time it takes for serum concentrations to decrease by half is measured and is 14 hours. The elimination rate constant is calculated using the following equation: $k_e = 0.693/t_{1/2} = 0.693/14\ h = 0.0495\ h^{-1}$. The concentration–time line can be extrapolated to the y-axis, where time = 0. Since this was the first dose of valproic acid, the extrapolated concentration at time = 0 (C_0 = 70 mg/L) is used to estimate the hybrid volume of distribution/bioavailability (V/F) parameter: $V/F = D/C_0 = 750\ mg/70\ L = 10.7\ L$. Even though the absolute volume of distribution and bioavailability cannot be computed without the administration of intravenous drug, the hybrid constant can be used in extravascular equations in place of V/F.

An alternative approach is to directly calculate the parameters without plotting the con-

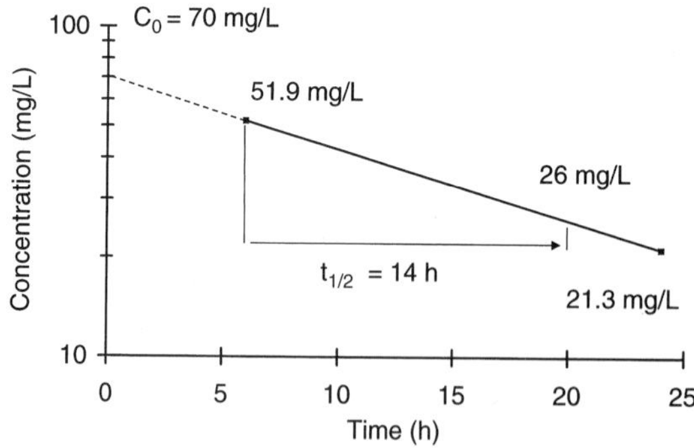

FIGURE 2-8 Valproic acid concentrations are plotted on semilogarithmic axes, and a straight line is drawn connecting the concentrations. Half-life ($t_{1/2}$) is determined by measuring the time needed for serum concentrations to decline by half (i.e., from 51.9 mg/L to 26 mg/L) and is converted to the elimination rate constant ($k_e = 0.693/t_{1/2} = 0.693/14\ h = 0.0495\ h^{-1}$). The concentration–time line can be extrapolated to the concentration axis to derive the concentration at time zero (C_0 = 70 mg/L) and used to compute the hybrid constant volume of distribution/bioavailability fraction ($V/F = D/C_0$).

centrations. The elimination rate constant (k_e) is computed using the following relationship: $k_e = -(\ln C_1 - \ln C_2)/(t_1 - t_2)$, where C_1 is the first concentration at time = t_1, and C_2 is the second concentration at time = t_2; $k_e = -[\ln (51.9 \text{ mg/L}) - \ln (21.3 \text{ mg/L})]/(6 \text{ h} - 24 \text{ h}) = 0.0495 \text{ h}^{-1}$. The elimination rate constant can be translated into the half-life using the following equation: $t_{1/2} = 0.693/k_e = 0.693/0.0495 \text{ h}^{-1} = 14$ h. The hybrid constant volume of distribution/bioavailability (V/F) is computed by taking the quotient of the dose and the extrapolated serum concentration at time = 0. The extrapolated serum concentration at time = 0 is calculated using a variation of the intravenous bolus equation: $C_0 = C/e^{-k_e t}$, where t and C are a time–concentration pair that occur after administration of the extravascular dose in the postabsorption and postdistribution phases. Either valproic acid concentration can be used to compute C_0. In this situation, the time–concentration pair at 24 hours will be used (time = 24 hours, concentration = 21.3 mg/L): $C_0 = C/e^{-k_e t} = (21.3 \text{ mg/L})/e^{-(0.0495 \text{ h}^{-1})(24 \text{ h})} = 70$ mg/L. The hybrid volume of distribution/bioavailability constant (V/F) is then computed: $V/F = D/C_0 = 750 \text{ mg}/(70 \text{ mg/L}) = 10.7$ L.

Multiple-Dose and Steady-State Equations

Medications are usually administered to patients as multiple doses, and drug serum concentrations for therapeutic drug monitoring are not obtained until steady state is achieved. For these reasons, multiple-dose equations that reflect steady-state conditions are usually more useful in clinical settings than are single-dose equations. Fortunately, it is simple to convert single-dose compartment model equations to their multiple-dose and steady-state counterparts.[7] To change a single-dose equation to the multiple-dose version, it is necessary to multiply each exponential term in the equation by the multiple dosing factor: $(1 - e^{-nk_i\tau})/(1 - e^{-k_i\tau})$, where n is the number of doses administered, k_i is the rate constant found in the exponential of the single-dose equation, and τ is the dosage interval. At steady state, the number of doses is large, the exponential term in the numerator of the multiple dosing factor ($-nk_e\tau$) becomes a larger negative number, and the exponent approaches zero. Therefore, the steady-state version of the multiple dosing factor becomes the following: $1/(1 - e^{-k_e\tau})$, where k_e is the elimination rate constant and τ is the dosage interval. Whenever the multiple dosing factor is used to change a single-dose equation to the multiple-dose or steady-state versions, the time variable in the equation resets to zero at the beginning of each dosage interval.

As an example of the conversion of a single-dose equation to the steady-state variant, the one-compartment model intravenous bolus equation is $C = (D/V)e^{-k_e t}$, where C is the concentration at time = t, D is the dose, V is the volume of distribution, k_e is the elimination rate constant, and t is time after the dose is administered. Since there is only one exponential in the equation, the multiple dosing factor at steady state is multiplied into the expression at only one place, substituting the elimination rate constant (k_e) for the rate constant in the multiple dosing factor: $C = (D/V)[e^{-k_e t}/(1 - e^{-k_e\tau})]$, where C is the steady-state concentration at any postdose time (t) after the dose (D) is given, V is the volume of distribution, k_e is the elimination rate constant, and τ is the dosage interval. Table 2-1 lists the one-compartment model equations for the various routes of administration under single-dose, multiple-dose, and steady-state conditions.

The following are examples of steady-state one-compartment model equations for intravenous, intermittent intravenous infusions, and extravascular routes of administration:

TABLE 2-1 Single-Dose, Multiple-Dose, and Steady-State One-Compartment Model Equations

ROUTE OF ADMINISTRATION	SINGLE DOSE	MULTIPLE DOSE	STEADY STATE
Intravenous bolus	$C = (D/V)e^{-k_e t}$	$C = (D/V)e^{-k_e t}[(1 - e^{-nk_e \tau})/(1 - e^{-k_e \tau})]$	$C = (D/V)[e^{-k_e t}/(1 - e^{-k_e \tau})]$
Continuous intravenous infusion	$C = [k_0/(k_e V)](1 - e^{-k_e t})$	N/A	$Css = k_0/Cl = k_0/(k_e V)$
Intermittent intravenous infusion	$C = [k_0/(k_e V)](1 - e^{-k_e t'})$	$C = [k_0/(k_e V)](1 - e^{-k_e t'})[(1 - e^{-nk_e \tau})/(1 - e^{-k_e \tau})]$	$C = [k_0/(k_e V)][(1 - e^{-k_e t'})/(1 - e^{-k_e \tau})]$
Extravascular (postabsorption, postdistribution)	$C = [(FD)/V]e^{-k_e t}$	$C = [(FD)/V]e^{-k_e t}[(1 - e^{-nk_e \tau})/(1 - e^{-k_e \tau})]$	$C = (FD/V)[e^{-k_e t}/(1 - e^{-k_e \tau})]$
Average steady-state concentration (any route of administration)	N/A	N/A	$Css = [F(D/\tau)]/Cl$

C = drug serum concentration at time = t; Cl = clearance; D = dose; k_e = the elimination rate constant; k_0 = infusion rate; n = number of administered doses; N/A = not available; τ = the dosage interval; V = volume of distribution.

Intravenous bolus. A patient with tonic-clonic seizures is given phenobarbital 100 mg intravenously daily until steady state occurs. Pharmacokinetic constants for phenobarbital in the patient are $k_e = 0.116\ d^{-1}$, V = 75 L. The steady-state concentration 23 hours [(23 h)/(24 h/d) = 0.96 d] after the last dose equals $C = (D/V)[e^{-k_e t}/(1 - e^{-k_e \tau})] = (100\ mg/75\ L)[e^{-(0.116\ d^{-1})(0.96\ d)}/(1 - e^{-(0.116\ d^{-1})(1\ d)}] = 10.9\ mg/L$.

Intermittent intravenous infusion. A patient with gram-negative pneumonia is administered tobramycin 140 mg every 8 hours until steady state is achieved. Pharmacokinetic parameters for tobramycin in the patient are V = 16 L, $k_e = 0.30\ h^{-1}$. The steady-state concentration immediately after a 1-hour infusion equals $C = [k_0/(k_e V)][(1 - e^{-k_e t'})/(1 - e^{-k_e \tau})] = [(140\ mg/h)/(0.30\ h^{-1} \cdot 16\ L)][(1 - e^{-(0.30\ h^{-1} \cdot 1\ h)})/(1 - e^{-(0.30\ h^{-1} \cdot 8\ h)})] = 8.3$ mg/L.

Extravascular. A patient with an arrhythmia is administered 250 mg of quinidine orally (as 300-mg quinidine sulfate tablets) every 6 hours until steady state occurs. Pharmacokinetic constants for quinidine in the patient are V = 180 L, $k_e = 0.0693\ h^{-1}$, F = 0.7. The postabsorption, postdistribution steady-state concentration just before the next dose (t = 6 h) equals $C = (FD/V)[e^{-k_e t}/(1 - e^{-k_e \tau})] = [(0.7 \cdot 250\ mg)/180\ L][e^{-(0.0693\ h^{-1} \cdot 6\ h)}/(1 - e^{-(0.0693\ h^{-1} \cdot 6\ h)})] = 1.9\ mg/L$.

It is also possible to compute pharmacokinetic parameters under multiple-dose and steady-state conditions. Table 2-2 lists the methods to compute pharmacokinetic constants using a one-compartment model for different routes of administration under single-dose, multiple-dose, and steady-state conditions. The main difference between single-dose and

TABLE 2-2 Single-Dose, Multiple-Dose, and Steady-State Pharmacokinetic Constant Computations Using a One-Compartment Model

ROUTE OF ADMINISTRATION	SINGLE DOSE	MULTIPLE DOSE	STEADY STATE
Intravenous bolus	$k_e = (\ln C_1 - \ln C_2)/(t_1 - t_2)$ $t_{1/2} = 0.693/k_e$ $V = D/C_0$ $Cl = k_eV$	$k_e = (\ln C_1 - \ln C_2)/(t_1 - t_2)$ $t_{1/2} = 0.693/k_e$ $V = D/(C_0 - C_{predose})$ $Cl = k_eV$	$k_e = (\ln C_1 - \ln C_2)/(t_1 - t_2)$ $t_{1/2} = 0.693/k_e$ $V = D/(C_0 - C_{predose})$ $Cl = k_eV$
Continuous intravenous infusion	N/A	N/A	$Cl = k_0/Css$
Intermittent intravenous infusion	$k_e = (\ln C_1 - \ln C_2)/(t_1 - t_2)$ $t_{1/2} = 0.693/k_e$ $V = [k_0(1 - e^{-k_et'})]/\{k_e[C_{max} - (C_{predose}e^{-k_et'})]\}$ $Cl = k_eV$	$k_e = (\ln C_1 - \ln C_2)/(t_1 - t_2)$ $t_{1/2} = 0.693/k_e$ $V = [k_0(1 - e^{-k_et'})]/\{k_e[C_{max} - (C_{predose}e^{-k_et'})]\}$ $Cl = k_eV$	$k_e = (\ln C_1 - \ln C_2)/(t_1 - t_2)$ $t_{1/2} = 0.693/k_e$ $V = [k_0(1 - e^{-k_et'})]/\{k_e[C_{max} - (C_{predose}e^{-k_et'})]\}$ $Cl = k_eV$
Extravascular (postabsorption, postdistribution)	$k_e = (\ln C_1 - \ln C_2)/(t_1 - t_2)$ $t_{1/2} = 0.693/k_e$ $V/F = D/C_0$ $Cl/F = k_e(V/F)$	$k_e = (\ln C_1 - \ln C_2)/(t_1 - t_2)$ $t_{1/2} = 0.693/k_e$ $V/F = D/(C_0 - C_{predose})$ $Cl/F = k_e(V/F)$	$k_e = (\ln C_1 - \ln C_2)/(t_1 - t_2)$ $t_{1/2} = 0.693/k_e$ $V/F = D/(C_0 - C_{predose})$ $Cl/F = k_e(V/F)$
Average steady-state concentration (any route of administration)	N/A	N/A	$Cl/F = (D/\tau)/Css$

C_0 = concentration at time = 0; C_1 = drug serum concentration at time = t_1; C_2 = drug serum concentration at time = t_2; Cl = drug clearance; Cl/F = hybrid constant clearance–bioavailability fraction; $C_{predose}$ = predose concentration; Css = steady-state concentration; D = dose; k_e = elimination rate constant; k_0 = continuous infusion rate; N/A = not available; t′ = infusion time; $t_{1/2}$ = half-life; V = volume of distribution; V/F = hybrid constant volume of distribution–bioavailability fraction.

multiple-dose calculations is in the computation of the volume of distribution. When a single dose of medication is given, the predose concentration is assumed to be zero. However, when multiple doses are given, the predose concentration is not usually zero, and the volume of distribution equation needs to have the baseline, predose concentration ($C_{predose}$) subtracted from the extrapolated drug concentration at time = 0 (C_0) for the intravenous bolus ($V = D/[C_0 - C_{predose}]$, where D is dose) and extravascular ($V/F = D/[C_0 - C_{predose}]$, where F is the bioavailability fraction) cases. In the case of intermittent intravenous infusions, the volume of distribution equation already has a parameter for the predose concentration in it[4]:

$$V = \frac{k_0(1 - e^{-k_et'})}{k_e[C_{max} - (C_{predose}e^{-k_et'})]}$$

where k_0 is the infusion rate, k_e is the elimination rate constant, t′ = infusion time, C_{max} is the maximum concentration at the end of infusion, and $C_{predose}$ is the predose concentration. For each route of administration, the elimination rate constant (k_e) is computed using the same equation as the single-dose situation: $k_e = -(\ln C_1 - \ln C_2)/(t_1 - t_2)$, where C_1 is the first concentration at time = t_1, and C_2 is the second concentration at time = t_2.

The following are examples of multiple-dose and steady-state computations of pharmacokinetic parameters using a one-compartment model for intravenous, intermittent intravenous infusions, and extravascular routes of administration:

Intravenous bolus. A patient receiving theophylline 300 mg intravenously every 6 hours has a predose concentration of 2.5 mg/L and postdose concentrations of 9.2 mg/L 1 hour and 4.5 mg/L 5 hours after the second dose is given. The patient has an elimination rate constant (k_e) of: $k_e = -(\ln C_1 - \ln C_2)/(t_1 - t_2) = -[(\ln 9.2 \text{ mg/L}) - (\ln 4.5 \text{ mg/L})]/(1 \text{ h} - 5 \text{ h}) = 0.179 \text{ h}^{-1}$. The volume of distribution of theophylline for the patient is $C_0 = C/e^{-k_e t} = (9.2 \text{ mg/L})/e^{-(0.179 \text{ h}^{-1})(1 \text{ h})} = 11.0$ mg/L and $V = D/[C_0 - C_{predose}] = (300 \text{ mg})/(11.0 \text{ mg/L} - 2.5 \text{ mg/L}) = 35.3$ L.

Intermittent intravenous infusion. A patient receives gentamicin 100 mg infused over 60 minutes every 12 hours. A predose steady-state concentration ($C_{predose}$) is drawn before a dose and is 2.5 mg/L. After the 1-hour infusion, a steady-state maximum concentration (C_{max}) is obtained and is 7.9 mg/L. Since the patient is at steady state, it can be assumed that all predose steady-state concentrations are equal. Because of this, the predose steady-state concentration 12 hours after the dose can also be considered equal to 2.5 mg/L and used to compute the elimination rate constant (k_e) of gentamicin for the patient: $k_e = -(\ln C_1 - \ln C_2)/(t_1 - t_2) = -[(\ln 7.9 \text{ mg/L}) - (\ln 2.5 \text{ mg/L})]/(1 \text{ h} - 12 \text{ h}) = 0.105 \text{ h}^{-1}$. The volume of distribution of gentamicin for the patient is:

$$V = \frac{k_0(1 - e^{-k_e t'})}{k_e[C_{max} - (C_{predose} e^{-k_e t'})]}$$

where k_0 is the infusion rate, k_e is the elimination rate constant, t' = infusion time, C_{max} is the maximum concentration at the end of infusion, and $C_{predose}$ is the predose concentration. In this example, volume of distribution is:

$$V = \frac{(100 \text{ mg/1 h})(1 - e^{-(0.105 \text{ h}^{-1})(1 \text{ h})})}{0.105 \text{ h}^{-1}[(7.9 \text{ mg/L}) - (2.5 \text{ mg/L} \cdot e^{-(0.105 \text{ h}^{-1})(1 \text{ h})})]} = 16.8 \text{ L}$$

Extravascular. A patient is given procainamide capsules 750 mg every 6 hours. The following concentrations are obtained before and after the second dose: $C_{predose}$ = 1.1 mg/L, concentrations 2 hours and 6 hours postdose equal 4.6 mg/L and 2.9 mg/L. The patient has an elimination rate constant (k_e) of: $k_e = -(\ln C_1 - \ln C_2)/(t_1 - t_2) = -[(\ln 4.6 \text{ mg/L}) - (\ln 2.9 \text{ mg/L})]/(2 \text{ h} - 6 \text{ h}) = 0.115 \text{ h}^{-1}$. The hybrid volume of distribution/bioavailability constant (V/F) of procainamide for the patient is: $C_0 = C/e^{-k_e t} = (2.9 \text{ mg/L})/e^{-(0.115 \text{ h}^{-1})(6 \text{ h})} = 5.8$ mg/L and $V/F = D/[C_0 - C_{predose}] = (750 \text{ mg})/(5.8 \text{ mg/L} - 1.1 \text{ mg/L}) = 160$ L.

Average Steady-State Concentration Equation

A very useful and easy equation can be used to compute the average steady-state concentration (Css) of a drug: $Css = [F(D/\tau)]/Cl$, where F is the bioavailability fraction, D is the dose, τ is the dosage interval, and Cl is the drug clearance.[8] This equation works for any single- or multiple-compartment model, and because of this it is deemed a model-independent equation. The steady-state concentration computed by this equation is the concentration that would have occurred if the dose, adjusted for bioavailability, was given as a continuous intravenous infusion. For example, 600 mg of theophylline tablets given orally every 12 hours (F = 1.0) would be equivalent to a 50 mg/h (600 mg/12 h = 50 mg/h) continuous intravenous infusion of theophylline. The average steady-state concentration equation is very useful when the half-life of the drug is long compared with the dosage interval or if a sustained-release dosage form is used. Examples of both situations follow:

Long half-life compared with dosage interval. A patient is administered 250 μg of digoxin tablets daily for heart failure until steady state. The pharmacokinetic constants for digoxin in the patient are F = 0.7, Cl = 120 L/d. The average steady-state concentration would be $Css = [F(D/\tau)]/Cl = [0.7(250\ \mu g/d)]/(120\ L/d) = 1.5\ \mu g/L$.

Sustained-release dosage form. A patient is given 1500 mg of procainamide sustained-release tablets every 12 hours until steady state for the treatment of an arrhythmia. The pharmacokinetic parameters for procainamide in the patient are F = 0.85, Cl = 30 L/h. The average steady-state concentration would be $Css = [F(D/\tau)]/Cl = [0.85(1500\ mg/12\ h)]/(30\ L/h) = 3.5\ mg/L$.

If an average steady-state concentration is known for a drug, the hybrid pharmacokinetic constant clearance/bioavailability (Cl/F) can be computed: $Cl/F = (D/\tau)/Css$, where D is dose and τ is the dosage interval. For example, a patient receiving 600 mg of sustained-release theophylline every 12 hours has a steady-state concentration of 11.2 mg/L. The clearance/bioavailability constant for theophylline in this patient would be $Cl/F = (D/\tau)/Css = (600\ mg/12\ h)/11.2\ mg/L = 4.5\ L/h$.

DESIGNING INDIVIDUALIZED DOSAGE REGIMENS USING ONE-COMPARTMENT MODEL EQUATIONS

The goal of therapeutic drug monitoring is to customize medication dosages that provide the optimal drug efficacy without adverse reactions. One-compartment model equations can be used to compute initial drug doses using population pharmacokinetic parameters that estimate the constants for a patient.[4,5,9] The patient's own unique pharmacokinetic parameters can be computed after doses have been administered and drug serum concentrations measured. At that time, individualized dosage regimens at steady state can be designed for a patient. Table 2-3 lists the equations used to customize doses for the various routes of administration.

Intravenous Bolus

If the volume of distribution and elimination rate constant can be estimated for a patient, a loading dose and initial maintenance dose can be computed. To design these doses, estimates of pharmacokinetic constants are obtained using patient characteristics such as weight, age, gender, renal and liver function, and other disease states and condi-

TABLE 2-3 Equations for Computing Individualized Dosage Regimens for Various Routes of Administration

ROUTE OF ADMINISTRATION	DOSAGE INTERVAL (τ), MAINTENANCE DOSE (MD OR K_0), AND LOADING DOSE (LD) EQUATIONS
Intravenous bolus	$\tau = (\ln C_{max,ss} - \ln C_{min,ss})/k_e$ $D = C_{max,ss} V(1 - e^{-k_e\tau})$ $LD = C_{max,ss} V$
Continuous intravenous infusion	$k_0 = CssCl = Cssk_eV$ $LD = CssV$
Intermittent intravenous infusion	$\tau = [(\ln C_{max,ss} - \ln C_{min,ss})/k_e] + t'$ $k_0 = C_{max,ss}k_eV[(1 - e^{-k_e\tau})/(1 - e^{-k_et'})]$ $LD = k_0/(1 - e^{-k_e\tau})$
Extravascular (postabsorption, postdistribution)	$\tau = [(\ln C_{max,ss} - \ln C_{min,ss})/k_e] + T_{max}$ $D = [(C_{max,ss}V)/F][(1 - e^{-k_e\tau})/e^{-k_eT_{max}}]$ $LD = D/(1 - e^{-k_e\tau})$
Average steady-state concentration (any route of administration)	$D = (CssCl\tau)/F = (Cssk_eV\tau)/F$ $LD = CssV$

Css = steady-state concentration; $C_{max,ss}$ and $C_{min,ss}$ = maximum and minimum steady-state concentrations; F = bioavailability fraction; k_e = elimination rate constant; k_0 = continuous infusion rate; t′ = infusion time; T_{max} = the time that $C_{max,ss}$ occurs; V = volume of distribution.

tions that are known to affect the disposition and elimination of the drug. When the actual elimination rate constant and volume of distribution are measured for the medication, a maintenance dose to achieve any target steady-state concentrations can be designed.

Desired maximum and minimum steady-state concentrations are chosen for the patient. If the patient has not received the drug before, the therapeutic range can be used to choose starting concentrations. If the patient has taken the drug on previous occasions, safe and effective concentrations may be known. The dosage interval (τ) can be computed using the desired maximum ($C_{max,ss}$) and minimum ($C_{min,ss}$) steady-state concentrations: $\tau = (\ln C_{max,ss} - \ln C_{min,ss})/k_e$, where k_e is the elimination rate constant. The maintenance dose is then computed using the one-compartment model equation for intravenous bolus administration at the time $C_{max,ss}$ occurs (t = 0 h after the bolus is given) solved for dose: $D = [C_{max,ss} V(1 - e^{-k_e\tau})]/e^{-k_e(0\ h)} = C_{max,ss} V(1 - e^{-k_e\tau})$. If a loading dose is necessary, it is computed using the following equation: $LD = C_{max,ss} V$.

An example of this approach is with a patient who needs to be treated for complex partial seizures with intravenous phenobarbital. An initial dosage regimen is designed using population pharmacokinetic parameters ($k_e = 0.139\ d^{-1}$, V = 50 L) to achieve maximum ($C_{max,ss}$) and minimum ($C_{min,ss}$) steady-state concentrations of 30 mg/L and 25 mg/L, respectively: $\tau = (\ln C_{max,ss} - \ln C_{min,ss})/k_e = [\ln (30\ mg/L) - \ln (25\ mg/L)]\ /0.139\ d^{-1} = 1.3\ d$, round to a practical dosage interval of 1 d; $D = C_{max,ss} V(1 - e^{-k_e\tau}) = (30\ mg/L \cdot 50\ L)(1 - e^{-(0.139\ d^{-1})(1\ d)}) = 195\ mg$, round to a practical dose of 200 mg. The patient would be prescribed intravenous phenobarbital 200 mg daily.

Continuous and Intermittent Intravenous Infusion

The dosage regimen for a continuous intravenous infusion is computed using the following equation: k_0 = CssCl = Cssk_eV, where k_0 is the infusion rate, Css is the steady-state drug concentration, Cl is the drug clearance, k_e is the elimination rate constant, and V is the volume of distribution. A loading dose is computed using the following expression: LD = CssV. An example using this method is a patient with a ventricular arrhythmia after a myocardial infarction needing treatment with lidocaine at a Css of 3.0 mg/L (population pharmacokinetic parameters used: V = 50 L, Cl = 1.0 L/min): LD = CssV = (3 mg/L)(50 L) = 150 mg; k_0 = CssCl = (3 mg/L)(1.0 L/min) = 3 mg/min. The patient would be prescribed lidocaine 150 mg intravenously followed by a 3-mg/min continuous infusion.

For intermittent intravenous infusions, the dosage interval (τ) is computed by choosing minimum ($C_{min,ss}$) and maximum ($C_{max,ss}$) steady-state concentrations: $\tau = [(\ln C_{max,ss} - \ln C_{min,ss})/k_e] + t'$, where k_e is the elimination rate constant, and t′ is the infusion time. The maintenance dose is calculated using the one-compartment model equation for intermittent intravenous infusions at the time $C_{max,ss}$ occurs solved for infusion rate (k_0): $k_0 = C_{max,ss}k_eV[(1 - e^{-k_e\tau})/(1 - e^{-k_et'})]$, where k_e is the elimination rate constant and V is the volume of distribution. A loading dose can be calculated using the following formula, which takes into account the amount of drug eliminated during the infusion time: $LD = k_0/(1 - e^{-k_e\tau})$.

An example using these techniques is a patient receiving tobramycin for the treatment of intra-abdominal sepsis. Using pharmacokinetic parameters (V = 20 L, k_e = 0.087 h^{-1}) previously measured in the patient using serum concentrations, compute a tobramycin dose (infused over 1 hour) that would provide maximum ($C_{max,ss}$) and minimum ($C_{min,ss}$) steady-state concentrations of 6 mg/L and 1 mg/L, respectively: $\tau = [(\ln C_{max,ss} - \ln C_{min,ss})/k_e] + t'$ = [(ln 6 mg/L − ln 1 mg/L)/0.087 h^{-1}] + 1 h = 22 h, round to practical dosage interval of 24 h; $k_0 = C_{max,ss}k_eV[(1 - e^{-k_e\tau})/(1 - e^{-k_et'})]$ = [(6 mg/L)(0.087 h^{-1})(20 L)][(1 − $e^{-(0.087\ h^{-1})(24\ h)}$)/(1 − $e^{-(0.087\ h^{-1})(1\ h)}$)] = 110 mg. The patient would be prescribed tobramycin 110 mg infused over 1 hour every 24 hours.

Extravascular

The dosage regimen for extravascular doses is determined by choosing maximum ($C_{max,ss}$) and minimum ($C_{min,ss}$) steady-state concentrations: $\tau = [(\ln C_{max,ss} - \ln C_{min,ss})/k_e] + T_{max}$, where k_e is the elimination rate constant and T_{max} is the time that the maximum concentration occurs. The maintenance dose is computed using the one-compartment model equation for extravascular doses at the time $C_{max,ss}$ occurs ($t = T_{max}$) solved for dose (D): $D = [(C_{max,ss}V)/F][(1 - e^{-k_e\tau})/e^{-k_eT_{max}}]$, where V is the volume of distribution and F is the bioavailability fraction. A loading dose can be computed using the following equation: $LD = D/(1 - e^{-k_e\tau})$.

An example of these computations is for a patient with simple partial seizures who needs to receive valproic acid capsules (population pharmacokinetic parameters are V = 12 L, k_e = 0.05 h^{-1}, T_{max} = 3 h, F = 1.0) and maintain steady-state maximum ($C_{max,ss}$) and minimum ($C_{min,ss}$) concentrations of 80 mg/L and 50 mg/L, respectively: $\tau = [(\ln C_{max,ss} - \ln C_{min,ss})/k_e] + T_{max}$ = [(ln 80 mg/L − ln 50 mg/L)/0.05 h^{-1}] + 3 h = 12.4 h, rounded to a practical dosage interval of 12 h; $D = [(C_{max,ss}V)/F][(1 - e^{-k_e\tau})/e^{-k_eT_{max}}]$ = [(80 mg/L · 12 L)/1.0)]

$[(1 - e^{(-0.05\ h^{-1})(12\ h)})/e^{(-0.05\ h^{-1})(3\ h)}]$ = 503 mg, rounded to a practical dose of 500 mg. The patient would be prescribed valproic acid capsules 500 mg orally every 12 hours.

Average Steady-State Concentration

If the drug is administered as a sustained-release dosage form or if the half-life is long compared with the dosage interval, the average steady-state concentration equation can be used to individualize doses. The dosage regimen is computed using the following equation: $D = (CssCl\tau)/F = (Cssk_eV\tau)/F$, where D is the dose, Css is the steady-state drug concentration, Cl is the drug clearance, τ is the dosage interval, k_e is the elimination rate constant, and V is the volume of distribution. A loading dose is computed using the following expression: LD = CssV.

An example of this technique is with a patient with an atrial arrhythmia needing treatment with procainamide sustained-release tablets (clearance is 24 L/h based on current procainamide continuous infusion; F = 0.85, τ = 12 h for sustained-release tablet) and an average steady-state procainamide concentration of 5 mg/L: $D = (CssCl\tau)/F$ = (5 mg/L · 24 L/h · 12 h)/0.85 = 1694 mg, rounded to a practical dose of 1500 mg. The patient would be prescribed procainamide sustained-release tablets 1500 mg orally every 12 hours.

MULTICOMPARTMENT MODELS

When serum concentrations decrease in a rapid fashion initially and then decline at a slower rate later (see Figure 2-2), a multicompartment model can be used to describe the serum concentration–time curve[1] (see Figure 2-1). Serum concentrations drop so rapidly after the dose is given because all of the drug is in the bloodstream initially and drug is leaving the vascular system by distribution to tissues and by hepatic metabolism or renal elimination or both. This portion of the curve is called the *distribution phase.* After this phase of the curve is finished, drug distribution is nearly complete and a pseudoequilibrium is established between the blood and the tissues. During the final part of the curve, serum concentrations drop more slowly, since only metabolism or elimination or both are taking place. This portion of the curve is called the *elimination phase,* and the elimination half-life of the drug is measured in this part of the serum concentration–time graph. Digoxin, vancomycin, and lidocaine are drugs that follow multicompartment pharmacokinetics.

A two-compartment model is the simplest of the multicompartment models. The following equation describes a two-compartment model after an intravenous bolus: $C = \{[D(\alpha - k_{21})]/[V_1(\alpha - \beta)]\}e^{-\alpha t} + \{[D(k_{21} - \beta)]/[V_1(\alpha - \beta)]\}e^{-\beta t}$, where C is the drug serum concentration, D is the intravenous bolus dose, k_{21} is the rate constant that describes the transfer of drug from compartment 2 to compartment 1, α is the distribution rate constant, β is the elimination rate constant, V_1 is the volume of distribution for compartment 1, and t is the time after the dose was administered. Similar equations for a two-compartment model are available for intravenous infusions and extravascular doses. To get accurate values for the pharmacokinetic constants in the equation, three to five serum concentrations for each phase of the curve need to be obtained after a dose is given to a patient. Because of the cost and time involved in obtaining six to ten serum concentrations after a dose, multicompartment models are rarely used in patient care situations. If a drug follows multicompartment pharmacokinetics, serum concentrations are usually not drawn for clinical use until the distribution phase is over and the elimination phase has been established. In these cases, simpler one-compartment model equations can be used to compute doses with an acceptable degree of accuracy.

MICHAELIS-MENTEN EQUATIONS FOR SATURABLE PHARMACOKINETICS

When the dose of a drug is increased and steady-state serum concentrations do not increase in a proportional fashion, but, rather, increase more than expected, Michaelis-Menten or saturable pharmacokinetics may be taking place. This situation occurs when the serum concentration of the drug approaches or exceeds the Km value for the enzyme system that is responsible for its metabolism. The Michaelis-Menten expression describes the dose required to attain a given steady-state drug concentration: MD = (V_{max} · Css)/(Km + Css), where MD is the maintenance dose, Css is the steady-state drug concentration, V_{max} is the maximum rate of drug metabolism, and Km is the concentration where the rate of metabolism is $V_{max}/2$. Phenytoin is an example of a drug that follows saturable pharmacokinetics.[10]

Computing the Michaelis-Menten constants for a drug is not as straightforward as the calculation of pharmacokinetic parameters for a one-compartment linear pharmacokinetic model. The calculation of V_{max} and Km requires a graphical solution.[10] The Michaelis-Menten equation is rearranged into the following formula: MD = V_{max} – [Km (MD/Css)]. This version of the function takes the form of the equation of a straight line: *y* = y-intercept + [(slope)*x*]. A plot of dose (MD) versus dose divided by the steady-state concentration (MD/Css) yields a straight line with a slope equal to –Km and a y-intercept of V_{max}. To use this approach, a patient is placed on an initial dose (MD_1) of the medication, a steady-state concentration is obtained (Css_1), and the dose–steady-state concentration ratio determined (MD_1/Css_1). The dose of the medication is changed (MD_2), a second steady-state concentration is measured (Css_2), and the new dose–steady-state concentration ratio is computed (MD_2/Css_2). The maintenance dose and maintenance dose–steady-state concentration pairs are plotted on a graph so that V_{max} (the y-intercept) and Km (the –slope) can be determined (Figure 2-9). If additional doses are administered until steady state has been achieved, they can also be added to the same plot and the best straight line computed using linear regression. Once V_{max} and Km are known, the Michaelis-Menten expression can be used to compute a dose to reach any steady-state concentration.

An example is a patient receiving phenytoin for the treatment of tonic-clonic seizures. The patient received a dose of 300 mg/d with a steady-state concentration of 8 mg/L and a dose of 500 mg/d with a steady-state concentration of 22 mg/L. The dose–steady-state concentration ratios are 37.5 L/d and 22.7 L/d for the first and second doses, respectively ([300 mg/d]/8 mg/L = 37.5 L/d; [500 mg/d]/22 mg/L = 22.7 L/d). A plot of these data yields a V_{max} = 807 mg/d and a Km = 13.5 mg/L (see Figure 2-9). The phenytoin dose to reach a steady-state concentration equal to 13 mg/L is MD = (V_{max} · Css)/(Km + Css) = (807 mg/d · 13 mg/L)/(13.5 mg/L + 13 mg/L) = 396 mg/d, rounded to a practical dose of 400 mg/d.

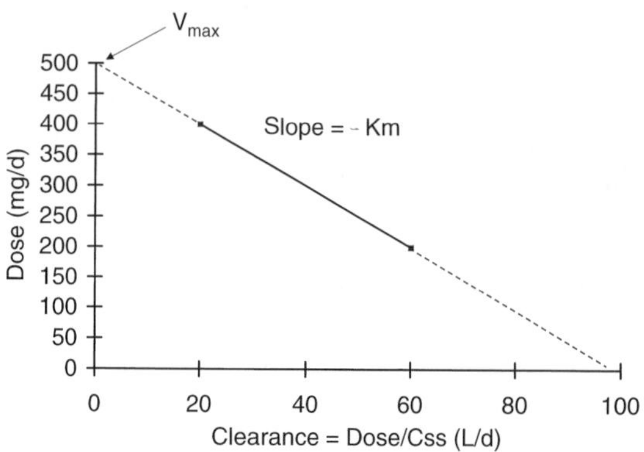

FIGURE 2-9 Michaelis-Menten plot for phenytoin. Dose is plotted versus the ratio of dose and steady-state concentration (*D/Css*) for two or more different doses, and a straight line is drawn connecting the points. The slope of the line is –Km, and the y-intercept is V_{max}. The Michaelis-Menten constants are then used to compute the dose needed to achieve a new desired steady-state concentration.

CALCULATION OF CLEARANCE, VOLUME OF DISTRIBUTION, AND HALF-LIFE IN PHARMACOKINETIC RESEARCH STUDIES

It is important to understand the methods used to compute the three principal pharmacokinetic parameters in research studies, because these will be used by clinicians to determine population pharmacokinetic parameters for initial dosage regimen design.[11] The typical pharmacokinetic research study administers a single dose of the medication and measures 10 to 15 serum concentrations for an estimated 3 to 5 half-lives or gives the drug until steady state is achieved and obtains 10 to 15 serum concentrations over a dosage interval. In either case, the serum concentration–time plot is used to compute the area under the serum concentration–time curve (AUC). For drugs that follow linear pharmacokinetics, the AUC extrapolated to infinity after a single dose equals the AUC over the dosage interval at steady state for a dose of the same size so that either can be used to compute pharmacokinetic constants.

Clearance (Cl) is computed by taking the ratio of the dose (D) and area under the serum concentration–time curve for a drug that is administered intravenously: Cl = D/AUC. If the dose is administered extravascularly, the bioavailability fraction (F) must be included to compensate for drug that does not reach the systemic vascular system: Cl = (FD)/AUC.

Of the three volumes of distribution typically computed in a pharmacokinetic experiment, the one most useful in clinical situations is the volume of distribution, calculated using the area under the serum concentration–time curve: $V = D/(k_eAUC)$, where k_e is the elimination rate constant. For doses administered extravascularly, the bioavailability fraction must be included to compensate for drug that does not reach the systemic vascular system: $V = (FD)/(k_eAUC)$.

Half-life is determined by plotting the serum concentration–time curve and computing the time it takes for serum concentrations to decrease by half in the postabsorption, postdistribution phase of the graph. To get the most accurate measurement of half-life, five to seven serum concentrations are usually measured during the terminal portion of the curve, and nonlinear regression is used to compute the best value for the parameter. Alternatively, the data can be plotted on semilogarithmic axes and linear regression used to compute the terminal half-life.

PROBLEMS

1. PZ is a 35-year-old, 60-kg female with a *Staphylococcus aureus* wound infection. While receiving vancomycin 1 g every 12 hours (infused over 1 hour), the steady-state peak concentration (obtained 30 minutes after the end of infusion) was 35 mg/L, and the steady-state trough concentration (obtained immediately predose) was 15 mg/L. (A) Using one-compartment intravenous bolus equations, compute the pharmacokinetic parameters for this patient. (B) Using the patient-specific pharmacokinetic parameters calculated in A, compute a new vancomycin dose that will achieve a $C_{max,ss}$ of 30 mg/L and a $C_{min,ss}$ of 7.5 mg/L.

2. Negamycin is a new antibiotic with an average volume of distribution of 0.35 L/kg and a half-life of 2 hours in patients with cystic fibrosis. Compute a dosage regimen for JM, a 22-year-old, 45-kg female cystic fibrosis patient with *Pseudomonas aeruginosa* in her sputum, which will achieve steady-state peak concentrations of 10 mg/L and trough concentrations of 0.6 mg/L, using one-compartment model intravenous bolus equations (assume that the drug is given as an intravenous bolus).

3. KL is a 65-year-old, 60-kg female being treated for septic shock. In addition to other antibiotics, she is being treated with tobramycin 60 mg every 8 hours (infused over 1 hour). Steady-state serum concentrations are $C_{max,ss}$ = 7.1 mg/L, $C_{min,ss}$ = 3.1 mg/L. Using one-compartment intermittent intravenous infusion equations, compute the pharmacokinetic parameters for this patient and use them to individualize the tobramycin dose to achieve a $C_{max,ss}$ of 8 mg/L and a $C_{min,ss}$ of 1.0 mg/L.

4. JB is a 52-year-old, 72-kg male being treated for gram-negative pneumonia. Assuming a V of 18 L and a $t_{1/2}$ of 8 hours, design a gentamicin dosage (infused over 1 hour) to achieve a $C_{max,ss}$ of 10 mg/L and a $C_{min,ss}$ of 1.2 mg/L, using one-compartment intermittent intravenous infusion equations.

5. EV is a 42-year-old, 84-kg male suffering from an acute asthma attack. Using one-compartment model equations, compute a theophylline intravenous bolus loading dose (to be administered over 20 minutes) and continuous infusion to achieve a Css of 12 mg/L. Assume a V of 40 L and $t_{1/2}$ of 5 hours.

6. BJ is a 62-year-old, 70-kg female with a ventricular arrhythmia. Assuming a V of 33 L and a Cl of 0.5 L/min, use one-compartment model equations to compute a lidocaine intravenous bolus loading dose (to be administered over 1 to 2 minutes) and continuous infusion to achieve a Css of 3 mg/L.

7. MM is a 54-year-old, 68-kg male being treated with procainamide 750-mg regular-release capsules every 6 hours for an arrhythmia. The following steady-state concen-

tration is available: $C_{min,ss}$ = 1.5 mg/L (obtained immediately predose). Calculate a dose that will achieve a $C_{min,ss}$ of 2.5 mg/L.

8. LM is a 59-year-old, 85-kg male needing treatment with oral quinidine for an arrhythmia. Assuming F = 0.7, T_{max} = 2 h, V = 200 L, and $t_{1/2}$ = 8 h, compute $C_{min,ss}$ for oral quinidine 400 mg every 6 hours.

9. JB is a 78-year-old, 100-kg male being treated with digoxin for heart failure. While the patient is receiving digoxin tablets 125 μg daily, a steady-state digoxin concentration of 0.6 μg/L is obtained. (A) Assuming F = 0.7, compute digoxin clearance for the patient using the average steady-state concentration equation. (B) Compute a new digoxin tablet dose for the patient, which will achieve a Css of 1.2 μg/L.

10. QJ is a 67-year-old, 80-kg male being treated for chronic obstructive pulmonary disease. Sustained-release oral theophylline is being added to his drug regimen. Assuming F = 1.0, V = 40 L, and $t_{1/2}$ = 5 hours, compute an oral theophylline dose to be administered every 12 hours that will achieve a Css of 8 mg/L, using the average steady-state concentration equation.

11. TD is a 32-year-old, 70-kg male with generalized tonic-clonic seizures. Assuming Michaelis-Menten parameters of V_{max} = 500 mg/d and Km = 4 mg/L, calculate a dose of phenytoin that will achieve a Css of 15 mg/L.

12. OP is a 28-year-old, 55-kg female with complex partial seizures. She has the following information available: Css = 8 mg/L while receiving phenytoin 300 mg at bedtime and Css = 22 mg/L while receiving phenytoin 400 mg at bedtime. Compute the patient's Michaelis-Menten parameters for phenytoin and the phenytoin dose that will achieve a Css of 15 mg/L.

ANSWERS TO PROBLEMS

1. (A) $k_e = -(\ln C_1 - \ln C_2)/(t_1 - t_2) = -[(\ln 35 \text{ mg/L}) - (\ln 15 \text{ mg/L})]/(1.5 \text{ h} - 12 \text{ h}) = 0.081 \text{ h}^{-1}$

$$t_{1/2} = 0.693/k_e = 0.693/0.081 \text{ h}^{-1}$$

$$C_0 = C/e^{-k_e t} = (35 \text{ mg/L})/e^{(-0.081 \text{ h}^{-1})(1.5 \text{ h})} = 39.5 \text{ mg/L}$$

$$V = D/[C_0 - C_{predose}] = (1000 \text{ mg})/(39.5 \text{ mg/L} - 15 \text{ mg/L}) = 41 \text{ L}$$

(B) $\tau = [(\ln C_{max,ss} - \ln C_{min,ss})/k_e] = [\ln (30 \text{ mg/L}) - \ln (7.5 \text{ mg/L})]/0.081 \text{ h}^{-1}$ = 17.1 h, rounded to a dosage interval of 18 hours

$D = C_{max,ss} V(1 - e^{-k_e \tau}) = (30 \text{ mg/L} \cdot 41 \text{ L})(1 - e^{(-0.081 \text{ d}^{-1})(18 \text{ h})})$ = 944 mg, rounded to a dose of 1000 mg

Recommended dosage: 1000 mg every 18 hours.

2. Estimated V = 0.35 L/kg (45 kg) = 15.8 L

Estimated $k_e = 0.693/t_{1/2} = 0.693/2 \text{ h} = 0.347 \text{ h}^{-1}$

$\tau = [(\ln C_{max,ss} - \ln C_{min,ss})/k_e] = [\ln (10 \text{ mg/L}) - \ln (0.6 \text{ mg/L})]/0.347 \text{ h}^{-1} = 8.1$ h, rounded to a dosage interval of 8 hours

$D = C_{max,ss} V(1 - e^{-k_e\tau}) = (10 \text{ mg/L} \cdot 15.8 \text{ L})(1 - e^{(-0.347 \text{ d}^{-1})(8 \text{ h})}) = 148$ mg, rounded to a dose of 150 mg

Recommended dosage: 150 mg every 8 hours.

If desired, a loading dose can be calculated: $LD = C_{max,ss} V = (10 \text{ mg/L})(15.8 \text{ L}) =$ 158 mg, rounded to a dose of 160 mg.

3. $k_e = -(\ln C_1 - \ln C_2)/(t_1 - t_2) = -[(\ln 7.1 \text{ mg/L}) - (\ln 3.1 \text{ mg/L})]/(1 \text{ h} - 8 \text{ h}) =$ 0.118 h^{-1}

$$V = \frac{k_0(1 - e^{-k_e t'})}{k_e [C_{max} - (C_{predose} e^{-k_e t'})]}$$

$$V = \frac{(60 \text{ mg/1 h})(1 - e^{(-0.118 \text{ h}^{-1})(1 \text{ h})})}{0.118 \text{ h}^{-1}[(7.1 \text{ mg/L}) - (3.1 \text{ mg/L} \cdot e^{(-0.118 \text{ h}^{-1})(1 \text{ h})})]} = 13 \text{ L}$$

$\tau = [(\ln C_{max,ss} - \ln C_{min,ss})/k_e] + t' = [(\ln 8 \text{ mg/L} - \ln 1 \text{ mg/L})/0.118 \text{ h}^{-1}] + 1 \text{ h} =$ 18.6 h, rounded to a dosage interval of 18 h

$k_0 = C_{max,ss} k_e V[(1 - e^{-k_e\tau})/(1 - e^{-k_e t'})] = [(8 \text{ mg/L})(0.118 \text{ h}^{-1})(13 \text{ L})]$ $[(1 - e^{(-0.118 \text{ h}^{-1}(18 \text{ h})})/(1 - e^{(-0.118 \text{ h}^{-1})(1 \text{ h})})] = 97$ mg, rounded to a dose of 100 mg

Recommended dosage: 100 mg every 18 hours.

4. $k_e = 0.693/t_{1/2} = 0.693/8 \text{ h} = 0.087 \text{ h}^{-1}$, $V = 18$ L

$\tau = [(\ln C_{max,ss} - \ln C_{min,ss})/k_e] + t' = [(\ln 10 \text{ mg/L} - \ln 1.2 \text{ mg/L})/0.087 \text{ h}^{-1}] + 1 \text{ h} =$ 25.4 h, rounded to a dosage interval of 24 hours

$k_0 = C_{max,ss} k_e V[(1 - e^{-k_e\tau})/(1 - e^{-k_e t'})] = [(10 \text{ mg/L})(0.087 \text{ h}^{-1})(18 \text{ L})]$ $[(1 - e^{(-0.087 \text{ h}^{-1})(24 \text{ h})})/(1 - e^{(-0.087 \text{ h}^{-1})(1 \text{ h})})] = 165$ mg

Recommended dosage: 165 mg every 24 hours.

5. $k_e = 0.693/t_{1/2} = 0.693/5 \text{ h} = 0.139 \text{ h}^{-1}$

$$V = 40 \text{ L}, Cl = k_e V = (0.139 \text{ h}^{-1})(40 \text{ L}) = 5.56 \text{ L/h}$$

$LD = Css\ V = (12 \text{ mg/L})(40 \text{ L}) = 480$ mg, rounded to 500 mg IV over 20 minutes

$k_0 = Css\ Cl = (12 \text{ mg/L})(5.56 \text{ L/h}) = 67$ mg/h, rounded to 70 mg/h

6. $LD = Css\ V = (3 \text{ mg/L})(33 \text{ L}) = 99$ mg, rounded to 100 mg IV over 2 minutes

$$k_0 = Css\ Cl = (3 \text{ mg/L})(0.5 \text{ L/min}) = 1.5 \text{ mg/min}$$

7. $D_{new}/D_{old} = Css_{new}/Css_{old}$

$$D_{new} = D_{old}(Css_{new}/Css_{old}) = 750 \text{ mg } [(2.5 \text{ mg/L})/(1.5 \text{ mg/L})] = 1250 \text{ mg}$$

Recommended dosage: 1250 mg every 6 hours.

8. $k_e = 0.693/t_{1/2} = 0.693/8\ h = 0.087\ h^{-1}$

$$C_{max,ss} = [(FD)/V][e^{-k_eT_{max}}/(1 - e^{-k_e\tau})]$$

$$C_{max,ss} = [(0.7 \cdot 400\ mg)/200\ L][e^{-(0.087\ h^{-1})(2\ h)}/(1 - e^{-(0.087\ h^{-1})(6\ h)})] = 2.9\ mg/L$$

$$C_{min,ss} = C_{max,ss}e^{-k_e(\tau - T_{max})} = (2.9\ mg/L)e^{-(0.087\ h^{-1})(6\ h - 2\ h)} = 2.0\ mg/L$$

9. (A) $Css = F(D/\tau)/Cl$

$$Cl = F(D/\tau)/Css = [0.7(125\ \mu g/1\ d)]/(0.6\ \mu g/L) = 146\ L/d$$

(B) $D_{new} = D_{old}(Css_{new}/Css_{old}) = 125\ \mu g[(1.2\ \mu g/L)/(0.6\ \mu g/L)] = 250\ \mu g$

Recommended dosage: 250 μg daily.

10. $k_e = 0.693/t_{1/2} = 0.693/5\ h = 0.139\ h^{-1}$

$$Cl = k_eV = (0.139\ h^{-1})(40\ L) = 5.56\ L/h$$

$$Css = F(D/\tau)/Cl$$

$D = (Css \cdot Cl \cdot \tau)/F = (8\ mg/L \cdot 5.56\ L/h \cdot 12\ h)/1.0 = 534\ mg$, rounded to 500 mg

Recommended dosage 500 mg every 12 hours.

11. $MD = (V_{max} \cdot Css)/(Km + Css) = (500\ mg/d \cdot 15\ mg/L)/(4\ mg/L + 15\ mg/L) = 395\ mg$, rounded to 400 mg

Recommended dosage: 400 mg daily at bedtime.

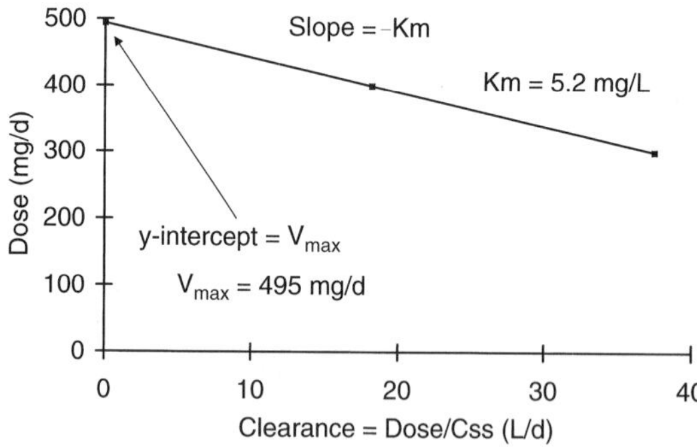

12. Graph data (see above graph): Km = 5.2 mg/L, V_{max} = 495 mg/d

$MD = (V_{max} \cdot Css)/(Km + Css) = (495\ mg/d \cdot 15\ mg/L)/(5.2\ mg/L + 15\ mg/L) = 367\ mg$, rounded to 375 mg

Recommended dosage: 375 mg daily at bedtime.

REFERENCES

1. Riegelman S, Loo JCK, Rowland M. Shortcomings in pharmacokinetic analysis by conceiving the body to exhibit properties of a single compartment. J Pharm Sci 1968;57:117–123.
2. Teorell T. Kinetics of distribution of substances administered to the body: I. The extravascular modes of administration. Arch Int Pharmacodyn Ther 1937;57:205–225.
3. Teorell T. Kinetics of distribution of substances administered to the body: II. The intravascular modes of administration. Arch Int Pharmacodyn Ther 1937;57:226–240.
4. Sawchuk RJ, Zaske DE, Cipolle RJ, Wargin WA, Strate RG. Kinetic model for gentamicin dosing with the use of individual patient parameters. Clin Pharmacol Ther 1977;21:362–365.
5. Matzke GR, McGory RW, Halstenson CE, Keane WF. Pharmacokinetics of vancomycin in patients with various degrees of renal function. Antimicrob Agents Chemother 1984;25:433–437.
6. Murphy JE, Winter ME. Clinical pharmacokinetics perals: bolus versus infusion equations. Pharmacother 1996;16:698–700.
7. Benet LZ. General treatment of linear mammillary models with elimination from any compartment as used in pharmacokinetics. J Pharm Sci 1972;61:536–541.
8. Wagner JG, Northam JI, Alway CD, Carpenter OS. Blood levels of drug at the equilibrium state after multiple dosing. Nature 1965;207:1301–1302.
9. Jusko WJ, Koup JR, Vance JW, Schentag JJ, Kuritzky P. Intravenous theophylline therapy: nomogram guidelines. Ann Intern Med 1977;86:400–404.
10. Ludden TM, Allen JP, Valutsky WA, et al. Individualization of phenytoin dosage regimens. Clin Pharmacol Ther 1977;21:287–293.
11. Shargel L, Yu ABC. Applied biopharmaceutics and pharmacokinetics. East Norwalk, CT: Appleton & Lange, 1999:67.

3

DRUG DOSING IN SPECIAL POPULATIONS: RENAL AND HEPATIC DISEASE, DIALYSIS, HEART FAILURE, OBESITY, AND DRUG INTERACTIONS

INTRODUCTION

All medications have specific disease states and conditions that change the pharmacokinetics of the drug and warrant dosage modification. However, the dosing of most drugs is altered by one or more of the important factors discussed in this chapter. Renal disease and hepatic disease decrease the elimination or metabolism of most drugs and change the clearance of the agent. Dialysis procedures, conducted using artificial kidneys in patients with renal failure, remove some medications from the body, whereas the pharmacokinetics of other drugs are not changed. Heart failure results in low cardiac output, which decreases blood flow to eliminating organs, and the clearance rate of drugs with moderate to high extraction ratios are particularly sensitive to alterations in organ blood flow. Obesity adds excessive adipose tissue to the body, which may change how drugs distribute in the body and alter the volume of distribution for the medication. Finally, drug interactions can inhibit or induce drug metabolism, alter drug protein binding, or change blood flow to organs that eliminate or metabolize the drug.

RENAL DISEASE

Most water-soluble drugs are eliminated unchanged to some extent by the kidney. In addition, drug metabolites that were made more water-soluble through oxidation or conjugation are typically removed by renal elimination. The nephron is the functional unit of the kidney that is responsible for waste product removal from the body and also eliminates drug molecules (Figure 3-1). Unbound drug molecules that are relatively small are filtered at the glomerulus. Glomerular filtration is the primary elimination route for many medica-

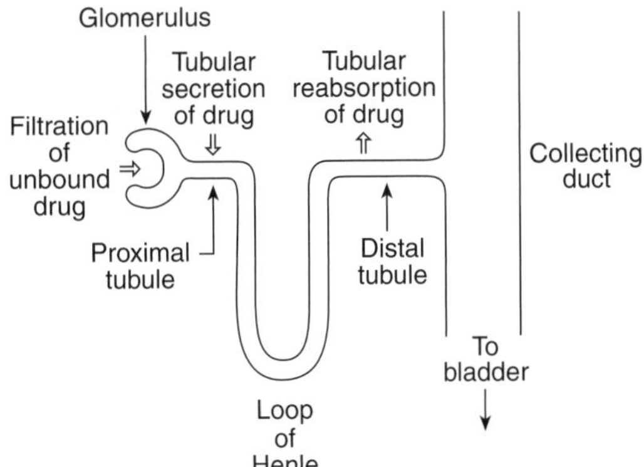

FIGURE 3-1 The nephron is the functional unit of the kidney responsible for drug elimination. Unbound drug is filtered freely at the glomerulus (*arrow at upper left*). Active tubular secretion of drug (*down arrow into nephron at top*) usually occurs in the proximal tubule of the nephron. Passive tubular reabsorption (*arrow out of nephron at top*) usually occurs in the distal tubule of the nephron. Tubular reabsorption requires un-ionized drug molecules so that the molecules can pass through the lipid membranes of the nephron and surrounding capillaries.

tions. Drugs can be actively secreted into the urine; this process usually takes place in the proximal tubules. Tubular secretion is an active process conducted by relatively specific carriers or pumps that move the drug from blood vessels in close proximity to the nephron into the proximal tubule. In addition, some medications may be reabsorbed from the urine back into the blood by the kidney. Reabsorption is usually a passive process and requires a degree of lipid solubility for the drug molecule. Thus, tubular reabsorption is influenced by the pH of the urine, the pKa of the drug molecule, and the resulting extent of molecular ionization. Compounds that are not ionized in the urine are more lipid-soluble, better able to pass through lipid membranes, and more prone to renal tubular reabsorption. The equation that describes these various routes of renal elimination is:

$$Cl_R = [(f_B \cdot GFR) + \frac{RBF \cdot (f_B Cl'_{sec})}{RBF + (f_B Cl'_{sec})}](1 - FR)$$

where f_B is the free fraction of drug in the blood, GFR is glomerular filtration rate, RBF is renal blood flow, Cl'_{sec} is the intrinsic clearance for tubular secretion of unbound drug, and FR is the fraction reabsorbed.[1]

When infants are born, renal function is not completely developed in full-term neonates (~40 weeks' gestational age). Kidney development is complete and renal function stabilizes 3 to 6 months after birth. In premature infants (<35 weeks), kidney development may take even longer during the postpartum period. Kidney function, as measured by glomerular filtration rate, typically averages ~120 to 140 mL/min in young, healthy adults between the ages of 18 and 22 years. As humans age, glomerular function gradually declines so that when a person is 65 years of age, the average glomerular filtration rate is ~50 to 60 mL/min. The expected glomerular filtration rate for otherwise healthy, normal 80-year-old adults is ~30 to 40 mL/min. A glomerular filtration rate of 80 to 120 mL/min is usually considered the normal range by most clinical laboratories.

Patients with renal disease have a functional loss of nephrons. Depending on the cause of the renal disease, patients with acute kidney failure may recoup their baseline renal function after a period of supportive care and dialysis long enough for their kidneys to recover. Patients with acute renal failure due to a sudden decrease in renal blood flow, such as that seen during hypotension, shock, or hypovolemia, or due to nephrotoxic drug therapy, such as aminoglycoside antibiotics or vancomycin, often experience a return of kidney function to preinsult level if they survive the underlying causes of the renal dysfunction. Patients with chronic renal failure sustain permanent loss of functional nephrons owing to irreversible damage, and they do not recover lost kidney function.

Measurement and Estimation of Creatinine Clearance

Glomerular filtration rate can be determined by administration of special test compounds; this is sometimes done by nephrologists when precise determination of renal function is needed. However, the most common method of estimating glomerular filtration for the purposes of drug dosing is to measure or estimate creatinine clearance (CrCl). Creatinine is a by-product of muscle metabolism that is primarily eliminated by glomerular filtration. Because of this property, it is used as a surrogate measurement of glomerular filtration rate. Creatinine clearance rates can be measured by collecting urine for a specified period and collecting a blood sample for determination of serum creatinine at the midpoint of the concurrent urine collection time: CrCl (in mL/min) = $(U_{Cr} \cdot V_{urine})/(S_{Cr} \cdot T)$, where U_{Cr} is the urine creatinine concentration in mg/dL, V_{urine} is the volume of urine collected in mL, S_{Cr} is the serum creatinine collected at the midpoint of the urine collection in mg/dL, and T is the time in minutes of the urine collection. Because creatinine renal secretion exhibits diurnal variation, most nephrologists use a 24-hour urine collection period for the determination of creatinine clearance. For example, a 24-hour urine was collected for a patient with the following results: U_{Cr} = 55 mg/dL, V_{urine} = 1000 mL, S_{Cr} = 1.0 mg/dL, T = 24 h × 60 min/h = 1440 min, and CrCl (in mL/min) = $(U_{Cr} \cdot V_{urine})/(S_{Cr} \cdot T)$ = (55 mg/dL · 1000 mL)/(1.0 mg/dL · 1440 min) = 38 mL/min. However, for the purpose of drug dosing, collection periods of 8 to 12 hours have been sufficient and provide a quicker turnaround time in emergency situations. Also, if renal function is stable, the blood sample for determination of serum creatinine may not need to be collected at the precise midpoint of the urine collection.

Routine measurement of creatinine clearances in patients has been fraught with problems. Incomplete urine collections, serum creatinine concentrations obtained at incorrect times, and collection time errors can produce erroneous measured creatinine clearance values. This realization has prompted investigators to derive methods that estimate creatinine clearance from serum creatinine values and other patient characteristics in various populations. The most widely used of these formulas for adults aged 18 years and older is the method suggested by Cockcroft and Gault[2]: for men, $CrCl_{est} = [(140 - age)BW]/(72 \cdot S_{Cr})$; for women, $CrCl_{est} = [0.85(140 - age)BW]/(72 \cdot S_{Cr})$, where $CrCl_{est}$ is estimated creatinine clearance in mL/min, age is in years, BW is body weight in kilograms, S_{Cr} is serum creatinine in mg/dL. The Cockcroft-Gault method should be used only in patients ≥18 years old, actual weight within 30% of their ideal body weight [IBW_{men} (in kg) = 50 + 2.3(Ht − 60) or IBW_{women} (in kg) = 45 + 2.3(Ht − 60), where Ht is height in inches], and stable serum creatinine concentrations. The 0.85 correction factor for women is present because they have smaller muscle mass than men and therefore produce less creatinine per day. For example, a 55-year-old, 80-kg, 71-inch man has a serum creatinine of 1.9 mg/dL. The estimated creatinine clearance would be: $IBW_{males} = 50 + 2.3(Ht - 60) = 50 + 2.3(71 - 60) = 75$ kg, so the patient is within 30% of his ideal body weight and the Cockcroft-Gault method can be used, $CrCl_{est} = [(140 - age)BW]/(72 \cdot S_{Cr}) = [(140 - 55\ y)80\ kg]/(72 \cdot 1.9\ mg/dL) = 50$ mL/min.

Some patients have decreased muscle mass because of disease states and conditions that affect muscle or prevent exercise. Examples are patients with spinal cord injury, cancer patients with muscle wasting, HIV-infected patients, cachectic patients, and patients with poor nutrition, whose muscle mass may be very small and so may have low creatinine production. In these cases, serum creatinine concentrations are low because of the low creatinine production rate and not because of the high renal clearance of creatinine. Investigators have suggested that if a patient's serum creatinine values are <1.0 mg/dL, then an arbitrary value of 1 mg/dL can be used in the Cockcroft-Gault formula to estimate creatinine clearance.[3–5] Although the resulting estimate of creatinine clearance appears to be closer to the actual creatinine clearance in these patients, it can still result in misestimates. It may be necessary to measure creatinine clearance in these patients if an accurate reflection of glomerular filtration rate is needed.

If serum creatinine values are not stable but are increasing or decreasing in a patient, the Cockcroft-Gault equation cannot be used to estimate creatinine clearance. Therefore, an alternate method must be used, as suggested by Jelliffe and Jelliffe.[6] The first step in this method is to estimate creatinine production. The formula for this is different for men and women because of gender-dependent differences in muscle mass: $Ess_{males} = IBW[29.3 - (0.203 \cdot age)]$; $Ess_{females} = IBW[25.1 - (0.175 \cdot age)]$, where Ess is the excretion of creatinine, IBW is ideal body weight in kilograms, and age is in years. The remainder of the equations correct creatinine production for renal function and adjust the estimated creatinine clearance value according to whether the renal function is getting better or worse:

$$Ess_{corrected} = Ess[1.035 - (0.0337 \cdot Scr_{ave})]$$

$$E = Ess_{corrected} - \frac{[4IBW(Scr_2 - Scr_1)]}{\Delta t}$$

$$CrCl\ (\text{in mL/min/1.73 m}^2) = E/(14.4 \cdot Scr_{ave})$$

where Scr_{ave} is the average of the two serum creatinine determinations in mg/dL, Scr_1 is the first serum creatinine and Scr_2 is the second serum creatinine both in mg/dL, and Δt is the time that expired between the measurement of Scr_1 and Scr_2 in minutes.

If patients are not within 30% of their ideal body weight, other methods of estimating creatinine clearance should be used.[7] Some clinicians suggest that ideal body weight rather than actual body weight used in the Cockcroft-Gault equation gives an adequate estimate of creatinine clearance for obese persons. However, a specific method suggested by Salazar and Corcoran[8] for estimating creatinine clearance for obese patients has been shown to be generally superior:

$$CrCl_{est(males)} = \frac{(137 - age)[(0.285 \cdot Wt) + (12.1 \cdot Ht^2)]}{(51 \cdot S_{Cr})}$$

$$CrCl_{est(females)} = \frac{(146 - age)[(0.287 \cdot Wt) + (9.74 \cdot Ht^2)]}{(60 \cdot S_{Cr})}$$

where age is in years, Wt is weight in kilograms, Ht is height in meters, and S_{Cr} is serum creatinine in mg/dL.

Methods of estimating creatinine clearance for children and young adults are also available according to their age[9]: age 0 to 1 year, $CrCl_{est}$ (in mL/min/1.73 m^2) = $(0.45 \cdot Ht)/S_{Cr}$; age 1 to 20 years, $CrCl_{est}$ (in mL/min/1.73 m^2) = $(0.55 \cdot Ht)/S_{Cr}$, where Ht is in centimeters and S_{Cr} is in mg/dL. Note that for these formulas, estimated creatinine clearance is normalized to 1.73 m^2, which is the body surface area of a male adult with a height and weight of approximately 178 cm (70 in) and 70 kg, respectively.

Estimation of Drug Dosing and Pharmacokinetic Parameters Using Creatinine Clearance

It is common to base initial doses of drugs that are renally eliminated on creatinine clearance. The basis for this is that renal clearance of the drug is less in patients with a reduced glomerular filtration rate, and measured or estimated creatinine clearance is a surrogate marker for glomerular filtration rate. An assumption made in this approach is that all drug-excreting processes of the kidney, including tubular secretion and reabsorption, decline parallel with glomerular filtration. The basis of this assumption is the intact nephron theory. Although tubular secretion and reabsorption may not always decline in proportion to glomerular filtration, this approach approximates the decline in tubular function and is a useful approach to initial drug dosing in patients with renal dysfunction. However, clinicians should bear in mind that the suggested doses for patients with renal impairment constitute an initial guideline only, and doses may need to be increased in patients who exhibit suboptimal drug response and decreased in patients who have adverse effects.

Breakpoints to consider altering drug doses are useful for clinicians to keep in mind. Generally, one should consider a possible *modest* decrease in drug doses when creatinine clearance is <50 to 60 mL/min, a *moderate* decrease in drug doses when creatinine clearance is <25 to 30 mL/min, and a *substantial* decrease in drug doses when creatinine clearance is ≤15 mL/min. To modify doses for patients with renal impairment, it is possible to decrease the drug dose and retain the usual dosage interval, retain the usual dose and increase the dosage interval, or simultaneously decrease the dosage and prolong the dosage interval. The approach depends on the route of administration, the dosage forms available, and the pharmacodynamic response to the drug. For example, if the drug is prescribed orally and only a limited number of solid dosage forms are available, one can usually administer the usual dose and increase the dosage interval. If the drug is given parenterally, a smaller dose can be administered, and it is more likely that the usual dosage interval will be retained. Finally, for drugs with narrow therapeutic ranges such as aminoglycoside antibiotics and vancomycin, in which target serum concentrations for maximum and minimum steady-state concentrations are established, both the dose and the dosage interval can be manipulated to achieve the targeted drug levels. If the drug dose is reduced and the dosage interval remains unaltered in patients with decreased renal function, maximum drug concentrations are usually lower and minimum drug concentrations higher than those encountered in patients with normal renal function receiving the typical drug dose (Figure 3-2). If the dosage interval is prolonged and the drug dosage remains the same, maximum and minimum drug concentrations are usually about the same as in patients with good renal function receiving the usual drug dose.

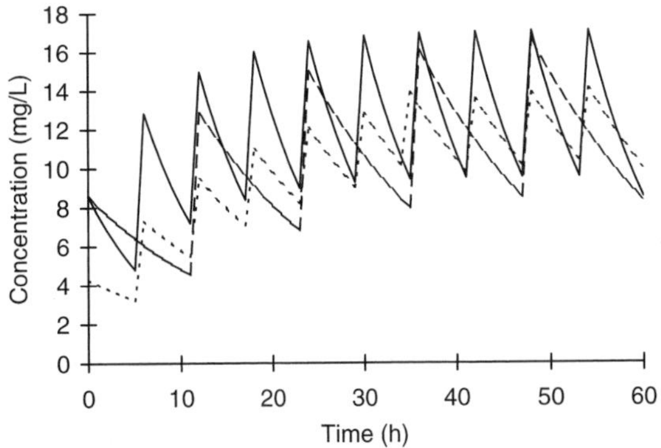

FIGURE 3-2 Serum concentration versus time profile for a patient with normal kidney function receiving a renally eliminated drug at the dose of 300 mg every 6 hours (*solid line*). In a patient with renal dysfunction, it is possible to give the same dose and prolong the dosage interval (300 mg every 12 hours, *dashed line*) or a reduced dose at the same dosage interval (150 mg every 6 hours, *dotted line*). Giving the same dose at a longer dosage interval in the patient with renal disease usually results in a concentration–time profile similar to that seen in a normal patient receiving the normal dose. However, giving a smaller dose and keeping the dosage interval the same usually produce a concentration–time profile with a lower peak steady-state concentration and a higher trough steady-state concentration. Note that since the total daily dose is the same for both renal disease dosage regimens (600 mg/d), the average steady-state concentration is identical for both dosage schemes. The same dosing options are available for liver-metabolizing drugs for patients with hepatic dysfunction.

Since the mid-1980s, the Food and Drug Administration (FDA) has required pharmacokinetic studies to be done for agents that are renally eliminated in patients with decreased creatinine clearance rates before receiving agency approval. In these cases, the package insert for the drug probably contains reasonable initial dosage guidelines. For example, the manufacturer's suggested guidelines for the dosing of gabapentin in patients with renal dysfunction are listed in Table 3-1. Guidelines for changing drug dosages for patients with decreased renal function are available for older drugs as well as updated

TABLE 3-1 Manufacturer's Recommended Dosing Schedule for Renal Dysfunction and Hemodialysis Patients Receiving Gabapentin

CRCL (mL/min)	TOTAL DAILY DOSE (mg/day)	DOSAGE REGIMEN (mg)
>60	1200	400 three times daily
30–60	600	300 twice daily
15–30	300	300 daily
<15	150	300 every other day
Hemodialysis	—	200–300 after each 4-hour hemodialysis period

guidelines for newer drugs that may not be included in the package insert.[10–14] Also, the primary literature should be consulted to ensure that the newest guidelines are used for all drugs. If no specific information is available for a medication, it is possible to calculate modified initial drug doses using the method described by Dettli.[15]

For drugs with narrow therapeutic indexes, measured or estimated creatinine clearance may be used to estimate pharmacokinetic parameters for a patient based on prior studies conducted in other patients with renal dysfunction. Estimated pharmacokinetic parameters are then used in pharmacokinetic dosing equations to compute initial doses for patients. Clearance is the best pharmacokinetic parameter to estimate using creatinine clearance because it is an independent parameter that deals solely with drug elimination. The relationship between drug clearance and creatinine clearance is usually approximated by a straight line with a slope that is a function of the renal clearance for the drug and an intercept that is related to the nonrenal clearance of the drug (Figure 3-3). For digoxin, an equation that describes the relationship between digoxin clearance and creatinine clearance (CrCl in mL/min) is Cl (in mL/min) = 1.303 · CrCl + Cl_{NR}, where Cl_{NR} is nonrenal clearance and is 20 mL/min in patients with moderate to severe heart failure and 40 mL/min in patients with no or mild heart failure.[16]

Elimination rate constant (k_e) can also be estimated using creatinine clearance, but it is a dependent pharmacokinetic parameter whose result relies on the relative values of clearance and volume of distribution (k_e = Cl/V). Because of this, changes in elimination rate constant may not always be due to changes in the renal elimination of the drug. The relationship between elimination rate constant and creatinine clearance is usually approximated by a straight line with a slope that is a function of renal elimination for the agent and an intercept that is related to the elimination of drug in functionally anephric patients (glomerular filtration rate ≈0; Figure 3-4). For the aminoglycoside antibiotics, an equation that represents the relationship between aminoglycoside antibiotic elimination rate constant (k_e) and creatinine clearance (CrCl in mL/min)[17] is k_e (in h^{-1}) = 0.00293 · CrCl + 0.014.

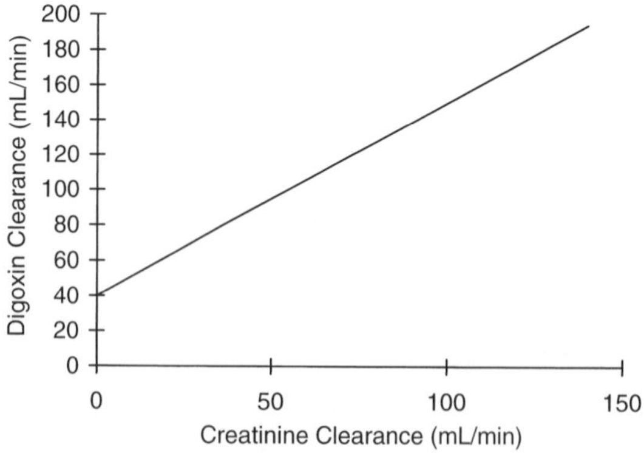

FIGURE 3-3 Relationship between creatinine clearance and digoxin clearance to estimate initial digoxin clearance when no drug concentrations are available. The y-axis intercept (40 mL/min) is nonrenal clearance for digoxin in patients with no or mild heart failure. If the patient has moderate to severe heart failure, nonrenal clearance is set to a value of 20 mL/min.

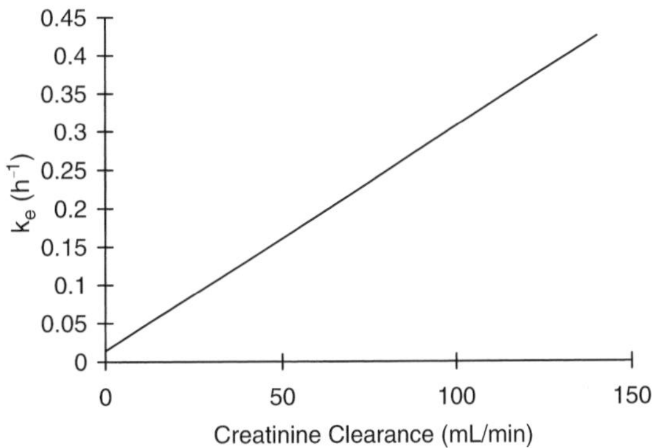

FIGURE 3-4 Relationship between creatinine clearance and aminoglycoside elimination rate constant (k_e) to estimate initial aminoglycoside elimination when no drug concentrations are available. The y-axis intercept (0.014 h^{-1}) is nonrenal elimination for aminoglycosides.

Volume of distribution can also change in patients with decreased renal function. Plasma protein binding displacement of drug by endogenous or exogenous substances that would normally be eliminated by the kidney but accumulate in the blood of patients with poor kidney function can increase the volume of distribution of drugs. Conversely, the volume of distribution of a drug can decrease if compounds normally excreted by the kidney accumulate to the extent that displacement of drug from tissue binding sites occurs. Digoxin volume of distribution decreases in patients with decreased renal function according to the following equation[18]: $V \text{ (in L)} = 226 + [(298 \cdot CrCl)/(29.1 + CrCl)]$, where CrCl is in mL/min. The decline in volume of distribution presumably occurs because of displacement of tissue-bound digoxin.

HEPATIC DISEASE

Most lipid-soluble drugs are metabolized to some degree by the liver. Phase I type reactions, such as oxidation, hydrolysis, and reduction, are often mediated by the cytochrome P-450 enzyme system (CYP), which is bound to the membrane of the endoplasmic reticulum inside hepatocytes. Phase II type reactions, including conjugation to form glucuronides, acetates, or sulfates, may also be mediated in the liver by cytosolic enzymes contained in hepatocytes. Phase I and Phase II drug metabolism generally results in metabolites that are more water-soluble and prone to elimination by the kidney. The liver receives its blood supply through the hepatic artery, which contains oxygenated blood from the aorta via the superior mesenteric artery, and the portal vein, which drains the gastrointestinal tract (Figure 3-5). Liver blood flow averages 1 to 1.5 L/min in adults with about one-third coming from the hepatic artery and about two-thirds coming from the portal vein. Orally administered medications must pass through the liver before entering the systemic circulation, so if the drug is metabolized by the liver, a portion of the dose may be inactivated by the hepatic first-pass effect before having a chance to exert a phar-

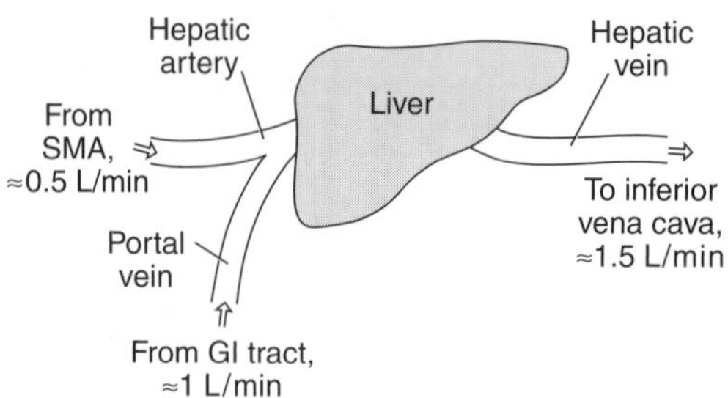

FIGURE 3-5 Schematic representation of the liver. Liver blood flow to the organ is supplied by the hepatic artery and the portal vein. The hepatic artery branches off of the superior mesenteric artery (*SMA*) and provides oxygenated blood to the liver at the rate of ~0.5 L/min. The portal vein drains blood from the gastrointestinal tract (*GI*) at the rate of ~1 L/min and passes its contents to the liver. Any chemical, including orally administered drugs, must pass through the liver before it enters the systemic circulation. The hepatic vein drains the liver of blood and empties into the inferior vena cava.

macologic effect. In addition to hepatic metabolism, drugs can be eliminated unchanged by the liver into the bile. The equation that describes hepatic drug metabolism is[19]:

$$Cl_H = \frac{LBF \cdot (f_B \cdot Cl'_{int})}{LBF + (f_B \cdot Cl'_{int})}$$

where LBF is liver blood flow, f_B is the fraction of unbound drug in the blood, and Cl'_{int} is intrinsic clearance.

Hepatic metabolism of drugs is not completely developed in neonates (~40 weeks' gestational age) and continues to increase so that by age 3 to 6 months it is stable. In premature infants (<35 weeks), hepatic metabolism may take even longer to develop in the postpartum period. On a per-kilogram basis, drug metabolism is more rapid in children until puberty. At that point, metabolic rate gradually decreases to adult values. The effect of advanced age on hepatic drug metabolism is variable. Patients over the age of 65 years may have decreased hepatic clearance of some drugs, but often concurrent disease states and conditions that affect drug pharmacokinetics obscure the influence of age in these older individuals. Elderly persons have decreased liver mass, and hepatocytes that are still present appear to have decreased ability to metabolize drugs.

There are two major types of liver disease: hepatitis and cirrhosis. Patients with hepatitis experience an inflammation of the liver, and, as a result, hepatocytes may experience decreased ability to function or die. Patients with acute hepatitis usually experience mild, transient decreases in drug metabolism that require no or minor changes in drug dosing. If the patient develops chronic hepatitis, irreversible hepatocyte damage is likely to be more widespread, and drug dosage changes will be required at some point. Patients with hepatic cirrhosis experience a permanent loss of functional hepatocytes. Drug dosage schedules usually need to be modified in patients with severe cirrhosis. With sufficient long-term hepatocyte damage, patients with chronic hepatitis can progress to hepatic cirrhosis.

When hepatocytes are damaged, they are no longer able to metabolize drugs efficiently, and intrinsic clearance decreases, which reduces the hepatic clearance of the drug.

If the drug experiences a hepatic first-pass effect, less drug will be lost by presystemic metabolism and bioavailability will increase. A simultaneous decrease in hepatic clearance and liver first-pass effect results in extremely large increases in steady-state concentrations for orally administered drugs. Liver blood flow also decreases in patients with cirrhosis because hepatocytes are replaced by nonfunctional connective tissue, which increases intraorgan pressure and causes portal vein hypertension and shunting of blood flow around the liver. The decrease in liver blood flow results in less drug delivery to still-functioning hepatocytes and depresses hepatic drug clearance even further. The liver produces albumin and probably α_1-acid glycoprotein, the two major proteins that bind acidic and basic drugs, respectively, in the blood. In patients with cirrhosis, the production of these proteins decline. When this is the case, the free fraction of drugs in the blood increases because of a lack of binding proteins. In addition, high concentrations of endogenous substances in the blood that are normally eliminated by the liver, such as bilirubin, can displace drugs from plasma protein binding sites. The increased free fraction in the blood alters hepatic and renal drug clearance as well as the volume of distribution for drugs that are highly protein-bound [$V = V_B + (f_B/f_T)V_T$, where V is the volume of distribution, V_B and V_T are the physiologic volumes of blood and tissues, respectively, and f_B and f_T are the free fraction of drug in the blood and tissues, respectively]. Since clearance typically decreases and volume of distribution usually increases or does not appreciably change for a drug in patients with liver disease, the elimination rate constant (k_e) almost always decreases in patients with decreased liver function ($k_e = Cl/V$, where Cl is clearance and V is volume of distribution).

Determination of Child-Pugh Scores

Unfortunately, there is no single laboratory test that can be used to assess liver function in the same way that measured or estimated creatinine clearance is used to measure renal function. The most common way to estimate the ability of the liver to metabolize drug is to determine the Child-Pugh score.[20] The Child-Pugh score consists of five laboratory tests or clinical symptoms: serum albumin, total bilirubin, prothrombin time, ascites, and hepatic encephalopathy. Each of these areas is given a score of 1 (normal) to 3 (severely abnormal; Table 3-2), and the scores for the five areas are totaled. The Child-Pugh score for a patient with normal liver function is 5, whereas the score for a patient with grossly abnormal serum albumin, total bilirubin, and prothrombin time values in addition to severe ascites and hepatic encephalopathy is 15. A Child-Pugh score of 8 to 9 is grounds for a moderate decrease (~25%) in initial daily drug dose for agents that are primarily (≥60%) hepatically metabolized, and a score of 10 or greater indicates that a significant decrease in initial daily dose (~50%) is required for drugs that are mostly liver-metabolized. As in any patient with or without liver dysfunction, initial doses are meant as starting points for dosage titration based on patient response and avoidance of adverse effects.

For example, the usual dose of a medication that is 95% liver-metabolized is 500 mg every 6 hours, and the total daily dose is 2000 mg/d. For a patient with hepatic cirrhosis with a Child-Pugh score of 12, an appropriate initial dose would be 50% of the usual dose or 1000 mg/d. The drug could be prescribed to the patient as 250 mg every 6 hours or 500 mg every 12 hours. The patient would need to be closely monitored for pharmacologic and toxic effects due to the medication, and the dose should be modified as needed.

TABLE 3-2 Child-Pugh Scores for Patients with Liver Disease

TEST/SYMPTOM	SCORE 1 POINT	SCORE 2 POINTS	SCORE 3 POINTS
Total bilirubin (mg/dL)	<2.0	2.0–3.0	>3.0
Serum albumin (g/dL)	>3.5	2.8–3.5	<2.8
Prothrombin time (seconds prolonged over control)	<4	4–6	>6
Ascites	Absent	Slight	Moderate
Hepatic encephalopathy	None	Moderate	Severe

From Pugh RN, Murray-Lyon IM, Dawson JL, Pietroni MC, Williams R. Transection of the oesophagus for bleeding oesophageal varices. Br J Surg 1973;60:646–649.

Estimation of Drug Dosing and Pharmacokinetic Parameters for Liver-Metabolized Drugs

For drugs that are primarily liver-metabolized, pharmacokinetic parameters are assigned to patients with liver disease by assessing values previously measured in patients with the same type of liver disease (e.g., hepatitis or cirrhosis) and a similar degree of liver dysfunction. Table 3-3 gives values for theophylline clearance in a variety of patients, including patients with cirrhosis.[21] The dose and dosing interval needed to achieve steady-state concentrations in the lower end of the therapeutic range using pharmacokinetic parameters measured in patients with liver disease are computed using pharmacokinetic equations. For example, the theophylline dosage rates listed in Table 3-3 are de-

TABLE 3-3 Theophylline Clearance and Dosage Rates for Patients with Various Disease States and Conditions

DISEASE STATE/CONDITION	MEAN CLEARANCE (mL/min/kg)	MEAN DOSE (mg/kg/h)
Children 1–9 years	1.4	0.8
Children 9–12 years or adult smokers	1.25	0.7
Adolescents 12–16 years or elderly smokers (>65 years)	0.9	0.5
Adult nonsmokers	0.7	0.4
Elderly nonsmokers (>65 years)	0.5	0.3
Decompensated congestive heart failure, cor pulmonale, cirrhosis	0.35	0.2

Mean volume of distribution = 0.5 L/kg.
From Edwards DJ, Zarowitz BJ, Slaughter RL. Theophylline. In: Evans WE, Schentag JJ, Jusko WJ, eds. Applied pharmacokinetics: principles of therapeutic drug monitoring. Vancouver, WA: Applied Therapeutics, Inc, 1992:557.

signed to produce steady-state theophylline concentrations between 8 and 12 mg/L. They were computed by multiplying theophylline clearance and the desired steady-state concentration (MD = Css · Cl, where MD is the maintenance dose, Css is the steady-state concentration, and Cl is drug clearance). Average theophylline clearance is about 50% less in adults with liver cirrhosis compared with adults with normal hepatic function. Because of this, initial theophylline doses for patients with hepatic cirrhosis are half the usual dose for adult patients with normal liver function.

When prescribing medications that are principally eliminated by the liver in patients with liver dysfunction, it is possible to decrease the dose while retaining the normal dosage interval, retain the normal dose and prolong the dosage interval, or modify both the dose and the dosage interval. Compared with persons with normal liver function receiving a drug at the usual dose and dosage interval, patients with hepatic disease who receive a normal dose but a prolonged dosage interval will have similar maximum and minimum steady-state serum concentrations (see Figure 3-2). However, if the dose is decreased but the dosage interval is kept at the usual frequency, maximum steady-state concentrations will be lower and minimum steady-state concentrations will be higher for patients with liver disease than for patients with normal hepatic function. The actual method used to reduce the dose for patients with liver dysfunction depends on the route of administration and the available dosage forms. For example, if the medication is available only as an oral capsule, the usual dose will be given to a patient with liver disease, but the dosage interval is likely to be prolonged. However, if the drug is given parenterally, it may be possible to simultaneously modify the dose and dosage interval to attain the same maximum and minimum steady-state concentrations in patients with hepatic dysfunction as those encountered in patients with normal liver function.

Implications of Hepatic Disease on Serum Drug Concentration Monitoring and Drug Effects

The pharmacokinetic alterations that occur with hepatic disease result in complex changes for total and unbound steady-state concentrations and drug response. The changes that occur depend on whether the drug has a low or high hepatic extraction ratio. As previously discussed, hepatic drug metabolism is described by the following equation[19]:

$$Cl_H = \frac{LBF \cdot (f_B \cdot Cl'_{int})}{LBF + (f_B \cdot Cl'_{int})}$$

where LBF is liver blood flow, f_B is the fraction of unbound drug in the blood, and Cl'_{int} is intrinsic clearance. For drugs with a low hepatic extraction ratio (≤30%), the numeric value of liver blood flow is much greater than the product of unbound fraction of drug in the blood and the intrinsic clearance of the compound ($LBF >> f_B \cdot Cl'_{int}$), and the sum in the denominator of the hepatic clearance equation is almost equal to liver blood flow [$LBF \approx LBF + (f_B \cdot Cl'_{int})$]. When this substitution is made into the hepatic clearance equation, hepatic clearance is equal to the product of free fraction in the blood and the intrinsic clearance of the drug for a drug with a low hepatic extraction ratio:

$$Cl_H = \frac{LBF \cdot (f_B \cdot Cl'_{int})}{LBF} = f_B \cdot Cl'_{int}$$

Similarly, for drugs with a high hepatic extraction ratio (≥70%), the numeric value of liver blood flow is much less than the product of unbound fraction of drug in the blood and the intrinsic clearance of the agent ($LBF << f_B \cdot Cl'_{int}$), and the sum in the denominator of the hepatic clearance equation is almost equal to the product of free fraction of drug in the blood and intrinsic clearance [$f_B \cdot Cl'_{int} \approx LBF + (f_B \cdot Cl'_{int})$]. When this substitution is made into the hepatic clearance equation, hepatic clearance is equal to liver blood flow for a drug with a high hepatic extraction ratio:

$$Cl_H = \frac{LBF \cdot (f_B \cdot Cl'_{int})}{f_B \cdot Cl'_{int}} = LBF$$

For drugs with intermediate hepatic extraction ratios, the entire liver clearance equation must be used and all three factors, liver blood flow, free fraction of drug in the blood, and intrinsic clearance, are important parameters that must be taken into account. An extremely important point for clinicians to understand is that the factors that are important determinants of hepatic clearance are different, depending on the liver extraction ratio for the drug.

To illustrate the differences that may occur in steady-state drug concentrations and pharmacologic effects for patients with liver disease, a graphic technique is used (Figure 3-6). The example assumes that a low hepatic extraction ratio drug (100% liver-metabolized) is being given to a patient as a continuous intravenous infusion and that all physiologic, pharmacokinetic, and drug effect parameters (shown on the y-axis) are initially stable. On the x-axis, an arrow indicates that intrinsic clearance decreases because of hepatic cirrhosis in the patient; an assumption made for this illustration is that any changes in the parameters are instantaneous. An increase in the parameter is denoted as an uptick in the line, whereas a decrease in the parameter is shown as a downtick in the line. The first three parameters are physiologic values (LBF, f_B, and Cl'_{int}) that will change in response to the development of hepatic dysfunction. In this case, only intrinsic clearance decreased due to the destruction of hepatocytes, and liver blood flow and free fraction of drug in the blood were not altered (see Figure 3-6). This change decreases the hepatic clearance of the drug, volume of distribution is not modified because blood and tissue volume or plasma protein and tissue binding did not change, and half-life increases because of the decrease in clearance [$t_{1/2} = (0.693 \cdot V)/Cl$, where $t_{1/2}$ is half-life, Cl is clearance, and V is volume of distribution]. Total and unbound steady-state drug concentrations increase in tandem because of the decrease in clearance and intrinsic clearance, and the pharmacologic response increases because of the increase in unbound serum concentration.

Using the same baseline conditions as in the previous example, it is possible to examine what would happen if the major change in a similar patient receiving the same drug was decreased plasma protein binding due to hypoalbuminemia and hyperbilirubinemia (Figure 3-7). Under these circumstances, liver blood flow and intrinsic clearance would not change, but free fraction of drug in the blood would increase. Because of the increased free fraction of drug in the blood, both clearance and volume of distribution would simultaneously increase. Clearance increases for a low hepatic extraction ratio drug because more is free to leave the bloodstream and enter hepatocytes, where it can be metabolized. Volume of distribution increases because more drug is free to leave the vascular system and enter various tissues. Depending on the relative changes in clearance and volume of distribution, half-life could increase, decrease, or not change; for the pur-

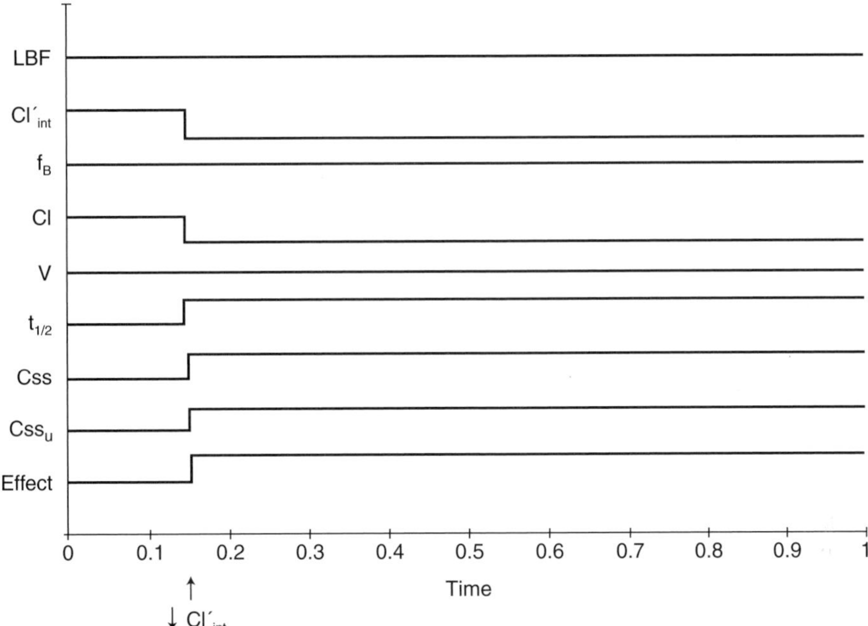

FIGURE 3-6 Changes in physiologic parameters (*LBF* = liver blood flow, Cl'_{int} = intrinsic clearance, f_B = free fraction of drug in the blood), pharmacokinetic parameters (*Cl* = clearance, *V* = volume of distribution, $t_{1/2}$ = half-life), and drug concentration and effect (*Css* = total steady-state concentration; Css_u = unbound steady-state concentration; *effect* = pharmacologic effect) for a low hepatic extraction ratio drug if intrinsic clearance decreases (*arrow*). An uptick in the line indicates an increase in the value of the parameter; a downtick in the line indicates a decrease in the value of the parameter. Intrinsic clearance could decrease owing to loss of functional hepatocytes secondary to liver cirrhosis or a drug interaction that inhibits drug-metabolizing enzymes.

pose of this example, the assumption is that alterations in these independent parameters are similar, so half-life does not change. The total steady-state concentration would decrease because total clearance increased, but the unbound steady-state concentration would remain unchanged because the decrease in total concentration is offset by the increase in free fraction of unbound drug. Finally, the pharmacologic effect of the drug is the same because free steady-state concentrations of the drug did not change. This can be an unexpected outcome for the decrease in protein binding, especially because the total steady-state concentration of the drug decreased. Clinicians need to be on the lookout for situations like this, because the total drug concentration (bound + unbound) can be misleading and cause an unwarranted increase in drug dosage. Unbound drug concentrations are available for several agents that are highly plasma protein–bound, such as phenytoin, valproic acid, and carbamazepine, and are valuable tools to guide drug dosage in liver disease patients.

Finally, decreases in liver blood flow need to be considered for drugs with low hepatic extraction ratios. A decrease in liver blood flow does not change intrinsic clearance, plasma protein binding, clearance, or volume of distribution under usual circumstances

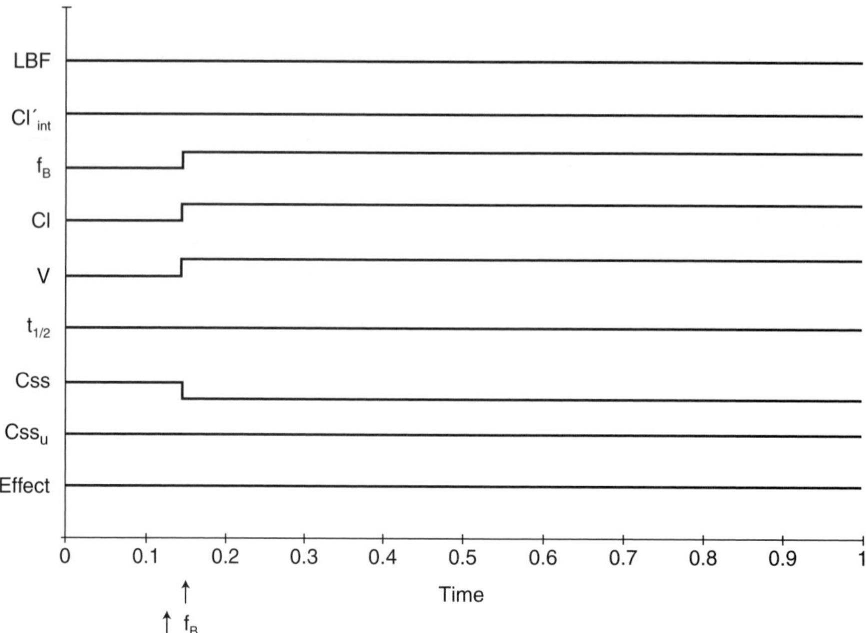

FIGURE 3-7 Changes in physiologic parameters (*LBF* = liver blood flow, Cl'_{int} = intrinsic clearance, f_B = free fraction of drug in the blood), pharmacokinetic parameters (*Cl* = clearance, *V* = volume of distribution, $t_{1/2}$ = half-life), and drug concentration and effect (*Css* = total steady-state concentration; Css_u = unbound steady-state concentration; *effect* = pharmacologic effect) for a low hepatic extraction ratio drug if decreased protein binding occurred (↑f_B, indicated by *arrow*). An uptick in the line indicates an increase in the value of the parameter; a downtick in the line indicates a decrease in the value of the parameter. Increased free fraction of drug in the blood secondary to decreased plasma protein binding could happen during liver dysfunction because of hypoalbuminemia or hyperbilirubinemia. Increased free fraction of drug can occur in patients with normal liver function secondary to a plasma protein binding displacement drug interaction.

and thus does not change total steady-state concentrations, unbound steady-state concentrations, or the pharmacologic effects of the drug. However, a drastic decrease in liver blood flow can effectively stop delivery of drug to the liver and change liver clearance even for compounds with low hepatic extraction ratios.

For drugs with high hepatic extraction ratios, the pattern of changes using the model previously mentioned is entirely different. If intrinsic clearance changes due to hepatocyte destruction for a high hepatic extraction ratio drug, liver blood flow and unbound fraction of drug in the blood remain unaltered (Figure 3-8). Pharmacokinetic constants also do not change, because none are influenced by intrinsic clearance. Because of this, unbound and total steady-state drug concentrations and pharmacologic effect are unchanged. If the drug were administered orally, the hepatic first-pass effect would be decreased, which would increase the bioavailability of the drug. Since this is effectively an increase in drug dosage, average total and unbound drug concentrations and pharmacologic effect would increase for this route of administration ($Css = [F(D/\tau)/Cl]$, where F is

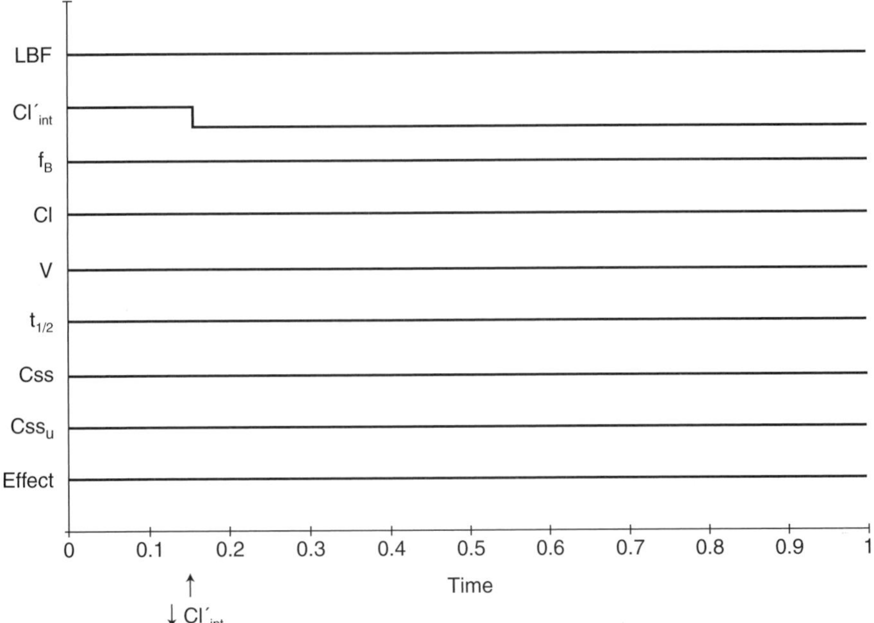

FIGURE 3-8 Changes in physiologic parameters (*LBF* = liver blood flow, Cl'_{int} = intrinsic clearance, f_B = free fraction of drug in the blood), pharmacokinetic parameters (*Cl* = clearance, *V* = volume of distribution, $t_{1/2}$ = half-life), and drug concentration and effect (*Css* = total steady-state concentration; Css_u = unbound steady-state concentration; *effect* = pharmacologic effect) for a high hepatic extraction ratio drug if intrinsic clearance decreases (indicated by *arrow*). An uptick in the line indicates an increase in the value of the parameter; a downtick in the line indicates a decrease in the value of the parameter. Intrinsic clearance could decrease owing to loss of functional hepatocytes secondary to liver cirrhosis or a drug interaction that inhibits drug-metabolizing enzymes.

the bioavailability fraction, Css is the total steady-state drug concentration, D is dose, τ is the dosage interval, and Cl is clearance).

A decrease in plasma protein binding due to lack of binding protein or displacement from binding sites causes severe problems for high hepatic extraction ratio drugs (Figure 3-9). Decreased plasma protein binding results in an increased free fraction of drug in the blood but no change in liver blood flow or intrinsic clearance. Since clearance is a function of liver blood flow, it does not change. However, a higher free fraction of drug in the blood increases the volume of distribution, and this change causes a longer half-life for the drug. Total steady-state concentration does not change because clearance did not change. But unbound steady-state concentration increases because of the increased free fraction of drug in the blood. Pharmacologic effect increases because of the increased unbound steady-state concentration. This is a very subtle change in drug metabolism, because total steady-state concentrations do not change, but the pharmacologic effect is augmented. Clinicians need to keep this possible change in mind and order unbound drug concentrations, if available, when they suspect that this phenomenon may be taking place.

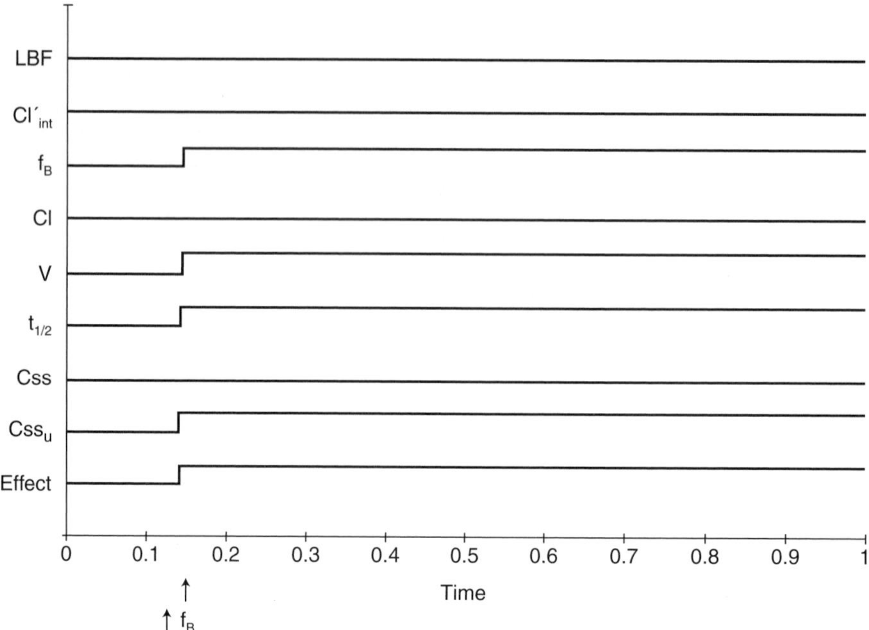

FIGURE 3-9 Changes in physiologic parameters (*LBF* = liver blood flow, Cl'_{int} = intrinsic clearance, f_B = free fraction of drug in the blood), pharmacokinetic parameters (*Cl* = clearance, *V* = volume of distribution, $t_{1/2}$ = half-life), and drug concentration and effect (*Css* = total steady-state concentration; Css_u = unbound steady-state concentration; *effect* = pharmacologic effect) for a high hepatic extraction ratio drug if decreased protein binding occurred (↑f_B, indicated by *arrow*). An uptick in the line indicates an increase in the value of the parameter; a downtick in the line indicates a decrease in the value of the parameter. Increased free fraction of drug in the blood secondary to decreased plasma protein binding could happen during liver dysfunction because of hypoalbuminemia or hyperbilirubinemia. Increased free fraction of drug can occur in patients with normal liver function secondary to a plasma protein binding displacement drug interaction.

If unbound drug concentrations (or no drug concentrations) are available, a trial decrease in dose may be warranted. Orally administered drug would result in a similar pattern of change, but the increased free fraction of drug in the blood would result in a larger hepatic first-pass effect and an effective reduction in dose, which would partially offset the increase in unbound steady-state concentration.

If liver blood flow decreases, the pharmacokinetic and pharmacologic changes are more straightforward for medications with large hepatic extraction ratios (Figure 3-10). Decreased liver blood flow does not change intrinsic clearance or the unbound fraction of drug in the blood. Clearance decreases because it depends on liver blood flow for drugs with a high hepatic extraction ratio. Volume of distribution remains constant, but half-life increases because of the decrease in clearance. Total steady-state concentration increases because of the decrease in clearance, free steady-state concentration rises because of the increase in total steady-state concentration, and the increase in pharmacologic effect tracks the change in free concentration. If the drug is given orally, the first-pass effect

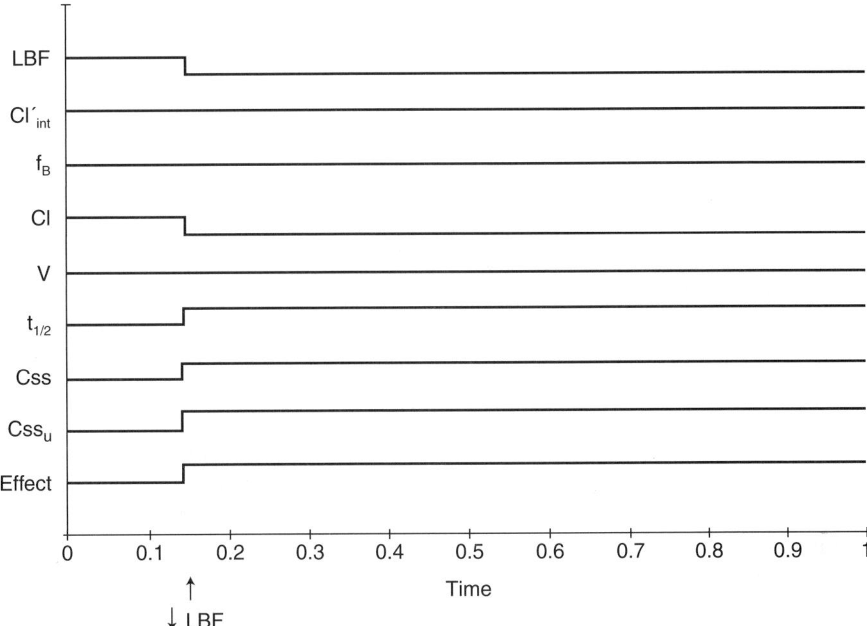

FIGURE 3-10 Changes in physiologic parameters (*LBF* = liver blood flow, Cl'_{int} = intrinsic clearance, f_B = free fraction of drug in the blood), pharmacokinetic parameters (*Cl* = clearance, *V* = volume of distribution, $t_{1/2}$ = half-life), and drug concentration and effect (*Css* = total steady-state concentration; Css_u = unbound steady-state concentration; *effect* = pharmacologic effect) for a high hepatic extraction ratio drug if liver blood flow decreases (↓LBF, indicated by *arrow*). An uptick in the line indicates an increase in the value of the parameter; a downtick in the line indicates a decrease in the value of the parameter. Decreased liver blood flow can occur because of portal hypertension secondary to hepatic cirrhosis. It can occur in patients with normal liver function secondary to a drug interaction with an agent that decreases cardiac output such as β-blockers.

would increase, and bioavailability would decrease, partially offsetting the increase in total and unbound steady-state concentrations.

HEART FAILURE

Heart failure is accompanied by a decrease in cardiac output, which results in lower liver and renal blood flow. Changes in drug pharmacokinetics due to decreased renal blood flow are not widely reported. However, declines in hepatic clearance, especially for compounds with moderate to high hepatic extraction ratios, are reported for many drugs. In addition, decreased drug bioavailability has been reported in patients with heart failure. The proposed mechanisms for decreased bioavailability are collection of edema fluid in the gastrointestinal tract, which makes absorption of drug molecules more difficult, and decreased blood flow to the gastrointestinal tract. The volume of distribution for some drugs decreases in patients with heart failure. Because clearance and volume of distribution may or may not simultaneously change, the alteration in half-life, if any, is difficult to predict in patients with heart failure.

DIALYSIS

Dialysis is a process whereby substances move via a concentration gradient across a semipermeable membrane (Figure 3-11). Artificial kidneys (also known as dialysis coils or filters) are available for use in hemodialysis, which use a synthetic semipermeable membrane to remove waste products from the blood. Also, physiologic membranes, such as those in the peritoneal cavity in the lower abdomen, can be used with peritoneal dialysis as an endogenous semipermeable membrane. Substances that are small enough to pass through the pores in the semipermeable membrane can pass out of the blood into the dialysis fluid. Once in the dialysis fluid, waste products and other compounds can be removed from the body. In some cases, dialysis is used to remove drugs from patients who have taken drug overdoses or are experiencing severe adverse effects from the drug. However, in most cases drug molecules are removed from the blood coincidental to the removal of toxic waste products that would usually be eliminated by the kidney.

Because drugs can be removed by dialysis, it is important to understand when drug dosing needs to be modified in patients with renal failure undergoing the procedure. Often, dialysis removes enough drug from a patient's body that supplemental doses need to be given after dialysis has been completed (Figure 3-12). In a patient with renal failure, the only clearance mechanism available to remove drugs from the body is nonrenal ($Cl = Cl_{NR}$, where Cl is total clearance and Cl_{NR} is nonrenal clearance). When the patient is receiving dialysis, clearance from both nonrenal routes and dialysis are present, which ac-

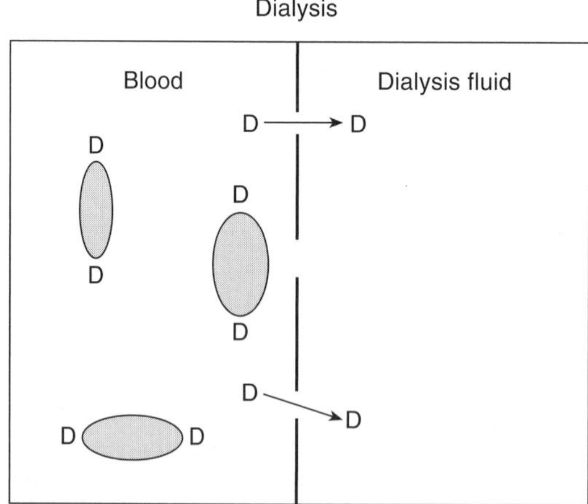

FIGURE 3-11 Dialysis removal of drug can occur when a patient's blood comes in contact with a semipermeable membrane that has drug-free dialysis fluid on the other side. In this schematic representation, the semipermeable membrane is shown to have pores large enough for unbound drug to pass through (*D*), but not for protein-bound drug to pass through (*Ds attached to ovals* representing plasma proteins).

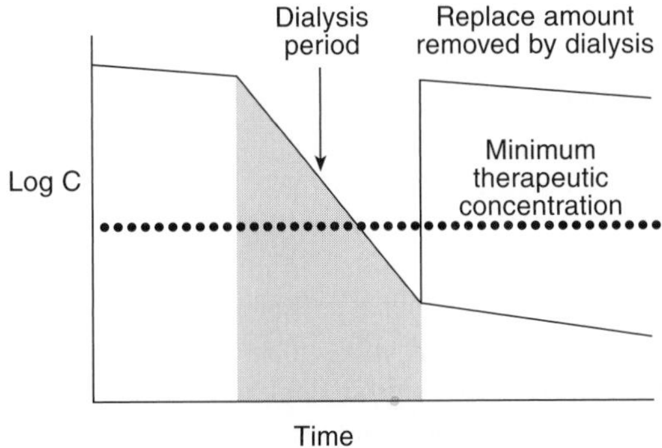

FIGURE 3-12 Concentration–time graph for a drug removed by dialysis. The *shaded area* indicates the time period in which a dialysis procedure was conducted. Because extra drug was removed from the blood during dialysis, concentrations dropped much faster during that period. After dialysis is finished, the concentrations again drop at the predialysis rate. If drug concentrations drop below the minimum therapeutic concentration (*dark, dotted horizontal line*), it may be necessary to give a supplemental dose to retain the pharmacologic effect of the drug (indicated by increase in drug concentration after dialysis).

celerate drug removal from the body during the dialysis procedure if the compound is significantly removed by dialysis ($Cl = Cl_{NR} + Cl_D$, where Cl_D is dialysis clearance). To determine whether dialysis clearance is significant, one should consider the absolute value of dialysis clearance and its relative contribution to total clearance. In addition, if dialysis clearance is ≥30% of total clearance or if the total amount of drug removed by the dialysis procedure is enough to warrant a postdialysis replacement dose, dialysis clearance is considered to be significant.

Drug Characteristics That Affect Dialysis Removal

MOLECULAR SIZE

Molecular size relative to pore size in the semipermeable membrane is a factor that influences dialysis clearance of a compound. Most hemodialysis procedures are conducted using "low-flux" artificial kidneys, which have relatively small pores in the semipermeable membranes. However, "high-flux" filters are now available and widely used in some patients. The semipermeable membranes of these artificial kidneys have much larger pore sizes and larger surface areas so that large drug molecules, such as vancomycin, which were previously considered unable to be removed by hemodialysis, can be cleared by high-flux filters. It is important that clinicians know which type of artificial kidney is used for a patient before assessing its potential to remove drug molecules.

For low-flux filters, small drug molecules (molecular mass <500 daltons, such as theophylline, lidocaine, and procainamide) relative to the pore size of the semipermeable membrane tend to be readily eliminated by dialysis and have high extraction ratios for the artificial kidney. In this case, "dialyzability" of the drug is influenced by blood flow to the artificial kidney, dialysis fluid flow rate to the artificial kidney, and the surface area of the semipermeable membrane inside the artificial kidney. Increased blood flow delivers more drug to the dialysis coil, increased dialysis fluid flow rate removes drug that entered the dialysis fluid more quickly from the artificial kidney and increases the concentration gradient across the semipermeable membrane, and increased semipermeable membrane surface area increases the number of pores that a drug molecule will encounter, thus making it easier for drug molecules to pass from the blood into the dialysis fluid.

Drug molecules with moderate molecular mass [500 to 1000 daltons, such as aminoglycoside antibiotics (~400 to 500 daltons) and digoxin] have a decreased ability to pass through the semipermeable membrane contained in low-flux filters. However, many drugs that fall in this intermediate category have sufficient dialysis clearances to require postdialysis replacement doses. Large drug molecules (molecular mass >1000 daltons, such as vancomycin) are not removed to a significant extent when low-flux filters are used for dialysis, because pore sizes in these artificial kidneys are too small for the molecules to fit through. However, many large-molecular-weight drugs can be removed by dialysis when high-flux filters are used, and, in some cases, supplemental postdialysis drug doses are needed to maintain therapeutic amounts of drug in the body.

WATER/LIPID SOLUBILITY

Drugs that have a high degree of water solubility tend to partition into the water-based dialysis fluid, whereas lipid-soluble drugs tend to remain in the blood.

PLASMA PROTEIN BINDING

Only unbound drug molecules are able to pass through the pores in the semipermeable membrane; drug–plasma protein complexes are too large to pass through the pores and gain access to the dialysis fluid side of the semipermeable membrane. Drugs that are not highly plasma protein-bound have high free fractions of drug in the blood and are prone to better dialysis clearance. Drugs that are highly bound to plasma proteins have low free fractions of drug in the blood and poor dialysis clearance rates.

VOLUME OF DISTRIBUTION

The volume of distribution of a drug is a function of blood volume (V_B), organ size (V_T), drug plasma protein binding (f_B, free fraction of drug in the blood), and drug tissue binding [f_T, free fraction of drug in the tissues; $V = V_B + (f_B/f_T)V_T$]. Medications with large volumes of distribution are principally located at tissue binding sites and not in the blood, where dialysis can remove the drug. Because of this, agents with large volumes of distribution are not easily removed from the body. In fact, some compounds such as digoxin, have good hemodialysis clearance rates, and drug contained in the bloodstream is very effectively eliminated. However, in this case most of the drug is in the tissues, and only a small amount of the total drug in the body is removed. If serum concentrations of these types of drugs are followed closely during hemodialysis, the concentrations decrease by a substantial amount. But when dialysis is completed, the blood and tissues have a chance to reequilibrate and serum concentrations increase, sometimes to their predialysis concentration. This "rebound" in serum concentration has been reported for several drugs.

Compounds with small volumes of distribution (<1 L/kg, such as the aminoglycoside antibiotics and theophylline) usually demonstrate high dialysis clearance rates. Drugs with moderate volumes of distribution (1 to 2 L/kg) have intermediate dialysis clearance values, whereas agents with large volumes of distribution (>2 L/kg, such as digoxin and tricyclic antidepressants) have poor dialysis characteristics.

HEMODIALYSIS

Hemodialysis is a very efficient procedure to remove toxic waste from the blood of renal failure patients (Figure 3-13). Blood is pumped out of the patient at 300 to 400 mL/min and through one side of the semipermeable membrane of the artificial kidney by the hemodialysis machine. Cleansed blood is then pumped back into the vascular system of the patient. In acute situations, vascular access can be obtained through centrally placed catheters. For patients with chronic renal failure, vascular shunts made of synthetic materials are surgically placed between a high blood flow artery and vein in the arm or in another site for the purpose of conducting hemodialysis. Dialysis fluid is pumped through the artificial kidney at 400 to 600 mL/min on the other side of the semipermeable membrane in the opposite direction of blood flow. This "countercurrent" flow is more efficient in removing waste products than in running the blood and dialysis fluid parallel with each other. Dialysis fluid is electrolyte and osmotically balanced for the individual patient. Serum electrolytes can be increased or decreased by increasing or decreasing the concentration of the ion in the dialysis fluid compared with the concurrent serum value. Also, by adding solutes to increase the osmolality of the dialysis fluid relative to the blood, it is possible to remove fluid from the patient's body by osmotic pressure across the semipermeable membrane of the artificial kidney. This process is known as *ultrafiltration*. Using low-flux filters, hemodialysis is usually performed for 3 to 4 hours three times weekly.

The FDA has required pharmacokinetic studies to be done for renally eliminated drugs in patients receiving chronic hemodialysis since the mid-1980s. Because of this, the package insert for the drug may include manufacturer-recommended doses to be administered to patients in the posthemodialysis period (see Table 3-1). Guidelines for the administration of posthemodialysis replacement doses are available for older drugs as well as updated guidelines for newer drugs that may not be included in the package insert.[10–13] Also,

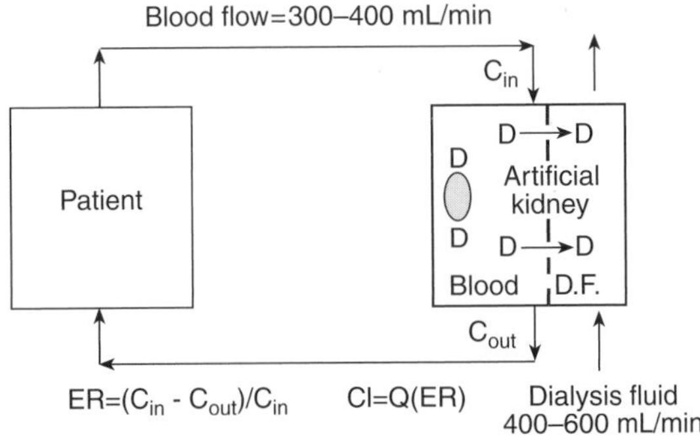

FIGURE 3-13 Hemodialysis removes blood from the patient's body (*arrows from patient to artificial kidney*) and passes it through an artificial kidney that contains a semipermeable membrane. Inside the artificial kidney, waste products pass into the dialysis fluid and are eliminated from the body. If drug molecules can pass through the pores in the semipermeable membrane, they will also be eliminated from the body. The extraction ratio (*ER*) of the artificial kidney can be computed using the concentration into (C_{in}) and out of (C_{out}) the device. Dialysis clearance (*Cl*) can be calculated by taking the product of the dialysis extraction ratio and blood flow to the dialysis machine (Q). *D* = drug; *D.F.* = dialysis fluid.

the primary literature should be consulted to ensure that the newest guidelines are used for all drugs. When one is assessing the hemodialysis removal characteristics of a drug and the need for postdialysis replacement doses, it should be recognized that most information available is for low-flux artificial kidneys. If a high-flux dialysis coil is used, the primary literature is probably the best source of information, but in many cases studies have not been conducted using this technology.

Computation of Initial Doses and Modification of Doses Using Drug Serum Concentrations

Initial drug doses of patients with renal failure undergoing hemodialysis can be based on expected pharmacokinetic parameters for this population when published information for a drug is inadequate or the agent has a very narrow therapeutic index. For example, an initial dosage regimen for tobramycin must be computed for a patient to achieve peak concentrations of 6 to 7 mg/L and postdialysis concentrations of 1 to 2 mg/L. The patient is a 62-year-old 173-cm (68-in) man who weighs 65 kg, has chronic renal failure, and receives hemodialysis three times weekly with a low-flux dialysis filter. Patients with renal failure are prone to poor fluid balance because their kidneys are not able to provide this important function. Because of this, this patient should be assessed for overhydration (due to renal failure) or underhydration (due to renal failure and increased loss from fever). Weight is a good indication of fluid status, and this patient's weight is less than his ideal weight [IBW_{men} = 50 kg + 2.3(Ht – 60 in) = 50 kg + 2.3(68 – 60) = 68 kg]. Other indications of state of hydration (e.g., skin turgor) indicate that the patient has normal fluid balance at this time. Because of this, the average volume of distribution for aminoglycoside antibiotics of 0.26 L/kg can be used.

A loading dose of tobramycin would be appropriate for this patient because the expected half-life is long (~50 h); administration of maintenance doses only might not result in therapeutic maximum concentrations for a considerable time period while drug accumulation is occurring. The loading dose is to be given after hemodialysis ends at 1300 H on Monday (hemodialysis conducted on Monday, Wednesday, and Friday from 0900 to 1300 H). Because the drug is expected to have a long half-life compared with the infusion time of the drug (1/2 to 1 hour), little drug will be eliminated from the patient during the infusion period, and intravenous bolus one-compartment model equations can be used. The loading dose for this patient is based on the expected volume of distribution: V = 0.26 L/kg · 65 kg = 16.9 L; LD = C_{max} · V = 6 mg/L · 16.9 L = 101 mg, rounded to 100 mg, where LD is loading dose and C_{max} is the maximum concentration after drug administration. This loading dose was given at 1400 H (Figure 3-14). Until the next dialysis period at 0900 H on Wednesday, tobramycin is cleared only by the patient's own body mechanisms. The expected elimination rate constant (k_e) for a patient with a creatinine clearance of approximately zero is k_e (in h^{-1}) = 0.00293 · CrCl + 0.014 = 0.00293 (0 mL/min) + 0.014 = 0.014 h^{-1}. The expected concentration at 0900 H on Wednesday is: $C = C_0 e^{-k_e t}$, where C is the concentration at t hours after the initial concentration of C_0; $C = (6\ mg/L)e^{-(0.014\ h^{-1})(43\ h)}$ = 3.3 mg/L.

While the patient is receiving hemodialysis, tobramycin is eliminated by the patient's own mechanisms and by dialysis clearance. During hemodialysis with a low-flux filter, the average half-life for aminoglycosides is 4 hours. Because the patient is on dialysis for 4 hours, the tobramycin serum concentration should decrease by half to 1.7 mg/L, or using

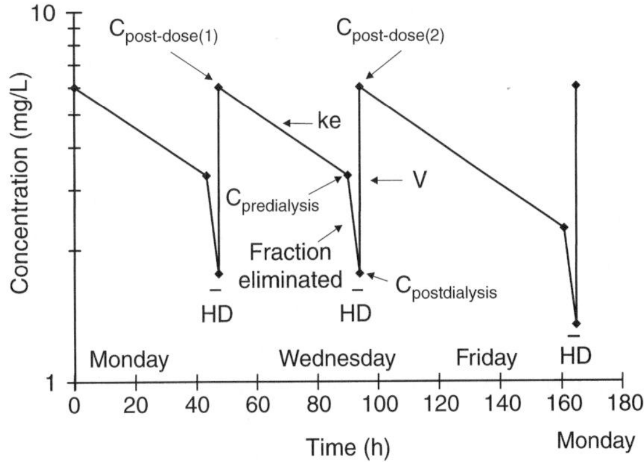

FIGURE 3-14 Concentration–time graph for tobramycin in a hemodialysis patient using estimated population pharmacokinetic parameters. The initial dose was given postdialysis at 1400 H on Monday (time = 0 hour). Hemodialysis periods are shown by small horizontal bars labeled *HD*, and days are indicated on the time line. To compute patient-specific pharmacokinetic parameters, four serum concentrations are measured. The elimination rate constant (k_e) is computed using two concentrations after dosage administration ($C_{postdose(1)}$ and $C_{predialysis}$), the fraction eliminated by dialysis by two concentrations ($C_{predialysis}$ and $C_{postdialysis}$) before and after dialysis, and the volume of distribution (*V*) using two concentrations ($C_{postdialysis}$ and $C_{postdose(2)}$) after another dosage administration.

formal computations: $k_e = 0.693/(t_{1/2}) = 0.693/4\ h = 0.173\ h^{-1}$; $C = C_0e^{-k_et} = (3.3\ mg/L)\ e^{-(0.173\ h^{-1})(4\ h)} = 1.7\ mg/L$. At this time, a postdialysis replacement dose could be given to increase the maximum concentration to its original value of 6 mg/L: Replacement dose = $(C_{max} - C_{baseline})V = (6\ mg/L - 1.7\ mg/L)16.9\ L = 73\ mg$, rounded to 75 mg, where C_{max} is the maximum postdose concentration and $C_{baseline}$ is the predose concentration. The postdialysis replacement dose of 75 mg was administered at 1400 H on Wednesday. Because all time frames and pharmacokinetic parameters are the same for Monday to Wednesday and Wednesday to Friday, the postdialysis replacement dose on Friday at 1400 H is also 75 mg. However, more time elapses from Friday after drug administration to Monday before dialysis (67 hours), the next day for hemodialysis to be conducted, and this needs to be accounted for: $C = C_0e^{-k_et} = (6\ mg/L)e^{-(0.014\ h^{-1})(67\ h)} = 2.3\ mg/L$. Again, a 4-hour hemodialysis period decreases serum concentrations by half to 1.2 mg/L: $C = C_0e^{-k_et} = (2.3\ mg/L)\ e^{-(0.173\ h^{-1})(4\ h)} = 1.2\ mg/L$. At this time, a postdialysis replacement dose can be given to increase the maximum concentration to the original value of 6 mg/L: Replacement dose = $(C_{max} - C_{baseline})V = (6\ mg/L - 1.2\ mg/L)16.9\ L = 81\ mg$, rounded to 80 mg, where C_{max} is the maximum postdose concentration and $C_{baseline}$ is the predose concentration. The postdialysis replacement dose of 80 mg was administered at 1400 H on Monday. Because all time frames and pharmacokinetic parameters are identical for subsequent weeks, the following postdialysis replacement doses are prescribed postdialysis at 1400 H: Wednesday and Friday 75 mg, Monday 80 mg. In this particular example, recommended daily doses are within 5 mg of each other, and, if the clinician wishes, the same postdialysis dose can be given on each day. However, this is not true in every case.

Since the initial dosage scheme outlined for this patient used average, estimated pharmacokinetic parameters, the patient probably has different pharmacokinetic characteristics. It is possible to measure the patient's unique pharmacokinetic parameters using four serum concentrations (see Figure 3-14). The intradialysis elimination rate constant can be determined by obtaining postdose ($C_{postdose(1)}$) and predialysis ($C_{predialysis}$) concentrations [$k_e = (C_{postdose} - C_{predialysis})/\Delta t$, where Δt is the time between the two concentrations], the fraction of drug eliminated by dialysis can be computed using predialysis and postdialysis ($C_{postdialysis}$) concentrations: Fraction eliminated = $[(C_{predialysis} - C_{postdialysis})/C_{predialysis}]$. The volume of distribution can be calculated using postdialysis and postdose concentrations: $V = D/(C_{postdose(2)} - C_{postdialysis})$. Note that if the drug demonstrates a postdialysis rebound in drug concentrations, postdialysis serum samples should be obtained after blood and tissue have had the opportunity to reequilibrate. In the case of aminoglycosides, postdialysis samples should be collected no sooner than 3 to 4 hours after the end of dialysis. After individualized pharmacokinetic parameters have been measured, they can be used in the same equations that were used to compute initial doses in the previous section in place of average population pharmacokinetic parameters, and they can be used to calculate individualized doses for dialysis patients. It is also possible to use a mixture of measured and population-estimated pharmacokinetic parameters. For instance, a clinician may wish to measure the elimination rate constant or volume of distribution for a patient but may elect to use an average population estimate for fraction of drug removed by the artificial kidney.

Methods to Measure Hemodialysis Clearance

If needed, hemodialysis clearance can be measured in patients. The extraction ratio method measures the extraction of drug across the artificial kidney by obtaining simultaneous blood samples on input (C_{in}) and outlet (C_{out}) sides of the dialysis coil (see Figure 3-13). The tubing carrying blood to and from the patient usually has injection ports that can be used as access points to get the necessary blood samples. The artificial kidney extraction ratio (ER) can be computed using drug concentrations measured from the blood samples: $ER = (C_{in} - C_{out})/C_{in}$. Blood flow from the hemodialysis machine (HDBF) is available as a continuous read-out on the pump, and hemodialysis clearance (Cl_{HD}) can be computed by taking the product of the extraction ratio and blood flow parameters: $Cl_{HD} = HDBF \cdot ER$. The advantage to this technique is that it is methodologically simple. The disadvantage is that if the dialysis extraction ratio is low, serum concentration differences between C_{in} and C_{out} will be small and difficult for the drug assay to determine. If serum concentrations of drug are measured, hemodialysis clearance should be corrected for the patient's hematocrit (Hct): $C1_{HD} = HDBF \cdot ER \cdot (1 - Hct)$.

Another method of measuring hemodialysis clearance is to collect the waste dialysis fluid used during the dialysis procedure and measure several serum drug concentrations during the same time interval (Figure 3-15). The amount of drug eliminated in the dialysis fluid ($A_{Dialysis}$) is determined by multiplying the volume of dialysis fluid ($V_{Dialysis}$) and the concentration of drug in the dialysis fluid ($C_{Dialysis}$): $A_{Dialysis} = V_{Dialysis} \cdot C_{Dialysis}$. Hemodialysis clearance (Cl_{HD}) is computed by dividing the amount of drug eliminated in the dialysis fluid by the area under the serum concentration–time curve during the dialysis period ($AUC_{Dialysis}$, calculated using the serum concentrations obtained during hemodialysis): $Cl_{HD} = A_{Dialysis}/AUC_{Dialysis}$. An advantage of this method is that hemodialysis clear-

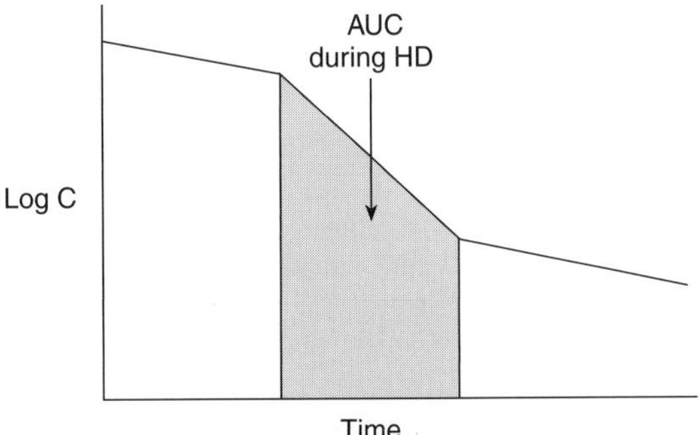

FIGURE 3-15 One method of measuring hemodialysis clearance is to take the quotient of the amount of drug eliminated by the dialysis procedure ($A_{Dialysis}$) and the area under the concentration–time curve (*AUC*) during the dialysis time period (*HD*, indicated by the *shaded area*).

ance is determined using multiple serum concentrations and may be more accurate. Disadvantages include collection of a large volume of dialysis fluid (~120 L) and the large number of serum concentrations needed to determine $AUC_{Dialysis}$.

The final method is to collect all the waste dialysis fluid used during the dialysis period and measure a single serum drug concentration at the midpoint of the procedure. Using this information, hemodialysis clearance (Cl_{HD}) can be computed using the following equation: $Cl_{HD} = (C_{Dialysis} \cdot V_{Dialysis})/(C_{Serum} \cdot T_{Dialysis})$, where $C_{Dialysis}$ is the drug concentration in the dialysis fluid, $V_{Dialysis}$ is the volume of dialysis fluid, C_{Serum} is the drug serum concentration, and $T_{Dialysis}$ is the duration of the hemodialysis procedure. An advantage of this technique is that it requires only one serum concentration. The chief disadvantage is that all dialysis fluid used during hemodialysis must be collected.

PERITONEAL DIALYSIS

Peritoneal dialysis is gaining in popularity as a method of removing waste substances from the blood of renal failure patients. This dialysis method involves the surgical insertion of a catheter in the lower abdomen into the peritoneal cavity (Figure 3-16). The peritoneal membrane covering the internal organs is highly vascularized, so that when dialysis fluid (1 to 3 L) is introduced into the peritoneal cavity using the catheter, waste products move from the blood vessels of the peritoneal membrane (a semipermeable membrane) into the dialysis fluid along a concentration gradient. The dialysis fluid is periodically removed from the peritoneal cavity and discarded. Outpatients undergoing chronic ambulatory peritoneal dialysis have dialysis fluid in their peritoneal cavities all day or most hours of a day.

Compared with hemodialysis, peritoneal dialysis removes drug much less efficiently. Therefore, replacement drug doses are less likely to be needed during intermittent peritoneal dialysis, and drug dosages will have to be increased while patients receive long-term peritoneal dialysis. For instance, in patients with end-stage renal disease, the half-life of aminoglycoside antibiotics is ~50 hours. During hemodialysis, the half-life reduces to ~4 hours, but during peritoneal dialysis in patients without peritonitis, the half-life de-

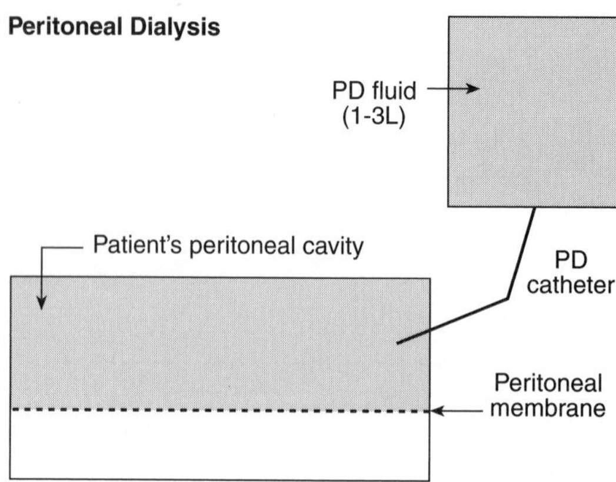

FIGURE 3-16 Schematic drawing of peritoneal dialysis procedure. A catheter (*PD catheter*) is surgically inserted into the patient's peritoneal cavity and used to introduce 1 to 3 L of dialysis fluid (*PD fluid*). The dialysis fluid comes into contact with capillaries in the peritoneal membrane, where waste products and drugs pass from the blood into the fluid. After the dwell time has concluded, the dialysis fluid is removed from the peritoneal cavity via the catheter and discarded.

creases to only ~36 hours. In patients receiving chronic peritoneal dialysis, dialysis removal of drug is simply another clearance mechanism taking place in the patient's body, so the usual methods of measuring serum concentrations and dosage adjustment require little or no modification. For patients undergoing peritoneal dialysis, clinicians should consult the manufacturer's package insert for drugs recently marketed (i.e., mid-1980s or later), reviews listing the peritoneal dialysis removal of older drugs and updated information on newer agents,[10–13] and the primary literature for the newest guidelines for all compounds.

Drugs can also be added to peritoneal dialysis fluid. If the agent is absorbed from the dialysis fluid into the body, systemic effects due to the drug may occur. Epoetin and insulin have been administered in this fashion to patients receiving peritoneal dialysis. Because the development of peritonitis is a common problem in patients receiving peritoneal dialysis, antibiotics have been administered intraperitoneally for local treatment of the infection using dialysis fluid as the delivery vehicle. In most cases, antibiotics are absorbed into the body when given this way, but therapeutic serum concentrations may not be achieved for all agents, making systemically administered doses necessary. Clinicians should pay particular attention to whether studies measuring peritoneal dialysis removal or absorption of drugs were conducted in patients with peritonitis. Peritonitis involves inflammation of the peritoneal membrane and increases its permeability. Increased permeability allows for greater flux of drug across the membrane, which allows more drug removal during dialysis or more drug absorption if the drug is added to the peritoneal dialysis fluid.

Methods of Measuring Peritoneal Dialysis Clearance

If necessary, peritoneal dialysis clearance can be measured in patients. One method is to collect the waste dialysis fluid used during a peritoneal dialysis period and measure several serum drug concentrations during the same time interval (see Figure 3-15). The amount of drug eliminated in the dialysis fluid ($A_{Dialysis}$) is calculated by multiplying the volume of dialysis fluid ($V_{Dialysis}$) and the concentration of drug in the dialysis fluid ($C_{Dialysis}$): $A_{Dialysis} = V_{Dialysis} \cdot C_{Dialysis}$. Peritoneal clearance ($Cl_{PD}$) is computed by dividing the amount of drug eliminated in the dialysis fluid by the area under the serum concentration–time curve during the dialysis period ($AUC_{Dialysis}$, calculated using the serum concentrations obtained during peritoneal dialysis): $Cl_{PD} = A_{Dialysis}/AUC_{Dialysis}$. An advantage of this method is that the dialysate volume is relatively small. Disadvantages are that a large number of serum concentrations are needed to determine $AUC_{Dialysis}$ and that, if only a small amount of drug is removed via dialysis, the drug assay may not be sensitive enough to measure a small concentration.

Another method of measuring peritoneal dialysis clearance is to collect all the waste dialysis fluid used during a dialysis period and measure a single serum drug concentration at the midpoint of the procedure. Using this information, peritoneal clearance (Cl_{PD}) can be computed using the following equation: $Cl_{PD} = (C_{Dialysis} \cdot V_{Dialysis})/(C_{Serum} \cdot T_{Dialysis})$, where $C_{Dialysis}$ is the drug concentration in the dialysis fluid, $V_{Dialysis}$ is the volume of dialysis fluid, C_{Serum} is the drug serum concentration, and $T_{Dialysis}$ is the duration in which dialysis fluid remained in the peritoneal cavity. Advantages of this technique are that it requires only one serum concentration and that the volume of dialysis fluid is relatively small. A disadvantage is that if only a small amount of drug is removed by dialysis, the drug assay may not be sensitive enough to measure a low concentration.

OBESITY

Excessive adipose tissue can alter the pharmacokinetics of drugs by changing the volume of distribution. The general physiologic equation for volume of distribution can be broken down into separate parameters for individual tissue types:

$$V = V_B + \frac{f_B}{f_T} V_T = V_B + \frac{f_B}{f_{heart}} V_{heart} + \frac{f_B}{f_{muscle}} V_{muscle} + \frac{f_B}{f_{fat}} V_{fat} + \ldots + \frac{f_B}{f_n} V_n$$

Because of this, the sheer amount of adipose tissue is a primary determinant of how much obesity will affect the volume of distribution of the drug. Also, the magnitude of effect that adipose tissue has on the volume of distribution for a drug depends on the binding of drug in the tissue itself. If the drug has a high affinity for adipose tissue and is highly bound there, the free fraction in adipose tissue will be small ($\downarrow f_{fat}$), and a large amount of drug will accumulate in that tissue.

Medications that have high lipid solubility tend to partition into adipose tissue, and the volume of distribution in obese patients for these drugs can be dramatically larger than in normal-weight patients. Examples of lipophilic drugs with larger volume of distribution values in obese individuals are diazepam,[22] carbamazepine,[23] and trazodone.[24] However, hydrophilic drugs tend not to distribute into adipose tissue, so that the volume of distribution for many water-soluble drugs is not significantly different in obese and normal-weight patients. The volumes of distribution for digoxin,[25] cimetidine,[26] and ranitidine[27] are similar in overweight and in normal-weight subjects.

Although excessive adipose tissue is the most obvious change that occurs in obese individuals, other physiologic changes are present. Although adipose cells contain >90% fat, additional supportive tissues, extracellular fluid, and blood are in adipose tissue. Also, some lean tissues undergo hypertrophy in obese persons. The net result of these changes is that hydrophilic drugs with small volumes of distribution may experience distribution alterations in obese patients. For example, the aminoglycoside antibiotics are water-soluble molecules that have relatively small volumes of distribution similar to the value of extracellular fluid (V = 0.26 L/kg). Since the volume of distribution is so small (~18 L in a 70-kg person), the addition of just a few liters of extracellular fluid can alter the pharmacokinetics of these antibiotics. The additional extracellular fluid contained in excessive adipose tissue and other organs that undergo hypertrophy in obese persons causes larger volumes of distribution for the aminoglycoside antibiotics. Formulas that correct aminoglycoside volume of distribution for obese persons are available.[28–30] However, if the volume of distribution of a hydrophilic drug is intermediate or large, the additional extracellular fluid contained in adipose tissue and other sources in obese persons may not significantly alter the distribution of the agent. Examples of medications that have larger and intermediate volumes of distribution are digoxin (V = 500 L) and vancomycin (V = 50 L); the addition of a few extra liters of extracellular fluid due to obesity does not substantially change the volume of distribution of these agents.[25,31]

Another change found in obese persons is increased glomerular filtration rates. This alteration primarily affects hydrophilic drug compounds that are renally eliminated and increases the renal clearance of the agent. Vancomycin,[31] the aminoglycosides,[28–30] and cimetidine[26] all have higher clearance rates in obese patients compared with those of normal-weight persons.

Obesity has variable effects on the metabolism of drugs. For many agents, such as carbamazepine[23] and cyclosporine,[32] obesity does not significantly affect hepatic clearance. For other drugs, obesity increases hepatic clearance, as with diazepam,[22] or decreases metabolic clearance, as with methylprednisolone.[33] Clinicians should be aware of this variability and prescribe hepatically metabolized drugs cautiously in obese persons without specific recommendations.

Half-life changes vary according to the relative alterations in clearance (Cl) and volume of distribution (V): $t_{1/2} = (0.693 \cdot V)/Cl$, where $t_{1/2}$ is half-life. In the case of the aminoglycoside antibiotics, clearance and volume of distribution increases are about the same magnitude in obese patients, so half-life does not change.[28–30] If the volume of distribution increases with obesity, but clearance is unaffected, half-life can increase dramatically, as with carbamazepine.[23] Finally, if clearance changes and volume of distribution remains constant, obesity may also cause a change in the half-life of a drug, as for methylprednisolone.[33]

DRUG INTERACTIONS

Pharmacokinetic drug interactions occur between drugs when one agent changes the clearance or volume of distribution of another medication. Several drug interaction mechanisms result in altered drug clearance. A drug can inhibit or induce the enzymes responsible for the metabolism of other drugs. Enzyme inhibition decreases intrinsic clearance, and enzyme induction increases intrinsic clearance. Another type of drug interaction displaces a drug from plasma protein-binding sites, because the two compounds share the same binding site and the two compete for the same area on plasma proteins. By virtue of its pharmacologic effect, a drug may increase or decrease blood flow to an organ that eliminates or metabolizes another medication and may thereby decrease the clearance of the medication. Two drugs eliminated by the same active renal tubular secretion mechanism can compete for the pathway and decrease the renal clearance of one or both agents.

Changes in plasma protein binding also cause alterations in volume of distribution. If two drugs share the same tissue binding sites, it is possible for tissue-binding displacement drug interactions to occur and change the volume of distribution for one of the medications. Half-life may change as a result of drug interactions, or, if clearance and volume of distribution alterations are about equal, half-life may remain constant even though a major drug interaction has occurred.

The same graphic scheme introduced in the hepatic disease section of this chapter can be used to understand the clinical impact of drug interactions (see Figures 3-6 through 3-10). To use these charts it is necessary to know whether the drug under discussion has a low extraction ratio or a high extraction ratio. The hepatic clearance of drugs with low hepatic extraction ratios equals the product of free fraction in the blood and intrinsic clearance ($Cl_H = f_B Cl'_{int}$), whereas the hepatic clearance of drugs with high hepatic extraction ratios equals liver blood flow ($Cl_H = LBF$). Whether a drug has a high or a low extraction ratio, the volume of distribution [$V = V_B + (f_B/f_T)V_T$] and half-life [$t_{1/2} = (0.693 \cdot V)/Cl$] relationships are the same. The unbound steady-state concentration of drug in the blood equals the product of the total steady-state concentration and the unbound fraction of drug in the blood: $Css_u = f_B Css$. The effect of the drug increases when the unbound steady-state concentration increases, and it decreases when Css_u declines.

Plasma Protein-Binding Displacement Drug Interactions

For a drug with a low hepatic extraction ratio, plasma protein-binding displacement drug interactions cause major pharmacokinetic alterations but are not clinically significant because the pharmacologic effect of the drug does not change (see Figure 3-7). Because the clearance of the drug depends on the fraction of unbound drug in the blood and intrinsic clearance for a low hepatic extraction ratio agent, addition of a plasma protein-binding displacement compound increases clearance ($\uparrow Cl = \uparrow f_B Cl'_{int}$) and volume of distribution [$\uparrow V = V_B + (\uparrow f_B/f_T)V_T$]. Since half-life depends on clearance and volume of distribution, it is likely that because both increase, half-life will not substantially change [$t_{1/2} = (0.693 \cdot \uparrow V)/\uparrow Cl$]. However, if either clearance or volume of distribution changes disproportionately, it is possible that half-life will change. The total steady-state concentration will decline because of the increase in clearance ($\downarrow Css = k_0/\uparrow Cl$, where k_0 is the infusion rate of drug). But the unbound steady-state concentration will remain unaltered because the free fraction of drug in the blood is higher than it was before the drug interaction occurred ($Css_u = \uparrow f_B \downarrow Css$).

The pharmacologic effect of the drug does not change because the free concentration of drug in the blood is unchanged. An example of this drug interaction is the addition of diflunisal to patients stabilized on warfarin therapy.[34] Diflunisal displaces warfarin from plasma protein-binding sites but does not augment the anticoagulant effect of warfarin. If drug concentrations are available for the medication, it can be difficult to convince clinicians that a drug dosage increase is not needed, even though total concentrations decline as a result of this interaction. When available, unbound drug concentrations can be used to document that no change in drug dosing is needed.

For drugs with high hepatic extraction ratios given intravenously, plasma protein-binding displacement drug interactions cause both major pharmacokinetic and pharmacodynamic changes (see Figure 3-9). Because the clearance of the drug depends solely on liver blood flow for an agent of this type, total clearance does not change. However, both volume of distribution [$\uparrow V = V_B + (\uparrow f_B/f_T)V_T$] and half-life [$\uparrow t_{1/2} = (0.693 \cdot \uparrow V)/Cl$] do increase because of plasma protein-binding displacement of the drug. Since total clearance did not change, the total steady-state concentration remains unaltered. However, the free concentration ($\uparrow Css_u = \uparrow f_B Css$) and pharmacologic effect ($\uparrow effect \propto \uparrow Css_u$) of the drug both increase. Currently, there are no clinically significant drug interactions of this type. But clinicians should be on the lookout for this profile for highly protein-bound drugs with high hepatic extraction ratios given intravenously, because the interaction is very subtle. Most noteworthy is the fact that although total concentrations remain unchanged, the pharmacologic effect of the drug is augmented. If available, unbound drug concentration can be used to document the drug interaction.

If a drug with a high hepatic extraction ratio is given orally, a plasma protein-binding displacement drug interaction causes a simultaneous increase in the unbound fraction of drug in the blood ($\uparrow f_B$) and the hepatic presystemic metabolism of the drug. Hepatic presystemic metabolism increases because the higher unbound fraction of drug in the blood allows more drug molecules to enter the liver, where they are ultimately metabolized. The increase in hepatic presystemic metabolism leads to an increased first-pass effect and decreased drug bioavailability ($\downarrow F$). Total steady-state drug concentrations are lower because of decreased drug bioavailability [$\downarrow Css = (\downarrow F[D/\tau])/Cl$]. However, the unbound steady-state drug concentration and pharmacologic effect remain unchanged owing to this type of drug interaction, because the increase in unbound fraction is offset by the decrease in the total steady-state concentration ($\sim Css_u = \uparrow f_B \downarrow Css$). Route of administration plays an important role in how important plasma protein-binding displacement drug interactions are for agents with high hepatic extraction ratios.

Inhibition Drug Interactions

Inhibition of hepatic drug metabolism is probably the most common drug interaction encountered in patients. For drugs with low hepatic extraction ratios, this type of drug interaction produces clinically significant changes in drug pharmacokinetics and effect (see Figure 3-6). The addition of a hepatic enzyme inhibitor decreases intrinsic clearance and total clearance for the drug ($\downarrow Cl = f_B \downarrow Cl'_{int}$). Since volume of distribution remains unaltered, the half-life of the drug increases [$\uparrow t_{1/2} = (0.693 \cdot V)/ \downarrow Cl$]. As a result of the total clearance decrease, total steady-state drug concentrations increase ($\uparrow Css = k_0/\downarrow Cl$). The rise in unbound steady-state drug concentration mirrors that seen with total drug concentration, and the effect of the drug increases in proportion to unbound concentration. An example of this drug interaction is the addition of ciprofloxacin to a patient stabilized on theophylline therapy.[35]

For drugs with high hepatic extraction ratios, inhibition drug interactions produce variable effects, depending on the route of administration of the drug. If the drug is given intravenously and an enzyme inhibitor is added, the decrease in intrinsic clearance is usually not substantial enough to cause major pharmacokinetic and pharmacodynamic effects, because clearance is a function of liver blood flow (see Figure 3-8). However, if the drug is given orally and an enzyme inhibitor is added to therapy, presystemic metabolism of the medication may be greatly depressed, and the first-pass effect can decrease dramatically, leading to improved drug bioavailability. This effective increase in administered oral dose increases the total and unbound steady-state drug concentrations and leads to an increase in the pharmacologic effect of the drug.

Induction Drug Interactions

Drugs with low hepatic extraction ratios exhibit clinically significant drug interactions that alter drug pharmacokinetics and pharmacologic response when hepatic enzyme inducers are co-administered (Figure 3-17). Enzyme inducers increase intrinsic clearance of the drug and thereby increase the total clearance of the medication ($\uparrow Cl = f_B \uparrow Cl'_{int}$). The increase in total clearance causes a shorter half-life, since volume of distribution remains

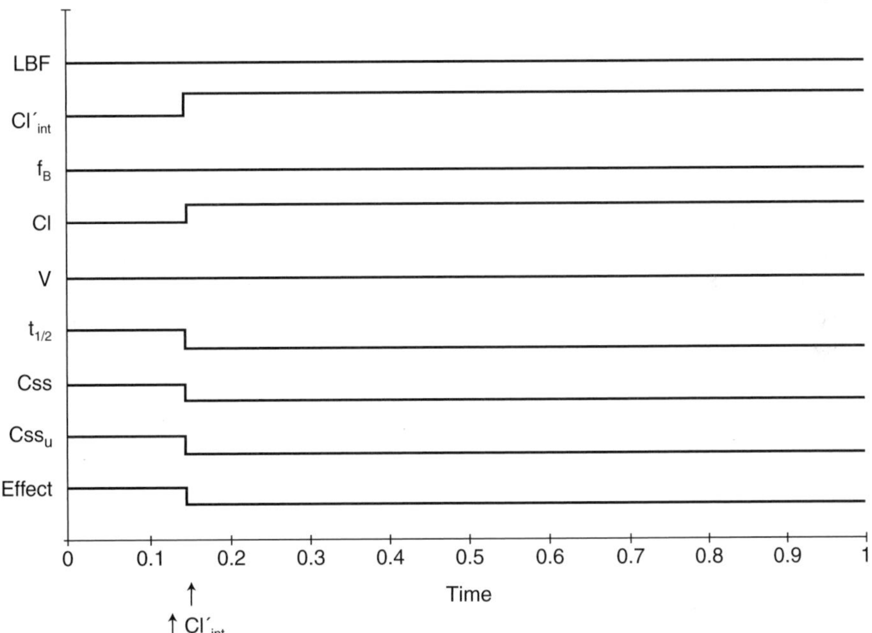

FIGURE 3-17 Changes in physiologic parameters (*LBF* = liver blood flow, Cl'_{int} = intrinsic clearance, f_B = free fraction of drug in the blood), pharmacokinetic parameters (*Cl* = clearance, *V* = volume of distribution, $t_{1/2}$ = half-life), and drug concentration and effect (*Css* = total steady-state concentration; Css_u = unbound steady-state concentration; *effect* = pharmacologic effect) for a low hepatic extraction ratio drug if intrinsic clearance increases (indicated by *arrow*). An uptick in the line indicates an increase in the value of the parameter; a downtick in the line indicates a decrease in the value of the parameter. Intrinsic clearance could increase owing to a drug interaction that induces drug-metabolizing enzymes.

unchanged ($\downarrow t_{1/2} = [0.693 \cdot V]/\uparrow Cl$). Increased total clearance also causes decreased total steady-state concentration ($\downarrow Css = k_0/\uparrow Cl$), unbound steady-state concentration ($\downarrow Css_u = f_B \downarrow Css$), and pharmacologic effect ($\downarrow effect \propto \downarrow Css_u$). Carbamazepine is a potent enzyme inducer, which, when added to a patient's therapy, can cause an induction drug interaction with many other medications, such as warfarin.[36]

For drugs with high hepatic extraction ratios, an induction drug interaction results in variable effects, depending on the route of administration of the drug. If the drug is given intravenously and an enzyme inducer is added, the increase in intrinsic clearance is usually not large enough to cause major pharmacokinetic and pharmacologic effect alterations, because total clearance is a function of liver blood flow (Figure 3-18). However, if the drug is given orally and an enzyme inducer is added to the treatment regimen, presystemic metabolism of the medication may be increased and the first-pass effect augmented, leading to decreased drug bioavailability. This effective decrease in administered oral dose decreases the total and unbound steady-state drug concentrations and leads to a decrease in the pharmacologic effect of the agent.

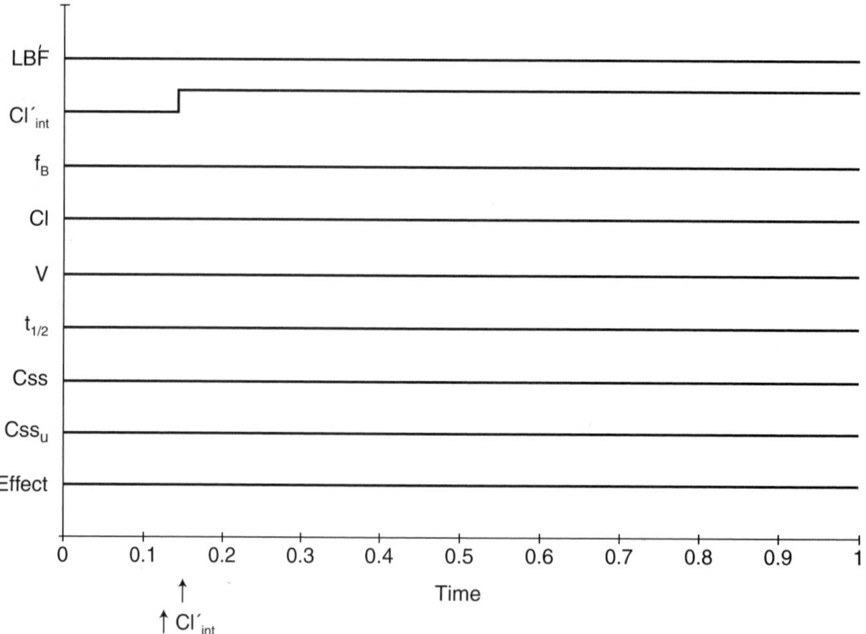

FIGURE 3-18 Changes in physiologic parameters (*LBF* = liver blood flow, Cl'_{int} = intrinsic clearance, f_B = free fraction of drug in the blood), pharmacokinetic parameters (*Cl* = clearance, *V* = volume of distribution, $t_{1/2}$ = half-life), and drug concentration and effect (*Css* = total steady-state concentration; Css_u = unbound steady-state concentration; *effect* = pharmacologic effect) for a high hepatic extraction ratio drug if intrinsic clearance increases (indicated by *arrow*). An uptick in the line indicates an increase in the value of the parameter; a downtick in the line indicates a decrease in the value of the parameter. Intrinsic clearance could increase owing to a drug interaction that induces drug-metabolizing enzymes.

Alteration in Organ Blood Flow

By virtue of the pharmacologic effect of a drug, it may be possible for an agent to change liver blood flow. For instance, β-blockers can decrease heart rate and cardiac output, which decreases liver blood flow. Because liver blood flow is the predominant factor that determines clearance for high hepatic extraction ratio drugs, this type of interaction is important only for this category of medication. β-Blockers decrease lidocaine clearance by decreasing liver blood flow.[37]

If a drug with a high hepatic extraction ratio is administered to a patient and another agent that decreases liver blood flow is then added to the patient's therapy, total clearance decreases (see Figure 3-10). Since volume of distribution remains unaltered, the half-life of the drug increases [$\uparrow t_{1/2} = (0.693 \cdot V)/\downarrow Cl$]. As a result of the total clearance decrease, total steady-state drug concentrations increase ($\uparrow Css = k_0/\downarrow Cl$). The rise in unbound steady-state drug concentration mirrors that seen with total drug concentration, and the effect of the drug increases in proportion to unbound concentration. If the co-administered drug increases liver blood flow, as may occur with vasodilators such as calcium channel blockers,[38,39] all the aforementioned changes will occur in the opposite direction [$\uparrow Cl = \uparrow LBF$; $\downarrow t_{1/2} = (0.693 \cdot V)/\uparrow Cl$; $\downarrow Css = k_0/\uparrow Cl$; $\downarrow Css_u = f_B \downarrow Css$], and the decline in unbound steady-state concentration will cause a decrease in pharmacologic effect of the drug.

PROBLEMS

1. A creatinine clearance is measured in a 75-year-old man with multiple myeloma to monitor changes in renal function. The serum creatinine, measured at the midpoint of the 24-hour urine collection, was 2.1 mg/dL. Urine creatinine concentration was 50 mg/dL, and urine volume was 1400 mL. Calculate this patient's creatinine clearance.

2. A 52-year-old woman, weighing 65 kg and 160 cm (63 in) tall, with a methacillin-resistant *Staphylococcus aureus* infection needs to have an initial vancomycin dose computed. To do this, an estimated creatinine clearance should be calculated. The patient has a serum creatinine value of 1.8 mg/dL. Calculate this patient's estimated creatinine clearance and estimated vancomycin clearance [assume that vancomycin clearance is Cl (in mL/min per kg) = 0.695 (CrCl in mL/min per kg) + 0.05].

3. A 70-year-old man, weighing 80 kg and 180 cm (71 in) tall, with a *Pseudomonas aeruginosa* infection needs to have an initial tobramycin dose computed. To do this, an estimated creatinine clearance must be calculated. The patient's current serum creatinine is 2.5 mg/dL and stable. Compute this patient's estimated creatinine clearance and estimated tobramycin elimination rate constant and half-life [assume that tobramycin elimination rate constant is k_e (in h^{-1}) = 0.00293 (CrCl in mL/min) + 0.014].

4. A 51-year-old woman, weighing 54 kg and 162 cm (64 in) tall, with worsening renal function needs a renal function assessment for drug dosage adjustment. Yesterday, at

0800 H, her serum creatinine was 1.3 mg/dL. Today at the same time, her serum creatinine was 2.1 mg/dL. Compute her estimated creatinine clearance.

5. A 66-year-old woman, weighing 120 kg and 157 cm (62 in) tall, has a serum creatinine of 3.1 mg/dL. Compute an estimated creatinine clearance for this patient.

6. A 59-year-old man, weighing 140 kg and 173 cm (68 in) tall, with severe heart failure has a serum creatinine of 2.4 mg/dL. Compute an estimated creatinine clearance, digoxin clearance, and digoxin volume of distribution for this patient. Assume estimated digoxin clearance in severe heart failure: Cl (in mL/min) = 1.303 (CrCl in mL/min) + 20; estimated digoxin volume of distribution: V (in L) = 226 + [(298 · CrCl)/(29.1 + CrCl)].

7. A 62-year-old, 65-kg man with hepatic cirrhosis (total bilirubin = 2.6 mg/dL, serum albumin = 2.5 mg/dL, prothrombin time prolonged over normal by 8 seconds, slight amount of ascitic fluid, no hepatic encephalopathy) and severe chronic obstructive pulmonary disease needs an initial theophylline dose to be computed. The patient is not a tobacco smoker and does not have heart failure. Compute the patient's Child-Pugh score, estimated theophylline clearance, and theophylline dose to achieve a steady-state concentration of 10 mg/L.

8. A 32-year-old woman, weighing 70 kg and 173 cm (68 in) tall, who has chronic renal failure and is receiving hemodialysis, developed atrial fibrillation. She is to receive a new antiarrhythmic agent, Defibfast, for the treatment of atrial fibrillation. The following average pharmacokinetic parameters were measured in six subjects with chronic renal failure: V = 0.5 L/kg, $t_{1/2}$ = 36 h. When these subjects received hemodialysis, the hemodialysis extraction ratio was 33%. The patient just completed a hemodialysis run (Monday 0800 to 1200 H). Compute a posthemodialysis loading dose to achieve a peak concentration of 50 mg/L. The next dialysis period is Wednesday at the same time. Calculate a posthemodialysis dose that will raise the patient's concentration to 50 mg/L.

9. A 47-year-old man, weighing 75 kg and 175 cm (69 in) tall, who is on hemodialysis with chronic renal failure, has a serious gram-negative infection being treated with a new antibiotic, Bactocidal. The following concentrations were obtained: Monday 1200 H (posthemodialysis) = 15 mg/L, Monday 1205 H (after intravenous 1000-mg bolus) = 65 mg/L, Wednesday 0800 H (prehemodialysis) = 32 mg/L, Wednesday 1200 H (posthemodialysis for 4 hours) = 8 mg/L. Compute volume of distribution, elimination rate constant and half-life for the interdialysis period, and the hemodialysis extraction ratio. What posthemodialysis dose on Wednesday would achieve a postdose concentration of 100 mg/L? What would be the pre- and posthemodialysis concentrations on Friday (hemodialysis from 0800 to 1200 H) if that dose was given?

10. A patient receiving hemodialysis has the following blood concentrations of drug during a hemodialysis run: concentration into artificial kidney = 75 mg/L, concentration leaving artificial kidney = 25 mg/L. Blood flow through the artificial kidney is 400 mL/min. Compute the hemodialysis extraction ratio and clearance.

11. A patient receiving peritoneal dialysis has the following drug concentrations: concentration in the dialysis fluid = 35 mg/L, concentration in serum at midpoint of peritoneal dialysis = 50 mg/L. The volume of dialysis fluid is 2 L, and the dwell time in the peritoneal cavity is 6 hours. Compute peritoneal dialysis for the drug.

12. A patient is receiving phenytoin (a low hepatic extraction ratio drug) for the treatment of tonic-clonic seizures. Because of continued seizure activity, valproic acid is added to the patient's drug regimen. Valproic acid inhibits the clearance of phenytoin and displaces phenytoin from plasma protein-binding sites. Assuming that these changes occur instantaneously with the institution of valproic acid therapy, diagram how the following parameters will change for phenytoin: liver blood flow, intrinsic clearance, free fraction of drug in the blood, clearance, volume of distribution, half-life, total steady-state concentration, unbound steady-state concentration, and drug effect.

ANSWERS TO PROBLEMS

1. $CrCl = (U_{Cr} \cdot V_{urine})/(S_{Cr} \cdot T) = (50\ mg/dL \cdot 1400\ mL)/(2.1\ mg/dL \cdot 1440\ min) = 23\ mL/min$

2. First, check the ideal body weight (IBW) of this patient to see whether she is obese.

   IBW = 45 kg + 2.3 (Ht – 60 in) = 45 kg + 2.3(63 – 60) = 52 kg; patient is within 30% of IBW (52 ± 16 kg)

   Calculate the estimated creatinine clearance:

   $CrCl_{est} = [0.85(140 - age)BW]/(72 \cdot S_{Cr}) = [0.85(140 - 52\ y)65\ kg]/(72 \cdot 1.8\ mg/dL) = 37\ mL/min$

   $$CrCl_{est} = (37\ mL/min)/65\ kg = 0.569\ mL/min/kg$$

   Calculate the estimated vancomycin clearance:

   Cl (in mL/min/kg) = 0.695 (CrCl in mL/min/kg) + 0.05 = 0.695(0.569 mL/min/kg) + 0.05 = 0.446 mL/min/kg

   $$Cl = 0.446\ mL/min/kg\ (65\ kg) = 29\ mL/min$$

3. First, check ideal body weight (IBW) of this patient to see whether he is obese.

   IBW = 50 kg + 2.3(Ht – 60 in) = 50 kg + 2.3(71 – 60) = 75 kg; patient is within 30% of IBW (75 ± 23 kg)

   Calculate the estimated creatinine clearance:

   $CrCl_{est} = [(140 - age)BW]/(72 \cdot S_{Cr}) = [(140 - 70\ y)80\ kg]/(72 \cdot 2.5\ mg/dL) = 31\ mL/min$

   Calculate estimated tobramycin elimination rate constant and half-life:

$$k_e(\text{in } h^{-1}) = 0.00293(\text{CrCl in mL/min}) + 0.014 = 0.00293(31 \text{ mL/min}) + 0.014 = 0.105 \text{ h}^{-1}$$

$$t_{1/2} = 0.693/k_e = 0.693/0.105 \text{ h}^{-1} = 6.6 \text{ h}$$

4. The Jelliffe method is used to estimate creatinine clearance in patients with changing renal function.

   Ideal body weight (IBW): IBW = 45 kg + 2.3(Ht – 60 in) = 45 kg + 2.3(64 – 60) = 54 kg

   $$Ess_{female} = IBW[25.1 - (0.175 \cdot age)] = 54 \text{ kg}[25.1 - (0.175 \cdot 51 \text{ y})] = 873.5$$

   Average serum creatinine (Scr): $Scr_{ave} = (1.3 \text{ mg/dL} + 2.1 \text{ mg/dL})/2 = 1.7 \text{ mg/dL}$

   $$Ess_{corrected} = Ess[1.035 - (0.0337 \cdot Scr_{ave})] = 873.5[1.035 - (0.0337 \cdot 1.7 \text{ mg/dL})] = 854.0$$

$$E = Ess_{corrected} - \frac{[4IBW(Scr_2 - Scr_1)]}{\Delta t} = 854 - \frac{[4 \cdot 54 \text{ kg}(2.1 \text{ mg/dL} - 1.3 \text{ mg/dL})]}{24 \text{ h} \cdot 60 \text{ min/h}} = 853.9$$

   $$CrCl = E/(14.4 \cdot Scr_{ave}) = 853.9/(14.4 \cdot 1.7 \text{ mg/dL}) = 35 \text{ mL/min per } 1.73 \text{ m}^2$$

5. This patient is obese, so the Salazar-Corcoran method is used.

   Height (Ht) is converted from inches to meters (m): Ht = (62 in · 2.54 cm/in)/(100 cm/m) = 1.57 m.

   $$CrCl_{est(females)} = \frac{(146 - age)[(0.287 \cdot Wt) + (9.74 \cdot Ht^2)]}{(60 \cdot S_{Cr})}$$

   $$CrCl_{est(females)} = \frac{(146 - 66 \text{ y})[(0.287 \cdot 120 \text{ kg}) + (9.74 \cdot \{1.57 \text{ m}\}^2)]}{(60 \cdot 3.1 \text{ mg/dL})} = 25 \text{ mL/min}$$

6. This patient is obese, so the Salazar-Corcoran method is used to estimate creatinine clearance.

   Height is converted from inches to meters: Ht = (68 in · 2.54 cm/in)/(100 cm/m) = 1.73 m.

   $$CrCl_{est(men)} = \frac{(137 - age)[(0.285 \cdot Wt) + (12.1 \cdot Ht^2)]}{(51 \cdot S_{Cr})}$$

   $$CrCl_{est(men)} = \frac{(137 - 59 \text{ y})[(0.285 \cdot 140 \text{ kg}) + (12.1 \cdot \{1.73 \text{ m}\}^2)]}{(51 \cdot 2.4 \text{ mg/dL})} = 49 \text{ mL/min}$$

   Calculate the estimated digoxin pharmacokinetic parameters:

   $$Cl (\text{in mL/min}) = 1.303(\text{CrCl in mL/min}) + 20 = 1.303(49 \text{ mL/min}) + 20 = 84 \text{ mL/min}$$

   $$V (\text{in L}) = 226 + [(298 \cdot CrCl)/(29.1 + CrCl)] = 226 + [(298 \cdot 49 \text{ mL/min})/(29.1 + 49 \text{ mL/min})] = 413 \text{ L}$$

7. Child-Pugh score (see Table 3-2): total bilirubin = 2 points, albumin = 3 points, prothrombin time = 3 points, ascites = 2 points, encephalopathy = 1 point. Total = 11 points, severe hepatic dysfunction.

Theophylline clearance (see Table 3-3): $Cl = 0.35$ mL/min/kg (65 kg) = 22.8 mL/min

$$Cl = (22.8 \text{ mL/min} \cdot 60 \text{ min/h})/1000 \text{ mL/L} = 1.37 \text{ L/h}$$

Theophylline maintenance dose (MD): $MD = Css \cdot Cl = (10 \text{ mg/L})(1.37 \text{ L/h}) =$ 14 mg/h of theophylline

8. Calculate the pharmacokinetic parameters:

$$V = 0.5 \text{ L/kg } (70 \text{ kg}) = 35 \text{ L}$$

$$k_e = 0.693/t_{1/2} = 0.693/36 \text{ h} = 0.0193 \text{ h}^{-1}$$

Calculate the loading dose (LD): $LD = C \cdot V = (50 \text{ mg/L})(35 \text{ L}) = 1750 \text{ mg}$

Calculate the predialysis concentration: $C = C_0 e^{-k_e t} = (50 \text{ mg/L})e^{-(0.0193 \text{ h}^{-1})(44 \text{ h})} =$ 21 mg/L

Calculate the posthemodialysis concentration: $C_{postdialysis} = C_{predialysis}(1 - ER_{HD}) =$ (21 mg/L)(1 – 0.33) = 14 mg/L

Calculate the postdialysis dose: $D = V(C_{postdose} - C_{predose}) = (35 \text{ L})(50 \text{ mg/L} - 14 \text{ mg/L}) = 1260 \text{ mg}$

9. Compute the pharmacokinetic parameters:

$$V = D/(C_{postdose} - C_{predose}) = 1000 \text{ mg}/(65 \text{ mg/L} - 15 \text{ mg/L}) = 20 \text{ L}$$

$$k_e = (\ln C_1 - \ln C_2)/\Delta t = (\ln 65 \text{ mg/L} - \ln 32 \text{ mg/L})/44 \text{ h} = 0.0161 \text{ h}^{-1}$$

$$t_{1/2} = 0.693/k_e = 0.693/0.0161 \text{ h}^{-1} = 43 \text{ h}$$

Calculate the hemodialysis extraction ratio (ER): $ER_{HD} = (C_{predialysis} - C_{postdialysis})/C_{predialysis} = (32 \text{ mg/L} - 8 \text{ mg/L})/32 \text{ mg/L} = 0.75$ or 75%

Compute the postdialysis dose for Wednesday: $D = V\ (C_{postdose} - C_{predose}) = (20 \text{ L})(100 \text{ mg/L} - 8 \text{ mg/L}) = 1840 \text{ mg}$

Calculate the predialysis concentration for Friday: $C = C_0 e^{-k_e t} = (100 \text{ mg/L})\, e^{-(0.0161 \text{ h}^{-1})(44 \text{ h})} = 49 \text{ mg/L}$

Calculate the postdialysis concentration for Friday: $C_{postdialysis} = C_{predialysis}(1 - ER_{HD}) = (49 \text{ mg/L})(1 - 0.75) = 12 \text{ mg/L}$

10. $ER_{HD} = (C_{predialysis} - C_{postdialysis})/C_{predialysis} = (75 \text{ mg/L} - 25 \text{ mg/L})/75 \text{ mg/L} = 0.67$ or 67%

$$Cl_{HD} = HDBF \cdot ER_{HD} = (400 \text{ mL/min})(0.67) = 268 \text{ mL/min}$$

11. $Cl_{PD} = (C_{Dialysis} \cdot V_{Dialysis})/(C_{Serum} \cdot T_{Dialysis}) = (35 \text{ mg/L} \cdot 2000 \text{ mL})/(50 \text{ mg/L} \cdot 360 \text{ min}) = 3.9 \text{ mL/min}$

12. See diagram in following figure. Addition of valproic acid increases the free fraction of phenytoin in the blood and decreases phenytoin intrinsic clearance. Because phenytoin is a low hepatic extraction ratio drug, clearance does not change ($Cl = \uparrow f_B \downarrow Cl'_{int}$). However, phenytoin volume of distribution does increase [$\uparrow V = V_B + (\uparrow f_B/f_T)V_T$], resulting in an increased half-life [$\uparrow t_{1/2} = (0.693 \cdot \uparrow V)/Cl$].

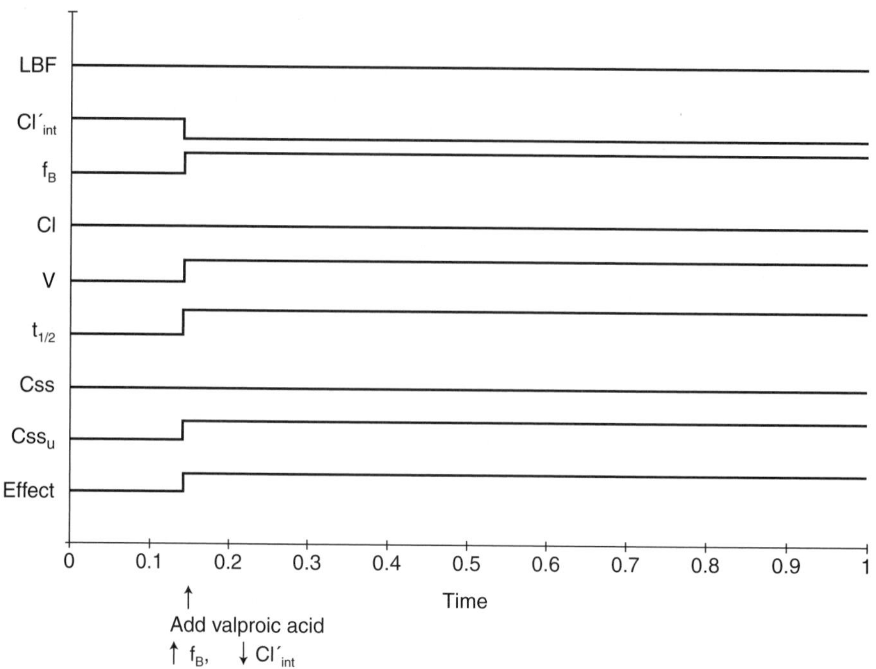

Total phenytoin concentration is unchanged, since clearance is stable. But because of the increase in free fraction, the unbound steady-state concentration rises ($\uparrow Css_u = \uparrow f_B Css$), and drug effect increases.

REFERENCES

1. Gibaldi M, Perrier D. Pharmacokinetics. In: Swarbrick J, ed. Drugs and the Pharmaceutical Sciences. Vol. 15. New York: Marcel Dekker, 1982:494.
2. Cockcroft DW, Gault MH. Prediction of creatinine clearance from serum creatinine. Nephron 1976;16:31–41.
3. Mohler JL, Barton SD, Blouin RA, Cowen DL, Flanigan RC. The evaluation of creatinine clearance in spinal cord injury patients. J Urol 1986;136:366–369.
4. Reichley RM, Ritchie DJ, Bailey TC. Analysis of various creatinine clearance formulas in predicting gentamicin elimination in patients with low serum creatinine. Pharmacotherapy 1995;15:625–630.
5. Smythe M, Hoffman J, Kizy K, Dmuchowshi C. Estimating creatinine clearance in elderly patients with low serum creatinine concentrations. Am J Hosp Pharm 1994;51:198–204.
6. Jelliffe RW, Jelliffe SM. A computer program for estimation of creatinine clearance from unstable serum creatinine levels, age, sex, and weight. Mathematical Biosciences 1972;14:17–24.
7. Dionne RE, Bauer LA, Gibson GA, Griffen WO, Blouin RA. Estimating creatinine clearance in morbidly obese patients. Am J Hosp Pharm 1981;38:841–844.
8. Salazar DE, Corcoran GB. Predicting creatinine clearance and renal drug clearance in obese patients from estimated fat-free body mass. Am J Med 1988;84:1053–1060.

9. Traub SL, Johnson CE. Comparison of methods of estimating creatinine clearance in children. Am J Hosp Pharm 1980;37:195–201.
10. Bennett WM. Guide to drug dosage in renal failure. Clin Pharmacokinet 1988;15:326–354.
11. Bennett WM, Aronoff GR, Golper TA. Drug prescribing in renal failure: dosing guidelines for adults. Philadelphia: American College of Physicians, 1994:253.
12. Fillastre JP, Singlas E. Pharmacokinetics of newer drugs in patients with renal impairment (part I). Clin Pharmacokinet 1991;20:293–310.
13. Singlas E, Fillastre JP. Pharmacokinetics of newer drugs in patients with renal impairment (part II). Clin Pharmacokinet 1991;20:389–410.
14. Lam YW, Banerji S, Hatfield C, Talbert RL. Principles of drug administration in renal insufficiency. Clin Pharmacokinet 1997;32:30–57.
15. Dettli L. Drug dosage in renal disease. Clin Pharmacokinet 1976;1:126–134.
16. Koup JR, Jusko WJ, Elwood CM, Kohli RK. Digoxin pharmacokinetics: role of renal failure in dosage regimen design. Clin Pharmacol Ther 1975;18:9–21.
17. DiPiro JT, Blouin RA, Pruemer JM, Spruill WJ. Concepts in clinical pharmacokinetics: a self instructional course. Bethesda: American Society of Hospital Pharmacists, Inc, 1988:158.
18. Jusko WJ, Szefler SJ, Goldfarb AL. Pharmacokinetic design of digoxin dosage regimens in relation to renal function. J Clin Pharmacol 1974;14:525–535.
19. Wilkinson GR, Shand DG. A physiological approach to hepatic drug clearance. Clin Pharmacol Ther 1975;18:377–390.
20. Pugh RN, Murray-Lyon IM, Dawson JL, Pietroni MC, Williams R. Transection of the oesophagus for bleeding oesophageal varices. Br J Surg 1973;60:646–649.
21. Edwards DJ, Zarowitz BJ, Slaughter RL. Theophylline. In: Evans WE, Schentag JJ, Jusko WJ, eds. Applied pharmacokinetics: principles of therapeutic drug monitoring. Vancouver, WA: Applied Therapeutics, Inc, 1992:557.
22. Abernethy DR, Greenblatt DJ, Divoll M, Harmatz JS, Shader RI. Alterations in drug distribution and clearance due to obesity. J Pharmacol Exp Ther 1981;217:681–685.
23. Caraco Y, Zylber-Katz E, Berry EM, Levy M. Significant weight reduction in obese subjects enhances carbamazepine elimination. Clin Pharmacol Ther 1992;51:501–506.
24. Greenblatt DJ, Friedman H, Burstein ES, Scavone JM, Blyden GT. Trazodone kinetics: effect of age, gender, and obesity. Clin Pharmacol Ther 1987;42:193–200.
25. Abernethy DR, Greenblatt DJ, Smith TW. Digoxin disposition in obesity: clinical pharmacokinetic investigation. Am Heart J 1981;102:740–744.
26. Bauer LA, Wareing-Tran C, Edwards WAD, Raisys V, Ferrer L. Cimetidine clearance in the obese. Clin Pharmacol Ther 1985;37:425–430.
27. Davis RL, Quenzer RW. Ranitidine pharmacokinetics in morbid obesity. Clin Pharmacol Ther 1990;47:154.
28. Blouin RA, Mann HJ, Griffen WO, Bauer LA, Record KE. Tobramycin pharmacokinetics in morbidly obese patients. Clin Pharmacol Ther 1979;26:508–512.
29. Bauer LA, Blouin RA, Griffen WO, Record KE, Bell RM. Amikacin pharmacokinetics in morbidly obese patients. Am J Hosp Pharm 1980;37:519–522.
30. Bauer LA, Edwards WAD, Dellinger EP, Simonowitz DA. Influence of weight on aminoglycoside pharmacokinetics in normal weight and morbidly obese patients. Eur J Clin Pharmacol 1983;24:643–647.
31. Blouin RA, Bauer LA, Miller DD, Record KE, Griffen WO. Vancomycin pharmacokinetics in normal and morbidly obese subjects. Antimicrob Agents Chemother 1982;21:575–580.
32. Flechner SM, Kolbeinsson ME, Tam J, Lum B. The impact of body weight on cyclosporine pharmacokinetics in renal transplant recipients. Transplantation 1989;47:806–810.
33. Dunn TE, Ludwig EA, Slaughter RI, Carara DJ, Jusko WJ. Pharmacokinetics and pharmacodynamics of methylprednisolone in obesity. Clin Pharmacol Ther 1991;49:536–549.

34. Serlin MJ, Mossman S, Sibeon RG, Tempero KF, Breckenridge AM. Interaction between diflunisal and warfarin. Clin Pharmacol Ther 1980;28:493–498.
35. Loi CM, Parker BM, Cusack BJ, Vestal R. Individual and combined effects of cimetidine and ciprofloxacin on theophylline metabolism in male nonsmokers. Br J Clin Pharmacol 1993;36:195–200.
36. Massey EW. Effect of carbamazepine on coumadin metabolism. Ann Neurol 1983;13:691–692.
37. Schneck DW, Luderer JR, Davis D, Vary J. Effects of nadolol and propranolol on plasma lidocaine clearance. Clin Pharmacol Ther 1984;36:584–587.
38. Bauer LA, Stenwall M, Horn JR, Davis R, Opheim K, Greene HL. Changes in antipyrine and indocyanine green kinetics during nifedipine, verapamil, and diltiazem therapy. Clin Pharmacol Ther 1986;40:239–242.
39. Reiss WG, Bauer LA, Horn JR, Zierler BK, Easterling TR, Strandness DE. The effects of oral nifedipine on hepatic blood flow in humans. Clin Pharmacol Ther 1991;50:379–384.

Part II

ANTIBIOTICS

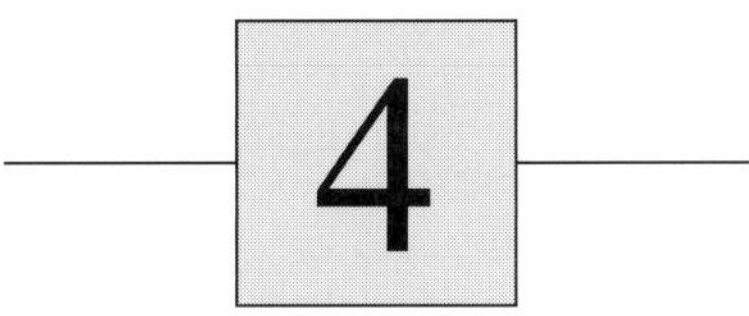

THE AMINOGLYCOSIDE ANTIBIOTICS

INTRODUCTION

The aminoglycoside antibiotics are widely used for the treatment of severe gram-negative infections such as pneumonia and bacteremia, often in combination with a β-lactam antibiotic. They are also used for gram-positive infections such as infective endocarditis in combination with penicillins when antibiotic synergy is required for optimal killing. Aminoglycoside antibiotics commonly available in the United States are gentamicin, tobramycin, netilmicin, and amikacin.

Aminoglycoside antibiotics are bactericidal, and the drugs exhibit concentration-dependent bacterial killing.[1] Antibiotics with concentration-dependent killing characteristically kill bacteria at a faster rate when drug concentrations are higher. Also, aminoglycosides have a concentration-dependent postantibiotic effect. This effect is the phenomenon of bacterial killing that continues even after serum concentrations have fallen below the minimum inhibitory concentration (MIC). Because the postantibiotic effect is concentration-dependent for the aminoglycosides, higher drug concentrations lead to a longer postantibiotic effect. The mechanisms of action for aminoglycosides are binding to the 30S ribosomal subunit, inhibiting protein synthesis and misreading of mRNA causing dysfunctional protein production.

THERAPEUTIC AND TOXIC CONCENTRATIONS

The MIC for susceptible bacteria is higher for amikacin than for the other aminoglycosides. Because all these drugs have similar pharmacokinetics, higher doses of amikacin are needed to treat infections. The conventional method of dosing aminoglycoside antibiotics is to administer multiple daily doses (usually every 8 hours).[2] To take advantage of concentration-dependent bacterial killing and the postantibiotic effect, extended-interval (usually the total daily dose given once per day) aminoglycoside administration is also a dosing option.[3] Because of these two different methods of dosage administration, it is important to identify which method is being used when discussing serum concentration monitoring.

Conventional Dosing

Aminoglycoside antibiotics are given as short-term (1/2- to 1-hour) infusions. If a 1-hour infusion is used, maximum end of infusion "peak" concentrations are measured when the infusion is completed (Figure 4-1). If a half-hour infusion is used, serum concentrations exhibit a distribution phase so that drug in the blood and in the tissues are not yet in equilibrium. Because of this, a half-hour waiting period is allowed for distribution to finish if a half-hour infusion is used before peak concentrations are measured. Therapeutic steady-state peak concentrations of gentamicin, tobramycin, and netilmicin are generally 5 to 10 μg/mL for gram-negative infections. Infection sites with more susceptible bacteria, such as intra-abdominal infections, usually can be treated with steady-state peak concentrations at the lower end of this range (typically 5 to 7 μg/mL). Infection sites that are difficult to penetrate and those with bacteria that have higher MIC values, such as pseudomonal pneumonia usually require steady-state peak concentrations in the higher end of the range (typically 8 to 10 μg/mL). When gentamicin, tobramycin, or netilmicin is used synergistically with penicillins or other antibiotics for the treatment of gram-positive infections such as infective endocarditis, steady-state peak concentrations of 3 to 5 μg/mL are often adequate. Therapeutic peak concentrations of amikacin are 15 to 30 μg/mL.

Exceeding peak steady-state concentrations of 12 to 14 μg/mL for gentamicin, to-

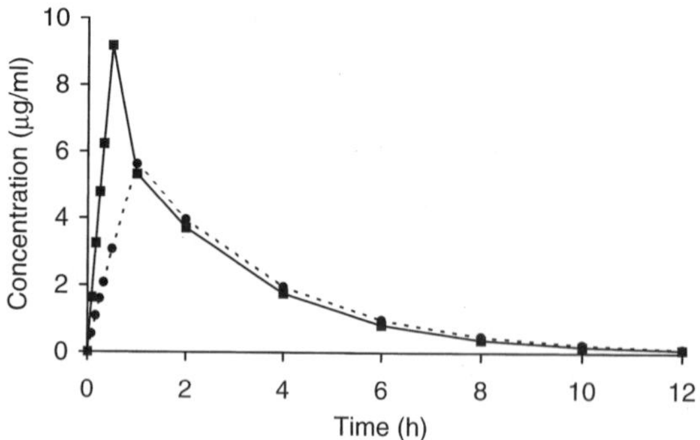

FIGURE 4-1 Concentration-time plot for gentamicin 120 mg given as a 1/2-hour infusion *(squares with solid line)* and as a 1-hour infusion *(circles with dashed line)*. When given as a 1/2-hour infusion, end of infusion concentrations are higher because the serum and tissues are not in equilibrium. A 1/2-hour waiting time for aminoglycoside distribution to tissues is allowed before peak concentrations are measured. If aminoglycosides are given as 1-hour infusions, distribution has an opportunity to occur during the infusion time, and peak concentrations can be obtained immediately. In either case, concentrations 1 hour after the infusion was initiated are similar.

bramycin, or netilmicin or 35 to 40 μg/mL for amikacin when using conventional dosing leads to an increased risk of *ototoxicity.*[4] The types of ototoxicity that aminoglycosides cause are auditory and vestibular, and the damage is permanent. Aminoglycosides accumulate in the lymph of the inner ear, causing ongoing damage to cochlear or vestibular sensory cells.[1] Auditory ototoxicity usually is first noted at high frequencies (>4000 Hz) and is difficult to detect using clinical means. Audiometry is required to detect high-tone hearing loss and is seldom done in patient care areas. Older patients may lose the ability to hear in this range for other reasons. If aminoglycoside treatment is not discontinued in persons with high-frequency auditory ototoxicity, hearing loss progresses to lower frequencies. As a result, aminoglycoside-induced hearing losses are not usually detected until the patient is unable to detect sounds in the conversational frequency zone (<4000 Hz). Often, the first sign of auditory ototoxicity is tinnitus. Vestibular ototoxicity results in a loss of balance. Again, this type of ototoxicity is difficult to detect because many patients treated with aminoglycosides are bed-bound. Moreover, loss of equilibrium, headache, ataxia, nausea, vomiting, nystagmus, and vertigo all can be signs of vestibular ototoxicity. Although this version of ototoxicity is also permanent, patients can often compensate using visual cues to maintain balance and avoid ataxia such as observing the horizon. Some studies have found predose ("trough") steady-state concentrations to be related to ototoxicity.[5,6] However, peak steady-state concentrations have also been elevated in these patients, which clouds the relationship between serum concentrations and this type of drug-induced adverse effect.

Trough steady-state concentrations (predose or minimum concentrations usually obtained within 30 minutes of the next dose) higher than 2 to 3 μg/mL for tobramycin, gentamicin, or netilmicin or 10 μg/mL for amikacin predispose patients to an increased risk of *nephrotoxicity.*[7,8] Aminoglycoside antibiotics accumulate in the proximal tubular cells of the kidney, decrease the ability of the kidney to concentrate urine, and ultimately decrease glomerular filtration.[9–11] Nephrotoxicity due to aminoglycoside therapy is unlikely to occur before 3 to 5 days of therapy with proper dosing of the antibiotic. Because many patients receiving aminoglycosides are critically ill, other sources of nephrotoxicity, such as hypotension or other nephrotoxic drug therapy, should be ruled out before a diagnosis of aminoglycoside renal damage is made. Unlike ototoxicity, aminoglycoside-induced nephrotoxicity is usually reversible with little, if any, residual damage if the antibiotic is withdrawn soon after renal function tests change. With proper patient monitoring, mild renal dysfunction resulting in serum creatinine increases of 0.5 to 2 mg/dL may be the only result of aminoglycoside nephrotoxicity. However, if the patient develops renal failure, the cost of maintaining the patient on dialysis until kidney function returns can exceed $50,000 to $100,000 and, if the patient is critically ill, may contribute to his or her death. In some investigations, peak concentrations have been related to nephrotoxicity.[12] But trough concentrations have also been high in these patients, which obscures the relationship between serum concentrations and nephrotoxicity.

Keeping peak and trough concentrations within the suggested ranges does not completely prevent nephrotoxicity and ototoxicity in patients but is hoped to decrease the likelihood of these serious adverse effects.[13] Also, even though serum concentrations are controlled within the suggested ranges, duration of therapy exceeding 14 days, large total cumulative doses, and concurrent therapy with other nephrotoxic drugs such as vancomycin can predispose patients to these side effects of aminoglycoside antibiotics.[14–17]

Extended-Interval Dosing

Because aminoglycoside antibiotics exhibit concentration-dependent bacterial killing and the postantibiotic effect is longer with higher concentrations, investigators began to study the possibility of giving a higher once-daily dose of aminoglycoside.[3,18,19] Generally, these studies have shown comparable microbiologic and clinical cure rates for many infections and about the same rate of nephrotoxicity (~5% to 10%) as with conventional dosing. Auditory ototoxicity has not been monitored using audiometry in most of these investigations, but loss of hearing in the conversational range as well as signs and symptoms of vestibular toxicity have usually been assessed and found to be similar to aminoglycoside therapy dosed conventionally. Based on these data, clinicians have begun using extended-interval dosing in selected patients. For *Pseudomonas aeruginosa* infections, in which the organism has an expected MIC ≈ 2 μg/mL, peak concentrations between 20 and 30 μg/mL and trough concentrations <1 μg/mL have been suggested.[3] At present, no consensus exists regarding how to approach concentration monitoring using this mode of administration.[20–26] However, a nomogram that adjusts doses based on a single postdose steady-state concentration to achieve these concentration goals has been proposed and is discussed in the dosing section of this chapter.[3]

Because of the extremely high peak concentrations obtained during extended-interval dosing of aminoglycosides, it may be difficult to understand why increased toxicity is not seen in patients. The reason may be that both nephrotoxicity and ototoxicity are due to accumulation of aminoglycoside in the relevant tissue. Because the dosage interval is prolonged in extended-interval administration, aminoglycoside concentrations are low for a long period of time and may allow for diffusion of drug out of tissue and into the blood, which avoids drug accumulation in the ear and kidney. Also, some of the uptake mechanisms into the ear and kidney may be saturable, so that high peak serum concentrations of aminoglycosides may not result in high renal or ear tissue concentrations.

Since large doses of aminoglycoside are given as a single dose with this mode of administration, two additional adverse effects are of concern. Because of the manufacturing process used to produce aminoglycoside antibiotics, very low residual amounts of gram-negative endotoxin are sometimes in the commercial product. Reports of infusion-related hypotension in patients receiving extended-interval aminoglycosides have been attributed to the amount of toxin administered at one time.[27,28] Acute neuromuscular blockade, usually associated with concurrent administration of anesthetics or neuromuscular blockers, is also a possible adverse effect of aminoglycosides associated with high drug concentrations. Because of the high peak concentrations achieved using extended-interval dosing, surgical and intensive care patients should be monitored for possible neuromuscular blockade.

Differential Toxicity Among Aminoglycosides

Studies are available that attempt to determine differences in nephrotoxicity among antibiotics. Gentamicin accumulates to a greater extent in kidney tissue compared with the accumulation of tobramycin.[11,13,16] Because doses of amikacin are larger than for gentamicin and tobramycin, amikacin renal accumulation must be adjusted for dosage differences.[9,13] When this is done, amikacin accumulation patterns are similar to those of gentamicin. Based on these accumulation profiles and associated clinical data and other trials, some clinicians believe that tobramycin is less nephrotoxic than gentamicin or amikacin.[29] Data are less conclusive for netilmicin. Other clinical trials that compare the nephrotoxicity potential of gentamicin and tobramycin indicate that the two drugs are similar in this area.[30,31] Generally, gentamicin is the most widely used aminoglycoside, followed by tobramycin and netilmicin. This usage pattern is due in part to the fact that gentamicin was the first aminoglycoside available generically and was much less expensive than the other drugs for a number of years. Amikacin is usually reserved for infections in which the organism is resistant to other aminoglycosides.

CLINICAL MONITORING PARAMETERS

Clinicians should always consult the patient's chart to confirm that antibiotic therapy is appropriate for current microbiologic cultures and sensitivities. Also, it should be confirmed that the patient is receiving other appropriate concurrent antibiotic therapy, such as β-lactam or anaerobic agents, when necessary to treat the infection. Patients with severe infections usually have elevated white blood cell count and body temperature. Measurement of serial white blood cell count and body temperature is useful to determine the efficacy of antibiotic therapy. A white blood cell count with a differential count can identify the types of white blood cells that are elevated. A large number of neutrophils and immature neutrophils, clinically known as a "shift to the left," can also be observed in patients with severe bacterial infections. Favorable response to antibiotic treatment is usually indicated by high white blood cell counts decreasing toward the normal range, the trend of body temperatures (plotted as body temperature versus time, also known as the "fever curve") approaching normal, and any specific infection site tests or procedures resolving. For instance, in patients with pneumonia chest x-ray findings should be resolving; in patients with an intra-abdominal infection abdominal pain and tenderness should be decreasing; and in patients with a wound infection the wound should be less inflamed with less purulent discharge. Clinicians should also be aware that immunocompromised patients with a bacterial infection may not be able to mount a fever or show an elevated white blood cell count.

Aminoglycoside steady-state peak and trough serum concentrations should be measured in 3 to 5 estimated half-lives when the drug is given using conventional dosage approaches. Methods of estimating this parameter are given in the initial dose calculation portion of this chapter. Because prolongation of the dosage interval is often used in patients with decreased elimination, a useful clinical rule is to measure serum concentrations after the third dose. If this approach is used, the dosage interval is increased in tandem with the increase in half-life so that 3 to 5 half-lives have elapsed by the time the third dose is administered. In addition, the third dose typically occurs 1 to 3 days after dosing has commenced, and this is also a good time to assess clinicial efficacy of the treatment. Steady-state serum concentrations, in conjunction with clinical response, are used to adjust the antibiotic dose, if necessary. Methods for adjusting aminoglycoside doses using serum concentrations are discussed later in this chapter. If the dosage is adjusted, aminoglycoside elimination changes, or laboratory and clinical monitoring indicate that the infection is not resolving or worsening, clinicians should consider rechecking steady-state drug concentrations. When extended-interval aminoglycoside therapy is used, an aminoglycoside serum concentration is measured 6 to 14 hours after a dose, and a dosage nomogram used to adjust the dosage interval or steady-state peak and trough concentrations can be measured and used to alter the dose and dosage interval.

Serial monitoring of serum creatinine concentrations should be used to detect nephrotoxicity. Ideally, a baseline serum creatinine concentration is obtained before aminoglycoside therapy is initiated and three times weekly during treatment. An increasing serum creatinine test on two or more consecutive measurement occasions indicates that more intensive monitoring of serum creatinine values—such as daily—is needed. If serum creatinine measurements increase more than 0.5 mg/dL over the baseline value (or >25% to 30% over baseline for serum creatinine values >2 mg/dL) and other causes of declining renal function have been ruled out (e.g., other nephrotoxic drugs or agents, hypotension), alternatives to aminoglycoside therapy or, if this option is not possible, intensive aminoglycoside serum concentration monitoring should be initiated to ensure that excessive amounts of aminoglycoside do not accumulate in the patient. In the clinical setting, audiometry is rarely used to detect ototoxicity because it is difficult to accomplish in severely ill patients. Instead, clinical signs and symptoms of auditory (decreased hearing acuity in the conversational range, feeling of fullness or pressure in the ears, tinnitus) or vestibular (loss of equilibrium, headache, nausea, vomiting, vertigo, nystagmus, ataxia) ototoxicity are monitored at the same time intervals as those of serum creatinine determination.

BASIC CLINICAL PHARMACOKINETIC PARAMETERS

The aminoglycosides are eliminated almost completely (≥90%) unchanged in the urine primarily by glomerular filtration[10,13,16] (Table 4-1). These antibiotics are usually given as short-term (1/2 to 1 hour) intermittent intravenous infusions, although they can be given intramuscularly. When given intramuscularly, they exhibit very good bioavailability (~100%) and are rapidly absorbed, with maximal concentrations occurring about 1 hour after injection. Exceptions to this situation are in patients who are hypotensive and those who are obese. Hypotensive patients shunt blood flow away from peripheral tissues such as muscle to provide maximal blood flow to internal organs. As a result, intramuscularly administered drugs may be malabsorbed in hypotensive patients, such as those with gram-negative sepsis. When administering aminoglycoside antibiotics to obese persons, care must be taken to use a needle long enough to penetrate subcutaneous fat and enter muscle tissue. Drug injected into poorly perfused fatty tissue is likely to be malabsorbed. Oral bioavailability is poor (<10%), so systemic infections cannot be treated by the oral route. Plasma protein binding is low (<10%).

Manufacturer-recommended doses for conventional dosing in patients with normal renal function are 3 to 5 mg/kg per day for gentamicin and tobramycin, 4 to 6 mg/kg per day for netilmicin, and 15 mg/kg per day for amikacin. These amounts are divided into three equal daily doses for gentamicin, tobramycin, and netilmicin, or two or three equal daily doses for amikacin. Extended-interval doses obtained from the literature for patients with normal renal function are 4 to 7 mg/kg per day for gentamicin, tobramycin, or netilmicin and 11 to 20 mg/kg per day for amikacin.[3,19–26,32–37]

TABLE 4-1 Disease States and Conditions That Alter Aminoglycoside Pharmacokinetics

DISEASE STATE/ CONDITION	HALF-LIFE (HOURS)	VOLUME OF DISTRIBUTION (L/kg)	COMMENTS
Adult, normal renal function	2 (range, 1.5–3)	0.26 (range, 0.2–0.3)	Usual doses are 3–5 mg/kg/d for gentamicin, tobramycin, netilmicin or 15 mg/kg/d for amikacin.
Adult, renal failure	50 (range, 36–72)	0.26	Renal failure patients commonly have fluid imbalances that may decrease (underhydration) or increase (overhydration) the volume of distribution and secondarily change half-life.
Burns	1.5	0.26	Burn patients commonly have fluid imbalances that may decrease (underhydration) or increase (overhydration) the volume of distribution and secondarily change half-life.
Penicillin therapy (patients with creatinine clearance <30 mL/min)	Variable	0.26	Some penicillins (penicillin G, ampicillin, nafcillin, carbenicillin, ticarcillin) can bind and inactivate aminoglycosides in vivo.
Obesity (>30% over IBW) with normal renal function	2–3	V (in L) = 0.26[IBW + 0.4 (TBW – IBW)]	Aminoglycosides enter the extracellular fluid contained in adipose tissue requiring a correction factor to estimate volume of distribution.
Cystic fibrosis	1.5	0.35	Larger volume of distribution and shorter half-life result in larger daily doses of 7.5–10 mg/kg/d for gentamicin, tobramycin, and netilmicin.
Acites/overhydration	Variable	V (in L) = (0.26 · DBW) + (TBW – DBW)	Aminoglycosides distribute to excess extracellular fluid; correction equation assumes that weight gain is due to fluid accumulation. Alterations in volume of distribution can cause secondary changes in half-life.

(continues)

TABLE 4-1 Disease States and Conditions That Alter Aminoglycoside Pharmacokinetics *(continued)*

DISEASE STATE/ CONDITION	HALF-LIFE (HOURS)	VOLUME OF DISTRIBUTION (L/kg)	COMMENTS
Hemodialysis	3–4	0.26	While receiving hemodialysis, aminoglycoside half-life decreases from ~50 h to ~4 h. Renal failure patients commonly have fluid imbalances that may decrease (underhydration) or increase (overhydration) the volume of distribution and secondarily change half-life.
Peritoneal dialysis	36	0.26	While receiving peritoneal dialysis, aminoglycoside half-life will decrease from ~50 h to ~36 h. Renal failure patients commonly have fluid imbalances that may decrease (underhydration) or increase (overhydration) the volume of distribution and secondarily change half-life.

DBW = dry body weight; IBW = ideal body weight; TBW = total body weight.

EFFECTS OF DISEASE STATES AND CONDITIONS ON AMINOGLYCOSIDE PHARMACOKINETICS AND DOSING

Nonobese adults with normal renal function (creatinine clearance >80 mL/min; see Table 4-1) have an average aminoglycoside half-life of 2 hours (range, 1.5 to 3 hours), and the average aminoglycoside volume of distribution is 0.26 L/kg (range, 0.2 to 0.3 L/kg) in this population.[38–41] The volume of distribution is similar to the extracellular fluid content of the body, and fluid balance is an important factor in estimating the aminoglycoside volume of distribution for a patient. Patients who have been febrile for 24 hours or more because of infections may be significantly dehydrated and have lower volumes of distribution until rehydrated.

Because aminoglycosides are eliminated primarily by glomerular filtration, renal dysfunction is the most important disease state that affects aminoglycoside pharmacokinetics.[42,43] The elimination rate constant decreases in proportion to creatinine clearance because of the decline in drug clearance[44,45] (Figure 4-2). This relationship between renal function and aminoglycoside elimination forms the basis of initial dosage computation, as seen later in this chapter. Because the kidney is responsible for maintaining fluid and electrolyte balance in the body, patients with renal failure are sometimes overhydrated. Body weight can be an effective way of detecting overhydration in a patient. If the usual weight of a certain patient is 70 kg in normal fluid balance, known as "dry weight," and the patient is 75 kg with signs and symptoms of overhydration (e.g., pedal edema, ex-

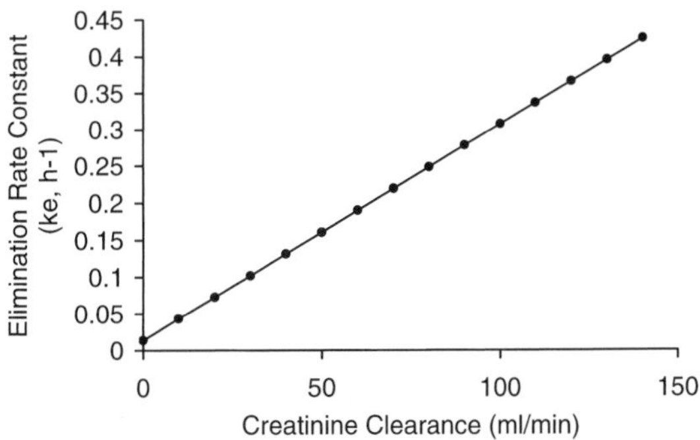

FIGURE 4-2 Relationship between renal function and aminoglycoside elimination. The elimination rate constant (k_e) for aminoglycoside antibiotics increases in proportion with creatinine clearance (CrCl). The equation for this relationship is k_e (in h^{-1}) = 0.00293(CrCl in mL/min) + 0.014. This equation is used to estimate the aminoglycoside elimination rate constant in patients for initial dosing purposes.

tended neck veins), the additional 5 kg of weight can be considered extra fluid and added to the estimated volume of distribution for the patient. Since 1 L of water weighs 1 kg, the estimated volume of distribution for this patient would be 18.2 L, using the patient's dry weight (V = 0.26 L/kg · 70 kg = 18.2 L) plus 5 L to account for the additional 5 kg of extra fluid, yielding a total volume of distribution of 23.2 L (V = 18.2 L + 5 L = 23.2 L). Care would be needed to alter the estimated volume of distribution toward normal, when the excess fluid was lost and the patient's weight returned to its usual value.

A major body burn (>40% body surface area) can cause large changes in aminoglycoside pharmacokinetics.[46–48] Forty-eight to 72 hours after a major burn, the basal metabolic rate of the patient increases to facilitate tissue repair. Because of the increase in basal metabolic rate, glomerular filtration rate increases, which increases aminoglycoside clearance. Because of the increase in drug clearance, the average half-life of aminoglycosides in burn patients is ~1.5 hours. If the patient is in normal fluid balance, the average volume of distribution is the same as in normal adults (0.26 L/kg). However, since the skin is the organ that prevents fluid evaporation from the body and since the integrity of the skin has been violated by thermal injury, burn patients can be dehydrated, especially if they have had a fever for more than 24 hours. The result is a lower volume of distribution for aminoglycosides. Alternatively, some burn patients may be overhydrated because of the vigorous fluid therapy used to treat hypotension. This results in a larger than expected aminoglycoside volume of distribution. Unfortunately, there is no precise way to correct fluid balance in these patients. Frequent use of aminoglycoside serum concentrations is used to guide therapy in this population.

Concurrent therapy with some penicillins can increase aminoglycoside clearance by chemically inactivating both the penicillin and aminoglycoside via formation of a covalent bond between the two antibiotic molecules.[49–53] Penicillin G, ampicillin, nafcillin, carbenicillin, and ticarcillin are the penicillins most likely to cause this interaction. Piperacillin and mezlocillin, as well as the cephalosporins, do not inactivate aminoglycosides to an appreciable extent. This in vivo interaction is most likely to occur in patients with poor renal function (creatinine clearance <30 mL/min) so that the elimination of both the aminoglycoside and penicillin is slower. Under these conditions, serum concentrations of both antibiotics are higher for a longer period of time and facilitate the inactivation process. In patients with renal failure who are receiving an aminoglycoside alone, the addition of one of the interacting penicillins can decrease the aminoglycoside half-life from ~50 hours when given alone to ~12 hours when given in combination and can result in a dosage increase for the aminoglycoside.

Another notable instance of this reduction of aminoglycoside concentration is in patients who are receiving concurrent therapy with one of the interacting penicillins and an aminoglycoside antibiotic when serum concentration monitoring of the aminoglycoside is planned. When a blood sample is obtained for measurement of the aminoglycoside serum concentration, penicillin contained in the blood collection tube can continue to inactivate aminoglycoside. This leads to spuriously low aminoglycoside concentration results, which can lead to dosing adjustment errors. For example, a peak gentamicin serum concentration is obtained in a patient receiving concurrent gentamicin and penicillin G therapy. When the blood sample was drawn from the patient, the gentamicin concentration was 8 μg/mL. By the time the sample is processed by the laboratory, 6 hours have expired because of transportation and other factors. Therefore, penicillin G inactivated aminoglycoside molecules, and the concentration of gentamicin decreased to 4 μg/mL. The laboratory measured this concentration and reported it to the clinicians caring for the patient. Because the desired peak concentration was 8 μg/mL, the dose of gentamicin was doubled so that the reported peak concentration of 4 μg/mL would increase to the target concentration. Of course, since the actual peak concentration was 8 μg/mL in the patient all along, the new peak concentration resulting from the dosage increase would be 16 μg/mL. To prevent this in vitro inactivation interaction in patients receiving concurrent penicillin and aminoglycoside treatment when the drug assay will not be run for longer than 1 to 2 hours after specimen collection, the serum should be separated from blood samples by means of centrifugation. The serum is removed and placed in a separate tube, then frozen to prevent the chemical reaction from occurring. Alternatively, a small amount of β-lactamase (<5% of total blood volume to prevent sample dilution) can be added to break the β-lactam bond of the penicillin and prevent inactivation of the aminoglycoside antibiotic.

Aminoglycosides are relatively polar molecules with good water solubility. Because of this, they do not enter adipose cells to any significant extent. However, in patients who weigh more than 30% over their ideal body weight, the volume of distribution for aminoglycosides increases because of the additional extracellular fluid contained in adipose tissue[54–56] (Figure 4-3). Aminoglycoside volume of distribution is affected by this relatively small amount of additional extracellular fluid in adipose tissue because the baseline volume of distribution of these drugs is relatively small to begin with (0.26 L/kg or ~18 L for a 70-kg person). For other water-soluble drugs with larger volumes of distribution, the additional extracellular fluid contained in adipose tissue may not be a significant factor. Adipose tissue contains ~40% of the extracellular fluid that is present in lean tissue. To compensate for the increased extracellular fluid of adipose tissue and the greater volume of distribution found in obese patients (>30% over ideal body weight), the following formula can be used to estimate aminoglycoside volume of distribution (V in L) for initial dosing purposes: $V = 0.26 \cdot [IBW + 0.4(TBW - IBW)]$, where IBW is ideal body weight and TBW is the patient's actual total body weight. In morbidly obese (>90% above ideal

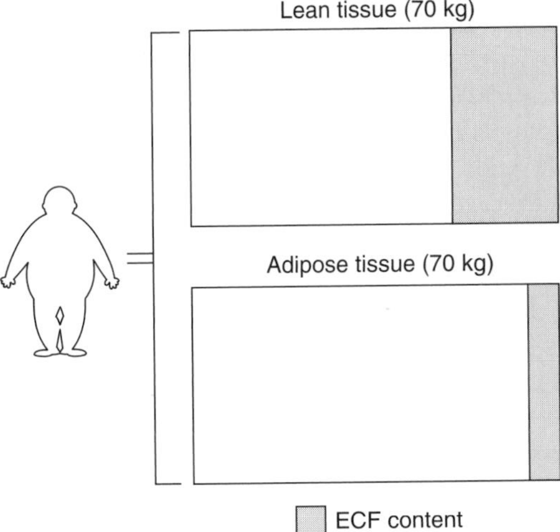

FIGURE 4-3 Schematic representation of extracellular fluid (ECF) content of lean and adipose tissue in a morbidly obese patient with an actual body weight of 140 kg and an ideal body weight of 70 kg. Lean tissue contains about 0.26 L/kg extracellular fluid, but adipose tissue has about 40% of the extracellular fluid content that lean tissue does. The equation that estimates volume of distribution for aminoglycosides in obese patients normalizes adipose tissue extracellular content into lean tissue equivalents.

body weight) patients with normal serum creatinine concentrations, the clearance of aminoglycoside antibiotics is also increased.[54–56] The reason for the increased drug clearance is larger kidneys, resulting in larger creatinine clearance rates. Because both volume of distribution and clearance simultaneously change in obese patients to about the same extent, the aminoglycoside half-life value is appropriate for the patient's renal function ($t_{1/2} = [0.693 \cdot V]/Cl$).

Cystic fibrosis is a disease state that affects exocrine glands. In the lung, the result is the production of thick, tenacious sputum that predisposes patients to pulmonary infections. Patients with cystic fibrosis have larger aminoglycoside volumes of distribution (0.35 L/kg) because body composition is altered.[32–35,57–60] Generally, patients with cystic fibrosis have decreased adipose tissue and increased extracellular fluid owing to disease state–induced gastrointestinal malabsorption. These patients also have higher aminoglycoside clearance values as a result of increased glomerular filtration rates. Because clearance rates tend to increase more than volume of distribution values, the average aminoglycoside half-life is typically shorter in patients with cystic fibrosis ($t_{1/2}$ = 1.5 hours). Aminoglycosides can also be administered by inhalation at a dose of 300 mg twice daily in a cyclic fashion (4 weeks on, 4 weeks off) for these patients.[61]

Patients with liver disease who have ascites have additional extracellular fluid because of accumulation of ascitic fluid.[62–64] Since aminoglycosides pass into ascitic fluid, the volume of distribution is increased in these patients. The approach to estimating an initial volume of distribution is similar to that used in patients with renal failure who are fluid-overloaded. The weight of the patient when ascitic fluid is not present is known as the patient's dry weight. If this value is not known and the patient is not obese, ideal body weight can be used as an estimate of dry weight. A reasonable estimate of the volume of distribution (V in L) of a patient with ascites or one who is overhydrated for other reasons can be estimated using the following equation: $V = (0.26 \cdot DBW) + (TBW - DBW)$, where DBW is the patient's dry body weight and TBW is the patient's actual total body weight. Because of the wide variation in aminoglycoside volume of distribution for patients with ascites or overhydration, dosing should be guided by aminoglycoside serum concentrations. Also, as excess fluid is lost, clinicians should anticipate a decrease in the volume of distribution for these drugs.

Premature infants (gestational age ≤34 weeks) have a larger amount of body water compared with that of adults.[36,65–67] Aminoglycoside volume of distribution is larger (0.5–0.6 L/kg) because of this physiologic difference. In addition, kidneys are not completely developed, so that glomerular filtration and aminoglycoside clearance are decreased. A larger volume of distribution and lower clearance rate result in a prolonged average half-life of 6 to 10 hours. Full-term neonates (gestational age ~40 weeks) also have a larger volume of distribution (mean V = 0.4 to 0.5 L/kg) and lower aminoglycoside clearance, resulting in longer half-life values ($t_{1/2}$ = 4 to 5 hours). By about 6 months, an infant's mean volume of distribution is still large (V = 0.3 to 0.4 L/kg), but kidney development is complete, aminoglycoside clearance increases, and half-life is shorter ($t_{1/2}$ = 2 to 3 hours). These values remain relatively constant until the child is about 2 years of age. At that time, aminoglycoside volume of distribution, clearance, and half-life gradually approach adult values at puberty (~12 to 14 years of age).

Hemodialysis efficiently removes aminoglycoside antibiotics from the body.[68–72] Gentamicin, tobramycin, netilmicin, and amikacin are relatively small molecules that are water-soluble and have a small volume of distribution and low plasma protein binding. All these characteristics lead to very good hemodialysis removal. The average aminoglycoside half-life in a patient with renal failure is 50 hours. During hemodialysis with a low-flux artificial kidney, half-life decreases to 4 hours and results in about 50% of the drug being removed during a typical dialysis period (3 to 4 hours). Similarly, hemodialysis performed with a high-flux filter decreases aminoglycoside half-life to 2 hours.[73] If the patient is properly hydrated, the volume of distribution for aminoglycosides is 0.26 L/kg. Hemodialysis procedures, such as ultrafiltration, can be used to assist in the maintenance of proper fluid balance. Because kidneys provide fluid and electrolyte balance, it is not unusual for patients with renal failure receiving hemodialysis to be over- or underhydrated. As previously discussed regarding renal failure, body weight is an effective way of assessing hydration status, and it can be used to adjust initial volume of distribution estimates.

Peritoneal dialysis is much less efficient in removing aminoglycosides from the body.[74–76] Peritoneal dialysis decreases the half-life of aminoglycosides in a renal failure patient from about 50 hours to about 36 hours during the dialysis procedure. If the patient is receiving peritoneal dialysis on an ongoing basis, such as continuous ambulatory peritoneal dialysis, aminoglycoside half-life will be shorter because of the additional dialysis clearance. Patients receiving continuous ambulatory peritoneal dialysis sometimes develop peritonitis, which can be treated by adding aminoglycoside or other antibiotics to the peritoneal dialysis fluid. Although about half of the intraperitoneal aminoglycoside dose is systemically absorbed during a 5- to 6-hour dwell time, a patient with peritonitis who develops secondary bacteremia may need parenteral antibiotics to cure the infection.[74–76] Peritonitis causes inflammation of the peritoneal membrane, which facilitates absorption of aminoglycoside administered via dialysis fluid and elimination of aminoglycoside in the body.

DRUG INTERACTIONS

Most important drug interactions are pharmacodynamic, not pharmacokinetic, in nature. Vancomycin,[14,17] amphotericin B,[17] cyclosporin,[77] and furosemide[12,16,17] enhance the nephrotoxicity potential of the aminoglycosides. Each of these agents can cause nephrotoxicity when administered alone. When these drugs are administered concurrently with an aminoglycoside, serum creatinine concentrations should be monitored on a daily basis. In addition, serum concentrations of vancomycin or cyclosporin, as well as the aminoglycoside, should be measured. Loop diuretics,[78,79] including furosemide, bumetanide, and ethacrynic acid, can cause ototoxicity, and reports of an increased incidence of this adverse effect have been reported when aminoglycosides have been co-administered. If aminoglycoside antibiotics are administered with loop diuretics, clinical signs and symptoms of ototoxicity (auditory: decreased hearing acuity in the conversational range, feeling of fullness or pressure in the ears, tinnitus; vestibular: loss of equilibrium, headache, nausea, vomiting, nystagmus, vertigo, ataxia) should be monitored daily.

Aminoglycosides have intrinsic nondepolarizing neuromuscular blocking activity and may prolong the effects of neuromuscular blocking agents such as succinylcholine.[80] Surgical and intensive care patients receiving neuromuscular blockers and aminoglycosides should be monitored for this potential adverse effect. As previously discussed, penicillins (primarily penicillin G, ampicillin, nafcillin, carbenicillin, ticarcillin) can inactivate aminoglycosides in vivo and in blood specimen tubes intended for the measurement of aminoglycoside serum concentrations.[49–53] These two classes of drugs can also inactivate each other in intravenous administration bags and syringes and should not be mixed together.

INITIAL DOSAGE DETERMINATION METHODS

Pharmacokinetic Dosing Method

The goal of initial dosing of aminoglycosides is to compute the best dose possible for the patient according to his or her set of disease states and conditions that influence aminoglycoside pharmacokinetics and the site and severity of the infection. To do this, pharmacokinetic parameters for the patient are estimated using average parameters measured in other patients with similar disease state and condition profiles.

ESTIMATE OF ELIMINATION RATE CONSTANT

Aminoglycosides are almost totally eliminated unchanged in the urine, and there is a good relationship between creatinine clearance and aminoglycoside elimination rate constant (see Figure 4-2). This relationship allows the estimation of the aminoglycoside elimination rate constant for a patient, which can be used to compute an initial dose of the antibiotic. Mathematically, the equation for the straight line shown in Figure 4-2 is k_e = 0.00293(CrCl) + 0.014, where k_e is the aminoglycoside elimination rate constant in h^{-1} and CrCl is creatinine clearance in mL/min. A limitation in using elimination rate constant as the elimination parameter in this relationship is that it is a hybrid pharmacokinetic constant whose value can be influenced by either clearance or volume of distribution (k_e = Cl/V). Because gentamicin, tobramycin, netilmicin, and amikacin have similar pharmacokinetic properties, the same elimination rate constant versus creatinine clearance relationship can be used for all of the antibiotics. For example, the estimated elimination rate constant for a person with a creatinine clearance of 10 mL/min is 0.043 h^{-1}, which yields an estimated half-life of 16 hours (k_e = 0.00293(CrCl) + 0.014 = 0.00293(10 mL/min) + 0.014 = 0.043 h^{-1}; $t_{1/2}$ = 0.693/(0.043 h^{-1}) = 16 h). Taking the patient's renal function into account when deriving initial doses of aminoglycoside antibiotics is the single most important characteristic to assess.

ESTIMATE OF VOLUME OF DISTRIBUTION

The average volume of distribution for patients without disease states and conditions that change this parameter is 0.26 L/kg. Thus, for a nonobese 70-kg patient, the estimated volume of distribution would be 18 L (V = 0.26 L/kg · 70 kg = 18 L). If a patient weighs less than his or her ideal body weight, actual body weight is used to estimate volume of distribution. For patients whose weight is between their ideal body weight and 30% over their ideal weight, actual body weight can be used to compute estimated volume of distribution, although some clinicians prefer to use ideal body weight for such patients. In patients who are more than 30% above their ideal body weight, volume of distribution (V) estimates should include both ideal and actual total body weights using the following equation: V = 0.26[IBW + 0.4(TBW – IBW)], where V is in L, IBW is ideal body weight in kilograms, and TBW is total body weight in kilograms. For an obese patient whose ideal body weight is 55 kg and total body weight is 95 kg, the estimated volume of distribution would be 18.5 L: V = 0.26[IBW + 0.4(TBW – IBW)] = 0.26[55kg + 0.4(95 kg – 55 kg)] = 18.5 L. In patients who are overhydrated or have ascites, their dry body weight (weight without the extra fluid) can be used to provide an improved volume of distribution estimate (V in L) using the following formula: V = (0.26 · DBW) + (TBW – DBW), where DBW is the patient's dry body weight and TBW is the patient's actual total body weight. For example, a patient with a significant amount of ascitic fluid currently weighs 80 kg. It is known from previous clinic visits and history that the patient usually weighs 70 kg without the additional fluid. The estimated volume of distribution for this patient would be 28.2 L: V = (0.26 · DBW) + (TBW – DBW) = (0.26 · 70 kg) + (80 kg – 70 kg) = 28.2 L. Other disease states and conditions influence aminoglycoside volume of distribution, and the values of this parameter given in Table 4-1 are used when necessary. For instance, the average volume of distribution for cystic fibrosis patients is 0.35 L/kg. Therefore, the estimated volume of distribution for a 55-kg patient with cystic fibrosis is 19.3 L: V = 0.35 L/kg (55 kg) = 19.3 L.

SELECTION OF APPROPRIATE PHARMACOKINETIC MODEL AND EQUATIONS

When given by intravenous injection over less than 1 hour, aminoglycosides follow a three-compartment pharmacokinetic model (Figure 4-4). After the end of infusion, serum concentrations drop rapidly because of distribution of drug from blood to tissues (α or

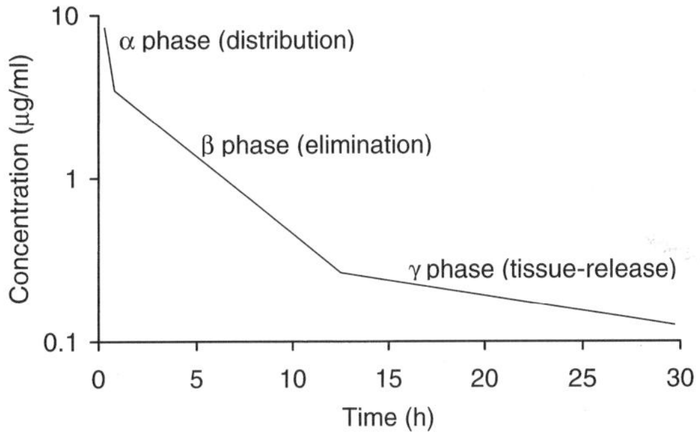

FIGURE 4-4 Multicompartment-model characteristics of aminoglycosides. If aminoglycoside antibiotics are given as an intravenous bolus injection, the serum concentration–time curve declines in three distinct phases. The first phase (α or distribution phase) occurs as antibiotic in the blood distributes into tissues, although drug is also cleared from the blood during this time, too. The second phase (β or elimination phase) begins when blood and tissues are in near equilibrium, and the predominate process is elimination from the body. The half-life for this phase of the curve is dramatically influenced by the patient's renal function ($t_{1/2}$ = 2 hours for normal renal function; $t_{1/2}$ = 50 hours for renal failure). The final phase (γ or tissue-release phase) occurs at very low serum concentrations (<0.5 μg/mL) and represents the release of tissue-bound aminoglycoside into the blood, where it will be cleared from the body.

distribution phase). If aminoglycosides are infused over 1 hour, the distribution phase is not usually observed. By about 1 hour after the beginning of the antibiotic infusion, drug concentrations decline more slowly, and the elimination rate constant for this segment of the concentration–time curve is the one that varies with renal function (β or elimination phase). Finally, at very low serum concentrations not detected by aminoglycoside concentration assays in clinical use (≤0.5 μg/mL), drug that was tissue-bound to various organs (especially the kidney) is released from tissue binding sites and eliminated (γ or tissue release phase). Although this model was instrumental in advancing current ideas regarding aminoglycoside tissue accumulation and nephrotoxicity, it cannot easily be used clinically because of its mathematical complexity.[9–11,13,16] Therefore, the simpler one-compartment model is widely used and allows accurate dosage calculation.[2,44,45,47,48,81]

Intavenously administered aminoglycosides are given over 1/2 to 1 hour as intermittent continuous infusions. Because drug is eliminated during the infusion time (and any waiting time that is necessary to allow for distribution to finish), pharmacokinetic equations that take into account this loss are preferred in patients with good renal function. If this is not done, a large amount of drug may be eliminated during infusion and waiting periods, and the peak concentration will be miscalculated. Generally, infusion equations should be used if the patient has a creatinine clearance greater than 30 mL/min. For creatinine clearances of 30 mL/min or less, very little aminoglycoside is eliminated during infusion and waiting period times, and intravenous bolus equations accurately compute peak concentrations.[82] Aminoglycoside steady-state peak ($C_{max,ss}$) and trough ($C_{min,ss}$) serum concentrations are chosen to treat the patient based on the type, site, and severity of infection as well as the infecting organism. Steady-state versions of one-compartment model intermittent intravenous infusion ($C_{max,ss} = [k_0/(k_eV)][(1 - e^{-k_et'})/(1 - e^{-k_e\tau})]$, $C_{min,ss} = C_{max,ss}e^{-[k_e(\tau-t')]}$, where k_0 is the infusion rate, k_e is the elimination rate constant, V is the volume of distribution, t′ is the drug infusion time, and τ is the dosage interval) or intravenous bolus ($C_{max,ss} = (D/V)[e^{-k_et}/(1 - e^{-k_e\tau})]$, $C_{min,ss} = C_{max,ss}e^{-k_e\tau}$, where D is the antibiotic dose, V is the volume of distribution, k_e is the elimination rate constant, t is time, and τ is the dosage interval) equations are chosen based on the patient's renal function to compute the required doses needed to achieve desired aminoglycoside concentrations. Note that intermittent intravenous infusion equations work well regardless of the patient's creatinine clearance. However, the intravenous bolus equations are easier to solve, save time, and are less likely to invoke a computational error, and for these reasons are recommended.

SELECTION OF STEADY-STATE CONCENTRATION

Aminoglycoside peak steady-state concentrations are selected based on site and severity of infection as well as the infecting organism. Severe infections, such as gram-negative pneumonia or septicemia or infections with organisms that have a high MIC such as *P. aeruginosa* (typical MIC ≈ 2 μg/mL for gentamicin, tobramycin, or netilmicin) generally require peak steady-state serum concentrations of 8 to 10 μg/mL for gentamicin, tobramycin, or netilmicin or 25 to 30 μg/mL for amikacin when using conventional dosing. Moderate infections at sites that are easier to penetrate or with organisms that display lower MIC values, such as intra-abdominal infections, are usually treated with peak gentamicin, tobramycin, or netilmicin steady-state serum concentrations of 5 to 7 μg/mL or with amikacin peak steady-state serum concentrations of 15 to 25 μg/mL. When treating urinary tract infections due to susceptible organisms or using aminoglycosides synergistically with penicillins or other antibiotics for the treatment of gram-positive infections such as infective endocarditis, steady-state peak concentrations of 3 to 5 μg/mL are usually adequate for gentamicin, tobramycin, and netilmicin and 12 to 15 μg/mL for amikacin. Pyelonephritis is considered a soft tissue infection, not a urinary tract infection, and requires higher peak steady-state concentrations to achieve a cure. Similar target peak steady-state concentrations for extended-interval aminoglycoside dosing are less established, although concentrations of 20 to 30 μg/mL have been suggested for *P. aeruginosa* and other serious infections. Desirable concentrations for steady-state trough concentrations are chosen based on avoidance of potential toxicity. For conventional dosing, steady-state trough concentrations should be maintained <2 μg/mL for tobramycin, gentamicin, and netilmicin or <5 to 7 μg/mL for amikacin. Using extended-interval dosing, steady-state trough concentrations should be <1 μg/mL for gentamicin, tobramycin, and netilmicin.

DOSAGE COMPUTATION

The equations given in Table 4-2A are used to compute aminoglycoside doses, depending on the renal function of the patient (intermittent intravenous infusion for creatinine clearances >30 mL/min, intravenous bolus for creatinine clearances ≤30 mL/min.

Example 1 JM is a 50-year-old, 70-kg, 178-cm (70-in) man with gram-negative pneumonia. His serum creatinine is 0.9 mg/dL, which has been stable over the last 5 days since admission. Compute a gentamicin dose using conventional dosing.

1. *Estimate the creatinine clearance.*

This patient has a stable serum creatinine and is not obese. The Cockcroft–Gault equation can be used to estimate creatinine clearance:

$$CrCl_{est} = [(140 - age)BW]/(72 \cdot S_{Cr}) = [(140 - 50\ y)70\ kg]/(72 \cdot 0.9\ mg/dL)$$

$$CrCl_{est} = 97\ mL/min$$

2. *Estimate the elimination rate constant (k_e) and half-life ($t_{1/2}$).*

The elimination rate constant versus creatinine clearance relationship is used to estimate the gentamicin elimination rate:

$$k_e = 0.00293(CrCl) + 0.014 = 0.00293(97\ mL/min) + 0.014 = 0.298\ h^{-1}$$

$$t_{1/2} = 0.693/k_e = 0.693/0.298\ h^{-1} = 2.3\ h$$

3. *Estimate the volume of distribution.*

The patient has no disease states or conditions that will alter the volume of distribution (V) from the normal value of 0.26 L/kg:

$$V = 0.26\ L/kg\ (70\ kg) = 18.2\ L$$

4. *Choose the desired steady-state serum concentrations.*

Patients with gram-negative pneumonia being treated with aminoglycoside antibiotics require steady-state peak concentrations ($C_{max,ss}$) of 8 to 10 μg/mL; steady-state trough ($C_{min,ss}$) concentrations should be <2 μg/mL to avoid toxicity. Set $C_{max,ss}$ = 9 μg/mL and $C_{min,ss}$ = 1 μg/mL.

5. *Use the intermittent intravenous infusion equations to compute the dose (Table 4-2C).*

Calculate the required dosage interval (τ) using a 1-hour infusion:

$$\tau = [(\ln C_{max,ss} - \ln C_{min,ss})/k_e] + t' = [(\ln 9\ \mu g/mL - \ln 1\ \mu g/mL)/0.298\ h^{-1}] + 1\ h = 8.4\ h$$

Dosage intervals should be rounded to clinically acceptable intervals of 8 hours, 12 hours, 18 hours, 24 hours, 36 hours, 48 hours, 72 hours, and multiples of 24 hours thereafter, whenever possible. In this case, the dosage interval is rounded to 8 hours. Also, steady-state peak concentrations are similar if drawn immediately after 1-hour infusion or 30 minutes after a 30-minute infusion, so the dose can be administered either way.

$$k_0 = C_{max,ss}k_eV[(1 - e^{-k_e\tau})/(1 - e^{-k_et'})]$$

$$k_0 = (9\ mg/L \cdot 0.298\ h^{-1} \cdot 18.2\ L)[(1 - e^{-(0.298\ h^{-1})(8\ h)})/(1 - e^{-(0.298\ h^{-1})(1\ h)})] = 172\ mg$$

Aminoglycoside doses should be rounded to the nearest 5 to 10 mg. This dose is rounded to 170 mg. (Note: μg/mL = mg/L, and this concentration unit was substituted for $C_{max,ss}$ to avoid unnecessary unit conversion.)

The prescribed maintenance dose is 170 mg every 8 hours.

6. *Compute the loading dose, if needed.*

Loading doses should be considered for patients with creatinine clearance values lower than 60 mL/min. The administration of a loading dose in these patients allows achieve-

TABLE 4-2A One-Compartment Model Equations Used with Aminoglycoside Antibiotics

ROUTE OF ADMINISTRATION	SINGLE DOSE	MULTIPLE DOSE	STEADY STATE
Intravenous bolus	$C = (D/V)e^{-k_e t}$	$C = (D/V)e^{-k_e t}[(1 - e^{-nk_e \tau})/(1 - e^{-k_e \tau})]$	$C = (D/V)[e^{-k_e t}/(1 - e^{-k_e \tau})]$
Intermittent intravenous infusion	$C = [k_0/(k_e V)](1 - e^{-k_e t'})$	$C = [k_0/(k_e V)](1 - e^{-k_e t'})$ $[(1 - e^{-nk_e \tau})/(1 - e^{-k_e \tau})]$	$C = [k_0/(k_e V)][(1 - e^{-k_e t'})/(1 - e^{-k_e \tau})]$

Symbol key: C is drug serum concentration at time = t, D is dose, V is volume of distribution, k_e is the elimination rate constant, n is the number of administered doses, τ is the dosage interval, k_0 is the infusion rate.

ment of therapeutic peak concentrations more quickly than if maintenance doses alone are given. However, since the pharmacokinetic parameters used to compute these initial doses are *estimated* values and not *actual* values, the patient's own parameters may be much different from the estimated constants and steady state will not be achieved until 3 to 5 half-lives have passed.

$$LD = k_0/(1 - e^{-k_e \tau}) = 170 \text{ mg}/(1 - e^{-(0.298 \text{ h}^{-1})(8 \text{ h})}) = 187 \text{ mg}$$

As noted, this loading dose is only about 10% greater than the maintenance dose and would not be given to the patient. Because the expected half-life is 2.3 hours, the patient should be at steady state after the second dose is given.

Example 2 Same patient profile as in example 1, but serum creatinine is 3.5 mg/dL, indicating renal impairment.

1. *Estimate the creatinine clearance.*

This patient has a stable serum creatinine and is not obese. The Cockcroft–Gault equation can be used to estimate creatinine clearance:

$$CrCl_{est} = [(140 - age)BW]/(72 \cdot S_{Cr}) = [(140 - 50 \text{ y})70 \text{ kg}]/(72 \cdot 3.5 \text{ mg/dL})$$

$$CrCl_{est} = 25 \text{ mL/min}$$

2. *Estimate the elimination rate constant (k_e) and half-life ($t_{1/2}$).*

The elimination rate constant versus creatinine clearance relationship is used to estimate the gentamicin elimination rate for this patient:

$$k_e = 0.00293(CrCl) + 0.014 = 0.00293(25 \text{ mL/min}) + 0.014 = 0.087 \text{ h}^{-1}$$

$$t_{1/2} = 0.693/k_e = 0.693/0.087 \text{ h}^{-1} = 8 \text{ h}$$

3. *Estimate the volume of distribution.*

The patient has no disease states or conditions that will alter the volume of distribution (V) from the normal value of 0.26 L/kg:

$$V = 0.26 \text{ L/kg } (70 \text{ kg}) = 18.2 \text{ L}$$

4. *Choose the desired steady-state serum concentrations.*

Patients with gram-negative pneumonia who are being treated with aminoglycoside antibiotics require steady-state peak concentrations ($C_{max,ss}$) of 8 to 10 μg/mL; steady-state trough ($C_{min,ss}$) concentrations should be <2 μg/mL to avoid toxicity. Set $C_{max,ss}$ = 9 μg/mL and $C_{min,ss}$ = 1 μg/mL.

5. *Use the intravenous bolus equations to compute the dose (see Table 4-2B).*

Calculate the required dosage interval (τ):

$$\tau = [(\ln C_{max,ss} - \ln C_{min,ss})/k_e] = (\ln 9\ \mu g/mL - \ln 1\ \mu g/mL)/0.087\ h^{-1} = 25\ h$$

Dosage intervals should be rounded to clinically acceptable intervals of 8 hours, 12 hours, 18 hours, 24 hours, 36 hours, 48 hours, 72 hours, and multiples of 24 hours thereafter, whenever possible. In this case, the dosage interval is rounded to 24 hours. Also, steady-state peak concentrations are similar if drawn immediately after a 1-hour infusion or 30 minutes after a 30-minute infusion, so the dose can be administered either way.

$$D = C_{max,ss} V(1 - e^{-k_e \tau})$$

$$D = 9\ mg/L \cdot 18.2\ L(1 - e^{-(0.087\ h^{-1})(24\ h)}) = 143\ mg$$

Aminoglycoside doses should be rounded to the nearest 5 to 10 mg. This dose is rounded to 145 mg. (Note: μg/mL = mg/L, and this concentration unit was substituted for $C_{max,ss}$ to avoid unnecessary unit conversion.)

TABLE 4-2B Pharmacokinetic Constant Computations Using a One-Compartment Model Used with Aminoglycoside Antibiotics

ROUTE OF ADMINISTRATION	SINGLE DOSE	MULTIPLE DOSE	STEADY STATE
Intravenous bolus	$k_e = (\ln C_1 - \ln C_2)/(t_1 - t_2)$ $t_{1/2} = 0.693/k_e$ $V = D/C_0$ $Cl = k_eV$	$k_e = (\ln C_1 - \ln C_2)/(t_1 - t_2)$ $t_{1/2} = 0.693/k_e$ $V = D/(C_0 - C_{predose})$ $Cl = k_eV$	$k_e = (\ln C_1 - \ln C_2)/(t_1 - t_2)$ $t_{1/2} = 0.693/k_e$ $V = D/(C_0 - C_{predose})$ $Cl = k_eV$
Intermittent intravenous infusion	$k_e = (\ln C_1 - \ln C_2)/(t_1 - t_2)$ $t_{1/2} = 0.693/k_e$ $V = [k_0(1 - e^{-k_e t'})]/\{k_e[C_{max} - (C_{predose}e^{-k_e t'})]\}$ $Cl = k_eV$	$k_e = (\ln C_1 - \ln C_2)/(t_1 - t_2)$ $t_{1/2} = 0.693/k_e$ $V = [k_0(1 - e^{-k_e t'})]/\{k_e[C_{max} - (C_{predose}e^{-k_e t'})]\}$ $Cl = k_eV$	$k_e = (\ln C_1 - \ln C_2)/(t_1 - t_2)$ $t_{1/2} = 0.693/k_e$ $V = [k_0(1 - e^{-k_e t'})]/\{k_e[C_{max} - (C_{predose}e^{-k_e t'})]\}$ $Cl = k_eV$

Symbol key: C_1 is drug serum concentration at time = t_1, C_2 is drug serum concentration at time = t_2, k_e is the elimination rate constant, $t_{1/2}$ is the half-life, V is the volume of distribution, k_0 is the continuous infusion rate, t′ is the infusion time, D is dose, C_0 is the concentration at time = 0, Cl is drug clearance, $C_{predose}$ is the predose concentration.

The prescribed maintenance dose is 145 mg every 24 hours. Although this dose is given once daily, it is not extended-interval dosing because desired serum concentrations are within the conventional range.

6. *Compute the loading dose, if needed.*

Loading doses should be considered for patients with creatinine clearance values lower than 60 mL/min. The administration of a loading dose in these patients allows achievement of therapeutic peak concentrations more quickly than if maintenance doses alone are given. However, because the pharmacokinetic parameters used to compute these initial doses are *estimated* values and not *actual* values, the patient's own parameters may be much different from the estimated constants and steady state will not be achieved until 3 to 5 half-lives have passed.

$$LD = C_{max,ss} V = 9 \text{ mg/L} \cdot 18.2 \text{ L} = 164 \text{ mg}$$

Round the loading dose to 165 mg. It is given as the first dose. The next dose is a maintenance dose given a dosage interval away from the loading dose—in this case 24 hours later.

Example 3 ZW is a 35-year-old, 150-kg, 165-cm (65-in) woman with an intra-abdominal infection. Her serum creatinine is 1.1 mg/dL and stable. Compute a tobramycin dose using conventional dosing.

1. *Estimate the creatinine clearance.*

This patient has a stable serum creatinine and is obese (IBW_{women} (in kg) = 45 + 2.3 (Ht − 60 in) = 45 + 2.3(65 − 60) = 57 kg). The Salazar and Corcoran equation can be used to estimate creatinine clearance:

$$CrCl_{est(females)} = \frac{(146 - age)[(0.287 \cdot Wt) + (9.74 \cdot Ht^2)]}{(60 \cdot S_{Cr})}$$

$$CrCl_{est(females)} = \frac{(146 - 35 \text{ y})\{(0.287 \cdot 150 \text{ kg}) + [9.74 \cdot (1.65 \text{ m})^2]\}}{(60 \cdot 1.1 \text{ mg/dL})} = 117 \text{ mL/min}$$

Note: Height is converted from inches to meters: Ht = (65 in · 2.54 cm/in)/(100 cm/m) = 1.65 m.

2. *Estimate the elimination rate constant (k_e) and half-life ($t_{1/2}$).*

The elimination rate constant versus creatinine clearance relationship is used to estimate the gentamicin elimination rate for this patient:

$$k_e = 0.00293(CrCl) + 0.014 = 0.00293(117 \text{ mL/min}) + 0.014 = 0.357 \text{ h}^{-1}$$

$$t_{1/2} = 0.693/k_e = 0.693/0.357 \text{ h}^{-1} = 1.9 \text{ h}$$

3. *Estimate the volume of distribution.*

The patient is obese, so the volume of distribution (V) is estimated using the following formula:

$$V = 0.26[IBW + 0.4(TBW - IBW)] = 0.26[57 \text{ kg} + 0.4(150 \text{ kg} - 57 \text{ kg})] = 24.5 \text{ L}$$

4. *Choose desired steady-state serum concentrations.*

Patients with intra-abdominal infection being treated with aminoglycoside antibiotics require steady-state peak concentrations ($C_{max,ss}$) of 5 to 7 μg/mL; steady-state trough ($C_{min,ss}$) concentrations should be <2 μg/mL to avoid toxicity. Set $C_{max,ss}$ = 6 μg/mL and $C_{min,ss}$ = 0.5 μg/mL.

5. *Use the intermittent intravenous infusion equations to compute the dose (see Table 4-2C).*

Calculate the required dosage interval (τ) using a 1-hour infusion:

$$\tau = [(\ln C_{max,ss} - \ln C_{min,ss})/k_e] + t' = [(\ln 6\ \mu g/mL - \ln 0.5\ \mu g/mL)/0.357\ h^{-1}] + 1\ h = 8\ h$$

Dosage intervals should be rounded to clinically acceptable intervals of 8 hours, 12 hours, 18 hours, 24 hours, 36 hours, 48 hours, 72 hours, and multiples of 24 hours thereafter, whenever possible. In this case, the dosage interval is 8 hours. Also, steady-state peak concentrations are similar if drawn immediately after a 1-hour infusion or 30 minutes after a 30-minute infusion, so the dose can be administered either way.

$$k_0 = C_{max,ss} k_e V[(1 - e^{-k_e\tau})/(1 - e^{-k_e t'})]$$

$$k_0 = (6\ mg/L \cdot 0.357\ h^{-1} \cdot 24.5\ L)[(1 - e^{-(0.357\ h^{-1})(8\ h)})/(1 - e^{-(0.357\ h^{-1})(1\ h)})] = 165\ mg$$

Aminoglycoside doses should be rounded to the nearest 5 to 10 mg. This dose does not need to be rounded. (Note: μg/mL = mg/L, and this concentration unit was substituted for $C_{max,ss}$ to avoid unnecessary unit conversion.)

The prescribed maintenance dose is 165 mg every 8 hours.

6. *Compute the loading dose, if needed.*

Loading doses should be considered for patients with creatinine clearance values lower than 60 mL/min. The administration of a loading dose in these patients allows achieve-

TABLE 4-2C Equations Used to Compute Individualized Dosage Regimens for Various Routes of Administration Used with Aminoglycoside Antibiotics

ROUTE OF ADMINISTRATION	DOSAGE INTERVAL (τ), MAINTENANCE DOSE (D OR K_0), AND LOADING DOSE (LD) EQUATIONS
Intravenous bolus	$\tau = (\ln C_{max,ss} - \ln C_{min,ss})/k_e$ $D = C_{max,ss} V(1 - e^{-k_e\tau})$ $LD = C_{max,ss} V$
Intermittent intravenous infusion	$\tau = [(\ln C_{max,ss} - \ln C_{min,ss})/k_e] + t'$ $k_0 = C_{max,ss} k_e V[(1 - e^{-k_e\tau})/(1 - e^{-k_e t'})]$ $LD = k_0/(1 - e^{-k_e\tau})$

$C_{max,ss}$ and $C_{min,ss}$ = maximum and minimum steady-state concentrations; V = volume of distribution; k_e = elimination rate constant; k_0 = infusion rate; t′ = infusion time; $t_{1/2}$ = half-life; τ = dosage interval; D = dose; LD = loading dose.

ment of therapeutic peak concentrations more quickly than if maintenance doses alone are given. However, since the pharmacokinetic parameters used to compute these initial doses are *estimated* values and not *actual* values, the patient's own parameters may be much different from the estimated constants and steady state will not be achieved until 3 to 5 half-lives have passed.

$$LD = k_0/(1 - e^{-k_e\tau}) = 165 \text{ mg}/(1 - e^{-(0.357 \text{ h}^{-1})(8 \text{ h})}) = 175 \text{ mg}$$

As noted, this loading dose is <10% greater than the maintenance dose and is not given to the patient. Because the expected half-life is 1.9 hours, the patient should be at steady state after the second dose is given.

Example 4 JM is a 20-year-old, 60-kg, 173-cm (68-in) man with a cystic fibrosis pulmonary exacerbation. His serum creatinine is 0.6 mg/dL, which has been the same at several clinic visits. Compute a tobramycin dose using conventional dosing.

1. *Estimate the creatinine clearance.*

This patient has a stable serum creatinine and is not obese. The Cockcroft–Gault equation can be used to estimate creatinine clearance:

$$CrCl_{est} = [(140 - age)BW]/(72 \cdot S_{Cr}) = [(140 - 20 \text{ y})60 \text{ kg}]/(72 \cdot 0.6 \text{ mg/dL})$$

$$CrCl_{est} = 167 \text{ mL/min}$$

This is a high creatinine clearance value, but the patient is young and has cystic fibrosis. Both of these situations can result in higher than expected creatinine clearance rates.

2. *Estimate the elimination rate constant (k_e) and half-life ($t_{1/2}$).*

The elimination rate constant versus creatinine clearance relationship is used to estimate the gentamicin elimination rate:

$$k_e = 0.00293(CrCl) + 0.014 = 0.00293(167 \text{ mL/min}) + 0.014 = 0.503 \text{ h}^{-1}$$

$$t_{1/2} = 0.693/k_e = 0.693/0.503 \text{ h}^{-1} = 1.4 \text{ h}$$

Patients with cystic fibrosis who have good renal function are expected to have short aminoglycoside half-lives.

3. *Estimate the volume of distribution.*

Patients with cystic fibrosis have average volume of distribution (V) values of 0.35 L/kg:

$$V = 0.35 \text{ L/kg } (60 \text{ kg}) = 21 \text{ L}$$

4. *Choose desired steady-state serum concentrations.*

Cystic fibrosis patients with a pulmonary exacerbation being treated with aminoglycoside antibiotics require steady-state peak concentrations ($C_{max,ss}$) of 8 to 10 μg/mL; steady-state trough ($C_{min,ss}$) concentrations should be <2 μg/mL to avoid toxicity. Set $C_{max,ss}$ = 8 μg/mL and $C_{min,ss}$ = 1 μg/mL.

5. *Use the intermittent intravenous infusion equations to compute the dose (see Table 4-2C).*

Calculate the required dosage interval (τ) using a 1-hour infusion:

$$\tau = [(\ln C_{max,ss} - \ln C_{min,ss})/k_e] + t' = [(\ln 8\ \mu g/mL - \ln 1\ \mu g/mL)/0.503\ h^{-1}] + 1\ h = 5.1\ h$$

Dosage intervals should be rounded to clinically acceptable intervals of 8 hours, 12 hours, 18 hours, 24 hours, 36 hours, 48 hours, 72 hours, and multiples of 24 hours thereafter, whenever possible. Some cystic fibrosis treatment centers prefer to administer aminoglycosides every 6 hours. In this case, the patient's clinical condition is not severe, so that the dosage interval is rounded to 8 hours. Because of this, the steady-state trough concentration is expected to fall below 1 μg/mL. Also, steady-state peak concentrations are similar if drawn immediately after a 1-hour infusion or 30 minutes after a 30-minute infusion, so the dose can be administered either way.

$$k_0 = C_{max,ss} k_e V[(1 - e^{-k_e \tau})/(1 - e^{-k_e t'})]$$

$$k_0 = (8\ mg/L \cdot 0.503\ h^{-1} \cdot 21\ L)[(1 - e^{-(0.503\ h^{-1})(8\ h)})/(1 - e^{-(0.503\ h^{-1})(1\ h)})] = 210\ mg$$

Aminoglycoside doses should be rounded to the nearest 5 to 10 mg. This dose of 210 mg does not need to be rounded. (Note: μg/mL = mg/L, and this concentration unit was substituted for $C_{max,ss}$ to avoid unnecessary unit conversion.)

The prescribed maintenance dose is 210 mg every 8 hours.

6. *Compute the loading dose, if needed.*

Loading doses should be considered for patients with creatinine clearance values lower than 60 mL/min. The administration of a loading dose in these patients allows achievement of therapeutic peak concentrations more quickly than if maintenance doses alone are given. However, because the pharmacokinetic parameters used to compute these initial doses are *estimated* values and not *actual* values, the patient's own parameters may be much different from the estimated constants and steady state will not be achieved until 3 to 5 half-lives have passed.

$$LD = k_0/(1 - e^{-k_e \tau}) = 210\ mg/(1 - e^{-(0.503\ h^{-1})(8\ h)}) = 214\ mg$$

As noted, this loading dose is <10% greater than the maintenance dose and is not given to the patient. Because the expected half-life is 1.4 hours, the patient should be at steady state after the second dose is given.

Example 5 JM is an 80-year-old, 80-kg, 173-cm (68-in) man with *Streptococcus viridans* endocarditis. His serum creatinine is 1.5 mg/dL and stable. Ampicillin and gentamicin are to be used to treat the infection. Compute a gentamicin dose using conventional dosing.

1. *Estimate the creatinine clearance.*

This patient has a stable serum creatinine and is not obese (IBW_{males} = 50 + 2.3(Ht – 60 in) = 50 + 2.3(68 – 60) = 68 kg; % overweight = {100[80 kg–68 kg]}/68 kg = 18%). The Cockcroft–Gault equation can be used to estimate creatinine clearance:

$$CrCl_{est} = [(140 - age)BW]/(72 \cdot S_{Cr}) = [(140 - 80\ y)80\ kg]/(72 \cdot 1.5\ mg/dL)$$

$$CrCl_{est} = 44\ mL/min$$

2. *Estimate the elimination rate constant (k_e) and half-life ($t_{1/2}$).*

The elimination rate constant versus creatinine clearance relationship is used to estimate the gentamicin elimination rate:

$$k_e = 0.00293(\text{CrCl}) + 0.014 = 0.00293(44 \text{ mL/min}) + 0.014 = 0.143 \text{ h}^{-1}$$

$$t_{1/2} = 0.693/k_e = 0.693/0.143 \text{ h}^{-1} = 4.8 \text{ h}$$

3. *Estimate the volume of distribution.*

The patient has no disease states or conditions that will alter the volume of distribution (V) from the normal value of 0.26 L/kg:

$$V = 0.26 \text{ L/kg } (80 \text{ kg}) = 20.8 \text{ L}$$

4. *Choose the desired steady-state serum concentrations.*

Patients with *S. viridans* endocarditis being treated with aminoglycoside antibiotics require steady-state peak concentrations ($C_{max,ss}$) of 3 to 5 μg/mL; steady-state trough ($C_{min,ss}$) concentrations should be <2 μg/mL to avoid toxicity. Set $C_{max,ss}$ = 4 μg/mL and $C_{min,ss}$ = 1 μg/mL.

5. *Use the intermittent intravenous infusion equations to compute the dose (see Table 4-2C).*

Calculate the required dosage interval (τ) using a 1-hour infusion:

$$\tau = [(\ln C_{max,ss} - \ln C_{min,ss})/k_e] + t' = [(\ln 4 \text{ μg/mL} - \ln 1 \text{ μg/mL})/0.143 \text{ h}^{-1}] + 1 \text{ h} = 11 \text{ h}$$

Dosage intervals should be rounded to clinically acceptable intervals of 8 hours, 12 hours, 18 hours, 24 hours, 36 hours, 48 hours, 72 hours, and multiples of 24 hours thereafter, whenever possible. In this case, the dosage interval is rounded to 12 hours. Also, steady-state peak concentrations are similar if drawn immediately after a 1-hour infusion or 30 minutes after a 30-minute infusion, so the dose can be administered either way.

$$k_0 = C_{max,ss} k_e V[(1 - e^{-k_e \tau})/(1 - e^{-k_e t'})]$$

$$k_0 = (4 \text{ mg/L} \cdot 0.143 \text{ h}^{-1} \cdot 20.8 \text{ L})[(1 - e^{-(0.143 \text{ h}^{-1})(12 \text{ h})})/(1 - e^{-(0.143 \text{ h}^{-1})(1 \text{ h})})] = 73 \text{ mg}$$

Aminoglycoside doses should be rounded to the nearest 5 to 10 mg. This dose is rounded to 70 mg. (Note: μg/mL = mg/L, and this concentration unit was substituted for $C_{max,ss}$ to avoid unnecessary unit conversion.)

The prescribed maintenance dose is 70 mg every 12 hours.

Because the patient is receiving concurrent treatment with ampicillin, care would be taken to avoid in vitro inactivation in blood sample tubes intended for the determination of aminoglycoside serum concentrations.

6. *Compute the gentamicin loading dose, if needed.*

Loading doses should be considered for patients with creatinine clearance values lower than 60 mL/min. The administration of a loading dose in these patients allows achievement of therapeutic peak concentrations more quickly than if maintenance doses alone are given. However, since the pharmacokinetic parameters used to compute these initial doses are *estimated* values and not *actual* values, the patient's own parameters may be much different from the estimated constants and steady state will not be achieved until 3 to 5 half-lives have passed.

$$LD = k_0/(1 - e^{-k_e\tau}) = 70\ mg/(1 - e^{-(0.143\ h^{-1})(12\ h)}) = 85\ mg$$

The loading dose should be given as the first dose. The next dose is a maintenance dose given a dosage interval away from the loading dose—in this case 12 hours later.

Example 6 Same patient profile as in example 2, but *extended-interval dosing* is used.

1. *Estimate the creatinine clearance.*

This patient has a stable serum creatinine and is not obese. The Cockcroft-Gault equation can be used to estimate creatinine clearance:

$$CrCl_{est} = [(140 - age)BW]/(72 \cdot S_{Cr}) = [(140 - 50\ y)70\ kg]/(72 \cdot 3.5\ mg/dL)$$

$$CrCl_{est} = 25\ mL/min$$

2. *Estimate the elimination rate constant (k_e) and half-life ($t_{1/2}$).*

The elimination rate constant versus creatinine clearance relationship is used to estimate the gentamicin elimination rate:

$$k_e = 0.00293(CrCl) + 0.014 = 0.00293(25\ mL/min) + 0.014 = 0.087\ h^{-1}$$

$$t_{1/2} = 0.693/k_e = 0.693/0.087\ h^{-1} = 8\ h$$

3. *Estimate the volume of distribution.*

The patient has no disease states or conditions that will alter the volume of distribution from the normal value of 0.26 L/kg:

$$V = 0.26\ L/kg\ (70\ kg) = 18.2\ L$$

4. *Choose the desired steady-state serum concentrations.*

Patients with gram-negative pneumonia being treated with aminoglycoside antibiotics require steady-state peak concentrations ($C_{max,ss}$) >20 μg/mL; steady-state trough ($C_{min,ss}$) concentrations should be <1 μg/mL to avoid toxicity. Set $C_{max,ss}$ = 20 μg/mL and $C_{min,ss}$ = 0.5 μg/mL.

5. *Use the intravenous bolus equations to compute the gentamicin dose (see Table 4-2C).*

Calculate the required dosage interval (τ):

$$\tau = [(\ln C_{max,ss} - \ln C_{min,ss})/k_e] = (\ln 20\ \mu g/mL - \ln 0.5\ \mu g/mL)/0.087\ h^{-1} = 42\ h$$

Dosage intervals should be rounded to clinically acceptable intervals of 24 hours, 36 hours, 48 hours, 60 hours, 72 hours, and multiples of 12 hours thereafter, whenever possible. In this case, the dosage interval is rounded to 48 hours. Also, steady-state peak concentrations are similar if drawn immediately after a 1-hour infusion or 30 minutes after a 30-minute infusion, so the dose can be administered either way.

$$D = C_{max,ss} V(1 - e^{-k_e \tau})$$

$$D = 20 \text{ mg/L} \cdot 18.2 \text{ L}(1 - e^{-(0.087 \text{ h}^{-1})(48 \text{ h})}) = 358 \text{ mg}$$

Aminoglycoside doses should be rounded to the nearest 5 to 10 mg. This dose is rounded to 360 mg. (Note: μg/mL = mg/L, and this concentration unit was substituted for $C_{max,ss}$ to avoid unnecessary unit conversion.)

The prescribed maintenance dose is 360 mg gentamicin every 48 hours.

Hull and Sarubbi Nomogram Method

For patients who do not have disease states or conditions that alter volume of distribution, the only two patient-specific factors that change when using the pharmacokinetic dosing method is patient weight and creatinine clearance. Because of this, it is possible to make a simple nomogram to handle uncomplicated patients with a standard volume of distribution (Table 4-3). The Hull and Sarubbi aminoglycoside dosing nomogram is a quick and efficient way to apply pharmacokinetic dosing concepts without using complicated pharmacokinetic equations.[44,45] With a simple modification, it can also be used for obese patients. If the patient is ≥30% above ideal body weight, an adjusted body weight (ABW) can be calculated and used as the weight factor (ABW (in kg) = IBW + 0.4[TBW – IBW], where IBW is ideal body weight in kilograms and TBW is actual total body weight in kilograms).[54–56] As can be seen, this equation is derived from the computation for volume of distribution in obese patients. Also, the Salazar and Corcoran method of estimating creatinine clearance in obese patients should be used to compute renal function.[83,84]

Steady-state peak concentrations are selected as discussed in the pharmacokinetic dosing method section and are used to determine a loading dose from the nomogram (see Table 4-3). Logically, lower loading doses produce lower expected peak concentrations, and higher loading doses result in higher expected peak concentrations. After the loading dose is found, the patient's creatinine clearance is used to estimate the half-life, dosage interval, and maintenance dose (as a percent of the administered loading dose). The maintenance dose supplied by the nomogram is the percent of the loading dose that was eliminated during the different dosage interval time frames and will therefore provide the same estimated peak concentration at steady state as that supplied by the loading dose. To illustrate how the nomogram is used, the same patient examples used in the previous section are repeated for this dosage approach, using the same example number. Since the nomogram uses slightly different estimates for volume of distribution and elimination rate constant, some minor differences in suggested doses are expected. Because the cystic fibrosis case example requires a different volume of distribution (0.35 L/kg), the Hull and Sarubbi nomogram cannot be used.

Example 1 JM is a 50-year-old, 70-kg, 178-cm (70-in) man with gram-negative pneumonia. His serum creatinine is 0.9 mg/dL, which has been stable over the last 5 days since admission. Compute a gentamicin dose using conventional dosing.

1. *Estimate the creatinine clearance.*

This patient has a stable serum creatinine and is not obese. The Cockcroft–Gault equation can be used to estimate creatinine clearance:

TABLE 4-3 Aminoglycoside Dosage Chart

1. Compute patient's creatinine clearance (CrCl) using Cockcroft-Gault method: CrCl = $[(140 - \text{age})\text{BW}]/(S_{Cr} \times 72)$. Multiply by 0.85 for women.
2. Use patient's weight if within 30% of ideal body weight (IBW); otherwise use adjusted dosing weight = IBW + [0.40(TBW – IBW)], where TBW = total body weight.
3. Select loading dose in mg/kg to provide peak serum concentrations in range listed in box for the desired aminoglycoside antibiotic:

AMINOGLYCOSIDE	USUAL LOADING DOSES (mg/kg)	EXPECTED PEAK SERUM CONCENTRATIONS (μg/mL)
Tobramycin Gentamicin Netilmicin	1.5–2.0	4–10
Amikacin Kanamycin	5.0–7.5	15–30

4. Select maintenance dose (as percentage of loading dose) to continue peak serum concentrations indicated in box according to desired dosage interval and the patient's creatinine clearance. To maintain usual peak/trough ratio, use dosage intervals in clear areas.

Percentage of Loading Dose Required for Dosage Interval Selected

CrCl (mL/min)	EST. HALF-LIFE (H)	8 HOURS (%)	12 HOURS (%)	24 HOURS (%)
>90	2–3	90	–	–
90	3.1	84	–	–
80	3.4	80	91	–
70	3.9	76	88	–
60	4.5	71	84	–
50	5.3	65	79	–
40	6.5	57	72	92
30	8.4	48	63	86
25	9.9	43	57	81
20	11.9	37	50	75
17	13.6	33	46	70
15	15.1	31	42	67
12	17.9	27	37	61
10*	20.4	24	34	56
7*	25.9	19	28	47
5*	31.5	16	23	41
2*	46.8	11	16	30
0*	69.3	8	11	21

* Dosing for patients with CrCl ≤10 mL/min should be assisted by measuring serum concentrations.
Adapted from Sarubbi FA, Jr, Hull JH. Amikacin serum concentrations: prediction of levels and dosage guidelines. Ann Intern Med 1978;89:612–618.

$$CrCl_{est} = [(140 - age)BW]/(72 \cdot S_{Cr}) = [(140 - 50\ y)70\ kg]/(72 \cdot 0.9\ mg/dL)$$

$$CrCl_{est} = 97\ mL/min$$

2. *Choose the desired steady-state serum concentrations.*

Patients with gram-negative pneumonia being treated with aminoglycoside antibiotics require steady-state peak concentrations ($C_{max,ss}$) of 8 to 10 μg/mL.

3. *Select the loading dose (see Table 4-3).*

A loading dose of 2 mg/kg provides a peak concentration of 8 to 10 μg/mL.

$$LD = 2\ mg/kg(70\ kg) = 140\ mg$$

4. *Determine the estimated half-life, maintenance dose, and dosage interval.*

From the nomogram, the estimated half-life is 2 to 3 hours, the maintenance dose (MD) is 90% of the loading dose (MD = 0.90[140 mg] = 126 mg), and the dosage interval is 8 hours.

Aminoglycoside doses should be rounded to the nearest 5 to 10 mg. Steady-state peak concentrations are similar if drawn immediately after a 1-hour infusion or 30 minutes after a 30-minute infusion, so the dose can be administered either way.

The prescribed maintenance dose is 125 mg gentamicin every 8 hours.

Example 2 Same patient profile as in example 1, but serum creatinine is 3.5 mg/dL, indicating renal impairment.

1. *Estimate the creatinine clearance.*

This patient has a stable serum creatinine and is not obese. The Cockcroft–Gault equation can be used to estimate creatinine clearance:

$$CrCl_{est} = [(140 - age)BW]/(72 \cdot S_{Cr}) = [(140 - 50\ y)70\ kg]/(72 \cdot 3.5\ mg/dL)$$

$$CrCl_{est} = 25\ mL/min$$

2. *Choose the desired steady-state serum concentrations.*

Patients with gram-negative pneumonia being treated with aminoglycoside antibiotics require steady-state peak concentrations ($C_{max,ss}$) of 8 to 10 μg/mL.

3. *Select the loading dose (see Table 4-3).*

A loading dose of 2 mg/kg provides a peak concentration of 8 to 10 μg/mL.

$$LD = 2\ mg/kg(70\ kg) = 140\ mg$$

4. *Determine the estimated half-life, maintenance dose, and dosage interval.*

From the nomogram, the estimated half-life is 9.9 hours, the maintenance dose (MD) is 81% of the loading dose (MD = 0.81[140 mg] = 113 mg), and the dosage interval is 24 hours. Note: Because of the $C_{max,ss}$ and $C_{min,ss}$ chosen for this patient, the 24-hour dosage interval was used.

Aminoglycoside doses should be rounded to the nearest 5 to 10 mg. Steady-state peak concentrations are similar if drawn immediately after a 1-hour infusion or 30 minutes after a 30-minute infusion, so the dose can be administered either way.

The prescribed maintenance dose is 115 mg gentamicin every 24 hours.

Example 3 ZW is a 35-year-old, 150-kg, 165-cm (65-in) woman with an intra-abdominal infection. Her serum creatinine is 1.1 mg/dL and stable. Compute a tobramycin dose using conventional dosing.

1. *Estimate the creatinine clearance.*

This patient has a stable serum creatinine and is obese (IBW_{women} (in kg) = 45 + 2.3 (Ht – 60 in) = 45 + 2.3(65 – 60) = 57 kg). The Salazar and Corcoran equation can be used to estimate creatinine clearance:

$$CrCl_{est(females)} = \frac{(146 - age)[(0.287 \cdot Wt) + (9.74 \cdot Ht^2)]}{(60 \cdot S_{Cr})}$$

$$CrCl_{est(females)} = \frac{(146\text{–}35\ y)\{(0.287 \cdot 150\ kg) + [9.74 \cdot (1.65\ m)^2]\}}{(60 \cdot 1.1\ mg/dL)} = 117\ mL/min$$

Note: Height is converted from inches to meters: Ht = (65 in · 2.54 cm/in)/(100 cm/m) = 1.65 m.

2. *Choose the desired steady-state serum concentrations.*

Patients with intra-abdominal infection being treated with aminoglycoside antibiotics require steady-state peak concentrations ($C_{max,ss}$) of 5 to 7 μg/mL.

3. *Select the loading dose (see Table 4-3).*

A loading dose of 1.7 mg/kg provides a peak concentration of 5 to 7 μg/mL.

Because the patient is obese, adjusted body weight (ABW) is used to compute the dose: ABW = IBW + 0.4[TBW – IBW] = 57 kg + 0.4[150 kg – 57 kg] = 94 kg.

$$LD = 1.7\ mg/kg(94\ kg) = 160\ mg$$

4. *Determine the estimated half-life, maintenance dose, and dosage interval.*

From the nomogram, the estimated half-life is 2 to 3 hours, the maintenance dose (MD) is 90% of the loading dose (MD = 0.90[160 mg] = 144 mg), and the dosage interval is 8 hours.

Aminoglycoside doses should be rounded to the nearest 5 to 10 mg. Steady-state peak concentrations are similar if drawn immediately after a 1-hour infusion or 30 minutes after a 30-minute infusion, so the dose can be administered either way.

The prescribed maintenance dose is 145 mg tobramycin every 8 hours.

Example 5 JM is an 80-year-old, 80-kg, 173-cm (68-in) man with *S. viridans* endocarditis. His serum creatinine is 1.5 mg/dL and stable. Ampicillin and gentamicin are used to treat the infection. Compute a gentamicin dose using conventional dosing.

1. *Estimate the creatinine clearance.*

This patient has a stable serum creatinine and is not obese (IBW_{man} = 50 + 2.3(Ht – 60 in) = 50 + 2.3(68 – 60) = 68 kg; % overweight = {100[80kg – 68 kg]}/68 kg = 18%). The Cockcroft–Gault equation can be used to estimate creatinine clearance:

$$CrCl_{est} = [(140 - age)BW]/(72 \cdot S_{Cr}) = [(140 - 80\ y)80\ kg]/(72 \cdot 1.5\ mg/dL)$$

$$CrCl_{est} = 44\ mL/min$$

2. *Choose desired steady-state serum concentrations.*

Patients with *S. viridans* endocarditis being treated with aminoglycoside antibiotics require steady-state peak concentrations ($C_{max,ss}$) of 3 to 5 μg/mL.

3. *Select the loading dose (see Table 4-3).*

A loading dose of 1.5 mg/kg provides a peak concentration of 5 to 7 μg/mL. This is the lowest dose suggested by the nomogram and is used in this example. However, some clinicians may substitute a loading dose of 1 to 1.2 mg/kg, designed to produce a steady-state peak concentration of 3 to 4 μg/mL.

LD = 1.5 mg/kg(80 kg) = 120 mg or LD = 1.2 mg/kg (80 kg) = 96 mg, rounded to 95 mg

4. *Determine the estimated half-life, maintenance dose, and dosage interval.*

From the nomogram, the estimated half-life is 6.5 hours, suggesting that a 12-dosage interval is appropriate. The maintenance dose (MD) is 72% of the loading dose (MD = 0.72[120 mg] = 86 mg or MD = 0.72[95 mg] = 68 mg), and the dosage interval is 12 hours.

Aminoglycoside doses should be rounded to the nearest 5 to 10 mg. Steady-state peak concentrations are similar if drawn immediately after a 1-hour infusion or 30 minutes after a 30-minute infusion, so the dose can be administered either way.

The prescribed maintenance dose is 85 mg gentamicin every 12 hours or 70 mg every 12 hours, depending on the loading dose chosen.

Because the patient is receiving concurrent treatment with ampicillin, care must be taken to avoid in vitro inactivation in blood sample tubes intended for the determination of aminoglycoside serum concentrations.

Hartford Nomogram Method for Extended-Interval Dosing

Interest is increasing in the use of extended-interval aminoglycoside dosing. Extended-interval doses obtained from the literature for patients with normal renal function are 4 to 7 mg/kg per day for gentamicin, tobramycin, or netilmicin and 11 to 20 mg/kg per day for amikacin.[3,19–26,32–37] To date, the only extended-interval aminoglycoside dosage approach for patients with renal dysfunction is the Hartford nomogram, which uses a 7-mg/kg dose[3] (Table 4-4). Although this nomogram was used in over 2000 patients, it has not been independently verified by investigators other than the originators and cannot be used for other dosage rates. The initial dose is 7 mg/kg of gentamicin or tobramycin. (Although it has not been tested with netilmicin, because of the pharmacokinetic similarity among

TABLE 4-4 Hartford Nomogram for Extended-Interval Aminoglycosides

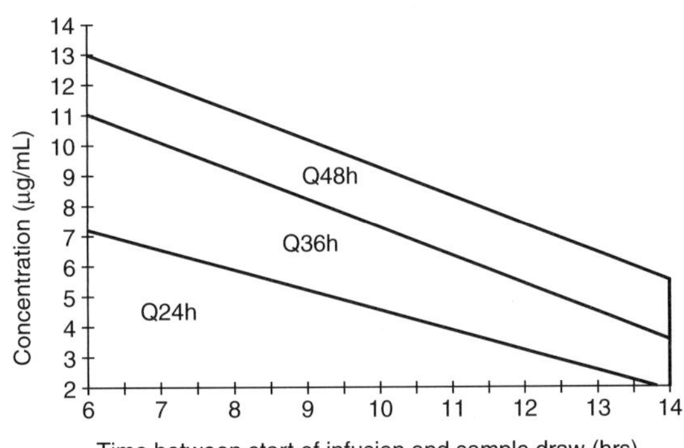

ODA nomogram for gentamicin and tobramycin at 7 mg kg.

1. Administer 7 mg/kg gentamicin or tobramycin with initial dosage interval:

ESTIMATED CrCl (mL/min)	INITIAL DOSAGE INTERVAL
≥60	q24h
40–59	q36h
20–39	q48h
<20	Monitor serial concentrations administer next dose when <1 μg/mL

2. Obtain timed serum concentration, 6–14 hours after dose (ideally first dose).
3. Alter dosage interval to that indicated by the nomogram zone (above q48h zone, monitor serial concentrations, and administer next dose when <1 μg/mL.

Adapted from Nicolau DP, Freeman CD, Belliveau PP, Nightingale CH, Ross JW, Quintilliani R. Experience with a once-daily aminoglycoside program administered to 2,184 adult patients. Antimicrob Agent Chemother 1995;39:650–655.

the antibiotics, it should be possible to use this aminoglycoside as well.) The dosage interval is set according to the patient's creatinine clearance (see Table 4-4).

The Hartford nomogram includes a method for adjusting doses based on gentamicin or tobramycin serum concentrations. This portion of the nomogram contains average serum concentration–time lines for gentamicin or tobramycin in patients with creatinine clearances of 60 mL/min, 40 mL/min, and 20 mL/min. A gentamicin or tobramycin serum concentration is measured 6 to 14 hours after the first dose is given, and this concentration–time point is plotted on the graph (see Table 4-4). The suggested dosage interval is indicated by which zone the serum concentration–time point falls in. To illustrate how the nomogram is used, the same patient examples used in the pharmacokinetic dosing section are repeated for this dosage approach using the same example number. Because the cystic fibrosis case example requires a different volume of distribution (0.35 L/kg) and extended-interval dosing has not been adequately tested in patients with endocarditis, the Hartford nomogram should not be used in these situations.

Example 1 JM is a 50-year-old, 70-kg, 178-cm (70-in) man with gram-negative pneumonia. His serum creatinine is 0.9 mg/dL, which has been stable over the last 5 days since admission. Compute a gentamicin dose using extended-interval dosing.

1. *Estimate the creatinine clearance.*

This patient has a stable serum creatinine and is not obese. The Cockcroft–Gault equation can be used to estimate creatinine clearance:

$$CrCl_{est} = [(140 - age)BW]/(72 \cdot S_{Cr}) = [(140 - 50\ y)70\ kg]/(72 \cdot 0.9\ mg/dL)$$

$$CrCl_{est} = 97\ mL/min$$

2. *Compute the initial dose and dosage interval (see Table 4-4).*

A dose (D) of 7 mg/kg provides a peak concentration >20 μg/mL.

$$D = 7\ mg/kg(70\ kg) = 490\ mg$$

Dosage interval is 24 hours using the nomogram. Aminoglycoside doses should be rounded to the nearest 5 to 10 mg.

The prescribed maintenance dose is 490 mg every 24 hours.

3. *Determine the dosage interval using serum concentration monitoring.*

A gentamicin serum concentration measured 10 hours after the dose is 3 μg/mL. Based on the nomogram, a dosage interval of 24 hours is the correct value and does not need to be altered.

Example 2 Same patient profile as in example 1, but serum creatinine is 3.5 mg/dL, indicating renal impairment.

1. *Estimate the creatinine clearance.*

This patient has a stable serum creatinine and is not obese. The Cockcroft–Gault equation can be used to estimate creatinine clearance:

$$CrCl_{est} = [(140 - age)BW]/(72 \cdot S_{Cr}) = [(140 - 50\ y)70\ kg]/(72 \cdot 3.5\ mg/dL)$$

$$CrCl_{est} = 25\ mL/min$$

2. *Compute the initial dose and dosage interval (see Table 4-4).*

A dose (D) of 7 mg/kg provides a peak concentration >20 μg/mL.

$$D = 7\ mg/kg(70\ kg) = 490\ mg$$

Dosage interval is 48 hours using the nomogram. Aminoglycoside doses should be rounded to the nearest 5 to 10 mg.

The prescribed maintenance dose is 490 mg gentamicin every 48 hours.

3. *Determine the dosage interval using serum concentration monitoring.*

A gentamicin serum concentration measured 13 hours after the dose is 9 μg/mL. Based on the nomogram, a dosage interval of 48 hours is too short, and serial concentrations should be monitored. When the gentamicin serum concentration is <1 μg/mL, the next dose can be given. Based on the patient's estimated elimination rate constant (k_e = 0.00293(CrCl) + 0.014 = 0.00293(25 mL/min) + 0.014 = 0.087 h^{-1}; $t_{1/2}$ = 0.693/k_e = 0.693/0.087 h^{-1} = 8 h), it will take approximately 3 to 4 half-lives or about an additional 24 to 32 hours after the gentamicin serum concentration for the value to drop below 1 μg/mL.

Example 3 ZW is a 35-year-old, 150-kg, 165-cm (65-in) woman with an intra-abdominal infection. Her serum creatinine is 1.1 mg/dL and stable. Compute a tobramycin dose using extended-interval dosing.

1. *Estimate the creatinine clearance.*

This patient has a stable serum creatinine and is obese ($IBW_{females}$ (in kg) = 45 + 2.3(Ht − 60 in) = 45 + 2.3(65 − 60) = 57 kg). The Salazar and Corcoran equation can be used to estimate creatinine clearance:

$$CrCl_{est(females)} = \frac{(146 - age)[(0.287 \cdot Wt) + (9.74 \cdot Ht^2)]}{(60 \cdot S_{Cr})}$$

$$CrCl_{est(females)} = \frac{(146 - 35\ y)\{(0.287 \cdot 150\ kg) + [9.74 \cdot (1.65\ m)^2]\}}{(60 \cdot 1.1\ mg/dL)} = 117\ mL/min$$

Note: Height is converted from inches to meters: Ht = (65 in · 2.54 cm/in)/(100 cm/m) = 1.65 m.

2. *Compute the initial dose and dosage interval (see Table 4-4).*

A dose (D) of 7 mg/kg provides a peak concentration >20 μg/mL. Because the patient is obese, adjusted body weight (ABW) is used to compute the dose: ABW = IBW + 0.4[TBW − IBW] = 57 kg + 0.4[150 kg − 57 kg] = 94 kg.

$$D = 7\ mg/kg(94\ kg) = 658\ mg$$

Dosage interval is 24 hours using the nomogram. Aminoglycoside doses should be rounded to the nearest 5 to 10 mg.

The prescribed maintenance dose is 660 mg tobramycin every 24 hours.

3. *Determine the dosage interval using serum concentration monitoring.*

A gentamicin serum concentration measured 8 hours after the dose is 4 μg/mL. Based on the nomogram, a dosage interval of 24 hours is the correct value and does not need to be altered.

Assuming linear pharmacokinetics, clinicians have begun to use the Hartford nomogram for doses other than 7 mg/kg. Because this approach has not been formally evaluated, extreme care should be exercised when using this approach. For example, if the clinical situation warrants it, a dose of 5 mg/kg can be administered to a patient, the initial dosage intervals suggested in the Hartford nomogram used, and a serum concentration measured to confirm the dosage interval. Assuming linear pharmacokinetics, the critical concentrations for changing dosage intervals on the Hartford nomogram graph can be decreased by 5/7 (the ratio of the 5 mg/kg dose administered to the 7 mg/kg dose suggested by the nomogram).

USE OF AMINOGLYCOSIDE SERUM CONCENTRATIONS TO ALTER DOSAGES

Because of pharmacokinetic variability among patients, doses computed using patient population characteristics are not likely to always produce expected aminoglycoside serum concentrations. Therefore, aminoglycoside serum concentrations are measured in many patients to ensure that therapeutic, nontoxic levels are present. However, not all patients require serum concentration monitoring. For example, if only a limited number of doses are expected to be administered, as in surgical prophylaxis or in a situation in which an appropriate dose for the patient's renal function and concurrent disease states is prescribed (e.g., 1 mg/kg every 8 hours for 3 to 5 days in a patient with a creatinine clearance of 80 to 120 mL/min for antibiotic synergy in the treatment of *Streptococcus aureus* aortic or mitral valve endocarditis), aminoglycoside serum concentration monitoring may not be necessary. Whether or not aminoglycoside concentrations are measured, important patient parameters (e.g., fever curves, white blood cell counts, and serum creatinine concentrations) should be monitored to confirm that the patient is responding to treatment and not developing adverse drug reactions.

When aminoglycoside serum concentrations are measured and a dosage change is necessary, clinicians should seek to use the simplest, most straightforward method of determining a dose that will provide safe and effective treatment. In most cases, a simple dosage ratio can be used to change aminoglycoside doses, because these antibiotics follow *linear pharmacokinetics.* Sometimes it is not possible to simply change the dose; the dosage interval must also be changed to achieve desired serum concentrations. In this case, it may be possible to use *pharmacokinetic concepts* to alter the aminoglycoside dose that the patient needs. In some situations, it may be necessary to compute the aminoglycoside pharmacokinetic parameters for the patient using the *Sawchuk-Zaske method* and to use these to calculate the best drug dose. Finally, computerized methods that incorporate expected population pharmacokinetic characteristics (*Bayesian pharmacokinetics computer programs*) can be used in difficult cases in which renal function is changing, serum concentrations are obtained at suboptimal times, or the patient was not at steady state when serum concentrations were measured.

Linear Pharmacokinetics Method

Because aminoglycoside antibiotics follow linear, dose-proportional pharmacokinetics, steady-state serum concentrations change in proportion to dose according to the following equation: $D_{new}/C_{ss,new} = D_{old}/C_{ss,old}$ or $D_{new} = (C_{ss,new}/C_{ss,old})D_{old}$, where D is the dose, Css is the steady-state peak or trough concentration, old indicates the dose that produced the steady-state concentration that the patient is currently receiving, and new denotes the dose necessary to produce the desired steady-state concentration. The advantage of this method is that it is both quick and simple. The disadvantages are that steady-state concentrations are required, and it may not be possible to attain desired serum concentrations by changing only the dosage.

Example 1 JM is a 50-year-old, 70-kg, 178-cm (70-in) man with gram-negative pneumonia. His serum creatinine is 0.9 mg/dL, which has been stable over the last 5 days since admission. Gentamicin 170 mg every 8 hours was prescribed and expected to achieve steady-state peak and trough concentrations of 9 μg/mL and 1 μg/mL, respectively. After the third dose, steady-state peak and trough concentrations were measured and were 12 μg/mL and 1.4 μg/mL, respectively. Calculate a new gentamicin dose that will provide a steady-state peak of 9 μg/mL.

1. *Estimate the creatinine clearance.*

This patient has a stable serum creatinine and is not obese. The Cockcroft–Gault equation can be used to estimate creatinine clearance:

$$CrCl_{est} = [(140 - age)BW]/(72 \cdot S_{Cr}) = [(140 - 50\ y)70\ kg]/(72 \cdot 0.9\ mg/dL)$$

$$CrCl_{est} = 97\ mL/min$$

2. *Estimate the elimination rate constant (k_e) and half-life ($t_{1/2}$).*

The elimination rate constant versus creatinine clearance relationship is used to estimate the gentamicin elimination rate for this patient:

$$k_e = 0.00293(CrCl) + 0.014 = 0.00293(97\ mL/min) + 0.014 = 0.298\ h^{-1}$$

$$t_{1/2} = 0.693/k_e = 0.693/0.298\ h^{-1} = 2.3\ h$$

Because the patient has been receiving gentamicin for more than 3 to 5 estimated half-lives, it is likely that the measured serum concentrations are steady-state values.

3. *Compute the new dose to achieve desired serum concentration.*

Using linear pharmacokinetics, the new dose to attain the desired concentration should be proportional to the old dose that produced the measured concentration:

$$D_{new} = (C_{ss,new}/C_{ss,old})D_{old} = [(9\ \mu g/mL)/(12\ \mu g/mL)]\ 170\ mg = 128\ mg, \text{ rounded to } 130\ mg$$

The new suggested dose is 130 mg every 8 hours to be started at the next scheduled dosing time.

4. *Check the steady-state trough concentration for new dosage regimen.*

Using linear pharmacokinetics, the new steady-state concentration can be estimated and should be proportional to the old dose that produced the measured concentration:

$$C_{ss,new} = (D_{new}/D_{old})C_{ss,old} = (130\ mg/170\ mg)\ 1.4\ \mu g/mL = 1.1\ \mu g/mL$$

This steady-state trough concentration should be safe and effective for the infection that is being treated.

Example 2 ZW is a 35-year-old, 150-kg, 165-cm (65-in) woman with an intra-abdominal infection. Her serum creatinine is 1.1 mg/dL and stable. Tobramycin 165 mg every 8 hours was prescribed and expected to achieve steady-state peak and trough concentrations of 6 μg/mL and 0.5 μg/mL, respectively. After the fifth dose, steady-state peak and trough concentrations were measured and were 4 μg/mL and <0.5 μg/mL (e.g., below assay limits), respectively. Calculate a new tobramycin dose that will provide a steady-state peak of 6 μg/mL.

1. *Estimate the creatinine clearance.*

This patient has a stable serum creatinine and is obese ($IBW_{females}$ (in kg) = 45 + 2.3(Ht – 60 in) = 45 + 2.3(65 – 60) = 57 kg). The Salazar and Corcoran equation can be used to estimate creatinine clearance:

$$CrCl_{est(females)} = \frac{(146 - age)[(0.287 \cdot Wt) + (9.74 \cdot Ht^2)]}{(60 \cdot S_{Cr})}$$

$$CrCl_{est(females)} = \frac{(146 - 35\ y)\{(0.287 \cdot 150\ kg) + [9.74 \cdot (1.65\ m)^2]\}}{(60 \cdot 1.1\ mg/dL)} = 117\ mL/min$$

Note: Height is converted from inches to meters: Ht = (65 in · 2.54 cm/in)/(100 cm/m) = 1.65 m.

2. *Estimate the elimination rate constant (k_e) and half-life ($t_{1/2}$).*

The elimination rate constant versus creatinine clearance relationship is used to estimate the gentamicin elimination rate:

$$k_e = 0.00293(CrCl) + 0.014 = 0.00293(117\ mL/min) + 0.014 = 0.357\ h^{-1}$$

$$t_{1/2} = 0.693/k_e = 0.693/0.357\ h^{-1} = 1.9\ h$$

Because the patient has been receiving tobramycin for more than 3 to 5 estimated half-lives, the measured serum concentrations are likely steady-state values.

3. *Compute the new dose to achieve desired serum concentration.*

Using linear pharmacokinetics, the new dose to attain the desired concentration should be proportional to the old dose that produced the measured concentration:

$$D_{new} = (C_{ss,new}/C_{ss,old})D_{old} = [(6\ \mu g/mL)/(4\ \mu g/mL)]\ 165\ mg = 247\ mg, \text{ rounded to } 250\ mg$$

The new suggested dose is 250 mg every 8 hours to be started at the next scheduled dosing time.

4. *Check the steady-state trough concentration for new dosage regimen.*

Using linear pharmacokinetics, the new steady-state concentration can be estimated and should be proportional to the old dose that produced the measured concentration. However, in this situation the trough concentration is below assay limits and was reported as <0.5 μg/mL. Because of this, the maximum value that the steady-state trough can be is 0.5 μg/mL, and this value can be used to compute a rough approximation of the expected concentration:

$$C_{ss,new} = (D_{new}/D_{old})C_{ss,old} = (250\ mg/165\ mg)\ 0.5\ \mu g/mL = 0.8\ \mu g/mL$$

Thus, the steady-state trough concentration should be no greater than 0.8 μg/mL. This steady-state trough concentration should be safe and effective for the infection that is being treated.

Pharmacokinetic Concepts Method

As implied by the name, the pharmacokinetic concepts technique derives alternate doses by estimating actual pharmacokinetic parameters or surrogates for pharmacokinetic parameters.[85] It is a very useful way of calculating drug doses when the linear pharmacokinetic method is not sufficient because a dosage change that produces a proportional change in steady-state peak and trough concentrations is not appropriate. The only requirement is a steady-state peak and trough aminoglycoside serum concentration pair obtained before and after a dose (Figure 4-5). The following steps are used to compute new aminoglycoside doses:

1. *Draw a rough sketch of the serum log concentration–time curve by hand, keeping track of the relative time between the serum concentrations (see Figure 4-5).*

2. *Because the patient is at steady state, the trough concentration can be extrapolated to the next trough value time (see Figure 4-5).*

3. *Draw the elimination curve between the steady-state peak concentration and the extrapolated trough concentration. Use this line to estimate half-life.* For example, a patient receives gentamicin 80 mg given every 8 hours that produces a steady-state peak of 7 μg/mL and a steady-state trough of 3.2 μg/mL. The dose is infused over 30 minutes with the peak concentration drawn 30 minutes later (see Figure 4-5). The time between the measured steady-state peak and the extrapolated trough concentration is 7 hours (the 8-hour dosage interval minus the 1-hour combined infusion and waiting time). The definition of half-life is the time needed for serum concentrations to decrease by half. Because the serum concentration declined by approximately half from the peak concentration to the trough concentration, the aminoglycoside half-life for this patient is approximately 7 hours. This information is used to set the new dosage interval for the patient.

4. *Determine the difference in concentration between the steady-state peak and trough concentrations. The difference in concentration changes proportionally with the dose size.* In this example, the patient is receiving a gentamicin dose of 80 mg every 8 hours, which produced steady-state peak and trough concentrations of 7 μg/mL and 3.2 μg/mL, respectively. The difference between the peak and trough values is 3.8 μg/mL. The change in serum concentration is proportional to the dose, and this information is used to set a new dose for the patient.

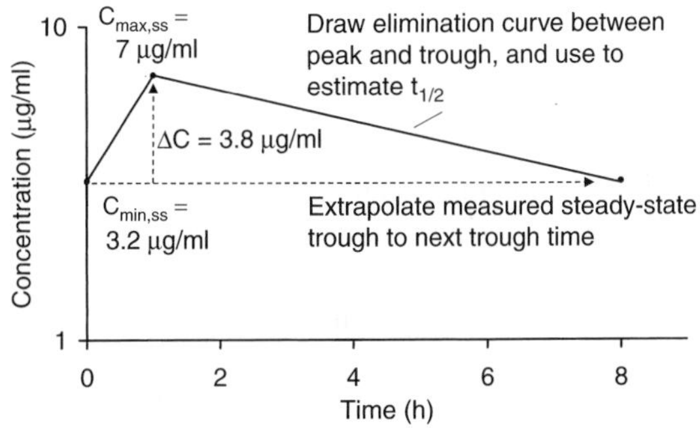

FIGURE 4-5 Graphic representation of the pharmacokinetic concepts method in which steady-state peak ($C_{max,ss}$) and trough ($C_{min,ss}$) concentration pair is used to individualize aminoglycoside therapy. Because the patient is at steady state, consecutive trough concentrations are identical, so the trough concentration can be extrapolated to the next predose time. The change in concentration after a dose is given *(ΔC)* is a surrogate measure of the volume of distribution and is used to compute the new dose for the patient.

5. *Choose new steady-state peak and trough concentrations.* For this example, the desired steady-state peak and trough concentrations are approximately 7 μg/mL and 1 μg/mL, respectively.

6. *Determine the new dosage interval for the desired concentrations.* In this example, the patient currently has the desired peak concentration of 7 μg/mL. In 1 half-life, the serum concentration declines to 3.5 μg/mL, in an additional half-life the gentamicin concentration decreases to 1.8 μg/mL, and in still another half-life the concentration declines to 0.9 μg/mL (Figure 4-6). Because the approximate half-life is 7 hours and 3 half-lives are required for serum concentrations to decrease from the desired peak concentration to the desired trough concentration, the dosage interval should be 21 hours (7 hours × 3 half-lives). This value is rounded to the clinically acceptable value of 24 hours, and the actual trough concentration is expected to be slightly lower than 0.9 μg/mL.

7. *Determine the new dose for the desired concentrations.* The desired peak concentration is 7 μg/mL, and the expected trough concentration is 0.9 μg/mL. The change in concentration between these values is 6.1 μg/mL. It is known from measured serum concentrations that administration of 80 mg changes serum concentrations by 3.8 μg/mL and that the change in serum concentration between the peak and trough values is proportional to the size of the dose. Therefore, a simple ratio is used to compute the required dose: $D_{new} = (\Delta C_{new}/\Delta C_{old})D_{old}$, where D_{new} and D_{old} are the new and old doses, respectively; ΔC_{new} is the change in concentration between the peak and trough for the new dose; and ΔC_{old} is the change in concentration between the peak and trough for the old dose (Note: This relationship is appropriate because doses are given into a fixed, constant volume of distribution—not because the drug follows linear pharmacokinetics. Therefore, this method works whether the agent follows nonlinear or linear pharmacokinetics). For this example: D_{new} = [(6.1 μg/mL)/(3.8 μg/mL)] 80 mg = 128 mg, which is rounded to 130 mg. Gentamicin 130 mg every 24 hours is started 24 hours after the last dose of the previous dosage regimen.

Once the pharmacokinetic concept method is mastered, it can be used without a calculator. The following are examples that use the *pharmacokinetic concepts method* to change aminoglycoside doses.

Example 1 JM is a 50-year-old, 70-kg, 178-cm (70-in) man with gram-negative pneumonia. His serum creatinine is 3.5 mg/dL, which has been stable over the last 5 days since admission. Gentamicin 115 mg every 24 hours was prescribed and is expected to achieve steady-state peak and trough concentrations of 8 to 10 μg/mL and <2 μg/mL, respectively. After the third dose, steady-state peak and trough concentrations were measured and were 12 μg/mL and 3.5 μg/mL, respectively. Calculate a new gentamicin dose that will provide a steady-state peak of 9 μg/mL and a trough between <2 μg/mL.

1. *Estimate the creatinine clearance.*

This patient has a stable serum creatinine and is not obese. The Cockcroft–Gault equation can be used to estimate creatinine clearance:

$$CrCl_{est} = [(140 - age)BW]/(72 \cdot S_{Cr}) = [(140 - 50\ y)70\ kg]/(72 \cdot 3.5\ mg/dL)$$

$$CrCl_{est} = 25\ mL/min$$

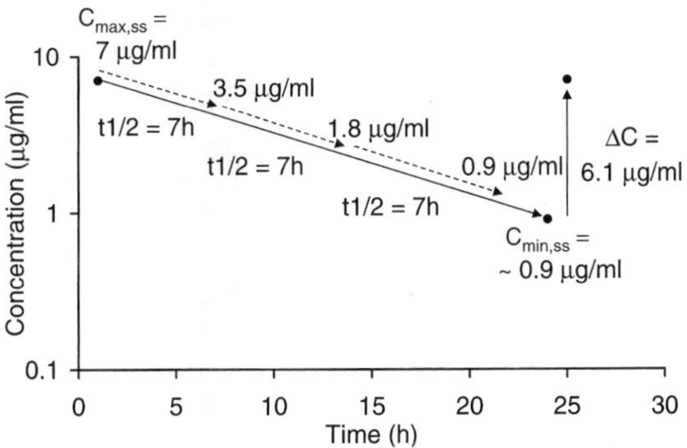

FIGURE 4-6 The pharmacokinetic concepts method uses the estimated half-life to graphically compute the new dosage interval and the change in concentration to calculate the aminoglycoside dose for an individual patient.

2. *Estimate the elimination rate constant (k_e) and half-life ($t_{1/2}$).*

The elimination rate constant versus creatinine clearance relationship is used to estimate the gentamicin elimination rate for this patient:

$$k_e = 0.00293(\text{CrCl}) + 0.014 = 0.00293(25 \text{ mL/min}) + 0.014 = 0.087 \text{ h}^{-1}$$

$$t_{1/2} = 0.693/k_e = 0.693/0.087 \text{ h}^{-1} = 8 \text{ h}$$

Because the patient has been receiving gentamicin for more than 3 to 5 estimated half-lives, it is likely that the measured serum concentrations are steady-state values. Use the *pharmacokinetics concepts method* to compute a new dose.

1. *Draw a rough sketch of the serum log concentration–time curve by hand, keeping track of the relative time between the serum concentrations (Figure 4-7).*

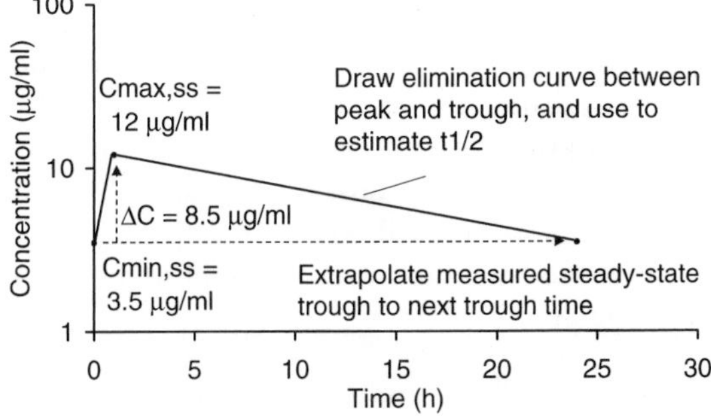

FIGURE 4-7 Graphic representation of the pharmacokinetic concepts method in which a steady-state peak ($C_{max,ss}$) and trough ($C_{min,ss}$) concentration pair is used to individualize aminoglycoside therapy. Because the patient is at steady state, consecutive trough concentrations are identical, so the trough concentration can be extrapolated to the next predose time. The change in concentration after a dose is given (ΔC) is a surrogate measure of the volume of distribution and is used to compute the new dose for the patient.

2. *Because the patient is at steady-state, the trough concentration can be extrapolated to the next trough value time (see Figure 4-7).*

3. *Draw the elimination curve between the steady-state peak concentration and the extrapolated trough concentration. Use this line to estimate half-life.* The patient is receiving gentamicin 115 mg every 24 hours, which produces a steady-state peak of 12 μg/mL and a steady-state trough of 3.5 μg/mL. The dose is infused over 30 minutes, and the peak concentration is drawn 30-minutes later (see Figure 4-7). The time between the measured steady-state peak and the extrapolated trough concentration is 23 hours (the 24-hour dosage interval minus the 1 hour combined infusion and waiting time). The definition of half-life is the time needed for serum concentrations to decrease by half. It takes 1 half-life for the peak serum concentration to decline from 12 μg/mL to 6 μg/mL and an additional half-life for the serum concentration to decrease from 6 μg/mL to 3 μg/mL. The concentration of 3 μg/mL is very close to the extrapolated trough value of 3.5 μg/mL. Therefore, 2 half-lives expired during the 23-hour time period between the peak concentration and the extrapolated trough concentration, and the estimated half-life is 12 hours (23 hours/2 half-lives = ~12 hours). This information can be used to set the new dosage interval for the patient.

4. *Determine the difference in concentration between the steady-state peak and trough concentrations. The difference in concentration changes proportionally with the dose size.* In this example, the patient is receiving gentamicin 115 mg every 24 hours, which produced steady-state peak and trough concentrations of 12 μg/mL and 3.5 μg/mL, respectively. The difference between the peak and trough values is 8.5 μg/mL. The change in serum concentration is proportional to the dose, and this information is used to set a new dose for the patient.

5. *Choose new steady-state peak and trough concentrations.* For this example, the desired steady-state peak and trough concentrations are approximately 9 μg/mL and <2 μg/mL, respectively.

6. *Determine the new dosage interval for the desired concentrations (Figure 4-8).* Using the desired concentrations, it takes 1 half-life for the peak concentration of 9 μg/mL to decrease to 4.5 μg/mL, 1 more half-life for the serum concentration to decrease to 2.3 μg/mL, and an additional half-life for serum concentrations to decline to 1.2 μg/mL. Therefore, the dosage interval needs to be approximately 3 half-lives or 36 hours (12 hours × 3 half-lives = 36 hours). When a dosage interval such as 36 hours is used, care must be taken to ensure that the scheduled doses are actually administered. Because the drug is given only every other day, this type of administration schedule is sometimes overlooked and doses are missed.

7. *Determine the new dose for the desired concentrations (see Figure 4-8).* The desired peak concentration is 9 μg/mL, and the expected trough concentration is 1.2 μg/mL. The change in concentration between these values is 7.8 μg/mL. It is known from measured serum concentrations that administration of 115 mg changes serum concentrations by 8.5 μg/mL and that the change in serum concentration between the peak and trough values is proportional to the size of the dose. In this case, $D_{new} = (\Delta C_{new}/\Delta C_{old})D_{old}$ = [(7.8 μg/mL)/(8.5 μg/mL)] 115 mg = 105 mg. Gentamicin 105 mg every 36 hours is started 36 hours after the last dose of the previous dosage regimen.

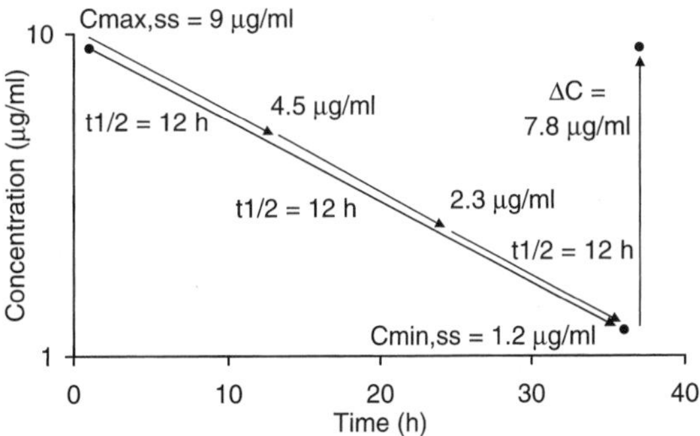

FIGURE 4-8 The pharmacokinetic concepts method uses the estimated half-life to graphically compute the new dosage interval and the change in concentration to calculate the aminoglycoside dose for an individual patient.

Example 2 ZW is a 35-year-old, 150-kg, 165-cm (65-in) woman with an intra-abdominal infection. Her serum creatinine is 1.1 mg/dL and stable. Tobramycin 165 mg every 8 hours was prescribed and expected to achieve steady-state peak and trough concentrations of 6 μg/mL and 0.5 μg/mL, respectively. After the fifth dose, steady-state peak and trough concentrations were measured and were 5 μg/mL and 2.6 μg/mL, respectively. Calculate a new tobramycin dose that will provide a steady-state peak of 6 μg/mL and a steady-state trough ≤1.

1. *Estimate the creatinine clearance.*

This patient has a stable serum creatinine and is obese ($IBW_{females}$ (in kg) = 45 + 2.3(Ht − 60 in) = 45 + 2.3(65 − 60) = 57 kg. The Salazar and Corcoran equation can be used to estimate creatinine clearance:

$$CrCl_{est(females)} = \frac{(146 - age)[(0.287 \cdot Wt) + (9.74 \cdot Ht^2)]}{(60 \cdot S_{Cr})}$$

$$CrCl_{est(females)} = \frac{(146 - 35\ y)\{(0.287 \cdot 150\ kg) + [9.74 \cdot (1.65\ m)^2]\}}{(60 \cdot 1.1\ mg/dL)} = 117\ mL/min$$

Note: Height is converted from inches to meters: Ht = (65 in · 2.54 cm/in)/(100 cm/m) = 1.65 m.

2. *Estimate the elimination rate constant (k_e) and half-life ($t_{1/2}$).*

The elimination rate constant versus creatinine clearance relationship is used to estimate the tobramycin elimination rate for this patient:

$$k_e = 0.00293(CrCl) + 0.014 = 0.00293(117\ mL/min) + 0.014 = 0.357\ h^{-1}$$

$$t_{1/2} = 0.693/k_e = 0.693/0.357\ h^{-1} = 1.9\ h$$

Because the patient has been receiving tobramycin for more than 3 to 5 estimated half-lives, it is likely that the measured serum concentrations are steady-state values. Use the *pharmacokinetic concepts method* to compute a new dose.

1. *Draw a rough sketch of the serum log concentration–time curve by hand, keeping track of the relative time between the serum concentrations (Figure 4-9).*

2. *Because the patient is at steady state, the trough concentration can be extrapolated to the next trough value time (see Figure 4-9).*

3. *Draw the elimination curve between the steady-state peak concentration and the extrapolated trough concentration. Use this line to estimate half-life.* The patient is receiving tobramycin 165 mg given every 8 hours, which produces a steady-state peak of 5 μg/mL and a steady-state trough of 2.6 μg/mL. The dose is infused over 30 minutes, and the peak concentration is drawn 30 minutes later (see Figure 4-9). The time between the measured steady-state peak and the extrapolated trough concentration is 7 hours (the 8-hour dosage interval minus the 1-hour combined infusion and waiting time). The definition of half-life is the time needed for serum concentrations to decrease by half. It takes 1 half-life for the peak serum concentration to decline from 5 μg/mL to 2.5 μg/mL. The concentration of 2.6 μg/mL is very close to the extrapolated trough value of 2.5 μg/mL. Therefore, 1 half-life expired during the 7-hour time period between the peak concentration and extrapolated trough concentration, and the estimated half-life is 7 hours. This information is used to set the new dosage interval for the patient.

4. *Determine the difference in concentration between the steady-state peak and trough concentrations. The difference in concentration changes proportionally with the dose size.* In this example, the patient is receiving tobramycin 165 mg every 8 hours, which produced steady-state peak and trough concentrations of 5 μg/mL and 2.6 μg/mL, respectively. The difference between the peak and trough values is 2.4 μg/mL. The change in serum concentration is proportional to the dose, and this information is used to set a new dose for the patient.

5. *Choose new steady-state peak and trough concentrations.* For this example, the desired steady-state peak and trough concentrations are approximately 6 μg/mL and ≤1 μg/mL, respectively.

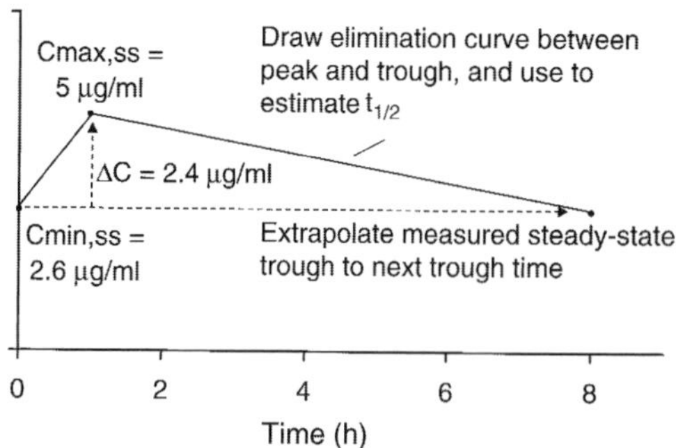

FIGURE 4-9 Graphic representation of the pharmacokinetic concepts method in which a steady-state peak ($C_{max,ss}$) and trough ($C_{min,ss}$) concentration pair is used to individualize aminoglycoside therapy. Because the patient is at steady state, consecutive trough concentrations are identical, so the trough concentration can be extrapolated to the next predose time. The change in concentration after a dose is given (ΔC) is a surrogate measure of the volume of distribution and is used to compute the new dose for the patient.

6. *Determine the new dosage interval for the desired concentrations.* Using the desired concentrations, it takes 1 half-life for the peak concentration of 6 μg/mL to decrease to 3 μg/mL, 1 more half-life for the serum concentration to decrease to 1.5 μg/mL, and an additional half-life for serum concentrations to decline to 0.8 μg/mL. Therefore, the dosage interval needs to be approximately 3 half-lives or 21 hours (7 hours × 3 half-lives = 21 hours), which is rounded to 24 hours.

7. *Determine the new dose for the desired concentrations.* The desired peak concentration is 6 μg/mL, and the expected trough concentration is 0.8 μg/mL. The change in concentration between these values is 5.2 μg/mL. It is known from measured serum concentrations that administration of 165 mg changes serum concentrations by 2.4 μg/mL and that the change in serum concentration between the peak and trough values is proportional to the size of the dose. In this case, $D_{new} = (\Delta C_{new}/\Delta C_{old})D_{old}$ = [(5.2 μg/mL)/(2.4 μg/mL)] 165 mg = 358 mg, rounded to 360 mg. Tobramycin 360 mg every 24 hours is started 24 hours after the last dose of the previous dosage regimen.

Sawchuk-Zaske Method

The Sawchuk-Zaske method of adjusting aminoglycoside doses was among the first techniques available to change doses using serum concentrations.[2,46–48,81] It allows the computation of an individual's unique pharmacokinetic constants and uses these to calculate a dose to achieve desired aminoglycoside concentrations. The standard Sawchuk-Zaske method conducts a small pharmacokinetic experiment using three to four aminoglycoside serum concentrations obtained during a dosage interval and does not require steady-state conditions. The modified Sawchuk-Zaske method assumes that steady state has been achieved and requires only a steady-state peak and trough concentration pair obtained before and after a dose. The Sawchuk-Zaske method has also been successfully used to dose vancomycin and theophylline.

STANDARD SAWCHUK-ZASKE METHOD

The standard version of the Sawchuk-Zaske method does not require steady-state concentrations. A trough aminoglycoside concentration is obtained before a dose, a peak aminoglycoside concentration is obtained after the dose is infused (immediately after a 1-hour infusion or 30 minutes after a 30-minute infusion), and one to two additional postdose serum aminoglycoside concentrations are obtained (Figure 4-10). Ideally, the one to two postdose concentrations should be obtained at least 1 estimated half-life from each other to minimize the influence of assay error. The postdose serum concentrations are used to calculate the aminoglycoside elimination rate constant and half-life (see Figure 4-10). The half-life can be computed by graphing the postdose concentrations on semilogarithmic paper, drawing the best straight line through the data points, and determining the time needed for serum concentrations to decline by half. After the half-life is known, the elimination rate constant (k_e) can be computed: $k_e = 0.693/t_{1/2}$. Alternatively, the elimination rate constant can be directly calculated using the postdose serum concentrations (k_e = [$\ln C_1 - \ln C_2$]/Δt, where C_1 and C_2 are postdose serum concentrations and Δt is the time that expired between the times that C_1 and C_2 were obtained), and the half-life can be computed using the elimination rate constant ($t_{1/2} = 0.693/k_e$). The volume of distribution is calculated using the following equation:

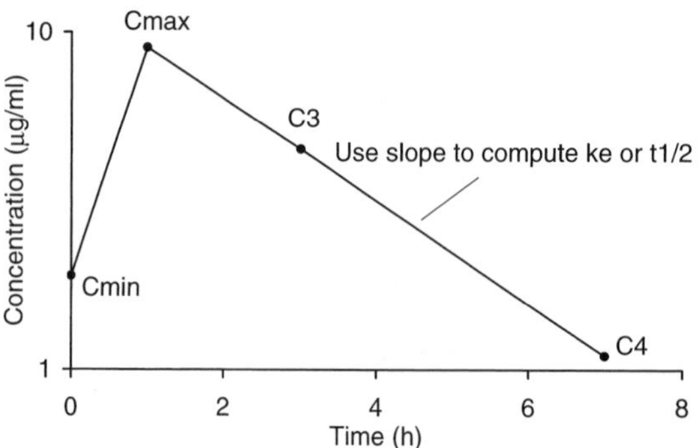

FIGURE 4-10 The Sawchuk-Zaske method for individualization of aminoglycoside doses uses a trough (C_{min}), peak (C_{max}), and one to two additional postdose concentrations (C_3, C_4) to compute a patient's unique pharmacokinetic parameters. This version of the Sawchuk-Zaske method does not require steady-state conditions. The peak and trough concentrations are used to calculate the volume of distribution, and the postdose concentrations (C_{max}, C_3, C_4) are used to compute half-life. After volume of distribution and half-life have been measured, they can be used to compute the exact dose needed to achieve desired aminoglycoside concentrations.

$$V = \frac{D/t'(1 - e^{-k_e t'})}{k_e[C_{max} - (C_{min} e^{-k_e t'})]}$$

where D is the aminoglycoside dose, t′ is the infusion time, k_e is the elimination rate constant, C_{max} is the peak concentration, and C_{min} is the trough concentration. The elimination rate constant and volume of distribution measured in this fashion are the patient's unique aminoglycoside pharmacokinetic constants and can be used in one-compartment model intravenous infusion equations to compute the required dose to achieve any desired serum concentration.

STEADY-STATE SAWCHUK-ZASKE METHOD

If a steady-state peak and trough aminoglycoside concentration pair is available for a patient, the Sawchuk-Zaske method can be used to compute patient pharmacokinetic parameters and aminoglycoside doses (Figure 4-11). Because the patient is at steady state, the measured trough concentration obtained before the dose was given can be extrapolated to the next dosage time and used to compute the aminoglycoside elimination rate constant ($k_e = [\ln C_{max,ss} - \ln C_{min,ss}]/\tau - t'$, where $C_{max,ss}$ and $C_{min,ss}$ are the steady-state peak and trough serum concentrations and t′ and τ are the infusion time and dosage interval), and the half-life can be computed using the elimination rate constant ($t_{1/2} = 0.693/k_e$). The volume of distribution is calculated using the following equation:

$$V = \frac{D/t'(1 - e^{-k_e t'})}{k_e[C_{max,ss} - (C_{min,ss}\, e^{-k_e t'})]}$$

where D is the aminoglycoside dose, t′ is the infusion time, k_e is the elimination rate constant, $C_{max,ss}$ is the steady-state peak concentration and $C_{min,ss}$ is the steady-state trough

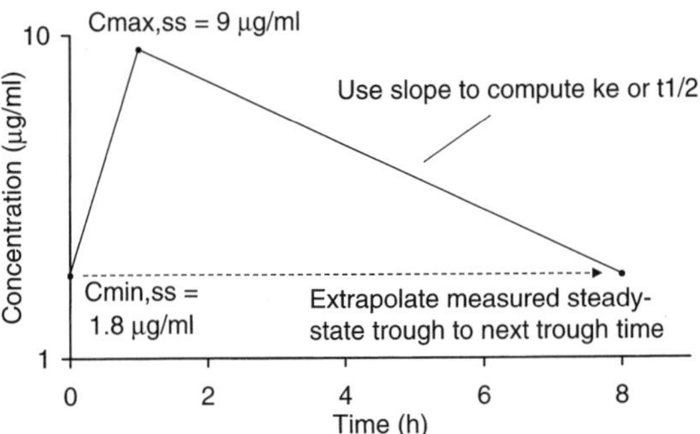

FIGURE 4-11 The steady-state version of the Sawchuk-Zaske method uses a steady-state peak ($C_{max,ss}$) and trough ($C_{min,ss}$) concentration pair to individualize aminoglycoside therapy. Because the patient is at steady state, consecutive trough concentrations are identical, so the trough concentration can be extrapolated to the next predose time. The steady-state peak and trough concentrations are used to calculate the volume of distribution and half-life. After volume of distribution and half-life have been measured, they can be used to compute the exact dose needed to achieve desired aminoglycoside concentrations.

concentration. The elimination rate constant and volume of distribution measured in this way are the patient's unique aminoglycoside pharmacokinetic constants and can be used in one-compartment model intravenous infusion equations to compute the required dose to achieve any desired serum concentration. The dosage calculations are similar to those done in the initial dosage section of this chapter, except that the patient's real pharmacokinetic parameters rather than population pharmacokinetic estimates are used in the equations.

To illustrate the similarities and differences between the *pharmacokinetic concepts method* and the *Sawchuk-Zaske method,* some of the same cases used in the previous section are used as examples here.

Example 1 JM is a 50-year-old, 70-kg, 178-cm (70-in) man with gram-negative pneumonia. His serum creatinine is 3.5 mg/dL, which has been stable over the last 5 days since admission. Gentamicin 115 mg every 24 hours was prescribed and expected to achieve steady-state peak and trough concentrations of 8 to 10 μg/mL and >2 μg/mL, respectively. After the third dose, steady-state peak and trough concentrations were measured and were 12 μg/mL and 3.5 μg/mL, respectively. Calculate a new gentamicin dose that will provide a steady-state peak of 9 μg/mL and a trough <2 μg/mL.

1. *Estimate the creatinine clearance.*

This patient has a stable serum creatinine and is not obese. The Cockcroft–Gault equation can be used to estimate creatinine clearance:

$$CrCl_{est} = [(140 - age)BW]/(72 \cdot S_{Cr}) = [(140 - 50\ y)70\ kg]/(72 \cdot 3.5\ mg/dL)$$

$$CrCl_{est} = 25\ mL/min$$

2. *Estimate the elimination rate constant (k_e) and half-life ($t_{1/2}$).*

The elimination rate constant versus creatinine clearance relationship is used to estimate the gentamicin elimination rate for this patient:

$$k_e = 0.00293(CrCl) + 0.014 = 0.00293(25 \text{ mL/min}) + 0.014 = 0.087 \text{ h}^{-1}$$

$$t_{1/2} = 0.693/k_e = 0.693/0.087 \text{ h}^{-1} = 8 \text{ h}$$

Because the patient has been receiving gentamicin for more than 3 to 5 estimated half-lives, the measured serum concentrations are likely to be steady-state values. Use the *steady-state Sawchuk-Zaske method* to compute a new dose.

1. *Compute the patient's elimination rate constant and half-life (note: for infusion times less than 1 hour, t′ is considered to be the sum of the infusion and waiting times).*

$$k_e = (\ln C_{max,ss} - \ln C_{min,ss})/\tau - t' = (\ln 12 \text{ μg/mL} - \ln 3.5 \text{ μg/mL})/(24 \text{ h} - 1 \text{ h}) = 0.054 \text{ h}^{-1}$$

$$t_{1/2} = 0.693/k_e = 0.693/0.054 \text{ h}^{-1} = 12.8 \text{ h}$$

2. *Compute the patient's volume of distribution.*

$$V = \frac{D/t'(1 - e^{-k_e t'})}{k_e[C_{max,ss} - (C_{min,ss}e^{-k_e t'})]} = \frac{(115 \text{ mg/1h})(1 - e^{-(0.054 \text{ h}^{-1})(1 \text{ h})})}{0.054 \text{ h}^{-1}[12 \text{ mg/L} - (3.5 \text{ mg/L } e^{-(0.054 \text{ h}^{-1})(1 \text{ h})})]}$$

$$V = 12.9 \text{ L}$$

3. *Choose new steady-state peak and trough concentrations.* For this example, the desired steady-state peak and trough concentrations are approximately 9 μg/mL and 1.5 μg/mL, respectively.

4. *Determine the new dosage interval for the desired concentrations.* As in the initial dosage section of this chapter, the dosage interval (τ) is computed using the following equation and a 1-hour infusion time (t′):

$$\tau = [(\ln C_{max,ss} - \ln C_{min,ss})/k_e] + t' = [(\ln 9 \text{ μg/mL} - \ln 1.5 \text{ μg/mL})/0.054 \text{ h}^{-1}] + 1 \text{ h} = 34 \text{ h, rounded to 36 h}$$

5. *Determine the new dose for the desired concentrations.* The dose is computed following the one-compartment model intravenous infusion equation used in the initial dosing section of this chapter:

$$k_0 = C_{max,ss}\, k_e V[(1 - e^{-k_e\tau})/(1 - e^{-k_e t'})]$$

$$k_0 = (9 \text{ mg/L} \cdot 0.054 \text{ h}^{-1} \cdot 12.8 \text{ L})[(1 - e^{-(0.054 \text{ h}^{-1})(36 \text{ h})})/(1 - e^{-(0.054 \text{ h}^{-1})(1 \text{ h})})] = 101 \text{ mg, rounded to 100 mg}$$

Gentamicin 100 mg every 36 hours is prescribed to begin 36 hours after the last dose of the previous regimen. This dose is very similar to that derived for the patient using the pharmacokinetic concepts method (105 mg every 36 hours).

Example 2 ZW is a 35-year-old, 150-kg, 165-cm (65-in) woman with an intra-abdominal infection. Her serum creatinine is 1.1 mg/dL and stable. Tobramycin 165 mg every 8 hours was prescribed and expected to achieve steady-state peak and trough concentrations of 6 μg/mL and 0.5 μg/mL, respectively. After the fifth dose, steady-state peak and trough concentrations were measured and were 5 μg/mL and 2.6 μg/mL, respectively. Calculate a new tobramycin dose that will provide a steady-state peak of 6 μg/mL and a steady-state trough ≤1.

1. *Estimate the creatinine clearance.*

This patient has a stable serum creatinine and is obese ($IBW_{females}$ (in kg) = 45 + 2.3 (Ht – 60 in) = 45 + 2.3(65 – 60) = 57 kg). The Salazar and Corcoran equation can be used to estimate creatinine clearance:

$$CrCl_{est(females)} = \frac{(146 - age)[(0.287 \cdot Wt) + (9.74 \cdot Ht^2)]}{(60 \cdot S_{Cr})}$$

$$CrCl_{est(females)} = \frac{(146 - 35\ y)\{(0.287 \cdot 150\ kg) + [9.74 \cdot (1.65\ m)^2]\}}{(60 \cdot 1.1\ mg/dL)} = 117\ mL/min$$

Note: Height is converted from inches to meters: Ht = (65 in · 2.54 cm/in)/(100 cm/m) = 165 m.

2. *Estimate the elimination rate constant (k_e) and half-life ($t_{1/2}$).*

The elimination rate constant versus creatinine clearance relationship is used to estimate the tobramycin elimination rate:

$$k_e = 0.00293(CrCl) + 0.014 = 0.00293(117\ mL/min) + 0.014 = 0.357\ h^{-1}$$

$$t_{1/2} = 0.693/k_e = 0.693/0.357\ h^{-1} = 1.9\ h$$

Because the patient has been receiving tobramycin for more than 3 to 5 estimated half-lives, the measured serum concentrations are likely to be steady-state values. Use the *steady-state Sawchuk-Zaske method* to compute a new dose.

1. *Compute the patient's elimination rate constant and half-life (note: for infusion times less than 1 hour, t′ is considered to be the sum of the infusion and waiting times).*

$$k_e = (\ln C_{max,ss} - \ln C_{min,ss})/\tau - t' = (\ln 5\ \mu g/mL - \ln 2.6\ \mu g/mL)/(8\ h - 1\ h) = 0.093\ h^{-1}$$

$$t_{1/2} = 0.693/k_e = 0.693/0.093\ h^{-1} = 7.5\ h$$

2. *Compute the patient's volume of distribution.*

$$V = \frac{D/t'\ (1 - e^{-k_e t'})}{k_e[C_{max,ss} - (C_{min,ss} e^{-k_e t'})]} = \frac{(165\ mg/1h)(1 - e^{-(0.093\ h^{-1})(1\ h)})}{0.093\ h^{-1}[5\ mg/L - (2.6\ mg/L\ e^{-(0.093\ h^{-1})(1\ h)})]}$$

$$V = 59.9\ L$$

3. *Choose new steady-state peak and trough concentrations.* For this example, the desired steady-state peak and trough concentrations are 6 μg/mL and 0.8 μg/mL, respectively.

4. *Determine the new dosage interval for the desired concentrations.* As in the initial dosage section of this chapter, the dosage interval (τ) is computed using the following equation with a 1-hour infusion time (t′):

$$\tau = [(\ln C_{max,ss} - \ln C_{min,ss})/k_e] + t' = [(\ln 6\ \mu g/mL - \ln 0.8\ \mu g/mL)/0.093\ h^{-1}] + 1\ h = 23\ h, \text{ rounded to } 24\ h$$

5. *Determine the new dose for the desired concentrations.* The dose is computed following the one-compartment model intravenous infusion equation used in the initial dosing section of this chapter:

$$k_0 = C_{max,ss} k_e V[(1 - e^{-k_e \tau})/(1 - e^{-k_e t'})]$$

$$k_0 = (6\ mg/L \cdot 0.093\ h^{-1} \cdot 59.9\ L)[(1 - e^{-(0.093\ h^{-1})(24\ h)})/(1 - e^{-(0.093\ h^{-1})(1\ h)})]$$
$$= 336\ mg, \text{ rounded to } 335\ mg$$

Gentamicin 335 mg every 24 hours is prescribed to begin 24 hours after the last dose of the previous regimen. This dose is very similar to that derived for the patient using the pharmacokinetic concepts method (360 mg every 24 hours).

Example 3 JH is a 24-year-old, 70-kg, 183-cm (72-in) man with gram-negative pneumonia. His serum creatinine is 1.0 mg/dL, which has been stable over the last 7 days since admission. Amikacin 400 mg every 8 hours was prescribed. After the third dose, the following amikacin serum concentrations were obtained:

TIME	AMIKACIN CONCENTRATION (μg/mL)
0800 H	2.0
0800–0900 H	Amikacin 400 mg administered to patient
0900 H	22.1
1100 H	11.9
1600 H	2.5

Medication administration sheets were checked, and the previous dose was given 2 hours early (2200 H the previous day). Because of this, it is known that the patient is not at steady state. Calculate a new amikacin dose that will provide a steady-state peak of 28 μg/mL and a trough of 3 μg/mL. Use the *Sawchuk-Zaske method* to compute a new dose.

1. *Plot the serum concentration–time data (Figure 4-12). Because serum concentrations decrease in a straight line, use any two postdose concentrations to compute the patient's elimination rate constant and half-life.*

$$k_e = (\ln C_{max,ss} - \ln C_{min,ss})/\tau - t' = (\ln 22.1\ \mu g/mL - \ln 2.5\ \mu g/mL)/(16 - 09) = 0.311\ h^{-1}$$

$$t_{1/2} = 0.693/k_e = 0.693/0.311\ h^{-1} = 2.2\ h$$

2. *Compute the patient's volume of distribution.*

$$V = \frac{D/t'\ (1 - e^{-k_e t'})}{k_e[C_{max,ss} - (C_{min,ss} e^{-k_e t'})]} = \frac{(400\ mg/1\ h)(1 - e^{-(0.311\ h^{-1})(1\ h)})}{0.311\ h^{-1}[22.1\ mg/L - (2.0\ mg/L\ e^{-(0.311\ h^{-1})(1\ h)})]}$$

$$V = 16.7\ L$$

3. *Choose new steady-state peak and trough concentrations.* For this example, the desired steady-state peak and trough concentrations are 28 μg/mL and 3 μg/mL, respectively.

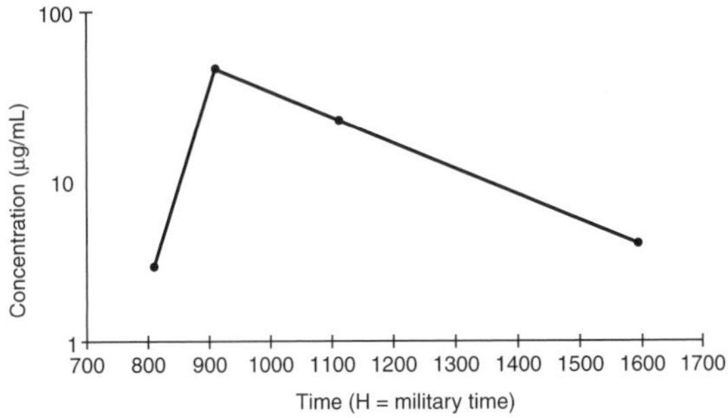

FIGURE 4-12 Graph of amikacin serum concentrations used in the Sawchuk-Zaske method example.

4. *Determine the new dosage interval for the desired concentrations.* As in the initial dosage section of this chapter, the dosage interval (τ) is computed by means of the following equation using a 1-hour infusion time (t'):

$$\tau = [(\ln C_{max,ss} - \ln C_{min,ss})/k_e] + t' = [(\ln 28\ \mu g/mL - \ln 3\ \mu g/mL)/0.311\ h^{-1}] + 1\ h = 8\ h$$

5. *Determine the new dose for the desired concentrations.* The dose is computed following the one-compartment model intravenous infusion equation used in the initial dosing section of this chapter:

$$k_0 = C_{max,ss} k_e V[(1 - e^{-k_e \tau})/(1 - e^{-k_e t'})]$$

$$k_0 = (28\ mg/L \cdot 0.311\ h^{-1} \cdot 16.7\ L)[(1 - e^{-(0.311\ h^{-1})(8\ h)})/(1 - e^{-(0.311\ h^{-1})(1\ h)})]$$
$$= 499\ mg,\ \text{rounded to}\ 500\ mg$$

Amikacin 500 mg every 8 hours is prescribed to begin 8 hours after the last dose of the previous regimen.

Bayesian Pharmacokinetics Computer Programs

Computer programs are available to assist in the computation of pharmacokinetic parameters for patients.[86–90] The most reliable computer programs use a nonlinear regression algorithm that incorporates components of Bayes' theorem. Nonlinear regression is a statistical technique that uses an iterative process to compute the best pharmacokinetic parameters for a concentration–time data set. Briefly, the patient's drug dosage schedule and serum concentrations are entered into the computer. The computer program has a pharmacokinetic equation preprogrammed for the drug and administration method (e.g., oral, intravenous bolus, and intravenous infusion). Typically, a one-compartment model is used, although some programs allow the user to choose among several different equations. Using population estimates based on demographic information for the patient (e.g., age, weight, gender, and renal function) supplied by the user, the computer program then computes estimated serum concentrations at each time there are actual serum concentrations. Kinetic parameters are then changed by the computer program, and a new set of estimated serum concentrations are computed. The pharmacokinetic parameters that generated the estimated serum concentrations closest to the actual values are remembered by the computer program, and the process is repeated until the set of pharmacokinetic parameters that result in estimated serum concentrations statistically closest to the actual serum concentrations are generated. These pharmacokinetic parameters can then be used to compute improved dosing schedules for patients.

Bayes' theorem is used in the computer algorithm to balance the results of the computations between values based solely on the patient's serum drug concentrations and those based only on patient population parameters. Results from studies that compare various methods of dosage adjustment have consistently found that these types of computer dosing programs perform at least as well as experienced clinical pharmacokineticists and clinicians and better than inexperienced clinicians.

Some clinicians use Bayesian pharmacokinetics computer programs exclusively to alter drug doses based on serum concentrations. An advantage of this approach is that consistent dosage recommendations are made when several different practitioners are involved in therapeutic drug monitoring programs. However, because simpler dosing methods work just as well for patients with stable pharmacokinetic parameters and steady-state drug concentrations, many clinicians reserve the use of computer programs for more difficult situations. Such situations include serum concentrations that are not at steady state, serum concentrations not obtained at the specific times needed to use simpler methods, and unstable pharmacokinetic parameters. Many Bayesian pharmacokinetics computer programs are available to users, and most provide answers similar to the one used in the following examples. The program used to solve problems in this book is DrugCalc, written by Dr. Dennis Mungall, and is available on his Internet web site, (http://members.aol.com/thertch/index.htm).[91]

Example 1 JM is a 50-year-old, 70-kg, 178-cm (70-in) man with gram-negative pneumonia. His serum creatinine is 0.9 mg/dL, which has been stable over the last 5 days since admission. Gentamicin 170 mg every 8 hours was prescribed and expected to produce steady-state peak and trough concentrations of 9 μg/mL and 1 μg/mL, respectively. After the third dose, steady-state peak and trough concentrations were measured and were 12 μg/mL and 1.4 μg/mL, respectively. Calculate a new gentamicin dose that will provide a steady-state peak of 9 μg/mL and a steady-state trough of 1 μg/mL.

1. *Enter the patient's demographic, drug dosing, and serum concentration–time data into the computer program.*

2. *Compute the pharmacokinetic parameters for the patient using the Bayesian pharmacokinetics computer program.*

The pharmacokinetic parameters computed by the program are a volume of distribution of 13.5 L, a half-life of 2.1 hours, and an elimination rate constant of 0.326 h^{-1}.

3. *Compute the dose required to achieve desired aminoglycoside serum concentrations.*

The one-compartment model intravenous infusion equations used by the program to compute doses indicate that 135 mg gentamicin every 8 hours produces a steady-state peak concentration of 9.2 μg/mL and a steady-state trough concentration of 0.9 μg/mL. By means of the simpler linear pharmacokinetics method previously described in this chapter, a similar dose of 140 mg every 8 hours was computed.

Example 2 JM is a 50-year-old, 70-kg, 178-cm (70-in) man with gram-negative pneumonia. His serum creatinine is 3.5 mg/dL, which has been stable over the last 5 days since admission. Gentamicin 115 mg every 24 hours was prescribed and expected to achieve steady-state peak and trough concentrations of 8 to 10 μg/mL and <2 μg/mL, respectively. After the third dose, steady-state peak and trough concentrations were measured and were 12 μg/mL and 3.5 μg/mL, respectively. Calculate a new gentamicin dose that will provide a steady-state peak of 9 μg/mL and a steady-state trough of 1.5 μg/mL.

1. *Enter the patient demographic, drug dosing, and serum concentration–time data into the computer program.*

2. *Compute the pharmacokinetic parameters for the patient using the Bayesian pharmacokinetics computer program.*

The pharmacokinetic parameters computed by the program are a volume of distribution of 14.6 L, a half-life of 14.7 hours, and an elimination rate constant of 0.047 h^{-1}. These values are slightly different from those computed using the steady-state Sawchuk-Zaske method (V = 12.9 L, $t_{1/2}$ = 12.8 h, k_e = 0.054 h^{-1}) because the patient probably was not at steady state when the serum concentrations were drawn.

3. *Compute the dose required to achieve desired aminoglycoside serum concentrations.*

The one-compartment model intravenous infusion equations used by the program to compute doses indicate that a 110-mg dose of gentamicin every 36 hours produces a steady-state peak concentration of 9 μg/mL and a steady-state trough concentration of 1.7 μg/mL. By means of the steady-state Sawchuk-Zaske and pharmacokinetic concepts methods previously described, similar doses of 100 mg every 36 hours and 105 mg every 36 hours, respectively, were computed.

Example 3 JH is a 24-year-old, 70-kg, 183-cm (72-in) man with gram-negative pneumonia. His serum creatinine is 1.0 mg/dL, which has been stable over the last 7 days since admission. Amikacin 400 mg every 8 hours was prescribed. After the third dose, the following amikacin serum concentrations were obtained:

TIME	AMIKACIN CONCENTRATION (μg/mL)
0800 H	2.0
0800–0900 H	Amikacin 400 mg administered to patient
0900 H	22.1
1100 H	11.9
1600 H	2.5

Medication administration sheets were checked, and the previous dose was given 2 hours early (2200 H the previous day). Because of this, it is known that the patient is not at steady state. Calculate a new amikacin dose that will provide a steady-state peak of 28 μg/mL and a trough between 3 and 5 μg/mL.

1. *Enter the patient's demographic, drug dosing, and serum concentration–time data into the computer program.*

2. *Compute the pharmacokinetic parameters for the patient using the Bayesian pharmacokinetics computer program.*

The pharmacokinetic parameters computed by the program are volume of distribution of 17.1 L, a half-life of 2.4 hours, and an elimination rate constant of 0.292 h^{-1}. These values are similar to those computed using the Sawchuk-Zaske method ($V = 17.0$ L, $t_{1/2} = 2.2$ h, $k_e = 0.311\ h^{-1}$).

3. *Compute the dose required to achieve desired aminoglycoside serum concentrations.*

The one-compartment model intravenous infusion equations used by the program to compute doses indicate that a dose of 500 mg every 8 hours produces a steady-state peak concentration of 28 μg/mL and a steady-state trough concentration of 3.6 μg/mL. Using the Sawchuk-Zaske method previously described in the chapter, the identical dose of 500 mg every 8 hours was computed.

SPECIAL DOSING CONSIDERATIONS

Aminoglycoside antibiotics are eliminated by dialysis, so renal failure patients receiving hemodialysis must have aminoglycoside dosage regimens that take dialysis clearance into account. Methods of computing aminoglycoside doses for hemodialysis patients are presented in Chapter 3 in Computation of Initial Doses and Modification of Doses Using Drug Serum Concentrations. Additional cases for this patient population are provided in the problem section of this chapter.

PROBLEMS

The following problems are intended to emphasize the computation of initial and individualized doses using clinical pharmacokinetic techniques. Clinicians should always consult the patient's chart to confirm that antibiotic therapy is appropriate for current microbiologic cultures and sensitivities. Also, the clinician should confirm that the patient is receiving other appropriate concurrent antibiotic therapy, such as β-lactam or anaerobic agents, when it is necessary to treat the infection.

1. PQ is a 75-year-old, 62-kg, 175-cm (69-in) man with gram-negative sepsis. His serum creatinine is 1.3 mg/dL, which has been stable since hospital admission. Compute a gentamicin dose to provide a steady-state peak concentration of 8 μg/mL and a steady-state trough concentration of 1.5 μg/mL using conventional dosing.
2. Patient PQ (see problem 1) was prescribed gentamicin 110 mg every 12 hours. Steady-state gentamicin concentrations were obtained before and after the fourth dose, and the peak concentration (obtained 30 minutes after a 30-minute infusion of gentamicin) was 9.5 μg/mL, whereas the trough concentration (obtained within 30 minutes before dosage administration) was 3.0 μg/mL. Compute a revised gentamicin dose to provide a steady-state peak concentration of 8 μg/mL and a steady-state trough concentration of 1 μg/mL using conventional dosing.

3. ZW is a 35-year-old, 75-kg, 170-cm (67-in) woman with gram-negative pneumonia and chronic renal failure. Her serum creatinine is 3.7 mg/dL, which has been stable since admission. Compute a gentamicin dose to provide a steady-state peak concentration of 10 μg/mL and a steady-state trough concentration of 1.0 μg/mL using conventional dosing.

4. Patient ZW (see problem 3) was prescribed gentamicin 120 mg every 24 hours. Steady-state gentamicin concentrations were obtained before and after the fourth dose, and the peak concentration (obtained 30 minutes after a 30-minute infusion of gentamicin) was 7 μg/mL, whereas the trough concentration (obtained within 30 minutes before dosage administration) was <0.5 μg/mL. Compute a revised gentamicin dose to provide a steady-state peak concentration of 10 μg/mL and a steady-state trough concentration of <2 μg/mL using conventional dosing.

5. JK is a 55-year-old, 140-kg, 173-cm (68-in) man with an intra-abdominal infection secondary to a knife wound. His serum creatinine is 0.9 mg/dL, which has been stable since admission. Compute a gentamicin dose to provide a steady-state peak concentration of 6 μg/mL and a steady-state trough concentration of 0.5 μg/mL using conventional dosing.

6. Patient JK (see problem 5) was prescribed gentamicin 120 mg every 8 hours. Steady-state gentamicin concentrations were obtained before and after the fourth dose, and the peak concentration (obtained 30 minutes after a 30-minute infusion of gentamicin) was 5.9 μg/mL, whereas the trough concentration (obtained within 30 minutes before dosage administration) was 2.5 μg/mL. Compute a revised gentamicin dose to provide a steady-state peak concentration of 6 μg/mL and a steady-state trough concentration of <1 μg/mL using conventional dosing.

7. AF is a 45-year-old, 140-kg, 157-cm (62-in) woman with a *Streptococcus viridans* endocarditis. Her current serum creatinine is 2.4 mg/dL and stable. Compute a tobramycin dose to provide a steady-state peak concentration of 4 μg/mL and a steady-state trough concentration of 0.5 μg/mL using conventional dosing.

8. Patient AF (see problem 7) was prescribed 100 mg tobramycin every 12 hours. Steady-state tobramycin concentrations were obtained before and after the fourth dose, and the peak concentration (obtained 30 minutes after a 30-minute infusion of tobramycin) was 6.2 μg/mL, whereas the trough concentration (obtained within 30 minutes before dosage administration) was 1.5 μg/mL. Compute a revised tobramycin dose to provide a steady-state peak concentration of 4 μg/mL and a steady-state trough concentration of ≤1 μg/mL using conventional dosing.

9. FH is a 24-year-old, 60-kg, 170-cm (67-in) man with cystic fibrosis and *Pseudomonas aeruginosa* cultured from a sputum culture. He was hospitalized because of worsening pulmonary function tests. His serum creatinine is 0.7 mg/dL. Compute a tobramycin dose to provide a steady-state peak concentration of 10 μg/mL and a steady-state trough concentration of <2 μg/mL using conventional dosing.

10. Patient FH (see problem 9) was prescribed 250 mg tobramycin every 8 hours. Steady-state tobramycin concentrations were obtained before and after the fourth dose, and the peak concentration (obtained 30 minutes after a 30-minute infusion of tobramycin) was 7.9 μg/mL, whereas the trough concentration (obtained within 30

minutes before dosage administration) was 1 μg/mL. Compute a revised tobramycin dose to provide a steady-state peak concentration of 10 μg/mL and a steady-state trough concentration of 1 to 2 μg/mL using conventional dosing.

11. TY is a 66-year-old, 65-kg, 165-cm (65 in) woman with a suspected tubo-ovarian abscess secondary to hysterectomy surgery. While in the hospital, she developed ascites because of preexisting liver cirrhosis, and her current weight is 72 kg. Her serum creatinine is 1.4 mg/dL. Compute a gentamicin dose to provide a steady-state peak concentration of 6 μg/mL and a steady-state trough concentration of <2 μg/mL using conventional dosing.

12. Patient TY (see problem 11) was prescribed gentamicin 120 mg every 12 hours. Steady-state gentamicin concentrations were obtained before and after the fourth dose, and the peak concentration (obtained 30 minutes after a 30-minute infusion of gentamicin) was 4 μg/mL, whereas the trough concentration (obtained within 30 minutes before dosage administration) was 0.8 μg/mL. Compute a revised gentamicin dose to provide a steady-state peak concentration of 6 μg/mL and a steady-state trough concentration of 1 μg/mL using conventional dosing.

13. UQ is a 27-year-old, 85-kg, 188-cm (74-in) male trauma patient with a gram-negative pneumonia. He is currently on a respirator. He sustained multiple injuries secondary to a motor vehicle accident 2 weeks ago and lost a large amount of blood at the accident site. He developed acute renal failure from prolonged hypotension and poor perfusion of his kidneys (postdialysis serum creatinine, 5.3 mg/dL). He is receiving hemodialysis on Mondays, Wednesdays, and Fridays from 0800 to 1200 H using a low-flux dialysis filter. Recommend a gentamicin dosage regimen that will achieve peak concentrations of 8 μg/mL and postdialysis concentrations of ~2 μg/mL. The first dose of the regimen is to be given immediately after hemodialysis is finished on Wednesday at 1200 H.

14. Patient UQ (see problem 13) was prescribed gentamicin 180 mg loading dose and 130 mg after each dialysis. The following serum concentrations were obtained:

DATE/TIME	DESCRIPTION	CONCENTRATION
Friday at 1200 H	Postdose (130 mg)	6.4 μg/mL
Monday at 0800 H	Predialysis	2.2 μg/mL
Monday at 1300 H	Postdialysis (1 hour after end of dialysis to allow for rebound in serum concentrations)	0.7 μg/mL
Monday at 1400 H	Postdose (130 mg)	6.9 μg/mL

Use these serum concentrations to compute the patient's own pharmacokinetic parameters for gentamicin and a new dosage schedule that will achieve peak concentrations of 8 μg/mL and postdialysis concentrations of <2 μg/mL.

15. LS is a 67-year-old, 60-kg, 157-cm (62-in) woman with a serum creatinine of 1.8 mg/dL. She is placed on tobramycin for a hospital-acquired gram-negative pneumonia. The prescribed dose was tobramycin 80 mg every 8 hours (infused over 1 hour), and two doses have been given at 0800 and 1600 H. A trough concentration of 2.9 μg/mL was obtained at 1530 H (30 minutes before the second dose), and a peak concentration of 5.2 μg/mL was obtained at 1705 H (5 minutes after infusion of the second dose). Compute the dose to give $C_{max,ss}$ = 8 μg/mL and $C_{min,ss}$ = 1.5 μg/mL.

16. KK is a 52-year-old, 87-kg, 188-cm (74-in) man who developed a fever after an appendectomy, and had elevated white blood cell count and abdominal pain 24 hours after surgery. His serum creatinine is 1.4 mg/dL and stable. (A) Compute an initial extended-interval gentamicin dose for this patient. (B) Nine hours after the second dose of gentamicin 610 mg every 24 hours, a gentamicin serum concentration of 8.2 μg/mL is measured. Compute a revised gentamicin dose to provide steady-state peak concentrations higher than 20 μg/mL and steady-state trough concentrations lower than 1 μg/mL.

17. XS is a 45-year-old, 65-kg, 162-cm (64-in) female bone marrow transplant recipient who develops a neutropenic fever. Her serum creatinine is 1.1 mg/dL. She is administered tobramycin 5 mg/kg daily (325 mg) as part of her antibiotic therapy. A tobramycin serum concentration of 19 μg/mL was obtained 5 hours after the first dose. Compute a revised tobramycin dose to provide steady-state peak concentrations higher than 25 μg/mL and steady-state trough concentrations lower than 1 μg/mL.

ANSWERS TO PROBLEMS

1. The initial gentamicin dose for patient PQ is calculated as follows.

1. *Estimate the creatinine clearance.*

This patient has a stable serum creatinine and is not obese. The Cockcroft–Gault equation can be used to estimate creatinine clearance:

$$CrCl_{est} = [(140 - age)BW]/(72 \cdot S_{Cr}) = [(140 - 75\ y)62\ kg]/(72 \cdot 1.3\ mg/dL)$$

$$CrCl_{est} = 43\ mL/min$$

2. *Estimate the elimination rate constant (k_e) and half-life ($t_{1/2}$).*

The elimination rate constant versus creatinine clearance relationship is used to estimate the gentamicin elimination rate for this patient:

$$k_e = 0.00293(CrCl) + 0.014 = 0.00293(43\ mL/min) + 0.014 = 0.140\ h^{-1}$$

$$t_{1/2} = 0.693/k_e = 0.693/0.140\ h^{-1} = 4.9\ h$$

3. *Estimate the volume of distribution.*

The patient has no disease states or conditions that would alter the volume of distribution from the normal value of 0.26 L/kg:

$$V = 0.26\ L/kg\ (62\ kg) = 16.1\ L$$

4. *Choose the desired steady-state serum concentrations.*

Patients with gram-negative sepsis being treated with aminoglycoside antibiotics require steady-state peak concentrations ($C_{max,ss}$) of 8 to 10 μg/mL; steady-state trough ($C_{min,ss}$) concentrations should be <2 μg/mL to avoid toxicity. Set $C_{max,ss}$ = 8 μg/mL and $C_{min,ss}$ = 1.5 μg/mL.

5. *Use the intermittent intravenous infusion equations to compute the dose.*

Calculate the required dosage interval (τ) using a 1-hour infusion:

$$\tau = [(\ln C_{max,ss} - \ln C_{min,ss})/k_e] + t' = [(\ln 8\ \mu g/mL - \ln 1.5\ \mu g/mL)/0.140\ h^{-1}] + 1\ h = 12.9\ h$$

Dosage intervals should be rounded to clinically acceptable intervals of 8 hours, 12 hours, 18 hours, 24 hours, 36 hours, 48 hours, 72 hours, and multiples of 24 hours thereafter, whenever possible. In this case, the dosage interval is rounded to 12 hours. Also, steady-state peak concentrations are similar if drawn immediately after a 1-hour infusion or 30 minutes after a 30-minute infusion, so the dose can be administered either way.

$$k_0 = C_{max,ss} k_e V[(1 - e^{-k_e \tau})/(1 - e^{-k_e t'})]$$

$$k_0 = (8\ mg/L \cdot 0.140\ h^{-1} \cdot 16.1\ L)[(1 - e^{-(0.140\ h^{-1})(12\ h)})/(1 - e^{-(0.140\ h^{-1})(1\ h)})] = 112\ mg$$

Aminoglycoside doses should be rounded to the nearest 5 to 10 mg. This dose is rounded to 110 mg. (Note: μg/mL = mg/L and this concentration unit was substituted for $C_{max,ss}$ to avoid unnecessary unit conversion.)

The prescribed maintenance dose is 110 mg gentamicin every 12 hours.

6. *Compute the loading dose, if needed.*

Loading doses should be considered for patients with creatinine clearance values lower than 60 mL/min. The administration of a loading dose in these patients allows achievement of therapeutic peak concentrations more quickly than if maintenance doses alone are given. However, because the pharmacokinetic parameters used to compute these initial doses are *estimated* values and not *actual* values, the patient's own parameters may be much different from the estimated constants, and steady-state will not be achieved until 3 to 5 half-lives have passed.

$$LD = k_0/(1 - e^{-k_e \tau}) = 110\ mg/(1 - e^{-(0.140\ h^{-1})(12\ h)}) = 135\ mg$$

Hull and Sarubbi Nomogram

1. *Estimate the creatinine clearance.*

This patient has a stable serum creatinine and is not obese. The Cockcroft–Gault equation can be used to estimate creatinine clearance:

$$CrCl_{est} = [(140 - age)BW]/(72 \cdot S_{Cr}) = [(140 - 75\ y)62\ kg]/(72 \cdot 1.3\ mg/dL)$$

$$CrCl_{est} = 43\ mL/min$$

2. *Choose the desired steady-state serum concentrations.*

Patients with gram-negative sepsis being treated with gentamicin require steady-state peak concentrations ($C_{max,ss}$) of 8 to 10 μg/mL.

3. *Select the loading dose (see Table 4-3).*

A loading dose (LD) of 2 mg/kg provides a peak concentration of 8 to 10 μg/mL.

$$LD = 2\ mg/kg(62\ kg) = 124\ mg, \text{ rounded to } 125\ mg$$

4. *Determine the estimated half-life, maintenance dose, and dosage interval.*

From the nomogram, the estimated half-life is 6.5 hours (suggesting that a 12-hour dosage interval is appropriate), the maintenance dose (MD) is 72% of the loading dose (MD = 0.72[125 mg] = 90 mg), and the dosage interval is 12 hours.

Aminoglycoside doses should be rounded to the nearest 5 to 10 mg. Steady-state peak concentrations are similar if drawn immediately after 1-hour infusion or 30 minutes after a 30-minute infusion, so the dose can be administered either way.

The prescribed maintenance dose is 90 mg every 12 hours.

2. The revised gentamicin dose for patient PQ is calculated as follows.

Pharmacokinetics Concepts Method

1. *Draw a rough sketch of the serum log concentration–time curve by hand, keeping track of the relative time between the serum concentrations (Figure 4-13).*

2. *Because the patient is at steady state, the trough concentration can be extrapolated to the next trough value time (see Figure 4-13).*

3. *Draw the elimination curve between the steady-state peak concentration and the extrapolated trough concentration. Use this line to estimate half-life.* The patient is receiving gentamicin 110 mg every 12 hours, which produces a steady-state peak of 9.5 μg/mL and a steady-state trough of 3.0 μg/mL. The dose is infused over 30 minutes, and the peak concentration is drawn 30 minutes later (see Figure 4-13). The time between the measured steady-state peak and the extrapolated trough concentration is 11 hours (the 12-hour dosage interval minus the 1 hour combined infusion and waiting time). The definition of half-life is the time needed for serum concentrations

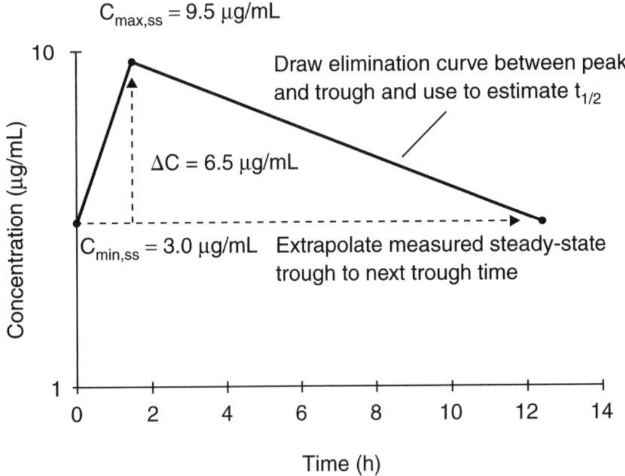

FIGURE 4-13 Solution to problem 2 using the pharmacokinetic concepts method.

to decrease by half. It takes 1 half-life for the peak serum concentration to decline from 9.5 μg/mL to 4.8 μg/mL and an additional half-life for the serum concentration to decrease from 4.8 μg/mL to 2.4 μg/mL. The concentration of 3.0 μg/mL is close to, but slightly higher than, the extrapolated trough value of 2.4 μg/mL. Therefore, 1.75 half-lives expired during the 11-hour time period between the peak concentration and extrapolated trough concentration, and the estimated half-life is 7 hours (11 hours/1.75 half-lives = ~7 hours). This information is used to set the new dosage interval for the patient.

4. *Determine the difference in concentration between the steady-state peak and trough concentrations. The difference in concentration changes proportionally with the dose size.* In this example, the patient is receiving a gentamicin dose of 110 mg every 12 hours, which produced steady-state peak and trough concentrations of 9.5 μg/mL and 3 μg/mL, respectively. The difference between the peak and trough values is 6.5 μg/mL. The change in serum concentration is proportional to the dose, and this information is used to set a new dose for the patient.

5. *Choose new steady-state peak and trough concentrations.* For this example, the desired steady-state peak and trough concentrations is approximately 8 μg/mL and 1 μg/mL, respectively.

6. *Determine the new dosage interval for the desired concentrations.* With the desired concentrations, it will take 1 half-life for the peak concentration of 8 μg/mL to decrease to 4 μg/mL, 1 more half-life for the serum concentration to decrease to 2 μg/mL, and an additional half-life for serum concentrations to decline to 1 μg/mL. Therefore, the dosage interval needs to be approximately 3 half-lives or 21 hours (7 hours × 3 half-lives = 21 hours). The dosage interval is rounded to the clinically acceptable value of 24 hours.

7. *Determine the new dose for the desired concentrations.* The desired peak concentrations is 8 μg/mL, and the expected trough concentration is 1 μg/mL. The change in concentration between these values is 7 μg/mL. It is known from measured serum concentrations that administration of 110 mg changes serum concentrations by 6.5 μg/mL and that the change in serum concentration between the peak and trough values is proportional to the size of the dose. In this case, $D_{new} = (\Delta C_{new}/\Delta C_{old})D_{old}$ = [(7 μg/mL)/(6.5 μg/mL)] 110 mg = 118 mg, rounded to 120 mg. Gentamicin 120 mg every 24 hours is started 24 hours after the last dose of the previous dosage regimen.

Steady-State Sawchuk-Zaske Method

1. *Compute the patient's elimination rate constant and half-life (note: for infusion times less than 1 hour, t′ is considered to be the sum of the infusion and waiting times).*

$$k_e = (\ln C_{max,ss} - \ln C_{min,ss})/\tau - t' = (\ln 9.5\ \mu g/mL - \ln 3\ \mu g/mL)/(12\ h - 1\ h) = 0.105\ h^{-1}$$

$$t_{1/2} = 0.693/k_e = 0.693/0.105\ h^{-1} = 6.6\ h$$

2. *Compute the patient's volume of distribution.*

$$V = \frac{D/t' (1 - e^{-k_e t'})}{k_e[C_{max,ss} - (C_{min,ss} e^{-k_e t'})]} = \frac{(110 \text{ mg}/1 \text{ h})(1 - e^{-(0.105 \text{ h}^{-1})(1 \text{ h})})}{0.105 \text{ h}^{-1}[9.5 \text{ mg/L} - (3 \text{ mg/L } e^{-(0.105 \text{ h}^{-1})(1 \text{ h})})]}$$

$V = 15.4$ L

3. *Choose new steady-state peak and trough concentrations.* For this example, the desired steady-state peak and trough concentrations are approximately 8 μg/mL and 1 μg/mL, respectively.

4. *Determine the new dosage interval for the desired concentrations.* As in the initial dosage section of this chapter, the dosage interval (τ) is computed according to the following equation using a 1-hour infusion time (t′):

$$\tau = [(\ln C_{max,ss} - \ln C_{min,ss})/k_e] + t' = [(\ln 8 \text{ μg/mL} - \ln 1 \text{ μg/mL})/0.105 \text{ h}^{-1}] + 1 \text{ h}$$
$$= 21 \text{ h, rounded to } 24 \text{ h}$$

5. *Determine the new dose for the desired concentrations.* The dose is computed according to the one-compartment model intravenous infusion equation used in the initial dosing section of this chapter:

$$k_0 = C_{max,ss} k_e V[(1 - e^{-k_e \tau})/(1 - e^{-k_e t'})]$$

$$k_0 = (8 \text{ mg/L} \cdot 0.105 \text{ h}^{-1} \cdot 15.4 \text{ L})[(1 - e^{-(0.105 \text{ h}^{-1})(24 \text{ h})})/(1 - e^{-(0.105 \text{ h}^{-1})(1 \text{ h})})]$$
$$= 119 \text{ mg, rounded to } 120 \text{ mg}$$

Gentamicin 120 mg every 24 hours is prescribed to begin 24 hours after the last dose of the previous regimen. This dose is identical with that derived for the patient using the pharmacokinetic concepts method (120 mg every 24 hours).

3. The initial gentamicin dose for patient ZW is calculated as follows.

1. *Estimate the creatinine clearance.*

Patient ZW has a stable serum creatinine and is not obese. The Cockcroft–Gault equation can be used to estimate creatinine clearance:

$$CrCl_{est} = \{[(140 - age)BW]/(72 \cdot S_{Cr})\}\ 0.85 = \{[(140 - 35 \text{ y})75 \text{ kg}]/(72 \cdot 3.7 \text{ mg/dL})\}0.85$$

$CrCl_{est} = 25$ mL/min

2. *Estimate the elimination rate constant (k_e) and half-life ($t_{1/2}$).*

The elimination rate constant versus creatinine clearance relationship is used to estimate the gentamicin elimination rate for this patient:

$$k_e = 0.00293(CrCl) + 0.014 = 0.00293(25 \text{ mL/min}) + 0.014 = 0.088 \text{ h}^{-1}$$

$$t_{1/2} = 0.693/k_e = 0.693/0.088 \text{ h}^{-1} = 7.9 \text{ h}$$

3. *Estimate the volume of distribution.*

The patient has no disease states or conditions that would alter the volume of distribution from the normal value of 0.26 L/kg.

$$V = 0.26 \text{ L/kg } (75 \text{ kg}) = 19.5 \text{ L}$$

4. *Choose the desired steady-state serum concentrations.*

Patients with gram-negative pneumonia being treated with aminolgycoside antibiotics require steady-state peak concentrations ($C_{max,ss}$) of 8 to 10 μg/mL; steady-state trough ($C_{min,ss}$) concentrations should be <2 μg/mL to avoid toxicity. Set $C_{max,ss}$ = 10 μg/mL and $C_{min,ss}$ = 1 μg/mL.

5. *Use the intermittent intravenous infusion equations to compute the dose.*

Calculate the required dosage interval (τ) using a 1-hour infusion:

$$\tau = [(\ln C_{max,ss} - \ln C_{min,ss})/k_e] + t' = [(\ln 10\ \mu g/mL - \ln 1\ \mu g/mL)/0.088\ h^{-1}] + 1\ h = 27\ h$$

Dosage intervals should be rounded to clinically acceptable intervals of 8 hours, 12 hours, 18 hours, 24 hours, 36 hours, 48 hours, 72 hours, and multiples of 24 hours thereafter, whenever possible. In this case, the dosage interval is rounded to 24 hours. Also, steady-state peak concentrations are similar if drawn immediately after a 1-hour infusion or 30 minutes after a 30-minute infusion, so the dose can be administered either way.

$$k_0 = C_{max,ss} k_e V[(1 - e^{-k_e \tau})/(1 - e^{-k_e t'})]$$

$$k_0 = (10\ mg/L \cdot 0.088\ h^{-1} \cdot 19.5\ L)[(1 - e^{-(0.088\ h^{-1})(24\ h)})/(1 - e^{-(0.088\ h^{-1})(1\ h)})] = 179\ mg$$

Aminoglycoside doses should be rounded to the nearest 5 to 10 mg. This dose is rounded to 180 mg. (Note: μg/mL = mg/L, and this concentration unit was substituted for $C_{max,ss}$ to avoid unnecessary unit conversion.)

The prescribed maintenance dose is 180 mg gentamicin every 24 hours.

6. *Compute the loading dose, if needed.*

Loading doses should be considered for patients with creatinine clearance values lower than 60 mL/min. The administration of a loading dose in these patients allows achievement of therapeutic peak concentrations more quickly than if maintenance doses alone are given. However, because the pharmacokinetic parameters used to compute these initial doses are *estimated* values and not *actual* values, the patient's own parameters may be much different from the estimated constants, and steady state cannot be achieved until 3 to 5 half-lives have passed.

$$LD = k_0/(1 - e^{-k_e \tau}) = 180\ mg/(1 - e^{-(0.088\ h^{-1})(24\ h)}) = 205\ mg$$

Hull and Sarubbi Nomogram

1. *Estimate the creatinine clearance.*

This patient has a stable serum creatinine and is not obese. The Cockcroft–Gault equation can be used to estimate creatinine clearance:

$$CrCl_{est} = \{[(140 - age)BW]/(72 \cdot S_{Cr})\}\ 0.85 = \{[(140 - 35\ y)75\ kg]/(72 \cdot 3.7\ mg/dL)\}0.85$$

$$CrCl_{est} = 25\ mL/min$$

2. *Choose the desired steady-state serum concentrations.*

Patients with gram-negative sepsis being treated with gentamicin require steady-state peak concentrations ($C_{max,ss}$) of 8 to 10 μg/mL.

3. *Select the loading dose (see Table 4-3).*

A loading dose (LD) of 2 mg/kg provides a peak concentration of 8 to 10 μg/mL.

$$LD = 2 \text{ mg/kg}(75 \text{ kg}) = 150 \text{ mg}$$

4. *Determine the estimated half-life, maintenance dose, and dosage interval.*

As calculated from the nomogram, the estimated half-life is 9.9 hours (suggesting that a 24-hour dosage interval is appropriate), the maintenance dose (MD) is 81% of the loading dose (MD = 0.81[150 mg] = 122 mg), and the dosage interval is 24 hours. Note: 24-hour dosage interval chosen because longer time period needed for concentrations to drop from 10 μg/mL to 1 μg/mL.

Aminoglycoside doses should be rounded to the nearest 5 to 10 mg. Steady-state peak concentrations are similar if drawn immediately after a 1-hour infusion or 30 minutes after a 30-minute infusion, so the dose can be administered either way.

The prescribed maintenance dose is 120 mg gentamicin every 24 hours.

4. Compute a modified dose of gentamicin for ZW using linear pharmacokinetics.

1. *Compute the new dose to achieve desired serum concentration.*

Using linear pharmacokinetics, the new dose to attain the desired concentration should be proportional to the old dose that produced the measured concentration.

$$D_{new} = (C_{ss,new}/C_{ss,old})D_{old} = [(10\ \mu\text{g/mL})/(7\ \mu\text{g/mL})]\ 120 \text{ mg}$$
$$= 171 \text{ mg rounded to } 170 \text{ mg}$$

The new suggested dose would be 170 mg every 24 hours to be started at the next scheduled dosing time.

2. *Check the steady-state trough concentration for the new dosage regimen.*

Using linear pharmacokinetics, the new steady-state concentration can be estimated and should be proportional to the old dose that produced the measured concentration. The measured trough concentration was below assay limits (<0.5 μg/mL), so the maximum value it can be is 0.5 μg/mL:

$$C_{ss,new} = (D_{new}/D_{old})C_{ss,old} = (170 \text{ mg}/120 \text{ mg})\ 0.5\ \mu\text{g/mL} = 0.7\ \mu\text{g/mL}$$

The steady-state trough concentration is expected to be no greater than 0.7 μg/mL and should be safe and effective for the infection that is being treated.

5. The initial gentamicin dose for patient JK is calculated as follows.

1. *Estimate the creatinine clearance.*

This patient has a stable serum creatinine and is obese (IBW_{men} (in kg) = 50 + 2.3(Ht − 60 in) = 50 + 2.3(68 − 60) = 68.4 kg). The Salazar and Corcoran equation can be used to estimate creatinine clearance:

$$CrCl_{est(males)} = \frac{(137 - age)[(0.285 \cdot Wt) + (12.1 \cdot Ht^2)]}{(51 \cdot S_{Cr})}$$

$$CrCl_{est(males)} = \frac{(137 - 55\ y)\{(0.285 \cdot 140\ kg) + [12.1 \cdot (1.73\ m)^2]\}}{(51 \cdot 0.9\ mg/dL)} = 136\ mL/min$$

Note: Height is converted from inches to meters: Ht = (68 in · 2.54 cm/in)/(100 cm/m) = 1.73 m.

2. *Estimate the elimination rate constant (k_e) and half-life ($t_{1/2}$).*

The elimination rate constant versus creatinine clearance relationship is used to estimate the gentamicin elimination rate for this patient.

$$k_e = 0.00293(CrCl) + 0.014 = 0.00293(136\ mL/min) + 0.014 = 0.412\ h^{-1}$$

$$t_{1/2} = 0.693/k_e = 0.693/0.412\ h^{-1} = 1.7\ h$$

3. *Estimate the volume of distribution.*

The patient is overweight so the volume of distribution is estimated using the equation that corrects for obesity:

$$V = 0.26\ L/kg\ [IBW + 0.4(TBW - IBW)] = 0.26\ L/kg[68.4\ kg + 0.4(140\ kg - 68.4\ kg)] = 25.2\ L$$

4. *Choose desired steady-state serum concentrations.*

Patients with intra-abdominal sepsis being treated with aminoglycoside antibiotics require steady-state peak concentrations ($C_{max,ss}$) of 5 to 6 μg/mL; steady-state trough ($C_{min,ss}$) concentrations should be <2 μg/mL to prevent toxicity. Set $C_{max,ss}$ = 6 μg/mL and $C_{min,ss}$ = 0.5 μg/mL.

5. *Use the intermittent intravenous infusion equations to compute dose.*

Calculate the required dosage interval (τ) using a 1-hour infusion:

$$\tau = [(\ln C_{max,ss} - \ln C_{min,ss})/k_e] + t' = [(\ln 6\ \mu g/mL - \ln 0.5\ \mu g/mL)/0.412\ h^{-1}] + 1\ h = 7\ h$$

Dosage intervals should be rounded to clinically acceptable intervals of 8 hours, 12 hours, 18 hours, 24 hours, 36 hours, 48 hours, 72 hours, and multiples of 24 hours thereafter, whenever possible. In this case, the dosage interval is rounded to 8 hours. Also, steady-state peak concentrations are similar if drawn immediately after a 1-hour infusion or 30 minutes after a 30-minute infusion, so the dose can be administered either way.

$$k_0 = C_{max,ss} k_e V[(1 - e^{-k_e \tau})/(1 - e^{-k_e t'})]$$

$$k_0 = (6\ mg/L \cdot 0.412\ h^{-1} \cdot 25.2\ L)[(1 - e^{-(0.412\ h^{-1})(8\ h)})/(1 - e^{-(0.412\ h^{-1})(1\ h)})] = 178\ mg$$

Aminoglycoside doses should be rounded to the nearest 5 to 10 mg. This dose is rounded to 180 mg. (Note: μg/mL = mg/L, and this concentration unit was substituted for $C_{max,ss}$ to avoid unnecessary unit conversion.)

The prescribed maintenance dose is 180 mg gentamicin every 8 hours.

6. *Compute the loading dose, if needed.*

Loading doses should be considered for patients with creatinine clearance values lower than 60 mL/min. The administration of a loading dose in these patients allows achievement of therapeutic peak concentrations more quickly than if maintenance doses alone are given. However, because the pharmacokinetic parameters used to compute these initial doses are *estimated* values and not *actual* values, the patient's own parameters may be much different from the estimated constants, and steady-state will not be achieved until 3 to 5 half-lives have passed.

$$LD = k_0/(1 - e^{-k_e \tau}) = 180 \text{ mg}/(1 - e^{-(0.412 \text{ h}^{-1})(8 \text{ h})}) = 187 \text{ mg}$$

Because the patient has a short aminoglycoside half-life, the loading dose is similar to the maintenance dose, and the loading dose is omitted.

Hull and Sarubbi Nomogram

1. *Estimate the creatinine clearance.*

This patient has a stable serum creatinine and is obese (IBW_{males} (in kg) = 50 + 2.3(Ht – 60 in) = 50 + 2.3(68 – 60) = 68.4 kg). The Salazar and Corcoran equation can be used to estimate creatinine clearance:

$$CrCl_{est(males)} = \frac{(137 - age)[(0.285 \cdot Wt) + (12.1 \cdot Ht^2)]}{(51 \cdot S_{Cr})}$$

$$CrCl_{est(males)} = \frac{(137 - 55 \text{ y})\{(0.285 \cdot 140 \text{ kg}) + [12.1 \cdot (1.73 \text{ m})^2]\}}{(51 \cdot 0.9 \text{ mg/dL})} = 136 \text{ mL/min}$$

Note: Height is converted from inches to meters: Ht = (68 in · 2.54 cm/in)/(100 cm/m) = 1.73 m.

2. *Choose the desired steady-state serum concentrations.*

Patients with intra-abdominal sepsis being treated with gentamicin require steady-state peak concentrations ($C_{max,ss}$) of 5 to 6 μg/mL.

3. *Select the loading dose (see Table 4-3).*

A loading dose (LD) of 1.5 mg/kg provides a peak concentration of 5 to 6 μg/mL. The patient is obese, so the patient's adjusted body weight (ABW) is used as the weight factor in the nomogram.

$$ABW \text{ (in kg)} = IBW + 0.4(TBW - IBW) = 68.4 \text{ kg} + 0.4(140 \text{ kg} - 68.4 \text{ kg}) = 97 \text{ kg}$$

$$LD = 1.5 \text{ mg/kg}(97 \text{ kg}) = 146 \text{ mg, rounded to } 145 \text{ mg}$$

4. *Determine the estimated half-life, maintenance dose, and dosage interval.*

From the nomogram, the estimated half-life is 2 to 3 hours (suggesting that an 8-hour dosage interval is appropriate), the maintenance dose (MD) is 90% of the loading dose (MD = 0.90[145 mg] = 131 mg), and the dosage interval is 8 hours.

Aminoglycoside doses should be rounded to the nearest 5 to 10 mg. Steady-state peak concentrations are similar if drawn immediately after a 1-hour infusion or 30 minutes after a 30-minute infusion, so the dose can be administered either way.

The prescribed maintenance dose is 130 mg gentamicin every 8 hours.

6. The revised gentamicin dose for patient JK is calculated as follows.

Pharmacokinetic Concepts Method

1. *Draw a rough sketch of the serum log concentration–time curve by hand, keeping track of the relative time between serum concentrations (Figure 4-14).*

2. *Since the patient is at steady state, the trough concentration can be extrapolated to the next trough value time (see Figure 4-14).*

3. *Draw the elimination curve between the steady-state peak concentration and the extrapolated trough concentration. Use this line to estimate half-life.* The patient is receiving a gentamicin dose of 120 mg every 8 hours, which produces a steady-state peak of 5.9 μg/mL and a steady-state trough of 2.5 μg/mL. The dose is infused over 30 minutes and the peak concentration is drawn 30 minutes later (see Figure 4-13). The time between the measured steady-state peak and the extrapolated trough concentration is 7 hours (the 8-hour dosage interval minus the 1-hour combined infusion and waiting time). The definition of half-life is the time needed for serum concentrations to decrease by half. It takes 1 half-life for the peak serum concentration to decline from 5.9 μg/mL to 3.0 μg/mL, and about one-fourth of an additional half-life for the serum concentration to decrease from 3.0 μg/mL to 2.5 μg/mL. Therefore, 1.25 half-lives expired during the 7-hour time period between the peak and extrapolated trough concentration and the estimated half-life is 6 hours (7 hours/1.25 half-lives = ~6 hours). This information is used to set the new dosage interval for the patient.

4. *Determine the difference in concentration between the steady-state peak and trough concentrations. The difference in concentration changes proportionally with*

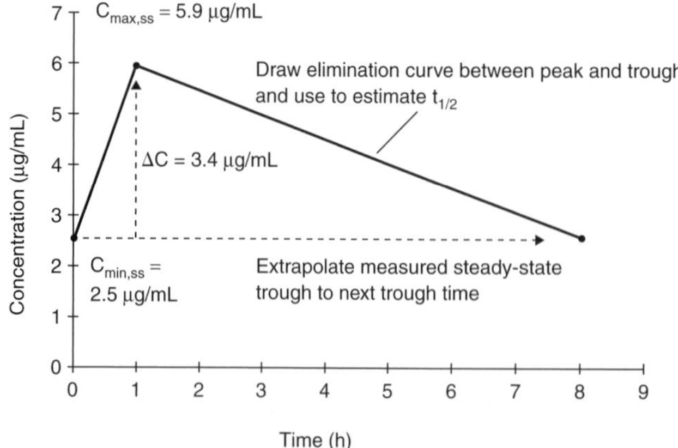

FIGURE 4-14 Solution to problem 6 using pharmacokinetic concepts method.

the dose size. In this example, the patient is receiving a gentamicin dose of 120 mg every 8 hours, which produced steady-state peak and trough concentrations of 5.9 μg/mL and 2.5 μg/mL, respectively. The difference between the peak and trough values is 3.4 μg/mL. The change in serum concentration is proportional to the dose, and this information is used to set a new dose for the patient.

5. *Choose new steady-state peak and trough concentrations.* For this example, the desired steady-state peak and trough concentrations are approximately 6 μg/mL and <1 μg/mL, respectively.

6. *Determine the new dosage interval for the desired concentrations.* Using the desired concentrations, it takes 1 half-life for the peak concentration of 6 μg/mL to decrease to 3 μg/mL, 1 more half-life for the serum concentration to decrease to 1.5 μg/mL, and an additional half-life for serum concentrations to decline to 0.8 μg/mL. Therefore, the dosage interval needs to be approximately 3 half-lives or 18 hours (6 hours × 3 half-lives = 18 hours).

7. *Determine the new dose for the desired concentrations.* The desired peak concentration is 6 μg/mL, and the expected trough concentration is 0.8 μg/mL. The change in concentration between these values is 5.2 μg/mL. It is known from measured serum concentrations that administration of 120 mg gentamicin changes serum concentrations by 3.4 μg/mL and that the change in serum concentration between the peak and trough values is proportional to the size of the dose. In this case, $D_{new} = (\Delta C_{new}/\Delta C_{old})D_{old}$ = [(5.2 μg/mL)/(3.4 μg/mL)] 120 mg = 184 mg. Gentamicin 185 mg every 18 hours is started 18 hours after the last dose of the previous dosage regimen.

Steady-State Sawchuk-Zaske Method

1. *Compute the patient's elimination rate constant and half-life (note: for infusion times less than 1 hour, t′ is considered to be the sum of the infusion and waiting times).*

$$k_e = (\ln C_{max,ss} - \ln C_{min,ss})/\tau - t' = (\ln 5.9\ \mu g/mL - \ln 2.5\ \mu g/mL)/(8\ h - 1\ h) = 0.123\ h^{-1}$$

$$t_{1/2} = 0.693/k_e = 0.693/0.123\ h^{-1} = 5.6\ h$$

2. *Compute the patient's volume of distribution.*

$$V = \frac{D/t'\ (1 - e^{-k_e t'})}{k_e[C_{max,ss} - (C_{min,ss}e^{-k_e t'})]} = \frac{(120\ mg/1\ h)(1 - e^{-(0.123\ h^{-1})(1\ h)})}{0.123\ h^{-1}[5.9\ mg/L - (2.5\ mg/L\ e^{-(0.123\ h^{-1})(1\ h)})}$$

$$V = 30.6\ L$$

3. *Choose new steady-state peak and trough concentrations.* For this example, the desired steady-state peak and trough concentrations are approximately 6 μg/mL and 0.8 μg/mL, respectively.

4. *Determine the new gentamicin dosage interval for the desired concentrations.* As in the initial dosage section of this chapter, the dosage interval (τ) is computed by means of the following equation using a 1-hour infusion time (t′):

$$\tau = [(\ln C_{max,ss} - \ln C_{min,ss})/k_e] + t' = [(\ln 6\ \mu g/mL - \ln 0.8\ \mu g/mL)/0.123\ h^{-1}] + 1\ h = 17\ h, \text{ rounded to } 18\ h$$

5. *Determine the new dose for the desired concentrations.* The gentamicin dose is computed using the one-compartment model intravenous infusion equation that is used in the initial dosing section of this chapter:

$$k_0 = C_{max,ss} k_e V[(1 - e^{-k_e \tau})/(1 - e^{-k_e t'})]$$

$$k_0 = (6\ mg/L \cdot 0.123\ h^{-1} \cdot 30.6\ L)[(1 - e^{-(0.123\ h^{-1})(18\ h)})/(1 - e^{-(0.123\ h^{-1})(1\ h)})]$$
$$= 174\ mg, \text{ rounded to } 175\ mg$$

Gentamicin 175 mg every 18 hours is prescribed to begin 18 hours after the last dose of the previous regimen. This dose is very similar to that derived for the patient using the pharmacokinetic concepts method (185 mg every 18 hours).

7. The initial tobramycin dose for patient AF is calculated as follows.

1. *Estimate the creatinine clearance.*

This patient has a stable serum creatinine and is obese ($IBW_{females}$ (in kg) = 45 + 2.3(Ht – 60 in) = 45 + 2.3(62 – 60) = 50 kg). The Salazar and Corcoran equation can be used to estimate creatinine clearance:

$$CrCl_{est(females)} = \frac{(146 - age)[(0.287 \cdot Wt) + (9.74 \cdot Ht^2)]}{(60 \cdot S_{Cr})}$$

$$CrCl_{est(females)} = \frac{(146 - 45\ y)\{(0.287 \cdot 140\ kg) + [9.74 \cdot (1.57\ m)^2]\}}{(60 \cdot 2.4\ mg/dL)} = 45\ mL/min$$

Note: Height is converted from inches to meters: Ht = (62 in · 2.54 cm/in)/(100 cm/m) = 1.57 m.

2. *Estimate the elimination rate constant (k_e) and half-life ($t_{1/2}$).*

The elimination rate constant versus creatinine clearance relationship is used to estimate the tobramycin elimination rate for this patient:

$$k_e = 0.00293(CrCl) + 0.014 = 0.00293(45\ mL/min) + 0.014 = 0.146\ h^{-1}$$

$$t_{1/2} = 0.693/k_e = 0.693/0.146\ h^{-1} = 4.7\ h$$

3. *Estimate the volume of distribution.*

The patient is obese, so the volume of distribution is estimated using the following formula:

$$V = 0.26[IBW + 0.4(TBW - IBW)] = 0.26[50\ kg + 0.4(140\ kg - 50\ kg)] = 22.3\ L$$

4. *Choose the desired steady-state serum concentrations.*

Endocarditis patients treated with aminoglycoside antibiotics for gram-positive synergy require steady-state peak concentrations ($C_{max,ss}$) of 3 to 4 μg/mL; steady-state trough ($C_{min,ss}$) concentrations should be <1 μg/mL to avoid toxicity. Set $C_{max,ss}$ = 4 μg/mL and $C_{min,ss}$ = 0.5 μg/mL.

5. *Use intermittent intravenous infusion equations to compute the tobramycin dose (see Table 4-2C).*

Calculate the required dosage interval (τ) using a 1-hour infusion:

$$\tau = [(\ln C_{max,ss} - \ln C_{min,ss})/k_e] + t' = [(\ln 4\ \mu g/mL - \ln 0.5\ \mu g/mL)/0.146\ h^{-1}] + 1\ h = 15\ h$$

Dosage intervals should be rounded to clinically acceptable intervals of 8 hours, 12 hours, 18 hours, 24 hours, 36 hours, 48 hours, 72 hours, and multiples of 24 hours thereafter, whenever possible. In this case, the dosage interval is rounded to 12 hours. Also, steady-state peak concentrations are similar if drawn immediately after a 1-hour infusion or 30 minutes after a 30-minute infusion, so the dose can be administered either way.

$$k_0 = C_{max,ss} k_e V[(1 - e^{-k_e \tau})/(1 - e^{-k_e t'})]$$

$$k_0 = (4\ mg/L \cdot 0.146\ h^{-1} \cdot 22.3\ L)[(1 - e^{-(0.146\ h^{-1})(12\ h)})/(1 - e^{-(0.146\ h^{-1})(1\ h)})] = 79\ mg$$

Aminoglycoside doses should be rounded to the nearest 5 to 10 mg. This dose is rounded to 80 mg. (Note: μg/mL = mg/L, and this concentration unit was substituted for $C_{max,ss}$ to avoid unnecessary unit conversion.)

The prescribed maintenance dose of tobramycin is 80 mg every 12 hours.

6. *Compute the loading dose (LD), if needed.*

Loading doses should be considered for patients with creatinine clearance values lower than 60 mL/min. The administration of a loading dose in these patients allows achievement of therapeutic peak concentrations more quickly than if maintenance doses alone are given. However, because the pharmacokinetic parameters used to compute these initial doses are *estimated* values and not *actual* values, the patient's own parameters may be much different from the estimated constants, and steady state is not achieved until 3 to 5 half-lives have passed.

$$LD = k_0/(1 - e^{-k_e \tau}) = 80\ mg/(1 - e^{-(0.146\ h^{-1})(12\ h)}) = 97\ mg$$

This loading dose is rounded to 100 mg and given as the first dose. The first maintenance dose is given 12 hours later.

Hull and Sarubbi Nomogram

1. *Estimate the creatinine clearance.*

This patient has a stable serum creatinine and is obese ($IBW_{females}$ (in kg) = 45 + 2.3(Ht – 60 in) = 45 + 2.3(62 – 60) = 50 kg). The Salazar and Corcoran equation can be used to estimate creatinine clearance:

$$CrCl_{est(females)} = \frac{(146 - age)[(0.287 \cdot Wt) + (9.74 \cdot Ht^2)]}{(60 \cdot S_{Cr})}$$

$$CrCl_{est(females)} = \frac{(146 - 45\ y)\{(0.287 \cdot 140\ kg) + [9.74 \cdot (1.57\ m)^2]\}}{(60 \cdot 2.4\ mg/dL)} = 45\ mL/min$$

Note: Height is converted from inches to meters: Ht = (62 in · 2.54 cm/in)/(100 cm/m) = 1.57 m.

2. *Choose the desired steady-state serum concentrations.*

Patients with gram-positive endocarditis being treated with aminoglycoside antibiotics for synergy require steady-state peak concentrations ($C_{max,ss}$) of 3 to 4 μg/mL.

3. *Select the loading dose (see Table 4-3).*

A loading dose (LD) of 1.5 mg/kg tobramycin provides a peak concentration of 5 to 7 μg/mL. This is the lowest dose suggested by the nomogram and is used in this example. However, some clinicians may substitute a loading dose of 1 to 1.2 mg/kg designed to produce a steady-state peak concentration of 3 to 4 μg/mL.

Because the patient is obese, adjusted body weight (ABW) is used to compute the dose: ABW = IBW + 0.4[TBW – IBW] = 50 kg + 0.4[140 kg – 50 kg] = 86 kg

LD = 1.5 mg/kg(86 kg) = 129 mg, rounded to 130 mg or LD = 1.2 mg/kg (86 kg)
= 103 mg, rounded to 100 mg

4. *Determine the estimated half-life, maintenance dose, and dosage interval.*

From the nomogram, the estimated half-life is ~6 hours, suggesting that a 12-dosage interval is appropriate. The maintenance dose (MD) is 72% of the loading dose (MD = 0.72[130 mg] = 94 mg or MD = 0.72[100 mg] = 72 mg), and the dosage interval is 12 hours.

Aminoglycoside doses should be rounded to the nearest 5 to 10 mg. Steady-state peak concentrations are similar if drawn immediately after a 1-hour infusion or 30 minutes after a 30-minute infusion, so the dose can be administered either way.

The prescribed maintenance dose is tobramycin 95 mg every 12 hours or 70 mg every 12 hours, depending on the loading dose chosen.

8. The modified dose of tobramycin for patient AF is calculated as follows.

Linear Pharmacokinetics Method

1. *Compute the new dose to achieve desired serum concentration.*

With the use of linear pharmacokinetics, the new dose to attain the desired concentration should be proportional to the old dose that produced the measured concentration:

$$D_{new} = (C_{ss,new}/C_{ss,old})D_{old} = [(4\ \mu g/mL)/(6.2\ \mu g/mL)]\ 100\ mg = 65\ mg$$

The new suggested dose is 65 mg every 12 hours to be started at the next scheduled dosing time.

2. *Check the steady-state trough concentration for the new dosage regimen.*

Using linear pharmacokinetics, the new steady-state concentration can be estimated and should be proportional to the old dose that produced the measured concentration.

$$C_{ss,new} = (D_{new}/D_{old})C_{ss,old} = (65\ mg/100\ mg)\ 1.5\ \mu g/mL = 1\ \mu g/mL$$

This steady-state trough concentration should be safe and effective for the infection that is being treated.

Pharmacokinetics Concepts Method

1. *Draw a rough sketch of the serum log concentration–time curve by hand, keeping track of the relative time between the serum concentrations (Figure 4-15).*

2. *Since the patient is at steady-state, the trough concentration can be extrapolated to the next trough value time (see Figure 4-15).*

3. *Draw the elimination curve between the steady-state peak concentration and the extrapolated trough concentration. Use this line to estimate half-life.* The patient is receiving tobramycin 100 mg every 12 hours, which produces a steady-state peak of 6.2 μg/mL and a steady-state trough of 1.5 μg/mL. The dose is infused over 30 minutes, and the peak concentration is drawn 30 minutes later (see Figure 4-15). The time between the measured steady-state peak and the extrapolated trough concentration is 11 hours (the 12-hour dosage interval minus the 1-hour combined infusion and waiting time). The definition of half-life is the time needed for serum concentrations to decrease by half. It takes 1 half-life for the peak serum concentration to decline from 6.2 μg/mL to 3.1 μg/mL and an additional half-life for the concentration to decrease from 3.1 μg/mL to 1.6 μg/mL. The concentration of 1.5 μg/mL is very close to the extrapolated trough value of 1.6 μg/mL. Therefore, 2 half-lives expired during the 11-hour time period between the peak concentration and extrapolated trough concentration, and the estimated half-life is ~6 hours. This information is used to set the new dosage interval for the patient.

4. *Determine the difference in concentration between the steady-state peak and trough concentrations. The difference changes proportionally with the dose size.* In this example, the patient is receiving tobramycin 100 mg every 12 hours, which produced steady-state peak and trough concentrations of 6.2 μg/mL and 1.5 μg/mL, respectively. The difference between the peak and trough values is 4.7 μg/mL. The change in serum concentration is proportional to the dose, and this information is used to set a new dose for the patient.

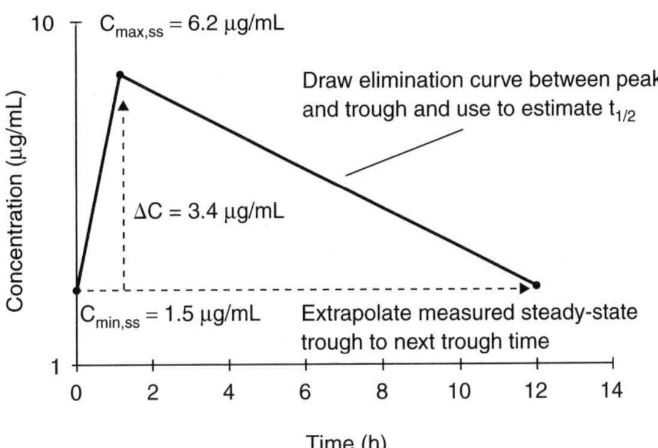

FIGURE 4-15 Solution to problem 8 using the pharmacokinetic concepts method.

5. *Choose new steady-state peak and trough concentrations.* For this example, the desired steady-state peak and trough concentrations are approximately 4 μg/mL and ≤1 μg/mL, respectively.

6. *Determine the new dosage interval for the desired concentrations.* With use of the desired concentrations, it will take 1 half-life for the peak concentration of 4 μg/mL to decrease to 2 μg/mL and 1 more half-life for the serum concentration to decrease to 1 μg/mL. Therefore, the dosage interval needs to be approximately 2 half-lives or 12 hours (6 hours × 2 half-lives = 12 hours).

7. *Determine the new tobramycin dose for the desired concentrations.* The desired peak concentration is 4 μg/mL, and the expected trough concentration is 1 μg/mL. The change in concentration between these values is 3.0 μg/mL. It is known from measured serum concentrations that administration of 100 mg changes serum concentrations by 4.7 μg/mL and that the change in serum concentration between the peak and trough values is proportional to the size of the dose. In this case, $D_{new} = (\Delta C_{new}/\Delta C_{old})D_{old}$ = [(3.0 μg/mL)/(4.7 μg/mL)] 100 mg = 64 mg, rounded to 65 mg. Tobramycin 65 mg every 12 hours is started 12 hours after the last dose of the previous dosage regimen,

Steady-State Sawchuk-Zaske Method

1. *Compute the patient's elimination rate constant and half-life (note: for infusion times less than 1 hour, t′ is considered to be the sum of the infusion and waiting times).*

$$k_e = (\ln C_{max,ss} - \ln C_{min,ss})/\tau - t' = (\ln 6.2\ \mu g/mL - \ln 1.5\ \mu g/mL)/(12\ h - 1\ h) = 0.129\ h^{-1}$$

$$t_{1/2} = 0.693/k_e = 0.693/0.129\ h^{-1} = 5.4\ h$$

2. *Compute the patient's volume of distribution.*

$$V = \frac{D/t'(1 - e^{-k_e t'})}{k_e[C_{max,ss} - (C_{min,ss}e^{-k_e t'})]} = \frac{(100\ mg/1\ h)(1 - e^{-(0.129\ h^{-1})(1\ h)})}{0.129\ h^{-1}[6.2\ mg/L - (1.5\ mg/L\ e^{-(0.129\ h^{-1})(1\ h)})]}$$

$$V = 19.2\ L$$

3. *Choose new steady-state peak and trough concentrations.* For this example, the desired steady-state peak and trough concentrations are 4 μg/mL and ≤1 μg/mL, respectively.

4. *Determine the new dosage interval for the desired concentrations.* As in the initial dosage section of this chapter, the dosage interval (τ) is computed by means of the following equation using a 1-hour infusion time (t′):

$$\tau = [(\ln C_{max,ss} - \ln C_{min,ss})/k_e] + t' = [(\ln 4\ \mu g/mL - \ln 1\ \mu g/mL)/0.129\ h^{-1}] + 1\ h = 12\ h$$

5. *Determine the new dose for the desired concentrations.* The dose is computed according to the one-compartment model intravenous infusion equation used in the initial dosing section of this chapter.

$k_0 = C_{max,ss} k_e V[(1 - e^{-k_e \tau})/(1 - e^{-k_e t'})]$

$k_0 = (4\ mg/L \cdot 0.129\ h^{-1} \cdot 19.2\ L)[(1 - e^{-(0.129\ h^{-1})(12\ h)})/(1 - e^{-(0.129\ h^{-1})(1\ h)})] = 65\ mg$

Tobramycin 65 mg every 12 hours is prescribed to begin 12 hours after the last dose of the previous regimen. This dose is identical with that derived for the patient using the linear pharmacokinetics method and the pharmacokinetic concepts method (65 mg every 12 hours).

9. The initial tobramycin dose for patient FH is calculated as follows.

1. *Estimate the creatinine clearance.*

This patient has a stable serum creatinine and is not obese. The Cockcroft–Gault equation can be used to estimate creatinine clearance:

$$CrCl_{est} = [(140 - age)BW]/(72 \cdot S_{Cr}) = [(140 - 24\ y)60\ kg]/(72 \cdot 0.7\ mg/dL)$$

$$CrCl_{est} = 138\ mL/min$$

2. *Estimate the elimination rate constant (k_e) and half-life ($t_{1/2}$).*

The elimination rate constant versus creatinine clearance relationship is used to estimate the tobramycin elimination rate for this patient:

$$k_e = 0.00293(CrCl) + 0.014 = 0.00293(138\ mL/min) + 0.014 = 0.419\ h^{-1}$$

$$t_{1/2} = 0.693/k_e = 0.693/0.419\ h^{-1} = 1.7\ h$$

3. *Estimate the volume of distribution.*

The patient has no disease states or conditions that would alter the volume of distribution from the normal value of 0.35 L/kg for cystic fibrosis patients.

$$V = 0.35\ L/kg\ (60\ kg) = 21\ L$$

4. *Choose the desired steady-state serum concentrations.*

Patients with cystic fibrosis who have a sputum culture positive for *Pseudomonas aeruginosa* and a pulmonary exacerbation treated with aminoglycoside antibiotics require steady-state peak concentrations ($C_{max,ss}$) of 8 to 10 μg/mL; steady-state trough ($C_{min,ss}$) concentrations should be <2 μg/mL to avoid toxicity. Set $C_{max,ss}$ = 10 μg/mL and $C_{min,ss}$ = 1 μg/mL.

5. *Use the intermittent intravenous infusion equations to compute the dose.*

Calculate the required dosage interval (τ) using a 1-hour infusion:

$$\tau = [(\ln C_{max,ss} - \ln C_{min,ss})/k_e] + t' = [(\ln 10\ \mu g/mL - \ln 1\ \mu g/mL)/0.419\ h^{-1}] + 1\ h = 6.5\ h$$

Dosage intervals should be rounded to clinically acceptable intervals of 8 hours, 12 hours, 18 hours, 24 hours, 36 hours, 48 hours, 72 hours, and multiples of 24 hours thereafter, whenever possible. In this case, the dosage interval is rounded to 8 hours. Also, steady-state peak concentrations are similar if drawn immediately after a

1-hour infusion or 30 minutes after a 30-minute infusion, so the dose can be administered either way.

$$k_0 = C_{max,ss} k_e V[(1 - e^{-k_e \tau})/(1 - e^{-k_e t'})]$$

$$k_0 = (10\ mg/L \cdot 0.419\ h^{-1} \cdot 21\ L)[(1 - e^{-(0.419\ h^{-1})(8\ h)})/(1 - e^{-(0.419\ h^{-1})(1\ h)})] = 248\ mg$$

Aminoglycoside doses should be rounded to the nearest 5 to 10 mg. This dose is rounded to 250 mg. (Note: μg/mL = mg/L, and this concentration unit was substituted for $C_{max,ss}$ to avoid unnecessary unit conversion.)

The prescribed maintenance dose is 250 mg tobramycin every 8 hours.

6. *Compute the loading dose, if needed.*

Loading doses for patients with creatinine clearance values higher than 60 mL/min are usually close to maintenance doses, so that they are often not given to this patient population.

$$LD = k_0/(1 - e^{-k_e \tau}) = 250\ mg/(1 - e^{-(0.419\ h^{-1})(8\ h)}) = 259\ mg\text{, rounded to } 260$$

10. The modified dose of tobramycin for patient FH is calculated as follows.

Linear Pharmacokinetics Method

1. *Compute a new dose to achieve the desired serum concentration.*

Using linear pharmacokinetics, the new dose to attain the desired concentration should be proportional to the old dose that produced the measured concentration:

$$D_{new} = (C_{ss,new}/C_{ss,old})D_{old} = [(10\ \mu g/mL)/(7.9\ \mu g/mL)]\ 250\ mg = 316\ mg$$

The new suggested dose is 315 mg tobramycin every 8 hours to be started at the next scheduled dosing time.

2. *Check the steady-state trough concentration for new dosage regimen.*

Using linear pharmacokinetics, the new steady-state concentration can be estimated and should be proportional to the old dose that produced the measured concentration:

$$C_{ss,new} = (D_{new}/D_{old})C_{ss,old} = (315\ mg/250\ mg)\ 1\ \mu g/mL = 1.3\ \mu g/mL$$

This steady-state trough concentration should be safe and effective for the infection that is being treated.

Pharmacokinetics Concept Method

1. *Draw a rough sketch of the serum log concentration–time curve by hand, keeping track of the relative time between the serum concentrations (Figure 4-16).*

2. *Since the patient is at steady state, the trough concentration can be extrapolated to the next trough value time (see Figure 4-16).*

3. *Draw the elimination curve between the steady-state peak concentration and the extrapolated trough concentration. Use this line to estimate half-life.* The patient is receiving tobramycin 250 mg every 8 hours, which produces a steady-state peak of

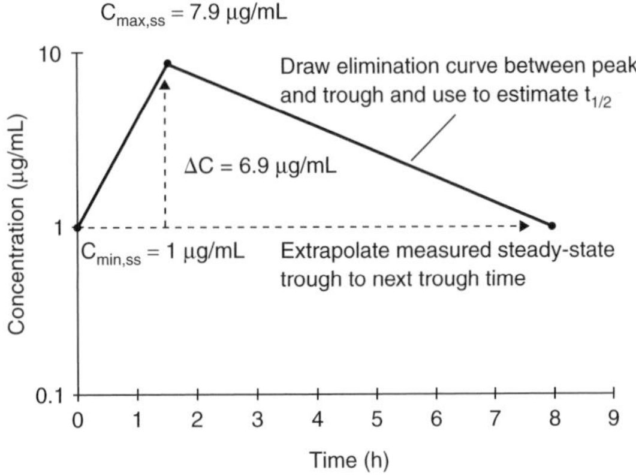

FIGURE 4-16 Solution to problem 10 using the pharmacokinetic concepts method.

7.9 μg/mL and a steady-state trough of 1 μg/mL. The dose is infused over 30 minutes, and the peak concentration is drawn 30 minutes later (see Figure 4-16). The time between the measured steady-state peak and the extrapolated trough concentration is 7 hours (the 8-hour dosage interval minus the 1-hour combined infusion and waiting time). The definition of half-life is the time needed for serum concentrations to decrease by half. It takes 1 half-life for the peak serum concentration to decline from 7.9 μg/mL to 4 μg/mL, an additional half-life for the serum concentration to decrease from 4 μg/mL to 2 μg/mL, and another half-life for the concentration to decline from 2 μg/mL to 1 μg/mL. Therefore, 3 half-lives expired during the 7-hour time period between the peak concentration and extrapolated trough concentration, and the estimated half-life is 2 hours (7 hours/3 half-lives = ~2 hours). This information is used to set the new dosage interval for the patient.

4. *Determine the difference in concentration between the steady-state peak and trough concentrations. The difference in concentration changes proportionally with the dose size.* In this example, the patient is receiving tobramycin 250 mg every 8 hours, which produced steady-state peak and trough concentrations of 7.9 μg/mL and 1 μg/mL, respectively. The difference between the peak and trough values is 6.9 μg/mL. The change in serum concentration is proportional to the dose, and this information is used to set a new dose for the patient.

5. *Choose new steady-state peak and trough concentrations.* For this example, the desired steady-state peak and trough concentrations are approximately 10 μg/mL and 1 μg/mL, respectively.

6. *Determine the new dosage interval for the desired concentrations.* Using the desired concentrations, it will take 1 half-life for the peak concentration of 10 μg/mL to decrease to 5 μg/mL, 1 more half-life for the serum concentration to decrease to 2.5 μg/mL, an additional half-life for serum concentrations to decline from 2.5 μg/mL to 1.3 μg/mL, and a final half-life for serum concentrations to reach 0.7 μg/mL. Therefore, the dosage interval needs to be approximately 4 half-lives or 8 hours (2 hours × 4 half-lives = 8 hours).

7. *Determine the new dose of tobramycin for the desired concentrations.* The desired peak concentration is 10 μg/mL, and the expected trough concentration is 0.7 μg/mL. The change in concentration between these values is 9.3 μg/mL. It is known from measured serum concentrations that administration of 250 mg changes serum concentrations by 6.9 μg/mL and that the change in serum concentration between the peak and trough values is proportional to the size of the dose. In this case, $D_{new} = (\Delta C_{new}/\Delta C_{old})D_{old}$ = [(9.3 μg/mL)/(6.9 μg/mL)] 250 mg = 336 mg, rounded to 335 mg. Tobramycin 335 mg every 8 hours is started 8 hours after the last dose of the previous dosage regimen.

Steady-State Sawchuk-Zaske Method

1. *Compute the patient's elimination rate constant and half-life (note: for infusion times less than 1 hour, t′ is considered to be the sum of the infusion and waiting times.)*

$$k_e = (\ln C_{max,ss} - \ln C_{min,ss})/\tau - t' = (\ln 7.9\ \mu g/mL - \ln 1\ \mu g/mL)/(8\ h - 1\ h) = 0.295\ h^{-1}$$

$$t_{1/2} = 0.693/k_e = 0.693/0.295\ h^{-1} = 2.3\ h$$

2. *Compute the patient's volume of distribution.*

$$V = \frac{D/t'(1 - e^{-k_e t'})}{k_e[C_{max,ss} - (C_{min,ss}e^{-k_e t'})]} = \frac{(250\ mg/1\ h)(1 - e^{-(0.295\ h^{-1})(1\ h)})}{0.295\ h^{-1}[7.9\ mg/L - (1\ mg/L\ e^{-(0.295\ h^{-1})(1\ h)})]}$$

$$V = 30.3\ L$$

3. *Choose new steady-state peak and trough concentrations.* For this example, the desired steady-state peak and trough concentrations are 10 μg/mL and 1 μg/mL, respectively.

4. *Determine the new dosage interval for the desired concentrations.* As in the initial dosage section of this chapter, the dosage interval (τ) is computed by means of the following equation using a 1-hour infusion time (t′):

$$\tau = [(\ln C_{max,ss} - \ln C_{min,ss})/k_e] + t' = [(\ln 10\ \mu g/mL - \ln 1\ \mu g/mL)/0.295\ h^{-1}] + 1\ h = 8.8\ h, \text{ rounded to } 8\ h$$

5. *Determine the new dose of tobramycin for the desired concentrations.* The dose is computed according to the one-compartment model intravenous infusion equation used in the initial dosing section of this chapter:

$$k_0 = C_{max,ss} k_e V[(1 - e^{-k_e \tau})/(1 - e^{-k_e t'})]$$

$$k_0 = (10\ mg/L \cdot 0.295\ h^{-1} \cdot 30.3\ L)[(1 - e^{-(0.295\ h^{-1})(8\ h)})/(1 - e^{-(0.295\ h^{-1})(1\ h)})] = 316\ mg, \text{ rounded to } 315\ mg$$

Tobramycin 315 mg every 8 hours is prescribed to begin 8 hours after the last dose of the previous regimen. This dose is identical with that derived for the patient using the linear pharmacokinetics method (315 mg every 8 hours) and is very similar to that calculated by the pharmacokinetic concepts method (335 mg every 8 hours).

11. The initial gentamicin dose for patient TY is calculated as follows.

1. *Estimate the creatinine clearance.*

This patient has a stable serum creatinine and is not obese. The Cockcroft–Gault equation can be used to estimate creatinine clearance:

$$CrCl_{est} = \{[(140 - age)BW] \cdot 0.85\}/(72 \cdot S_{Cr}) = \{[(140 - 66\ y)65\ kg] \cdot 0.85\}/(72 \cdot 1.4\ mg/dL)$$

$$CrCl_{est} = 41\ mL/min$$

2. *Estimate the elimination rate constant (k_e) and half-life ($t_{1/2}$).*

The elimination rate constant versus creatinine clearance relationship is used to estimate the gentamicin elimination rate for this patient:

$$k_e = 0.00293(CrCl) + 0.014 = 0.00293(41\ mL/min) + 0.014 = 0.133\ h^{-1}$$

$$t_{1/2} = 0.693/k_e = 0.693/0.133\ h^{-1} = 5.2\ h$$

3. *Estimate the volume of distribution.*

The patient has excess extracellular fluid due to ascites, and the formula will be used to take this into account. The patient's dry weight (DBW) before accumulation of ascitic fluid was 65 kg, and her current weight (TBW) has increased to 72 kg.

$$V = (0.26 \cdot DBW) + (TBW - DBW) = (0.26 \cdot 65\ kg) + (72\ kg - 65\ kg) = 23.9\ L$$

4. *Choose the desired steady-state serum concentrations.*

For this example, a steady-state peak concentration ($C_{max,ss}$) of 6 μg/mL and steady-state trough ($C_{min,ss}$) concentration of 1 μg/mL is used to design the dosage regimen.

5. *Use the intermittent intravenous infusion equations to compute the dose.*

Calculate the required dosage interval (τ) using a 1-hour infusion:

$$\tau = [(\ln C_{max,ss} - \ln C_{min,ss})/k_e] + t' = [(\ln 6\ \mu g/mL - \ln 1\ \mu g/mL)/0.133\ h^{-1}] + 1\ h = 14.5\ h$$

Dosage intervals should be rounded to clinically acceptable intervals of 8 hours, 12 hours, 18 hours, 24 hours, 36 hours, 48 hours, 72 hours, and multiples of 24 hours thereafter, whenever possible. In this case, the dosage interval is rounded to 12 hours. Also, steady-state peak concentrations are similar if drawn immediately after a 1-hour infusion or 30 minutes after a 30-minute infusion, so the dose can be administered either way.

$$k_0 = C_{max,ss} k_e V[(1 - e^{-k_e \tau})/(1 - e^{-k_e t'})]$$

$$k_0 = (6\ mg/L \cdot 0.133\ h^{-1} \cdot 23.9\ L)[(1 - e^{-(0.133\ h^{-1})(12\ h)})/(1 - e^{-(0.133\ h^{-1})(1\ h)})] = 122\ mg$$

Aminoglycoside doses should be rounded to the nearest 5 to 10 mg. This dose is rounded to 120 mg. (Note: μg/mL = mg/L, and this concentration unit was substituted for $C_{max,ss}$ to avoid unnecessary unit conversion.)

The prescribed maintenance dose is 120 mg gentamicin every 12 hours.

6. *Compute the loading dose, if needed.*

Loading doses for patients with creatinine clearance values lower than 60 mL/min can be given:

$$LD = k_0/(1 - e^{-k_e\tau}) = 120\ mg/(1 - e^{-(0.133\ h^{-1})(12\ h)}) = 151\ mg, \text{ rounded to } 150\ mg$$

The loading dose should be given as the first dose, and subsequent doses are maintenance doses.

12. The modified dose of gentamicin for patient TY is calculated as follows.

Linear Pharmacokinetics Method

1. *Compute the new dose to achieve the desired serum concentration.*

Calculated by linear pharmacokinetics, the new dose to attain the desired concentration should be proportional to the old dose that produced the measured concentration:

$$D_{new} = (C_{ss,new}/C_{ss,old})D_{old} = [(6\ \mu g/mL)/(4\ \mu g/mL)]\ 120\ mg = 180\ mg$$

The new suggested dose is 180 mg gentamicin every 12 hours to be started at next scheduled dosing time.

2. *Check the steady-state trough concentration for the new dosage regimen.*

By using linear pharmacokinetics, the new steady-state concentration can be estimated and should be proportional to the old dose that produced the measured concentration:

$$C_{ss,new} = (D_{new}/D_{old})C_{ss,old} = (180\ mg/120\ mg)\ 0.8\ \mu g/mL = 1.2\ \mu g/mL$$

This steady-state trough concentration should be safe and effective for the infection that is being treated.

Pharmacokinetic Concepts Method

1. *Draw a rough sketch of the serum log concentration–time curve by hand, keeping track of the relative time between the serum concentrations (Figure 4-17).*

2. *Since the patient is at steady state, the trough concentration can be extrapolated to the next trough value time (see Figure 4-17).*

3. *Draw the elimination curve between the steady-state peak concentration and the extrapolated trough concentration. Use this line to estimate half-life.* The patient is receiving 120 mg gentamicin every 12 hours, which produces a steady-state peak of 4 μg/mL and a steady-state trough of 0.8 μg/mL. The dose is infused over 30 minutes, and the peak concentration is drawn 30 minutes later (see Figure 4-17). The time between the measured steady-state peak and the extrapolated trough concentration is 11 hours (the 12-hour dosage interval minus the 1-hour combined infusion and waiting time). The definition of half-life is the time needed for serum concentrations to decrease by half. It takes 1 half-life for the peak serum concentration to decline from 4 μg/mL to 2 μg/mL and an additional half-life for the serum concentration to decrease from 2 μg/mL to 1 μg/mL. The concentration of 1 μg/mL is close to the ob-

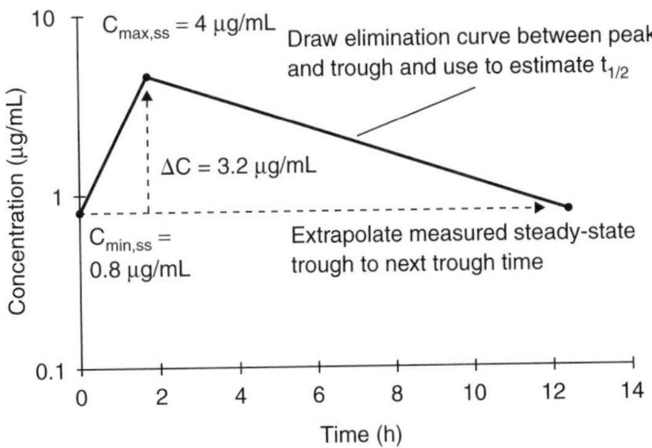

FIGURE 4-17 Solution to problem 12 using the pharmacokinetic concepts method.

served value of 0.8 μg/mL. Therefore, 2 half-lives expired during the 11-hour time period between the peak concentration and the extrapolated trough concentration, and the estimated half-life is 6 hours (11 hours/2 half-lives = ~6 hours). This information is used to set the new dosage interval for the patient.

4. *Determine the difference in concentration between the steady-state peak and trough concentrations. The difference in concentration changes proportionally with the dose size.* In this example, the patient is receiving a gentamicin dose of 120 mg every 12 hours, which produced steady-state peak and trough concentrations of 4 μg/mL and 0.8 μg/mL, respectively. The difference between the peak and trough values is 3.2 μg/mL. The change in serum concentration is proportional to the dose, and this information is used to set a new dose for the patient.

5. *Choose new steady-state peak and trough concentrations.* For this example, the desired steady-state peak and trough concentrations are approximately 6 μg/mL and 1 μg/mL, respectively.

6. *Determine the new dosage interval for the desired concentrations.* Using the desired concentrations, it will take 1 half-life for the peak concentration of 6 μg/mL to decrease to 3 μg/mL and an additional half-life for serum concentrations to decline from 3 μg/mL to 1.5 μg/mL. This concentration is close to the desired trough concentration of 1 μg/mL. Therefore, the dosage interval needs to be approximately 2 half-lives or 12 hours (6 hours × 2 half-lives = 12 hours).

7. *Determine the new dose of gentamicin for the desired concentrations.* The desired peak concentration is 6 μg/mL, and the expected trough concentration is 1.5 μg/mL. The change in concentration between these values is 4.5 μg/mL. It is known from measured serum concentrations that administration of 120 mg changes serum concentrations by 3.2 μg/mL and that the change in serum concentration between the peak and trough values is proportional to the size of the dose. In this case, $D_{new} = (\Delta C_{new}/\Delta C_{old})D_{old}$ = [(4.5 μg/mL)/(3.2 μg/mL)] 120 mg = 168 mg, rounded to 170 mg. Gentamicin 170 mg every 12 hours is started 12 hours after the last dose of the previous dosage regimen.

Steady-State Sawchuk-Zaske Method

1. *Compute the patient's elimination rate constant and half-life (note: for infusion times of less than 1 hour, t′ is considered to be the sum of the infusion and waiting times).*

$$k_e = (\ln C_{max,ss} - \ln C_{min,ss})/\tau - t' = (\ln 4\ \mu g/mL - \ln 0.8\ \mu g/mL)/(12\ h - 1\ h) = 0.146\ h^{-1}$$

$$t_{1/2} = 0.693/k_e = 0.693/0.146\ h^{-1} = 4.7\ h$$

2. *Compute the patient's volume of distribution.*

$$V = \frac{D/t'(1 - e^{-k_e t'})}{k_e[C_{max,ss} - (C_{min,ss}e^{-k_e t'})]} = \frac{(120\ mg/1\ h)(1 - e^{-(0.146\ h^{-1})(1\ h)})}{0.146\ h^{-1}[4\ mg/L - (0.8\ mg/L\ e^{-(0.146\ h^{-1})(1\ h)})]}$$

$$V = 33.7\ L$$

3. *Choose new steady-state peak and trough concentrations.* For this example, the desired steady-state peak and trough concentrations are 6 μg/mL and 1 μg/mL, respectively.

4. *Determine the new dosage interval for the desired concentrations.* As in the initial dosage section of this chapter, the dosage interval (τ) is computed using the following equation with a 1-hour infusion time (t′):

$$\tau = [(\ln C_{max,ss} - \ln C_{min,ss})/k_e] + t' = [(\ln 6\ \mu g/mL - \ln 1.0\ \mu g/mL)/0.146\ h^{-1}] + 1\ h = 13.3\ h, \text{ rounded to } 12\ h$$

5. *Determine the new dose for the desired concentrations.* The gentamicin dose is computed according to the one-compartment model intravenous infusion equation used in the initial dosing section of this chapter:

$$k_0 = C_{max,ss} k_e V[(1 - e^{-k_e \tau})/(1 - e^{-k_e t'})]$$

$$k_0 = (6\ mg/L \cdot 0.146\ h^{-1} \cdot 33.7\ L)[(1 - e^{-(0.146\ h^{-1})(12\ h)})/(1 - e^{-(0.146\ h^{-1})(1\ h)})] = 180\ mg$$

Gentamicin 180 mg every 12 hours is prescribed to begin 12 hours after the last dose of the previous regimen. This dose is identical with that derived for the patient using the linear pharmacokinetics method (180 mg every 12 hours) and is very similar to that derived by the pharmacokinetic concepts method (170 mg every 12 hours).

13. The initial gentamicin dose for patient UQ is calculated as follows.

1. *Estimate the creatinine clearance.*

This patient is not obese. The patient is in acute renal failure and is receiving hemodialysis. Because dialysis removes creatinine, the serum creatinine cannot be used to estimate creatinine clearance for the patient. Since the patient's renal function is poor enough to require dialysis, the creatinine clearance is assumed to be zero.

2. *Estimate the elimination rate constant (k_e) and half-life ($t_{1/2}$).*

The elimination rate constant versus creatinine clearance relationship is used to estimate the gentamicin elimination rate for this patient:

$$k_e = 0.00293(\text{CrCl}) + 0.014 = 0.00293(0 \text{ mL/min}) + 0.014 = 0.014 \text{ h}^{-1}$$

$$t_{1/2} = 0.693/k_e = 0.693/0.014 \text{ h}^{-1} = 50 \text{ h}$$

3. *Estimate the volume of distribution.*

The patient has renal failure and needs to be assessed for volume status to rule out over- and underhydration. In this case, the patient is in good fluid balance, and the volume of distribution from the normal value of 0.26 L/kg is used:

$$V = 0.26 \text{ L/kg } (85 \text{ kg}) = 22.1 \text{ L}$$

4. *Choose the desired steady-state serum concentrations.*

Patients with gram-negative pneumonia being treated with aminoglycoside antibiotics require steady-state peak concentrations ($C_{max,ss}$) of 8 to 10 μg/mL; steady-state trough ($C_{min,ss}$) concentrations should be <2 μg/mL to avoid toxicity. Set $C_{max,ss}$ = 8 μg/mL and $C_{min,ss}$ ~2 μg/mL.

5. *Compute the first dose.*

Because the patient has renal failure with a gentamicin half-life of ~50 hours, very little antibiotic is eliminated during the 1/2- to 1-hour infusion time. Simple intravenous bolus equations can be used to compute doses in this case.

$$LD = C_{max} V = 8 \text{ mg/L} \cdot 22.1 \text{ L} = 177 \text{ mg}$$

Aminoglycoside doses should be rounded to the nearest 5 to 10 mg. This dose is rounded to 180 mg. (Note: μg/mL = mg/L, and this concentration unit was substituted for C_{max} to avoid unnecessary unit conversion.

The prescribed maintenance dose is 180 mg gentamicin postdialysis at 1200 H on Wednesday.

6. *Estimate the predialysis and postdialysis aminoglycoside concentrations.*

The next dialysis session is on Friday at 0800 H. The time expired between the dose given on Wednesday at 1200 H and this hemodialysis period is 44 hours (Figure 4-18). During the interdialysis time period only the patient's own endogenous clearance will eliminate gentamicin. The predialysis serum concentration will be:

$$C = C_0 e^{-k_e t} = (8 \text{ μg/mL}) e^{-(0.014 \text{ h}^{-1})(44 \text{ h})} = 4.3 \text{ μg/mL}$$

The average half-life of aminoglycosides during hemodialysis with a low-flux membrane is 4 hours. Because the usual dialysis time is 3 to 4 hours with a low-flux filter, intradialysis elimination can be computed:

$$k_e = 0.693/t_{1/2} = 0.693/4 \text{ h} = 0.173 \text{ h}^{-1}$$

$$C = C_0 e^{-k_e t} = (4.3 \text{ μg/mL}) e^{-(0.173 \text{ h}^{-1})(4 \text{ h})} = 2.2 \text{ μg/mL}$$

Alternatively, because aminoglycoside half-life on dialysis is 4 hours and the dialysis period is 4 hours, one can deduce that the postdialysis serum concentration will be half the predialysis value.

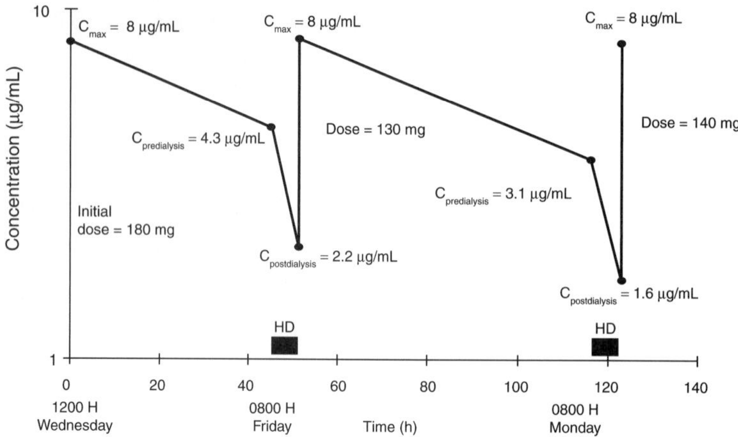

FIGURE 4-18 Solution to problem 13.

7. *Calculate the postdialysis replacement dose.*

The postdialysis serum concentration of 2.2 µg/mL is an estimate of the actual gentamicin serum concentration and is close enough to the target concentration that a postdialysis dose will be administered immediately at the end of the procedure.

$$\text{Replacement dose} = (C_{max} - C_{baseline})V = (8 \text{ mg/L} - 2.2 \text{ mg/L})\ 22.1 \text{ L}$$
$$= 128 \text{ mg, rounded to } 130 \text{ mg}$$

8. *Compute the predialysis and postdialysis concentrations plus the postdialysis dose for next dialysis cycle.*

The Friday-to-Monday dialysis cycle includes an extra day, so the concentration profile for that time period is estimated (see Figure 4-18). The time between the gentamicin dose given at 1200 H on Friday, and the next dialysis period at 0800 H on Monday is 68 hours.

$$C = C_0e^{-k_et} = (8\ \mu g/mL)e^{-(0.014\ h^{-1})(68\ h)} = 3.1\ \mu g/mL \text{ predialysis on Monday}$$

$$C = C_0e^{-k_et} = (3.1\ \mu g/mL)e^{-(0.173\ h^{-1})(4\ h)} = 1.6\ \mu g/mL \text{ postdialysis on Monday}$$

Replacement dose = $(C_{max} - C_{baseline})V = (8 \text{ mg/L} - 1.6 \text{ mg/L})\ 22.1 \text{ L} = 141$ mg, rounded to 140 mg. The dialysis periods for this patient are scheduled, and because the dosage recommendation is based on estimated pharmacokinetic parameters, a postdialysis dose of 130 mg gentamicin can be suggested so that all doses are uniform.

14. The revised gentamicin dose for patient UQ using *intravenous bolus equations* is calculated as follows.

1. *Compute the patient's elimination rate constant and half-life.*

$$k_e = (\ln C_{postdose} - \ln C_{predialysis})/\Delta t = (\ln 6.4\ \mu g/mL - \ln 2.2\ \mu g/mL)/(68\ h) = 0.0157\ h^{-1}$$

$$t_{1/2} = 0.693/k_e = 0.693/0.0157\ h^{-1} = 44\ h$$

2. *Compute the patient's volume of distribution.*

$$V = \frac{D}{C_{postdose(2)} - C_{predialysis}} = \frac{130\ mg}{6.9\ mg/L - 0.7\ mg/L}$$

$$V = 21\ L$$

3. *Compute the fraction of gentamicin eliminated by the dialysis procedure.*

Fraction eliminated = $(C_{predialysis} - C_{postdialysis})/C_{predialysis}$ = (2.2 μg/mL – 0.7 μg/mL)/2.2 μg/mL = 0.68 or 68%

The fraction remaining after hemodialysis is 1 – fraction eliminated or 1 – 0.68 = 0.32 or 32%.

4. *Compute predialysis and postdialysis concentrations plus postdialysis dose for next dialysis cycle using patient's own pharmacokinetic parameters.*

The time between the gentamicin concentration obtained at 1400 H on Monday and the next dialysis period at 0800 H on Wednesday is 42 hours.

$C = C_0e^{-k_et} = (6.9\ \mu g/mL)e^{-(0.0157\ h^{-1})(42\ h)} = 3.6\ \mu g/mL$ predialysis on Wednesday

The fraction remaining after hemodialysis is 0.32.

Fraction remaining = 0.32 · 3.6 μg/mL = 1.2 μg/mL

Replacement dose = $(C_{max} - C_{baseline})V$ = (8 mg/L – 1.2 mg/L) 21 L = 143 mg, rounded to 145 mg

15. This patient is an older person with poor renal function ($CrCl_{est}$ = {[(140 – age)BW] · 0.85}/(72 · S_{Cr}) = {[(140 – 67 y)60 kg] · 0.85}/(72 · 1.8 mg/dL) = 29 mL/min) and is not at steady state when the serum concentrations were obtained. Because of this, a Bayesian pharmacokinetics computer program is the best method for computing revised doses for this patient.

1. *Enter the patient's demographic, drug dosing, and serum concentration–time data into the computer program.*

2. *Compute the pharmacokinetic parameters for the patient using the Bayesian pharmacokinetics computer program.*

The pharmacokinetic parameters computed by the program are a volume of distribution of 21.4 L, a half-life of 13.5 hours, and an elimination rate constant of 0.051 h^{-1}.

3. *Compute the dose required to achieve desired aminoglycoside serum concentrations.*

The one-compartment model intravenous infusion equations used by the program to compute doses indicate that a dose of 150 mg every 36 hours produces steady-state peak concentration of 8.1 μg/mL and a steady-state trough concentration of 1.3 μg/mL.

16. Patient KK could receive an extended-interval gentamicin dose between 5 and 7 mg/kg.

(A) Hartford Nomogram for Initial Dosing Guidelines

1. *Estimate the creatinine clearance.*

Patient KK has a stable serum creatinine and is not obese. The Cockcroft–Gault equation can be used to estimate creatinine clearance:

$$CrCl_{est} = [(140 - \text{age})BW]/(72 \cdot S_{Cr}) = [(140 - 52\text{ y})87\text{ kg}]/(72 \cdot 1.4\text{ mg/dL})$$

$$CrCl_{est} = 76\text{ mL/min}$$

2. *Compute the initial dose and the dosage interval (see Table 4-4).*

A dose (D) of 7 mg/kg provides a peak concentration >20 μg/mL.

$$D = 7\text{ mg/kg}(87\text{ kg}) = 609\text{ mg, rounded to }610\text{ mg}$$

Since the patient's estimated creatinine clearance is >60 mL/min, a dosage interval of 24 hours is chosen.

The prescribed maintenance dose is 610 mg gentamicin every 24 hours.

(B) Hartford Nomogram for Individualizing Dosage Interval

3. *Determine the dosage interval using serum concentration monitoring (see Table 4-4).*

A gentamicin serum concentration measured 9 hours after the dose is 8.2 μg/mL. Based on the nomogram, a dosage interval of 36 hours is the correct value and is instituted with the next dose: 610 mg every 36 hours.

Bayesian Pharmacokinetics Computer Dosing Program for Individualizing Dose and Dosage Interval

1. *Enter the patient's demographic, drug dosing, and serum concentration–time data into the computer program.*

2. *Compute the pharmacokinetic parameters for the patient using a Bayesian pharmacokinetics computer program.*

The pharmacokinetic parameters computed by the program are a volume of distribution of 21.5 L, a half-life of 4.7 hours, and an elimination rate constant of 0.149 h^{-1}.

3. *Compute the dose required to achieve desired aminoglycoside serum concentrations.*

The one-compartment model intravenous infusion equations used by the program to compute doses indicate that a dose of 550 mg gentamicin every 24 hours produces a steady-state peak concentration of 24.4 μg/mL and a steady-state trough concentration of 0.8 μg/mL.

17. Patient XS had extended-interval tobramycin therapy instituted by other clinicians at a rate of 5 mg/kg per day. The tobramycin dose is less than 7 mg/kg, and the serum concentration was not obtained 6 to 14 hours after the dose. For these reasons, the

Hartford nomogram cannot be used, and a Bayesian pharmacokinetics computer program is the best method to compute revised doses for this patient.

1. *Enter the patient's demographic, drug dosing, and serum concentration–time data into the computer program.*

2. *Compute the pharmacokinetic parameters for the patient using the Bayesian pharmacokinetics computer program.*

The pharmacokinetic parameters computed by the program are a volume of distribution of 11.6 L, a half-life of 6.6 hours, and an elimination rate constant of 0.105 h^{-1}.

3. *Compute the dose required to achieve desired aminoglycoside serum concentrations.*

If the patient continues to receive the prescribed dose, the estimated steady-state peak and trough concentrations are 28.9 μg/mL and 2.6 μg/mL. The one-compartment model intravenous infusion equations used by the program to compute doses indicate that a dose of 300 mg every 36 hours will produce a steady-state peak concentration of 25.1 μg/mL and a steady-state trough concentration of 0.6 μg/mL.

REFERENCES

1. Chambers HF, Sande MA. Antimicrobial agents: the aminoglycosides. In: Hardman JG, Limbird LE, Molinoff PB, Ruddon RW, Gilman AG, eds. Goodman and Gilman's The Pharmacological Basis of Therapeutics. New York: McGraw-Hill, 1996:1103–1122.
2. Zaske DE, Cipolle RJ, Rotschafer JC, Solem LD, Mosier NR, Strate RG. Gentamicin pharmacokinetics in 1,640 patients: method for control of serum concentrations. Antimicrob Agents Chemother 1982;21:407–411.
3. Nicolau DP, Freeman CD, Belliveau PP, Nightingale CH, Ross JW, Quintilliani R. Experience with a once-daily aminoglycoside program administered to 2,184 adult patients. Antimicrob Agent Chemother 1995;39:650–655.
4. Jackson GG, Arcieri G. Ototoxicity of gentamicin in man: a survey and controlled analysis of clinical experience in the United States. J Infect Dis 1971;124(suppl):130–137.
5. Black RE, Lau WK, Weinstein RJ, Young LS, Hewitt WL. Ototoxicity of amikacin. Antimicrob Agents Chemother 1976;9:956–961.
6. Mawer GE, Ahmad R, Dobbs SM, Tooth JA. Prescribing aids for gentamicin. Br J Clin Pharmacol 1974;1:45–50.
7. Smith CR, Maxwell RR, Edwards CQ, Rogers JF, Lietman PS. Nephrotoxicity induced by gentamicin and amikacin. Johns Hopkins Med J 1978;142:85–90.
8. Dahlgren JG, Anderson ET, Hewitt WL. Gentamicin blood levels: a guide to nephrotoxicity. Antimicrob Agents Chemother 1975;8:58–62.
9. French MA, Cerra FB, Plaut ME, Schentag JJ. Amikacin and gentamicin accumulation pharmacokinetics and nephrotoxicity in critically ill patients. Antimicrob Agents Chemother 1981;19:147–152.
10. Schentag JJ, Jusko WJ. Renal clearance and tissue accumulation of gentamicin. Clin Pharmacol Ther 1977;22:364–370.
11. Schentag JJ, Plaut ME, Cerra FB. Comparative nephrotoxicity of gentamicin and tobramycin: pharmacokinetic and clinical studies in 201 patients. Antimicrob Agents Chemother 1981;19:859–866.

12. Moore RD, Smith CR, Lipsky JJ, Mellits ED, Lietman PS. Risk factors for nephrotoxicity in patients treated with aminoglycosides. Ann Intern Med 1984;100:352–357.
13. Schentag JJ, Plaut ME, Cerra FB, Wels PB, Walczak P, Buckley RJ. Aminoglycoside nephrotoxicity in critically ill surgical patients. J Surg Res 1979;26:270–279.
14. Rybak MJ, Albrecht LM, Boike SC, Chandrasekar PH. Nephrotoxicity of vancomycin, alone and with an aminoglycoside. J Antimicrob Chemother 1990;25:679–687.
15. Lane AZ, Wright GE, Blair DC. Ototoxicity and nephrotoxicity of amikacin: an overview of phase II and phase III experience in the United States. Am J Med 1977;62:911–918.
16. Schentag JJ, Cerra FB, Plaut ME. Clinical and pharmacokinetic characteristics of aminoglycoside nephrotoxicity in 201 critically ill patients. Antimicrob Agents Chemother 1982; 21:721–726.
17. Bertino JS, Jr, Booker LA, Franck PA, Jenkins PL, Franck KR, Nafziger AN. Incidence of and significant risk factors for aminoglycoside-associated nephrotoxicity in patients dosed by using individualized pharmacokinetic monitoring [see comments]. J Infect Dis 1993;167:173–179.
18. Prins JM, Buller HR, Kuijper EJ, Tange RA, Speelman P. Once versus thrice daily gentamicin in patients with serious infections [see comments]. Lancet 1993;341:335–339.
19. Maller R, Ahrne H, Holmen C, Lausen I, Nilsson LE, Smedjegard J. Once- versus twice-daily amikacin regimen: efficacy and safety in systemic gram-negative infections. Scandinavian Amikacin Once Daily Study Group. J Antimicrob Chemother 1993;31:939–948.
20. Barclay ML, Begg EJ, Hickling KG. What is the evidence for once-daily aminoglycoside therapy? Clin Pharmacokinet 1994;27:32–48.
21. Barclay ML, Duffull SB, Begg EJ, Buttimore RC. Experience of once-daily aminoglycoside dosing using a target area under the concentration–time curve. Aust N Z J Med 1995;25:230–235.
22. Barclay ML, Kirkpatrick CM, Begg EJ. Once daily aminoglycoside therapy. Is it less toxic than multiple daily doses and how should it be monitored? Clin Pharmacokinet 1999;36:89–98.
23. Begg EJ, Barclay ML, Duffull SB. A suggested approach to once-daily aminoglycoside dosing. Br J Clin Pharmacol 1995;39:605–609.
24. Blaser J, Konig C, Simmen HP, Thurnheer U. Monitoring serum concentrations for once-daily netilmicin dosing regimens. J Antimicrob Chemother 1994;33:341–348.
25. Janknegt R. Aminoglycoside monitoring in the once- or twice-daily era. The Dutch situation considered. Pharm World Sci 1993;15:151–155.
26. Prins JM, Koopmans RP, Buller HR, Kuijper EJ, Speelman P. Easier monitoring of aminoglycoside therapy with once-daily dosing schedules. Eur J Clin Microbiol Infect Dis 1995; 14:531–535.
27. Anon. Endotoxin-like reactions associated with intravenous gentamicin—California, 1998. MMWR Morb Mortal Wkly Rep 1998;47:877–880.
28. Krieger JA, Duncan L. Gentamicin contaminated with endotoxin [letter]. N Engl J Med 1999;340:1122.
29. Smith CR, Lipsky JJ, Laskin OL, et al. Double-blind comparison of the nephrotoxicity and auditory toxicity of gentamicin and tobramycin. N Engl J Med 1980;302:1106–1109.
30. Feig PU, Mitchell PP, Abrutyn E, et al. Aminoglycoside nephrotoxicity: a double blind prospective randomized study of gentamicin and tobramycin. J Antimicrob Chemother 1982; 10:217–226.
31. Kahlmeter G, Hallberg T, Kamme C. Gentamicin and tobramycin in patients with various infections—nephrotoxicity. J Antimicrob Chemother 1978;(4 Suppl A):47–52.
32. Vic P, Ategbo S, Turck D, et al. Efficacy, tolerance, and pharmacokinetics of once daily tobramycin for pseudomonas exacerbations in cystic fibrosis. Arch Dis Child 1998;78:536–539.
33. Bragonier R, Brown NM. The pharmacokinetics and toxicity of once-daily tobramycin therapy in children with cystic fibrosis. J Antimicrob Chemother 1998;42:103–106.

34. Bates RD, Nahata MC, Jones JW, et al. Pharmacokinetics and safety of tobramcyin after once-daily administration in patients with cystic fibrosis. Chest 1997;112:1208–1213.
35. Bass KD, Larkin SE, Paap C, Haase GM. Pharmacokinetics of once-daily gentamicin dosing in pediatric patients. J Pediatr Surg 1998;33:1104–1107.
36. Weber W, Kewitz G, Rost KL, Looby M, Nitz M, Harnisch L. Population kinetics of gentamicin in neonates. Eur J Clin Pharmacol 1993;44:S23–S25.
37. Demczar DJ, Nafziger AN, Bertino JS, Jr. Pharmacokinetics of gentamicin at traditional versus high doses: implications for once-daily aminoglycoside dosing. Antimicrob Agents Chemother 1997;41:1115–1159.
38. Bauer LA, Blouin RA. Amikacin pharmacokinetics in young men with pneumonia. Clin Pharm 1982;1:353–355.
39. Bauer LA, Blouin RA. Influence of age on tobramycin pharmacokinetics in patients with normal renal function. Antimicrob Agents Chemother 1981;20:587–589.
40. Bauer LA, Blouin RA. Gentamicin pharmacokinetics: effect of aging in patients with normal renal function. J Am Geriatr Soc 1982;30:309–311.
41. Bauer LA, Blouin RA. Influence of age on amikacin pharmacokinetics in patients without renal disease. Comparison with gentamicin and tobramycin. Eur J Clin Pharmacol 1983;24:639–642.
42. Barza M, Brown RB, Shen D, Gibaldi M, Weinstein L. Predictability of blood levels of gentamicin in man. J Infect Dis 1975;132:165–174.
43. Kaye D, Levison ME, Labovitz ED. The unpredictability of serum concentrations of gentamicin: pharmacokinetics of gentamicin in patients with normal and abnormal renal function. J Infect Dis 1974;130:150–154.
44. Sarubbi FA, Jr, Hull JH. Amikacin serum concentrations: prediction of levels and dosage guidelines. Ann Intern Med 1978;89:612–618.
45. Hull JH, Sarubbi FA, Jr. Gentamicin serum concentrations: pharmacokinetic predictions. Ann Intern Med 1976;85:183–189.
46. Bootman JL, Wertheimer AI, Zaske D, Rowland C. Individualizing gentamicin dosage regimens in burn patients with gram-negative septicemia: a cost-benefit analysis. J Pharm Sci 1979;68:267–272.
47. Zaske DE, Sawchuk RJ, Gerding DN, Strate RG. Increased dosage requirements of gentamicin in burn patients. J Trauma 1976;16:824–828.
48. Zaske DE, Sawchuk RJ, Strate RG. The necessity of increased doses of amikacin in burn patients. Surgery 1978;84:603–608.
49. Tindula RJ, Ambrose PJ, Harralson AF. Aminoglycoside inactivation by penicillins and cephalosporins and its impact on drug-level monitoring. Drug Intell Clin Pharm 1983; 17:906–908.
50. Wallace SM, Chan LY. In vitro interaction of aminoglycosides with beta-lactam penicillins. Antimicrob Agents Chemother 1985;28:274–281.
51. Henderson JL, Polk RE, Kline BJ. In vitro inactivation of gentamicin, tobramycin, and netilmicin by carbenicillin, azlocillin, or mezlocillin. Am J Hosp Pharm 1981;38:1167–1170.
52. Pickering LK, Rutherford I. Effect of concentration and time upon inactivation of tobramycin, gentamicin, netilmicin and amikacin by azlocillin, carbenicillin, mecillinam, mezlocillin and piperacillin. J Pharmacol Exp Ther 1981;217:345–349.
53. Hale DC, Jenkins R, Matsen JM. In-vitro inactivation of aminoglycoside antibiotics by piperacillin and carbenicillin. Am J Clin Pathol 1980;74:316–319.
54. Bauer LA, Blouin RA, Griffen WO, Jr, Record KE, Bell RM. Amikacin pharmacokinetics in morbidly obese patients. Am J Hosp Pharm 1980;37:519–522.
55. Bauer LA, Edwards WA, Dellinger EP, Simonowitz DA. Influence of weight on aminoglycoside pharmacokinetics in normal weight and mobidly obese patients. Eur J Clin Pharmacol 1983;24:643–647.

56. Blouin RA, Mann HJ, Griffen WO, Jr, Bauer LA, Record KE. Tobramycin pharmacokinetics in morbidly obese patients. Clin Pharmacol Ther 1979;26:508–512.
57. Bauer LA, Piecoro JJ, Jr, Wilson HD, Blouin RA. Gentamicin and tobramycin pharmacokinetics in patients with cystic fibrosis. Clin Pharm 1983;2:262–264.
58. Bosso JA, Townsend PL, Herbst JJ, Matsen JM. Pharmacokinetics and dosage requirements of netilmicin in cystic fibrosis patients. Antimicrob Agents Chemother 1985;28:829–831.
59. Kearns GL, Hilman BC, Wilson JT. Dosing implications of altered gentamicin disposition in patients with cystic fibrosis. J Pediatr 1982;100:312–318.
60. Kelly HB, Menendez R, Fan L, Murphy S. Pharmacokinetics of tobramycin in cystic fibrosis. J Pediatr 1982;100:318–321.
61. Ramsey BW, Pepe MS, Quan JM, et al. Intermittent administration of inhaled tobramycin in patients with cystic fibrosis. Cystic Fibrosis Inhaled Tobramycin Study Group. N Engl J Med 1999;340:23–30.
62. Lanao JM, Dominguez-Gil A, Macias JG, Diez JL, Nieto MJ. The influence of ascites on the pharmacokinetics of amikacin. Int J Clin Pharmacol Ther Toxicol 1980;18:57–61.
63. Gill MA, Kern JW. Altered gentamicin distribution in ascitic patients. Am J Hosp Pharm 1979;36:1704–1706.
64. Sampliner R, Perrier D, Powell R, Finley P. Influence of ascites on tobramycin pharmacokinetics. J Clin Pharmacol 1984;24:43–46.
65. Izquierdo M, Lanao JM, Cervero L, Jimenez NV, Dominguez-Gil A. Population pharmacokinetics of gentamicin in premature infants. Ther Drug Monit 1992;14:177–183.
66. Hindmarsh KW, Nation RL, Williams GL, John E, French JN. Pharmacokinetics of gentamicin in very low birth weight preterm infants. Eur J Clin Pharmacol 1983;24:649–653.
67. Rameis H, Popow C, Graninger W. Gentamicin monitoring in low-birth-weight newborns. Biol Res Pregnancy Perinatol 1983;4:123–126.
68. Madhavan T, Yaremchuk K, Levin N, et al. Effect of renal failure and dialysis on the serum concentration of the aminoglycoside amikacin. Antimicrob Agents Chemother 1976; 10:464–466.
69. Armstrong DK, Hodgman T, Visconti JA, Reilley TE, Garner WL, Dasta JF. Hemodialysis of amikacin in critically ill patients. Crit Care Med 1988;16:517–520.
70. Herrero A, Rius Alarco F, Garcia Diez JM, Mahiques E, Domingo JV. Pharmacokinetics of netilmicin in renal insufficiency and hemodialysis. Int J Clin Pharmacol Ther Toxicol 1988;26:84–87.
71. Halstenson CE, Berkseth RO, Mann HJ, Matzke GR. Aminoglycoside redistribution phenomenon after hemodialysis: netilmicin and tobramycin. Int J Clin Pharmacol Ther Toxicol 1987; 25:50–55.
72. Matzke GR, Halstenson CE, Keane WF. Hemodialysis elimination rates and clearance of gentamicin and tobramycin. Antimicrob Agents Chemother 1984;25:128–130.
73. Basile C, Di Maggio A, Curino E, Scatizzi A. Pharmacokinetics of netilmicin in hypertonic hemodiafiltration and standard hemodialysis. Clin Nephrol 1985;24:305–309.
74. Smeltzer BD, Schwartzman MS, Bertino JS, Jr. Amikacin pharmacokinetics during continuous ambulatory peritoneal dialysis. Antimicrob Agents Chemother 1988;32:236–240.
75. Pancorbo S, Comty C. Pharmacokinetics of gentamicin in patients undergoing continuous ambulatory peritoneal dialysis. Antimicrob Agents Chemother 1981;19:605–607.
76. Bunke CM, Aronoff GR, Brier ME, Sloan RS, Luft FC. Tobramycin kinetics during continuous ambulatory peritoneal dialysis. Clin Pharmacol Ther 1983;34:110–116.
77. Chandrasekar PH, Cronin SM. Nephrotoxicity in bone marrow transplant recipients receiving aminoglycoside plus cyclosporine or aminoglycoside alone. J Antimicrob Chemother 1991; 27:845–849.
78. Harpur ES. The pharmacology of ototoxic drugs. Br J Audiol 1982;16:81–93.

79. Mathog RH, Klein WJ, Jr. Ototoxicity of ethacrynic acid and aminoglycoside antibiotics in uremia. N Engl J Med 1969;280:1223–1224.

80. Paradelis AG, Triantaphyllidis C, Giala MM. Neuromuscular blocking activity of aminoglycoside antibiotics. Methods Find Exp Clin Pharmacol 1980;2:45–51.

81. Sawchuk RJ, Zaske DE, Cipolle RJ, Wargin WA, Strate RG. Kinetic model for gentamicin dosing with the use of individual patient parameters. Clin Pharmacol Ther 1977;21:362–369.

82. Murphy JE, Winter ME. Clinical pharmacokinetic pearls: bolus verus infusion equations. Pharmacotherapy 1996;16:698–700.

83. Spinler SA, Nawarskas JJ, Boyce EG, Connors JE, Charland SL, Goldfarb S. Predictive performance of ten equations for estimating creatinine clearance in cardiac patients. Iohexol Cooperative Study Group. Ann Pharmacother 1998;32:1275–1283.

84. Salazar DE, Corcoran GB. Predicting creatinine clearance and renal drug clearance in obese patients from estimated fat-free body mass. Am J Med 1988;84:1053–1060.

85. McCormack JP, Carleton B. A simpler approach to pharmacokinetic dosage adjustments. Pharmacotherapy 1997;17:1349–1351.

86. Burton ME, Brater DC, Chen PS, Day RB, Huber PJ, Vasko MR. A Bayesian feedback method of aminoglycoside dosing. Clin Pharmacol Ther 1985;37:349–357.

87. Burton ME, Chow MS, Platt DR, Day RB, Brater DC, Vasko MR. Accuracy of Bayesian and Sawchuk-Zaske dosing methods for gentamicin. Clin Pharm 1986;5:143–149.

88. Rodvold KA, Blum RA. Predictive performance of Sawchuk-Zaske and Bayesian dosing methods for tobramycin. J Clin Pharmacol 1987;27:419–424.

89. Murray KM, Bauer LA, Koup JR. Predictive performance of computer dosing methods for tobramycin using two pharmacokinetic models and two weighting algorithms. Clin Pharm 1986;5:411–414.

90. Koup JR, Killen T, Bauer LA. Multiple-dose non-linear regression analysis program. Aminoglycoside dose prediction. Clin Pharmacokinet 1983;8:456–462.

91. Wandell M, Mungall D. Computer assisted drug interpretation and drug regimen optimization. Amer Assoc Clin Chem 1984;6:1–11.

5

VANCOMYCIN

INTRODUCTION

Vancomycin is a glycopeptide antibiotic used to treat severe gram-positive infections due to organisms that are resistant to other antibiotics such as methicillin-resistant staphylococci and ampicillin-resistant enterococci. It is also used to treat infections caused by other sensitive gram-positive organisms in patients who are allergic to penicillins.

Vancomycin is bactericidal and exhibits time-dependent or concentration-independent bacterial killing.[1] Antibiotics with time-dependent killing characteristically kill bacteria most effectively when drug concentrations are a multiple (usually three to five times) of the minimum inhibitory concentration (MIC) for the bacteria.[1,2] The mechanism of action for vancomycin is inhibition of cell wall synthesis in susceptible bacteria by binding to the D-alanyl-D-alanine terminal end of cell wall precursor units.[3] Many strains of enterococcus have high MIC values for vancomycin; for these bacteria, vancomycin may demonstrate only bacteriostatic properties.

THERAPEUTIC AND TOXIC CONCENTRATIONS

Vancomycin is administered as a short-term (1-hour) intravenous infusion. Infusion rate–related side effects have been noted when shorter infusion times (~30 minutes or less) have been used. Urticarial or erythematous reactions, intense flushing (known as "red-man" or "red-neck" syndrome), tachycardia, and hypotension all have been reported and can be largely avoided with the longer infusion time. Even with a 1-hour infusion time, vancomycin serum concentrations exhibit a distribution phase, so that drug in the blood and in the tissues are not yet in equilibrium (Figure 5-1). Because of this, a 1/2- to

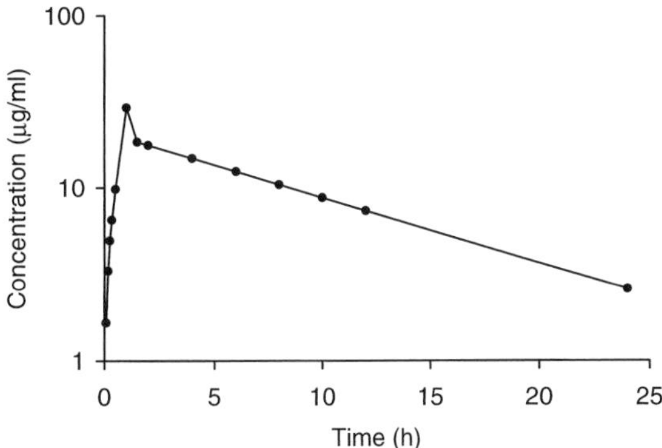

FIGURE 5-1 Concentration–time plot for vancomycin 1000 mg given as a 1-hour infusion (*circles with dashed line*). When vancomycin is given as a 1-hour infusion, end of infusion concentrations are higher because the serum and tissues are not in equilibrium. A 1/2- to 1-hour waiting time for vancomycin distribution to tissues is allowed before peak concentrations are measured.

1-hour waiting period is allowed for distribution to finish before maximum or peak concentrations are measured. Since vancomycin exhibits time-dependent killing, microbiologic or clinical cure rates are not closely associated with peak serum concentrations. However, ototoxicity has been reported when vancomycin serum concentrations exceed 80 μg/mL,[4,5] so the therapeutic range for steady-state peak concentrations is usually considered to be 20 to 40 μg/mL. Because vancomycin does not enter the central nervous system in appreciable amounts when given intravenously,[3] steady-state peak concentrations of 40 to 60 μg/mL or direct administration into the cerebrospinal fluid may be necessary.[6,7]

Vancomycin-associated ototoxicity is usually first noted by the appearance of tinnitus, dizziness, or high-frequency hearing loss (>4000 Hz).[4,7,8] Because the hearing loss is initially at high frequencies, the auditory deficit can be challenging to detect unless audiometry is conducted at baseline before drug is administered and during vancomycin treatment. Since audiometry is difficult to conduct in seriously ill patients, it is rarely done in patients receiving ototoxic drugs. Therefore, clinicians should monitor for signs and symptoms that may indicate ototoxicity in a patient (auditory: tinnitus, feelings of fullness or pressure in the ears, loss of hearing acuity in the conversational range; vestibular: loss of equilibrium, headache, nausea, vomiting, vertigo, dizziness, nystagmus, ataxia). Ototoxicity can be permanent if appropriate changes in vancomycin dosing are not made.[4,7–9] In some reports of vancomycin-induced ototoxicity, it is unclear when vancomycin serum concentrations were obtained during the dosage interval; thus, the exact association between peak concentrations and ototoxicity is uncertain.

Trough concentrations (predose or minimum concentrations usually obtained within 30 minutes of the next dose) are usually related to therapeutic outcome for vancomycin because the antibiotic follows time-dependent bacterial killing.[1] Optimal bactericidal effects are found at concentrations three to five times the organism's MIC.[1,2] Because the average vancomycin MICs for *Staphylococcus aureus* and *Staphylococcus epidermidis* are 1 to 2 μg/mL, minimum predose or trough steady-state concentrations of 5 to 10 μg/mL are usually adequate to resolve infections with susceptible organisms. Trough vancomycin steady-state concentrations above 15 μg/mL are related to an increased incidence of nephrotoxicity.[10,11] Many patients receiving vancomycin are critically ill; thus, other sources of renal dysfunction, such as hypotension or other nephrotoxic drug therapy, should be ruled out before the diagnosis of vancomycin-induced renal damage is made in a patient. Compared with aminoglycoside antibiotics, vancomycin is usually considered to have less potential for nephrotoxicity.[12] In contrast to ototoxicity, vancomycin-related nephrotoxicity is usually reversible, with a low incidence of residual damage if the antibiotic is withdrawn or if doses are appropriately adjusted soon after renal function tests change. With adequate patient monitoring, the only result of vancomycin nephrotoxicity may be transient serum creatinine increases of 0.5 to 2.0 mg/dL. However, if kidney damage progresses to renal failure, the cost of maintaining the patient on dialysis until kidney function returns can exceed $50,000 to $100,000 and, if the patient is critically ill, may contribute to his or her death.

Nephrotoxicity and ototoxicity cannot be completely prevented when using vancomycin by keeping serum concentrations within the suggested ranges. However, by adjusting vancomycin dosage regimens so that potentially toxic serum concentrations are prevented, drug concentration–related adverse effects should be held to an absolute minimum.

CLINICAL MONITORING PARAMETERS

Clinicians should always consult the patient's chart to confirm that antibiotic therapy is appropriate for current microbiologic cultures and sensitivities. Also, it should be confirmed that the patient is receiving other appropriate concurrent antibiotic therapy, such as aminoglycosides, when necessary to treat the infection. Patients with severe infections usually have elevated white blood cell counts and body temperatures. Measurement of serial white blood cell counts and body temperatures are useful to determine the efficacy of antibiotic therapy. A white blood cell count with a differential identifies the types of white blood cells that are elevated. A large number of neutrophils and immature neutrophils, clinically known as a "shift to the left," can also be observed in patients with severe bacterial infections. Favorable response to antibiotic treatment is usually indicated by high white blood cell counts decreasing toward the normal range, the trend of body temperatures (plotted as body temperature versus time, also known as the "fever curve") approaching normal, and any specific infection site tests or procedures resolving. For instance, in patients with pneumonia the chest x-ray should be resolving, in patients with infective endocarditis the size of the bacterial vegetation on the heart valve should be decreasing, and in patients with a wound infection the wound should be less inflamed with less purulent discharge. Clinicians should also be aware that an immunocompromised patient with a bacterial infection may not be able to mount a fever or have an elevated white blood cell count.

Vancomycin steady-state serum concentrations should be measured in 3 to 5 estimated half-lives. Methods of estimating this parameter are given in the initial dose calculation section of this chapter. Since prolongation of the dosage interval is often used in patients with decreased elimination, a useful clinical rule is to measure serum concentrations after the third dose. If this approach is used, the dosage interval is increased in tandem with the increase in half-life, so that 3 to 5 half-lives have elapsed by the time the third dose is administered. In addition, the third dose typically occurs 1.5 to 3 days after dosing has commenced, and this is a good time to also assess clinical efficacy of the treatment. Steady-state serum concentrations, in conjunction with clinical response, are used to adjust the antibiotic dose, if necessary. Methods of adjusting vancomycin doses using serum concentrations are discussed later in this chapter. If the dosage is adjusted, vancomycin elimination changes or if laboratory and clinical monitoring indicates that the infection is not resolving or worsening, clinicians should consider rechecking steady-state drug concentrations.

Although many clinicians continue to monitor both steady-state peak and trough vancomycin serum concentrations, some individuals advocate the measurement of just a steady-state trough concentration.[13] The reasoning behind this approach is that vancomycin follows time-dependent bacterial killing, and the efficacy of the drug should be most closely related to the minimum serum concentration encountered over the dosage interval. Since nephrotoxicity is related to high trough concentrations, measurement of this value should ensure therapeutic, nonnephrotoxic drug concentrations. Vancomycin has a moderate-sized volume of distribution (~0.7 L/kg) and does not significantly change for most disease states or conditions. Based on this, the argument has been made that if a patient has a therapeutic steady-state trough concentration (5 to 10 μg/mL) and the dose is in the usual range (500 to 1500 mg with the most typical value being 1000 mg), it is difficult to produce a steady-state peak concentration that would be higher than the accepted toxic range (>80 μg/mL).[14] Although these arguments are intellectually sound and appealing, one of the reasons for measuring drug serum concentrations is pharmacokinetic variability. If a patient develops ototoxicity while receiving vancomycin, it can be difficult to prove that steady-state peak concentrations were in the acceptable range if no serum concentrations were obtained at the time.

Serial monitoring of serum creatinine concentrations should be used to detect nephrotoxicity. Ideally, a baseline serum creatinine concentration is obtained before vancomycin therapy is initiated and obtained three times weekly during treatment. An increasing serum creatinine test on two or more consecutive measurement occasions indicates that more intensive monitoring of serum creatinine values—such as daily—is needed. If serum creatinine measurements increase more than 0.5 mg/dL over the baseline value (or >25% to 30% over baseline for serum creatinine values >2 mg/dL) and other causes of declining renal function have been ruled out (e.g., other nephrotoxic drugs or agents, hypotension), alternatives to vancomycin therapy or, if not possible, intensive vancomycin serum concentration monitoring should be initiated to ensure that excessive amounts of vancomycin do not accumulate in the patient. In the clinical setting, audiometry is rarely used to detect ototoxicity because it is difficult to accomplish in severely ill patients. Instead, clinical signs and symptoms of auditory (decreased hearing acuity in the conversational range, feeling of fullness or pressure in the ears, tinnitus) or vestibular (loss of equilibrium, headache, nausea, vomiting, vertigo, nystagmus, ataxia) ototoxicity are monitored at the same time intervals as serum creatinine determination. Vancomycin can also cause allergic symptoms such as chills, fever, skin rashes, and anaphylactoid reactions.

BASIC CLINICAL PHARMACOKINETIC PARAMETERS

Vancomycin is almost completely eliminated unchanged in the urine primarily by glomerular filtration (≥90%; Table 5-1).[15] This antibiotic is given by short-term (1-hour) intermittent intravenous infusion. Intramuscular administration is usually avoided because this route has been reported to cause tissue necrosis at the site of injection. Oral bioavailability is poor (<10%), so systemic infections cannot be treated by this route of administration.[5] However, patients with renal failure who have been given oral vancomycin for the treatment of antibiotic-associated colitis have accumulated therapeutic concentrations because gut wall inflammation increased vancomycin bioavailability and renal dysfunction decreased drug clearance.[16–19] Plasma protein binding is ~55%.[20] The recommended dose for vancomycin in patients with normal renal function is 30 mg/kg per day given as two or four divided daily doses. In adults of normal weight with good renal function, the dose is usually 2 gm per day given as 1000 mg every 12 hours.

TABLE 5-1 Disease States and Conditions That Alter Vancomycin Pharmacokinetics

DISEASE STATE/ CONDITION	HALF-LIFE (HOURS)	VOLUME OF DISTRIBUTION (L/kg)	COMMENTS
Adult, normal renal function	8 (range, 7–9)	0.7 (range, 0.5–1.0)	Usual dose 30 mg/kg/d in two divided doses
Adult, renal failure	130 (range, 120–140)	0.7 (range, 0.5–1.0)	Underhydration or overhydration does not affect the volume of distribution as much as with aminoglycosides.
Burns	4	0.7	Because of shorter half-life, some patients may need every 6- to 8-hour dosage interval to maintain therapeutic trough concentrations.
Obesity (>30% over IBW) with normal renal function	3–4	V = 0.7 IBW	Total daily doses are based on TBW, V estimates based on IBW. Because of shorter half-life, some patients may require every-8-hour dosage interval to maintain therapeutic trough concentrations.

IBW = ideal body weight; TBW = total body weight; V = volume of distribution.

EFFECTS OF DISEASE STATES AND CONDITIONS ON VANCOMYCIN PHARMACOKINETICS AND DOSING

In nonobese adults with normal renal function (creatinine clearance >80 mL/min; see Table 5-1) vancomycin has an average half-life of 8 hours (range, 7 to 9 hours), and its average volume of distribution is 0.7 L/kg (range, 0.5 to 1.0 L/kg) in this population.[21,22] Because of the moderate size of the volume of distribution, fluid balance and thus under- or overhydration are less of an issue with vancomycin compared with the aminoglycoside antibiotics.

Because vancomycin is eliminated principally by glomerular filtration, renal dysfunction is the most important disease state that influences vancomycin pharmacokinetics.[23–25] Vancomycin total clearance decreases proportionally with decreases in creatinine clearance[23] (Figure 5-2). The relationship between renal function and vancomycin clearance forms the basis for initial dosage computation methods presented later in this chapter.

Major body burns (over 30% to 40% of body surface area) can cause large changes in vancomycin pharmacokinetics.[26] Forty-eight to 72 hours after a major burn, the basal metabolic rate of the patient increases to facilitate tissue repair. The increase in basal metabolic rate causes an increase in glomerular filtration rate, which increases vancomycin clearance. Because of the increase in drug clearance, the average half-life of vancomycin in burn patients is 4 hours.

Obese persons with normal serum creatinine concentrations have increased vancomycin clearance because of increased glomerular filtration rate and are best dosed with vancomycin using total body weight.[21,22,27,28] Kidney hypertrophy is the reason for the increased drug clearance, which results in larger glomerular filtration rates. Volume of distribution does not significantly change with obesity and is best estimated using ideal body weight (IBW) in patients more than 30% overweight (>30% over IBW; V = 0.7 L/kg IBW).[21,22,28] Because the primary pharmacokinetic change in vancomycin in obese patients is increased drug clearance with a negligible change in volume of distribution, average half-life decreases to 3.3 hours ($t_{1/2} = [0.693 \cdot V]/Cl$). Although the average dose in

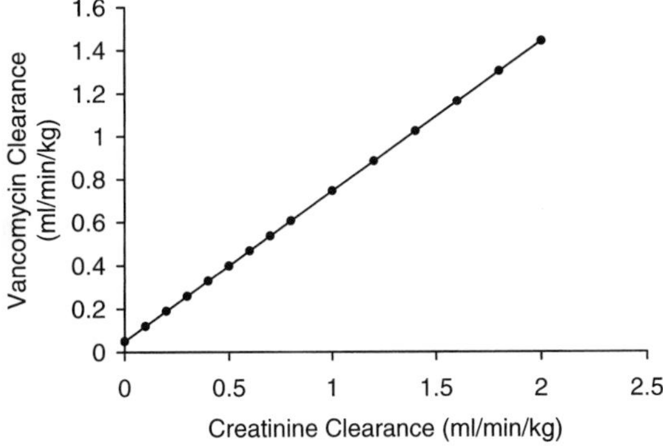

FIGURE 5-2 The clearance rate for vancomycin increases in proportion to creatinine clearance (CrCl). The equation for this relationship is Cl (in mL/min/kg) = 0.695(CrCl in mL/min/kg) + 0.05. This equation is used to estimate vancomycin clearance in patients for initial dosing purposes.

morbidly obese and normal-weight patients with normal serum creatinine concentrations was ~30 mg/kg per day using total body weight in both populations, some morbidly obese patients required every-8-hour dosing to maintain vancomycin steady-state trough concentrations higher than 5 μg/mL.[21]

Premature infants (gestational age 32 weeks) have a greater amount of body water compared with that in adults. However, vancomycin's volume of distribution (V = 0.7 L/kg) is not greatly affected by greater amounts of body water, as is the case with aminoglycoside antibiotics.[29] Kidneys are not completely developed at this early age, so glomerular filtration and vancomycin clearance (15 mL/min) are decreased.[29] A lower clearance rate with about the same volume of distribution as adults results in a longer average half-life for vancomycin in premature babies (10 hours). In full-term neonates (gestational age ~40 weeks), vancomycin has a similar volume of distribution compared with that in premature infants, but vancomycin clearance rate is twice that in infants born prematurely (30 mL/min). The increase in drug clearance is due to additional renal development that occurred in utero. The vancomycin half-life in full-term infants is about 7 hours. At about 3 months of age, vancomycin clearance has nearly doubled again (50 mL/min), resulting in a half-life of approximately 4 hours. The increase in vancomycin clearance continues until the child reaches 4 to 8 years of age, when clearance is 130 to 160 mL/min and volume of distribution remains ~0.7 L/kg, so that half-life is 2 to 3 hours. At that time, vancomycin clearance and half-life gradually approach adult values as puberty approaches in children (~12 to 14 years of age).

The effect of hemodialysis on vancomycin pharmacokinetics depends on the type of artificial kidney used during the procedure. Vancomycin is a relatively large molecule with a moderate-sized volume of distribution and intermediate protein binding. These characteristics lead to poor removal of the drug from the body by hemodialysis. The mean vancomycin half-life in patients with renal failure is 120 to 140 hours.[25,30,31] Using traditional low-flux hemodialysis filters, an insignificant amount (<10%) of the total vancomycin body stores is removed during a 3- to 4-hour dialysis period.[24,25] When hemodialysis is performed with a high-flux filter, vancomycin serum concentrations decrease by one-third during the dialysis period, but then slowly rebound for the next 10 to 12 hours, reaching nearly 90% of predialysis values.[32] Postdialysis vancomycin serum concentrations should be measured after the rebound period in patients receiving hemodialysis with a high-flux filter to determine whether supplemental doses are needed.

Peritoneal dialysis removes only a negligible amount of vancomycin.[33–35] Patients who develop peritonitis while receiving peritoneal dialysis can be treated by placing vancomycin into the dialysis fluid. Over a 6-hour dwell time, approximately 50% of a vancomycin dose (1000 mg in 2 L dialysis fluid) is absorbed from the peritoneal cavity in patients with renal failure who do not have peritonitis.[33] Peritonitis causes inflammation of the peritoneal membrane, which facilitates absorption of vancomycin placed in the peritoneal dialysis fluid (up to 90% absorbed) and dialysis elimination of vancomycin from the body.[35]

DRUG INTERACTIONS

The most important drug interactions with vancomycin are pharmacodynamic, not pharmacokinetic, in nature. Co-administration of aminoglycoside antibiotics enhances the nephrotoxicity potential of vancomycin.[9,36,37] Aminoglycosides can cause nephrotoxicity when administered alone. When an aminoglycoside and vancomycin are administered concurrently, serum creatinine concentrations should be monitored on a daily basis. In addition, serum concentrations of the aminoglycoside, as well as vancomycin, should be measured.

When vancomycin is administered to patients being stabilized on warfarin therapy, the hypoprothrombinemic effect of the anticoagulant may be augmented.[38] The mechanism of this interaction is unknown, but resulted in a mean 45% increase in prothrombin time over baseline values when warfarin was given alone. In patients receiving warfarin therapy who require vancomycin treatment, a baseline prothrombin time ratio (INR) should be measured before the antibiotic is administered, and daily INR tests should be obtained until anticoagulation status is stable.

INITIAL DOSAGE DETERMINATION METHODS

Pharmacokinetic Dosing Method

The goal of initial dosing of vancomycin is to compute the best dose possible for the patient, given disease states and conditions that influence vancomycin pharmacokinetics and the site and severity of the infection. To do this, pharmacokinetic parameters are estimated in the patient by using mean parameters measured in other persons with similar disease state and condition profiles.

ESTIMATE OF CLEARANCE

Vancomycin is almost completely eliminated unchanged by the kidney, and there is a good relationship between creatinine clearance and vancomycin clearance[23] (see Figure 5-2). This relationship allows an estimation of vancomycin clearance, which can be used to calculate an initial dose of the drug. Mathematically, the equation for the straight line shown in Figure 5-2 is Cl = 0.695(CrCl) + 0.05, where Cl is vancomycin clearance in mL/min per kg and CrCl is creatinine clearance in mL/min per kg. Because each clearance value is normalized for the patient's weight, the estimated or measured creatinine clearance must be divided by the patient's weight in kilograms before using it in the equation, and the resulting vancomycin clearance must be multiplied by the patient's weight if the answer is needed in units of mL/min. The weight factor used for all individuals, including obese patients, is total body weight (TBW).[21,22,25,27,28] It is not possible to simply enter a patient's creatinine clearance in mL/min and expect the resulting vancomycin clearance to have the units of mL/min. This does not work because the y-intercept of creatinine clearance/vancomycin clearance equation, which represents nonrenal vancomycin clearance, is in mL/min per kg, so mathematical cancellation of the weight factor is not possible.

For example, the estimated clearance of vancomycin in an individual with a creatinine clearance of 100 mL/min who weighs 70 kg is 1.04 mL/min per kg or 73 mL/min: Cl = 0.695[(100 mL/min)/70 kg] + 0.05 = (1.04 mL/min/kg) or (1.04 mL/min/kg) · 70 kg = 73 mL/min. Taking the patient's renal function into account when deriving an initial dose of vancomycin is the single most important characteristic to assess.

ESTIMATE OF VOLUME OF DISTRIBUTION

The average volume of distribution of vancomycin is 0.7 L/kg.[21,22] The weight factor that is used to calculate vancomycin volume of distribution for obese patients is ideal body weight (IBW).[21,22,28] Thus, for an 80-kg patient, the estimated vancomycin volume of distribution would be 56 L: V = 0.7 L/kg · 80 kg = 56 L. For a 150-kg obese patient with an IBW of 60 kg, the estimated vancomycin volume of distribution is 42 L: V = 0.7 L/kg · 60 kg = 42 L.

ESTIMATES OF ELIMINATION RATE CONSTANT AND HALF-LIFE

The vancomycin elimination rate constant (k_e) is computed using the estimated clearance and volume of distribution values for the drug in the following equation: $k_e = Cl/V$. It is usually expressed using the unit of h^{-1}. For example, for a patient with a vancomycin clearance of 1.04 mL/min per kg and a vancomycin volume of distribution of 0.7 L/kg, the elimination rate constant (in h^{-1}) would be computed as follows: k_e = (1.04 mL/min/kg · 60 min/h)/(0.7 L/kg · 1000 mL/L) = 0.089 h^{-1}, where 60 min/h and 1000 mL/L are used as unit conversion factors for time and volume, respectively. Vancomycin half-life would be calculated using the equation that relates elimination rate constant and half-life: $t_{1/2} = 0.693/k_e = 0.693/0.089\ h^{-1} = 7.8\ h$.

SELECTION OF APPROPRIATE PHARMACOKINETIC MODEL AND EQUATIONS

When given by intravenous infusion over 1 hour, vancomycin serum concentrations follow a two- or three-compartment pharmacokinetic model (see Figure 5-1). After the end of infusion if a two-compartment model is followed, serum concentrations drop rapidly because of distribution of drug from blood to tissues (α or distribution phase). By about 30 to 60 minutes after the end of infusion, vancomycin serum concentrations decline more slowly, and the elimination rate constant for this portion of the concentration–time curve varies with renal function (β or elimination phase). In patients whose vancomycin serum concentration–time curve follows a three-compartment model, an intermediate distribution phase is found between the α and β portions of the graph. Although these models are important to understand conceptually, they cannot easily be used clinically because of their mathematical complexity. Because of this, the simpler one-compartment model is widely used and allows accurate dosage calculation when peak vancomycin serum concentrations are obtained after drug distribution is finished.[21,25]

Intravenously administered vancomycin is given over 1 hour as intermittent continuous infusions. Since the drug has a long half-life relative to the infusion time (1 hour) and waiting time (0.5 to 1 hour) necessary to allow for distribution to complete before peak concentrations are obtained, little of the drug is eliminated during this 1.5- to 2-hour time period. Intravenous infusion pharmacokinetic equations that take into account the loss of drug during the infusion time are not generally needed because so little vancomycin is eliminated during the infusion and waiting time periods. So, although the antibiotic is given as an intravenous infusion, intravenous bolus equations accurately predict peak vancomycin concentrations and are mathematically simpler.[39] For these reasons, intravenous bolus equations for computing vancomycin doses are preferred by many clinicians (Table 5-2A). Vancomycin steady-state peak ($C_{max,ss}$) and trough ($C_{min,ss}$) serum concentrations are chosen to treat the patient, based on the type, site, and severity of infection as well as the infecting organism. Steady-state versions of one-compartment model intra-

TABLE 5-2A Equations Used With Vancomycin Antibiotics

ROUTE OF ADMINISTRATION	SINGLE DOSE	MULTIPLE DOSE	STEADY STATE
ONE-COMPARTMENT MODEL			
Intravenous bolus	$C = (D/V)e^{-k_e t}$	$C = (D/V)e^{-k_e t}[(1 - e^{-nk_e \tau})/(1 - e^{-k_e \tau})]$	$C = (D/V)[e^{-k_e t}/(1 - e^{-k_e \tau})]$

Symbol key: C is drug serum concentration at time = t, D is dose, V is volume of distribution, k_e is the elimination rate constant, n is the number of administered doses, τ is the dosage interval.

venous bolus equations are as follows (see Tables 5-2A and B): $C_{max,ss} = (D/V)/(1 - e^{-k_e \tau})$, $C_{min,ss} = C_{max,ss}e^{-k_e \tau}$, where D is the antibiotic dose, V is the volume of distribution, k_e is the elimination rate constant, t is time, and τ is the dosage interval.

STEADY-STATE CONCENTRATION SELECTION

Vancomycin steady-state trough concentrations are selected based on the site and severity of infection in addition to the infecting organism. A commonly used therapeutic range for this value is 5 to 10 μg/mL. Far less clinical data are available to aid in the selection of vancomycin serum concentration compared with what is available for aminoglycoside serum concentrations. Severe, life-threatening infections should be treated with vancomycin trough steady-state concentrations in the upper end of this range (7.5 to 10 μg/mL). Recent data suggest that steady-state trough concentrations as high as 15 μg/mL may pose no greater risk of vancomycin-induced nephrotoxicity than those within the traditional therapeutic range.[10] If a patient does not respond adequately to vancomycin therapy that provides trough serum concentrations within the usual range, clinicians should consider prescribing an increased dose that produces a value as high as 15 μg/mL. In patients with sites of infection that are difficult to penetrate, such as the central nervous system, it may be necessary to exceed this value with caution to eradicate the infecting or-

TABLE 5-2B Pharmacokinetic Constant Computations Utilizing a One-Compartment Model Used With Vancomycin

ROUTE OF ADMINISTRATION	SINGLE DOSE	MULTIPLE DOSE	STEADY STATE
Intravenous bolus	$k_e = (\ln C_1 - \ln C_2)/(t_1 - t_2)$ $t_{1/2} = 0.693/k_e$ $V = D/C_{max}$ $Cl = k_eV$	$k_e = (\ln C_1 - \ln C_2)/(t_1 - t_2)$ $t_{1/2} = 0.693/k_e$ $V = D/(C_{max} - C_{min})$ $Cl = k_eV$	$k_e (\ln C_1 - \ln C_2)/(t_1 - t_2)$ $t_{1/2} = 0.693/k_e$ $V = D/(C_{max,ss} - C_{min,ss})$ $Cl = k_eV$

Symbol key: C_1 is drug serum concentration at time = t_1, C_2 is drug serum concentration at time = t_2, k_e is the elimination rate constant, $t_{1/2}$ is the half-life, V is the volume of distribution, D is dose, Cl is drug clearance, C_{min} is the predose trough concentration, C_{max} is the postdose peak concentration.

ganism. Whenever vancomycin doses that exceed steady-state trough concentrations of 10 μg/mL are used, serum creatinine concentrations should be monitored daily to detect early signs of nephrotoxicity.

Steady-state peak vancomycin concentrations are chosen to provide adequate antibiotic penetration to the site of infection and to avoid adverse drug reactions. A commonly used therapeutic range for this value is 20 to 40 μg/mL. In severe, life-threatening infections of the central nervous system, peak vancomycin serum concentrations as high as 60 mg/mL may be necessary to facilitate drug penetration. Whenever doses of vancomycin are used that exceed steady-state peak concentrations of 40 μg/mL, the patient should be monitored daily for early signs of ototoxicity (decreased hearing acuity in the conversational range, feeling of fullness or pressure in the ears, tinnitus, loss of equilibrium, headache, nausea, vomiting, vertigo, nystagmus, ataxia).

DOSAGE COMPUTATION

The equations given in Table 5-2C are used to compute vancomycin doses.

Example 1 JM is a 50-year-old, 70-kg, 178-cm (70-in) man with a methicillin-resistant *Staphylococcus aureus* wound infection. His serum creatinine is 0.9 mg/dL, which has been stable over the last 5 days since admission. Compute a vancomycin dose for this patient.

1. *Estimate the creatinine clearance.*

This patient has a stable serum creatinine and is not obese. The Cockcroft–Gault equation can be used to estimate creatinine clearance:

$$CrCl_{est} = [(140 - age)BW]/(72 \cdot S_{Cr}) = [(140 - 50\ y)70\ kg]/(72 \cdot 0.9\ mg/dL)$$

$$CrCl_{est} = 97\ mL/min$$

2. *Estimate the vancomycin clearance.*

The vancomycin clearance versus creatinine clearance relationship is used to estimate the vancomycin clearance for this patient:

$$Cl = 0.695(CrCl) + 0.05 = 0.695[(97\ mL/min)/70\ kg] + 0.05 = 1.013\ mL/min/kg$$

TABLE 5-2C Equations Used to Compute Individualized Dosage Regimens for Various Routes of Administration Used With Vancomycin

ROUTE OF ADMINISTRATION	DOSAGE INTERVAL (τ), MAINTENANCE DOSE (D), AND LOADING DOSE (LD) EQUATIONS
Intravenous bolus	$\tau = (\ln C_{max,ss} - \ln C_{min,ss})/k_e$ $D = C_{max,ss} V(1 - e^{-k_e\tau})$ $LD = C_{max,ss} V$

Symbol key: $C_{max,ss}$ and $C_{min,ss}$ are the maximum and minimum steady-state concentrations, k_e is the elimination rate constant, V is the volume of distribution.

3. *Estimate the vancomycin volume of distribution.*

The average volume of distribution for vancomycin is 0.7 L/kg:

$$V = 0.7 \text{ L/kg} \cdot 70 \text{ kg} = 49 \text{ L}$$

4. *Estimate the vancomycin elimination rate constant (k_e) and half-life ($t_{1/2}$).*

$$k_e = Cl/V = [(1.013 \text{ mL/min/kg})] \cdot 60 \text{ min/h})/(0.7 \text{ L/kg} \cdot 1000 \text{ ml/L}) = 0.087 \text{ h}^{-1}$$

$$t_{1/2} = 0.693/k_e = 0.693/0.087 \text{ h}^{-1} = 8 \text{ h}$$

5. *Choose the desired steady-state serum concentrations.*

Patients with *S. aureus* wound infections need to be carefully assessed. This patient did not appear to be in acute distress, with a normal temperature and a slightly elevated white blood cell count. The wound was warm and red with a slight purulent discharge. Because the infection was localized to the wound area, a $C_{min,ss}$ = 7 μg/mL and $C_{max,ss}$ = 20 μg/mL were chosen.

6. *Use the intravenous bolus equations to compute the dose (see Table 5-2C).*

Calculate the required dosage interval (τ):

$$\tau = (\ln C_{max,ss} - \ln C_{min,ss})/k_e = (\ln 20 \text{ μg/mL} - \ln 7 \text{ μg/mL})/0.087 \text{ h}^{-1} = 12.1 \text{ h}$$

Dosage intervals should be rounded to clinically acceptable intervals of 12 hours, 18 hours, 24 hours, 36 hours, 48 hours, 72 hours, and multiples of 24 hours thereafter, whenever possible. In this case, the dosage interval is rounded to 12 hours.

Calculate the required dose (D):

$$D = C_{max,ss} V(1 - e^{-k_e\tau}) = 20 \text{ mg/L} \cdot 49 \text{ L } (1 - e^{-(0.087 \text{ h}^{-1})(12 \text{ h})}) = 635 \text{ mg}$$

Vancomycin doses should be rounded to the nearest 100 to 250 mg. This dose is rounded to 750 mg. (Note: μg/mL = mg/L, and this concentration unit was substituted for $C_{max,ss}$ to avoid unnecessary unit conversion.)

The prescribed maintenance dosage is 750 mg every 12 hours.

7. *Compute the loading dose (LD), if needed.*

Loading doses should be considered for patients with creatinine clearance values lower than 60 mL/min. The administration of a loading dose allows achievement of therapeutic concentrations more quickly than if maintenance doses alone are given. However, since the pharmacokinetic parameters used to compute these initial doses are *estimated* values and not *actual* values, the patient's own parameters may be much different from the estimated constants and steady-state will not be achieved until 3 to 5 half-lives have passed.

$$LD = C_{max,ss} V = 20 \text{ mg/L} \cdot 49 \text{ L} = 980 \text{ mg}$$

As noted, this patient has good renal function (CrCl ≥60 mL/min), so a loading dose would not be prescribed.

Example 2 Same patient profile as in example 1, but serum creatinine is 3.5 mg/dL, indicating renal impairment.

1. *Estimate the creatinine clearance.*

This patient has a stable serum creatinine and is not obese. The Cockcroft–Gault equation can be used to estimate creatinine clearance:

$$CrCl_{est} = [(140 - age)BW]/(72 \cdot S_{Cr}) = [(140 - 50\ y)70\ kg]/(72 \cdot 3.5\ mg/dL)$$

$$CrCl_{est} = 25\ mL/min$$

2. *Estimate the vancomycin clearance.*

The vancomycin clearance versus creatinine clearance relationship is used to estimate the vancomycin clearance for this patient:

$$Cl = 0.695(CrCl) + 0.05 = 0.695[(25\ mL/min)/70\ kg] + 0.05 = 0.298\ mL/min/kg$$

3. *Estimate the vancomycin volume of distribution.*

The average volume of distribution for vancomycin is 0.7 L/kg:

$$V = 0.7\ L/kg \cdot 70\ kg = 49\ L$$

4. *Estimate the vancomycin elimination rate constant (k_e) and half-life ($t_{1/2}$).*

$$k_e = Cl/V = [(0.298\ mL/min/kg) \cdot (60\ min/h)]/(0.7\ L/kg \cdot 1000\ mL/L) = 0.0256\ h^{-1}$$

$$t_{1/2} = 0.693/k_e = 0.693/0.0256\ h^{-1} = 27\ h$$

5. *Choose the desired steady-state serum concentrations.*

Patients with *S. aureus* wound infections must be carefully assessed. This patient did not appear to be in acute distress, with a normal temperature and a slightly elevated white blood cell count. The wound was warm and red with a slight amount of purulent discharge. Because the infection was localized to the wound area, a $C_{min,ss}$ = 7 μg/mL and $C_{max,ss}$ = 20 μg/mL were chosen.

6. *Use the intravenous bolus equations to compute the dose (see Table 5-2C).*

Calculate the required dosage interval (τ):

$$\tau = (\ln C_{max,ss} - \ln C_{min,ss})/k_e = (\ln 20\ \mu g/mL - \ln 7\ \mu g/mL)/0.0256\ h^{-1} = 41\ h$$

Dosage intervals should be rounded to clinically acceptable intervals of 12 hours, 18 hours, 24 hours, 36 hours, 48 hours, 72 hours, and multiples of 24 hours thereafter, whenever possible. In this case, the dosage interval is rounded to 48 hours.

Calculate the required dose (D):

$$D = C_{max,ss}\,V(1 - e^{-k_e\tau}) = 20\ mg/L \cdot 49\ L\ (1 - e^{-(0.0256\ h^{-1})(48\ h)}) = 693\ mg$$

Vancomycin doses should be rounded to the nearest 100 to 250 mg. This dose is rounded to 750 mg. (Note: μg/mL = mg/L, and this concentration unit was substituted for $C_{max,ss}$ to avoid unnecessary unit conversion.)

The prescribed maintenance dosage is 750 mg every 48 hours.

7. *Compute the loading dose (LD), if needed.*

Loading doses should be considered for patients with creatinine clearance values lower than 60 mL/min. The administration of a loading dose allows achievement of therapeutic concentrations more quickly than if maintenance doses alone are given. However, since the pharmacokinetic parameters used to compute these initial doses are *estimated* values and not *actual* values, the patient's own parameters may be much different from the estimated constants, and steady-state will not be achieved until 3 to 5 half-lives have passed.

$$LD = C_{max,ss} V = 20 \text{ mg/L} \cdot 49 \text{ L} = 980 \text{ mg}$$

As noted, patient JM has poor renal function (CrCl <60 mL/min), so a loading dose is prescribed and given as the first dose. Vancomycin doses should be rounded to the nearest 100 to 250 mg. This dose is rounded to 1000 mg. (Note: μg/mL = mg/L, and this concentration unit was substituted for $C_{max,ss}$ to avoid unnecessary unit conversion.) The first maintenance dose is given one dosage interval (48 hours) after the loading dose was administered.

Example 3 ZW is a 35-year-old, 150-kg, 165-cm (65-in) woman with *S. epidermidis* infection of a prosthetic knee joint. Her serum creatinine is 0.7 mg/dL and stable. Compute a vancomycin dose for this patient.

1. *Estimate the creatinine clearance.*

This patient has a stable serum creatinine and is obese ($IBW_{females}$ (in kg) = 45 + 2.3(Ht − 60 in) = 45 + 2.3(65 − 60 in) = 57 kg). The Salazar-Corcoran equation can be used to estimate creatinine clearance:

$$CrCl_{est(females)} = \frac{(146 - age)[(0.287 \cdot Wt) + (9.74 \cdot Ht^2)]}{(60 \cdot S_{Cr})}$$

$$CrCl_{est(females)} = \frac{(146 - 35 \text{ y})\{(0.287 \cdot 150 \text{ kg}) + [9.74 \cdot (1.65 \text{ m})^2]\}}{(60 \cdot 0.7 \text{ mg/dL})} = 184 \text{ mL/min}$$

Note: Height is converted from inches to meters: Ht = (65 in · 2.54 cm/in)/(100 cm/m) = 1.65 m.

2. *Estimate the vancomycin clearance.*

The vancomycin clearance versus creatinine clearance relationship is used to estimate the vancomycin clearance for this patient. Because maintenance doses are based on total body weight (TBW), this weight factor is used to compute clearance:

$$Cl = 0.695(CrCl) + 0.05 = 0.695[(184 \text{ mL/min})/150 \text{ kg}] + 0.05 = 0.902 \text{ mL/min/kg TBW}$$

3. *Estimate the vancomycin volume of distribution.*

The average volume of distribution for vancomycin is 0.7 L/kg and is computed using the patient's ideal body weight because obesity does not significantly alter this parameter:

$$V = 0.7 \text{ L/kg} \cdot 57 \text{ kg} = 40 \text{ L}$$

4. *Estimate the vancomycin elimination rate constant (k_e) and half-life ($t_{1/2}$).*

Note that in obese persons, different weight factors are needed for vancomycin clearance and volume of distribution, so these weights are included in the equation for elimination rate constant:

$k_e = Cl/V = (0.902 \text{ mL/min/kg TBW} \cdot 150 \text{ kg TBW} \cdot 60 \text{ min/h})/(0.7 \text{ L/kg IBW} \cdot 57 \text{ kg IBW} \cdot 1000 \text{ mL/L}) = 0.205 \text{ h}^{-1}$

$t_{1/2} = 0.693/k_e = 0.693/0.205 \text{ h}^{-1} = 3.4 \text{ h}$

5. *Choose the desired steady-state serum concentrations.*

A $C_{min,ss} = 7.5$ μg/mL and $C_{max,ss} = 35$ μg/mL were chosen for this patient with a *S. epidermidis* prosthetic joint infection.

6. *Use the intravenous bolus equations to compute the dose (see Table 5-2C).*

Calculate the required dosage interval (τ):

$$\tau = (\ln C_{max,ss} - \ln C_{min,ss})/k_e = (\ln 35 \text{ μg/mL} - \ln 7.5 \text{ μg/mL})/0.205 \text{ h}^{-1} = 7.5 \text{ h}$$

Dosage intervals in obese persons should be rounded to clinically acceptable intervals of 8 hours, 12 hours, 18 hours, 24 hours, 36 hours, 48 hours, 72 hours, and multiples of 24 hours thereafter, whenever possible. In this patient, the dosage interval is rounded to 8 hours.

Calculate the required dose (D):

$$D = C_{max,ss} V(1 - e^{-k_e\tau}) = 35 \text{ mg/L} \cdot 40 \text{ L } (1 - e^{-(0.205 \text{ h}^{-1})(8 \text{ h})}) = 1128 \text{ mg}$$

Vancomycin doses should be rounded to the nearest 100 to 250 mg. This dose is rounded to 1250 mg. (Note: μg/mL = mg/L, and this concentration unit was substituted for $C_{max,ss}$ to avoid unnecessary unit conversion.)

The prescribed maintenance dosage is 1250 mg every 8 hours.

7. *Compute the loading dose (LD), if needed.*

Loading doses should be considered for patients with creatinine clearance values lower than 60 mL/min. The administration of a loading dose allows achievement of therapeutic concentrations more quickly than if maintenance doses alone are given. However, since the pharmacokinetic parameters used to compute these initial doses are *estimated* values and not *actual* values, the patient's own parameters may be much different from the estimated constants, and steady-state will not be achieved until 3 to 5 half-lives have passed.

$$LD = C_{max,ss} V = 35 \text{ mg/L} \cdot 40 \text{ L} = 1400 \text{ mg}$$

As noted, this patient has good renal function (CrCl ≥60 mL/min), so a loading dose is not prescribed.

Example 4 JM is an 80-year-old, 80-kg, 173-cm (68-in) man with *Streptococcus viridans* endocarditis. He is allergic to penicillins and cephalosporins. His serum creatinine is 1.5 mg/dL and stable. Compute a vancomycin dose for this patient.

1. *Estimate the creatinine clearance.*

This patient has a stable serum creatinine and is not obese (IBW_{men} = 50 + 2.3(Ht – 60 in) = 50 + 2.3 (68 – 60) = 68 kg; % overweight = {100[80 kg – 68 kg]}/68 kg = 18%). The Cockcroft-Gault equation can be used to estimate creatinine clearance:

$$CrCl_{est} = [(140 - \text{age})BW]/(72 \cdot S_{Cr}) = [(140 - 80 \text{ y})80 \text{ kg}]/(72 \cdot 1.5 \text{ mg/dL})$$

$$CrCl_{est} = 44 \text{ mL/min}$$

2. *Estimate the vancomycin clearance.*

The vancomycin clearance versus creatinine clearance relationship is used to estimate the vancomycin clearance for this patient:

$$Cl = 0.695(CrCl) + 0.05 = 0.695[(44 \text{ mL/min})/80 \text{ kg}] + 0.05 = 0.432 \text{ mL/min per kg.}$$

3. *Estimate the vancomycin volume of distribution.*

The average volume of distribution for vancomycin is 0.7 L/kg:

$$V = 0.7 \text{ L/kg} \cdot 80 \text{ kg} = 56 \text{ L}$$

4. *Estimate the vancomycin elimination rate constant (k_e) and half-life ($t_{1/2}$).*

$$k_e = Cl/V = [(0.432 \text{ mL/min/kg}) \cdot (60 \text{ min/h})]/(0.7 \text{ L/kg} \cdot 1000 \text{ mL/L}) = 0.0370 \text{ h}^{-1}$$

$$t_{1/2} = 0.693/k_e = 0.693/0.0370 \text{ h}^{-1} = 18.7 \text{ h}$$

5. *Choose the desired steady-state serum concentrations.*

Steady-state vancomycin serum concentrations of $C_{min,ss}$ = 5 μg/mL and $C_{max,ss}$ = 25 μg/mL were chosen to treat this patient.

6. *Use intravenous bolus equations to compute dose (see Table 5-2C).*

Calculate the required dosage interval (τ):

$$\tau = (\ln C_{max,ss} - \ln C_{min,ss})/k_e = (\ln 25 \text{ μg/mL} - \ln 5 \text{ μg/mL})/0.0370 \text{ h}^{-1} = 43 \text{ h}$$

Dosage intervals should be rounded to clinically acceptable intervals of 12 hours, 18 hours, 24 hours, 36 hours, 48 hours, 72 hours, and multiples of 24 hours thereafter, whenever possible. In this patient, the dosage interval is rounded to 48 hours.

Calculate the required dose (D):

$$D = C_{max,ss} V(1 - e^{-k_e\tau}) = 25 \text{ mg/L} \cdot 56 \text{ L } (1 - e^{-(0.0370 \text{ h}^{-1})(48 \text{ h})}) = 1163 \text{ mg}$$

Vancomycin doses should be rounded to the nearest 100 to 250 mg. This dose is rounded to 1250 mg. (Note: μg/mL = mg/L, and this concentration unit was substituted for $C_{max,ss}$ to avoid unnecessary unit conversion.)

The prescribed maintenance dosage is 1250 mg every 48 hours.

7. *Compute the loading dose (LD), if needed.*

Loading doses should be considered for patients with creatinine clearance values lower than 60 mL/min. The administration of a loading dose allows achievement of therapeutic concentrations more quickly than if maintenance doses alone are given. However, because the pharmacokinetic parameters used to compute these initial doses are *estimated* values and not *actual* values, the patient's own parameters may be much different from the estimated constants, and steady-state is not achieved until 3 to 5 half-lives have passed.

$$LD = C_{max,ss} V = 25 \text{ mg/L} \cdot 56 \text{ L} = 1400 \text{ mg}$$

As noted, patient JM has poor renal function (CrCl <60 mL/min), so a loading dose is prescribed and given as the first dose. Vancomycin doses are rounded to the nearest 100 to 250 mg. This dose is rounded to 1500 mg. (Note: μg/mL = mg/L, and this concentration unit was substituted for $C_{max,ss}$ to avoid unnecessary unit conversion.) The first maintenance dose is given one dosage interval (48 hours) after the loading dose was administered.

Moellering Nomogram Method

Because the only two patient-specific factors that change when using the pharmacokinetic dosing method are patient weight and creatinine clearance, a simple nomogram can be made to handle uncomplicated patients. The Moellering dosage nomogram was the first widely used approach that incorporated pharmacokinetic concepts to compute doses of vancomycin for patients with compromised renal function[23] (Table 5-3). The stated goal of the nomogram is to provide average steady-state vancomycin concentrations of 15 μg/mL (or 15 mg/L). To use the nomogram, the patient's creatinine clearance is computed and divided by body weight, so that the units for creatinine clearance are mL/min per kg. This value is converted to a vancomycin maintenance dose in terms of mg/kg per 24 hours. If the patient has renal impairment, a loading dose of 15 mg/kg is suggested. The nomogram does not provide a value for dosage interval.

The relationship between vancomycin clearance and creatinine clearance in the pharmacokinetic dosing method is the one used to construct the Moellering nomogram. Hence, the dosage recommendations made by both these methods are generally similar, though not identical, because vancomycin peak and trough concentrations cannot be specified using the nomogram. A modification of the vancomycin clearance–creatinine clearance equation can be made, which provides a direct calculation of the vancomycin maintenance dose.[40] Because the equation computes vancomycin clearance, it can be converted to the maintenance dose required to provide an average steady-state concentration of 15 mg/L by multiplying the equation by the concentration (MD = Css · Cl, where MD is maintenance dose) and appropriate unit conversion constants:

$$\text{Cl (in mL/min/kg)} = 0.695(\text{CrCl in mL/min/kg}) + 0.05$$

$$\text{D (in mg/h/kg)} = [(15\ \text{mg/L} \cdot 60\ \text{min/h})/1000\ \text{mL/L}][0.695(\text{CrCl in mL/min/kg}) + 0.05]$$

$$\text{D (in mg/h/kg)} = 0.626(\text{CrCl in mL/min/kg}) + 0.05$$

The use of this modification is straightforward. The patient's creatinine clearance is estimated using an appropriate technique (Cockcroft–Gault method[41] for normal weight patients, Salazar-Corcoran method[42] for obese patients). The vancomycin maintenance dose is directly computed using the dosing equation and multiplied by the patient's weight to convert the answer into the units of mg/h. Guidance to the appropriate dosage interval (in hours) can be gained by dividing this dosage rate into a clinically acceptable dose such as 1000 mg. To illustrate how this dosing approach is used, the same patient examples used in the previous section are repeated for this dosage approach.

Example 1 JM is a 50-year-old, 70-kg, 178-cm (70-in) man with a methicillin-resistant *S. aureus* wound infection. His serum creatinine is 0.9 mg/dL, which has been stable over the last 5 days since admission. Compute a vancomycin dose for this patient.

TABLE 5-3 Moellering Nomogram Vancomycin Dosage Chart

1. Compute patient's creatinine clearance (CrCl) using Cockcroft–Gault method for normal weight or Salazar-Corcoran method for obese patients.
2. Divide CrCl by patient's weight.
3. Compute 24-hour maintenance dose for CrCl value.
4. Loading dose of 15 mg/kg should be given in patients with significant renal function impairment.

CREATININE CLEARANCE (mL/min/kg)*	VANCOMYCIN DOSE (mg/kg/24 h)
2	30.9
1.9	29.3
1.8	27.8
1.7	26.3
1.6	24.7
1.5	23.2
1.4	21.6
1.3	20.1
1.2	18.5
1.1	17
1.0	15.4
0.9	13.9
0.8	12.4
0.7	10.8
0.6	9.3
0.5	7.7
0.4	6.2
0.3	4.6
0.2	3.1
0.1	1.5

* Dose for functionally anephric patients is 1.9 mg/kg/24 h.
Adapted from Moellering RC, Jr, Krogstad DJ, Greenblatt DJ. Vancomycin therapy in patients with impaired renal function: a nomogram for dosage. Ann Intern Med 1981;94:343–346.

1. *Estimate the creatinine clearance.*

This patient has a stable serum creatinine and is not obese. The Cockcroft–Gault equation can be used to estimate creatinine clearance:

$$CrCl_{est} = [(140 - age)BW]/(72 \cdot S_{Cr}) = [(140 - 50\ y)70\ kg]/(72 \cdot 0.9\ mg/dL)$$

$$CrCl_{est} = 97\ mL/min$$

2. *Determine the dosage interval and maintenance dosage.*

The maintenance dosage is calculated using the modified vancomycin dosing equation:

$$\text{D (in mg/h/kg)} = 0.626(\text{CrCl in mL/min/kg}) + 0.05$$

$$\text{D} = 0.626[(97 \text{ mL/min})/70 \text{ kg}] + 0.05 = 0.918 \text{ mg/h/kg}$$

$$\text{D} = 0.918 \text{ mg/h/kg} \cdot 70 \text{ kg} = 64.2 \text{ mg/h}$$

Because the patient has good renal function, the typical dosage interval of 12 hours is used:

$$\text{D} = 64.2 \text{ mg/h} \cdot 12 \text{ h} = 770 \text{ mg}$$

Vancomycin doses should be rounded to the nearest 100 to 250 mg. This dose is rounded to 750 mg. The prescribed maintenance dosage is 750 mg every 12 hours.

3. *Compute the loading dose.*

A loading dose (LD) of 15 mg/kg is suggested by the Moellering nomogram:

$$\text{LD} = 15 \text{ mg/kg}(70 \text{ mg}) = 1050 \text{ mg}$$

As noted, this patient has good renal function (CrCl ≥60 mL/min), so a loading dose can be optionally prescribed.

Example 2 Same patient profile as in example 1, but serum creatinine is 3.5 mg/dL, indicating renal impairment.

1. *Estimate the creatinine clearance.*

This patient has a stable serum creatinine and is not obese. The Cockcroft–Gault equation can be used to estimate creatinine clearance:

$$\text{CrCl}_{\text{est}} = [(140 - \text{age})\text{BW}]/(72 \cdot \text{S}_{\text{Cr}}) = [(140 - 50 \text{ y})70 \text{ kg}]/(72 \cdot 3.5 \text{ mg/dL})$$

$$\text{CrCl}_{\text{est}} = 25 \text{ mL/min}$$

2. *Determine the dosage interval and maintenance dosage.*

The maintenance dosage is calculated using the modified vancomycin dosing equation:

$$\text{D (in mg/h/kg)} = 0.626(\text{CrCl in mL/min/kg}) + 0.05$$

$$\text{D} = 0.626[(25 \text{ mL/min})/70 \text{ kg}] + 0.05 = 0.274 \text{ mg/h/kg}$$

$$\text{D} = [(0.274 \text{ mg/h/kg}) \cdot (70 \text{ kg})] = 19.2 \text{ mg/h}$$

The standard dose of vancomycin 1000 mg can be used to gain an approximation for an acceptable dosage interval (τ):

$$\tau = 1000 \text{ mg}/(19.2 \text{ mg/h}) = 52 \text{ h}$$

Dosage intervals should be rounded to clinically acceptable intervals of 12 hours, 18 hours, 24 hours, 36 hours, 48 hours, 72 hours, and multiples of 24 hours thereafter, whenever possible. In this case, the dosage interval is rounded to 48 hours.

$$D = 19.2\ \text{mg/h} \cdot 48\ \text{h} = 922\ \text{mg}$$

Vancomycin doses should be rounded to the nearest 100 to 250 mg. This dose is rounded to 1000 mg. The prescribed maintenance dosage is 1000 mg every 48 hours.

3. *Compute the loading dose.*

A loading dose (LD) of 15 mg/kg is suggested by the Moellering nomogram:

$$LD = 15\ \text{mg/kg}(70\ \text{kg}) = 1050\ \text{mg}$$

The patient has poor renal function (CrCl <60 mL/min), so a loading dose could be prescribed and given as the first dose. However, in this case the loading dose is nearly identical to the maintenance dose and would not be given.

Example 3 ZW is a 35-year-old, 150-kg, 165-cm (65-in) woman with a *S. epidermidis* infection of a prosthetic knee joint. Her serum creatinine is 0.7 mg/dL and stable. Compute a vancomycin dose for this patient.

1. *Estimate the creatinine clearance.*

This patient has a stable serum creatinine and is obese ($IBW_{females}$ (in kg) = 45 + 2.3(Ht – 60 in) = 45 + 2.3(65 – 60) = 57 kg). The Salazar-Corcoran equation can be used to estimate creatinine clearance:

$$CrCl_{est(females)} = \frac{(146 - \text{age})[(0.287 \cdot \text{Wt}) + (9.74 \cdot \text{Ht}^2)]}{(60 \cdot S_{Cr})}$$

$$CrCl_{est(females)} = \frac{(146 - 35\ \text{y})\{(0.287 \cdot 150\ \text{kg}) + [9.74 \cdot (1.65\ \text{m})^2]\}}{(60 \cdot 0.7\ \text{mg/dL})} = 184\ \text{mL/min}$$

Note: Height is converted from inches to meters: Ht = (65 in · 2.54 cm/in)/(100 cm/m) = 1.65 m.

2. *Determine the dosage interval and maintenance dosage.*

The maintenance dosage is calculated using the modified vancomycin dosing equation:

$$D\ (\text{in mg/h/kg}) = 0.626(\text{CrCl in mL/min/kg}) + 0.05$$

$$D = 0.626[(184\ \text{mL/min})/150\ \text{kg}] + 0.05 = 0.818\ \text{mg/h/kg}$$

$$D = 0.818\ \text{mg/h/kg} \cdot 150\ \text{kg} = 122.7\ \text{mg/h}$$

Because the patient has excellent renal function and is obese, a dosage interval of 8 hours is used:

$$D = 122.7\ \text{mg/h} \cdot 8\ \text{h} = 981\ \text{mg}$$

Vancomycin doses should be rounded to the nearest 100 to 250 mg. This dose is rounded to 1000 mg. The prescribed maintenance dosage is 1000 mg every 8 hours.

3. *Compute the loading dose.*

A loading dose (LD) of 15 mg/kg is suggested by the Moellering nomogram. As noted, this patient has good renal function (CrCl ≥60 mL/min), so a loading dose would probably not be prescribed for this patient.

Example 4 JM is an 80-year-old, 80-kg, 173-cm (68-in) man with *S. viridans* endocarditis. He is allergic to penicillins and cephalosporins. His serum creatinine is 1.5 mg/dL and stable. Compute a vancomycin dose for this patient.

1. *Estimate the creatinine clearance.*

This patient has a stable serum creatinine and is not obese (IBW_{males} = 50 + 2.3(Ht – 60 in) = 50 + 2.3(68 – 60) = 68 kg; % overweight = {100[80 kg–68 kg]}/68 kg = 18%). The Cockcroft–Gault equation can be used to estimate creatinine clearance:

$$CrCl_{est} = [(140 - age)BW]/(72 \cdot S_{Cr}) = [(140 - 80\ y)80\ kg]/(72 \cdot 1.5\ mg/dL)$$

$$CrCl_{est} = 44\ mL/min$$

2. *Determine the dosage interval and the maintenance dosage.*

The maintenance dose is calculated using the modified vancomycin dosing equation:

$$D\ (in\ mg/h/kg) = 0.626(CrCl\ in\ mL/min/kg) + 0.05$$

$$D = 0.626[(44\ mL/min)/80\ kg] + 0.05 = 0.394\ mg/h/kg$$

$$D = 0.394\ mg/h/kg \cdot 80\ kg = 31.5\ mg/h$$

The standard dose of 1000 mg can be used to gain an approximation for an acceptable dosage interval (τ):

$$\tau = 1000\ mg/(31.5\ mg/h) = 31.7\ h$$

Dosage intervals should be rounded to clinically acceptable intervals of 12 hours, 18 hours, 24 hours, 36 hours, 48 hours, 72 hours, and multiples of 24 hours thereafter, whenever possible. In this case, the dosage interval is rounded to 36 hours.

$$D = 31.5\ mg/h \cdot 36\ h = 1134\ mg$$

Vancomycin doses should be rounded to the nearest 100 to 250 mg. This dose is rounded to 1250 mg. The prescribed maintenance dosage is 1250 mg every 36 hours.

3. *Compute the loading dose.*

A loading dose (LD) of 15 mg/kg is suggested by the Moellering nomogram:

$$LD = 15\ mg/kg(80\ kg) = 1200\ mg$$

This patient has poor renal function (CrCl <60 mL/min), so a loading dose could be prescribed and given as the first dose. However, in this case the loading dose is nearly identical to the maintenance dose and would not be given.

Matzke Nomogram Method

The Matzke dosing nomogram is a quick and efficient way to apply pharmacokinetic dosing concepts without using complicated pharmacokinetic equations[25] (Table 5-4). The nomogram has not been tested in obese subjects (>30% over ideal body weight) and should not be used in this patient population. In addition, the authors suggest that the nomogram should not be used in patients undergoing peritoneal dialysis.

The nomogram is constructed to produce steady-state vancomycin peak and trough concentrations of 30 μg/mL and 7.5 μg/mL, respectively. A loading dose of 25 mg/kg is given as the first dose, and subsequent maintenance doses of 19 mg/kg are given according to a dosage interval that varies by the patient's creatinine clearance. The dosage interval supplied by the nomogram is the time needed for 19 mg/kg of vancomycin to be eliminated from the body. By replacing the amount eliminated over the dosage interval with a maintenance dose of the same magnitude, the same peak and trough vancomycin concentration–time profile is reproduced after each dose. To illustrate how the nomogram is used, the same patient examples used in the previous section (omitting the obese patient) are repeated for this dosage approach. Because the nomogram uses slightly different estimates for volume of distribution and elimination rate constant as well as fixed steady-state peak and trough drug concentrations, differences in suggested doses are expected.

TABLE 5-4 Matzke Nomogram Vancomycin Dosage Chart

1. Compute patient's creatinine clearance (CrCl) using Cockcroft–Gault method: CrCl = [(140 – age)BW]/(S_{cr} × 72). Multiply by 0.85 for females.
2. Nomogram is not verified in obese persons.
3. Dosage chart is designed to achieve peak serum concentrations of 30 μg/mL and trough concentrations of 7.5 μg/mL.
4. Compute loading dose of 25 mg/kg.
5. Compute maintenance dose of 19 mg/kg given at the dosage interval listed in the following chart for the patient's CrCl:

CrCl (mL/min)	DOSAGE INTERVAL (DAYS)
≥120	0.5
100	0.6
80	0.75
60	1.0
40	1.5
30	2.0
20	2.5
10	4.0
5	6.0
0	12.0

Adapted from Matzke GR, Halstenson CE, Olson PL, Collins AJ, Abraham PA. Systemic absorption of oral vancomycin in patients with renal insufficiency and antibiotic-associated colitis. Am J Kidney Dis 1987;9:422–425.

Although the Matzke nomogram has been shown to provide precise and unbiased dosage recommendations, it does supply relatively large doses because expected peak and trough concentrations are in the middle of their respective therapeutic ranges.

Example 1 JM is a 50-year-old, 70-kg, 178-cm (70-in) man with a methicillin-resistant *Staphylococcus aureus* (MRSA) wound infection. His serum creatinine is 0.9 mg/dL, which has been stable over the last 5 days since admission. Compute a vancomycin dose for this patient.

1. *Estimate the creatinine clearance.*

This patient has a stable serum creatinine and is not obese. The Cockcroft–Gault equation can be used to estimate creatinine clearance:

$$CrCl_{est} = [(140 - age)BW]/(72 \cdot S_{Cr}) = [(140 - 50\ y)70\ kg]/(72 \cdot 0.9\ mg/dL)$$

$$CrCl_{est} = 97\ mL/min$$

2. *Compute the loading dose (see Table 5-4).*

A loading dose of 25 mg/kg provides a peak concentration of 30 μg/mL.

$$LD = 25\ mg/kg(70\ kg) = 1750\ mg$$

3. *Determine the dosage interval and the maintenance dosage.*

As determined from the nomogram, the dosage interval is 0.6 days, which should be rounded to every 12 hours. The maintenance dose is 19 mg/kg · 70 kg = 1330 mg. Vancomycin doses should be rounded to the nearest 100 to 250 mg. This dose is rounded to 1250 mg and given one dosage interval (12 hours) after the loading dose.

The prescribed maintenance dosage is 1250 mg every 12 hours.

Example 2 Same patient profile as in example 1, but serum creatinine is 3.5 mg/dL, indicating renal impairment.

1. *Estimate the creatinine clearance.*

This patient has a stable serum creatinine and is not obese. The Cockcroft–Gault equation can be used to estimate creatinine clearance:

$$CrCl_{est} = [(140 - age)BW]/(72 \cdot S_{Cr}) = [(140 - 50\ y)70\ kg]/(72 \cdot 3.5\ mg/dL)$$

$$CrCl_{est} = 25\ mL/min$$

2. *Compute the loading dose (see Table 5-4).*

A loading dose of 25 mg/kg provides a peak concentration of 30 μg/mL.

$$LD = 25\ mg/kg(70\ kg) = 1750\ mg$$

3. *Determine the dosage interval and the maintenance dosage.*

After rounding creatinine clearance to 30 mL/min, the nomogram suggests a dosage interval of 2 days. The maintenance dose would be 19 mg/kg · 70 kg = 1330 mg. Vancomycin doses should be rounded to the nearest 100 to 250 mg. This dose is rounded to 1250 mg and given one dosage interval (2 days × 24 hours/day = 48 hours) after the loading dose.

The prescribed maintenance dosage is 1250 mg every 48 hours.

Example 3 JM is an 80-year-old, 80-kg, 173-cm (68-in) man with *Streptococcus viridans* endocarditis who is allergic to penicillins and cephalosporins. His serum creatinine is 1.5 mg/dL and stable. Compute a vancomycin dose for this patient.

1. *Estimate the creatinine clearance.*

This patient has a stable serum creatinine and is not obese (IBW_{men} = 50 + 2.3(Ht – 60 in) = 50 + 2.3(68 – 60) = 68 kg; % overweight = {100[80 kg – 68 kg]}/68 kg = 18%). The Cockcroft–Gault equation can be used to estimate creatinine clearance:

$$CrCl_{est} = [(140 - age)BW]/(72 \cdot S_{Cr}) = [(140 - 80\ y)80\ kg]/(72 \cdot 1.5\ mg/dL)$$

$$CrCl_{est} = 44\ mL/min$$

2. *Compute the loading dose (see Table 5-4).*

A loading dose of 25 mg/kg provides a peak concentration of 30 μg/mL.

$$LD = 25\ mg/kg(80\ kg) = 2000\ mg$$

3. *Determine the dosage interval and maintenance dose.*

After rounding creatinine clearance to 40 mL/min, the nomogram suggests a dosage interval of 1.5 days. The maintenance dose is 19 mg/kg · 80 kg = 1520 mg. Vancomycin doses should be rounded to the nearest 100 to 250 mg. This dose is rounded to 1500 mg and started one dosage interval (1.5 days × 24 hours/day = 36 hours) after the loading dose.

The prescribed maintenance dosage is 1500 mg every 36 hours.

USE OF VANCOMYCIN SERUM CONCENTRATIONS TO ALTER DOSAGES

Because of pharmacokinetic variability among patients, it is likely that doses calculated using patient population characteristics will not always produce vancomycin serum concentrations that are expected. Because of this, vancomycin serum concentrations are measured in many patients to ensure that therapeutic, nontoxic levels are present. However, not all patients may require serum concentration monitoring. For example, if only a limited number of doses are expected to be administered, as is the case for surgical prophylaxis, or if an appropriate dose for the renal function and concurrent disease states of the patient is prescribed (e.g., 15 mg/kg every 12 hours for a patient with a creatinine clearance of 80 to 120 mL/min), vancomycin serum concentration monitoring may not be necessary. Whether or not vancomycin concentrations are measured, important patient parameters (e.g., fever curves, white blood cell counts, serum creatinine concentrations) should be monitored to confirm that the patient is responding to treatment and not developing adverse drug reactions.

When vancomycin serum concentrations are measured in patients and a dosage change is necessary, clinicians should seek the simplest, most straightforward method available to determine a dose that will provide safe and effective treatment. In most cases, a simple dosage ratio can be used to change vancomycin doses, since these antibiotics follow *linear pharmacokinetics*. Sometimes it is not possible to simply change the dose, and the dosage interval must also be changed to achieve desired serum concentrations. In this case, it may be possible to use *pharmacokinetic concepts* to alter the vancomycin dose. In some situations, it may be necessary to compute the vancomycin pharmacokinetic parameters for the patient using the *one-compartment model parameter method* and to use these parameters to calculate the best drug dose. Finally, computerized methods that incorporate expected population pharmacokinetic characteristics (*Bayesian pharmacokinetics computer programs*) can be used in difficult cases in which renal function is changing, serum concentrations are obtained at suboptimal times, or the patient was not at steady state when serum concentrations were measured.

Linear Pharmacokinetics Method

Because vancomycin antibiotics follow linear, dose-proportional pharmacokinetics, steady-state serum concentrations change in proportion to dose according to the following equation: $D_{new}/C_{ss,new} = D_{old}/C_{ss,old}$ or $D_{new} = (C_{ss,new}/C_{ss,old})D_{old}$, where D is the dose, Css is the steady-state peak or trough concentration, old indicates the dose that produced the steady-state concentration that the patient is currently receiving, and new denotes the dose necessary to produce the desired steady-state concentration. The advantages of this method are that it is quick and simple. The disadvantages are steady-state concentrations are required, and it may not be possible to attain desired serum concentrations by only changing the dose.

Example 1 JM is a 50-year-old, 70-kg, 178-cm (70-in) man with a methicillin-resistant *S. aureus* pneumonia. His serum creatinine is 0.9 mg/dL, which has been stable over the last 5 days since admission. Vancomycin 1000 mg every 12 hours was prescribed and expected to achieve steady-state peak and trough concentrations of 25 μg/mL and 7 μg/mL, respectively. After the third dose, steady-state peak and trough concentrations were measured and were 45 μg/mL and 12 μg/mL, respectively. Calculate a new vancomycin dose that will provide a steady-state trough of 7 μg/mL.

1. *Estimate the creatinine clearance.*

This patient has a stable serum creatinine and is not obese. The Cockcroft–Gault equation can be used to estimate creatinine clearance:

$$CrCl_{est} = [(140 - age)BW]/(72 \cdot S_{Cr}) = [(140 - 50\ y)70\ kg]/(72 \cdot 0.9\ mg/dL)$$

$$CrCl_{est} = 97\ mL/min$$

2. *Estimate the elimination rate constant (k_e) and half-life ($t_{1/2}$).*

The vancomycin clearance versus creatinine clearance relationship is used to estimate drug clearance for this patient:

$$Cl = 0.695(CrCl) + 0.05 = 0.695[(97 \text{ mL/min})/70 \text{ kg}] + 0.05 = 1.013 \text{ mL/min/kg}$$

The average volume of distribution for vancomycin is 0.7 L/kg:

$$V = 0.7 \text{ L/kg} \cdot 70 \text{ kg} = 49 \text{ L}$$

$$k_e = Cl/V = (1.013 \text{ mL/min/kg} \cdot 60 \text{ min/h})/(0.7 \text{ L/kg} \cdot 1000 \text{ mL/L}) = 0.0868 \text{ h}^{-1}$$

$$t_{1/2} = 0.693/k_e = 0.693/0.0868 \text{ h}^{-1} = 8 \text{ h}$$

Because the patient has been receiving vancomycin for ~3 estimated half-lives, it is likely that the measured serum concentrations are steady-state values.

3. *Compute the new dose to achieve desired serum concentration.*

By using linear pharmacokinetics, the new dose to attain the desired concentration should be proportional to the old dose that produced the measured concentration:

$$D_{new} = (C_{ss,new}/C_{ss,old})D_{old} = [(7 \text{ μg/mL})/(12 \text{ μg/mL})]\ 1000 \text{ mg} = 583 \text{ mg, round to 500 mg}$$

The new suggested dose is vancomycin 500 mg every 12 hours to be started at the next scheduled dosing time.

4. *Check the steady-state peak concentration for a new dosage regimen.*

By using linear pharmacokinetics, the new steady-state concentration can be estimated and should be proportional to the old dose that produced the measured concentration:

$$C_{ss,new} = (D_{new}/D_{old})C_{ss,old} = (500 \text{ mg}/1000 \text{ mg})\ 45 \text{ μg/mL} = 22.5 \text{ μg/mL}$$

This steady-state peak concentration should be safe and effective for the infection that is being treated.

Example 2 ZW is a 35-year-old, 150-kg, 165-cm (65-in) woman with an enterococcal endocarditis. Her serum creatinine is 1.1 mg/dL and stable. Vancomycin 1400 mg every 12 hours was prescribed and expected to achieve steady-state peak and trough concentrations of 30 μg/mL and 7 μg/mL, respectively. After the fifth dose, steady-state peak and trough concentrations were measured and were 19 μg/mL and 4 μg/mL, respectively. Calculate a new vancomycin dose that will provide a steady-state trough of 7 μg/mL.

1. *Estimate the creatinine clearance.*

This patient has a stable serum creatinine and is obese ($IBW_{females}$ (in kg) = 45 + 2.3(Ht − 60 in) = 45 + 2.3(65 − 60) = 57 kg). The Salazar-Corcoran equation can be used to estimate creatinine clearance:

$$CrCl_{est(females)} = \frac{(146 - \text{age})[(0.287 \cdot Wt) + (9.74 \cdot Ht^2)]}{(60 \cdot S_{Cr})}$$

$$CrCl_{est(females)} = \frac{(146 - 35 \text{ y})\{(0.287 \cdot 150 \text{ kg}) + [9.74 \cdot (1.65 \text{ m})^2]\}}{(60 \cdot 1.1 \text{ mg/dL})} = 117 \text{ mL/min}$$

Note: Height is converted from inches to meters: Ht = (65 in · 2.54 cm/in)/(100 cm/m) = 1.65 m.

2. *Estimate the elimination rate constant (k_e) and half-life ($t_{1/2}$).*

The vancomycin clearance versus creatinine clearance relationship is used to estimate drug clearance for this patient:

$$Cl = 0.695(CrCl) + 0.05 = 0.695[(117\ mL/min)/150\ kg] + 0.05 = 0.592\ mL/min/kg$$

The average volume of distribution for vancomycin is 0.7 L/kg IBW:

$$V = 0.7\ L/kg \cdot 57\ kg = 40\ L$$

$$k_e = Cl/V = (0.592\ mL/min/kg \cdot 150\ kg \cdot 60\ min/h)/(0.7\ L/kg \cdot 57\ kg \cdot 1000\ mL/L) = 0.134\ h^{-1}$$

$$t_{1/2} = 0.693/k_e = 0.693/0.134\ h^{-1} = 5.2\ h$$

Because the patient has been receiving vancomycin for more than 3 to 5 estimated half-lives, it is likely that the measured serum concentrations are steady-state values.

3. *Compute the new dose to achieve desired serum concentration.*

With the use of linear pharmacokinetics, the new dose to attain the desired concentration should be proportional to the old dose that produced the measured concentration:

$$D_{new} = (C_{ss,new}/C_{ss,old})D_{old} = [(7\ \mu g/mL)/(4\ \mu g/mL)]\ 1400\ mg = 2450\ mg, \text{ rounded to } 2500\ mg$$

The new suggested dose is 2500 mg every 12 hours to be started at the next scheduled dosing time.

4. *Check the steady-state peak concentration for the new dosage regimen.*

By using linear pharmacokinetics, the new steady-state concentration can be estimated and should be proportional to the old dose that produced the measured concentration:

$$C_{ss,new} = (D_{new}/D_{old})C_{ss,old} = (2500\ mg/1400\ mg)\ 19\ \mu g/mL = 34\ \mu g/mL$$

This steady-state peak concentration should be safe and effective for the infection that is being treated.

Pharmacokinetic Concepts Method

As implied by the name, the pharmacokinetic concepts method derives alternate doses by estimating actual pharmacokinetic parameters or surrogates for pharmacokinetic parameters.[43] It is a very useful way to calculate drug doses when the linear pharmacokinetic method is not sufficient because a dosage change that will produce a proportional change in steady-state peak and trough concentrations is not appropriate. The only requirement is a steady-state peak and trough vancomycin serum concentration pair obtained before and after a dose (see Figure 5-3). The following steps are used to compute new vancomycin doses:

1. *Draw a rough sketch of the serum log concentration–time curve by hand, keeping track of the relative time between the serum concentrations (see Figure 5-3).*

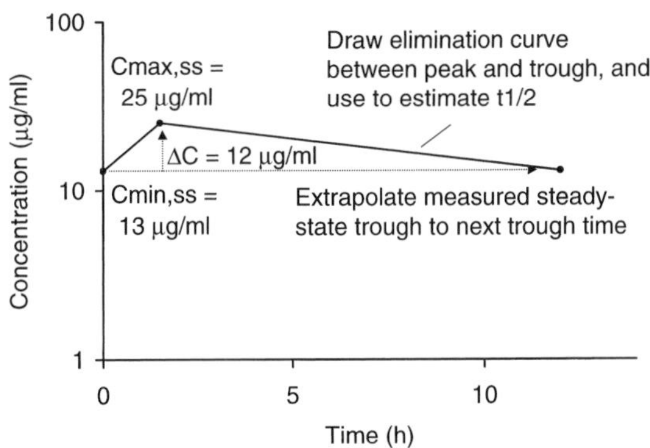

FIGURE 5-3 Graphic representation of the pharmacokinetic concepts method in which a steady-state peak ($C_{max,ss}$) and trough ($C_{min,ss}$) concentration pair is used to individualize vancomycin therapy. Because the patient is at steady state, consecutive trough concentrations are identical, so the trough concentration can be extrapolated to the next predose time. The change in concentration after a dose is given (ΔC) is a surrogate measure of the volume of distribution and is used to compute the new dose for the patient.

2. *Since the patient is at steady state, the trough concentration can be extrapolated to the next trough value time (see Figure 5-3).*

3. *Draw the elimination curve between the steady-state peak concentration and the extrapolated trough concentration. Use this line to estimate half-life.* For example, a patient receives a vancomycin 1000 mg every 12 hours, which produces a steady-state peak of 25 μg/mL and a steady-state trough of 13 μg/mL. The dose is infused over 1 hour, and the peak concentration is drawn 30 minutes later (see Figure 5-3). The time between the measured steady-state peak and the extrapolated trough concentration is 10.5 hours (the 12-hour dosage interval minus the 1.5-hour combined infusion and waiting time). The definition of half-life is the time needed for serum concentrations to decrease by half. Because the serum concentration declined by approximately half from the peak concentration to the trough concentration, the vancomycin half-life for this patient is approximately 10.5 hours. This information is used to set the new dosage interval for the patient.

4. *Determine the difference in concentration between the steady-state peak and trough concentrations. The difference in concentration changes proportionally with the dose size.* In this example, the patient is receiving a vancomycin dose of 1000 mg every 12 hours, which produced steady-state peak and trough concentrations of 25 μg/mL and 13 μg/mL, respectively. The difference between the peak and trough values is 12 μg/mL. The change in serum concentration is proportional to the dose, and this information is used to set a new dose for the patient.

5. *Choose new steady-state peak and trough concentrations.* For this example, the desired steady-state peak and trough concentrations are approximately 30 μg/mL and 7 μg/mL, respectively.

6. *Determine the new dosage interval for the desired concentrations.* This patient has a desired peak concentration of 30 μg/mL. In 1 half-life, the serum concentration will decline to 15 μg/mL, and in an additional half-life the vancomycin concentration will decrease to 7.5 μg/mL (see Figure 5-4). Since the approximate half-life is 10.5 hours and 2 half-lives are required for serum concentrations to decrease from the desired peak concentration to the desired trough concentration, the dosage interval should be 21 hours (10.5 hours × 2 half-lives). This value is rounded to the clinically acceptable value of 24 hours, and the actual trough concentration is expected to be slightly lower than 7.5 μg/mL.

7. *Determine the new dose for the desired concentrations.* The desired peak concentration is 30 μg/mL, and the expected trough concentration is 7.5 μg/mL. The change in concentration between these values is 22.5 μg/mL. It is known from measured serum concentrations that administration of 1000 mg changes serum concentrations by 13 μg/mL and that the change in serum concentration between the peak and trough values is proportional to the size of the dose. Therefore, a simple ratio is used to compute the required dose: $D_{new} = (\Delta C_{new}/\Delta C_{old})D_{old}$, where D_{new} and D_{old} are the new and old doses, respectively; ΔC_{new} is the change in concentration between the peak and trough for the new dose; and ΔC_{old} is the change in concentration between the peak and trough for the old dose. (Note: This relationship is appropriate because doses are given into a fixed, constant volume of distribution; it is not because the drug follows linear pharmacokinetics. Therefore, this method works whether the agent follows nonlinear or linear pharmacokinetics.) For this example: D_{new} = [(22.5 μg/mL)/(13 μg/mL)] 1000 mg = 1731 mg, which is rounded to 1750 mg. Vancomycin 1750 mg every 24 hours is started 24 hours after the last dose of the previous dosage regimen.

Once the pharmacokinetic concepts method is mastered, it can be used without the need for a calculator. Following are examples that use this to change vancomycin doses.

Example 1 JM is a 50-year-old, 70-kg, 178-cm (70-in) man with a methicillin-resistant *S. aureus* wound infection. His serum creatinine is 3.5 mg/dL, which has been stable over the last 5 days since admission. Vancomycin 800 mg every 24 hours was pre-

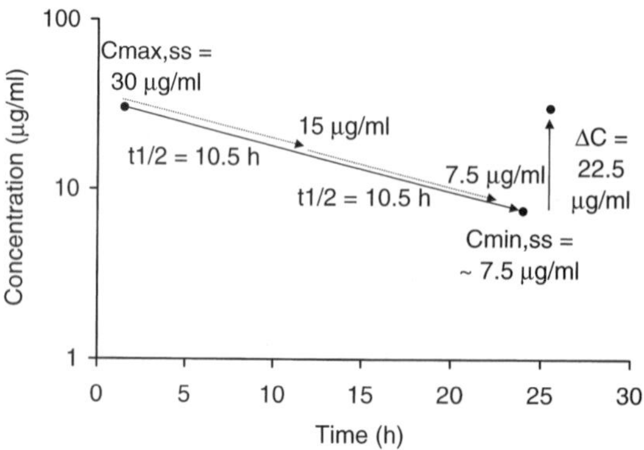

FIGURE 5-4 The pharmacokinetic concepts method uses the estimated half-life to graphically compute the new dosage interval and the change in concentration to calculate the dose.

scribed and expected to achieve steady-state peak and trough concentrations of 20 μg/mL and 5 μg/mL, respectively. After the fourth dose, steady-state peak and trough concentrations were measured and were 25 μg/mL and 12 μg/mL, respectively. Calculate a new vancomycin dose that will provide a steady-state peak of 20 μg/mL and a trough of 5 μg/mL.

1. *Estimate the creatinine clearance.*

This patient has a stable serum creatinine and is not obese. The Cockcroft–Gault equation can be used to estimate creatinine clearance:

$$CrCl_{est} = [(140 - age)BW]/(72 \cdot S_{Cr}) = [(140 - 50\ y)70\ kg]/(72 \cdot 3.5\ mg/dL)$$

$$CrCl_{est} = 25\ mL/min$$

2. *Estimate the elimination rate constant (k_e) and half-life ($t_{1/2}$).*

The vancomycin clearance versus creatinine clearance relationship is used to estimate drug clearance for this patient:

$$Cl = 0.695(CrCl) + 0.05 = 0.695[(25\ mL/min)/70\ kg] + 0.05 = 0.298\ mL/min/kg$$

The average volume of distribution for vancomycin is 0.7 L/kg:

$$V = 0.7\ L/kg \cdot 70\ kg = 49\ L$$

$$k_e = Cl/V = (0.298\ mL/min/kg \cdot 60\ min/h)/(0.7\ L/kg \cdot 1000\ mL/L) = 0.0255\ h^{-1}$$

$$t_{1/2} = 0.693/k_e = 0.693/0.0255\ h^{-1} = 27\ h$$

Because the patient has been receiving vancomycin for ~3 estimated half-lives, the measured serum concentrations are likely to be close to steady-state values. This steady-state concentration pair can be used to compute the patient's unique pharmacokinetic parameters, which in turn can be used to calculate individualized doses.

Pharmacokinetic Concepts Method

1. *Draw a rough sketch of the serum log concentration–time curve by hand, keeping track of the relative time between the serum concentrations (Figure 5-5).*

2. *Since the patient is at steady state, the trough concentration can be extrapolated to the next trough value time (see Figure 5-5).*

3. *Draw the elimination curve between the steady-state peak concentration and the extrapolated trough concentration. Use this line to estimate half-life.* The patient is receiving vancomycin 800 mg every 24 hours, which produced a steady-state peak of 25 μg/mL and a steady-state trough of 12 μg/mL. The dose is infused over 1 hour and the peak concentration is drawn 30 minutes later (see Figure 5-5). The time between the measured steady-state peak and the extrapolated trough concentration is 22.5 hours (the 24-hour dosage interval minus the 1.5-hour combined infusion and waiting time). The definition of half-life is the time needed for serum concentrations to decrease by half. It takes 1 half-life for the peak serum concentration to decline from 25 μg/mL to 12.5 μg/mL. The concentration of 12 μg/mL is very close to the extrapolated trough value of 12.5 μg/mL. Therefore, 1 half-life expired during the 22.5-hour time period between the peak concentration and extrapolated trough concentration, and the estimated half-life is 22.5 hours. This information is used to set the new dosage interval for the patient.

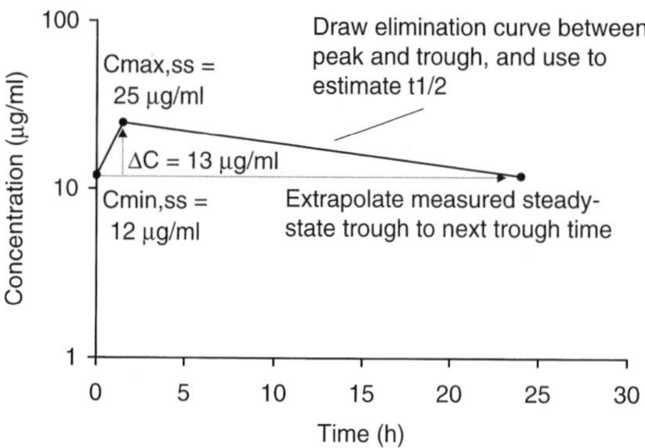

FIGURE 5-5 Graphic representation of the pharmacokinetic concepts method in which a steady-state peak ($C_{max,ss}$) and trough ($C_{min,ss}$) concentration pair is used to individualize vancomycin therapy. Because the patient is at steady state, consecutive trough concentrations are identical, so the trough concentration can be extrapolated to the next predose time. The change in concentration after a dose is given (ΔC) is a surrogate measure of the volume of distribution and is used to compute the new dose for the patient.

4. *Determine the difference in concentration between the steady-state peak and trough concentrations. The difference in concentration changes proportionally with the dose size.* In this example, the patient is receiving a vancomycin dose of 800 mg every 24 hours, which produced steady-state peak and trough concentrations of 25 μg/mL and 12 μg/mL, respectively. The difference between the peak and trough values is 13 μg/mL. The change in serum concentration is proportional to the dose, and this information is used to set a new dose for the patient.

5. *Choose the new steady-state peak and trough concentrations.* For this example, the desired steady-state peak and trough concentrations are 20 μg/mL and 5 μg/mL, respectively.

6. *Determine the new dosage interval for the desired concentrations (Figure 5-6).* With the desired concentrations, it will take 1 half-life for the peak concentration of 20 μg/mL to decrease to 10 μg/mL, and an additional half-life for serum concentrations to decline from 10 μg/mL to 5 μg/mL. Therefore, the dosage interval needs to be approximately 2 half-lives or 43 hours (22.5 hours × 2 half-lives = 45 hours). This dosage interval is rounded to 48 hours.

7. *Determine the new dose for the desired concentrations (see Figure 5-6).* The desired peak concentration is 20 μg/mL, and the expected trough concentration is 5 μg/mL. The change in concentration between these values is 15 μg/mL. It is known from measured serum concentrations that administration of 800 mg changes serum concentrations by 13 μg/mL and that the change in serum concentration between the peak and trough values is proportional to the size of the dose. In this case, $D_{new} = (\Delta C_{new}/\Delta C_{old})D_{old}$ = [(15 μg/mL)/(13 μg/mL)] 800 mg = 923 mg, rounded to 1000 mg. Vancomycin 1000 mg every 48 hours is started 48 hours after the last dose of the previous dosage regimen.

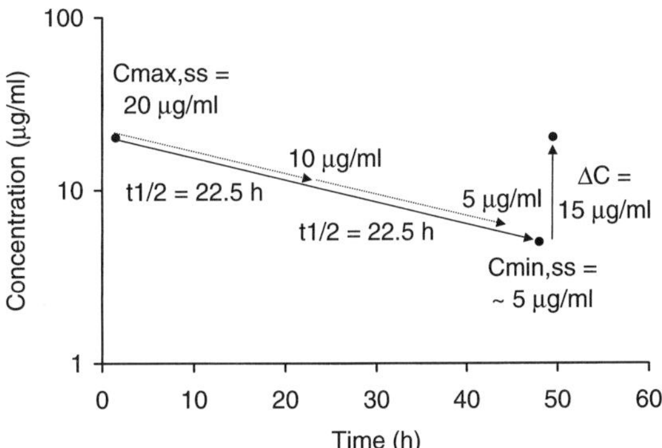

FIGURE 5-6 The pharmacokinetic concepts method uses the estimated half-life to graphically compute the new dosage interval and the change in concentration to calculate the dose for a patient.

Example 2 ZW is a 35-year-old, 150-kg, 165-cm (65-in) woman with a *S. epidermidis* infection of a prosthetic knee joint. Her serum creatinine is 1.1 mg/dL and stable. Vancomycin 2500 mg every 18 hours was prescribed and expected to achieve steady-state peak and trough concentrations of 30 µg/mL and 10 µg/mL, respectively. After the fifth dose, steady-state peak and trough concentrations were measured and were 40 µg/mL and 3 µg/mL, respectively. Calculate a new vancomycin dose that will provide a steady-state peak of 30 µg/mL and a steady-state trough 10 µg/mL.

1. *Estimate the creatinine clearance.*

This patient has a stable serum creatinine and is obese ($IBW_{females}$ (in kg) = 45 + 2.3(Ht − 60 in) = 45 + 2.3(65 − 60) = 57 kg. The Salazar-Corcoran equation can be used to estimate creatinine clearance:

$$CrCl_{est(females)} = \frac{(146 - age)[(0.287 \cdot Wt) + (9.74 \cdot Ht^2)]}{(60 \cdot S_{Cr})}$$

$$CrCl_{est(females)} = \frac{(146 - 35\ y)\{(0.287 \cdot 150\ kg) + [9.74 \cdot (1.65\ m)^2]\}}{(60 \cdot 1.1\ mg/dL)} = 117\ mL/min$$

Note: Height is converted from inches to meters: Ht = (65 in · 2.54 cm/in)/(100 cm/m) = 1.65 m.

2. *Estimate the elimination rate constant (k_e) and half-life ($t_{1/2}$).*

The vancomycin clearance versus creatinine clearance relationship is used to estimate drug clearance for this patient:

$$Cl = 0.695(CrCl) + 0.05 = 0.695[(117\ mL/min)/150\ kg] + 0.05 = 0.592\ mL/min/kg\ TBW$$

The average volume of distribution for vancomycin is 0.7 L/kg IBW:

$$V = 0.7\ L/kg \cdot 57\ kg = 40\ L$$

$$k_e = Cl/V = (0.592\ mL/min/kg\ TBW \cdot 150\ kg \cdot 60\ min/h)/(0.7\ L/kg\ IBW \cdot 57\ kg \cdot 1000\ mL/L) = 0.134\ h^{-1}$$

$$t_{1/2} = 0.693/k_e = 0.693/0.134\ h^{-1} = 5.2\ h$$

Because the patient has been receiving vancomycin for >5 estimated half-lives, it is likely that the measured serum concentrations are steady-state values.

Pharmacokinetics Concepts Method

1. *Draw a rough sketch of the serum log concentration–time curve by hand, keeping track of the relative time between the serum concentrations (Figure 5-7).*

2. *Since the patient is at steady state, the trough concentration can be extrapolated to the next trough value time (see Figure 5-7).*

3. *Draw the elimination curve between the steady-state peak concentration and the extrapolated trough concentration. Use this line to estimate half-life.* The patient is receiving vancomycin 2500 mg every 18 hours, which produces a steady-state peak of 40 μg/mL and a steady-state trough of 3 μg/mL. The dose is infused over 1 hour, and the peak concentration is drawn 30 minutes later (see Figure 5-7). The time between the measured steady-state peak and the extrapolated trough concentration is 16.5 hours (the 18-hour dosage interval minus the 1.5-hour combined infusion and waiting time). The definition of half-life is the time needed for serum concentrations to decrease by half. It takes 1 half-life for the peak serum concentration to decline from 40 μg/mL to 20 μg/mL, another half-life to decrease from 20 μg/mL to 10 μg/mL, an additional half-life to decrease from 10 μg/mL to 5 μg/mL, and a final half-life to decrease from 5 μg/mL to 2.5 μg/mL. The concentration of 3 μg/mL is very close to the extrapolated trough value of 2.5 μg/mL. Therefore, 4 half-lives expired during the 16.5-hour time period between peak concentration and extrapolated trough concentration, and the estimated half-life is 4.1 hours (16.5 hours/4 half-lives = 4.1 h). This information is used to set the new dosage interval for the patient.

4. *Determine the difference in concentration between the steady-state peak and trough concentrations. The difference in concentration changes proportionally with the dose size.*

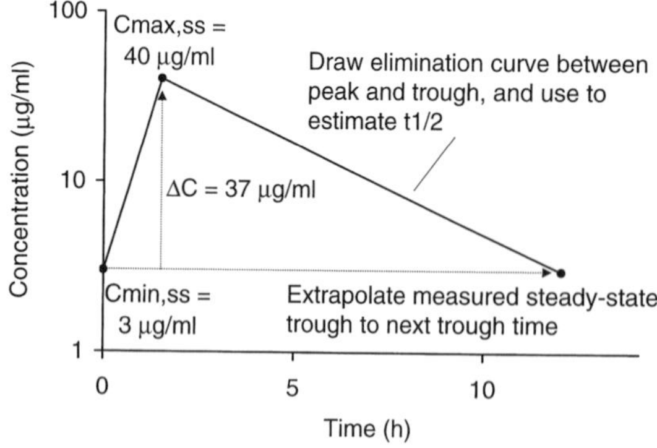

FIGURE 5-7 Graphic representation of the pharmacokinetic concepts method in which a steady-state peak ($C_{max,ss}$) and trough ($C_{min,ss}$) concentration pair is used to individualize vancomycin therapy. Because the patient is at steady state, consecutive trough concentrations are identical, so the trough concentration can be extrapolated to the next predose time. The change in concentration after a dose is given (ΔC) is a surrogate measure of the volume of distribution and is used to compute the new dose for the patient.

In this example, the patient is receiving a vancomycin dose of 2500 mg every 18 hours, which produced steady-state peak and trough concentrations of 40 μg/mL and 3 μg/mL, respectively. The difference between the peak and trough values is 37 μg/mL. The change in serum concentration is proportional to the dose, and this information is used to set a new dose for the patient.

5. *Choose new steady-state peak and trough concentrations.* For this example, the desired steady-state peak and trough concentrations are 30 μg/mL and 10 μg/mL, respectively.

6. *Determine the new dosage interval for the desired concentrations (Figure 5-8).* Using the desired concentrations, it will take 1 half-life for the peak concentration of 30 μg/mL to decrease to 15 μg/mL, and an additional half-life for serum concentrations to decline from 15 μg/mL to 8 μg/mL. This concentration is close to the desired trough concentration of 10 μg/mL. Therefore, the dosage interval needs to be approximately 2 half-lives or 8.2 hours (4.1 hours × 2 half-lives = 4.1 hours). This dosage interval is rounded to 8 hours.

7. *Determine the new dose for the desired concentrations (see Figure 5-8).* The desired peak concentration is 30 μg/mL, and the expected trough concentration is 8 μg/mL. The change in concentration between these values is 22 μg/mL. It is known from measured serum concentrations that administration of 2500 mg vancomycin changes serum concentrations by 37 μg/mL and that the change in serum concentration between the peak and trough values is proportional to the size of the dose. In this case, $D_{new} = (\Delta C_{new}/\Delta C_{old})D_{old}$ = [(22 μg/mL)/(37 μg/mL)] 2500 mg = 1486 mg, rounded to 1500 mg. Vancomycin 1500 mg every 8 hours is started 8 hours after the last dose of the previous dosage regimen.

One-Compartment Model Parameter Method

The one-compartment model parameter method of adjusting drug doses was among the first techniques available to change doses using serum concentrations.[44] It allows the computation of an individual's unique pharmacokinetic constants and uses them to calculate a dose that achieves desired vancomycin concentrations. The standard one-compart-

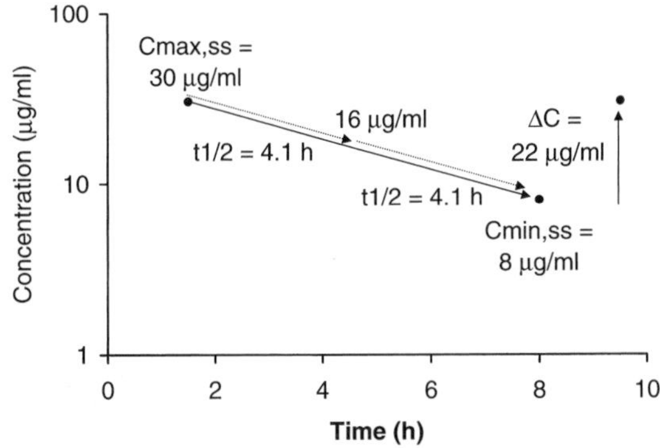

FIGURE 5-8 The pharmacokinetic concepts method uses the estimated half-life to graphically compute the new dosage interval and the change in concentration to calculate the dose for a patient.

ment model parameter method conducts a small pharmacokinetic experiment using three to four vancomycin serum concentrations obtained during a dosage interval and does not require steady-state conditions. The steady-state one-compartment model parameter method assumes that steady state has been achieved and requires only a steady-state peak and trough concentration pair obtained before and after a dose. One-compartment model intravenous bolus equations are used successfully to dose drugs that are given by infusion when the infusion time is less than the drug half-life.[39]

STANDARD ONE-COMPARTMENT MODEL

The standard version of the one-compartment model parameter method does not require steady-state concentrations. A trough vancomycin concentration is obtained before a dose, a peak vancomycin concentration is obtained after the dose is infused (1/2 to 1 hour after a 1-hour infusion), and one to two additional postdose serum vancomycin concentrations are obtained (Figure 5-9). Ideally, one to two postdose concentrations should be obtained at least 1 estimated half-life from each other to minimize the influence of assay error. The postdose serum concentrations are used to calculate the vancomycin elimination rate constant and half-life (see Figure 5-9). The half-life can be computed by graphing the postdose concentrations on semilogarithmic paper, drawing the best straight line through the data points, and determining the time needed for serum concentrations to decline by half. After the half-life is known, the elimination rate constant (k_e) can be computed: $k_e = 0.693/t_{1/2}$. Alternatively, the elimination rate constant can be directly calculated using the postdose serum concentrations ($k_e = [\ln C_1 - \ln C_2]/\Delta t$, where C_1 and C_2 are postdose serum concentrations and Δt is the time that expired between the times that C_1 and C_2 were obtained), and the half-life can be computed using the elimination rate constant ($t_{1/2} = 0.693/k_e$). The volume of distribution (V) is calculated using the following

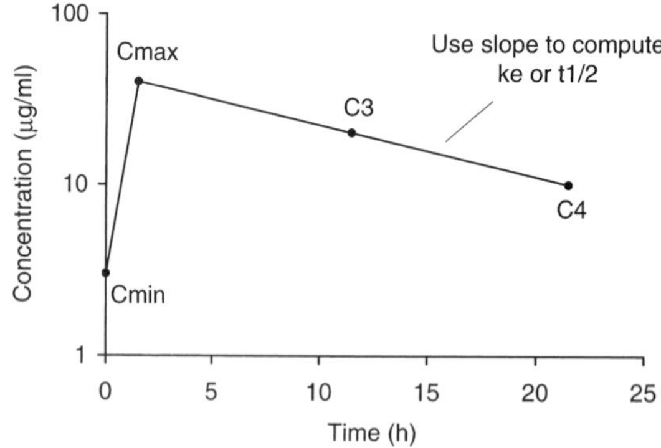

FIGURE 5-9 The one-compartment model parameter method for individualization of vancomycin doses uses a trough (C_{min}), peak (C_{max}), and one to two additional postdose concentrations (C_3, C_4) to compute a patient's unique pharmacokinetic parameters. This version of the one-compartment model parameter method does not require steady-state conditions. The peak and trough concentrations are used to calculate the volume of distribution, and the postdose concentrations (C_{max}, C_3, C_4) are used to compute half-life. After the volume of distribution and half-life have been measured, they can be used to compute the exact dose needed to achieve desired vancomycin concentrations.

equation: $V = D/(C_{max} - C_{min})$, where D is the vancomycin dose, C_{max} is the peak concentration and C_{min} is the trough concentration. The elimination rate constant and volume of distribution measured in this fashion are the patient's unique vancomycin pharmacokinetic constants and can be used in one-compartment model intravenous bolus equations to compute the required dose to achieve any desired serum concentration.

STEADY-STATE ONE-COMPARTMENT MODEL

If a steady-state peak and trough vancomycin concentration pair is available for a patient, the one-compartment model parameter method can be used to compute patient pharmacokinetic parameters and vancomycin doses (Figure 5-10). Because the patient is at steady state, the measured trough concentration obtained before the dose was given can be extrapolated to the next dosage time and used to compute the vancomycin elimination rate constant ($k_e = [\ln C_{max,ss} - \ln C_{min,ss}]/\tau - t'$, where $C_{max,ss}$ and $C_{min,ss}$ are the steady-state peak and trough serum concentrations and t′ and τ are the infusion time and dosage interval), and the half-life can be computed using the elimination rate constant ($t_{1/2} = 0.693/k_e$). The volume of distribution (V) is calculated using the following equation: $V = D/(C_{max,ss} - C_{min,ss})$, where D is the vancomycin dose, $C_{max,ss}$ is the steady-state peak concentration, and $C_{min,ss}$ is the steady-state trough concentration. The elimination rate constant and volume of distribution measured in this way are the patient's unique vancomycin pharmacokinetic constants and can be used in one-compartment model intravenous bolus equations to compute the required dose to achieve any desired serum concentration. The dosage calculations are similar to those done in the initial dosage section of this chapter, except that the patient's real pharmacokinetic parameters are used in the equations rather than population pharmacokinetic estimates.

To illustrate the similarities and differences between the pharmacokinetic concepts and the one-compartment model parameter methods, some of the same cases used in the previous section are used as examples here.

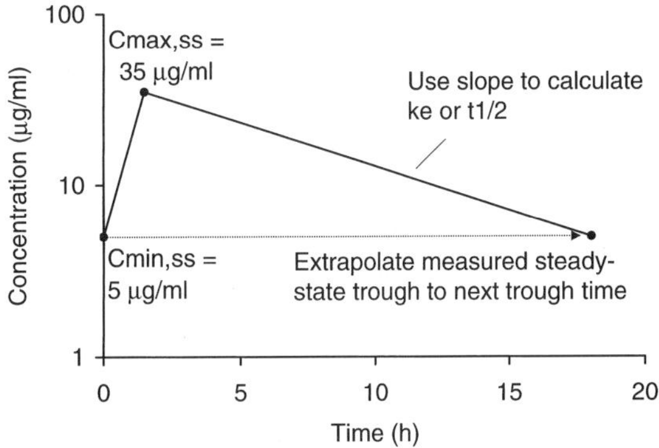

FIGURE 5-10 The steady-state version of the one-compartment model parameter method uses a steady-state peak ($C_{max,ss}$) and trough ($C_{min,ss}$) concentration pair to individualize vancomycin therapy. Because the patient is at steady state, consecutive trough concentrations are identical, so the trough concentration can be extrapolated to the next predose time. The steady-state peak and trough concentrations are used to calculate the volume of distribution and half-life. After the volume of distribution and half-life have been measured, they can be used to compute the exact dose needed to achieve desired vancomycin concentrations.

Example 1 JM is a 50-year-old, 70-kg, 178-cm (70-in) man with a methicillin-resistant *S. aureus* wound infection. His serum creatinine is 3.5 mg/dL, which has been stable over the last 5 days since admission. Vancomycin 800 mg every 24 hours was prescribed and expected to achieve steady-state peak and trough concentrations of 20 μg/mL and 5 μg/mL, respectively. After the fourth dose, steady-state peak and trough concentrations were measured and were 25 μg/mL and 12 μg/mL, respectively. Calculate a new vancomycin dose that will provide a steady-state peak of 20 μg/mL and a trough of 5 μg/mL.

1. *Estimate the creatinine clearance.*

This patient has a stable serum creatinine and is not obese. The Cockcroft–Gault equation can be used to estimate creatinine clearance:

$$CrCl_{est} = [(140 - age)BW]/(72 \cdot S_{Cr}) = [(140 - 50\ y)70\ kg]/(72 \cdot 3.5\ mg/dL)$$

$$CrCl_{est} = 25\ mL/min$$

2. *Estimate the elimination rate constant (k_e) and half-life ($t_{1/2}$).*

The vancomycin clearance versus creatinine clearance relationship is used to estimate drug clearance for this patient:

$$Cl = 0.695(CrCl) + 0.05 = 0.695[(25\ mL/min)/70\ kg] + 0.05 = 0.298\ mL/min/kg$$

The average volume of distribution for vancomycin is 0.7 L/kg:

$$V = 0.7\ L/kg \cdot 70\ kg = 49\ L$$

$$k_e = Cl/V = (0.298\ mL/min/kg \cdot 60\ min/h)/(0.7\ L/kg \cdot 1000\ mL/L) = 0.0255\ h^{-1}$$

$$t_{1/2} = 0.693/k_e = 0.693/0.0255\ h^{-1} = 27\ h$$

Because the patient has been receiving vancomycin for ~3 estimated half-lives, it is likely that the measured serum concentrations are close to steady-state values. This steady-state concentration pair can be used to compute the patient's unique pharmacokinetic parameters, which in turn can be used to calculate individualized doses.

One-Compartment Model Parameter Method

1. *Compute the patient's elimination rate constant and half-life (note: t′ = infusion time + waiting time of 1 hour and 1/2 hour, respectively).*

$$k_e = (\ln C_{max,ss} - \ln C_{min,ss})/\tau - t' = (\ln 25\ \mu g/mL - \ln 12\ \mu g/mL)/(24\ h - 1.5\ h) = 0.0326\ h^{-1}$$

$$t_{1/2} = 0.693/k_e = 0.693/0.0326\ h^{-1} = 21.2\ h$$

2. *Compute the patient's volume of distribution.*

$$V = D/(C_{max,ss} - C_{min,ss}) = 800\ mg/(25\ mg/L - 12\ mg/L) = 61.5\ L$$

3. *Choose new steady-state peak and trough concentrations.* For this example, the desired steady-state peak and trough concentrations are 20 μg/mL and 5 μg/mL, respectively.

4. *Determine the new dosage interval for the desired concentrations.* As in the initial dosage section of this chapter, the dosage interval (τ) is computed using the following equation:

$\tau = (\ln C_{max,ss} - \ln C_{min,ss})/k_e = (\ln 20\ \mu g/mL - \ln 5\ \mu g/mL)/0.0326\ h^{-1}$
$= 42$ h, rounded to 48 h

5. *Determine the new dose for the desired concentrations.* The dose is computed following the one-compartment model intravenous bolus equation used in the initial dosing section of this chapter:

$D = C_{max,ss}\ V\ (1 - e^{-k_e\tau}) = 20\ mg/L \cdot 61.5\ L\ (1 - e^{-(0.0326\ h^{-1})(48\ h)})$
$= 973$ mg, rounded to 1000 mg

Vancomycin 1000 mg every 48 hours is prescribed to begin 48 hours after the last dose of the previous regimen. This dosage is identical to that derived for the patient using the pharmacokinetic concepts method.

Example 2 ZW is a 35-year-old, 150-kg, 165-cm (65-in) woman with a *S. epidermidis* infection of a prosthetic knee joint. Her serum creatinine is 1.1 mg/dL and stable. A vancomycin dose of 2500 mg every 18 hours was prescribed and expected to achieve steady-state peak and trough concentrations of 30 μg/mL and 10 μg/mL, respectively. After the fifth dose, steady-state peak and trough concentrations were measured and were 40 μg/mL and 3 μg/mL, respectively. Calculate a new vancomycin dose that will provide a steady-state peak of 30 μg/mL and a steady-state trough of 10 μg/mL.

1. *Estimate the creatinine clearance.*

This patient has a stable serum creatinine and is obese ($IBW_{females}$ (in kg) = 45 + 2.3(Ht − 60 in) = 45 + 2.3(65 − 60) = 57 kg). The Salazar-Corcoran equation can be used to estimate creatinine clearance:

$$CrCl_{est(females)} = \frac{(146 - age)[(0.287 \cdot Wt) + (9.74 \cdot Ht^2)]}{(60 \cdot S_{Cr})}$$

$$CrCl_{est(females)} = \frac{(146 - 35\ y)\{(0.287 \cdot 150\ kg) + [9.74 \cdot (1.65\ m)^2]\}}{(60 \cdot 1.1\ mg/dL)} = 117\ mL/min$$

Note: Height is converted from inches to meters: Ht = (65 in · 2.54 cm/in)/(100 cm/m) = 1.65 m.

2. *Estimate the elimination rate constant (k_e) and half-life ($t_{1/2}$).*

The vancomycin clearance versus creatinine clearance relationship is used to estimate drug clearance for this patient:

$Cl = 0.695(CrCl) + 0.05 = 0.695[(117\ mL/min)/150\ kg] + 0.05 = 0.592\ mL/min/kg\ TBW$

The average volume of distribution for vancomycin is 0.7 L/kg IBW:

$V = 0.7\ L/kg \cdot 57\ kg = 40\ L$

$k_e = Cl/V = (0.592\ mL/min/kg\ TBW \cdot 150\ kg \cdot 60\ min/h)/$
$(0.7\ L/kg\ IBW \cdot 57\ kg \cdot 1000\ mL/L) = 0.134\ h^{-1}$

$t_{1/2} = 0.693/k_e = 0.693/0.134\ h^{-1} = 5.2\ h$

Because the patient has been receiving vancomycin for >5 estimated half-lives, it is likely that the measured serum concentrations are steady-state values.

One-Compartment Model Parameter Method

1. *Compute the patient's elimination rate constant and half-life (note: assumed infusion time and waiting time are 1 hour and 1/2 hour, respectively).*

$k_e = (\ln C_{max,ss} - \ln C_{min,ss})/\tau - t' = (\ln 40\ \mu g/mL - \ln 3\ \mu g/mL)/(18\ h - 1.5\ h) = 0.157\ h^{-1}$

$t_{1/2} = 0.693/k_e = 0.693/0.157\ h^{-1} = 4.4\ h$

2. *Compute the patient's volume of distribution.*

$$V = D/(C_{max,ss} - C_{min,ss}) = 2500\ mg/(40\ mg/L - 3\ mg/L) = 67.6\ L$$

3. *Choose new steady-state peak and trough concentrations.* For this example, the desired steady-state peak and trough concentrations are 30 μg/mL and 10 μg/mL, respectively.

4. *Determine the new dosage interval for the desired concentrations.* As in the initial dosage section of this chapter, the dosage interval (τ) is computed using the following equation:

$$\tau = (\ln C_{max,ss} - \ln C_{min,ss})/k_e = (\ln 30\ \mu g/mL - \ln 10\ \mu g/mL)/0.157\ h^{-1}$$
$$= 7\ h\text{, rounded to } 8\ h$$

5. *Determine the new dose for the desired concentrations.* The dose is computed following the one-compartment model intravenous bolus equation used in the initial dosing section of this chapter:

$$D = C_{max,ss}\ V(1 - e^{-k_e\tau}) = 30\ mg/L \cdot 67.6\ L\ (1 - e^{-(0.157\ h^{-1})(8\ h)})$$
$$= 1450\ mg\text{, rounded to } 1500\ mg$$

Vancomycin 1500 mg every 8 hours is prescribed to begin 8 hours after the last dose of the previous regimen. This dosage is identical to that derived for the patient using the pharmacokinetic concepts method.

Example 3 JH is a 24-year-old, 70-kg, 183-cm (72-in) man with methicillin-resistant *S. aureus* endocarditis. His serum creatinine is 1.0 mg/dL, which has been stable over the last 7 days since admission. Vancomycin 1000 mg every 12 hours was prescribed. After the third dose, the following vancomycin serum concentrations were obtained:

TIME	VANCOMYCIN CONCENTRATION (μg/mL)
0800 H	2.0
0800–0900 H	Vancomycin 1000 mg administered over 1 hour
1000 H	18.0
1500 H	10.1
2000 H	5.7

Medication administration sheets were checked, and the previous dose was given 2 hours early (1800 H the previous day). Because of this, it is known that the patient is not at steady state. Calculate a new vancomycin dose that will provide a steady-state peak of 30 μg/mL and a trough between 10 μg/mL.

One-Compartment Model Parameter Method

1. *Plot the serum concentration–time data (Figure 5-11). Because serum concentrations decrease in a straight line, use any two postdose concentrations to compute the patient's elimination rate constant and half-life.*

$$k_e = (\ln C_{max} - \ln C_{min})/\Delta t = (\ln 18\ \mu g/mL - \ln 5.7\ \mu g/mL)/(10\ h) = 0.115\ h^{-1}$$

$$t_{1/2} = 0.693/k_e = 0.693/0.115\ h^{-1} = 6\ h$$

2. *Compute the patient's volume of distribution.*

$$V = D/(C_{max} - C_{min}) = 1000\ mg/(18\ mg/L - 2.0\ mg/L) = 62.5\ L$$

3. *Choose new steady-state peak and trough concentrations.* For this example, the desired steady-state peak and trough concentrations are 30 μg/mL and 10 μg/mL, respectively.

4. *Determine the new dosage interval for the desired concentrations.* As in the initial dosage section of this chapter, the dosage interval (τ) is computed using the following equation:

$$\tau = (\ln C_{max,ss} - \ln C_{min,ss})/k_e = (\ln 30\ \mu g/mL - \ln 10\ \mu g/mL)/0.115\ h^{-1} = 10\ h, \text{ rounded to } 12\ h$$

5. *Determine the new dose for the desired concentrations.* The dose is computed following the one-compartment model intravenous bolus equation used in the initial dosing section of this chapter:

$$D = C_{max,ss} V(1 - e^{-k_e\tau}) = 30\ mg/L \cdot 62.5\ L\ (1 - e^{-(0.115\ h^{-1})(12\ h)}) = 1403\ mg, \text{ rounded to } 1500\ mg$$

Vancomycin 1500 mg every 12 hours is prescribed to begin 12 hours after the last dose of the previous regimen.

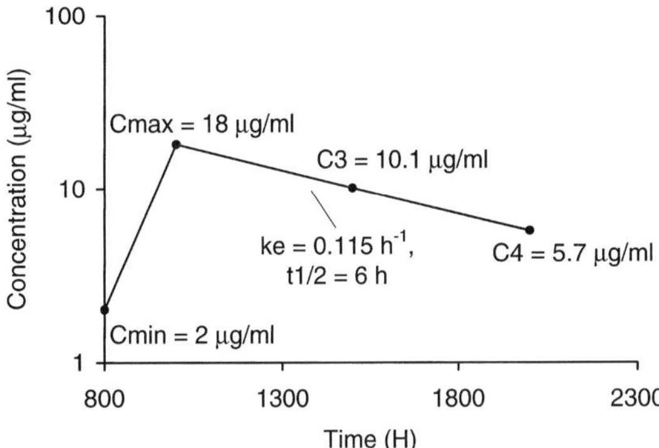

FIGURE 5-11 Graph of vancomycin serum concentrations used in one-compartment model parameter method example.

BAYESIAN PHARMACOKINETICS COMPUTER PROGRAMS

Computer programs are available that can assist in the computation of pharmacokinetic parameters for patients.[45–47] The most reliable computer programs use a nonlinear regression algorithm that incorporates components of Bayes' theorem. Nonlinear regression is a statistical technique that uses an iterative process to compute the best pharmacokinetic parameters for a concentration–time data set. Briefly, the patient's drug dosage schedule and serum concentrations are entered into the computer. The computer program has a pharmacokinetic equation preprogrammed for the drug and administration method (e.g., oral, intravenous bolus, intravenous infusion). Typically, a one-compartment model is used, although some programs allow the user to choose among several different equations. Using population estimates based on demographic information for the patient (e.g., age, weight, gender, renal function) supplied by the user, the computer program then computes estimated serum concentrations at each time there are actual serum concentrations. Kinetic parameters are then changed by the computer program, and a new set of estimated serum concentrations are computed.

The pharmacokinetic parameters that generated the estimated serum concentrations closest to the actual values are remembered by the computer program, and the process is repeated until the set of pharmacokinetic parameters that result in estimated serum concentrations that are statistically closest to the actual serum concentrations are generated. These pharmacokinetic parameters can then be used to compute improved dosing schedules for patients. Bayes' theorem is used in the computer algorithm to balance the results of the computations between values based solely on the patient's serum drug concentrations and those based only on patient population parameters. Results from studies that compare various methods of dosage adjustment have consistently found that these types of computer dosing programs perform at least as well as experienced clinical pharmacokineticists and clinicians and better than inexperienced clinicians.

Some clinicians use Bayesian pharmacokinetics computer programs exclusively to alter drug doses based on serum concentrations. An advantage of this approach is that consistent dosage recommendations are made when several different practitioners are involved in therapeutic drug monitoring programs. However, since simpler dosing methods work just as well for patients with stable pharmacokinetic parameters and steady-state drug concentrations, many clinicians reserve the use of computer programs for more difficult situations. Such situations include serum concentrations that are not at steady state, serum concentrations not obtained at the specific times needed to use simpler methods, and unstable pharmacokinetic parameters. Many Bayesian pharmacokinetics computer programs are available to users, and most provide answers similar to the ones used in the following examples. The program used to solve problems in this book is DrugCalc, written by Dr. Dennis Mungall and available on his Internet web site[48] (http://members. aol. com/thertch/index.htm).

Example 1 JM is a 50-year-old, 70-kg, 178-cm (70-in) man with a methicillin-resistant *S. aureus* wound infection. His serum creatinine is 3.5 mg/dL, which has been stable over the last 5 days since admission. Vancomycin 800 mg every 24 hours was prescribed and expected to achieve steady-state peak and trough concentrations of 20 μg/mL and 5 μg/mL, respectively. After the fourth dose, steady-state peak and trough concentrations were measured and were 25 μg/mL and 12 μg/mL, respectively. Calculate a new vancomycin dose that will provide a steady-state peak of 20 μg/mL and a trough of 5 μg/mL.

1. *Enter the patient's demographic, drug dosing, and serum concentration–time data into the computer program.*

2. *Compute the pharmacokinetic parameters for the patient using the Bayesian pharmacokinetics computer program.*

The pharmacokinetic parameters computed by the program are a volume of distribution of 57.4 L, a half-life of 24.2 hours, and an elimination rate constant of 0.0286 h^{-1}.

3. *Compute the dose required to achieve desired vancomycin serum concentrations.*

The one-compartment model intravenous infusion equations used by the program to compute doses indicate that a dose of 1000 mg every 48 hours will produce a steady-state peak concentration of 23 μg/mL and a steady-state trough concentration of 6 μg/mL. Use of the pharmacokinetic concepts method and the one-compartment model parameter method produced the same answer for this patient.

Example 2 ZW is a 35-year-old, 150-kg, 165-cm (65-in) woman with a *S. epidermidis* infection of a prosthetic knee joint. Her serum creatinine is 1.1 mg/dL and stable. Vancomycin 2500 mg every 18 hours was prescribed and expected to achieve steady-state peak and trough concentrations of 30 μg/mL and 10 μg/mL, respectively. After the fifth dose, steady-state peak and trough concentrations were measured and were 40 μg/mL and 3 μg/mL, respectively. Calculate a new vancomycin dose that will provide a steady-state peak of 30 μg/mL and a steady-state trough 10 μg/mL.

1. *Enter the patient's demographic, drug dosing, and serum concentration–time data into the computer program.*

2. *Compute the pharmacokinetic parameters for the patient using the Bayesian pharmacokinetics computer program.*

The pharmacokinetic parameters computed by the program are a volume of distribution of 55.9 L, a half-life of 4.4 hours, and an elimination rate constant of 0.158 h^{-1}.

3. *Compute the dose required to achieve desired vancomycin serum concentrations.*

The one-compartment model intravenous infusion equations used by the program to compute doses indicate that a dose of 1250 mg every 8 hours will produce a steady-state peak concentration of 28.8 μg/mL and a steady-state trough concentration of 9.6 μg/mL. Use of the pharmacokinetic concepts method and the one-compartment model parameter method produced a comparable answer for this patient (1500 mg every 8 hours).

Example 3 KU is an 80-year-old, 65-kg, 173-cm (68-in) man with *S. viridans* endocarditis who is allergic to penicillins and cephalosporins. His serum creatinine is 1.9 mg/dL, which has been stable. Vancomycin 1000 mg every 12 hours was prescribed with the expectation that it would produce steady-state peak and trough concentrations of 30 μg/mL and 10 μg/mL, respectively. After the third dose, a trough concentration was measured and was 17.5 μg/mL. Calculate a new vancomycin dose that will provide a steady-state peak of 30 μg/mL and a steady-state trough 10 μg/mL.

1. *Enter the patient's demographic, drug dosing, and serum concentration–time data into the computer program.* In this case, it is unlikely that the patient is at steady state, so the linear pharmacokinetics method cannot be used.

2. *Compute the pharmacokinetic parameters for the patient using the Bayesian pharmacokinetics computer program.*

The pharmacokinetic parameters computed by the program are a volume of distribution of 74.8 L, a half-life of 33.6 hours, and an elimination rate constant of 0.0206 h^{-1}.

3. *Compute the dose required to achieve desired vancomycin serum concentrations.*

The one-compartment model intravenous infusion equations used by the program to compute doses indicate that 1250 mg every 48 hours will produce a steady-state peak concentration of 26 μg/mL and a steady-state trough concentration of 10 μg/mL.

PROBLEMS

The following problems are intended to emphasize the computation of initial and individualized doses using clinical pharmacokinetic techniques. Clinicians should always consult the patient's chart to confirm that antibiotic therapy is appropriate for current microbiologic cultures and sensitivities. Also, it should be confirmed that the patient is receiving other appropriate concurrent antibiotic therapy, such as aminoglycoside antibiotics, when necessary to treat the infection.

1. KI is a 75-year-old, 62-kg, 175-cm (69-in) man with *S. epidermidis* sepsis. His serum creatinine is 1.3 mg/dL, which has been stable since admission. Compute a vancomycin dose for this patient to provide a steady-state peak concentration of 30 μg/mL and a steady-state trough concentration of 10 μg/mL.
2. Patient KI (see problem 1) was prescribed vancomycin 1000 mg every 36 hours. Steady-state vancomycin concentrations were obtained before and after the fourth dose. The peak concentration (obtained 30 minutes after a 1-hour infusion of vancomycin) was 34 μg/mL, and the trough concentration (obtained immediately before dosage administration) was 2.5 μg/mL. Compute a revised vancomycin dose for this patient to provide a steady-state peak concentration of 30 μg/mL and a steady-state trough concentration of 7 μg/mL.
3. HT is a 35-year-old, 75-kg, 170-cm (67-in) woman with a methicillin-resistant *S. aureus* wound infection and chronic renal failure. Her serum creatinine is 3.7 mg/dL, which has been stable since admission. Compute a vancomycin dose for this patient to provide a steady-state peak concentration of 25 μg/mL and a steady-state trough concentration of 5 μg/mL.
4. Patient HT (see problem 3) was prescribed vancomycin 1200 mg every 48 hours. Steady-state vancomycin concentrations were obtained before and after the fourth dose. The peak concentration (obtained 30 minutes after a 1-hour infusion of vancomycin) was 55 μg/mL, whereas the trough concentration (obtained within 30 min-

utes before dosage administration) was 18 μg/mL. Compute a revised vancomycin dose for this patient to provide a steady-state peak concentration of 25 μg/mL and a steady-state trough concentration of 5 μg/mL.

5. LK is a 55-year-old, 140-kg, 173-cm (68-in) man with a penicillin-resistant enterococcal endocarditis. His serum creatinine is 0.9 mg/dL, which has been stable since admission. Compute a vancomycin dose for this patient to provide a steady-state peak concentration of 40 μg/mL and a steady-state trough concentration of 10 μg/mL.

6. Patient LK (see problem 5) was prescribed vancomycin 1000 mg every 8 hours. Steady-state vancomycin concentrations were obtained before and after the fourth dose. The peak concentration (obtained 30 minutes after a 1-hour infusion of vancomycin) was 42 μg/mL, whereas the trough concentration (obtained within 30 minutes before dosage administration) was 18 μg/mL. Compute a revised vancomycin dose for this patient to provide a steady-state peak concentration of 40 μg/mL and a steady-state trough concentration of 10 μg/mL.

7. AF is a 45-year-old, 140-kg, 157-cm (62-in) woman with *S. viridans* endocarditis who is allergic to penicillins and cephalosporins. Her serum creatinine is 2.4 mg/dL and stable. Compute a vancomycin dose for this patient to provide a steady-state peak concentration of 25 μg/mL and a steady-state trough concentration of 7 μg/mL.

8. Patient AF (see problem 7) was prescribed 1300 mg every 24 hours. Steady-state vancomycin concentrations were obtained before and after the fourth dose. The peak concentration (obtained 30 minutes after a 1-hour infusion of vancomycin) was 30 μg/mL, whereas the trough concentration (obtained within 30 minutes before dosage administration) was 2.5 μg/mL. Compute a revised vancomycin dose for this patient to provide a steady-state peak concentration of 25 μg/mL and a steady-state trough concentration of 7 μg/mL.

9. DG is a 66-year-old, 65-kg, 165-cm (65-in) woman with methicillin-resistant *S. aureus* sternal osteomyelitis secondary to coronary artery bypass graft surgery. While in the hospital, she developed ascites as a result of hepatorenal syndrome, and her current weight is 72 kg. Her serum creatinine is 1.4 mg/dL and stable. Compute a vancomycin dose for this patient to provide a steady-state peak concentration of 30 μg/mL and a steady-state trough concentration of 7 μg/mL.

10. Patient DG (see problem 9) was prescribed 1200 mg every 36 hours. Steady-state vancomycin concentrations were obtained before and after the fifth dose. The peak concentration (obtained 30 minutes after a 1-hour infusion of vancomycin) was 17 μg/mL, whereas the trough concentration (obtained within 30 minutes before dosage administration) was 4 μg/mL. Compute a revised vancomycin dose for this patient to provide a steady-state peak concentration of 30 μg/mL and a steady-state trough concentration of 7 μg/mL.

11. GG is a 27-year-old, 85-kg, 188-cm (74-in) male trauma patient with a penicillin-resistant enterococcal pneumonia who is currently on a respirator. He sustained multiple injuries as a result of a motor vehicle accident 2 weeks earlier and lost a large amount of blood at the accident site. He developed acute renal failure owing to prolonged hypotension and poor kidney perfusion (postdialysis serum creatinine is 5.3 mg/dL). He is receiving hemodialysis on Mondays, Wednesdays, and Fridays from 0800 to 1200 H, using a low-flux dialysis filter. Recommend a vancomycin dosage regimen that will achieve peak concentrations of 40 μg/mL and trough concentrations of 10 μg/mL. The first dose of the regimen will be given immediately after hemodialysis is finished on Wednesday at 1200 H.

12. Patient GG (see problem 11) was prescribed vancomycin 1600 mg loading dose on Wednesday at 1200 H, and the following vancomycin serum concentrations were obtained:

Use these serum concentrations to compute the patient's own pharmacokinetic parameters for vancomycin and a new dosage schedule that will achieve peak concentrations of 40 μg/mL and trough concentrations of 10 μg/mL.

DATE/TIME	DESCRIPTION	CONCENTRATION (μg/mL)
Friday at 0800 H	Predialysis	20
Monday at 0800 H	Predialysis	12.1

13. FD is a 67-year-old, 60-kg, 157-cm (62-in) woman with a serum creatinine of 1.8 mg/dL who was placed on vancomycin for a postsurgical brain abscess. The prescribed dose was vancomycin 900 mg every 12 hours (infused over 1 hour), and two doses have been given at 0800 and 2000 H. A trough concentration of 20 μg/mL was obtained at 0730 H the next morning (30 minutes before the third dose). Compute the dose to give $C_{max,ss}$ = 40 μg/mL and $C_{min,ss}$ = 15 μg/mL.

14. OI is a 52-year-old, 87-kg, 188-cm (74-in) man with postoperative *S. epidermidis* septic arthritis. His serum creatinine is 1.4 mg/dL and stable. Nine hours after the second dose of vancomycin 1000 mg every 12 hours, a vancomycin serum concentration of 5 μg/mL is measured. Compute a revised vancomycin dose for this patient to provide steady-state peak concentrations of 30 μg/mL and steady-state trough concentrations of 7 μg/mL.

15. HY is a 45-year-old, 65-kg, 162-cm (64-in) female bone marrow transplant recipient who develops methicillin-resistant *S. aureus* sepsis. Her serum creatinine is 1.1 mg/dL. She is administered vancomycin 750 mg every 12 hours. A vancomycin serum concentration was obtained 5 hours after the first dose and was 15 μg/mL. Compute a revised vancomycin dose for this patient to provide steady-state peak concentrations of 35 μg/mL and steady-state trough concentrations of 10 μg/mL.

ANSWERS TO PROBLEMS

1. The initial vancomycin dose for patient KI is calculated as follows.

Pharmacokinetic Dosing Method

1. *Estimate the creatinine clearance.*

This patient has a stable serum creatinine and is not obese. The Cockcroft–Gault equation can be used to estimate creatinine clearance:

$$CrCl_{est} = [(140 - age)BW]/(72 \cdot S_{Cr}) = [(140 - 75\ y)62\ kg]/(72 \cdot 1.3\ mg/dL)$$

$$CrCl_{est} = 43\ mL/min$$

2. *Estimate the vancomycin clearance.*

The vancomycin clearance versus creatinine clearance relationship is used to estimate the vancomycin clearance for this patient:

$$Cl = 0.695(CrCl) + 0.05 = 0.695[(43\ mL/min)/62\ kg] + 0.05 = 0.533\ mL/min/kg$$

3. *Estimate the vancomycin volume of distribution.*

The average volume of distribution for vancomycin is 0.7 L/kg:

$$V = 0.7\ L/kg \cdot 62\ kg = 43.4\ L$$

4. *Estimate the vancomycin elimination rate constant (k_e) and half-life ($t_{1/2}$).*

$$k_e = Cl/V = (0.533\ mL/min/kg \cdot 60\ min/h)/(0.7\ L/kg \cdot 1000\ mL/L) = 0.0457\ h^{-1}$$

$$t_{1/2} = 0.693/k_e = 0.693/0.0457\ h^{-1} = 15.2\ h$$

5. *Choose desired steady-state serum concentrations.*

A $C_{min,ss}$ = 10 μg/mL and $C_{max,ss}$ = 30 μg/mL were chosen to treat this patient.

6. *Use the intravenous bolus equations to compute the dose (see Table 5-2).*

Calculate the required dosage interval (τ):

$$\tau = (\ln C_{max,ss} - \ln C_{min,ss})/k_e = (\ln 30\ \mu g/mL - \ln 10\ \mu g/mL)/0.0457\ h^{-1} = 24.1\ h$$

Dosage intervals should be rounded to clinically acceptable intervals of 12 hours, 18 hours, 24 hours, 36 hours, 48 hours, 72 hours, and multiples of 24 hours thereafter, whenever possible. In this case, the dosage interval is rounded to 24 hours.

Calculate the required dose (D):

$$D = C_{max,ss} V(1 - e^{-k_e\tau}) = 30\ mg/L \cdot 43.4\ L\ (1 - e^{-(0.0457\ h^{-1})(24\ h)}) = 867\ mg$$

Vancomycin doses should be rounded to the nearest 100 to 250 mg. This dose is rounded to 750 mg. (Note: μg/mL = mg/L, and this concentration unit was substituted for $C_{max,ss}$ to avoid unnecessary unit conversion.)

The prescribed maintenance dose is 750 mg every 24 hours.

7. *Compute the loading dose, if needed.*

Loading doses should be considered for patients with creatinine clearance values lower than 60 mL/min. The administration of a loading dose allows achievement of therapeutic concentrations more quickly than if maintenance doses alone are given. However, since the pharmacokinetic parameters used to compute these initial doses are *estimated* values and not *actual* values, the patient's own parameters may be much different from the estimated constants and steady-state will not be achieved until 3 to 5 half-lives have passed.

$$LD = C_{max,ss} V = 30 \text{ mg/L} \cdot 43.4 \text{ L} = 1302 \text{ mg}$$

As noted, this patient has poor renal function (CrCl <60 mL/min), so a loading dose is prescribed and given as the first dose. Vancomycin doses should be rounded to the nearest 100 to 250 mg. This dose is rounded to 1250 mg. (Note: μg/mL = mg/L, and this concentration unit was substituted for $C_{max,ss}$ to avoid unnecessary unit conversion.) The first maintenance dose is given one dosage interval (24 hours) after the loading dose is administered.

Moellering Nomogram Method

1. *Estimate the creatinine clearance.*

This patient has a stable serum creatinine and is not obese. The Cockcroft–Gault equation can be used to estimate creatinine clearance:

$$CrCl_{est} = [(140 - \text{age})BW]/(72 \cdot S_{Cr}) = [(140 - 75 \text{ y})62 \text{ kg}]/(72 \cdot 1.3 \text{ mg/dL})$$

$$CrCl_{est} = 43 \text{ mL/min}$$

2. *Determine the dosage interval and maintenance dosage.*

The maintenance dosage is calculated using the modified vancomycin dosing equation:

$$D \text{ (in mg/h/kg)} = 0.626(\text{CrCl in mL/min/kg}) + 0.05$$

$$D = 0.626[(43 \text{ mL/min})/62 \text{ kg}] + 0.05 = 0.484 \text{ mg/h/kg}$$

$$D = 0.484 \text{ mg/h/kg} \cdot 62 \text{ kg} = 30 \text{ mg/h}$$

The standard dose of vancomycin 1000 mg can be used to gain an approximation for an acceptable dosage interval (τ):

$$\tau = 1000 \text{ mg}/(30 \text{ mg/h}) = 33 \text{ h}$$

Dosage intervals should be rounded to clinically acceptable intervals of 12 hours, 18 hours, 24 hours, 36 hours, 48 hours, 72 hours, and multiples of 24 hours thereafter, whenever possible. In this case, the dosage interval is rounded to 36 hours.

$$D = 30 \text{ mg/h} \cdot 36 \text{ h} = 1080 \text{ mg}$$

Vancomycin doses should be rounded to the nearest 100 to 250 mg. This dose is rounded to 1000 mg. The prescribed maintenance dosage is 1000 mg every 36 hours.

3. *Compute the loading dose.*

A loading dose of 15 mg/kg is suggested by the Moellering nomogram:

$$LD = 15 \text{ mg/kg}(62 \text{ kg}) = 930 \text{ mg}$$

This loading dose is less than the suggested maintenance dose, so it is not prescribed.

Matzke Nomogram Method

1. *Estimate the creatinine clearance.*

This patient has a stable serum creatinine and is not obese. The Cockcroft–Gault equation can be used to estimate creatinine clearance:

$$CrCl_{est} = [(140 - age)BW]/(72 \cdot S_{Cr}) = [(140 - 75\ y)62\ kg]/(72 \cdot 1.3\ mg/dL)$$

$$CrCl_{est} = 43\ mL/min$$

2. *Compute the loading dose (see Table 5-4).*

A loading dose of 25 mg/kg provides a peak concentration of 30 μg/mL.

$$LD = 25\ mg/kg(62\ kg) = 1550\ mg,\ \text{rounded to}\ 1500\ mg$$

3. *Determine the dosage interval and maintenance dose.*

According to the nomogram, the dosage interval is 1.5 days or 36 hours. The maintenance dose is 19 mg/kg · 62 kg = 1178 mg. Vancomycin doses should be rounded to the nearest 100 to 250 mg. This dose is rounded to 1250 mg and given one dosage interval (36 hours) after the loading dose.

The prescribed maintenance dosage is 1250 mg every 36 hours.

2. The revised vancomycin dose for patient KI is calculated as follows.

Pharmacokinetic Concepts Method

1. *Estimate the creatinine clearance.*

This patient has a stable serum creatinine and is not obese. The Cockcroft–Gault equation can be used to estimate creatinine clearance:

$$CrCl_{est} = [(140 - age)BW]/(72 \cdot S_{Cr}) = [(140 - 75\ y)62\ kg]/(72 \cdot 1.3\ mg/dL)$$

$$CrCl_{est} = 43\ mL/min$$

2. *Estimate the elimination rate constant (k_e) and half-life ($t_{1/2}$).*

The vancomycin clearance versus creatinine clearance relationship is used to estimate drug clearance for this patient:

$$Cl = 0.695(CrCl) + 0.05 = 0.695[(43\ mL/min)/62\ kg] + 0.05 = 0.533\ mL/min/kg$$

The average volume of distribution for vancomycin is 0.7 L/kg:

$$V = 0.7\ L/kg \cdot 62\ kg = 43.4\ L$$

$$k_e = Cl/V = (0.533\ mL/min/kg \cdot 60\ min/h)/(0.7\ L/kg \cdot 1000\ mL/L) = 0.0457\ h^{-1}$$

$$t_{1/2} = 0.693/k_e = 0.693/0.0457\ h^{-1} = 15.2\ h$$

Because the patient has been receiving vancomycin for >3 to 5 estimated half-lives, it is likely that the measured serum concentrations are close to steady-state values. This steady-state concentration pair can be used to compute the patient's unique pharmacokinetic parameters, which in turn can be used to calculate individualized doses. Use the *pharmacokinetic concepts method* to compute a new dose.

1. *Draw a rough sketch of the serum log concentration–time curve by hand, keeping track of the relative time between the serum concentrations (Figure 5-12).*

2. *Because the patient is at steady state, the trough concentration can be extrapolated to the next trough value time (see Figure 5-12).*

3. *Draw the elimination curve between the steady-state peak concentration and the extrapolated trough concentration. Use this line to estimate half-life.* The patient is receiving vancomycin 1000 mg every 36 hours, which produces a steady-state peak of 34 μg/mL and a steady-state trough of 3 μg/mL. The dose is infused over 1 hour, and the peak concentration is drawn 30 minutes later (see Figure 5-12). The time between the measured steady-state peak and the extrapolated trough concentration is 34.5 hours (the 36-hour dosage interval minus the 1.5-hour combined infusion and waiting time). The definition of half-life is the time needed for serum concentrations to decrease by half. It takes 1 half-life for the peak serum concentration to decline from 34 μg/mL to 17 μg/mL, another half-life for concentrations to decrease from 17 μg/mL to 8.5 μg/mL, an additional half-life for concentrations to drop from ~8 μg/mL to 4 μg/mL, and a final half-life for the concentration to decrease to 2 μg/mL. The concentration of 2 μg/mL is very close to the extrapolated trough value of 2.5 μg/mL. Therefore, 4 half-lives expired during the 34.5-hour time period between the peak concentration and the extrapolated trough concentration, and the estimated half-life is 9 hours (34.5 h/4 half-lives = ~9 h). This information is used to set the new dosage interval for the patient.

4. *Determine the difference in concentration between the steady-state peak and trough concentrations. The difference in concentration changes proportionally with the dose size.* In this example, the patient is receiving a vancomycin dose of 1000 mg every 36 hours, which produced steady-state peak and trough concentrations of 34

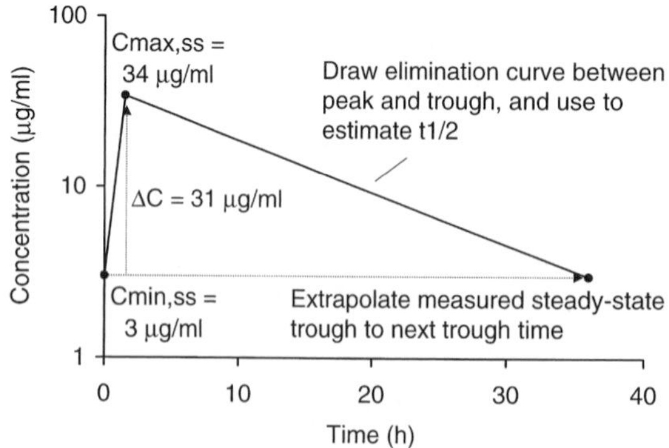

FIGURE 5-12 Solution to problem 2 using the pharmacokinetic concepts method.

μg/mL and 2.5 μg/mL, respectively. The difference between the peak and trough values is 31.5 μg/mL. The change in vancomycin serum concentration is proportional to the dose, and this information is used to set a new dose for the patient.

5. *Choose new steady-state peak and trough concentrations.* For this example, the desired steady-state peak and trough concentrations are 30 μg/mL and 7 μg/mL, respectively.

6. *Determine the new dosage interval for the desired concentrations.* Using the desired concentrations, it will take 1 half-life for the peak concentration of 30 μg/mL to decrease to 15 μg/mL and an additional half-life for serum concentrations to decline from 15 μg/mL to 7.5 μg/mL. Therefore, the dosage interval needs to be approximately 2 half-lives or 18 hours (9 hours × 2 half-lives = 18 hours).

7. *Determine the new dose for the desired concentrations.* The desired peak concentration is 30 μg/mL, and the expected trough concentration is 7 μg/mL. The change in concentration between these values is 23 μg/mL. It is known from measured serum concentrations that administration of 1000 mg vancomycin changes serum concentrations by 31.5 μg/mL and that the change in serum concentration between the peak and trough values is proportional to the size of the dose. In this case, $D_{new} = (\Delta C_{new}/\Delta C_{old})D_{old}$ = [(23 μg/mL)/(31.5 μg/mL)] 1000 mg = 730 mg, rounded to 750 mg. Vancomycin 750 mg every 18 hours is started 18 hours after the last dose of the previous dosage regimen.

One-Compartment Model Parameter Method

1. *Estimate the creatinine clearance.*

This patient has a stable serum creatinine and is not obese. The Cockcroft–Gault equation can be used to estimate creatinine clearance:

$$CrCl_{est} = [(140 - age)BW]/(72 \cdot S_{Cr}) = [(140 - 75\ y)62\ kg]/(72 \cdot 1.3\ mg/dL)$$

$$CrCl_{est} = 43\ mL/min$$

2. *Estimate the elimination rate constant (k_e) and half-life ($t_{1/2}$).*

The vancomycin clearance versus creatinine clearance relationship is used to estimate drug clearance for this patient:

$$Cl = 0.695(CrCl) + 0.05 = 0.695[(43\ mL/min)/62\ kg] + 0.05 = 0.533\ mL/min/kg$$

The average volume of distribution for vancomycin is 0.7 L/kg:

$$V = 0.7\ L/kg \cdot 62\ kg = 43.4\ L$$

$$k_e = Cl/V = (0.533\ mL/min/kg \cdot 60\ min/h)/(0.7\ L/kg \cdot 1000\ mL/L) = 0.0457\ h^{-1}$$

$$t_{1/2} = 0.693/k_e = 0.693/0.0457\ h^{-1} = 15.2\ h$$

Because the patient has been receiving vancomycin for >3 to 5 estimated half-lives, it is likely that the measured serum concentrations are close to steady-state values. This steady-state concentration pair can be used to compute the patient's unique pharmacokinetic parameters, which can be used to calculate individualized doses. Use the *one-compartment model parameter method* to compute a new dose.

1. *Compute the patient's elimination rate constant and half-life (note: t′ = infusion time + waiting time of 1 hour and 1/2 hour, respectively).*

$$k_e = (\ln C_{max,ss} - \ln C_{min,ss})/\tau - t' = (\ln 34\ \mu g/mL - \ln 2.5\ \mu g/mL)/(36\ h - 1.5\ h) = 0.0757\ h^{-1}$$

$$t_{1/2} = 0.693/k_e = 0.693/0.0757\ h^{-1} = 9.2\ h$$

2. *Compute the patient's volume of distribution.*

$$V = D/(C_{max,ss} - C_{min,ss}) = 1000\ mg/(34\ mg/L - 2.5\ mg/L) = 31.7\ L$$

3. *Choose new steady-state peak and trough concentrations.* For this example, the desired steady-state peak and trough concentrations are 30 μg/mL and 7 μg/mL, respectively.

4. *Determine the new dosage interval for the desired concentrations.* As in the initial dosage section of this chapter, the dosage interval (τ) is computed using the following equation:

$$\tau = (\ln C_{max,ss} - \ln C_{min,ss})/k_e = (\ln 30\ \mu g/mL - \ln 7\ \mu g/mL)/0.0757\ h^{-1} = 19\ h, \text{ rounded to } 18\ h$$

5. *Determine the new dose for the desired concentrations.* The dose is computed following the one-compartment model intravenous bolus equation used in the initial dosing section of this chapter:

$$D = C_{max,ss}\, V(1 - e^{-k_e \tau}) = 30\ mg/L \cdot 31.7\ L\ (1 - e^{-(0.0757\ h^{-1})(18\ h)}) = 708\ mg, \text{ rounded to } 750\ mg$$

Vancomycin 750 mg every 18 hours is prescribed to begin 18 hours after the last dose of the previous regimen. This dose is identical to that derived for the patient using the pharmacokinetic concepts method.

Bayesian Pharmacokinetics Computer Program Method

1. *Enter the patient's demographic, drug dosing, and serum concentration–time data into the computer program.*

2. *Compute pharmacokinetic parameters for the patient using the Bayesian pharmacokinetics computer program.*

The pharmacokinetic parameters computed by the program are a volume of distribution of 33.5 L, a half-life of 9.6 hours, and an elimination rate constant of 0.0720 h^{-1}.

3. *Compute the dose required to achieve desired vancomycin serum concentrations.*

The one-compartment model intravenous infusion equations used by the program to compute doses indicate that 750 mg every 18 hours will produce a steady-state peak concentration of 29.6 μg/mL and a steady-state trough concentration of 8.6

μg/mL. The pharmacokinetic concepts method and the one-compartment model parameter method produced the identical answer for this patient.

3. The initial vancomycin dose for patient HT is calculated as follows.

Pharmacokinetic Dosing Method

1. *Estimate the creatinine clearance.*

This patient has a stable serum creatinine and is not obese. The Cockcroft–Gault equation can be used to estimate creatinine clearance:

$$CrCl_{est} = \{[(140 - age)BW]/(72 \cdot S_{Cr})\}0.85 = \{[(140 - 35\ y)75\ kg]/(72 \cdot 3.7\ mg/dL)\}0.85$$

$$CrCl_{est} = 25\ mL/min$$

2. *Estimate the vancomycin clearance.*

The vancomycin clearance versus creatinine clearance relationship is used to estimate the vancomycin clearance for this patient:

$$Cl = 0.695(CrCl) + 0.05 = 0.695[(25\ mL/min)/75\ kg] + 0.05 = 0.283\ mL/min/kg$$

3. *Estimate the vancomycin volume of distribution.*

The average volume of distribution for vancomycin is 0.7 L/kg:

$$V = 0.7\ L/kg \cdot 75\ kg = 52.5\ L$$

4. *Estimate the vancomycin elimination rate constant (k_e) and half-life ($t_{1/2}$).*

$$k_e = Cl/V = (0.283\ mL/min/kg \cdot 60\ min/h)/(0.7\ L/kg \cdot 1000\ mL/L) = 0.0242\ h^{-1}$$

$$t_{1/2} = 0.693/k_e = 0.693/0.0242\ h^{-1} = 28.6\ h$$

5. *Choose the desired steady-state serum concentrations.*

A $C_{min,ss}$ = 5 μg/mL and $C_{max,ss}$ = 25 μg/mL were chosen to treat this patient.

6. *Use the intravenous bolus equations to compute dose (see Table 5-2).*

Calculate the required dosage interval (τ):

$$\tau = (\ln C_{max,ss} - \ln C_{min,ss})/k_e = (\ln 25\ \mu g/mL - \ln 5\ \mu g/mL)/0.0242\ h^{-1} = 66\ h$$

Dosage intervals should be rounded to clinically acceptable intervals of 12 hours, 18 hours, 24 hours, 36 hours, 48 hours, 72 hours, and multiples of 24 hours thereafter, whenever possible. In this case, the dosage interval is rounded to 72 hours.

Calculate the required dose (D):

$$D = C_{max,ss} V(1 - e^{-k_e\tau}) = 25\ mg/L \cdot 52.5\ L\ (1 - e^{-(0.0242\ h^{-1})(72\ h)}) = 1083\ mg$$

Vancomycin doses should be rounded to the nearest 100 to 250 mg. This dose is rounded to 1000 mg. (Note: μg/mL = mg/L, and this concentration unit was substituted for $C_{max,ss}$ to avoid unnecessary unit conversion.)

The prescribed maintenance dose is 1000 mg every 72 hours.

7. *Compute the loading dose, if needed.*

Loading doses should be considered for patients with creatinine clearance values lower than 60 mL/min. The administration of a loading dose in these patients allows achievement of therapeutic concentrations more quickly than if maintenance doses alone are given. However, because the pharmacokinetic parameters used to compute these initial doses are *estimated* values and not *actual* values, the patient's own parameters may be much different from the estimated constants, and steady-state is not achieved until 3 to 5 half-lives have passed.

$$LD = C_{max,ss} V = 25 \text{ mg/L} \cdot 52.5 \text{ L} = 1313 \text{ mg}$$

As noted, this patient has poor renal function (CrCl <60 mL/min), so a loading dose is prescribed and given as the first dose. Vancomycin doses should be rounded to the nearest 100 to 250 mg. This dose is rounded to 1250 mg. (Note: μg/mL = mg/L, and this concentration unit was substituted for $C_{max,ss}$ to avoid unnecessary unit conversion.) The first maintenance dose is given one dosage interval (72 hours) after the loading dose was administered.

Moellering Nomogram Method

1. *Estimate the creatinine clearance.*

This patient has a stable serum creatinine and is not obese. The Cockcroft–Gault equation can be used to estimate creatinine clearance:

$$CrCl_{est} = \{[(140 - age)BW]/(72 \cdot S_{Cr})\}0.85 = \{[(140 - 35 \text{ y})75 \text{ kg}]/(72 \cdot 3.7 \text{ mg/dL})\}0.85$$

$$CrCl_{est} = 25 \text{ mL/min}$$

2. *Determine the dosage interval and the maintenance dosage.*

The maintenance dosage is calculated using the modified vancomycin dosing equation:

$$D \text{ (in mg/h/kg)} = 0.626(CrCl \text{ in mL/min/kg}) + 0.05$$

$$D = 0.626[(25 \text{ mL/min})/75 \text{ kg}] + 0.05 = 0.260 \text{ mg/h/kg}$$

$$D = 0.260 \text{ mg/h/kg} \cdot 75 \text{ kg} = 19.5 \text{ mg/h}$$

The standard dose of 1000 mg can be used to gain an approximation for an acceptable dosage interval (τ):

$$\tau = 1000 \text{ mg}/(19.5 \text{ mg/h}) = 51 \text{ h}$$

Dosage intervals should be rounded to clinically acceptable intervals of 12 hours, 18 hours, 24 hours, 36 hours, 48 hours, 72 hours, and multiples of 24 hours thereafter, whenever possible. In this case, the dosage interval is rounded to 48 hours.

$$D = 19.5 \text{ mg/h} \cdot 48 \text{ h} = 936 \text{ mg}$$

Vancomycin doses should be rounded to the nearest 100 to 250 mg. This dose is rounded to 1000 mg. The prescribed maintenance dosage is 1000 mg every 48 hours.

3. *Compute the loading dose.*

A loading dose of 15 mg/kg is suggested by the Moellering nomogram:

$$LD = 15 \text{ mg/kg}(75 \text{ kg}) = 1125 \text{ mg}$$

This loading dose is rounded to 1250 mg and given as the first dose. The first maintenance dosage is given one dosage interval (48 hours) after the loading dose.

Matzke Nomogram Method

1. *Estimate the creatinine clearance.*

This patient has a stable serum creatinine and is not obese. The Cockcroft–Gault equation can be used to estimate creatinine clearance:

$$CrCl_{est} = \{[(140 - \text{age})BW]/(72 \cdot S_{Cr})\}0.85 = \{[(140 - 35 \text{ y})75 \text{ kg}]/(72 \cdot 3.7 \text{ mg/dL})\}0.85$$

$$CrCl_{est} = 25 \text{ mL/min}$$

2. *Compute the loading dose (see Table 5-4).*

A loading dose of 25 mg/kg provides a peak concentration of 30 μg/mL.

$$LD = 25 \text{ mg/kg}(75 \text{ kg}) = 1875 \text{ mg, rounded to } 1750 \text{ mg}$$

3. *Determine the dosage interval and maintenance dosage.*

Round the creatinine clearance value to 30 mL/min. From the nomogram, the dosage interval is 2 days or 48 hours. The maintenance dosage is:

$$19 \text{ mg/kg} \cdot 75 \text{ kg} = 1425 \text{ mg}$$

Vancomycin doses should be rounded to the nearest 100 to 250 mg. This dose is rounded to 1500 mg and is given one dosage interval (48 hours) after the loading dose.

The prescribed maintenance dosage is 1500 mg every 48 hours.

4. The revised vancomycin dose for patient HT is calculated as follows.

Pharmacokinetic Concepts Method

1. *Estimate the creatinine clearance.*

This patient has a stable serum creatinine and is not obese. The Cockcroft–Gault equation can be used to estimate creatinine clearance:

$$CrCl_{est} = \{[(140 - \text{age})BW]/(72 \cdot S_{Cr})\}0.85 = \{[(140 - 35 \text{ y})75 \text{ kg}]/(72 \cdot 3.7 \text{ mg/dL})\}0.85$$

$$CrCl_{est} = 25 \text{ mL/min}$$

2. *Estimate the elimination rate constant (k_e) and half-life ($t_{1/2}$).*

The vancomycin clearance versus creatinine clearance relationship is used to estimate drug clearance for this patient:

$$Cl = 0.695(CrCl) + 0.05 = 0.695[(25 \text{ mL/min})/75 \text{ kg}] + 0.05 = 0.283 \text{ mL/min/kg}$$

The average volume of distribution for vancomycin is 0.7 L/kg:

$$V = 0.7 \text{ L/kg} \cdot 75 \text{ kg} = 52.5 \text{ L}$$

$$k_e = Cl/V = (0.283 \text{ mL/min/kg} \cdot 60 \text{ min/h})/(0.7 \text{ L/kg} \cdot 1000 \text{ mL/L}) = 0.0242 \text{ h}^{-1}$$

$$t_{1/2} = 0.693/k_e = 0.693/0.0242 \text{ h}^{-1} = 28.6 \text{ h}$$

Because the patient has been receiving vancomycin for >3 to 5 estimated half-lives, it is likely that the measured serum concentrations are close to steady-state values. This steady-state concentration pair can be used to compute the patient's unique pharmacokinetic parameters, which in turn can be used to calculate individualized doses. Use the *pharmacokinetic concepts method* to compute a new dose.

1. *Draw a rough sketch of the serum log concentration–time curve by hand, keeping track of the relative time between the serum concentrations (Figure 5-13).*

2. *Because the patient is at steady state, the trough concentration can be extrapolated to the next trough value time (see Figure 5-13).*

3. *Draw the elimination curve between the steady-state peak concentration and the extrapolated trough concentration. Use this line to estimate half-life.* The patient is receiving vancomycin 1200 mg every 48 hours, which produces a steady-state peak of 55 μg/mL and a steady-state trough of 18 μg/mL. The dose is infused over 1 hour, and the peak concentration is drawn 30 minutes later (see Figure 5-13). The time between the measured steady-state peak and the extrapolated trough concentration is 46.5 hours (the 48-hour dosage interval minus the 1.5-hour combined infusion and waiting time). The definition of half-life is the time needed for serum concentrations to decrease by half. It takes 1 half-life for the peak serum concentration to decline from 55 μg/mL to 28 μg/mL and an additional half-life for concentrations to drop from 28 μg/mL to 14 μg/mL. The concentration of 18 μg/mL is close to the extrapolated trough value of 14 μg/mL. Therefore, ~1.5 half-lives expired during the 46.5-hour time period between the peak concentration and extrap-

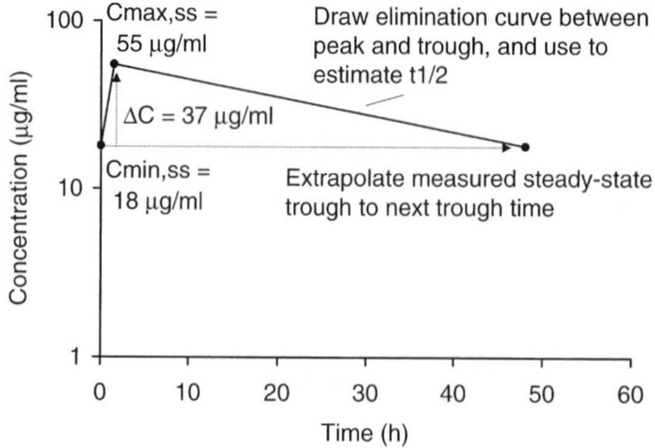

FIGURE 5-13 Solution to problem 4 using the pharmacokinetic concepts method.

olated trough concentration, and the estimated half-life is ~31 hours (46.5 h/1.5 half-lives = ~31 h). This information is used to set the new dosage interval for the patient.

4. *Determine the difference in concentration between the steady-state peak and trough concentrations. The difference in concentration changes proportionally with the dose size.* In this example, the patient is receiving vancomycin 1200 mg every 48 hours, which produced steady-state peak and trough concentrations of 55 μg/mL and 18 μg/mL, respectively. The difference between the peak and trough values is 37 μg/mL. The change in serum concentration is proportional to the dose, and this information is used to set a new dose for the patient.

5. *Choose new steady-state peak and trough concentrations.* For this example, the desired steady-state peak and trough concentrations are 25 μg/mL and 5 μg/mL, respectively.

6. *Determine the new dosage interval for the desired concentrations.* Using the desired concentrations, it will take 1 half-life for the peak concentration of 25 μg/mL to decrease to 12.5 μg/mL and an additional half-life for serum concentrations to decline from 12.5 μg/mL to 6 μg/mL. A concentration of 6 μg/mL is close to the desired concentration of 5 μg/mL. Therefore, the dosage interval needs to be approximately 2 half-lives or 72 hours (31 hours × 2 half-lives = 62 hours, rounded to 72 hours).

7. *Determine the new dose for the desired concentrations.* The desired peak concentration is 25 μg/mL, and the expected trough concentration is 6 μg/mL. The change in concentration between these values is 19 μg/mL. It is known from measured serum concentrations that administration of 1200 mg vancomycin changes serum concentrations by 37 μg/mL and that the change in serum concentration between the peak and trough values is proportional to the size of the dose. In this case, $D_{new} = (\Delta C_{new}/\Delta C_{old})D_{old}$ = [(19 μg/mL)/(37 μg/mL)] 1200 mg = 616 mg, rounded to 750 mg. Vancomycin 750 mg every 72 hours is started 72 hours after the last dose of the previous dosage regimen.

One-Compartment Model Parameter Method

1. *Estimate the creatinine clearance.*

This patient has a stable serum creatinine and is not obese. The Cockcroft–Gault equation can be used to estimate creatinine clearance:

$$CrCl_{est} = \{[(140 - age)BW]/(72 \cdot S_{Cr})\}\ 0.85 = \{[(140 - 35\ y)75\ kg]/(72 \cdot 3.7\ mg/dL)\}0.85$$

$$CrCl_{est} = 25\ mL/min$$

2. *Estimate the elimination rate constant (k_e) and half-life ($t_{1/2}$).*

The vancomycin clearance versus creatinine clearance relationship is used to estimate drug clearance for this patient:

$$Cl = 0.695(CrCl) + 0.05 = 0.695[(25\ mL/min)/75\ kg] + 0.05 = 0.283\ mL/min/kg$$

The average volume of distribution for vancomycin is 0.7 L/kg:

$$V = 0.7\ L/kg \cdot 75\ kg = 52.5\ L$$

$$k_e = Cl/V = (0.283\ mL/min/kg \cdot 60\ min/h)/(0.7\ L/kg \cdot 1000\ mL/L) = 0.0242\ h^{-1}$$

$$t_{1/2} = 0.693/k_e = 0.693/0.0242\ h^{-1} = 28.6\ h$$

Because the patient has been receiving vancomycin for >3 to 5 estimated half-lives, it is likely that the measured serum concentrations are close to steady-state values. This steady-state concentration pair can be used to compute the patient's unique pharmacokinetic parameters, which in turn can be used to calculate individualized doses. Use the *one-compartment model parameter method* to compute a new dose.

1. *Compute the patient's elimination rate constant and half-life (note: t′ = infusion time + waiting time of 1 hour and 1/2 hour, respectively).*

$$k_e = (\ln C_{max,ss} - \ln C_{min,ss})/\tau - t' = (\ln 55\ \mu g/mL - \ln 18\ \mu g/mL)/(48\ h - 1.5\ h) = 0.0240\ h^{-1}$$

$$t_{1/2} = 0.693/k_e = 0.693/0.0240\ h^{-1} = 28.9\ h$$

2. *Compute the patient's volume of distribution.*

$$V = D/(C_{max,ss} - C_{min,ss}) = 1200\ mg/(55\ mg/L - 18\ mg/L) = 32.4\ L$$

3. *Choose new steady-state peak and trough concentrations.* For this example, the desired steady-state peak and trough concentrations are 25 μg/mL and 5 μg/mL, respectively.

4. *Determine the new dosage interval for the desired concentrations.* As in the initial dosage section of this chapter, the dosage interval (τ) is computed using the following equation:

$$\tau = (\ln C_{max,ss} - \ln C_{min,ss})/k_e = (\ln 25\ \mu g/mL - \ln 5\ \mu g/mL)/0.0240\ h^{-1} = 67\ h, \text{ rounded to } 72\ h$$

5. *Determine the new dose for the desired concentrations.* The dose is computed using the one-compartment model intravenous bolus equation used in the initial dosing section of this chapter:

$$D = C_{max,ss}\ V(1 - e^{-k_e\tau}) = 25\ mg/L \cdot 32.4\ L\ (1 - e^{-(0.0240\ h^{-1})(72\ h)}) = 667\ mg, \text{ rounded to } 750\ mg$$

Vancomycin 750 mg every 72 hours is prescribed to begin 72 hours after the last dose of the previous regimen. This dose is identical to that derived for the patient using the pharmacokinetic concepts method.

Bayesian Pharmacokinetics Computer Program Method

1. *Enter the patient's demographic, drug dosing, and serum concentration–time data into the computer program.*

2. *Compute the pharmacokinetic parameters for the patient using the Bayesian pharmacokinetics computer program.*

The pharmacokinetic parameters computed by the program are a volume of distribution of 33.8 L, a half-life of 31.3 hours, and an elimination rate constant of 0.0221 h^{-1}.

3. *Compute the dose required to achieve desired vancomycin serum concentrations.*

The one-compartment model intravenous infusion equations used by the program to compute doses indicate that a dose of 750 mg every 72 hours produces a steady-state peak concentration of 27.7 μg/mL and a steady-state trough concentration of 5.8 μg/mL. The identical dose was computed using the one-compartment model parameter method and the pharmacokinetic concepts method.

5. The initial vancomycin dose for patient LK is calculated as follows.

Pharmacokinetic Dosing Method

1. *Estimate the creatinine clearance.*

This patient has a stable serum creatinine and is obese (IBW_{males} (in kg) = 50 + 2.3(Ht – 60 in) = 50 + 2.3(68 – 60) = 68.4 kg). The Salazar-Corcoran equation can be used to estimate creatinine clearance:

$$CrCl_{est(males)} = \frac{(137 - age)[(0.285 \cdot Wt) + (12.1 \cdot Ht^2)]}{(51 \cdot S_{Cr})}$$

$$CrCl_{est(males)} = \frac{(137 - 55\ y)\{(0.285 \cdot 140\ kg) + [12.1 \cdot (1.73\ m)^2]\}}{(51 \cdot 0.9\ mg/dL)} = 136\ mL/min$$

Note: Height is converted from inches to meters: Ht = (68 in · 2.54 cm/in)/(100 cm/m) = 1.73 m.

2. *Estimate the vancomycin clearance.*

The vancomycin clearance versus creatinine clearance relationship is used to estimate the vancomycin clearance for this patient:

$$Cl = 0.695(CrCl) + 0.05 = 0.695[(136\ mL/min)/140\ kg] + 0.05 = 0.724\ mL/min/kg\ TBW$$

3. *Estimate the vancomycin volume of distribution.*

The average volume of distribution for vancomycin is 0.7 L/kg IBW:

$$V = 0.7\ L/kg \cdot 68.4\ kg = 47.9\ L$$

4. *Estimate the vancomycin elimination rate constant (k_e) and half-life ($t_{1/2}$).*

$$k_e = Cl/V = (0.724\ mL/min/kg\ TBW \cdot 140\ kg \cdot 60\ min/h)/(0.7\ L/kg\ IBW \cdot 68.4\ kg \cdot 1000\ mL/L) = 0.127\ h^{-1}$$

$$t_{1/2} = 0.693/k_e = 0.693/0.127\ h^{-1} = 5.5\ h$$

5. *Choose the desired steady-state serum concentrations.*

A $C_{min,ss}$ = 10 μg/mL and $C_{max,ss}$ = 40 μg/mL were chosen to treat this patient.

6. *Use the intravenous bolus equations to compute the dose (see Table 5-2).*

Calculate the required dosage interval (τ):

$$\tau = (\ln C_{max,ss} - \ln C_{min,ss})/k_e = (\ln 40\ \mu g/mL - \ln 10\ \mu g/mL)/0.127\ h^{-1} = 11\ h$$

Dosage intervals should be rounded to clinically acceptable intervals of 12 hours, 18 hours, 24 hours, 36 hours, 48 hours, 72 hours, and multiples of 24 hours thereafter, whenever possible. In this case, the dosage interval is rounded to 12 hours.

Calculate the required dose (D):

$$D = C_{max,ss} V(1 - e^{-k_e\tau}) = 40\ mg/L \cdot 47.9\ L\ (1 - e^{-(0.127\ h^{-1})(12\ h)}) = 1498\ mg$$

Vancomycin doses should be rounded to the nearest 100 to 250 mg. This dose is rounded to 1500 mg. (Note: μg/mL = mg/L, and this concentration unit was substituted for $C_{max,ss}$ so that unnecessary unit conversion was not required.)

The prescribed maintenance dosage is 1500 mg every 12 hours.

7. *Compute the loading dose, if needed.*

Loading doses should be considered for patients with creatinine clearance values lower than 60 mL/min. The administration of a loading dose allows achievement of therapeutic concentrations more quickly than if maintenance doses alone are given. However, because the pharmacokinetic parameters used to compute these initial doses are *estimated* values and not *actual* values, the patient's own parameters may be much different from the estimated constants, and steady-state is not achieved until 3 to 5 half-lives have passed.

$$LD = C_{max,ss} V = 40\ mg/L \cdot 47.9\ L = 1915\ mg$$

As noted, this patient has good renal function (CrCl ≥60 mL/min), so a loading dose is not necessary. (Note: μg/mL = mg/L, and this concentration unit was substituted for $C_{max,ss}$ to avoid unnecessary unit conversion.)

Moellering Nomogram Method

1. *Estimate the creatinine clearance.*

This patient has a stable serum creatinine and is obese (IBW_{males} (in kg) = 50 + 2.3(Ht − 60 in) = 50 + 2.3(68 − 60) = 68.4 kg). The Salazar-Corcoran equation can be used to estimate creatinine clearance:

$$CrCl_{est(males)} = \frac{(137 - age)[(0.285 \cdot Wt) + (12.1 \cdot Ht^2)]}{(51 \cdot S_{Cr})}$$

$$CrCl_{est(males)} = \frac{(137 - 55\ y)\{(0.285 \cdot 140\ kg) + [12.1 \cdot (1.73\ m)^2]\}}{(51 \cdot 0.9\ mg/dL)} = 136\ mL/min$$

Note: Height is converted from inches to meters: Ht = (68 in · 2.54 cm/in)/(100 cm/m) = 1.73 m.

2. *Determine the dosage interval and maintenance dosage.*

The maintenance dosage is calculated using the modified vancomycin dosing equation:

$$D\ (in\ mg/h/kg) = 0.626(CrCl\ in\ mL/min/kg) + 0.05$$

$$D = 0.626[(136\ mL/min)/140\ kg] + 0.05 = 0.657\ mg/h/kg\ TBW$$

$$D = 0.657\ mg/h/kg \cdot 140\ kg = 92\ mg/h$$

The standard dose of vancomycin 1000 mg can be used to gain an approximation for an acceptable dosage interval (τ):

$$\tau = 1000\ mg/(92\ mg/h) = 11\ h$$

Dosage intervals should be rounded to clinically acceptable intervals of 12 hours, 18 hours, 24 hours, 36 hours, 48 hours, 72 hours, and multiples of 24 hours thereafter, whenever possible. In this case, the dosage interval is rounded to 12 hours.

$$D = 92\ mg/h \cdot 12\ h = 1104\ mg$$

Vancomycin doses should be rounded to the nearest 50 to 100 mg. This dose is rounded to 1000 mg. The prescribed maintenance dosage is 1000 mg every 12 hours.

3. *Compute the loading dose.*

A loading dose of 15 mg/kg IBW is suggested by the Moellering nomogram.

$$LD = 15\ mg/kg(68.4\ kg) = 1026\ mg$$

This loading dose is smaller than the maintenance dose and would not be given.

6. The revised vancomycin dose for patient LK is calculated as follows.

Pharmacokinetic Concepts Method

1. *Estimate the creatinine clearance.*

This patient has a stable serum creatinine and is obese (IBW_{males} (in kg) = 50 + 2.3(Ht – 60 in) = 50 + 2.3(68 – 60) = 68.4 kg). The Salazar-Corcoran equation can be used to estimate creatinine clearance:

$$CrCl_{est(males)} = \frac{(137 - age)[(0.285 \cdot Wt) + (12.1 \cdot Ht^2)]}{(51 \cdot S_{Cr})}$$

$$CrCl_{est(males)} = \frac{(137 - 55\ y)\{(0.285 \cdot 140\ kg) + [12.1 \cdot (1.73\ m)^2]\}}{(51 \cdot 0.9\ mg/dL)} = 136\ mL/min$$

Note: Height is converted from inches to meters: Ht = (68 in · 2.54 cm/in)/(100 cm/m) = 1.73 m.

2. *Estimate the elimination rate constant (k_e) and half-life ($t_{1/2}$).*

The vancomycin clearance versus creatinine clearance relationship is used to estimate drug clearance for this patient:

$$Cl = 0.695(CrCl) + 0.05 = 0.695[(136\ mL/min)/140\ kg] + 0.05 = 0.724\ mL/min/kg\ TBW$$

The average volume of distribution for vancomycin is 0.7 L/kg IBW:

$$V = 0.7\ L/kg \cdot 68.4\ kg = 47.9\ L$$

$$k_e = Cl/V = (0.724\ mL/min/kg\ TBW \cdot 140\ kg \cdot 60\ min/h)/(0.7\ L/kg \cdot 68.4\ kg\ IBW \cdot 1000\ mL/L) = 0.127\ h^{-1}$$

$$t_{1/2} = 0.693/k_e = 0.693/0.127\ h^{-1} = 5.5\ h$$

Because the patient has been receiving vancomycin for >3 to 5 estimated half-lives, it is likely that the measured serum concentrations are close to steady-state values. This steady-state concentration pair can be used to compute the patient's unique pharmacokinetic parameters, which in turn can be used to calculate individualized doses. Use the *pharmacokinetic concepts method* to compute a new dose.

1. *Draw a rough sketch of the serum log concentration–time curve by hand, keeping track of the relative time between the serum concentrations (Figure 5-14).*

2. *Because the patient is at steady state, the trough concentration can be extrapolated to the next trough value time (see Figure 5-14).*

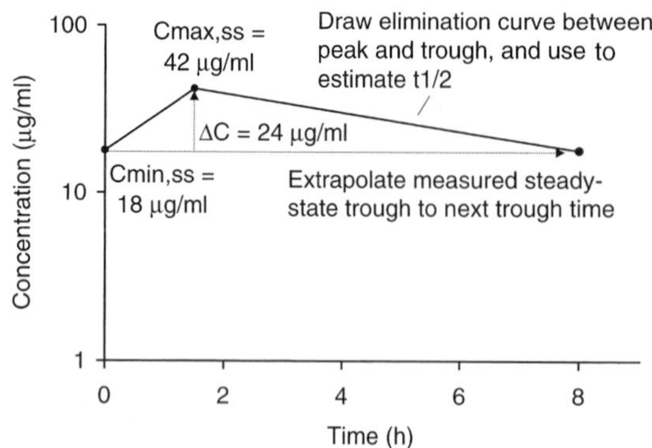

FIGURE 5-14 Solution to problem 6 using the pharmacokinetic concepts method.

3. *Draw the elimination curve between the steady-state peak concentration and the extrapolated trough concentration. Use this line to estimate half-life.* The patient is receiving vancomycin 1000 mg every 8 hours, which produces a steady-state peak of 42 μg/mL and a steady-state trough of 18 μg/mL. The dose is infused over 1 hour, and the peak concentration is drawn 30 minutes later (see Figure 5-14). The time between the measured steady-state peak and the extrapolated trough concentration is 6.5 hours (the 8-hour dosage interval minus the 1.5-hour combined infusion and waiting time). The definition of half-life is the time needed for serum concentrations to decrease by half. It takes 1 half-life for the peak serum concentration to decline from 42 μg/mL to 21 μg/mL. The concentration of 18 μg/mL is just slightly below 21 μg/mL. Therefore, ~1.25 half-lives expired during the 6.5-hour time period between the peak concentration and extrapolated trough concentration, and the estimated half-life is ~5 hours (6.5 h/1.25 half-lives = ~5 h). This information is used to set the new dosage interval for the patient.

4. *Determine the difference in concentration between the steady-state peak and trough concentrations. The difference in concentration changes proportionally with the dose size.* In this example, the patient is receiving vancomycin 1000 mg every 8 hours, which produced steady-state peak and trough concentrations of 42 μg/mL and 18 μg/mL, respectively. The difference between the peak and trough values is 24 μg/mL. The change in serum concentration is proportional to the dose, and this information is used to set a new dose for the patient.

5. *Choose new steady-state peak and trough concentrations.* For this example, the desired steady-state peak and trough concentrations are 40 μg/mL and 10 μg/mL, respectively.

6. *Determine the new dosage interval for the desired concentrations.* Using the desired concentrations, it will take 1 half-life for the peak concentration of 40 μg/mL to decrease to 20 μg/mL and an additional half-life for serum concentrations to decline from 20 μg/mL to 10 μg/mL. Therefore, the dosage interval needs to be approximately 2 half-lives or 12 hours (5 hours × 2 half-lives = 10 hours, rounded to 12 hours).

7. *Determine the new dose for the desired concentrations.* The desired peak concentration is 40 μg/mL, and the expected trough concentration is 10 μg/mL. The change in concentration between these values is 30 μg/mL. It is known from measured serum concentrations that administration of 1000 mg changes serum concentrations by 24 μg/mL and that the change in serum concentration between the peak and trough values is proportional to the size of the dose. In this case, $D_{new} = (\Delta C_{new}/\Delta C_{old})D_{old}$ = [(30 μg/mL)/(24 μg/mL)] 1000 mg = 1250 mg.

Vancomycin 1250 mg every 12 hours is started 12 hours after the last dose of the previous dosage regimen.

One-Compartment Model Parameter Method

1. *Estimate the creatinine clearance.*

This patient has a stable serum creatinine and is obese (IBW_{males} (in kg) = 50 +

2.3(Ht – 60 in) = 50 + 2.3(68 – 60) = 68.4 kg). The Salazar-Corcoran equation can be used to estimate creatinine clearance:

$$CrCl_{est(males)} = \frac{(137 - age)[(0.285 \cdot Wt) + (12.1 \cdot Ht^2)]}{(51 \cdot S_{Cr})}$$

$$CrCl_{est(males)} = \frac{(137 - 55\ y)\{(0.285 \cdot 140\ kg) + [12.1 \cdot (1.73\ m)^2]\}}{(51 \cdot 0.9\ mg/dL)} = 136\ mL/min$$

Note: Height is converted from inches to meters: Ht = (68 in · 2.54 cm/in)/(100 cm/m) = 1.73 m.

2. *Estimate the elimination rate constant (k_e) and half-life ($t_{1/2}$).*

The vancomycin clearance versus creatinine clearance relationship is used to estimate drug clearance for this patient:

$$Cl = 0.695(CrCl) + 0.05 = 0.695[(136\ mL/min)/140\ kg] + 0.05 = 0.724\ mL/min/kg\ TBW$$

The average volume of distribution for vancomycin is 0.7 L/kg IBW:

$$V = 0.7\ L/kg \cdot 68.4\ kg = 47.9\ L$$

$$k_e = Cl/V = (0.724\ mL/min/kg\ TBW \cdot 140\ kg \cdot 60\ min/h)/(0.7\ L/kg\ IBW \cdot 68.4\ kg \cdot 1000\ mL/L) = 0.127\ h^{-1}$$

$$t_{1/2} = 0.693/k_e = 0.693/0.127\ h^{-1} = 5.5\ h$$

Because the patient has been receiving vancomycin for >3 to 5 estimated half-lives, it is likely that the measured serum concentrations are close to steady-state values. This steady-state concentration pair can be used to compute the patient's own unique pharmacokinetic parameters, which in turn can be used to calculate individualized doses. Use the *one-compartment model parameter method* to compute a new dose.

1. *Compute the patient's elimination rate constant and half-life (note: t′ = infusion time + waiting time of 1 hour and 1/2 hour, respectively).*

$$k_e = (\ln C_{max,ss} - \ln C_{min,ss})/\tau - t' = (\ln 42\ \mu g/mL - \ln 18\ \mu g/mL)/(8\ h - 1.5\ h) = 0.130\ h^{-1}$$

$$t_{1/2} = 0.693/k_e = 0.693/0.130\ h^{-1} = 5.3\ h$$

2. *Compute the patient's volume of distribution.*

$$V = D/(C_{max,ss} - C_{min,ss}) = 1000\ mg/(42\ mg/L - 18\ mg/L) = 41.7\ L$$

3. *Choose new steady-state peak and trough concentrations.* For this example, the desired steady-state peak and trough concentrations are 40 μg/mL and 10 μg/mL, respectively.

4. *Determine the new dosage interval for the desired concentrations.* As in the initial dosage section of this chapter, the dosage interval (τ) is computed using the following equation:

$$\tau = (\ln C_{max,ss} - \ln C_{min,ss})/k_e = (\ln 40\ \mu g/mL - \ln 10\ \mu g/mL)/0.130\ h^{-1}$$
$$= 11\ h, \text{ rounded to } 12\ h$$

5. *Determine the new dose for the desired concentrations.* The dose is computed according to the one-compartment model intravenous bolus equation used in the initial dosing section of this chapter:

$$D = C_{max,ss}\ V(1 - e^{-k_e\tau}) = 40\ mg/L \cdot 41.7\ L\ (1 - e^{-(0.130\ h^{-1})(12\ h)})$$
$$= 1318\ mg, \text{ rounded to } 1250\ mg$$

Vancomycin 1250 mg every 12 hours is prescribed to begin 12 hours after the last dose of the previous regimen. This dose is identical to that derived for the patient using the pharmacokinetic concepts method.

Bayesian Pharmacokinetics Computer Program Method

1. *Enter the patient's demographic, drug dosing, and serum concentration–time data into the computer program.*

2. *Compute the pharmacokinetic parameters for the patient using the Bayesian pharmacokinetics computer program.*

The pharmacokinetic parameters computed by the program are a volume of distribution of 68.4 L, a half-life of 12.6 hours, and an elimination rate constant of 0.0551 h^{-1}.

3. *Compute the dose required to achieve desired vancomycin serum concentrations.*

The one-compartment model intravenous infusion equations used by the program to compute doses indicate that vancomycin 1750 mg every 24 hours will produce a steady-state peak concentration of 34 μg/mL and a steady-state trough concentration of 9.7 μg/mL. Use of the other dosing methods produced an answer for this patient of 1250 mg every 12 hours. The Bayesian computer program suggests a longer dosage interval and a larger dose because of the population pharmacokinetic parameter influence for volume of distribution on the dosing algorithm. If additional concentrations are entered into the program, the effect of the population parameters diminishes and eventually produces the same answer as the other two methods.

7. The initial vancomycin dose for patient AF is calculated as follows.

Pharmacokinetic Dosing Method

1. *Estimate the creatinine clearance.*

This patient has a stable serum creatinine and is obese ($IBW_{females}$ (in kg) = 45 + 2.3(Ht – 60 in) = 45 + 2.3(62 – 60) = 49.6 kg). The Salazar-Corcoran equation can be used to estimate creatinine clearance:

$$CrCl_{est(females)} = \frac{(146 - age)[(0.287 \cdot Wt) + (9.74 \cdot Ht^2)]}{(60 \cdot S_{Cr})}$$

$$CrCl_{est(females)} = \frac{(146 - 45\ y)\{(0.287 \cdot 140\ kg) + [9.74 \cdot (1.57\ m)^2]\}}{(60 \cdot 2.4\ mg/dL)} = 45\ mL/min$$

Note: Height is converted from inches to meters: Ht = (62 in · 2.54 cm/in)/(100 cm/m) = 1.57 m.

2. *Estimate the vancomycin clearance.*

The vancomycin clearance versus creatinine clearance relationship is used to estimate the vancomycin clearance for this patient:

$$Cl = 0.695(CrCl) + 0.05 = 0.695[(45\ mL/min)/140\ kg] + 0.05 = 0.274\ mL/min/kg\ TBW$$

3. *Estimate the vancomycin volume of distribution.*

The average volume of distribution for vancomycin is 0.7 L/kg IBW:

$$V = 0.7\ L/kg \cdot 49.6\ kg = 34.7\ L$$

4. *Estimate the vancomycin elimination rate constant (k_e) and half-life ($t_{1/2}$).*

$$k_e = Cl/V = (0.274\ mL/min/kg\ TBW \cdot 140\ kg \cdot 60\ min/h)/(0.7\ L/kg\ IBW \cdot 49.6\ kg \cdot 1000\ mL/L) = 0.0663\ h^{-1}$$

$$t_{1/2} = 0.693/0.0663\ h^{-1} = 10.5\ h$$

5. *Choose the desired steady-state serum concentrations.*

A $C_{min,ss}$ = 7 μg/mL and $C_{max,ss}$ = 25 μg/mL were chosen to treat this patient.

6. *Use the intravenous bolus equations to compute dose (see Table 5-2).*

Calculate the required dosage interval (τ):

$$\tau = (\ln C_{max,ss} - \ln C_{min,ss})/k_e = (\ln 25\ \mu g/mL - \ln 7\ \mu g/mL)/0.0663\ h^{-1} = 19.2\ h$$

Dosage intervals should be rounded to clinically acceptable intervals of 12 hours, 18 hours, 24 hours, 36 hours, 48 hours, 72 hours, and multiples of 24 hours thereafter, whenever possible. In this case, the dosage interval is rounded to 18 hours.

Calculate the required dose (D):

$$D = C_{max,ss}\, V(1 - e^{-k_e\tau}) = 25\ mg/L \cdot 34.7\ L\ (1 - e^{-(0.0663\ h^{-1})(18\ h)}) = 605\ mg$$

Vancomycin doses should be rounded to the nearest 100 to 250 mg. This dose is rounded to 500 mg. (Note: μg/mL = mg/L, and this concentration unit was substituted for $C_{max,ss}$ so that unnecessary unit conversion was not required.) The prescribed maintenance dose is 500 mg every 18 hours.

7. *Compute the loading dose, if needed.*

Loading doses should be considered for patients with creatinine clearance values lower than 60 mL/min. The administration of a loading dose allows achievement of therapeutic concentrations more quickly than if maintenance doses alone are given. However, because the pharmacokinetic parameters used to compute these initial doses are *estimated* values and not *actual* values, the patient's own parameters may be much different from the estimated constants, and steady-state will not be achieved until 3 to 5 half-lives have passed.

$$LD = C_{max,ss} V = 25 \text{ mg/L} \cdot 34.7 \text{ L} = 868 \text{ mg}$$

As noted, this patient has moderate renal function (CrCl <60 mL/min), so a loading dose is prescribed. The loading dose is rounded to 750 mg and given as the first dose. Maintenance doses begin one dosage interval after the loading dose was administered. (Note: μg/mL = mg/L, and this concentration unit was substituted for $C_{max,ss}$ so that unnecessary unit conversion was not required.)

Moellering Nomogram Method

1. *Estimate the creatinine clearance.*

This patient has a stable serum creatinine and is obese ($IBW_{females}$ (in kg) = 45 + 2.3(Ht – 60 in) = 45 + 2.3(62 – 60) = 49.6 kg). The Salazar-Corcoran equation can be used to estimate creatinine clearance:

$$CrCl_{est(females)} = \frac{(146 - \text{age})[(0.287 \cdot \text{Wt}) + (9.74 \cdot \text{Ht}^2)]}{(60 \cdot S_{Cr})}$$

$$CrCl_{est(females)} = \frac{(146 - 45 \text{ y})\{(0.287 \cdot 140 \text{ kg}) + [9.74 \cdot (1.57 \text{ m})^2]\}}{(60 \cdot 2.4 \text{ mg/dL})} = 45 \text{ mL/min}$$

Note: Height is converted from inches to meters: Ht = (62 in · 2.54 cm/in)/(100 cm/m) = 1.57 m.

2. *Determine the dosage interval and maintenance dosage.*

The maintenance dose is calculated using the modified vancomycin dosing equation:

$$D \text{ (in mg/h/kg)} = 0.626(\text{CrCl in mL/min/kg}) + 0.05$$

$$D = 0.626[(45 \text{ mL/min})/140 \text{ kg}] + 0.05 = 0.252 \text{ mg/h/kg TBW}$$

$$D = 0.252 \text{ mg/h/kg} \cdot 140 \text{ kg} = 35.2 \text{ mg/h}$$

The standard dose of 1000 mg can be used to gain an approximation for an acceptable dosage interval (τ):

$$\tau = 1000 \text{ mg}/(35.2 \text{ mg/h}) = 28.4 \text{ h}$$

Dosage intervals should be rounded to clinically acceptable intervals of 12 hours, 18 hours, 24 hours, 36 hours, 48 hours, 72 hours, and multiples of 24 hours thereafter, whenever possible. In this case, the dosage interval is rounded to 24 hours.

$$D = 35.2 \text{ mg/h} \cdot 24 \text{ h} = 845 \text{ mg}$$

Vancomycin doses should be rounded to the nearest 100 to 250 mg. This dose is rounded to 750 mg. The prescribed maintenance dosage is 750 mg every 24 hours.

3. *Compute the loading dose.*

A loading dose of 15 mg/kg IBW is suggested by the Moellering nomogram:

$$LD = 15 \text{ mg/kg}(49.6 \text{ kg}) = 744 \text{ mg}$$

This loading dose of 744 mg is smaller than the maintenance dose and would not be given.

8. The revised vancomycin dose for patient AF is calculated as follows.

Pharmacokinetic Concept Method

1. *Estimate the creatinine clearance.*

This patient has a stable serum creatinine and is obese ($IBW_{females}$ (in kg) = 45 + 2.3(Ht – 60 in) = 45 + 2.3(62 – 60) = 49.6 kg). The Salazar-Corcoran equation can be used to estimate creatinine clearance:

$$CrCl_{est(females)} = \frac{(146 - age)[(0.287 \cdot Wt) + (9.74 \cdot Ht^2)]}{(60 \cdot S_{Cr})}$$

$$CrCl_{est(females)} = \frac{(146 - 45 \text{ y})\{(0.287 \cdot 140 \text{ kg}) + [9.74 \cdot (1.57 \text{ m})^2]\}}{(60 \cdot 2.4 \text{ mg/dL})} = 45 \text{ mL/min}$$

Note: Height is converted from inches to meters: Ht = (62 in · 2.54 cm/in)/(100 cm/m) = 1.57 m.

2. *Estimate the elimination rate constant (k_e) and half-life ($t_{1/2}$).*

The vancomycin clearance versus creatinine clearance relationship is used to estimate drug clearance for this patient:

$$Cl = 0.695(CrCl) + 0.05 = 0.695[(45 \text{ mL/min})/140 \text{ kg}] + 0.05 = 0.274 \text{ mL/min/kg TBW}$$

The average volume of distribution for vancomycin is 0.7 L/kg IBW:

$$V = 0.7 \text{ L/kg} \cdot 49.6 \text{ kg} = 34.7 \text{ L}$$

$$k_e = Cl/V = (0.274 \text{ mL/min/kg TBW} \cdot 140 \text{ kg} \cdot 60 \text{ min/h})/(0.7 \text{ L/kg} \cdot 49.6 \text{ kg} \cdot 1000 \text{ ml/L}) = 0.0663 \text{ h}^{-1}$$

$$t_{1/2} = 0.693/k_e = 0.693/0.0663 \text{ h}^{-1} = 10.5 \text{ h}$$

Because the patient has been receiving vancomycin for >3 to 5 estimated half-lives, it is likely that the measured serum concentrations are close to steady-state values. This steady-state concentration pair can be used to compute the patient's unique pharmacokinetic parameters, which in turn can be used to calculate individualized doses. Use the *pharmacokinetic concepts method* to compute a new dose.

1. *Draw a rough sketch of the serum log concentration–time curve by hand, keeping track of the relative time between the serum concentrations (Figure 5-15).*

2. *Because the patient is at steady state, the trough concentration can be extrapolated to the next trough value time (see Figure 5-15).*

3. *Draw the elimination curve between the steady-state peak concentration and the extrapolated trough concentration. Use this line to estimate half-life.* The patient is receiving vancomycin 1300 mg every 24 hours, which produces a steady-state peak of 30 μg/mL and a steady-state trough of 2.5 μg/mL. The dose is infused over 1 hour,

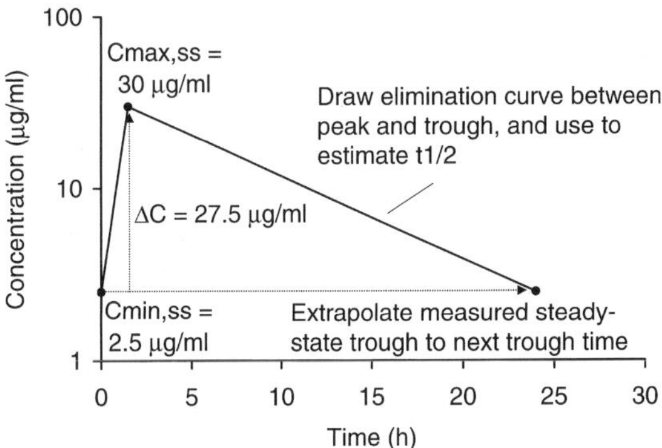

FIGURE 5-15 Solution to problem 8 using the pharmacokinetic concepts method.

and the peak concentration is drawn 30 minutes later (see Figure 5-15). The time between the measured steady-state peak and the extrapolated trough concentration is 22.5 hours (the 24-hour dosage interval minus the 1.5-hour combined infusion and waiting time). The definition of half-life is the time needed for serum concentrations to decrease by half. It takes 1 half-life for the peak serum concentration to decline from 30 μg/mL to 15 μg/mL, an additional half-life for the concentration to decrease from 15 μg/mL to 7.5 μg/mL, another half-life for the concentration to decline from 7.5 μg/mL to 4 μg/mL, and a final half-life for the concentration to reach 2 μg/mL. The concentration of 2 μg/mL is just slightly below 2.5 μg/mL. Therefore, 4 half-lives expired during the 22.5-hour time period between the peak concentration and the extrapolated trough concentration, and the estimated half-life is ~6 hours (22.5 h/4 half-lives = ~6 h). This information is used to set the new dosage interval for the patient.

4. *Determine the difference in concentration between the steady-state peak and trough concentrations. The difference in concentration changes proportionally with the dose size.* In this example, the patient is receiving a vancomycin dose of 1300 mg every 24 hours, which produced steady-state peak and trough concentrations of 30 μg/mL and 2.5 μg/mL, respectively. The difference between the peak and trough values is 27.5 μg/mL. The change in serum concentration is proportional to the dose, and this information is used to set a new dose for the patient.

5. *Choose new steady-state peak and trough concentrations.* For this example, the desired steady-state peak and trough concentrations are 25 μg/mL and 7 μg/mL, respectively.

6. *Determine the new dosage interval for the desired concentrations.* With the desired concentrations, it will take 1 half-life for the peak concentration of 25 μg/mL to decrease to 12.5 μg/mL, and an additional half-life for serum concentrations to decline from 12.5 μg/mL to 6 μg/mL. Therefore, the dosage interval needs to be approximately 2 half-lives or 12 hours (6 hours × 2 half-lives = 12 hours).

7. *Determine the new dose for the desired concentrations.* The desired peak concentration is 25 μg/mL, and the expected trough concentration is 6 μg/mL. The change in concentration between these values is 19 μg/mL. It is known from measured vancomycin serum concentrations that administration of 1300 mg vancomycin changes serum concentrations by 27.5 μg/mL and that the change in serum concentration between the peak and trough values is proportional to the size of the dose. In this case, $D_{new} = (\Delta C_{new}/\Delta C_{old})D_{old}$ = [(19 μg/mL)/(27.5 μg/mL)] 1300 mg = 898 mg, rounded to 1000 mg. Vancomycin 1000 mg every 12 hours is started 12 hours after the last dose of the previous dosage regimen.

One-Compartment Model Parameter Method

1. *Estimate the creatinine clearance.*

This patient has a stable serum creatinine and is obese ($IBW_{females}$ (in kg) = 45 + 2.3(Ht − 60 in) = 45 + 2.3(62 − 60) = 49.6 kg). The Salazar-Corcoran equation can be used to estimate creatinine clearance:

$$CrCl_{est(females)} = \frac{(146 - age)[(0.287 \cdot Wt) + (9.74 \cdot Ht^2)]}{(60 \cdot S_{Cr})}$$

$$CrCl_{est(females)} = \frac{(146 - 45\ y)\{(0.287 \cdot 140\ kg) + [9.74 \cdot (1.57\ m)^2]\}}{(60 \cdot 2.4\ mg/dL)} = 45\ mL/min$$

Note: Height is converted from inches to meters: Ht = (62 in · 2.54 cm/in)/(100 cm/m) = 1.57 m.

2. *Estimate the elimination rate constant (k_e) and half-life ($t_{1/2}$).*

The vancomycin clearance versus creatinine clearance relationship is used to estimate drug clearance for this patient:

$$Cl = 0.695(CrCl) + 0.05 = 0.695[(45\ mL/min)/140\ kg] + 0.05 = 0.274\ mL/min/kg\ TBW$$

The average volume of distribution for vancomycin is 0.7 L/kg IBW:

$$V = 0.7\ L/kg \cdot 49.6\ kg = 34.7\ L$$

$$k_e = Cl/V = (0.274\ mL/min/kg\ TBW \cdot 140\ kg \cdot 60\ min/h)/(0.7\ L/kg \cdot 49.6\ kg \cdot 1000\ mL/L) = 0.0663\ h^{-1}$$

$$t_{1/2} = 0.693/k_e = 0.693/0.0663\ h^{-1} = 10.5\ h$$

Because the patient has been receiving vancomycin for >3 to 5 estimated half-lives, it is likely that the measured serum concentrations are close to steady-state values. This steady-state concentration pair can be used to compute the patient's unique pharmacokinetic parameters, which in turn can be used to calculate individualized doses. Use the *one-compartment model parameter method* to compute a new dose.

1. *Compute the patient's elimination rate constant and half-life (note: t′ = infusion time + waiting time of 1 hour and 1/2 hour, respectively).*

$$k_e = (\ln C_{max,ss} - \ln C_{min,ss})/\tau - t' = (\ln 30\ \mu g/mL - \ln 2.5\ \mu g/mL)/(24\ h - 1.5\ h) = 0.110\ h^{-1}$$

$$t_{1/2} = 0.693/k_e = 0.693/0.110\ h^{-1} = 6.3\ h$$

2. *Compute the patient's volume of distribution.*

$$V = D/(C_{max,ss} - C_{min,ss}) = 1300 \text{ mg}/(30 \text{ mg/L} - 2.5 \text{ mg/L}) = 47.3 \text{ L}$$

3. *Choose new steady-state peak and trough concentrations.* For this example, the desired steady-state peak and trough concentrations are 25 μg/mL and 7 μg/mL, respectively.

4. *Determine the new dosage interval for the desired concentrations.* As in the initial dosage section of this chapter, the dosage interval (τ) is computed using the following equation:

$$\tau = (\ln C_{max,ss} - C_{min,ss})/k_e = (\ln 25 \text{ μg/mL} - \ln 7 \text{ μg/mL})/0.110 \text{ h}^{-1} = 12 \text{ h}$$

5. *Determine the new dose for the desired concentrations.* The dose is computed according to the one-compartment model intravenous bolus equation used in the initial dosing section of this chapter:

$$D = C_{max,ss} V(1 - e^{-k_e\tau}) = 25 \text{ mg/L} \cdot 47.3 \text{ L } (1 - e^{-(0.110 \text{ h}^{-1})(12 \text{ h})})$$
$$= 867 \text{ mg, rounded to } 750 \text{ mg}$$

Vancomycin 750 mg every 12 hours is prescribed to begin 12 hours after the last dose of the previous regimen. This dose is very similar to that derived for the patient using the pharmacokinetic concepts method (1000 mg every 12 hours).

Bayesian Pharmacokinetics Computer Program Method

1. *Enter the patient's demographic, drug dosing, and serum concentration–time data into the computer program.*

2. *Compute the pharmacokinetic parameters for the patient using the Bayesian pharmacokinetics computer program.*

The pharmacokinetic parameters computed by the program are a volume of distribution of 41.4 L, a half-life of 6.3 hours, and an elimination rate constant of 0.110 h^{-1}.

3. *Compute the dose required to achieve desired vancomycin serum concentrations.*

The one-compartment model intravenous infusion equations used by the program to compute doses indicate that a dose of vancomycin 750 mg every 12 hours will produce a steady-state peak concentration of 23.4 μg/mL and a steady-state trough concentration of 7 μg/mL. Using the pharmacokinetic concepts method produced an answer for this patient of 1000 mg every 12 hours, whereas a dose of vancomycin 750 mg every 12 hours was computed using the one-compartment model parameter method.

9. The initial vancomycin dose for patient DG is calculated as follows.

Pharmacokinetic Dosing Method

1. *Estimate the creatinine clearance.*

This patient has a stable serum creatinine and is not obese. The Cockcroft–Gault equation can be used to estimate creatinine clearance:

$$CrCl_{est} = \{[(140 - age)BW]/(72 \cdot S_{Cr})\}0.85 = \{[(140 - 66\ y)65\ kg]/(72 \cdot 1.4\ mg/dL)\}0.85$$

$$CrCl_{est} = 14\ mL/min$$

Note: The patient's weight before ascites was used to compute $CrCl_{est}$, but the weight after ascites was used in the drug dose calculations because the extra ascitic fluid contributes to the volume of distribution.

2. *Estimate the vancomycin clearance.*

The vancomycin clearance versus creatinine clearance relationship is used to estimate the vancomycin clearance for this patient:

$$Cl = 0.695(CrCl) + 0.05 = 0.695[(41\ mL/min)/72\ kg] + 0.05 = 0.446\ mL/min/kg$$

3. *Estimate the vancomycin volume of distribution.*

The average volume of distribution for vancomycin is 0.7 L/kg:

$$V = 0.7\ L/kg \cdot 72\ kg = 50.4\ L$$

4. *Estimate the vancomycin elimination rate constant (k_e) and half-life ($t_{1/2}$).*

$$k_e = Cl/V = (0.446\ mL/min/kg \cdot 60\ min/h)/(0.7\ L/kg \cdot 1000\ mL/L) = 0.0382\ h^{-1}$$

$$t_{1/2} = 0.693/k_e = 0.693/0.0382\ h^{-1} = 18.1\ h$$

5. *Choose desired steady-state serum concentrations.*

$C_{min,ss} = 7\ \mu g/mL$ and $C_{max,ss} = 30\ \mu g/mL$ were chosen to treat this patient.

6. *Use the intravenous bolus equations to compute dose (see Table 5-2).*

Calculate the required dosage interval (τ):

$$\tau = (\ln C_{max,ss} - \ln C_{min,ss})/k_e = (\ln 30\ \mu g/mL - \ln 7\ \mu g/mL)/0.0382\ h^{-1} = 38.1\ h$$

Dosage intervals should be rounded to clinically acceptable intervals of 12 hours, 18 hours, 24 hours, 36 hours, 48 hours, 72 hours, and multiples of 24 hours thereafter, whenever possible. In this case, the dosage interval is rounded to 36 hours.

Calculate the required dose (D):

$$D = C_{max,ss} V(1 - e^{-k_e\tau}) = 30\ mg/L \cdot 50.4\ L\ (1 - e^{-(0.0382\ h^{-1})(36\ h)}) = 1130\ mg$$

Vancomycin doses should be rounded to the nearest 100 to 250 mg. This dose is rounded to 1250 mg. (Note: $\mu g/mL = mg/L$, and this concentration unit was substituted for $C_{max,ss}$ to avoid unnecessary unit conversion.)

The prescribed maintenance dosage is 1250 mg every 36 hours.

7. *Compute the loading dose, if needed.*

Loading doses should be considered for patients with creatinine clearance values lower than 60 mL/min. The administration of a loading dose allows achievement of therapeutic concentrations more quickly than if maintenance doses alone are given. However, because the pharmacokinetic parameters used to compute these initial doses are *estimated* values and not *actual* values, the patient's own parameters may be much different from the estimated constants and steady state will not be achieved until 3 to 5 half-lives have passed.

$$LD = C_{max,ss}\,V = 30\ mg/L \cdot 50.4\ L = 1512\ mg$$

As noted, this patient has moderate renal function (CrCl <60 mL/min), so a loading dose is prescribed and given as the first dose. Vancomycin doses should be rounded to the nearest 100 to 250 mg. This dose is rounded to 1500 mg. (Note: μg/mL = mg/L, and this concentration unit was substituted for $C_{max,ss}$ to avoid unnecessary unit conversion.) The first maintenance dose is given one dosage interval (36 hours) after the loading dose was administered.

Moellering Nomogram Method

1. *Estimate the creatinine clearance.*

This patient has a stable serum creatinine and is not obese. The Cockcroft–Gault equation can be used to estimate creatinine clearance:

$$CrCl_{est} = \{[(140 - age)BW]/(72 \cdot S_{Cr})\}0.85 = \{[(140 - 66\ y)65\ kg]/(72 \cdot 1.4\ mg/dL)\}0.85$$

$$CrCl_{est} = 41\ mL/min$$

Note: The patient's weight before ascites was used to compute $CrCl_{est}$, but the weight after ascites was used in the drug dose calculations because the extra ascitic fluid contributes to the volume of distribution.

2. *Determine the dosage interval and maintenance dosage.*

The maintenance dosage is calculated using the modified vancomycin dosing equation:

$$D\ (in\ mg/h/kg) = 0.626(CrCl\ in\ mL/min/kg) + 0.05$$

$$D = 0.626[(41\ mL/min)/72\ kg] + 0.05 = 0.407\ mg/h/kg$$

$$D = 0.407\ mg/h/kg \cdot 72\ kg = 29.3\ mg/h$$

The standard dose of 1000 mg can be used to gain an approximation for an acceptable dosage interval (τ):

$$\tau = 1000\ mg/(29.3\ mg/h) = 34.1\ h$$

Dosage intervals should be rounded to clinically acceptable intervals of 12 hours, 18 hours, 24 hours, 36 hours, 48 hours, 72 hours, and multiples of 24 hours thereafter, whenever possible. In this case, the dosage interval is rounded to 36 hours.

$$D = 29.3\ mg/h \cdot 36\ h = 1055\ mg$$

Vancomycin doses should be rounded to the nearest 100 to 250 mg. This dose is rounded to 1000 mg. The prescribed maintenance dosage is 1000 mg every 36 hours.

3. *Compute the loading dose.*

A loading dose of 15 mg/kg is suggested by the Moellering nomogram:

$$LD = 15 \text{ mg/kg}(72 \text{ kg}) = 1080 \text{ mg}$$

This loading dose is similar to the suggested maintenance dose, so is not prescribed.

Matzke Nomogram Method

1. *Estimate the creatinine clearance.*

This patient has a stable serum creatinine and is not obese. The Cockcroft–Gault equation can be used to estimate creatinine clearance:

$$CrCl_{est} = \{[(140 - \text{age})BW]/(72 \cdot S_{Cr})\}0.85 = \{[(140 - 66 \text{ y})65 \text{ kg}]/(72 \cdot 1.4 \text{ mg/dL})\}0.85$$

$$CrCl_{est} = 41 \text{ mL/min}$$

Note: The patient's weight before ascites was used to compute $CrCl_{est}$, but the weight after ascites was used in the drug dose calculations because the extra ascitic fluid contributes to the volume of distribution.

2. *Compute the loading dose (see Table 5-4).*

A loading dose of 25 mg/kg provides a peak concentration of 30 μg/mL.

$$LD = 25 \text{ mg/kg}(72 \text{ kg}) = 1800 \text{ mg, rounded to } 1750$$

3. *Determine the dosage interval and maintenance dose.*

According to the nomogram, the dosage interval is 1.5 days or 36 hours. The maintenance dose is 19 mg/kg · 72 kg = 1368 mg. Vancomycin doses should be rounded to the nearest 100 to 250 mg. This dose is rounded to 1250 mg and given one dosage interval (36 hours) after the loading dose.

The prescribed maintenance dosage is 1250 mg every 36 hours.

10. The revised vancomycin dose for patient DG is calculated as follows.

Linear Pharmacokinetics Method

1. *Estimate the creatinine clearance.*

This patient has a stable serum creatinine and is not obese. The Cockcroft–Gault equation can be used to estimate creatinine clearance:

$$CrCl_{est} = \{[(140 - \text{age})BW]/(72 \cdot S_{Cr})\}0.85 = \{[(140 - 66 \text{ y})65 \text{ kg}]/(72 \cdot 1.4 \text{ mg/dL})\}0.85$$

$$CrCl_{est} = 41 \text{ mL/min}$$

Note: The patient's weight before ascites was used to compute $CrCl_{est}$, but the weight after ascites was used in the drug dose calculations because the extra ascitic fluid contributes to the volume of distribution.

2. *Estimate the elimination rate constant (k_e) and half-life ($t_{1/2}$).*

The vancomycin clearance versus creatinine clearance relationship is used to estimate drug clearance for this patient:

$$Cl = 0.695(CrCl) + 0.05 = 0.695[(41 \text{ mL/min})/72 \text{ kg}] + 0.05 = 0.446 \text{ mL/min/kg}$$

The average volume of distribution for vancomycin is 0.7 L/kg:

$$V = 0.7 \text{ L/kg} \cdot 72 \text{ kg} = 50.4 \text{ L}$$

$$k_e = Cl/V = (0.446 \text{ mL/min/kg} \cdot 60 \text{ min/h})/(0.7 \text{ L/kg} \cdot 1000 \text{ mL/L}) = 0.0382 \text{ h}^{-1}$$

$$t_{1/2} = 0.693/k_e = 0.693/0.0382 \text{ h}^{-1} = 18.1 \text{ h}$$

Because the patient has been receiving vancomycin for >3 to 5 estimated half-lives, it is likely that the measured serum concentrations are steady-state values.

3. *Compute the new dose to achieve desired serum concentration.*

Computed by linear pharmacokinetics, the new dose to attain the desired concentration should be proportional to the old dose that produced the measured concentration:

$$D_{new} = (C_{ss,new}/C_{ss,old})D_{old} = [(7 \text{ μg/mL})/(4 \text{ μg/mL})] \text{ 1200 mg}$$
$$= 2100 \text{ mg, rounded to 2000 mg}$$

The new suggested dose is 2000 mg every 36 hours to be started at next scheduled dosing time.

4. *Check the steady-state peak concentration for the new dosage regimen.*

Using linear pharmacokinetics, the new steady-state concentration can be estimated and should be proportional to the old dose that produced the measured concentration:

$$C_{ss,new} = (D_{new}/D_{old})C_{ss,old} = (2000 \text{ mg}/1200 \text{ mg}) \text{ 17 μg/mL} = 28.3 \text{ μg/mL}$$

This steady-state peak concentration is safe and effective for the infection that is being treated.

11. The initial vancomycin dose for patient GG is calculated as follows.

Pharmacokinetic Dosing Method

1. *Estimate the creatinine clearance.*

This patient is not obese, but is in acute renal failure and receiving hemodialysis. Because dialysis removes creatinine, the serum creatinine cannot be used to estimate creatinine clearance for the patient. Since the renal function is poor enough to require dialysis, the creatinine clearance is assumed to be zero.

2. *Estimate the vancomycin clearance.*

The vancomycin clearance versus creatinine clearance relationship is used to estimate the vancomycin clearance for this patient:

$$Cl = 0.695(CrCl) + 0.05 = 0.695[(0 \text{ mL/min})/85 \text{ kg}] + 0.05 = 0.05 \text{ mL/min/kg}$$

3. *Estimate the vancomycin volume of distribution.*

The average volume of distribution for vancomycin is 0.7 L/kg:

$$V = 0.7 \text{ L/kg} \cdot 85 \text{ kg} = 59.5 \text{ L}$$

4. *Estimate the vancomycin elimination rate constant (k_e) and half-life ($t_{1/2}$).*

$$k_e = Cl/V = (0.05 \text{ mL/min/kg} \cdot 60 \text{ min/h})/(0.7 \text{ L/kg} \cdot 1000 \text{ mL/L}) = 0.0043 \text{ h}^{-1}$$

$$t_{1/2} = 0.693/k_e = 0.693/0.0043 \text{ h}^{-1} = 161 \text{ h}$$

5. *Choose desired steady-state serum concentrations.*

A $C_{min,ss}$ = 10 μg/mL and $C_{max,ss}$ = 40 μg/mL were chosen to treat this patient.

6. *Use the intravenous bolus equations to compute the dose (see Table 5-2).*

Calculate the required dosage interval (τ):

$$\tau = (\ln C_{max,ss} - \ln C_{min,ss})/k_e = (\ln 40 \text{ μg/mL} - \ln 10 \text{ μg/mL})/0.0043 \text{ h}^{-1} = 322 \text{ h}$$

Dosage intervals should be rounded to clinically acceptable intervals of 12 hours, 18 hours, 24 hours, 36 hours, 48 hours, 72 hours, and multiples of 24 hours thereafter, whenever possible. In this case, the dosage interval is rounded to 312 hours or 13 days.

Calculate the required dose (D):

$$D = C_{max,ss} V(1 - e^{-k_e \tau}) = 40 \text{ mg/L} \cdot 59.5 \text{ L } (1 - e^{-(0.0043 \text{ h}^{-1})(312 \text{ h})}) = 1759 \text{ mg}$$

Vancomycin doses should be rounded to the nearest 100 to 250 mg. This dose is rounded to 1750 mg. (Note: μg/mL = mg/L, and this concentration unit was substituted for $C_{max,ss}$ to avoid unnecessary unit conversion.)

The prescribed maintenance dose is 1750 mg every 13 days.

7. *Compute the loading dose, if needed.*

Loading doses should be considered for patients with creatinine clearance values lower than 60 mL/min. The administration of a loading dose allows achievement of therapeutic concentrations more quickly than if maintenance doses alone are given. However, because the pharmacokinetic parameters used to compute these initial doses are *estimated* values and not *actual* values, the patient's own parameters may be much different from the estimated constants, and steady-state will not be achieved until 3 to 5 half-lives have passed.

$$LD = C_{max,ss} V = 40 \text{ mg/L} \cdot 59.5 \text{ L} = 2380 \text{ mg}$$

As noted, this patient has poor renal function (CrCl <60 mL/min), so a loading dose is prescribed and given as the first dose. Vancomycin doses should be rounded to the nearest 100 to 250 mg. This dose is rounded to 2250 mg. (Note: μg/mL = mg/L, and this concentration unit was substituted for $C_{max,ss}$ to avoid unnecessary unit conversion.) The first maintenance dose is given one dosage interval (13 days) after the loading dose was administered. In this patient, only one dose may be needed if the infection resolves before a maintenance dose is due.

Moellering Nomogram Method

1. *Estimate the creatinine clearance.*

This patient is not obese but is in acute renal failure and receiving hemodialysis. Because dialysis removes creatinine, the serum creatinine cannot be used to estimate creatinine clearance for the patient. Since the patient's renal function is poor enough to require dialysis, the creatinine clearance is assumed to be zero.

2. *Determine the dosage interval and maintenance dose.*

The maintenance dose is calculated using the nomogram suggested dose for functionally anephric patients:

$$D = 1.9 \text{ mg/kg/24 h} \cdot \text{Wt}$$

$$D = 1.9 \text{ mg/kg/24 h} \cdot 85 \text{ kg} = 162 \text{ mg/24 h}$$

The standard dose of 2000 mg/24 h in patients with normal renal function can be used to gain an approximation for an acceptable dosage interval (τ):

$$\tau = (2000 \text{ mg})/(162 \text{ mg/d}) = 12.3 \text{ d}$$

Dosage intervals should be rounded to clinically acceptable intervals of 12 hours, 18 hours, 24 hours, 36 hours, 48 hours, 72 hours, and multiples of 24 hours thereafter, whenever possible. In this case, the dosage interval is rounded to 12 days.

$$D = 162 \text{ mg/d} \cdot 12 \text{ d} = 1944 \text{ mg}$$

Vancomycin doses should be rounded to the nearest 100 to 250 mg. This dose is rounded to 2000 mg. The prescribed maintenance dosage is 2000 mg every 12 days.

3. *Compute the loading dose.*

A loading dose of 15 mg/kg is suggested by the Moellering nomogram:

$$LD = 15 \text{ mg/kg}(85 \text{ kg}) = 1275 \text{ mg}$$

This loading dose is less than the suggested maintenance dosage, so it is not prescribed.

Matzke Nomogram Method

1. *Estimate the creatinine clearance.*

This patient is not obese, is in acute renal failure, and is receiving hemodialysis. Because dialysis removes creatinine, the serum creatinine cannot be used to estimate creatinine clearance for the patient. Since the patient's renal function is poor enough to require dialysis, the creatinine clearance is assumed to be zero.

2. *Compute the loading dose (see Table 5-4).*

A loading dose of 25 mg/kg provides a peak concentration of 30 μg/mL.

$$LD = 25 \text{ mg/kg}(85 \text{ kg}) = 2125 \text{ mg, rounded to } 2000$$

3. *Determine the dosage interval and maintenance dose.*

According to the nomogram, the dosage interval is 12 days. The maintenance dose is 19 mg/kg · 85 kg = 1615 mg. Vancomycin doses should be rounded to the nearest 100 to 250 mg. This dose is rounded to 1500 mg and is given one dosage interval (12 days) after the loading dose. In this patient, only one dose may be needed if the infection resolves before a maintenance dose is due.

The prescribed maintenance dosage is 1500 mg every 12 days.

12. The revised vancomycin dose for patient GG is calculated as follows.

After the first dose, this patient is not at steady state so none of the steady-state dosing methods are valid. Also, hemodialysis with a low-flux filter will not effect the elimination of the drug and is not a factor in calculating the drug dose.

One-Compartment Model Parameter Method

1. *Compute the patient's elimination rate constant and half-life (Table 5-2, single-dose equations. Note t′ = infusion time + waiting time of 1 hour and ½ hour, respectively).*

$$k_e = (\ln C_1 - \ln C_2)/\Delta t = (\ln 20 \ \mu g/mL - \ln 12.1 \ \mu g/mL)/(72 \text{ h}) = 0.0070 \text{ h}^{-1}$$

$$t_{1/2} = 0.693/k_e = 0.693/0.0070\text{h}^{-1} = 99.2 \text{ h}$$

2. *Compute the patient's volume of distribution.*

The vancomycin serum concentration needs to be extrapolated to the immediate post-dose time 36 hours previous to the first measured concentration before the volume of distribution can be calculated:

$$C_{max} = C/e^{-k_e t} = (20 \ \mu g/mL)/e^{-(0.0070 \text{ h}^{-1})(36 \text{ h})} = 25.7 \ \mu g/mL$$

$$V = D/C_{max} = 1600 \text{ mg}/(25.7 \text{ mg/L}) = 62.3 \text{ L}$$

3. *Choose new steady-state peak and trough concentrations.* For this example, the desired steady-state peak and trough concentrations are 40 μg/mL and 10 μg/mL, respectively.

4. *Determine the new dosage interval for the desired concentrations.* As in the initial dosage section of this chapter, the dosage interval (τ) is computed using the following equation:

$$\tau = (\ln C_{max,ss} - \ln C_{min,ss})/k_e = (\ln 40 \ \mu g/mL - \ln 10 \ \mu g/mL)/0.0070 \text{ h}^{-1}$$
$$= 198 \text{ h, rounded to } 192 \text{ h or } 8 \text{ d}$$

5. *Determine the new dose for the desired concentrations.* The dose is computed according to the one-compartment model intravenous bolus equation used in the initial dosing section of this chapter:

$$D = C_{max,ss} V(1 - e^{-k_e\tau}) = 40 \text{ mg/L} \cdot 58.8 \text{ L } (1 - e^{-(0.0070 \text{ h}^{-1})(192 \text{ h})})$$
$$= 1739 \text{ mg, rounded to } 1750 \text{ mg}$$

Vancomycin 1750 mg every 8 days is prescribed to begin 8 days after the last dose of the previous regimen. In this patient, it may not be necessary to administer a maintenance dose if the infection resolves before the next dose is due.

Bayesian Pharmacokinetics Computer Program Method

1. *Enter the patient's demographic, drug dosing, and serum concentration–time data into the computer program.*

2. *Compute the pharmacokinetic parameters for the patient using the Bayesian pharmacokinetics computer program.*

The pharmacokinetic parameters computed by the program are a volume of distribution of 60.9 L, a half-life of 108 hours, and an elimination rate constant of 0.0064 h^{-1}.

3. *Compute the dose required to achieve the desired vancomycin serum concentrations.*

The one-compartment model intravenous infusion equations used by the program to compute doses indicate that vancomycin 1250 mg every 7 days will produce a steady-state peak concentration of 31.3 μg/mL and a steady-state trough concentration of 10.4 μg/mL.

13. The revised vancomycin dose for patient FD is calculated as follows.

Bayesian Pharmacokinetics Computer Program Method

After the second dose, this patient is not at steady state, so none of the steady-state dosing methods is valid.

1. *Enter the patient's demographic, drug dosing, and serum concentration–time data into the computer program.*

2. *Compute the pharmacokinetic parameters for the patient using the Bayesian pharmacokinetics computer program.*

The pharmacokinetic parameters computed by the program are a volume of distribution of 63.1 L, a half-life of 38.1 hours, and an elimination rate constant of 0.0182 h^{-1}.

3. *Compute the dose required to achieve the desired vancomycin serum concentrations.*

The one-compartment model intravenous infusion equations used by the program to compute doses indicate that a dose of 1250 mg every 48 hours will produce a steady-state peak concentration of 33.7 μg/mL and a steady-state trough concentration of 14.4 μg/mL. Because the trough concentration selected is higher than the typical therapeutic range to enhance central nervous system penetration, the patient needs to be carefully monitored for drug-induced nephrotoxicity and ototoxicity.

14. The revised vancomycin dose for patient OI is calculated as follows.

Bayesian Pharmacokinetics Computer Program Method

After the second dose, this patient is not at steady state, so none of the steady-state dosing methods is valid.

1. *Enter the patient's demographic, drug dosing, and serum concentration–time data into the computer program.*

2. *Compute the pharmacokinetic parameters for the patient using the Bayesian pharmacokinetics computer program.*

The pharmacokinetic parameters computed by the program are a volume of distribution of 38 L, a half-life of 3.4 hours and an elimination rate constant of 0.203 h^{-1}.

3. *Compute the dose required to achieve the desired vancomycin serum concentrations.*

The one-compartment model intravenous infusion equations used by the program to compute doses indicate that a dose of 1000 mg every 8 hours will produce a steady-state peak concentration of 30 μg/mL and a steady-state trough concentration of 7.2 μg/mL.

15. The revised vancomycin dose for patient HY is calculated as follows.

Bayesian Pharmacokinetics Computer Program Method

After the first dose, this patient is not at steady state, so none of the steady-state dosing methods is valid.

1. *Enter the patient's demographic, drug dosing, and serum concentration–time data into the computer program.*

2. *Compute the pharmacokinetic parameters for the patient using the Bayesian pharmacokinetics computer program.*

The pharmacokinetic parameters computed by the program are a volume of distribution of 40.2 L, a half-life of 13.4 hours, and an elimination rate constant of 0.0517 h^{-1}.

3. *Compute the dose required to achieve desired vancomycin serum concentrations.*

The one-compartment model intravenous infusion equations used by the program to compute doses indicate that a dose of 1000 mg every 24 hours will produce a steady-state peak concentration of 33.7 μg/mL and a steady-state trough concentration of 10.5 μg/mL.

REFERENCES

1. Ackerman BH, Vannier AM, Eudy EB. Analysis of vancomycin time-kill studies with *Staphylococcus* species by using a curve stripping program to describe the relationship between concentration and pharmacodynamic response. Antimicrob Agents Chemother 1992;36: 1766–1769.
2. Louria DB, Kaminski T, Buchman J. Vancomycin in severe staphylococcal infections. Arch Intern Med 1961;107:225–240.
3. Kapusnik-Uner JE, Sande MA, Chambers HF. Antimicrobial agents: tetracyclines, chloramphenicol, erythromycin, and miscellaneous antibacterial agents. In: Hardman JG, Limbird LE, eds. Goodman & Gilman's The Pharmacological Basis of Therapeutics. New York: McGraw-Hill, 1996:1123–1154.
4. Kirby WMM, Perry DM, Bauer AW. Treatment of staphylococcal septicemia with vancomycin. N Engl J Med 1960;262:49–55.
5. Geraci JE, Heilman FR, Nichols DR, Wellman WE, Ross GT. Some laboratory and clinical experience with a new antibiotic vancomycin. Antibiotics Annual 1956-1957:90–106.
6. Young EJ, Ratner RE, Clarridge JE. Staphylococcal ventriculitis treated with vancomycin. South Med J 1981;74:1014–1015.
7. Gump DW. Vancomycin for treatment of bacterial meningitis. Rev Infect Dis 1981;3(suppl):S289–S292.
8. Bailie GR, Neal D. Vancomycin ototoxicity and nephrotoxicity. A review. Med Toxicol Adverse Drug Exp 1988;3:376–386.
9. Mellor JA, Kingdom J, Cafferkey M, Keane C. Vancomycin ototoxicity in patients with normal renal function. Br J Audiol 1984;18:179–180.
10. Welty TE, Copa AK. Impact of vancomycin therapeutic drug monitoring on patient care. Ann Pharmacother 1994;28:1335–1359.
11. Zimmermann AE, Katona BG, Plaisance KI. Association of vancomycin serum concentrations with outcomes in patients with gram-positive bacteremia. Pharmacotherapy 1995;15:85–91.
12. Cantu TG, Yamanaka-Yuen NA, Lietman PS. Serum vancomycin concentrations: reappraisal of their clinical value. Clin Infect Dis 1994;18:533–543.
13. Karam CM, McKinnon PS, Neuhauser MM, Rybak MJ. Outcome assessment of minimizing vancomycin monitoring and dosing adjustments. Pharmacotherapy 1999;19:257–266.
14. Saunders NJ. Why monitor peak vancomycin concentrations? Lancet 1994;344:1748–1750.
15. Kirby WMM, Divelbiss CL. Vancomycin: clinical and laboratory studies. Antibiotics Annual 1956-1957:107–117.
16. Spitzer PG, Eliopoulos GM. Systemic absorption of enteral vancomycin in a patient with pseudomembranous colitis. Ann Intern Med 1984;100:533–534.
17. Dudley MN, Quintiliani R, Nightingale CH, Gontarz N. Absorption of vancomycin [letter]. Ann Intern Med 1984;101:144.
18. Thompson CM, Jr, Long SS, Gilligan PH, Prebis JW. Absorption of oral vancomycin—possible associated toxicity. Int J Pediatr Nephrol 1983;4:1–4.
19. Matzke GR, Halstenson CE, Olson PL, Collins AJ, Abraham PA. Systemic absorption of oral vancomycin in patients with renal insufficiency and antibiotic-associated colitis. Am J Kidney Dis 1987;9:422–425.
20. Krogstad DJ, Moellering RC, Jr, Greenblatt DJ. Single-dose kinetics of intravenous vancomycin. J Clin Pharmacol 1980;20:197–201.
21. Bauer LA, Black DJ, Lill JS. Vancomycin dosing in morbidly obese patients. Eur J Clin Pharmacol 1998;54:621–625.

22. Blouin RA, Bauer LA, Miller DD, Record KE, Griffen WO, Jr. Vancomycin pharmacokinetics in normal and morbidly obese subjects. Antimicrob Agents Chemother 1982;21:575–580.
23. Moellering RC, Jr, Krogstad DJ, Greenblatt DJ. Vancomycin therapy in patients with impaired renal function: a nomogram for dosage. Ann Intern Med 1981;94:343–346.
24. Matzke GR, Kovarik JM, Rybak MJ, Boike SC. Evaluation of the vancomycin-clearance:creatinine-clearance relationship for predicting vancomycin dosage. Clin Pharm 1985;4:311–315.
25. Matzke GR, McGory RW, Halstenson CE, Keane WF. Pharmacokinetics of vancomycin in patients with various degrees of renal function. Antimicrob Agents Chemother 1984; 25:433–437.
26. Rybak MJ, Albrecht LM, Berman JR, Warbasse LH, Svensson CK. Vancomycin pharmacokinetics in burn patients and intravenous drug abusers. Antimicrob Agents Chemother 1990; 34:792–795.
27. Vance-Bryan K, Guay DR, Gilliland SS, Rodvold KA, Rotschafer JC. Effect of obesity on vancomycin pharmacokinetic parameters as determined by using a Bayesian forecasting technique. Antimicrob Agents Chemother 1993;37:436–440.
28. Ducharme MP, Slaughter RL, Edwards DJ. Vancomycin pharmacokinetics in a patient population: effect of age, gender, and body weight. Ther Drug Monit 1994;16:513–518.
29. Schaad UB, McCracken GH, Jr, Nelson JD. Clinical pharmacology and efficacy of vancomycin in pediatric patients. J Pediatr 1980;96:119–126.
30. Rodvold KA, Blum RA, Fischer JH, et al. Vancomycin pharmacokinetics in patients with various degrees of renal function. Antimicrob Agents Chemother 1988;32:848–852.
31. Tan CC, Lee HS, Ti TY, Lee EJC. Pharmacokinetics of intravenous vancomycin in patients with end-stage renal disease. Ther Drug Monitor 1990;12:29–34.
32. Pollard TA, Lampasona V, Akkerman S, et al. Vancomycin redistribution: dosing recommendations following high-flux hemodialysis. Kidney Int 1994;45:232–237.
33. Pancorbo S, Comty C. Peritoneal transport of vancomycin in 4 patients undergoing continuous ambulatory peritoneal dialysis. Nephron 1982;31:37–39.
34. Bunke CM, Aronoff GR, Brier ME, Sloan RS, Luft FC. Vancomycin kinetics during continuous ambulatory peritoneal dialysis. Clin Pharmacol Ther 1983;34:631–637.
35. Morse GD, Nairn DK, Walshe JJ. Once weekly intraperitoneal therapy for gram-positive peritonitis. Am J Kidney Dis 1987;10:300–305.
36. Rybak MJ, Albrecht LM, Boike SC, Chandrasekar PH. Nephrotoxicity of vancomycin, alone and with an aminoglycoside. J Antimicrob Chemother 1990;25:679–687.
37. Farber BF, Moellering RC, Jr. Retrospective study of the toxicity of preparations of vancomycin from 1974 to 1981. Antimicrob Agents Chemother 1983;23:138–141.
38. Angaran DM, Dias VC, Arom KV, et al. The comparative influence of prophylactic antibiotics on the prothrombin response to warfarin in the postoperative prosthetic cardiac valve patient. Cefamandole, cefazolin, vancomycin. Ann Surg 1987;206:155–161.
39. Murphy JE, Winter ME. Clinical pharmacokinetic pearls: bolus versus infusion equations. Pharmacotherapy 1996;16:698–700.
40. Black DJ. Modification of Moellering vancomycin clearance/creatinine clearance relationship to allow direct calculation of vancomycin doses (personal communication), 1993.
41. Cockcroft DW, Gault MH. Prediction of creatinine clearance from serum creatinine. Nephron 1976;16:31–41.
42. Salazar DE, Corcoran GB. Predicting creatinine clearance and renal drug clearance in obese patients from estimated fat-free body mass. Am J Med 1988;84:1053–1060.
43. McCormack JP, Carleton B. A simpler approach to pharmacokinetic dosage adjustments. Pharmacotherapy 1997;17:1349–1351.
44. Shargel L, Yu ABC. Applied biopharmaceutics and pharmacokinetics. Stamford, CT: Appleton & Lange, 1999.

45. Pryka RD, Rodvold KA, Garrison M, Rotschafer JC. Individualizing vancomycin dosage regimens: one- versus two-compartment Bayesian models. Ther Drug Monit 1989;11:450–454.
46. Rodvold KA, Pryka RD, Garrison M, Rotschafer JC. Evaluation of a two-compartment Bayesian forecasting program for predicting vancomycin concentrations. Ther Drug Monit 1989;11:269–275.
47. Rodvold KA, Rotschafer JC, Gilliland SS, Guay DR, Vance-Bryan K. Bayesian forecasting of serum vancomycin concentrations with non-steady-state sampling strategies. Ther Drug Monit 1994;16:37–41.
48. Wandell M, Mungall D. Computer assisted drug interpretation and drug regimen optimization. Am Assoc Clin Chem 1984;6:1–11.

Part III

CARDIOVASCULAR AGENTS

6

DIGOXIN

INTRODUCTION

Digoxin is the primary cardiac glycoside in clinical use. It is used for the treatment of congestive heart failure (CHF) because of its inotropic effects on the myocardium and for the treatment of atrial fibrillation because of its chronotropic effects on the electrophysiologic system of the heart. The role of digoxin in the treatment of each of these disease states has changed in recent years, because a better understanding of the pathophysiology of these conditions has been gained and new drug therapies have been developed.[1,2] For the treatment of chronic CHF, angiotensin I-converting enzyme inhibitors (ACE inhibitors) and diuretics are the primary pharmacotherapeutic agents, whereas the roles of angiotensin II receptor antagonists, spironolactone, and β-blockers continue to be developed.[3] For the treatment of acute or severe heart failure, agents that decrease cardiac preload (diuretics, nitrates) or afterload (vasodilators) and ACE inhibitors (which decrease both preload and afterload) are used in conjunction with potent intravenously administered inotropic agents (dobutamine, dopamine, adrenergic agonists) to balance the current cardiovascular status of the patient.[3] In either the acute or the severe heart failure situation, digoxin can be used when a mild inotropic or oral agent is needed.

If a patient presents with severe cardiovascular symptoms due to atrial fibrillation, direct-current cardioversion is a treatment option.[4] For atrial fibrillation with mild or no cardiovascular symptoms, many clinicians prefer to prescribe intravenous calcium channel blockers (diltiazem or verapamil) for the control of ventricular rate.[4] If atrial fibrillation is due to excessive adrenergic tone, intravenous β-blockers can also be used. Digoxin continues to be widely prescribed for the control of ventricular rate in patients with atrial fibrillation and can be an excellent choice if the patient has concurrent heart failure. After ventricular rate is controlled, the patient's heart may spontaneously revert to normal sinus rhythm; otherwise, electrical or pharmacologic cardioversion of atrial fibrillation may be necessary.

The positive inotropic effect of digoxin is caused by binding to sodium- and potassium-activated adenosine triphosphatase, also known as Na^+, K^+-ATPase or the sodium pump.[5] Digoxin-induced inhibition of Na^+, K^+-ATPase leads to decreased transport of sodium out of myocardial cells and increased intracellular sodium concentrations that aid calcium entry and decrease calcium elimination via the sodium-calcium exchanger. The increased intracellular calcium is stored in the endoplasmic reticulum so that action potential–induced calcium release is augmented, causing enhanced myocardial contractility. The chronotropic effects of digoxin are mediated via increased parasympathetic activity and vagal tone.

THERAPEUTIC AND TOXIC CONCENTRATIONS

When given as oral or intravenous doses, the serum digoxin concentration–time curve follows a two-compartment model and exhibits a long and large distribution phase of 8 to 12 hours[6–8] (Figure 6-1). During the distribution phase, digoxin in the serum is not in equilibrium with digoxin in the tissues, so digoxin serum concentrations should not be measured until the distribution phase is finished. When drug distribution is complete, digoxin serum and tissue concentrations are proportional to each other, so that digoxin serum con-

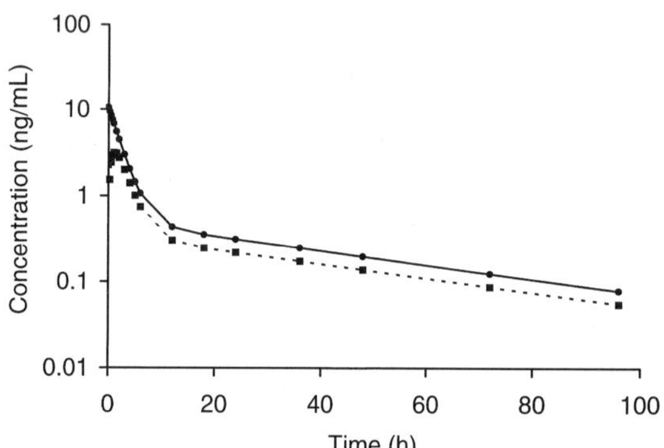

FIGURE 6-1 Digoxin serum concentrations after 250-μg doses given intravenously (*circles with solid line*) and orally as a tablet (*squares with dashed line*). After an intravenous dose, digoxin serum concentrations are very high, because all of the drug is initially contained in the blood. During the distribution phase, digoxin begins to move out of the vascular system into the tissues. It is also cleared from the body during this phase. Digoxin serum concentrations decline relatively rapidly over an 8- to 12-hour time period until the blood and tissues are in pseudoequilibrium with each other. During the elimination phase, digoxin serum concentrations in patients with good renal function (creatinine clearance >80 mL/min) decline with a half-life of about 36 hours. After oral tablet administration, about 70% of a digoxin dose is absorbed from the gastrointestinal tract. Maximum, or peak, concentrations occur about 1.5 to 2 hours after oral dosing with tablets, and the distribution phase still lasts 8 to 12 hours. During the elimination phase, intravenous and oral digoxin have the same terminal half-life.

centrations reflect concentrations at the site of action. When a digoxin serum concentration is very high but the patient is not exhibiting signs or symptoms of digitalis overdose, clinicians should consider the possibility that the blood sample for the determination of a digoxin serum concentration was obtained during the distribution phase, is too high because digoxin has not had the opportunity to diffuse out of the bloodstream into the myocardium, and is not reflective of myocardial tissue concentrations.

There is much inter- and intrapatient variability in the pharmacodynamic responses to digoxin. Clinically beneficial inotropic effects of digoxin are generally achieved at steady-state serum concentrations of 0.5 to 1 ng/mL.[9,10] Increasing steady-state serum concentrations to 1.2 to 1.5 ng/mL may provide some additional inotropic effect.[9,10] Chronotropic effects usually require higher digoxin steady-state serum concentrations of 0.8 to 1.5 ng/mL.[11,12] Additional chronotropic effects may be observed at digoxin steady-state serum concentrations as high as 2 ng/mL. Because of pharmacodynamic variability, clinicians should consider these ranges as initial guidelines and rely heavily on patient response to monitor digoxin therapy.

Steady-state digoxin serum concentrations higher than 2 ng/mL are associated with an increased incidence of adverse drug reactions. At digoxin concentrations of 2.5 ng/mL or higher, ~50% of all patients exhibit some form of digoxin toxicity.[13] Most digoxin side effects involve the gastrointestinal tract, central nervous system, or cardiovascular system.[14] Gastrointestinal-related adverse effects include anorexia, nausea, vomiting, diarrhea, abdominal pain, and constipation. Central nervous system side effects are headache, fatigue, insomnia, confusion, and vertigo. Visual disturbances can also occur and are manifested as blurred vision and changes in color vision or colored halos around objects, often involving the yellow-green spectrum. As can be appreciated, most of the gastrointestinal and central nervous system side effects of digoxin are nonspecific and could be caused by many different things. Because of this, clinicians should pay close attention to any new symptoms reported by patients receiving cardiac glycosides. Cardiac side effects commonly include second- or third-degree atrioventricular block, atrioventricular dissociation, bradycardia, premature ventricular contractions, and ventricular tachycardia. Rarely, almost every cardiac arrhythmia has been reported to occur because of digoxin toxicity. If a patient develops a new arrhythmia while receiving digoxin treatment, consideration should be given of the possibility that it is digoxin-induced. Also, note that relatively minor adverse effects such as nausea, headache, or changes in color vision may not occur in a patient before major cardiovascular side effects are found. In life-threatening digoxin overdose, digoxin antigen binding fragments or digoxin immune Fab (Digibind) are portions of digoxin-specific antibodies that can be used to rapidly reverse the adverse symptoms (see Special Dosing Considerations).

CLINICAL MONITORING PARAMETERS

In patients receiving digoxin for heart failure, the common signs and symptoms of CHF should be routinely monitored: left-sided failure—dyspnea on exertion, paroxysmal nocturnal dyspnea, orthopnea, tachypnea, cough, hemoptysis, pulmonary rales/edema, S_3 gallop, pleural effusion, Cheyne-Stokes respiration; right-sided failure—abdominal pain, anorexia, nausea, bloating, constipation, ascites, peripheral edema, jugular venous distention, hepatojugular reflux, hepatomegaly; general symptoms—fatigue, weakness, nocturia, central nervous system symptoms, tachycardia, pallor, digital cyanosis, cardiomegaly.[3] A very useful functional classification for heart failure patients proposed by the New York Heart Association (NYHA) is given in Table 6-1.

When used for the treatment of atrial fibrillation, digoxin does not stop atrial arrhythmia but is used to decrease or control the ventricular rate to an acceptable value (usually <100 beats/min).[4] The patient's pulse or ventricular rate should be monitored, and an electrocardiogram can be useful to clinicians who are able to interpret the output. Atrial fibrillation is characterized by 400 to 600 nonuniform atrial beats/min. Sinus rhythm is not restored with the use of digoxin alone, although atrial fibrillation can spontaneously remit. Depending on the symtomatology experienced by the patient, cardioversion can be attempted by using direct electrical current or by using an antiarrhythmic agent, such as quinidine, procainamide, or propafenone. Adequate anticoagulation to prevent thromboembolism is needed before cardioversion if atrial fibrillation has been present for longer than 48 hours. Before pharmacologic, also known as chemical, cardioversion is attempted, the patient should have received adequate digoxin therapy to control ventricular rate. Antiarrhythmic drugs alone to convert a patient from atrial fibrillation to normal sinus rhythm can result in a paroxysmal increase in aberrant impulses through the atrioventricular node and the development of ventricular arrhythmias.

Patients with severe heart disease such as coronary artery disease (angina, myocardial infarction) can have increased pharmacodynamic sensitivity to cardiac glycosides, and patients receiving these drugs should be monitored closely for adverse drug effects.[13,15] Also, augmented pharmacologic responses to digitalis derivatives occur with serum electrolyte disturbances such as hypokalemia, hypomagnesemia, and hypercalcemia, even though steady-state digoxin serum concentrations are in the therapeutic range.[5] Serum potassium concentrations should be routinely monitored in patients receiving digoxin and potassium-wasting diuretics. Potassium supplementation may be necessary in some of these patients. Also, many patients receiving digoxin and diuretics may be receiving ACE inhibitors, which can cause potassium retention. When a patient is receiving all three

TABLE 6-1 New York Heart Association (NYHA) Functional Classification for Heart Failure

CLASS	DESCRIPTION
I	Patients with cardiac disease but without limitations of physical activity. Ordinary physical activity does not cause undue fatigue, dyspnea, or palpitation.
II	Patients with cardiac disease that results in slight limitations of physical activity. Ordinary physical activity results in fatigue, palpitation, dyspnea, or angina.
III	Patients with cardiac disease that results in marked limitations of physical activity. Although patients are comfortable at rest, less than ordinary activity leads to symptoms.
IV	Patients with cardiac disease that results in an inability to carry on physical activity without discomfort. Symptoms of congestive heart failure are present even at rest. With any physical activity, increased discomfort is experienced.

From Johnson JA, Parker RB, Geraci SA. Heart failure. In: DiPiro JT, Talbert RL, Yee GC, Matzke GR, Wells BG, Posey LM, eds. Pharmacotherapy—a pathophysiologic approach. Stamford, CT: Appleton & Lange, 1999:153–181.

drugs, it can be difficult to reasonably ascertain what the patient's serum potassium status is without measuring it.

As an adjunct to the patient's clinical response, postdistribution (8 to 12 hours post-dose) steady-state digoxin serum concentrations can be measured 3 to 5 half-lives after a stable dose is initiated. Digoxin is primarily eliminated unchanged by the kidney (~75%), so its clearance is predominately influenced by renal function.[7,8] When stable, therapeutic steady-state digoxin serum concentrations and dosage levels have been established, serum creatinine measurements can be used to detect changes in renal function that may result in digoxin clearance and concentration alterations. Hospitalized patients with severe or acute heart failure may need to have serum creatinine determinations two to three times weekly to monitor renal function, whereas ambulatory patients with stable heart failure may need serum creatinine measurements yearly only.

BASIC CLINICAL PHARMACOKINETIC PARAMETERS

The primary route of digoxin elimination from the body is by the kidney via glomerular filtration as unchanged drug (~75%).[7,8] The remainder of a digoxin dose (~25%) is removed by hepatic metabolism or biliary excretion. Enterohepatic recirculation (reabsorption of drug from the gastrointestinal tract after elimination in the bile) of digoxin occurs.[16] Digoxin is given as an intravenous injection or orally as a tablet, capsule, or elixir. When given intravenously, digoxin doses should be infused over at least 5 to 10 minutes. Average bioavailability constants (F) for the tablet, capsule, and elixir are 0.7, 0.9, and 0.8, respectively.[17–22] P-glycoprotein appears to be involved as a transport protein in the renal tubular and biliary secretion of digoxin, and it may also interfere with the oral absorption of the drug. Digoxin is not usually administered intramuscularly owing to erratic absorption and severe pain at the injection site. Plasma protein binding is ~25% for digoxin.[23,24] Usual digoxin doses for adults are 250 μg/d (range, 125 to 500 μg/d) in patients with good renal function (creatinine clearance ≥80 mL/min) and 125 μg every 2 to 3 days in patients with renal dysfunction (creatinine clearance ≤15 mL/min).

EFFECTS OF DISEASE STATES AND CONDITIONS ON DIGOXIN PHARMACOKINETICS AND DOSING

Adults with normal renal function (creatinine clearance ≥80 mL/min; Table 6-2) have an average digoxin half-life of 36 hours (range, 24 to 48 hours) and volume of distribution of 7 L/kg (range, 5 to 9 L/kg).[25,26] The volume of distribution is large because of the extensive tissue binding of digoxin in the body. Digoxin pharmacokinetics are not effected by obesity (>30% over ideal body weight), so volume of distribution and dosage estimates should be based on ideal body weight.[27,28]

Because digoxin is principally eliminated by the kidney, renal dysfunction is the most important disease state that affects digoxin pharmacokinetics.[8] The digoxin clearance rate decreases in proportion to creatinine clearance, and this relationship is used to aid in the computation of initial doses later in this chapter (Figure 6-2). The equation that estimates digoxin clearance from creatinine clearance is $Cl = 1.303\ (CrCl) + Cl_{NR}$, where Cl is digoxin clearance in milliliters per minute (mL/min), CrCl is creatinine clearance in

TABLE 6-2 Disease States and Conditions That Alter Digoxin Pharmacokinetics

DISEASE STATE/ CONDITION	HALF-LIFE	VOLUME OF DISTRIBUTION (L/kg)	COMMENT
Adult, normal renal function	36 hours or 1.5 days (range, 24–48 hours)	7 (range, 5–9)	Usual dose 250 μg/d (range, 125–500 μg/d), resulting in total body stores of 8–12 μg/kg for heart failure or 13–15 μg/kg for atrial fibrillation. Digoxin is eliminated ~75% unchanged renally/~25% nonrenally.
Adult, renal failure	120 hours or 5 days	4.5 $V = \left(226 + \frac{298 \cdot CrCl}{29.1 + CrCl}\right) \cdot (Wt/70)$ where V is digoxin volume of distribution in L/70 kg, Wt is body weight in kg (use ideal body weight if >30% overweight) and CrCl is creatinine clearance in mL/min.	Renal failure patients have decreased digoxin clearance and volume of distribution. As a result, half-life is not as long as might be expected ($t_{1/2}$ = [0.693V]/Cl). Digoxin total body stores decrease to 6–10 μg/kg because of reduced volume of distribution.
Moderate to severe heart failure	See comments.	7	Heart failure patients (NYHA III–IV) have decreased cardiac output, which causes decreased liver blood flow and digoxin hepatic clearance. In patients with good renal function (creatinine clearance >80 mL/min), the effect on digoxin total clearance is negligible. But in patients with poor renal function (creatinine clearance <30 mL/min), nonrenal clearance is a primary elimination pathway.
Obesity (>30% over IBW) with normal renal function	36 hours or 1.5 days	V = 7 L/kg IBW	Digoxin does not distribute to adipose tissue, so volume of distribution calculations should be conducted with IBW.

TABLE 6-2 ***(Continued)***

DISEASE STATE/ CONDITION	HALF-LIFE	VOLUME OF DISTRIBUTION (L/kg)	COMMENT
Hyperthyroidism with normal renal function	24 hours or 1 day	7	Hyperthyroid patients are hypermetabolic and have higher digoxin renal and nonrenal clearances.

IBW = ideal body weight; NYHA = New York Heart Association.

mL/min, and Cl_{NR} is digoxin clearance by nonrenal routes of elimination of 40 mL/min in patients with no or mild heart failure (NYHA CHF class I or II; see Table 6-1).[8] Digoxin volume of distribution, in addition to clearance, decreases with declining renal function.[6,29] Although the mechanism for this change is not as well understood, digoxin is likely displaced from tissue binding sites by an unknown substance or substances in patients with renal dysfunction, so that drug that would have been bound to tissues becomes unbound. Unbound digoxin molecules displaced from tissue binding sites move into the blood causing the decreased volume of distribution [$\downarrow V = V_b + (f_b/\uparrow f_t)\ V_t$, where V is digoxin volume of distribution, V_b is blood volume, V_t is tissue volume, f_b is the unbound fraction of digoxin in the blood, and f_t is the unbound fraction of digoxin in the tissues]. The equation that estimates digoxin volume of distribution using creatinine clearance is:

$$V = (226 + \frac{298 \cdot CrCl}{29.1 + CrCl})\ (Wt/70)$$

where V is digoxin volume of distribution in liters per 70 kg, Wt is body weight in kg (use ideal body weight if >30% overweight), and CrCl is creatinine clearance in mL/min.[29] Because digoxin volume of distribution and clearance decrease simultaneously

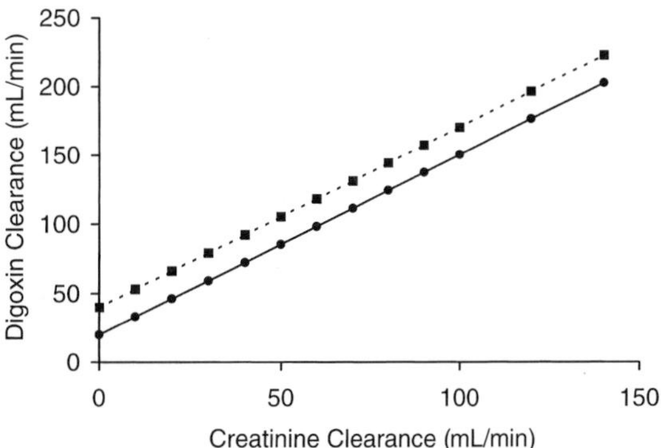

FIGURE 6-2 Digoxin clearance is proportional to creatinine clearance for patients with (*circles with solid line:* Cl = 1.303[CrCl] + 20) and without (*squares with dashed line:* Cl = 1.303[CrCl] + 40) moderate to severe (New York Heart Association class III or IV) heart failure. Nonrenal clearance (y-intercept) is lower for patients with moderate to severe heart failure, because reduced cardiac output results in decreased liver blood flow and digoxin hepatic clearance.

in patients with renal failure, the average half-life for digoxin of 5 days is shorter than what might be expected if clearance alone decreased [$t_{1/2} = (0.693 \cdot V)/Cl$]. Digoxin is not significantly eliminated by hemodialysis or peritoneal dialysis.[25,26]

Heart failure decreases cardiac output, which in turn decreases liver blood flow. Liver blood flow is an important factor in the determination of hepatic clearance for drugs, because it is the vehicle that delivers drug molecules to the liver for possible elimination. Moderate-severe heart failure (NYHA CHF class III or IV; see Table 6-1) decreases the hepatic clearance of digoxin by this mechanism.[8] When estimating digoxin clearance for computing initial drug doses, it is necessary to decrease the nonrenal clearance (Cl_{NR}) factor to 20 mL/min in the equation to compensate for decreased hepatic clearance: Cl = 1.303 (CrCl) + 20, where Cl is digoxin clearance in mL/min, CrCl is creatinine clearance in mL/min, and 20 is digoxin nonrenal clearance Cl_{NR} in mL/min.

Thyroid hormone regulates basal metabolic rate, and thyroid status influences every major organ system in the body, including the heart (heart rate and cardiac output), liver (liver blood flow and microsomal drug-metabolizing enzyme function), and kidney (renal blood flow and glomerular filtration rate). Patients who are hypothyroid have slower metabolic rates and eliminate digoxin more slowly than euthyroid patients ($t_{1/2}$ = 48 hours with normal renal function).[25,26,30–32] Hyperthyroid patients have faster metabolic rates and eliminate digoxin faster than euthyroid patients ($t_{1/2}$ = 24 hours with normal renal function).[25,26,30–32] Hyperthyroid patients can present with atrial fibrillation, which may be treated with digoxin. Generally, such patients require higher doses of digoxin to control ventricular rate because of the increase in digoxin clearance.

As with other drugs, digoxin clearance is lower in neonates and premature infants because renal and hepatic functions are not completely developed.[33,34] Premature infants and neonates have average digoxin half-lives of 60 hours and 45 hours, respectively. In older babies and young children (6 months to 8 years old), renal and hepatic functions are fully developed and half-lives can be as short as 18 hours. Older children (≥12 years old) have mean digoxin half-lives ($t_{1/2}$ = 36 hours) that are similar to those found in adults. Also, volume of distribution is larger in infants and children compared with that in adults, as found with many other drugs.

Malabsorption of oral digoxin has been reported in patients with severe diarrhea, radiation treatments to the abdomen, and gastrointestinal hypermotility.[30,35–39] In these cases, steady-state digoxin serum concentrations decrease because of poor bioavailability of the drug.

DRUG INTERACTIONS

Digoxin has numerous drug interactions with other agents. Because of this, only the most common and severe drug interactions are discussed. Clinicians should consult a current drug interaction reference when other medications are prescribed to patients receiving digoxin therapy. Quinidine decreases both the renal and nonrenal clearance of digoxin and also decreases the volume of distribution of digoxin.[40–45] Inhibition of P-glycoprotein, a drug efflux pump found in the kidney, liver, and intestine, may be involved in this interaction.[46] The result of this complex interaction is that concurrent quinidine therapy increases the average steady-state digoxin concentration by 30% to 70%. Verapamil, diltiazem, and bepridil inhibit digoxin clearance and increase mean digoxin steady-state concentrations by various degrees.[45,47–52] Of these calcium channel blockers, verapamil is the most potent inhibitor of digoxin clearance and increases digoxin steady-state serum concentrations up to 70%. Diltiazem and bepridil therapy each increase average digoxin steady-state serum concentrations by about 30%.

Amiodarone[53–56] and propafenone[57–59] are newer antiarrhythmic agents that decrease digoxin clearance. In addition to this drug interaction mechanism, amiodarone simultaneously increases digoxin oral bioavailability. Digoxin steady-state serum concentrations increase two to three times over baseline values with concomitant amiodarone therapy. Because amiodarone has a very long half-life (~50 days), the onset of the drug interaction with digoxin can be very long. As serum concentrations of amiodarone slowly increase and approach steady-state values, digoxin clearance and bioavailability are simultaneously slowly changing. The insidious nature of the amiodarone–digoxin drug interaction can make it difficult to detect in patients. Propafenone therapy increases mean digoxin steady-state concentrations by 30% to 60% in a dose-dependent fashion with propafenone doses of 450 mg/d, causing digoxin concentration changes in the lower end of the range, and propafenone doses of 900 mg/d, causing digoxin concentration changes in the upper end of the range.

Cyclosporine therapy has been reported to increase average steady-state digoxin concentrations up to 50%.[60] Although the mechanism is unknown, it is likely due to either a cyclosporine-induced decrease in glomerular filtration rate or hepatic enzyme inhibition.

About 10% of patients receiving digoxin therapy have significant amounts of *Eubacterium letum* in their gastrointestinal tract, which metabolizes orally administered digoxin before it can be absorbed.[61,62] Erythromycin, clarithromycin, and tetracycline can kill this bacterium.[63–68] Digoxin steady-state serum concentrations increase an average of 30% in these patients when one of the three latter antibiotics have been prescribed. P-glycoprotein inhibition may be one of the mechanisms involved with this interaction involving macrolide antibiotics.[68]

The absorption of oral digoxin from the gastrointestinal tract is influenced by many different compounds. Aluminum-containing antacids and kaolin-pectin physically adsorb digoxin and rend it unabsorbable.[69] These compounds should be administered no closer than 2 hours before or after an oral digoxin dose. Similarly, cholestyramine also reduces digoxin oral bioavailability by binding it in the gastrointestinal tract and should be given no closer than 8 hours before or after an oral digoxin dose.[70,71] Sulfasalazine and neomycin each decrease digoxin oral bioavailability by unknown mechanisms.[72,73] Propantheline increases oral digoxin bioavailability by prolonging gastrointestinal transit time, whereas metoclopramide and cisapride decreases oral digoxin bioavailability by decreasing gastrointestinal transit time.[71,74,75]

INITIAL DOSAGE DETERMINATION METHODS

Pharmacokinetic Dosing Method

The goal of initial dosing of digoxin is to compute the best dose possible for the patient given the set of disease states and conditions that influence digoxin pharmacokinetics and the cardiovascular disorder being treated. To do this, pharmacokinetic parameters for the patient are estimated using average parameters measured in other patients with similar disease states and condition profiles. This approach is also known as the Jusko-Koup method of digoxin dosing.[8,29]

ESTIMATE OF CLEARANCE

Digoxin is predominantly eliminated unchanged in the urine, and there is a good relationship between creatinine clearance and digoxin clearance (see Figure 6-2). This relationship allows digoxin clearance to be estimated for a patient, which can be used to compute an initial dose of the cardiac glycoside. Mathematically, the equation for the straight line shown in Figure 6-2 is $Cl = 1.303(CrCl) + Cl_{NR}$, where Cl is the digoxin clearance in mL/min, CrCl is creatinine clearance in mL/min, and Cl_{NR} is digoxin nonrenal clearance.[8] A digoxin nonrenal clearance value of 40 mL/min is used for patients who do not have heart failure or who have only mild signs and symptoms of heart failure (NYHA CHF class I or II). Patients with moderate or severe heart failure (NYHA CHF class III or IV) have significant decreases in cardiac output, which leads to a reduction in liver blood flow and digoxin hepatic clearance. In these cases, digoxin nonrenal clearance is set at 20 mL/min in the equation. For example, the estimated digoxin clearance for a person with a creatinine clearance of 10 mL/min is 53 mL/min if the patient has no or mild symptoms of heart failure [Cl = 1.303(10 mL/min) + 40 = 53 mL/min] or 33 mL/min if the patient has moderate to severe symptoms of heart failure [Cl = 1.303(10 mL/min) + 20 = 33 mL/min]. Taking a patient's renal function into account when deriving initial doses of digoxin is the single most important characteristic to assess.

ESTIMATE OF VOLUME OF DISTRIBUTION

The average volume of distribution for patients without disease states and conditions that change this parameter is 7 L/kg.[25,26] Because obesity does not change digoxin volume of distribution, the weight factor used in this calculation is ideal body weight (IBW) for patients who are significantly overweight (>30% over IBW).[27,28] Thus, for a 70-kg patient with good renal function, the estimated volume of distribution is 490 L (V = 7 L/kg · 70 kg = 490 L). If a patient weighs less than their ideal body weight, actual body weight is used to estimate volume of distribution. For patients whose weight is between their ideal body weight and 30% over ideal weight, actual body weight can be used to compute estimated volume of distribution, although some clinicians prefer to use ideal body weight. In patients who are more than 30% above their ideal body weight, volume of distribution (V) estimates should be based on ideal body weight. For an obese patient with normal renal function whose ideal body weight is 55 kg and total body weight is 95 kg, the estimated volume of distribution would be 385 L: V = 7 L/kg · IBW = 7 L/kg (55 kg) = 385 L.

For patients with renal dysfunction (creatinine clearance ≤30 mL/min), creatinine clearance should be used to provide an improved volume of distribution estimate (V in L) using the following formula:

$$V = \left(226 + \frac{298 \cdot CrCl}{29.1 + CrCl}\right)(Wt/70)$$

where CrCl is the patient's creatinine clearance in mL/min.[29] For example, a 70-kg patient with significant renal dysfunction (CrCl = 10 mL/min) is to receive a loading dose of digoxin, and an estimate of digoxin volume of distribution is needed. The estimated volume of distribution for this patient would be 302 L:

$$V = \left(226 + \frac{298 \cdot CrCl}{29.1 + CrCl}\right)(Wt/70) = \left(226 + \frac{298 \cdot 10\ mL/min}{29.1 + 10\ mL/min}\right)(70\ kg/70) = 302\ L$$

In patients who are more than 30% above their ideal body weight, volume of distribution (V) estimates should be based on ideal body weight, so the weight factor used in the equation would be IBW.

SELECTION OF APPROPRIATE PHARMACOKINETIC MODEL AND EQUATIONS

When given by intravenous injection or orally, digoxin follows a two-compartment pharmacokinetic model (see Figure 6-1). After the end of intravenous infusion or after peak concentration has been reached after an oral dose, serum concentrations drop over an 8- to 12-hour period because of distribution of drug from blood to tissues (α or distribution phase). After distribution of digoxin is complete, drug concentrations decline more slowly, and the elimination rate constant for this segment of the concentration–time curve is the one that varies with renal function (β or elimination phase). Although this model is the most correct from a strict pharmacokinetic viewpoint, it cannot easily be used clinically because of its mathematical complexity. During the elimination phase of the concentration–time curve, digoxin serum concentrations drop very slowly owing to the long elimination half-life (36 hours with normal renal function, 5 days with end-stage renal disease). Because of this, a very simple pharmacokinetic equation that computes the average digoxin steady-state serum concentration (Css in ng/mL = μg/L) is widely used and allows maintenance dosage calculation: $Css = [F(D/\tau)]/Cl$ or $D/\tau = (Css \cdot Cl)/F$, where F is the bioavailability fraction for the oral dosage form (F = 1 for intravenous digoxin), D is the digoxin dose in micrograms (μg), τ is the dosage interval in days, and Cl is digoxin clearance in L/d.[8,29]

The equation to calculate loading dose (LD in μg) is based on a simple one-compartment model: $LD = (Css \cdot V)/F$, where Css is the desired digoxin steady-state concentration in μg/L, which is equivalent to ng/mL; V is the digoxin volume of distribution; and F is the bioavailability fraction for the oral dosage form (F = 1 for intravenous digoxin). When digoxin loading doses are administered, they are usually given in divided doses separated by 4 to 6 hours (50% of dose first, followed by two additional doses of 25%). A portion of the loading dose can be withheld if the patient experiences any digoxin adverse effects, such as a low pulse rate. This technique is used to allow the assessment of clinical response before additional digoxin is given to avoid accidental overdosage.

STEADY-STATE CONCENTRATION SELECTION

Digoxin steady-state concentrations are selected based on the cardiovascular disease being treated. For heart failure, steady-state serum concentrations of 0.5 to 1 ng/mL are usually effective.[9,10] For initial dosing purposes, a target digoxin concentration of 0.8 ng/mL is reasonable. For patients with atrial fibrillation, steady-state serum concentrations of 0.8 to 1.5 ng/mL are usually needed to control the ventricular rate to 100 beats/min or less.[11,26] An initial target digoxin concentration of 1.2 ng/mL is reasonable for patients with this disease state.

Example 1 MJ is a 50-year-old, 70-kg, 178-cm (70-in) male with atrial fibrillation for less than 24 hours. His serum creatinine is 0.9 mg/dL, which has been stable over the last 5 days since admission. Compute an intravenous digoxin dose for this patient to control ventricular rate.

1. *Estimate the creatinine clearance.*

This patient has a stable serum creatinine and is not obese. The Cockcroft–Gault equation can be used to estimate creatinine clearance:

$$CrCl_{est} = [(140 - age)BW]/(72 \cdot S_{Cr}) = [(140 - 50\ y)70\ kg]/(72 \cdot 0.9\ mg/dL)$$

$$CrCl_{est} = 97\ mL/min$$

2. *Estimate the digoxin clearance.*

The drug clearance versus creatinine clearance relationship is used to estimate the digoxin clearance for this patient (Cl_{NR} = 40 mL/min, since the patient does not have moderate to severe heart failure):

$$Cl = 1.303\ (CrCl) + Cl_{NR} = 1.303(97\ mL/min) + 40\ mL/min = 167\ mL/min$$

3. *Use the average steady-state concentration equation to compute digoxin maintenance dose.*

For a patient with atrial fibrillation the desired digoxin concentration is 0.8 to 1.5 ng/mL. A serum concentration of 1.2 ng/mL is chosen for this patient, and intravenous digoxin is used (F = 1). Note that concentration units are ng/mL = μg/L, and this conversion is made before the equation is used. Also, conversion factors are needed to change milliliters to liters (1000 ml/L) and minutes to days (1440 min/d):

$$MD/\tau = (Css \cdot Cl)/F = (1.2\ \mu g/L \cdot 167\ mL/min \cdot 1440\ min/d)/(1 \cdot 1000\ mL/L)$$
$$= 288\ \mu g/d, \text{ rounded to } 250\ \mu g/d$$

4. *Use the loading dose equation to compute the digoxin loading dose (if needed).*

The patient has good renal function and is not obese. Therefore, a volume of distribution of 7 L/kg and actual body weight can be used to compute the digoxin loading dose. An intravenous loading dose (F = 1) can be used in this patient to achieve the desired pharmacologic effect quicker than would occur if maintenance doses alone were used and concentrations were allowed to accumulate over 3 to 5 half-lives.

$$V = 7\ L/kg \cdot 70\ kg = 490\ L$$

$$LD = (Css \cdot V)/F = (1.2\ \mu g/L \cdot 490\ L)/1 = 588\ \mu g, \text{ rounded to } 500\ \mu g$$

When digoxin loading doses are administered, they are usually given in divided doses separated by 4 to 6 hours (50% of dose at first, followed by two additional doses of 25%). In this case, an initial intravenous dose of 250 μg is given, followed by two additional intravenous doses of 125 μg each. One of the loading doses can be withheld if pulse rate is less than 50 to 60 beats/min or if other undesirable digoxin adverse effects are noted.

Example 2 Same patient profile as in example 1, but serum creatinine is 3.5 mg/dL, indicating renal impairment.

1. *Estimate the creatinine clearance.*

This patient has a stable serum creatinine and is not obese. The Cockcroft–Gault equation can be used to estimate creatinine clearance:

$$CrCl_{est} = [(140 - age)BW]/(72 \cdot S_{Cr}) = [(140 - 50\ y)70\ kg]/(72 \cdot 3.5\ mg/dL)$$

$$CrCl_{est} = 25\ mL/min$$

2. *Estimate the digoxin clearance.*

The drug clearance versus creatinine clearance relationship is used to estimate the digoxin clearance for this patient (Cl_{NR} = 40 mL/min, because the patient does not have moderate to severe heart failure):

$$Cl = 1.303\ (CrCl) + Cl_{NR} = 1.303(25\ mL/min) + 40\ mL/min = 73\ mL/min$$

3. *Use the average steady-state concentration equation to compute the digoxin maintenance dose.*

For a patient with atrial fibrillation, the desired digoxin concentration is 0.8 to 1.5 ng/mL. A serum concentration of 1.2 ng/mL is chosen for this patient, and intravenous digoxin is used (F = 1). Note that concentration units are ng/mL = μg/L, and this conversion is made before the equation is used. Also, conversion factors are needed to change milliliters to liters (1000 mL/L) and minutes to days (1440 min/d):

$$MD/\tau = (Css \cdot Cl)/F = (1.2\ \mu g/L \cdot 73\ mL/min \cdot 1440\ min/d)/(1 \cdot 1000\ mL/L) = 125\ \mu g/d$$

4. *Use the loading dose equation to compute the digoxin loading dose (if needed).*

The patient has poor renal function and is not obese. Therefore, the volume of distribution equation that adjusts the parameter estimate for renal dysfunction can be used to compute the digoxin loading dose. An intravenous loading dose (F = 1) can be given to achieve the desired pharmacologic effect more quickly than if maintenance doses alone were used to allow concentrations to accumulate over 3 to 5 half-lives.

$$V = (226 + \frac{298 \cdot CrCl}{29.1 + CrCl})\ (Wt/70) = (226 + \frac{298 \cdot 25\ mL/min}{29.1 + 25\ mL/min})(70\ kg/70) = 364\ L$$

$$LD = (Css \cdot V)/F = (1.2\ \mu g/L \cdot 364\ L)/1 = 437\ \mu g, \text{ rounded to } 400\ \mu g$$

When digoxin loading doses are administered, they are usually given in divided doses separated by 4 to 6 hours (50% of dose first, followed by two additional doses of 25%). In this case, an initial intravenous dose of 200 μg is given, followed by two additional intravenous doses of 100 μg each. One of the loading doses can be withheld if pulse rate is less than 50 to 60 beats/min or if other undesirable digoxin adverse effects are noted.

Example 3 Same patient profile as in example 1, but serum creatinine is 3.5 mg/dL, indicating renal impairment. In addition, the patient is being treated for NYHA class III moderate heart failure, not atrial fibrillation. Compute an oral digoxin tablet maintenance dose for this patient.

1. *Estimate the creatinine clearance.*

This patient has a stable serum creatinine and is not obese. The Cockcroft–Gault equation can be used to estimate creatinine clearance:

$$CrCl_{est} = [(140 - age)BW]/(72 \cdot S_{Cr}) = [(140 - 50\ y)70\ kg]/(72 \cdot 3.5\ mg/dL)$$

$$CrCl_{est} = 25\ mL/min$$

2. *Estimate the digoxin clearance.*

The drug clearance versus creatinine clearance relationship is used to estimate the digoxin clearance (Cl_{NR} = 20 mL/min, since the patient has moderate heart failure):

$$Cl = 1.303\ (CrCl) + Cl_{NR} = 1.303(25\ mL/min) + 20\ mL/min = 53\ mL/min$$

3. *Use the average steady-state concentration equation to compute the digoxin maintenance dose.*

For a patient with heart failure, the desired digoxin concentration is 0.5 to 1 ng/mL. A serum concentration of 0.8 ng/mL is chosen for this patient, and oral digoxin is used (F = 0.7). Note that concentration units are ng/mL = μg/L, and this conversion is made before the equation is used. Also, conversion factors are needed to change milliliters to liters (1000 mL/L) and minutes to days (1440 min/d):

$$MD/\tau = (Css \cdot Cl)/F = (0.8\ \mu g/L \cdot 53\ mL/min \cdot 1440\ min/d)/(0.7 \cdot 1000\ mL/L) = 87\ \mu g/d, \text{ or } 174\ \mu g \text{ every 2 days (i.e., } 87\ \mu g/d \cdot 2\ d = 174\ \mu g \text{ every 2 days).}$$

This oral tablet dose is rounded to 125 μg every other day.

Example 4 OI is a 65-year-old, 170-kg, 165-cm (65-in) female with NYHA class III moderate heart failure. Her serum creatinine is 4.7 mg/dL and stable. Compute an intravenous digoxin loading and maintenance dose for this patient.

1. *Estimate the creatinine clearance.*

This patient has a stable serum creatinine and is obese [$IBW_{females}$ (in kg) = 45 + 2.3(Ht – 60 in) = 45 + 2.3(65 – 60) = 57 kg]. The Salazar and Corcoran equation can be used to estimate creatinine clearance:

$$CrCl_{est(females)} = \frac{(146 - age)[(0.287 \cdot Wt) + (9.74 \cdot Ht^2)]}{(60 \cdot S_{Cr})}$$

$$CrCl_{est(females)} = \frac{(146 - 65\ y)\{(0.287 \cdot 170\ kg) + [9.74 \cdot (1.65\ m)^2]\}}{(60 \cdot 4.7\ mg/dL)} = 22\ mL/min$$

Note: Height is converted from inches to meters: Ht = (65 in · 2.54 cm/in)/(100 cm/m) = 1.65 m.

2. *Estimate the digoxin clearance.*

The drug clearance versus creatinine clearance relationship is used to estimate the digoxin clearance (Cl_{NR} = 20 mL/min, since the patient has moderate to severe heart failure):

$$Cl = 1.303\ (CrCl) + Cl_{NR} = 1.303(22\ mL/min) + 20\ mL/min = 48\ mL/min$$

3. *Use the average steady-state concentration equation to compute the digoxin maintenance dose.*

For a patient with heart failure, the desired digoxin concentration is 0.5 to 1 ng/mL. A serum concentration of 0.8 ng/mL is chosen, and intravenous digoxin is used (F = 1). Note that concentration units are ng/mL = μg/L, and this conversion is made before the equation is used. Also, conversion factors are needed to change milliliters to liters (1000 mL/L) and minutes to days (1440 min/d):

$$MD/\tau = (Css \cdot Cl)/F = (0.8\ \mu g/L \cdot 48\ mL/min \cdot 1440\ min/d)/(1 \cdot 1000\ mL/L) = 55\ \mu g/d, \text{ or } 110\ \mu g \text{ every 2 days (i.e., } 55\ \mu g/d \cdot 2\ d = 110\ \mu g \text{ every 2 days)}.$$

This intravenous dose is rounded to 125 μg every other day.

4. *Use the loading dose equation to compute the digoxin loading dose (if needed).*

The patient has poor renal function and is obese. Therefore, the volume of distribution equation that adjusts the parameter estimate for renal dysfunction can be used to compute the digoxin loading dose, and ideal body weight is used as the weight factor. An intravenous loading dose (F = 1) can be given to achieve the desired pharmacologic effect more quickly than if maintenance doses alone were used to allow concentrations to accumulate over 3 to 5 half-lives.

$$V = (226 + \frac{298 \cdot CrCl}{29.1 + CrCl})(Wt/70) = (226 + \frac{298 \cdot 22\ mL/min}{29.1 + 22\ mL/min})(57\ kg/70) = 288\ L$$

$$LD = (Css \cdot V)/F = (0.8\ \mu g/L \cdot 288\ L)/1 = 230\ \mu g, \text{ rounded to } 250\ \mu g$$

When digoxin loading doses are administered, they are usually given in divided doses separated by 4 to 6 hours (50% of dose first, followed by two additional doses of 25%). In this case, an initial intravenous dose of 125 μg is given, followed by two additional intravenous doses of 62.5 μg each. One of the loading doses can be withheld if pulse rate is less than 50 to 60 beats/min or other undesirable digoxin adverse effects are noted.

Jelliffe Method

Another approach to deriving initial doses of digoxin is to compute an appropriate loading dose that provides an amount of the drug in the body that evokes the appropriate pharmacologic response.[76,77] The amount of digoxin in the body that produces the desired effect is known as the total body stores (TBS) of digoxin. The percent of drug that is lost on a daily basis (%lost/d) is related to renal function according to the following equation: %lost/d = 14% + 0.20(CrCl), where 14% is the percent of digoxin eliminated per day by nonrenal routes and CrCl is creatinine clearance in mL/min.[77] Because the goal of therapy is to provide the total body stores of digoxin that cause the appropriate inotropic or chronotropic effect, the maintenance dose (MD in μg/d) is the amount of digoxin eliminated on a daily basis: MD = [TBS · (%lost/d)]/F, where TBS is total body stores in μg/d, %lost/d is the percent of digoxin TBS lost per day, F is the bioavailability factor for the dosage form, and 100 is a conversion factor to convert the percentage to a fraction. Combining the two equations produces the initial digoxin maintenance dose: MD = {TBS · [14% + 0.20(CrCl)]}/(F · 100).

For patients with creatinine clearance values higher than 30 mL/min, digoxin total body stores of 8 to 12 μg/kg are usually required to cause inotropic effects, whereas 13 to 15 μg/kg are generally needed to cause chronotropic effects.[78,79] Since renal disease (creatinine clearance <30 mL/min) decreases digoxin volume of distribution, initial digoxin total body stores of 6 to 10 μg/kg are recommended for patients with poor renal function.[79] Because obesity does not change digoxin volume of distribution, the weight factor used in this calculation is ideal body weight (IBW) for patients who are significantly overweight (>30% over IBW).[27,28] If a patient weighs less than his or her ideal body weight, actual body weight is used to calculate total body stores. For patients whose weight is between their ideal body weight and 30% over ideal weight, actual body weight can be used to compute total body stores, although some clinicians prefer to use ideal body weight for these persons. If a loading dose is required, the total body store (TBS in μg) is calculated and used to compute the loading dose (LD in μg) after correction for dosage form bioavailability (F): LD = TBS/F.[76,77]

To contrast the Jelliffe dosage method with the Jusko-Koup dosage method, the same patient cases are used as examples for this section.

Example 1 MJ is a 50-year-old, 70-kg, 178-cm (70-in) male with atrial fibrillation for less than 24 hours. His serum creatinine is 0.9 mg/dL, which has been stable over the last 5 days since admission. Compute an intravenous digoxin dose to control the ventricular rate.

1. *Estimate the creatinine clearance.*

This patient has a stable serum creatinine and is not obese. The Cockcroft–Gault equation can be used to estimate creatinine clearance:

$$CrCl_{est} = [(140 - age)BW]/(72 \cdot S_{Cr}) = [(140 - 50\ y)70\ kg]/(72 \cdot 0.9\ mg/dL)$$

$$CrCl_{est} = 97\ mL/min$$

2. *Estimate the total body store (TBS) and the maintenance dose (MD).*

The patient has good renal function and is not obese. Digoxin total body stores of 13 to 15 μg/kg are effective in the treatment of atrial fibrillation. A digoxin dose of 14 μg/kg is chosen for this patient.

$$TBS = 14\ \mu g/kg \cdot 70\ kg = 980\ \mu g$$

$$MD = \{TBS \cdot [14\% + 0.20(CrCl)]\}/(F \cdot 100) = \{980\ \mu g \cdot [14\% + 0.20(97\ mL/min)]\}/(1 \cdot 100) = 328\ \mu g/d, \text{ rounded to } 375\ \mu g/d$$

3. *Use the loading dose equation to compute the digoxin loading dose (if needed).*

Digoxin total body store is used to calculate the loading dose after correcting for bioavailability:

$$LD = TBS/F = 980\ \mu g/1 = 980\ \mu g, \text{ rounded to } 1000\ \mu g$$

When digoxin loading doses are administered, they are usually given in divided doses separated by 4 to 6 hours (50% of dose first, followed by two additional doses of 25%). In this case, an initial intravenous dose of 500 μg is given, followed by two additional intravenous doses of 250 μg each. One of the loading doses can be withheld if pulse rate is less than 50 to 60 beats/min or other undesirable digoxin adverse effects are noted.

Example 2 Same patient profile as in example 1, but serum creatinine is 3.5 mg/dL, indicating renal impairment.

1. *Estimate the creatinine clearance.*

This patient has a stable serum creatinine and is not obese. The Cockcroft–Gault equation can be used to estimate creatinine clearance:

$$CrCl_{est} = [(140 - age)BW]/(72 \cdot S_{Cr}) = [(140 - 50\ y)70\ kg]/(72 \cdot 3.5\ mg/dL)$$

$$CrCl_{est} = 25\ mL/min$$

2. *Estimate the total body store (TBS) and maintenance dose (MD).*

The patient has poor renal function and is not obese. Digoxin total body stores of 6 to 10 μg/kg are recommended for patients with renal dysfunction. A digoxin dose of 8 μg/kg is chosen for this patient.

$$TBS = 8\ \mu g/kg \cdot 70\ kg = 560\ \mu g$$

$$MD = \{TBS \cdot [14\% + 0.20(CrCl)]\}/(F \cdot 100) = \{560\ \mu g \cdot [14\% + 0.20(25\ mL/min)]\}/(1 \cdot 100) = 106\ \mu g/d, \text{ rounded to } 125\ \mu g/d$$

3. *Use the loading dose equation to compute the digoxin loading dose (if needed).*

Digoxin total body store is used to calculate the loading dose after correcting for bioavailability:

$$LD = TBS/F = 560\ \mu g/1 = 560\ \mu g, \text{ rounded to } 500\ \mu g$$

When digoxin loading doses are administered, they are usually given in divided doses separated by 4 to 6 hours (50% of dose at first, followed by two additional doses of 25%). In this case, an initial intravenous dose of 250 μg is given, followed by two additional intravenous doses of 125 μg each. One of the loading doses can be withheld if pulse rate is less than 50 to 60 beats/min or other undesirable digoxin adverse effects are noted.

Example 3 Same patient profile as in example 1, but serum creatinine is 3.5 mg/dL, indicating renal impairment. In addition, the patient is being treated for NYHA class III moderate heart failure, not atrial fibrillation. Compute an oral digoxin tablet maintenance dose for this patient.

1. *Estimate the creatinine clearance.*

This patient has a stable serum creatinine and is not obese. The Cockcroft–Gault equation can be used to estimate creatinine clearance:

$$CrCl_{est} = [(140 - age)BW]/(72 \cdot S_{Cr}) = [(140 - 50\ y)70\ kg]/(72 \cdot 3.5\ mg/dL)$$

$$CrCl_{est} = 25\ mL/min$$

2. *Estimate the total body store (TBS) and maintenance dose (MD).*

The patient has poor renal function and is not obese. Digoxin total body stores of 6 to 10 μg/kg are recommended for patients with renal dysfunction. A digoxin dose of 8 μg/kg is chosen for this patient.

$$TBS = 8\ \mu g/kg \cdot 70\ kg = 560\ \mu g$$

$$MD = \{TBS \cdot [14\% + 0.20(CrCl)]\}/(F \cdot 100) = \{560\ \mu g \cdot [14\% + 0.20(25\ mL/min)]\}/(0.7 \cdot 100) = 152\ \mu g/d, \text{ rounded to } 125\ \mu g/d$$

Example 4 OI is a 65-year-old, 170-kg, 165-cm (65-in) female with NYHA class III moderate heart failure. Her serum creatinine is 4.7 mg/dL and stable. Compute an intravenous digoxin loading and maintenance dose for this patient.

1. *Estimate the creatinine clearance.*

This patient has a stable serum creatinine and is obese [$IBW_{females}$ (in kg) = 45 + 2.3(Ht – 60 in) = 45 + 2.3(65 – 60) = 57 kg]. The Salazar and Corcoran equation can be used to estimate creatinine clearance:

$$CrCl_{est(females)} = \frac{(146 - age)[(0.287 \cdot Wt) + (9.74 \cdot Ht^2)]}{(60 \cdot S_{Cr})}$$

$$CrCl_{est(females)} = \frac{(146 - 65\ y)\{(0.287 \cdot 170\ kg) + [9.74 \cdot (1.65\ m)^2]\}}{(60 \cdot 4.7\ mg/dL)} = 22\ mL/min$$

Note: Height is converted from inches to meters: Ht = (65 in · 2.54 cm/in)/(100 cm/m) = 1.65 m.

2. *Estimate the total body store (TBS) and maintenance dose (MD).*

The patient has poor renal function and is obese. Digoxin total body stores of 6 to 10 μg/kg are recommended for patients with renal dysfunction, and ideal body weight (IBW) should be used in the computation. A digoxin dose of 8 μg/kg is chosen for this patient.

TBS = 8 μg/kg · 57 kg = 456 μg

MD = {TBS · [14% + 0.20(CrCl)]}/(F · 100) = {456 μg · [14% + 0.20(22 mL/min)]}/(1 · 100) = 84 μg/d, or 168 μg every 2 days (i.e., 84 μg/d · 2 days = 168 μg every 2 days).

This intravenous dose is rounded to 150 μg every other day.

3. *Use the loading dose equation to compute the digoxin loading dose (if needed).*

Digoxin total body store is used to calculate the loading dose after correcting for bioavailability:

LD = TBS/F = 456 μg/1 = 456 μg, rounded to 500 μg

When digoxin loading doses are administered, they are usually given in divided doses separated by 4 to 6 hours (50% of dose first, followed by two additional doses of 25%). In this case, an initial intravenous dose of 250 μg is given, followed by two additional intravenous doses of 125 μg each. One of the loading doses can be withheld if pulse rate is less than 50 to 60 beats/min or other undesirable digoxin adverse effects are noted.

USE OF DIGOXIN SERUM CONCENTRATIONS TO ALTER DOSAGES

Because of pharmacokinetic variability among patients, it is likely that doses computed using patient population characteristics do not always produce digoxin serum concentrations that are expected. Because of this, digoxin serum concentrations are measured in many patients to ensure that therapeutic, nontoxic levels are present and to check for compliance to dosage regimens. However, not all patients may require serum concentration monitoring. For example, if an appropriate dose for the patient's renal function and concurrent disease states is prescribed (e.g., 250 μg/d in a patient with a creatinine clearance of 80 to 100 mL/min for heart failure) and the desired clinical effect is achieved without adverse effects, digoxin serum concentration monitoring may not be necessary. Whether or not digoxin concentrations are measured, important patient parameters (e.g., dyspnea, orthopnea, tachypnea, cough, pulmonary rales/edema, S_3 gallop for heart failure) should be monitored to confirm that the patient is responding to treatment and not developing adverse drug reactions.

When digoxin serum concentrations are measured in patients and a dosage change is necessary, clinicians should seek to use the simplest, most straightforward method available to determine a dose that will provide safe and effective treatment. In most cases, a simple dosage ratio can be used to change digoxin doses, since digoxin follows *linear pharmacokinetics*. Sometimes, it is not possible to simply change the dose because of the limited number of oral dosage strengths, and the dosage interval must also be changed. Available digoxin tablet strengths are 125 μg, 250 μg, and 500 μg, whereas 50-, 100-, and 200-μg digoxin capsules are available. In some situations, it may be necessary to compute the digoxin pharmacokinetic parameters for the patient and use these to calculate the best drug dose. Finally, computerized methods that incorporate expected population pharmacokinetic characteristics (*Bayesian pharmacokinetics computer programs*) can be used in difficult cases in which renal function is changing, serum concentrations are obtained at suboptimal times, or the patient was not at steady state when serum concentrations were measured.

Linear Pharmacokinetics Method

Because digoxin follows linear, dose-proportional pharmacokinetics, steady-state serum concentrations change in proportion to dose according to the following equation: $D_{new}/Css_{new} = D_{old}/Css_{old}$ or $D_{new} = (Css_{new}/Css_{old})D_{old}$, where D is the dose in μg, Css is the steady-state concentration in ng/mL, old indicates the dose that produced the steady-state concentration that the patient is currently receiving, and new denotes the dose necessary to produce the desired steady-state concentration. The advantages of this method are that it is quick and simple. The disadvantage is that steady-state concentrations are required. Also, because of a limited number of solid oral dosage strengths, it may not be possible to attain desired serum concentrations by only changing the dose. In these cases, dosage intervals are extended for patients receiving tablets so that doses can be given as multiples of 125 μg and for patients receiving capsules so that doses can be given in multiples of 50 μg. The estimated times to achieve steady-state concentrations on a stable digoxin dosage regimen vary according to renal function and are listed in Table 6-3.[79] An alternative to this way of estimating time to steady state is to compute the expected digoxin half-life ($t_{1/2}$ in days) using digoxin clearance (Cl in L/d) and volume of distribution (V in L) and allow 3 to 5 half-lives to pass before obtaining digoxin serum concentrations: $t_{1/2} = (0.693 \cdot V)/Cl$.

Example 1 MJ is a 50-year-old, 70-kg, 178-cm (70-in) man with moderate heart failure. His serum creatinine is 0.9 mg/dL, which has been stable over the last 6 months. A digoxin dose of 250 μg/d using oral tablets was prescribed and expected to achieve steady-state concentrations of 0.8 ng/mL. After 1 week of treatment, a steady-state

TABLE 6-3 Estimated Time to Steady State for Digoxin Administration When a Stable Dosage Regimen Is Administered

CREATININE CLEARANCE (mL/min/70 kg)	NUMBER OF DAYS BEFORE STEADY STATE ACHIEVED
0	22
10	19
20	16
30	14
40	13
50	12
60	11
70	10
80	9
90	8
100	7

From Anon. Lanoxin (digoxin) tablets, U.S.P. monograph. In: Arky R, ed. Physicians' desk reference. Montvale, NJ: Medical Economics Company, 1999:1167–1171.

digoxin concentration was measured and was 0.6 ng/mL. Calculate a new digoxin dose that will provide a steady-state concentration of 0.9 ng/mL.

1. *Estimate the creatinine clearance.*

This patient has a stable serum creatinine and is not obese. The Cockcroft–Gault equation can be used to estimate creatinine clearance:

$$CrCl_{est} = [(140 - age)BW]/(72 \cdot S_{Cr}) = [(140 - 50\ y)70\ kg]/(72 \cdot 0.9\ mg/dL)$$

$$CrCl_{est} = 97\ mL/min$$

The patient has good renal function and is expected to have achieved steady state after 7 days of treatment.

2. *Compute the new dose to achieve desired serum concentration.*

Using linear pharmacokinetics, the new dose to attain the desired concentration should be proportional to the old dose that produced the measured concentration:

$$D_{new} = (Css_{new}/Css_{old})D_{old} = [(0.9\ \mu g/mL)/(0.6\ \mu g/mL)]\ 250\ \mu g/d = 375\ \mu g/d$$

The new suggested dose is 375 μg/d given as digoxin tablets to be started at the next scheduled dosing time.

Example 2 OI is a 65-year-old, 170-kg, 165-cm (65-in) woman with NYHA class III heart failure. Her serum creatinine is 4.7 mg/dL and stable. A digoxin dose of 125 μg/d given as tablets was prescribed and expected to achieve steady-state concentrations of 1 ng/mL. After the 3 weeks of therapy, a steady-state digoxin concentration was measured and was 2.5 ng/mL. Calculate a new digoxin dose that will provide a steady-state concentration of 1.2 μg/mL.

1. *Estimate the creatinine clearance.*

This patient has a stable serum creatinine and is obese [$IBW_{females}$ (in kg) = 45 + 2.3 (Ht – 60 in) = 45 + 2.3(65 – 60) = 57 kg]. The Salazar and Corcoran equation can be used to estimate creatinine clearance:

$$CrCl_{est(females)} = \frac{(146 - age)[(0.287 \cdot Wt) + (9.74 \cdot Ht^2)]}{(60 \cdot S_{Cr})}$$

$$CrCl_{est(females)} = \frac{(146 - 65\ y)\{(0.287 \cdot 170\ kg) + [9.74 \cdot (1.65\ m)^2]\}}{(60 \cdot 4.7\ mg/dL)} = 22\ mL/min$$

Note: Height is converted from inches to meters: Ht = (65 in · 2.54 cm/in)/(100 cm/m) = 1.65 m.

This patient has poor renal function but is expected to be at steady state with regard to digoxin serum concentrations after 3 weeks of treatment.

2. *Compute a new dose to achieve desired serum concentration.*

Using linear pharmacokinetics, compute the new dose to attain the desired concentration proportionally with the old dose that produced the measured concentration:

$D_{new} = (Css_{new}/Css_{old})D_{old}$ = [(1.2 ng/mL)/(2.5 ng/mL)] 125 μg/d = 60 μg/d, or 120 μg every other day (i.e., 60 μg/d · 2 days = 120 μg every 2 days).

This would be rounded to digoxin tablets 125 μg every other day.

The new suggested dose is 125 μg every other day given as digoxin tablets to be started at the next scheduled dosing time. Because the dosage interval is being changed, a day is skipped before the next dose is given.

Pharmacokinetic Parameter Method

The pharmacokinetic parameter method calculates the patient-specific drug clearance and uses it to design improved dosage regimens.[25,26] Digoxin clearance can be measured using a single steady-state digoxin concentration (Css) and the following formula: $Cl = [F(D/\tau)]/Css$, where Cl is digoxin clearance in liters per day, F is the bioavailability factor for the dosage form used, τ is the dosage interval in days, and Css is the digoxin steady-state concentration in ng/mL, which also is μg/L. Although this method does allow computation of digoxin clearance, it yields exactly the same digoxin dose as that supplied using linear pharmacokinetics. As a result, most clinicians prefer to directly calculate the new dose using the simpler linear pharmacokinetics method. To illustrate this point, the patient cases used to illustrate the linear pharmacokinetics method are used as examples for the pharmacokinetic parameter method.

Example 1 MJ is a 50-year-old, 70-kg, 178-cm (70-in) male with moderate heart failure. His serum creatinine is 0.9 mg/dL, which has been stable over the last 6 months. A digoxin dose of 250-μg/d oral tablets was prescribed and expected to achieve steady-state concentrations of 0.8 ng/mL. After 1 week of treatment, a steady-state digoxin concentration was measured as 0.6 ng/mL. Calculate a new digoxin dose that will provide a steady-state concentration of 0.9 ng/mL.

1. *Estimate the creatinine clearance.*

This patient has a stable serum creatinine and is not obese. The Cockcroft–Gault equation can be used to estimate creatinine clearance:

$$CrCl_{est} = [(140 - age)BW]/(72 \cdot S_{Cr}) = [(140 - 50\ y)70\ kg]/(72 \cdot 0.9\ mg/dL)$$

$$CrCl_{est} = 97\ mL/min$$

The patient has good renal function and is expected to achieve steady state after 7 days of treatment.

2. *Compute the drug clearance.*

Note that digoxin concentrations in ng/mL are the same as those for μg/L. This unit substitution is directly made to avoid conversion factors in the computation.

$$Cl = [F(D/\tau)]/Css = [0.7(250\ \mu g/d)]/0.6\ \mu g/L = 292\ L/d$$

3. *Compute the new dose to achieve desired serum concentration.*

The average steady-state equation is used to compute the new digoxin dose.

$$D/\tau = (Css \cdot Cl)/F = (0.9\ \mu g/L \cdot 292\ L/d)/0.7 = 375\ \mu g/d$$

The new suggested dose is 375 μg/d given as digoxin tablets to be started at the next scheduled dosing time.

Example 2 OI is a 65-year-old, 170-kg, 165-cm (65-in) female with NYHA class III heart failure. Her serum creatinine is 4.7 mg/dL and stable. A digoxin dose of 125 μg/d given as tablets was prescribed and expected to achieve steady-state concentrations of 1 ng/mL. After the 3 weeks of therapy, a steady-state digoxin concentration was measured at 2.5 ng/mL. Calculate a new digoxin dose that will provide a steady-state concentration of 1.2 ng/mL.

1. *Estimate the creatinine clearance.*

This patient has a stable serum creatinine and is obese [$IBW_{females}$ (in kg) = 45 + 2.3(Ht − 60 in) = 45 + 2.3(65 − 60 in) = 57 kg]. The Salazar and Corcoran equation can be used to estimate creatinine clearance.

$$CrCl_{est(females)} = \frac{(146 - age)[(0.287 \cdot Wt) + (9.74 \cdot Ht^2)]}{(60 \cdot S_{Cr})}$$

$$CrCl_{est(females)} = \frac{(146 - 65\ y)\{(0.287 \cdot 170\ kg) + [9.74 \cdot (1.65\ m)^2]\}}{(60 \cdot 4.7\ mg/dL)} = 22\ mL/min$$

Note: Height is converted from inches to meters: Ht = (65 in · 2.54 cm/in)/(100 cm/m) = 1.65 m.

This patient has poor renal function but is expected to be at steady state with regard to digoxin serum concentrations after 3 weeks of treatment.

2. *Compute the drug clearance.*

Note that digoxin concentrations in ng/mL are the same as those for μg/L. This unit substitution is directly made to avoid conversion factors in the computation.

$$Cl = [F(D/\tau)]/Css = [0.7(125\ \mu g/d)]/2.5\ \mu g/L = 35\ L/d$$

3. *Compute the new dose to achieve desired serum concentration.*

The average steady-state equation is used to compute the new digoxin dose.

$$D/\tau = (Css \cdot Cl)/F = (1.2\ \mu g/L \cdot 35\ L/d)/0.7 = 60\ \mu g/d, \text{ or } 120\ \mu g \text{ every other day}$$
$$(\text{i.e., } 60\ \mu g/d \cdot 2 \text{ days} = 120\ \mu g \text{ every 2 days}).$$

This would be rounded to digoxin tablets 125 μg every other day.

The new suggested dose is 125 μg every other day given as digoxin tablets to be started at the next scheduled dosing time. Because the dosage interval is being changed, a day is skipped before the next dose is given.

BAYESIAN PHARMACOKINETICS COMPUTER PROGRAMS

Computer programs are available to assist in the computation of pharmacokinetic parameters for patients.[80,81] The most reliable computer programs use a nonlinear regression algorithm that incorporates components of Bayes' theorem. Nonlinear regression is a statistical technique that uses an iterative process to compute the best pharmacokinetic parameters for a concentration–time data set. Briefly, the patient's drug dosage schedule and serum concentrations are entered into the computer. The computer program has a pharmacokinetic equation preprogrammed for the drug and administration method (e.g., oral, intravenous bolus, intravenous infusion). Typically, a one-compartment model is used, although some programs allow the user to choose among several different equations. Using population estimates based on demographic information for the patient (e.g., age, weight, gender, renal function) supplied by the user, the computer program then computes estimated serum concentrations at each time there are actual serum concentrations. Kinetic parameters are then changed by the computer program, and a new set of estimated serum concentrations are computed. The pharmacokinetic parameters that generated the estimated serum concentrations closest to the actual values are remembered by the computer program, and the process is repeated until the set of pharmacokinetic parameters are generated that result in estimated serum concentrations that are statistically closest to the actual serum concentrations. These pharmacokinetic parameters can then be used to compute improved dosing schedules for patients. Bayes' theorem is used in the computer algorithm to balance the results of the computations between values based solely on the patient's serum drug concentrations and those based only on patient population parameters. Results from studies that compare various methods of dosage adjustment have consistently found that these types of computer dosing programs perform at least as well as experienced clinical pharmacokineticists and clinicians and better than inexperienced clinicians.

Some clinicians use Bayesian pharmacokinetics computer programs exclusively to alter drug doses based on serum concentrations. An advantage of this approach is that consistent dosage recommendations are made when several different practitioners are involved in therapeutic drug monitoring programs. However, since simpler dosing methods work just as well for patients with stable pharmacokinetic parameters and steady-state drug concentrations, many clinicians reserve the use of computer programs for more difficult situations. Such situations include serum concentrations that are not at steady state, serum concentrations not obtained at the specific times needed to use simpler methods, and unstable pharmacokinetic parameters. Many Bayesian pharmacokinetics computer programs are available to users, and most should provide answers similar to the ones used in the following examples. The program used to solve problems in this book is DrugCalc, written by Dr. Dennis Mungall, and is available on his Internet web site (http://members.aol.com/thertch/index.htm).[82]

Example 1 MJ is a 50-year-old, 70-kg, 178-cm (70-in) male with moderate heart failure. His serum creatinine is 0.9 mg/dL, which has been stable over the last 6 months. A digoxin dose of 250 μg/d using oral tablets was prescribed and expected to achieve steady-state concentrations of 0.8 ng/mL. After 1 week of treatment, a steady-state digoxin concentration was measured at 0.6 ng/mL. Calculate a new digoxin dose that would provide a steady-state concentration of 0.9 ng/mL.

1. *Enter the patient's demographic, drug dosing, and serum concentration–time data into the computer program.*

2. *Compute the pharmacokinetic parameters for the patient using the Bayesian pharmacokinetics computer program.*

The pharmacokinetic parameters computed by the program are a clearance of 8.8 L/h, a volume of distribution of 578 L, and a half-life of 46 hours.

3. *Compute the dose required to achieve desired digoxin serum concentration.*

The one-compartment model equations used by the program to compute doses indicate that digoxin tablets 343 μg/d produce a steady-state concentration of 0.9 ng/mL. This dose is rounded to 375 μg/d. Using the simpler linear pharmacokinetics method previously described in this chapter, the identical dose of 375 μg/d was computed.

Example 2 OI is a 65-year-old, 170-kg, 165-cm (65-in) female with NYHA class III heart failure. Her serum creatinine is 4.7 mg/dL and stable. A digoxin dose of 125 μg/d given as tablets was prescribed and expected to achieve steady-state concentrations of 1 ng/mL. After the 3 weeks of therapy, a steady-state digoxin concentration was measured at 2.5 ng/mL. Calculate a new digoxin dose that will provide a steady-state concentration of 1.2 ng/mL.

1. *Enter the patient's demographic, drug dosing, and serum concentration–time data into the computer program.*

2. *Compute the pharmacokinetic parameters for the patient using the Bayesian pharmacokinetics computer program.*

The pharmacokinetic parameters computed by the program are a clearance of 1.4 L/h, a volume of distribution of 516 L, and a half-life of 249 hours. The clearance value is slightly different from that computed using the steady-state pharmacokinetic parameter method (35 L/d or 1.5 L/h), because the patient probably was not at steady state when the serum concentrations were drawn.

3. *Compute the dose required to achieve desired digoxin serum concentration.*

The one-compartment model equations used by the program to compute doses indicate that a dose of 141 μg every 3 days will produce a steady-state concentration of 1.2 ng/mL. This is rounded to 125 μg every 3 days. Using the steady-state pharmacokinetic parameter method previously described, a similar dose of 125 μg every other day was computed.

Example 3 JH is a 74-year-old, 85-kg, 173-cm (68-in) male with atrial fibrillation. His serum creatinine is 1.9 mg/dL, which has been stable over the last 7 days since admission. An intravenous digoxin loading dose of 500 μg was prescribed (given as doses of 250 μg, 125 μg, and 125 μg every 4 hours at 0800 H, 1200 H, and 1600 H, respectively). An oral maintenance dose of digoxin tablets 125 μg was given the next morning at 0800 H. Because the patient still had a rapid ventricular rate, a digoxin concentration was obtained at 1600 H and was 0.9 ng/mL. Recommend a stat intravenous digoxin dose to be given at 2300 H, which will achieve a digoxin serum concentration of 1.5 ng/mL, and an oral maintenance dose, which will provide a steady-state concentration of the same level.

1. *Enter the patient's demographic, drug dosing, and serum concentration–time data into the computer program.*

2. *Compute the pharmacokinetic parameters for the patient using the Bayesian pharmacokinetics computer program.*

The pharmacokinetic parameters computed by the program are a clearance of 4.8 L/h, a volume of distribution of 390 L, and a half-life of 57 hours.

3. *Compute the dose required to achieve the desired digoxin serum concentration.*

The stat intravenous digoxin dose is calculated using the volume of distribution supplied by the computer program. The booster dose (BD), which will change serum concentrations by the desired amount, is BD = [V(ΔC)]/F, where V is the volume of distribution in L, ΔC is the necessary change in digoxin serum concentration in μg/L, and F is the bioavailability for the dosage form.

$$BD = V(\Delta C) = [390\ L(1.5\ \mu g/L - 0.9\ \mu g/L)]/1 = 234\ \mu g, \text{ rounded to } 250\ \mu g \text{ intravenously stat}$$

The one-compartment model equations used by the program to compute doses indicate that a digoxin tablet dose of 273 μg/d will produce a steady-state concentration of 1.5 ng/mL. This dose is rounded to 250 μg/d of digoxin tablets and is started at 0800 H the next morning.

SPECIAL DOSING CONSIDERATIONS

Use of Digoxin Immune Fab in Digoxin Overdoses

Digoxin immune Fab (Digibind) are digoxin antibody molecule segments that bind and neutralize digoxin and can be used in digoxin overdose situations.[83,84] The antibody fragments are derived from antidigoxin antibodies formed in sheep. Improvements in digoxin adverse effects can be seen within 30 minutes of digoxin immune Fab administration. Digoxin serum concentrations are not useful after digoxin immune Fab has been given to a patient because pharmacologically inactive digoxin bound to the antibody segments is measured and produces falsely high results. The elimination half-life of digoxin immune Fab is 15 to 20 hours in patients with normal renal function, and it is eliminated by the kidney. The half-life of digoxin immune Fab is not known in patients with impaired renal function but is assumed to be prolonged. In functionally anephric patients, the Fab fragment–digoxin complex may not be readily cleared from the body, so these patients should be closely monitored in the event that digoxin dissociates from the Fab fragment and reintoxication occurs.

Because digoxin immune Fab is a foreign protein, allergic reactions can occur, including anaphylactic shock, so patient blood pressure and temperature should be closely monitored. In addition, the electrocardiogram and serum potassium concentration should be closely monitored for patients receiving this agent. Initially, patients may be hyperkalemic owing to digoxin-induced displacement of intracellular potassium. However, hypokalemia can occur rapidly as the Fab fragments bind digoxin. As a result, repeated measurements of serum potassium are necessary, especially after the first few hours of digoxin immune Fab. Because the pharmacologic effects of digoxin will be lost, heart failure may worsen or a rapid ventricular rate may develop in patients treated for atrial fibrillation. Readministration of Digibind may be necessary if digoxin adverse effects have not abated several hours after administration of the antibody fragments or if adverse effects recur. When patients do not respond to Digibind, clinicians should consider the possibility that the patient is not digoxin-toxic and seek other causes of the patients' clinical symptomatology.

If a digoxin serum concentration or an estimate of the number of tablets ingested is not available, 20 vials of Digibind are usually adequate for treatment of most life-threatening acute overdoses in children and adults, whereas six vials are usually adequate for treatment of chronic digoxin overdoses.[85] If digoxin serum concentrations are available or a reasonable estimate for the number of digoxin tablets acutely ingested is available, the Digibind dose should be computed using one of the two approaches outlined in the following text.[85] If it is possible to calculate a Digibind dose using both of the following methods, it is recommended that the higher dose be administered to the patient.

CHRONIC OVERDOSE OR ACUTE OVERDOSE 8 TO 12 HOURS AFTER INGESTION

In cases of chronic or acute overdose 8 to 12 hours after ingestion, a postabsorption, postdistribution digoxin concentration can be used to estimate the necessary dose of Digibind for a patient using the following formula: Digibind dose (in vials) = (digoxin concentration in ng/mL)(body weight in kg)/100.

Example HY is a 72-year-old, 80-kg, 170-cm (67-in) male who has accidentally been taking twice his prescribed dosage of digoxin tablets. The admitting digoxin serum concentration is 4.1 ng/mL. Compute an appropriate dose of Digibind for this patient.

Digibind dose (in vials) = (digoxin concentration in ng/mL)(body weight in kg)/100
= (4.1 ng/mL · 80 kg)/100 = 3.3 vials, rounded to 4 vials

ACUTE DIGOXIN OVERDOSE IN WHICH NUMBER OF TABLETS IS KNOWN OR CAN BE ESTIMATED

For a patient with an acute overdose of a known or estimable number of digoxin tablets, digoxin total body stores are estimated using the number of tablets ingested corrected for dosage form bioavailability: TBS = F(# dosage units)(dosage form strength), where TBS is digoxin total body stores in mg, F is the bioavailability for the dosage form (note: The suggested bioavailability constant of digoxin in the Digibind package insert is 0.8 for tablets and 1 for capsules, which allows for variability in the fraction of the dose that was absorbed), number of dosage units is the number of tablets or capsules, and dosage form strength is in mg (note: 250 μg = 0.25 mg). Each vial of Digibind inactivates approximately 0.5 mg of digoxin, so the dose of Digibind (in vials) can be calculated using the following equation: Digibind dose = TBS/(0.5 mg/vial), where TBS is digoxin total body stores in mg.

Example DL is a 22-year-old, 85-kg, 175-cm (69-in) male who took approximately 50 digoxin tablets of 0.25-mg strength about 4 hours ago. Compute an appropriate dose of Digibind for this patient.

TBS = F(# dosage units)(dosage form strength)
= 0.8 (50 tablets · 0.25 mg/tablet) = 10 mg

Digibind dose = TBS/(0.5 mg/vial) = 10 mg/(0.5 mg/vial) = 20 vials

Conversion of Patient Doses Between Dosage Forms

When patients are switched between digoxin dosage forms, differences in bioavailability should be accounted for within the limits of available oral dosage forms using the following equation: $D_{IV} = D_{PO} \cdot F$, where D_{IV} is the equivalent digoxin intravenous dose in μg, D_{PO} is the equivalent digoxin oral dose, and F is the bioavailability fraction appropriate for the oral dosage form (F = 0.7 for tablets, 0.8 for elixir, 0.9 for capsules). Whenever possible, digoxin tablet doses should be rounded to the nearest 125 μg to prevent having to break tablets in half. Similarly, digoxin capsule doses should be rounded to the nearest 50 μg, because that is the smallest dose size available. In either case, it is best to avoid mixing tablet or capsule dosage strengths, so that patients do not become confused with multiple prescription vials and take the wrong dose of medication. For example, if it were necessary to prescribe 375 μg/d of digoxin tablets, it would be preferable to have the patient take three 125-μg tablets daily or 1.5 250-μg tablets daily rather than a 125-μg and 250-μg tablet each day.

Example 1 YT is a 67-year-old, 60-kg, 165-cm (65-in) male with atrial fibrillation who is receiving 200 μg of intravenous digoxin daily, which produces a steady-state digoxin concentration of 1.3 ng/mL. Compute an oral tablet dose that will maintain steady-state digoxin concentrations at approximately the same level.

1. *Convert the current digoxin dose to the equivalent amount for the new dosage form/route.*

$$D_{PO} = D_{IV}/F = 200\ \mu g/0.7 = 286\text{-}\mu g \text{ digoxin tablets, rounded to } 250\ \mu g$$

2. *Estimate the change in digoxin steady-state concentration caused by rounding of the dose.*

The oral tablet dose of digoxin 286 μg would have produced a steady-state concentration similar to the intravenous dose of 200 μg. However, the dose had to be rounded to a dose that could be given as a tablet. The expected digoxin steady-state concentration from the rounded dose should be proportional to the ratio of the rounded dose and the actual computed dose:

$$Css_{new} = Css_{old}(D_{rounded}/D_{computed}) = 1.3\ ng/mL(250\ \mu g/286\ \mu g) = 1.1\ ng/mL$$

where Css_{new} is the new expected digoxin steady-state concentration due to tablet administration in ng/mL, Css_{old} is the measured digoxin steady-state concentration due to intravenous administration in ng/mL, $D_{rounded}$ is the oral dose rounded to account for dosage form strengths in μg, and $D_{computed}$ is the exact oral dose computed during the intravenous to oral conversion calculation in μg. However, the steady-state digoxin concentration after the dosage form change may not be exactly the value calculated owing to a variety of causes. Because of interindividual variations in digoxin bioavailability, the patient's actual bioavailability constant for oral tablets may be different from the average population bioavailability constant used to convert the dose. Also, there are day-to-day intrasubject variations in the rate and extent of digoxin absorption that affect the actual steady-state digoxin concentration obtained while taking the drug orally. Finally, other oral drug therapy that did not influence digoxin pharmacokinetics when given intravenously may alter the expected digoxin concentration.

Example 2 KL is an 82-year-old, 45-kg, 147-cm (58-in) female with heart failure who is receiving 125 μg of oral digoxin tablets daily, which produces a steady-state digoxin concentration of 1 ng/mL. Compute an intravenous dose that will maintain steady-state digoxin concentrations at approximately the same level.

1. *Convert the current digoxin dose to the equivalent amount for the new dosage form/route.*

$$D_{IV} = D_{PO} \cdot F = 125\ \mu g \cdot 0.7 = 87.5\ \mu g \text{ digoxin intravenously, rounded to } 90\ \mu g$$

2. *Estimate the change in digoxin steady-state concentration due to rounding of dose.*

The intravenous dose of 87.5 μg digoxin would have produced a steady-state concentration similar to the oral tablet dose of 125 μg. However, the dose was rounded to an amount that could reasonably be measured in a syringe. The expected digoxin steady-state concentration from the rounded dose should be proportional to the ratio of the rounded dose and the actual computed dose:

$$Css_{new} = Css_{old}(D_{rounded}/D_{computed}) = 1 \text{ ng/mL}(90 \text{ μg}/87.5 \text{ μg}) = 1 \text{ ng/mL}$$

where Css_{new} is the new expected digoxin steady-state concentration due to intravenous administration in ng/mL, Css_{old} is the measured digoxin steady-state concentration due to oral tablet administration in ng/mL, $D_{rounded}$ is the intravenous dose rounded to allow accurate dosage measurement in μg, and $D_{computed}$ is the exact intravenous dose computed during the intravenous to oral conversion calculation in μg. Since the rounded intravenous digoxin dose is so close to the exact dose needed, steady-state digoxin concentrations are not expected to change appreciably. However, the steady-state digoxin concentration after the dosage form change may not be exactly the value calculated for many reasons. Because of interindividual variations in digoxin bioavailability, the patient's actual bioavailability constant for oral tablets may be different from that of the average population's bioavailability constant used to convert the dose. Also, there are day-to-day intrasubject variations in the rate and extent of digoxin absorption that affect the steady-state digoxin concentration obtained with oral administration of digoxin that will not be present with intravenous administration of the drug. Finally, other drug therapies that influence digoxin pharmacokinetics when given orally, but not intravenously, may alter the expected digoxin concentration.

PROBLEMS

The following problems are intended to emphasize the computation of initial and individualized doses using clinical pharmacokinetic techniques. Clinicians should always consult the patient's chart to confirm that other drug therapy is appropriate for current disease state signs and symptoms. Also, it should be confirmed that the patient is receiving other appropriate concurrent therapy, when necessary, to treat the cardiovascular condition.

1. UV is a 75-year-old, 62-kg, 177-cm (69-in) male with atrial fibrillation. His serum creatinine is 1.3 mg/dL, which has been stable since admission. Compute an intravenous loading dose and maintenance digoxin dosage to provide a steady-state concentration of 1.5 ng/mL or digoxin total body store of 15 μg/kg.

2. Patient UV (see problem 1) was prescribed digoxin 200 μg/d intravenously, which has been given for 2 weeks. A steady-state digoxin concentration was 2.4 ng/mL. Compute a revised digoxin dose to provide a steady-state concentration of 1.5 ng/mL.

3. Patient UV (see problems 1 and 2) had a dosage change to digoxin 125 μg/d intravenously, which produced a steady-state concentration of 1.4 ng/mL. Compute an oral tablet digoxin dose that will provide about the same steady-state drug concentration as that found during intravenous therapy.

4. SD is a 35-year-old, 75-kg, 170-cm (67-in) female with NYHA class IV heart failure secondary to viral cardiomyopathy. Her serum creatinine is 3.7 mg/dL, which has been stable since admission. Compute oral digoxin loading and maintenance doses using tablets to provide a steady-state concentration of 1 ng/mL.

5. Patient SD (see problem 4) was prescribed digoxin 187.5 μg/d orally as tablets. A steady-state digoxin concentration was obtained at 0.7 ng/mL. Compute a revised digoxin dosage for this patient using oral tablets to provide a steady-state concentration of 1 ng/mL.

6. Patient SD (see problems 4 and 5) had a dosage change to digoxin 250 μg/d orally in tablet form, which produced a steady-state concentration of 1.2 ng/mL. Compute an intravenous digoxin dosage that will provide about the same steady-state drug concentration as that found during oral tablet therapy.

7. BN is a 55-year-old, 140-kg, 172-cm (68-in) man with atrial fibrillation. His serum creatinine is 0.9 mg/dL, which has been stable since admission. Compute an intravenous loading dose and oral tablet maintenance dosage of digoxin to provide a steady-state concentration of 1.2 ng/mL.

8. Patient BN (see problem 7) was prescribed digoxin tablets 500 μg/d. A steady-state digoxin concentration was obtained at 2.4 ng/mL. Compute a revised digoxin tablet dosage for this patient to provide a steady-state concentration of 1.5 ng/mL.

9. VG is a 75-year-old, 180-kg, 157-cm (62-in) female with NYHA class III heart failure. Her serum creatinine is 6 mg/dL and stable. Compute digoxin oral capsule loading dose and a maintenance dosage for this patient to provide a steady-state concentration of 1 ng/mL.

10. Patient VG (see problem 9) was prescribed digoxin capsules 150 μg every other day. Steady-state digoxin concentration was 0.7 ng/mL. Compute a revised digoxin capsule dosage for this patient to provide a steady-state concentration of 1 ng/mL.

11. QW is a 34-year-old, 50-kg, 162-cm (64-in) woman with atrial fibrillation secondary to hyperthyroidism. Her serum creatinine is 0.8 mg/dL and stable. Compute a digoxin intravenous loading dose and an oral capsule maintenance dosage to provide a steady-state concentration of 1.5 ng/mL.

12. RT is a 68-year-old, 88-kg, 180-cm (71-in) man with NYHA class II heart failure. His serum creatinine is 2.3 mg/dL and stable. Digoxin therapy was initiated, and after the third oral dose of digoxin tablets 250 μg/d, a digoxin serum concentration was obtained according to the following schedule:

DAY/TIME	DIGOXIN DOSE (μg)/CONCENTRATION (C)
Day 1/0800 H	250
Day 2/0800 H	250
Day 3/0800 H	250
Day 4/0730 H	C = 1 ng/mL

Calculate a digoxin tablet dose that will provide a steady-state digoxin concentration of 0.8 ng/mL.

13. LK is a 72-year-old, 68-kg, 155-cm (61-in) woman with NYHA class III heart failure. Her serum creatinine is 2.9 mg/dL and stable. Digoxin therapy was initiated, and after an intravenous loading dose of 500 μg plus two intravenous doses of digoxin 125 μg/d, a digoxin serum concentration was obtained according to the following schedule:

DAY/TIME	DIGOXIN DOSE (μg)/CONCENTRATION (C)
Day 1/0800 H	250
Day 1/1200 H	125
Day 1/1600 H	125
Day 2/0800 H	125
Day 3/0800 H	125
Day 4/0730 H	C = 2 ng/mL

Calculate a digoxin tablet dose that will provide a steady-state digoxin concentration of 1 ng/mL.

14. BH is a 61-year-old, 91-kg, 185-cm (73-in) man with atrial fibrillation. His serum creatinine is 1.9 mg/dL and stable. Digoxin therapy was initiated, and after an intravenous loading dose of 1000 μg plus three oral doses of digoxin tablets 125 μg/d, a digoxin serum concentration was obtained according to the following schedule:

DAY/TIME	DIGOXIN DOSE (μg)/CONCENTRATION (C)
Day 1/0800 H	500 IV
Day 1/1200 H	250 IV
Day 1/1600 H	250 IV
Day 2/0800 H	125 tablet
Day 3/0800 H	125 tablet
Day 4/0800 H	125 tablet
Day 5/0730 H	C = 0.9 ng/mL

Calculate a digoxin tablet dosage that will provide a steady-state digoxin concentration of 1.5 ng/mL.

ANSWERS TO PROBLEMS

1. The initial digoxin doses for patient UV are calculated as follows.

Pharmacokinetic Dosing Method

1. *Estimate the creatinine clearance.*

This patient has a stable serum creatinine and is not obese. The Cockcroft–Gault equation can be used to estimate creatinine clearance:

$$CrCl_{est} = [(140 - age)BW]/(72 \cdot S_{Cr}) = [(140 - 75\ y)62\ kg]/(72 \cdot 1.3\ mg/dL)$$

$$CrCl_{est} = 43\ mL/min$$

2. *Estimate the drug clearance.*

The drug clearance versus creatinine clearance relationship is used to estimate the digoxin clearance (Cl_{NR} = 40 mL/min, since the patient does not have moderate-severe heart failure):

$$Cl = 1.303\ (CrCl) + Cl_{NR} = 1.303(43\ mL/min) + 40\ mL/min = 96\ mL/min$$

3. *Use the average steady-state concentration equation to compute the digoxin maintenance dosage.*

For a patient with atrial fibrillation, the desired digoxin concentration is 0.8 to 1.5 ng/mL. A serum concentration of 1.5 ng/mL was chosen for this patient, and intravenous digoxin is to be used (F = 1). Note that for concentration units, ng/mL = μg/L, and this conversion is made before the equation is used. Also, conversion factors are needed to change milliliters to liters (1000 mL/L) and minutes to days (1440 min/d).

$$MD/\tau = (Css \cdot Cl)/F = (1.5\ \mu g/L \cdot 96\ mL/min \cdot 1440\ min/d)/(1 \cdot 1000\ mL/L)$$
$$= 208\ \mu g/d, \text{ rounded to } 200\ \mu g/d$$

4. *Use the loading dose equation to compute the digoxin loading dose (if needed).*

The patient has moderate renal function and is not obese. Therefore, a volume of distribution of 7 L/kg and actual body weight can be used to compute the digoxin loading dose. An intravenous loading dose (F = 1) can be given in this patient to achieve the desired pharmacologic effect more quickly than if maintenance doses alone are used and concentrations are allowed to accumulate over 3 to 5 half-lives.

$$V = 7\ L/kg \cdot 62\ kg = 434\ L$$

$$LD = (Css \cdot V)/F = (1.5\ \mu g/L \cdot 434\ L)/1 = 651\ \mu g, \text{ rounded to } 600\ \mu g$$

When digoxin loading doses are administered, they are usually given in divided doses separated by 4 to 6 hours (50% of dose first, followed by two additional doses of 25%). In this case, an initial intravenous dose of 300 μg is given, followed by two intravenous doses of 150 μg each. One of the loading doses can be withheld if pulse rate is less than 50 to 60 beats/min or if other undesirable digoxin adverse effects are noted.

Jelliffe Method

1. *Estimate the creatinine clearance.*

This patient has a stable serum creatinine and is not obese. The Cockcroft–Gault equation can be used to estimate creatinine clearance:

$CrCl_{est} = [(140 - age)BW]/(72 \cdot S_{Cr}) = [(140 - 75\ y)62\ kg]/(72 \cdot 1.3\ mg/dL)$

$CrCl_{est} = 43\ mL/min$

2. *Estimate the total body store (TBS) and maintenance dosage (MD).*

The patient has moderate renal function and is not obese. Digoxin total body stores of 13 to 15 μg/kg are effective in the treatment of atrial fibrillation. A digoxin dose of 15 μg/kg is chosen for this patient.

$TBS = 15\ \mu g/kg \cdot 62\ kg = 930\ \mu g$

$MD = \{TBS \cdot [14\% + 0.20(CrCl)]\}/(F \cdot 100)$
$= \{930\ \mu g \cdot [14\% + 0.20(43\ mL/min)]\}/(1 \cdot 100) = 210\ \mu g/d$, rounded to 200 μg/d

3. *Use the loading dose equation to compute the digoxin loading dose (if needed).*

Digoxin total body store is used to calculate the loading dose after correcting for bioavailability:

$$LD = TBS/F = 930\ \mu g/1 = 930\ \mu g, \text{ rounded to } 1000\ \mu g$$

When digoxin loading doses are administered, they are usually given in divided doses separated by 4 to 6 hours (50% of dose first, followed by two additional doses of 25%). In this case, an initial intravenous dose of 500 μg is given, followed by two intravenous doses of 250 μg each. One of the loading doses can be withheld if the pulse rate is less than 50 to 60 beats/min or other undesirable digoxin adverse effects are noted.

2. The revised digoxin dose for patient UV is calculated as follows.

Linear Pharmacokinetics Method

1. *Estimate the creatinine clearance.*

This patient has a stable serum creatinine and is not obese. The Cockcroft–Gault equation can be used to estimate creatinine clearance:

$CrCl_{est} = [(140 - age)BW]/(72 \cdot S_{Cr}) = [(140 - 75\ y)62\ kg]/(72 \cdot 1.3\ mg/dL)$

$CrCl_{est} = 43\ mL/min$

The patient has moderate renal function and is expected to achieve steady state after 14 days of treatment.

2. *Compute the new dosage to achieve the desired serum concentration.*

With linear pharmacokinetics, compute the new dose to attain the desired concentration proportional to the old dose that produced the measured concentration:

$$D_{new} = (Css_{new}/Css_{old})D_{old} = (1.5\ ng/mL/2.4\ ng/mL)\ 200\ \mu g/d = 125\ \mu g/d$$

The new dose is 125 μg/d, given as intravenous digoxin to be started at the next scheduled dosing time.

Pharmacokinetic Parameter Method

1. *Estimate the creatinine clearance.*

This patient has a stable serum creatinine and is not obese. The Cockcroft–Gault equation can be used to estimate creatinine clearance:

$$CrCl_{est} = [(140 - age)BW]/(72 \cdot S_{Cr}) = [(140 - 75\ y)62\ kg]/(72 \cdot 1.3\ mg/dL)$$

$$CrCl_{est} = 43\ mL/min$$

The patient has moderate renal function and is expected to achieve steady state after 14 days of treatment.

2. *Compute the drug clearance.*

Note that digoxin concentrations in ng/mL are the same as those for μg/L. This unit substitution is directly made to avoid conversion factors in the computation.

$$Cl = [F(D/\tau)]/Css = [1(200\ \mu g/d)]/2.4\ \mu g/L = 83\ L/d$$

3. *Compute the new dose to achieve the desired serum concentration.*

The average steady-state equation is used to compute the new digoxin dose.

$$D/\tau = (Css \cdot Cl)/F = (1.5\ \mu g/L \cdot 83\ L/d)/1 = 125\ \mu g/d$$

The new suggested dose is 125 μg/d, given as intravenous digoxin to be started at the next scheduled dosing time.

3. An equivalent oral dose for patient UV is computed as follows.

1. *Convert the current digoxin dose to the equivalent amount for the new dosage form/route.*

$D_{PO} = D_{IV}/F = 125\ \mu g/0.7 = 179$-μg digoxin tablets, rounded to 187.5 μg (1½ 125-μg tablets)

2. *Estimate the change in digoxin steady-state concentration caused by rounding of dose.*

The oral tablet dose of 179-μg digoxin would have produced a steady-state concentration similar to the intravenous dose of 125 μg. However, the dose had to be rounded to a dose that can be given as tablets. The expected digoxin steady-state concentration from the rounded dose should be proportional to the ratio of the rounded dose and the actual computed dose:

$$Css_{new} = Css_{old}(D_{rounded}/D_{computed}) = 1.4\ ng/mL(187.5\ \mu g/179\ \mu g) = 1.5\ ng/mL$$

4. The initial digoxin doses for patient SD are calculated as follows.

Pharmacokinetic Dosing Method

1. *Estimate the creatinine clearance.*

This patient has a stable serum creatinine and is not obese. The Cockcroft–Gault equation can be used to estimate creatinine clearance:

$CrCl_{est} = \{[(140 - age)BW]/(72 \cdot S_{Cr})\}0.85 = \{[(140 - 35\ y)75\ kg]/(72 \cdot 3.7\ mg/dL)\}0.85$

$CrCl_{est} = 25\ mL/min$

2. *Estimate the drug clearance.*

The drug clearance versus creatinine clearance relationship is used to estimate the digoxin clearance (Cl_{NR} = 20 mL/min, since the patient has moderate to severe heart failure):

$$Cl = 1.303\ (CrCl) + Cl_{NR} = 1.303(25\ mL/min) + 20\ mL/min = 53\ mL/min$$

3. *Use the average steady-state concentration equation to compute the digoxin maintenance dosage.*

For a patient with heart failure, the desired digoxin concentration is 0.5 to 1 ng/mL. A serum concentration of 1 ng/mL was chosen for this patient, and oral digoxin is used (F = 0.7). Note that for concentration units, ng/mL = μg/L, and this conversion is made before the equation is used. Also, conversion factors are needed to change milliliters to liters (1000 mL/L) and minutes to days (1440 min/d).

$$MD/\tau = (Css \cdot Cl)/F = (1\ \mu g/L \cdot 53\ mL/min \cdot 1440\ min/d)/(0.7 \cdot 1000\ mL/L) = 108\ \mu g/d\text{, rounded to } 125\ \mu g/d$$

4. *Use the loading dose equation to compute the digoxin loading dose (if needed).*

The patient has poor renal function. Therefore, the volume of distribution equation that adjusts the parameter estimate for renal dysfunction can be used to compute the digoxin loading dose. An oral loading dose (F = 0.7) can be given to achieve the desired pharmacologic effect more quickly than if maintenance doses alone are used to allow concentrations to accumulate over 3 to 5 half-lives.

$$V = (226 + \frac{298 \cdot CrCl}{29.1 + CrCl})(Wt/70) = (226 + \frac{298 \cdot 25\ mL/min}{29.1 + 25\ mL/min})(75\ kg/70) = 390\ L$$

$$LD = (Css \cdot V)/F = (1\ \mu g/L \cdot 390\ L)/0.7 = 557\ \mu g\text{, rounded to } 500\ \mu g$$

When digoxin loading doses are administered, they are usually given in divided doses separated by 4 to 6 hours (50% of dose first, followed by two additional doses of 25%). In this case, an initial oral dose of 250 μg is given, followed by two oral doses of 125 μg each. One of the loading doses can be withheld if pulse rate is less than 50 to 60 beats/min or other undesirable digoxin adverse effects are noted.

Jelliffe Method

1. *Estimate the creatinine clearance.*

This patient has a stable serum creatinine and is not obese. The Cockcroft–Gault equation can be used to estimate creatinine clearance:

$CrCl_{est} = \{[(140 - age)BW]/(72 \cdot S_{Cr})\}0.85 = \{[(140 - 35\ y)75\ kg]/(72 \cdot 3.7\ mg/dL)\}0.85$

$CrCl_{est} = 25\ mL/min$

2. *Estimate the total body store (TBS) and maintenance dosage (MD).*

The patient has poor renal function and is not obese. Digoxin total body stores of 6 to 10 μg/kg are effective in the treatment of heart failure in patients with poor renal function. A digoxin dose of 8 μg/kg is chosen for this patient.

$$TBS = 8\ \mu g/kg \cdot 75\ kg = 600\ \mu g$$

$$MD = \{TBS \cdot [14\% + 0.20(CrCl)]\}/(F \cdot 100)$$
$$= \{600\ \mu g \cdot [14\% + 0.20(25\ mL/min)]\}/(0.7 \cdot 100) = 163\ \mu g/d, \text{ rounded to } 187.5\ \mu g/d$$

3. *Use the loading dose equation to compute the digoxin loading dose (if needed).*

Digoxin total body store is used to calculate the loading dose after correcting for bioavailability:

$$LD = TBS/F = 600\ \mu g/0.7 = 857\ \mu g, \text{ rounded to } 750\ \mu g$$

When digoxin loading doses are administered, they are usually given in divided doses separated by 4 to 6 hours (50% of dose first, followed by two additional doses of 25%). In this case, an initial oral dose of 375 μg is given, followed by two oral doses of 187.5 μg each. One of the loading doses can be withheld if pulse rate is less than 50 to 60 beats/min or other undesirable digoxin adverse effects are noted.

5. The revised digoxin dose for patient SD is calculated as follows.

Linear Pharmacokinetics Method

1. *Estimate the creatinine clearance.*

This patient has a stable serum creatinine and is not obese. The Cockcroft–Gault equation can be used to estimate creatinine clearance:

$$CrCl_{est} = \{[(140 - age)BW]/(72 \cdot S_{Cr})\}\ 0.85 = \{[(140 - 35\ y)75\ kg]/(72 \cdot 3.7\ mg/dL)\}0.85$$

$$CrCl_{est} = 25\ mL/min$$

The patient has poor renal function and is expected to achieve steady state after 14 days of treatment.

2. *Compute the new dose to achieve the desired serum concentration.*

With linear pharmacokinetics, compute the new dose to attain the desired concentration that is proportional to the old dose that produced the measured concentration:

$$D_{new} = (Css_{new}/Css_{old})D_{old} = (1\ ng/mL\ /0.7\ ng/mL)\ 187.5\ \mu g/d$$
$$= 268\ \mu g/d, \text{ rounded to } 250\ \mu g/d$$

The new dose is 250 μg/d, given as oral digoxin tablets to be started at the next scheduled dosing time.

Pharmacokinetic Parameter Method

1. *Estimate the creatinine clearance.*

This patient has a stable serum creatinine and is not obese. The Cockcroft–Gault equation can be used to estimate creatinine clearance:

$$CrCl_{est} = \{[(140 - age)BW]/(72 \cdot S_{Cr})\}0.85 = \{[(140 - 35\ y)75\ kg]/(72 \cdot 3.7\ mg/dL)\}0.85$$

$$CrCl_{est} = 25\ mL/min$$

The patient has poor renal function and is expected to achieve steady state after 14 days of treatment.

2. *Compute the drug clearance.*

Note that digoxin concentrations in ng/mL are the same as those for μg/L. This unit substitution is directly made to avoid conversion factors in the computation.

$$Cl = [F(D/\tau)]/Css = [0.7(187.5\ \mu g/d)]/0.7\ \mu g/L = 188\ L/d$$

3. *Compute the new dose to achieve the desired serum concentration.*

The average steady-state equation is used to compute the new digoxin dose.

$$D/\tau = (Css \cdot Cl)/F = (1\ \mu g/L \cdot 188\ L/d)/0.7 = 268\ \mu g/d,\ \text{rounded to}\ 250\ \mu g/d$$

The new suggested dose is 250 μg/d, given as digoxin tablets to be started at the next scheduled dosing time.

6. An equivalent oral dosage for patient SD is computed as follows.

1. *Convert the current digoxin dose to the equivalent amount for the new dosage form/route.*

$$D_{IV} = D_{PO} \cdot F = 250\ \mu g/d \cdot 0.7 = 175\ \mu g/d\ \text{intravenous digoxin}$$

2. *Estimate the change in digoxin steady-state concentration caused by rounding of dose.*

This step is not necessary because the actual equivalent intravenous dose can be given without rounding.

7. The initial digoxin doses for patient BN are calculated as follows.

Pharmacokinetic Dosing Method

1. *Estimate the creatinine clearance.*

This patient has a stable serum creatinine and is obese [IBW_{males} (in kg) = 50 + 2.3(Ht − 60 in) = 50 + 2.3(68 − 60) = 68.4 kg]. The Salazar and Corcoran equation can be used to estimate creatinine clearance:

$$CrCl_{est(males)} = \frac{(137 - age)[(0.285 \cdot Wt) + (12.1 \cdot Ht^2)]}{(51 \cdot S_{Cr})}$$

$$CrCl_{est(males)} = \frac{(137 - 55\ y)\{(0.285 \cdot 140\ kg) + [12.1 \cdot (1.73\ m)^2]\}}{(51 \cdot 0.9\ mg/dL)} = 136\ mL/min$$

Note: Height is converted from inches to meters: Ht = (68 in · 2.54 cm/in)/(100 cm/m) = 1.73 m.

2. *Estimate the drug clearance.*

The drug clearance versus creatinine clearance relationship is used to estimate the digoxin clearance (Cl_{NR} = 40 mL/min, because the patient does not have moderate to severe heart failure).

$$Cl = 1.303\ (CrCl) + Cl_{NR} = 1.303(136\ mL/min) + 40\ mL/min = 217\ mL/min$$

3. *Use the average steady-state concentration equation to compute the digoxin maintenance dose.*

For a patient with atrial fibrillation, the desired digoxin concentration is 0.8 to 1.5 ng/mL. A serum concentration of 1.2 ng/mL is chosen for this patient, and oral digoxin tablets are used (F = 0.7). Note that for concentration units, ng/mL = μg/L, and this conversion is made before the equation is used. Also, conversion factors are needed to change milliliters to liters (1000 mL/L) and minutes to days (1440 min/d).

$$MD/\tau = (Css \cdot Cl)/F = (1.2\ \mu g/L \cdot 217\ mL/min \cdot 1440\ min/d)/(0.7 \cdot 1000\ mL/L)$$
$$= 535\ \mu g/d, \text{ rounded to } 500\ \mu g/d$$

4. *Use the loading dose equation to compute the digoxin loading dose (if needed).*

The patient has good renal function and is obese. Therefore, a volume of distribution of 7 L/kg and ideal body weight can be used to compute the digoxin loading dose. An intravenous loading dose (F = 1) can be given to achieve the desired pharmacologic effect more quickly than if maintenance doses alone are used and concentrations are allowed to accumulate over 3 to 5 half-lives.

$$V = 7\ L/kg \cdot 68.4\ kg = 479\ L$$

$$LD = (Css \cdot V)/F = (1.2\ \mu g/L \cdot 479\ L)/1 = 575\ \mu g, \text{ rounded to } 600\ \mu g$$

When digoxin loading doses are administered, they are usually given in divided doses separated by 4 to 6 hours (50% of dose first, followed by two additional doses of 25%). In this case, an initial intravenous dose of 300 μg is given, followed by two intravenous doses of 150 μg each. One of the loading doses can be withheld if pulse rate is less than 50 to 60 beats/min or other undesirable digoxin adverse effects are noted.

Jelliffe Method

1. *Estimate the creatinine clearance.*

This patient has a stable serum creatinine and is obese [IBW_{males} (in kg) = 50 + 2.3(Ht − 60 in) = 50 + 2.3(68 − 60) = 68.4 kg]. The Salazar and Corcoran equation can be used to estimate creatinine clearance:

$$CrCl_{est(males)} = \frac{(137 - age)[(0.285 \cdot Wt) + (12.1 \cdot Ht^2)]}{(51 \cdot S_{Cr})}$$

$$CrCl_{est(males)} = \frac{(137 - 55\ y)\{(0.285 \cdot 140\ kg) + [12.1 \cdot (1.73\ m)^2]\}}{(51 \cdot 0.9\ mg/dL)} = 136\ mL/min$$

Note: Height is converted from inches to meters: Ht = (68 in · 2.54 cm/in)/(100 cm/m) = 1.73 m.

2. *Estimate the total body store (TBS) and the maintenance dosage (MD).*

The patient has moderate renal function and is obese. Digoxin total body stores of 13 to 15 μg/kg are effective in the treatment of atrial fibrillation. A digoxin dose of 14 μg/kg is chosen for this patient, and ideal body weight is used to compute doses. Digoxin tablets are used as the dosage form for maintenance doses.

$$TBS = 14\ \mu g/kg \cdot 68.4\ kg = 958\ \mu g$$

$$MD = \{TBS \cdot [14\% + 0.20(CrCl)]\}/(F \cdot 100) = \{958\ \mu g \cdot [14\% + 0.20\ (136\ mL/min)]\}/(0.7 \cdot 100) = 563\ \mu g/d, \text{ rounded to } 500\ \mu g/d$$

3. *Use the loading dose equation to compute the digoxin loading dose (if needed).*

Digoxin total body store is used to calculate the loading dose after correcting for bioavailability:

$$LD = TBS/F = 958\ \mu g/1 = 958\ \mu g, \text{ rounded to } 1000\ \mu g$$

When digoxin loading doses are administered, they are usually given in divided doses separated by 4 to 6 hours (50% of dose first, followed by two additional doses of 25%). In this case, an initial intravenous dose of 500 μg is given, followed by two intravenous doses of 250 μg each. One of the loading doses can be withheld if the pulse rate is less than 50 to 60 beats/min or if other undesirable digoxin adverse effects are noted.

8. The revised digoxin dose for patient BN is calculated as follows.

Linear Pharmacokinetics Method

1. *Estimate the creatinine clearance.*

This patient has a stable serum creatinine and is obese [IBW_{males} (in kg) = 50 + 2.3(Ht – 60 in) = 50 + 2.3(68 – 60) = 68.4 kg]. The Salazar and Corcoran equation can be used to estimate creatinine clearance:

$$CrCl_{est(males)} = \frac{(137 - age)[(0.285 \cdot Wt) + (12.1 \cdot Ht^2)]}{(51 \cdot S_{Cr})}$$

$$CrCl_{est(males)} = \frac{(137 - 55\ y)\{(0.285 \cdot 140\ kg) + [12.1 \cdot (1.73\ m)^2]\}}{(51 \cdot 0.9\ mg/dL)} = 136\ mL/min$$

Note: Height is converted from inches to meters: Ht = (68 in · 2.54 cm/in)/(100 cm/m) = 1.73 m.

The patient has moderate renal function and is expected to achieve steady state after 7 days of treatment.

2. *Compute the new dose to achieve the desired serum concentration.*

With linear pharmacokinetics, compute the new dose to attain the desired concentration that is proportional to the old dose that produced the measured concentration:

$$D_{new} = (Css_{new}/Css_{old})D_{old} = [(1.5\ ng/mL)/(2.4\ ng/mL)]\ 500\ \mu g/d = 313\ \mu g/d, \text{ rounded to } 375\ \mu g/d$$

The new dose is 375 μg/d, given as digoxin tablets to be started at the next scheduled dosing time. If desired, one daily dose can be withheld to allow the digoxin concentration to decline, and the new dose can be started the following day.

Pharmacokinetic Parameter Method

1. *Estimate the creatinine clearance.*

This patient has a stable serum creatinine and is obese [IBW_{males} (in kg) = 50 + 2.3(Ht – 60 in) = 50 + 2.3(68 – 60) = 68.4 kg]. The Salazar and Corcoran equation can be used to estimate creatinine clearance:

$$CrCl_{est(males)} = \frac{(137 - age)[(0.285 \cdot Wt) + (12.1 \cdot Ht^2)]}{(51 \cdot S_{Cr})}$$

$$CrCl_{est(males)} = \frac{(137 - 55\ y)\{(0.285 \cdot 140\ kg) + [12.1 \cdot (1.73\ m)^2]\}}{(51 \cdot 0.9\ mg/dL)} = 136\ mL/min$$

Note: Height is converted from inches to meters: Ht = (68 in · 2.54 cm/in)/(100 cm/m) = 1.73 m.

The patient has good renal function and is expected to achieve steady state after 7 days of treatment.

2. *Compute the drug clearance.*

Note that digoxin concentrations in ng/mL are the same as those for μg/L. This unit substitution is directly made to avoid conversion factors in the computation.

$$Cl = [F(D/\tau)]/Css = [0.7(500\ \mu g/d)]/2.4\ \mu g/L = 146\ L/d$$

3. *Compute the new dose to achieve desired serum concentration.*

The average steady-state equation is used to compute the new digoxin dose.

$$D/\tau = (Css \cdot Cl)/F = (1.5\ \mu g/L \cdot 146\ L/d)/0.7 = 313\ \mu g/d, \text{ rounded to } 375\ \mu g/d$$

The new suggested dose is 375 μg/d, given as digoxin tablets to be started at the next scheduled dosing time. If desired, one daily dose can be withheld to allow the digoxin concentration to decline, and the new dose can be started the following day.

9. The initial digoxin doses for patient VG are calculated as follows.

Pharmacokinetic Dosing Method

1. *Estimate the creatinine clearance.*

This patient has a stable serum creatinine and is obese [$IBW_{females}$ (in kg) = 45 + 2.3(Ht – 60 in) = 45 + 2.3(62 – 60) = 50 kg]. The Salazar and Corcoran equation can be used to estimate creatinine clearance:

$$CrCl_{est(females)} = \frac{(146 - age)[(0.287 \cdot Wt) + (9.74 \cdot Ht^2)]}{(60 \cdot S_{Cr})}$$

$$CrCl_{est(females)} = \frac{(146 - 75\ y)\{(0.287 \cdot 180\ kg) + [9.74 \cdot (1.57\ m)^2]\}}{(60 \cdot 6\ mg/dL)} = 15\ mL/min$$

Note: Height is converted from inches to meters: Ht = (62 in · 2.54 cm/in)/(100 cm/m) = 1.57 m.

The patient has poor renal function and is expected to achieve steady state after ~20 days of treatment.

2. *Estimate the drug clearance.*

The drug clearance versus creatinine clearance relationship is used to estimate the digoxin clearance (Cl_{NR} = 20 mL/min, because the patient has moderate to severe heart failure):

$$Cl = 1.303\ (CrCl) + Cl_{NR} = 1.303(15\ mL/min) + 20\ mL/min = 39\ mL/min$$

3. *Use the average steady-state concentration equation to compute the digoxin maintenance dosage.*

For a patient with heart failure, the desired digoxin concentration is 0.5 to 1 ng/mL. A serum concentration of 1 ng/mL is chosen for this patient, and oral digoxin capsules are to be used (F = 0.9). Note that for concentration, units ng/mL = μg/L, and this conversion is made before the equation is used. Also, conversion factors are needed to change milliliters to liters (1000 mL/L) and minutes to days (1440 min/d).

$$MD/\tau = (Css \cdot Cl)/F = (1\ \mu g/L \cdot 39\ mL/min \cdot 1440\ min/d)/(0.9 \cdot 1000\ mL/L) = 63\ \mu g/d, \text{ rounded to } 50\ \mu g/d$$

4. *Use the loading dose equation to compute the digoxin loading dose (if needed).*

The patient has poor renal function and is obese. Therefore, the volume of distribution equation that adjusts the parameter estimate for renal dysfunction can be used to compute the digoxin loading dose, and ideal body weight is used as the weight factor. An oral loading dose using capsules (F = 0.9) can be given to achieve the desired pharmacologic effect more quickly than if maintenance doses alone are used to allow concentrations to accumulate over 3 to 5 half-lives.

$$V = \left(226 + \frac{298 \cdot CrCl}{29.1 + CrCl}\right)(Wt/70) = \left(226 + \frac{298 \cdot 15\ mL/min}{29.1 + 15\ mL/min}\right)(50\ kg/70) = 234\ L$$

$$LD = (Css \cdot V)/F = (1\ \mu g/L \cdot 234\ L)/0.9 = 260\ \mu g, \text{ rounded to } 300\ \mu g$$

When digoxin loading doses are administered, they are usually given in divided doses separated by 4 to 6 hours (50% of dose first, followed by two additional doses of 25%). In this case, an initial oral dose of 200 μg is given, followed by two oral doses of 50 μg each, so that available capsule strengths can be used. One of the loading doses can be withheld if pulse rate is less than 50 to 60 beats/min or other undesirable digoxin adverse effects are noted.

Jelliffe Method

1. *Estimate the creatinine clearance.*

This patient has a stable serum creatinine and is obese [$IBW_{females}$ (in kg) = 45 + 2.3(Ht − 60 in) = 45 + 2.3(62 − 60) = 50 kg]. The Salazar and Corcoran equation can be used to estimate creatinine clearance:

$$CrCl_{est(females)} = \frac{(146 - age)[(0.287 \cdot Wt) + (9.74 \cdot Ht^2)]}{(60 \cdot S_{Cr})}$$

$$CrCl_{est(females)} = \frac{(146 - 75\ y)\{(0.287 \cdot 180\ kg) + [9.74 \cdot (1.57\ m)^2]\}}{(60 \cdot 6\ mg/dL)} = 15\ mL/min$$

Note: Height is converted from inches to meters: Ht = (62 in · 2.54 cm/in)/(100 cm/m) = 1.57 m.

The patient has poor renal function and is expected to achieve steady state after ~20 days of treatment.

2. *Estimate the total body store (TBS) and maintenance dosage (MD).*

The patient has poor renal function and is obese. Digoxin total body stores of 6 to 10 μg/kg are effective in the treatment of heart failure in patients with poor renal function. A digoxin dose of 8 μg/kg is chosen, and ideal body weight is used to compute the dose.

TBS = 8 μg/kg · 50 kg = 400 μg

MD = {TBS · [14% + 0.20(CrCl)]}/(F · 100)
= {400 μg · [14% + 0.20(15 mL/min)]}/(0.9 · 100) = 75 μg/d or 150 μg every other day (i.e., 75 μg/d · 2 days = 150 μg every 2 days)

3. *Use the loading dose equation to compute the digoxin loading dose (if needed).*

Digoxin total body store is used to calculate the loading dose after correcting for bioavailability:

LD = TBS/F = 400 μg/0.9 = 444 μg, rounded to 400 μg

When digoxin loading doses are administered, they are usually given in divided doses separated by 4 to 6 hours (50% of dose first, followed by two additional doses of 25%). In this case, an initial oral dose of 200 μg is given, followed by two oral doses of 100 μg each. One of the loading doses can be withheld if pulse rate is less than 50 to 60 beats per/min or other undesirable digoxin adverse effects are noted.

10. The revised digoxin dose for patient VG is calculated as follows.

Linear Pharmacokinetics Method

1. *Estimate the creatinine clearance.*

This patient has a stable serum creatinine and is obese [$IBW_{females}$ (in kg) = 45 + 2.3(Ht – 60 in) = 45 + 2.3(62 – 60) = 50 kg]. The Salazar and Corcoran equation can be used to estimate creatinine clearance:

$$CrCl_{est(females)} = \frac{(146 - age)[(0.287 \cdot Wt) + (9.74 \cdot Ht^2)]}{(60 \cdot S_{Cr})}$$

$$CrCl_{est(females)} = \frac{(146 - 75\ y)\{(0.287 \cdot 180\ kg) + [9.74 \cdot (1.57\ m)^2]\}}{(60 \cdot 6\ mg/dL)} = 15\ mL/min$$

Note: Height is converted from inches to meters: Ht = (62 in · 2.54 cm/in)/(100 cm/m) = 1.57 m.

The patient has poor renal function and is expected to achieve steady state after ~21 days of treatment.

2. *Compute the new dose to achieve the desired serum concentration.*

With the use of linear pharmacokinetics, the new dose to attain the desired concentration should be proportional to the old dose that produced the measured concentration:

$$D_{new} = (Css_{new}/Css_{old})D_{old} = [(1\ ng/mL)/(0.7\ ng/mL)]\ 150\ \mu g/2\ d = 214\ \mu g/2\ d \text{ or } 107\ \mu g/d, \text{ rounded to } 100\ \mu g/d$$

The new dose is 100 μg/d, given as oral digoxin capsules to be started at the next scheduled dosing time.

Pharmacokinetic Parameter Method

1. *Estimate the creatinine clearance.*

This patient has a stable serum creatinine and is obese [$IBW_{females}$ (in kg) = 45 + 2.3(Ht – 60 in) = 45 + 2.3(62 – 60) = 50 kg]. The Salazar and Corcoran equation can be used to estimate creatinine clearance:

$$CrCl_{est(females)} = \frac{(146 - age)[(0.287 \cdot Wt) + (9.74 \cdot Ht^2)]}{(60 \cdot S_{Cr})}$$

$$CrCl_{est(females)} = \frac{(146 - 75\ y)\{(0.287 \cdot 180\ kg) + [9.74 \cdot (1.57\ m)^2]\}}{(60 \cdot 6\ mg/dL)} = 15\ mL/min$$

Note: Height is converted from inches to meters: Ht = (62 in · 2.54 cm/in)/(100 cm/m) = 1.57 m.

The patient has good renal function and is expected to achieve steady state after ~21 days of treatment.

2. *Compute the drug clearance.*

Note that digoxin concentrations in ng/mL are the same as those for μg/L. This unit substitution is directly made to avoid conversion factors in the computation.

$$Cl = [F(D/\tau)]/Css = [0.9(150\ \mu g/2\ d)]/0.7\ \mu g/L = 96\ L/d$$

3. *Compute the new dose to achieve the desired serum concentration.*

The average steady-state equation is used to compute the new digoxin dose:

$$D/\tau = (Css \cdot Cl)/F = (1\ \mu g/L \cdot 96\ L/d)/0.9 = 107\ \mu g/d, \text{ rounded to } 100\ \mu g/d$$

The new suggested dose is 100 μg/d, given as digoxin capsules to be started at the next scheduled dosing time.

11. The initial digoxin doses for patient QW are calculated as follows.

Pharmacokinetic Dosing Method

1. *Estimate the creatinine clearance.*

This patient has a stable serum creatinine and is not obese. The Cockcroft–Gault equation can be used to estimate creatinine clearance:

$$CrCl_{est} = \{[(140 - age)BW]/(72 \cdot S_{Cr})\}0.85 = \{[(140 - 34\ y)50\ kg]/(72 \cdot 0.8\ mg/dL)\}0.85$$

$$CrCl_{est} = 78\ mL/min$$

2. *Estimate the drug clearance.*

The drug clearance versus creatinine clearance relationship is used to estimate the digoxin clearance (Cl_{NR} = 40 mL/min, because the patient does not have moderate to severe heart failure):

$$Cl = 1.303\ (CrCl) + Cl_{NR} = 1.303(78\ mL/min) + 40\ mL/min = 142\ mL/min$$

However, this patient is hyperthyroid, which is a disease state known to increase digoxin metabolism and shorten half-life ($t_{1/2}$ = 1 d). Assuming a normal volume of distribution (7 L/kg) and this half-life allows the computation of the expected digoxin clearance rate for the patient:

$$V = 7\ L/kg \cdot 50\ kg = 350\ L$$

$k_e = 0.693/t_{1/2} = 0.693/1\ d = 0.693\ d^{-1}$, where k_e is the terminal elimination rate constant

$$Cl = k_eV = 0.693\ d^{-1} \cdot 350\ L = 243\ L/d$$

This clearance rate is probably more reflective of the patient's digoxin elimination status and is used to compute her digoxin dose.

3. *Use the average steady-state concentration equation to compute the digoxin maintenance dosage.*

For a patient with atrial fibrillation, the desired digoxin concentration is 0.8 to 1.5 ng/mL. A serum concentration of 1.2 ng/mL is chosen for this patient, and oral digoxin capsules are used (F = 0.9). Note that for concentration, units ng/mL = μg/L, and this conversion is made before the equation is used.

$MD/\tau = (Css \cdot Cl)/F = (1.2\ \mu g/L \cdot 243\ L/d)/0.9 = 324\ \mu g/d$, rounded to 300 μg/d.

This is a large dose of digoxin, but hyperthyroid patients have increased digoxin clearance rates and require larger doses. If this dose were administered to patient QW, she would need to be monitored several times daily for digoxin adverse effects, and digoxin concentrations should be used to help guide therapy.

4. *Use the loading dose equation to compute the digoxin loading dose (if needed).*

V = 350 L from previous calculation

$LD = (Css \cdot V)/F = (1.2\ \mu g/L \cdot 350\ L)/1 = 420\ \mu g$, rounded to 400 μg

When digoxin loading doses are administered, they are usually given in divided doses separated by 4 to 6 hours (50% of dose first, followed by two additional doses of 25%). In this case, an initial intravenous dose of 200 μg is given, followed by two intravenous doses of 100 μg each. One of the loading doses can be withheld if pulse rate is less than 50 to 60 beats/min or other undesirable digoxin adverse effects are noted.

Jelliffe Method

1. *Estimate the creatinine clearance.*

This patient has a stable serum creatinine and is not obese. The Cockcroft–Gault equation can be used to estimate creatinine clearance:

$$CrCl_{est} = \{[(140 - age)BW]/(72 \cdot S_{Cr})\}0.85 = \{[(140 - 34\ y)50\ kg]/(72 \cdot 0.8\ mg/dL)\}0.85$$

$$CrCl_{est} = 78\ mL/min$$

2. *Estimate the total body store (TBS) and the maintenance dosage (MD).*

The patient has good renal function and is not obese. Digoxin total body stores of 13 to 15 μg/kg are effective in the treatment of atrial fibrillation. A digoxin dose of 14 μg/kg is chosen for this patient. Digoxin capsules are used as the dosage form for maintenance doses. Note that this dosing method does not include a way to adjust dosage requirements for disease states that cause higher-than-average clearance rates.

$$TBS = 14\ \mu g/kg \cdot 50\ kg = 700\ \mu g$$

$$MD = \{TBS \cdot [14\% + 0.20(CrCl)]\}/(F \cdot 100) = \{700\ \mu g \cdot [14\% + 0.20(78\ mL/min)]\}/(0.9 \cdot 100) = 231\ \mu g/d, \text{ rounded to } 200\ \mu g/d$$

3. *Use the loading dose equation to compute the digoxin loading dose (if needed).*

Digoxin total body store is used to calculate the loading dose after correcting for bioavailability:

$$LD = TBS/F = 700\ \mu g/1 = 700\ \mu g, \text{ rounded to } 750\ \mu g$$

When digoxin loading doses are administered, they are usually given in divided doses separated by 4 to 6 hours (50% of dose first, followed by two additional doses of 25%). In this case, an initial intravenous dose of 375 μg is given, followed by two intravenous doses of 187.5 μg each. One of the loading doses can be withheld if the pulse rate is less than 50 to 60 beats/min or if other undesirable digoxin adverse effects are noted.

12. The digoxin doses for patient RT are calculated as follows.

1. *Enter the patient's demographic, drug dosing, and serum concentration–time data into the computer program.*

2. *Compute the pharmacokinetic parameters for the patient using the Bayesian pharmacokinetics computer program.*

The pharmacokinetic parameters computed by the program are a clearance of 3 L/h, a volume of distribution of 403 L, and a half-life of 92 hours.

3. *Compute the dose required to achieve the desired digoxin serum concentrations.*

The one-compartment model equations used by the program to compute doses indicate that digoxin tablets 185 μg every 2 days will produce a predose steady-state concentration of 0.8 ng/mL. This dose is rounded to 187.5 μg (1½ 125-μg tablets) every other day.

13. The digoxin doses for patient LK are calculated as follows.

1. *Enter the patient's demographic, drug dosing, and serum concentration–time data into the computer program.*

2. *Compute the pharmacokinetic parameters using the Bayesian pharmacokinetics computer program.*

The pharmacokinetic parameters computed by the program are a clearance of 1.5 L/h, a volume of distribution of 276 L, and a half-life of 124 hours.

3. *Compute the dose required to achieve the desired digoxin serum concentrations.*

The one-compartment model equations used by the program to compute doses indicate that digoxin tablets 193 μg every 3 days will produce a predose steady-state concentration of 1 ng/mL. This dose is rounded to 187.5 μg (1½ 125-μg tablets) every third day.

14. The digoxin doses for patient BH are calculated as follows.

1. *Enter the patient's demographic, drug dosing, and serum concentration–time data into the computer program.*

2. *Compute the pharmacokinetic parameters using the Bayesian pharmacokinetics computer program.*

The pharmacokinetic parameters computed by the program are a clearance of 6.5 L/h, a volume of distribution of 509 L, and a half-life of 54 hours.

3. *Compute the dose required to achieve the desired digoxin serum concentrations.*

The one-compartment model equations used by the program to compute doses indicate that digoxin tablets 383 μg/d will produce a predose steady-state concentration of 1.5 ng/mL. This dose is rounded to 375 μg/d.

REFERENCES

1. Packer M, Gheorghiade M, Young JB, et al. Withdrawal of digoxin from patients with chronic heart failure treated with angiotensin-converting-enzyme inhibitors. RADIANCE Study. N Engl J Med 1993;329:1–7.
2. The effect of digoxin on mortality and morbidity in patients with heart failure. The Digitalis Investigation Group. N Engl J Med 1997;336:525–533.

3. Johnson JA, Parker RB, Geraci SA. Heart failure. In: DiPiro JT, Talbert RL, Yee GC, Matzke GR, Wells BG, Posey LM, eds. Pharmacotherapy—a pathophysiologic approach. Stamford, CT: Appleton & Lange, 1999:153–181.
4. Bauman JL, Schoen MD. Arrhythmias. In: DiPiro JT, Talbert RL, Yee GC, Matzke GR, Wells BG, Posey LM, eds. Pharmacotherapy—a pathophysiologic approach. Stamford, CT: Appleton & Lange, 1999:232–264.
5. Kelly RA, Smith TW. Pharmacological treatment of heart failure. In: Hardman JG, Limbird LE, Molinoff PB, Ruddon RW, Gilman AG, eds. The pharmacologic basis of therapeutics. New York: McGraw-Hill, 1996:809–838.
6. Reuning RH, Sams RA, Notari RE. Role of pharmacokinetics in drug dosage adjustment: I. Pharmacologic effect kinetics and apparent volume of distribution of digoxin. J Clin Pharmacol New Drugs 1973;13:127–141.
7. Koup JR, Greenblatt DJ, Jusko WJ, Smith TW, Koch-Weser J. Pharmacokinetics of digoxin in normal subjects after intravenous bolus and infusion doses. J Pharmacokinet Biopharm 1975;3: 181–192.
8. Koup JR, Jusko WJ, Elwood CM, Kohli RK. Digoxin pharmacokinetics: role of renal failure in dosage regimen design. Clin Pharmacol Ther 1975;18:9–21.
9. Slatton ML, Irani WN, Hall SA, et al. Does digoxin provide additional hemodynamic and autonomic benefit at higher doses in patients with mild to moderate heart failure and normal sinus rhythm? J Am Coll Cardiol 1997;29:1206–1213.
10. Gheorghiade M, Hall VB, Jacobsen G, Alam M, Rosman H, Goldstein S. Effects of increasing maintenance dose of digoxin on left ventricular function and neurohormones in patients with chronic heart failure treated with diuretics and angiotensin-converting enzyme inhibitors. Circulation 1995;92:1801–1807.
11. Beasley R, Smith DA, McHaffie DJ. Exercise heart rates at different serum digoxin concentrations in patients with atrial fibrillation. Br Med J (Clin Res Ed) 1985;290:9–11.
12. Aronson JK, Hardman M. ABC of monitoring drug therapy. Digoxin. Br Med J 1992;305: 1149–1152.
13. Smith TW, Haber E. Digoxin intoxication: the relationship of clinical presentation to serum digoxin concentration. J Clin Invest 1970;49:2377–2386.
14. Chung EK. Digitalis intoxication. Postgrad Med J 1972;48:163–179.
15. Beller GA, Smith TW, Abelmann WH, Haber E, Hood WB, Jr. Digitalis intoxication. A prospective clinical study with serum level correlations. N Engl J Med 1971;284:989–997.
16. Norregaard-Hansen K, Klitgaard NA, Pedersen KE. The significance of the enterohepatic circulation on the metabolism of digoxin in patients with the ability of intestinal conversion of the drug. Acta Med Scand 1986;220:89–92.
17. Johnson BF, Smith G, French J. The comparability of dosage regimens of Lanoxin tablets and Lanoxicaps. Br J Clin Pharmacol 1977;4:209–211.
18. Johnson BF, Bye C, Jones G, Sabey GA. A completely absorbed oral preparation of digoxin. Clin Pharmacol Ther 1976;19:746–751.
19. Kramer WG, Reuning RH. Use of area under the curve to estimate absolute bioavailability of digoxin [letter]. J Pharm Sci 1978;67:141–142.
20. Beveridge T, Nuesch E, Ohnhaus EE. Absolute bioavailability of digoxin tablets. Arzneimittelforschung 1978;28:701–703.
21. Ohnhaus EE, Vozeh S, Nuesch E. Absolute bioavailability of digoxin in chronic renal failure. Clin Nephrol 1979;11:302–306.
22. Ohnhaus EE, Vozeh S, Nuesch E. Absorption of digoxin in severe right heart failure. Eur J Clin Pharmacol 1979;15:115–120.
23. Hinderling PH. Kinetics of partitioning and binding of digoxin and its analogues in the subcompartments of blood. J Pharm Sci 1984;73:1042–1053.

24. Storstein L. Studies on digitalis: V. The influence of impaired renal function, hemodialysis, and drug interaction on serum protein binding of digitoxin and digoxin. Clin Pharmacol Ther 1976;20:6–14.
25. Iisalo E. Clinical pharmacokinetics of digoxin. Clin Pharmacokinet 1977;2:1–16.
26. Aronson JK. Clinical pharmacokinetics of digoxin 1980. Clin Pharmacokinet 1980;5:137–149.
27. Ewy GA, Groves BM, Ball MF, Nimmo L, Jackson B, Marcus F. Digoxin metabolism in obesity. Circulation 1971;44:810–814.
28. Abernethy DR, Greenblatt DJ, Smith TW. Digoxin disposition in obesity: clinical pharmacokinetic investigation. Am Heart J 1981;102:740–744.
29. Jusko WJ, Szefler SJ, Goldfarb AL. Pharmacokinetic design of digoxin dosage regimens in relation to renal function. J Clin Pharmacol 1974;14:525–535.
30. Ochs HR, Greenblatt DJ, Bodem G, Dengler HJ. Disease-related alterations in cardiac glycoside disposition. Clin Pharmacokinet 1982;7:434–451.
31. Bonelli J, Haydl H, Hruby K, Kaik G. The pharmacokinetics of digoxin in patients with manifest hyperthyroidism and after normalization of thyroid function. Int J Clin Pharmacol Biopharm 1978;16:302–306.
32. Koup JR. Distribution of digoxin in hyperthyroid patients. Int J Clin Pharmacol Ther Toxicol 1980;18:236.
33. Nyberg L, Wettrell G. Pharmacokinetics and dosage of digoxin in neonates and infants. Eur J Clin Pharmacol 1980;18:69–74.
34. Nyberg L, Wettrell G. Digoxin dosage schedules for neonates and infants based on pharmacokinetic considerations. Clin Pharmacokinet 1978;3:453–461.
35. Heizer WD, Pittman AW, Hammond JE, Fitch DD, Bustrack JA, Hull JH. Absorption of digoxin from tablets and capsules in subjects with malabsorption syndromes. Drug Intell Clin Pharm 1989;23:764–769.
36. Heizer WD, Smith TW, Goldfinger SE. Absorption of digoxin in patients with malabsorption syndromes. N Engl J Med 1971;285:257–259.
37. Kolibash AJ, Kramer WG, Reuning RH, Caldwell JH. Marked decline in serum digoxin concentration during an episode of severe diarrhea. Am Heart J 1977;94:806–807.
38. Bjornsson TD, Huang AT, Roth P, Jacob DS, Christenson R. Effects of high-dose cancer chemotherapy on the absorption of digoxin in two different formulations. Clin Pharmacol Ther 1986;39:25–28.
39. Jusko WJ, Conti DR, Molson A, Kuritzky P, Giller J, Schultz R. Digoxin absorption from tablets and elixir. The effect of radiation-induced malabsorption. JAMA 1974;230:1554–1555.
40. Ejvinsson G. Effect of quinidine on plasma concentrations of digoxin. Br Med J 1978;1: 279–280.
41. Leahey EB, Jr, Reiffel JA, Drusin RE, Heissenbuttel RH, Lovejoy WP, Bigger JT, Jr. Interaction between quinidine and digoxin. JAMA 1978;240:533–534.
42. Reiffel JA, Leahey EB, Jr, Drusin RE, Heissenbuttel RH, Lovejoy W, Bigger JT, Jr. A previously unrecognized drug interaction between quinidine and digoxin. Clin Cardiol 1979;2:40–42.
43. Hager WD, Fenster P, Mayersohn M, et al. Digoxin-quinidine interaction: pharmacokinetic evaluation. N Engl J Med 1979;300:1238–1241.
44. Doering W. Quinidine-digoxin interaction: pharmacokinetics, underlying mechanism and clinical implications. N Engl J Med 1979;301:400–404.
45. Bauer LA, Horn JR, Pettit H. Mixed-effect modeling for detection and evaluation of drug interactions: digoxin-quinidine and digoxin-verapamil combinations. Ther Drug Monit 1996;18:46–52.
46. Fromm MF, Kim RB, Stein CM, Wilkinson GR, Roden DM. Inhibition of P-glycoprotein-mediated drug transport: a unifying mechanism to explain the interaction between digoxin and quinidine. Circulation 1999;99:552–557.

47. Pedersen KE, Dorph-Pedersen A, Hvidt S, Klitgaard NA, Nielsen-Kudsk F. Digoxin-verapamil interaction. Clin Pharmacol Ther 1981;30:311–316.
48. Klein HO, Lang R, Weiss E, et al. The influence of verapamil on serum digoxin concentration. Circulation 1982;65:998–1003.
49. Pedersen KE, Thayssen P, Klitgaard NA, Christiansen BD, Nielsen-Kudsk F. Influence of verapamil on the inotropism and pharmacokinetics of digoxin. Eur J Clin Pharmacol 1983;25: 199–206.
50. Yoshida A, Fujita M, Kurosawa N, et al. Effects of diltiazem on plasma level and urinary excretion of digoxin in healthy subjects. Clin Pharmacol Ther 1984;35:681–685.
51. Rameis H, Magometschnigg D, Ganzinger U. The diltiazem-digoxin interaction. Clin Pharmacol Ther 1984;36:183–189.
52. Belz GG, Wistuba S, Matthews JH. Digoxin and bepridil: pharmacokinetic and pharmacodynamic interactions. Clin Pharmacol Ther 1986;39:65–71.
53. Moysey JO, Jaggarao NS, Grundy EN, Chamberlain DA. Amiodarone increases plasma digoxin concentrations. Br Med J (Clin Res Ed) 1981;282:272.
54. Maragno I, Santostasi G, Gaion RM, Paleari C. Influence of amiodarone on oral digoxin bioavailability in healthy volunteers. Int J Clin Pharmacol Res 1984;4:149–153.
55. Nademanee K, Kannan R, Hendrickson J, Ookhtens M, Kay I, Singh BN. Amiodarone-digoxin interaction: clinical significance, time course of development, potential pharmacokinetic mechanisms and therapeutic implications. J Am Coll Cardiol 1984;4:111–116.
56. Robinson K, Johnston A, Walker S, Mulrow JP, McKenna WJ, Holt DW. The digoxin-amiodarone interaction. Cardiovasc Drugs Ther 1989;3:25–28.
57. Nolan PE, Jr., Marcus FI, Erstad BL, Hoyer GL, Furman C, Kirsten EB. Effects of coadministration of propafenone on the pharmacokinetics of digoxin in healthy volunteer subjects. J Clin Pharmacol 1989;29:46–52.
58. Bigot MC, Debruyne D, Bonnefoy L, Grollier G, Moulin M, Potier JC. Serum digoxin levels related to plasma propafenone levels during concomitant treatment. J Clin Pharmacol 1991;31:521–526.
59. Calvo MV, Martin-Suarez A, Martin Luengo C, Avila C, Cascon M, Dominguez-Gil Hurle A. Interaction between digoxin and propafenone. Ther Drug Monit 1989;11:10–15.
60. Dorian P, Strauss M, Cardella C, David T, East S, Ogilvie R. Digoxin-cyclosporine interaction: severe digitalis toxicity after cyclosporine treatment. Clin Invest Med 1988;11:108–112.
61. Dobkin JF, Saha JR, Butler VP, Jr, Neu HC, Lindenbaum J. Inactivation of digoxin by *Eubacterium lentum,* an anaerobe of the human gut flora. Trans Assoc Coll Am Physicians 1982;95: 22–29.
62. Saha JR, Butler VP, Jr, Neu HC, Lindenbaum J. Digoxin-inactivating bacteria: identification in human gut flora. Science 1983;220:325–327.
63. Lindenbaum J, Rund DG, Bulter VP, Jr, Tse-Eng D, Saha JR. Inactivation of digoxin by the gut flora: reversal by antibiotic therapy. N Engl J Med 1981;305:789–794.
64. Morton MR, Cooper JW. Erythromycin-induced digoxin toxicity. Drug Intell Clin Pharm 1989;23:668–670.
65. Maxwell DL, Gilmour-White SK, Hall MR. Digoxin toxicity due to interaction of digoxin with erythromycin. Br Med J 1989;298:572.
66. Brown BA, Wallace RJ, Jr, Griffith DE, Warden R. Clarithromycin-associated digoxin toxicity in the elderly. Clin Infect Dis 1997;24:92–93.
67. Nawarskas JJ, McCarthy DM, Spinler SA. Digoxin toxicity secondary to clarithromycin therapy. Ann Pharmacother 1997;31:864–866.
68. Wakasugi H, Yano I, Ito T, et al. Effect of clarithromycin on renal excretion of digoxin: interaction with P-glycoprotein. Clin Pharmacol Ther 1998;64:123–128.

69. Allen MD, Greenblatt DJ, Harmatz JS, Smith TW. Effect of magnesium—aluminum hydroxide and kaolin—pectin on absorption of digoxin from tablets and capsules. J Clin Pharmacol 1981; 21:26–30.
70. Hall WH, Shappell SD, Doherty JE. Effect of cholestyramine on digoxin absorption and excretion in man. Am J Cardiol 1977;39:213–216.
71. Brown DD, Schmid J, Long RA, Hull JH. A steady-state evaluation of the effects of propantheline bromide and cholestyramine on the bioavailability of digoxin when administered as tablets or capsules. J Clin Pharmacol 1985;25:360–364.
72. Juhl RP, Summers RW, Guillory JK, Blaug SM, Cheng FH, Brown DD. Effect of sulfasalazine on digoxin bioavailability. Clin Pharmacol Ther 1976;20:387–394.
73. Lindenbaum J, Maulitz RM, Butler VP, Jr. Inhibition of digoxin absorption by neomycin. Gastroenterology 1976;71:399–404.
74. Johnson BF, Bustrack JA, Urbach DR, Hull JH, Marwaha R. Effect of metoclopramide on digoxin absorption from tablets and capsules. Clin Pharmacol Ther 1984;36:724–730.
75. Kirch W, Janisch HD, Santos SR, Duhrsen U, Dylewicz P, Ohnhaus EE. Effect of cisapride and metoclopramide on digoxin bioavailability. Eur J Drug Metab Pharmacokinet 1986;11: 249–250.
76. Jelliffe RW, Brooker G. A nomogram for digoxin therapy. Am J Med 1974;57:63–68.
77. Jelliffe RW. An improved method of digoxin therapy. Ann Intern Med 1968;69:703–717.
78. Mutnick AH. Digoxin. In: Schumacher GE, ed. Therapeutic drug monitoring. Stamford, CT: Appleton & Lange, 1995:469–491.
79. Anon. Lanoxin (digoxin) tablets, U.S.P. monograph. In: Arky R, ed. Physicians' desk reference. Montvale, NJ: Medical Economics Company, 1999:1167–1171.
80. Sheiner LB, Halkin H, Peck C, Rosenberg B, Melmon KL. Improved computer-assisted digoxin therapy. A method using feedback of measured serum digoxin concentrations. Ann Intern Med 1975;82:619–627.
81. Peck CC, Sheiner LB, Martin CM, Combs DT, Melmon KL. Computer-assisted digoxin therapy. N Engl J Med 1973;289:441–446.
82. Wandell M, Mungall D. Computer assisted drug interpretation and drug regimen optimization. Am Assoc Clin Chem 1984;6:1–11.
83. Smith TW, Butler VP, Jr, Haber E, et al. Treatment of life-threatening digitalis intoxication with digoxin-specific Fab antibody fragments: experience in 26 cases. N Engl J Med 1982;307: 1357–1362.
84. Smolarz A, Roesch E, Lenz E, Neubert H, Abshagen P. Digoxin specific antibody (Fab) fragments in 34 cases of severe digitalis intoxication. J Toxicol Clin Toxicol 1985;23:327–340.
85. Anon. Digibind (digoxin immune FAB, ovine) monograph. In: Arky R, ed. Physicians' desk reference. Montvale, NJ: Medical Economics Company, 1999:1110–1112.

7

LIDOCAINE

INTRODUCTION

Lidocaine is a local anesthetic agent that also has antiarrhythmic effects. It is classified as a type IB antiarrhythmic agent and is a second-line drug for the treatment of ventricular tachycardia or ventricular fibrillation.[1,2] For episodes of sustained ventricular tachycardia (>30 seconds in duration, >150 beats/min) with serious signs or symptoms of hemodynamic instability (angina, pulmonary edema, hypotension, hemodynamic collapse), electrical cardioversion is the treatment of choice.[1] However, in patients who are more hemodynamically stable, sustained monomorphic or polymorphic ventricular tachycardia may be treated using lidocaine therapy. The primary treatment for ventricular fibrillation is also direct-current cardioversion. Lidocaine is an alternative antiarrhythmic agent for patients who are not converted by means of electrical shock and intravenous epinephrine or vasopressin.

Lidocaine inhibits transmembrane sodium influx into the His-Purkinje fiber conduction system, thereby decreasing conduction velocity.[2] It also decreases the duration of the action potential and, as a result, decreases the duration of the absolute refractory period in Purkinje fibers and bundle of His. Automaticity is decreased during lidocaine therapy. The net effect of these cellular changes is that lidocaine eradicates ventricular reentrant arrhythmias by abolishing unidirectional blocks via increased conduction through diseased fibers.

THERAPEUTIC AND TOXIC CONCENTRATIONS

When given intravenously, the serum lidocaine concentration–time curve follows a two-compartment model.[3,4] This is especially apparent when initial loading doses of lidocaine are given as rapid intravenous injections over 1 to 5 minutes (maximum rate: 25 to 50 mg/min), and a distribution phase of 30 to 40 minutes is observed after drug administration (Figure 7-1). Unlike digoxin, the myocardium responds to the higher concentrations achieved during the distribution phase because lidocaine moves rapidly from the blood into the heart, and its onset of action after a loading dose is within a few minutes after the intravenous injection is completed.[1,2] Because of these factors, the heart is considered to be located in the central compartment of the two-compartment model for lidocaine.

The generally accepted therapeutic range for lidocaine is 1.5 to 5 μg/mL. In the upper end of the therapeutic range (>3 μg/mL), some patients experience minor side effects, such as drowsiness, dizziness, paresthesias, and euphoria. Lidocaine serum concentrations higher than the therapeutic range can cause muscle twitching, confusion, agitation, dysarthria, psychosis, seizures, or coma. Cardiovascular adverse effects such as atrioventricular block, hypotension, and circulatory collapse have been reported at lidocaine concentrations higher than 6 μg/mL but are not strongly correlated with specific serum levels. Lidocaine-induced seizures are not as difficult to treat as theophylline-induced seizures and usually respond to traditional antiseizure medication therapy. Lidocaine metabolites (MEGX and GX; see Basic Clinical Pharmacokinetic Parameters) probably contribute to the central nervous system side effects attributed to lidocaine therapy.[5–7] Clinicians should understand that all patients with "toxic" lidocaine serum concentrations in the listed ranges do not exhibit signs or symptoms of lidocaine toxicity. Rather, lidocaine concentrations in the given ranges increase the likelihood that an adverse effect will occur.

For dose adjustment purposes, lidocaine serum concentrations are best measured at steady state after the patient has received a consistent dosage regimen for 3 to 5 drug half-lives. Lidocaine half-life varies from 1 to 1.5 hours in normal adults to 5 hours or more in

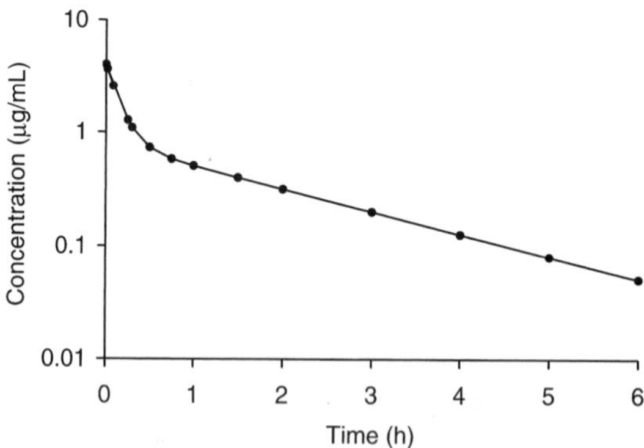

FIGURE 7-1 Lidocaine serum concentrations initially drop rapidly after an intravenous bolus as drug distributes from the blood into the tissues during the distribution phase. During the distribution phase, drug leaves the blood as a result of tissue distribution and elimination. After ½ to 1 hour, an equilibrium is established between the blood and tissues, and serum concentrations drop more slowly because elimination is the primary process removing drug from the blood. This type of serum concentration–time profile is described by a two-compartment model. The conduction system of the heart responds to the high concentrations of lidocaine present during the distribution phase, so lidocaine has a quick onset of action.

adult patients with liver failure. If lidocaine is given as a continuous intravenous infusion, it can take a considerable amount of time (3 to 5 half-lives, or 7.5 to 25 hours) for patients to achieve effective concentrations, so an intravenous loading dose is commonly administered to patients (Figure 7-2). The ideal situation is to administer an intravenous loading dose that will achieve the desired concentration immediately, then start an intravenous continuous infusion that will maintain that concentration (see Figure 7-2). To derive this perfect situation, the lidocaine volume of distribution for the central compartment (Vc in L) would have to be known to compute the loading dose (LD in mg): $LD = Css \cdot Vc$, where Css is the desired lidocaine concentration in mg/L. The volume of distribution for the central compartment of the two-compartment model is used to compute the loading dose, because lidocaine distributes rapidly to the myocardium and the heart is considered to reside in the central compartment of the model. However, this pharmacokinetic parameter is rarely, if ever, known for a patient, so a loading dose based on a population average central volume of distribution is used to calculate the amount of lidocaine needed. Since the patient's unique central volume of distribution is most likely greater (resulting in a loading dose that is too low) or lesser (resulting in a loading dose that is too large) than the population's average volume of distribution used to compute the loading dose, the desired steady-state lidocaine concentration will not be achieved. Because of this, it will still take 3 to 5 half-lives for the patient to reach steady-state conditions while receiving a constant intravenous infusion rate (Figure 7-3).

After a lidocaine loading dose is given, serum concentrations from this dose rapidly decline owing to distribution from blood to tissues, and serum concentrations due to the infusion are not able to increase rapidly enough to avoid a temporary decline or dip in lidocaine concentrations (see Figure 7-2). The decline may be severe enough that ventricular arrhythmias that were initially suppressed by lidocaine may recur because of subtherapeutic antiarrhythmic concentrations. Therefore, because of this dip in concentrations due to distribution of drug after the intravenous loading dose, an additional dose (50% of

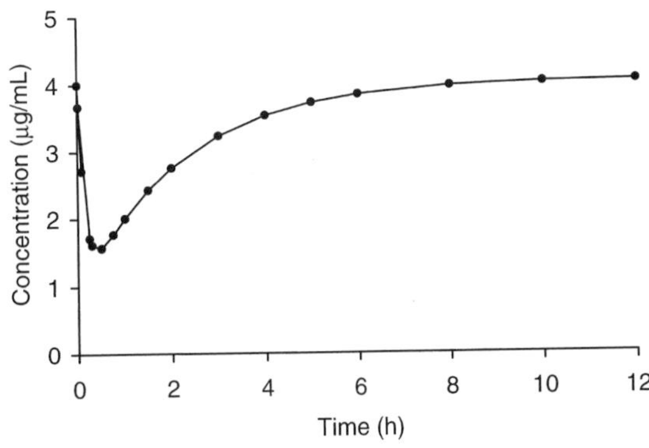

FIGURE 7-2 To maintain therapeutic lidocaine concentrations, an intravenous bolus (over 1 to 5 minutes) of lidocaine is followed by a continuous intravenous infusion of the drug. Even though the infusion is started immediately after the loading dose is given, serum concentrations due to the infusion cannot increase rapidly enough to counter the large decrease in concentrations during the distribution phase from the bolus dose. The dip in serum lidocaine concentrations below therapeutic amounts can allow previously treated arrhythmias to recur.

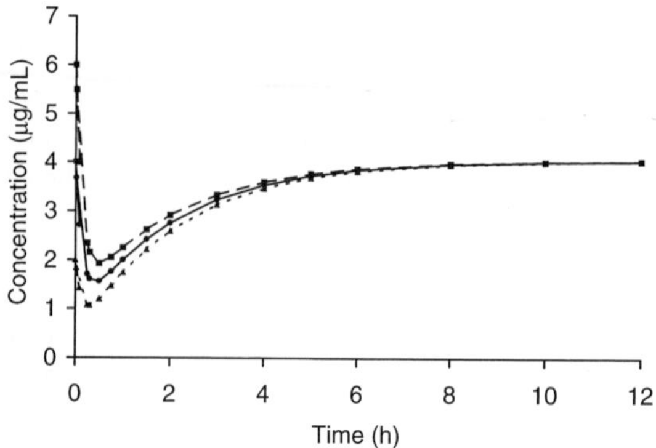

FIGURE 7-3 Because the central volume of distribution is not known at the time an intravenous loading dose of lidocaine is administered, average population parameters must be assumed and almost always result in initial lidocaine serum concentrations that are higher (*dashed line with squares*) or lower (*dotted line with triangles*) than those that were expected (*solid line with circles*). So the main clinical goal of administering loading doses of lidocaine is to achieve therapeutic concentrations as soon as possible, not to attain steady-state concentrations immediately after the loading dose is given.

original loading dose) can be given 20 to 30 minutes after the original loading dose or several additional doses (33% to 50% of original loading dose) can be given every 5 to 10 minutes to a total maximum of 3 mg/kg[4] (Figure 7-4). Thus, lidocaine intravenous loading doses do not usually achieve steady-state serum concentrations immediately, but it is hoped that they do result in therapeutic concentrations and response sooner than simply starting an intravenous infusion alone.

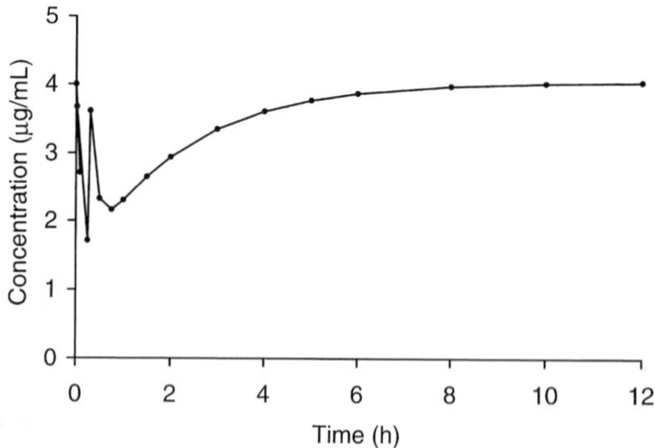

FIGURE 7-4 Because the dip in serum lidocaine concentrations below therapeutic amounts can allow previously treated arrhythmias to recur, a supplemental loading or "booster" dose is typically given 20 to 30 minutes after the initial loading dose. This prevents lidocaine serum concentrations from declining too far during the distribution phase of the intravenous bolus dose and before serum concentrations from the intravenous infusion have had an opportunity to attain therapeutic concentrations.

CLINICAL MONITORING PARAMETERS

The electrocardiogram (ECG or EKG) should be monitored to determine the response to lidocaine in patients with ventricular tachycardia or ventricular fibrillation. The goal of therapy is suppression of ventricular arrhythmias and avoidance of adverse drug reactions. Lidocaine therapy is often discontinued after 6 to 24 hours of treatment, so the need for long-term antiarrhythmic drug use can be assessed. However, longer-term infusions may be used in patients with persistent tachyarrhythmias. For long-term therapy, electrophysiologic studies using programmed stimulation to replicate the ventricular arrhythmia or 24-hour ECG monitoring using a Holter monitor can be performed in patients while receiving a variety of antiarrhythmic agents to determine effective antiarrhythmic drug therapy. Because lidocaine is administered only parenterally, it is rarely used for more than a few days unless oral antiarrhythmic agents are ineffective.

Because lidocaine is usually given for a short duration (<24 hours), often serum lidocaine concentrations do not have to be obtained in patients who are receiving appropriate doses and who currently have no ventricular arrhythmia or adverse drug effects. However, lidocaine serum concentrations should be obtained in patients who have a recurrence of ventricular tachyarrhythmias, are experiencing possible lidocaine side effects, or are receiving lidocaine doses not consistent with disease states and conditions known to alter lidocaine pharmacokinetics (see Effects of Disease States and Conditions on Lidocaine Pharmacokinetics and Dosing). Serum concentration monitoring can aid in the decision to increase or decrease the lidocaine dose. For instance, if the ventricular arrhythmia reappears and the lidocaine serum concentration is less than 5 μg/mL, increasing the lidocaine dose is a therapeutic option. However, if the lidocaine serum concentration is greater than 5 μg/mL, a dosage increase is unlikely to be effective in suppressing the arrhythmia; moreover, there is an increased likelihood that drug side effects may occur. Similarly, if a possible lidocaine adverse drug reaction is noted in a patient and the lidocaine serum concentration is less than 3 to 5 μg/mL, the observed problem may not be due to lidocaine treatment, and other sources can be investigated. Patients receiving lidocaine infusions for longer than 24 hours are prone to unexpected accumulation of lidocaine concentrations in the serum and should be closely monitored for lidocaine side effects.[8–11] While receiving lidocaine, patients should be monitored for the following adverse drug effects: drowsiness, dizziness, paresthesias, euphoria, muscle twitching, confusion, agitation, dysarthria, psychosis, sei-zures, coma, atrioventricular block, and hypotension.

BASIC CLINICAL PHARMACOKINETIC PARAMETERS

Lidocaine is almost completely eliminated by hepatic metabolism (>95%).[3,12] Hepatic metabolism is mainly via the CYP3A enzyme system. Monoethylglycinexylidide (MEGX) is the primary metabolite resulting from lidocaine metabolism.[5–7] Although a portion of MEGX is eliminated renally, most of the metabolite is further converted hepatically to glycinexylidide (GX) and other inactive metabolites. GX is primarily eliminated by the kidney. MEGX and GX have some antiarrhythmic activity (MEGX ~80% and GX ~10%, relative to lidocaine) but have also been implicated as the cause of some adverse effects attributed to lidocaine therapy.[5–7] Because both metabolites are eliminated by the kidney, patients with renal failure should be monitored for adverse effects due to metabolite accumulation, even though lidocaine serum concentrations are within the therapeutic range. The hepatic extraction ratio of lidocaine is about 70%, so lidocaine is typically classified as a high extraction ratio drug. Because of this, liver blood flow is expected to be the predominant factor influencing the clearance of lidocaine (Cl ≈ LBF, where Cl is lidocaine clearance and LBF is liver blood flow—both in L/min), and many disease states and conditions that alter lidocaine clearance do so through changes in liver blood flow. However, because a hepatic extraction ratio greater than 70% is the definition of a high extraction ratio agent and the extraction ratio for lidocaine is on the margin of this range, changes in lidocaine intrinsic clearance or plasma protein binding may very possibly change lidocaine clearance.

Lidocaine is usually given intravenously but may also be given intramuscularly.[13] After intramuscular injection, absorption is rapid and complete, with maximum concentrations occurring about 1 hour after administration and 100% bioavailability as long as the patient's peripheral circulation is not compromised from hypotension or shock. Intramuscular administration of medications can increase creatinine kinase (CK) concentrations because of minor skeletal muscle trauma inflicted by the injection, and this enzyme is monitored in patients who may have had a myocardial infarction. Thus, the creatinine kinase isozyme that is relatively specific to the heart (CK-MB) needs to be measured in patients with myocardial infarction who have received intramuscular injections. Oral absorption of lidocaine is nearly 100%.[3] However, lidocaine is extensively metabolized by the CYP3A enzymes contained in the intestinal wall and liver, resulting in a large first-pass effect and low, variable oral bioavailability (F ≈ 30%). Because roughly 70% of an oral dose is converted to metabolites, MEGX and GX concentrations are high after oral administration of lidocaine, resulting in a high incidence of adverse effects.

Plasma protein binding in healthy persons is about 70%.[14–16] Of this value, approximately 30% is due to drug binding to albumin, whereas 70% is due to lidocaine bound to α_1-acid glycoprotein (AAG).[8,10,11] AAG is classified as an acute-phase reactant protein present in lower amounts in all individuals but secreted in large amounts in response to certain stresses and disease states, such as trauma, heart failure, and myocardial infarction. In patients with these disease states, lidocaine binding to AAG can be even larger and may result in an unbound fraction as low as 10% to 15%. AAG concentrations continuously increase during the first 12 to 72 hours after a myocardial infarction, and, as a result, the lidocaine-unbound fraction decreases on average from about 30% to 20% during this time period. The continuous increase in protein binding due to AAG secretion causes a continuous decrease in lidocaine clearance in patients with myocardial infarction, and lidocaine concentrations can accumulate to unexpectedly high levels in patients receiving the drug for longer than 24 hours. Patients without myocardial infarction also experience accumulation of lidocaine concentrations during long-term (>24 hours) infusions because of competition for hepatic metabolism between parent drug and metabolites.[9,17] Thus, monitoring for adverse reactions in patients receiving long-term lidocaine infusions is important, and lidocaine serum concentrations can be useful adjuncts to prevent lidocaine toxicity.

The recommended dose of lidocaine is based on the concurrent disease states and conditions present in the patient that can influence lidocaine concentrations. Lidocaine pharmacokinetic parameters used to compute doses are given in the following section for specific patient profiles.

EFFECTS OF DISEASE STATES AND CONDITIONS ON LIDOCAINE PHARMACOKINETICS AND DOSING

In healthy adults without the disease states and conditions given later in this section and with normal liver function, an average lidocaine half-life is 1.5 hours (range, 1 to 2 hours), the mean central volume of distribution equals 0.5 L/kg (Vc = 0.4 – 0.6 L/kg), and the average volume of distribution for the entire body is 1.5 L/kg (V_{area} = 1 – 2 L/kg; Table 7-1).[3,9,18] Disease states and conditions that change lidocaine pharmacokinetics and dosage requirements may alter clearance, the central volume of distribution, and the volume of distribution for the entire body. The volume of distribution for the central compartment of the two-compartment model is used to compute the loading dose, because lidocaine distributes rapidly to the myocardium and the heart is considered to reside in the central compartment of the model. The elimination rate constant ($k = 0.693/t_{1/2}$, where $t_{1/2}$ is the half-life) and clearance ($Cl = kV_{area}$) can be computed from the aforementioned pharmacokinetic parameters.

Patients with liver cirrhosis or acute hepatitis have reduced lidocaine clearance, which results in a prolonged average lidocaine half-life of 5 hours.[12,19–22] The mechanisms for depressed clearance in patients with liver disease are destruction of liver parenchyma where hepatic drug-metabolizing enzymes are present and reduction of liver blood flow. The central volume of distribution and the volume of distribution for the entire body are larger in patients with liver disease because albumin and α_1-acid glycoprotein (AAG) concentrations are lower in these patients and result in reduced lidocaine plasma protein binding (average Vc = 0.6 L/kg, average V_{area} = 2.6 L/kg). However, the effect that liver disease has on lidocaine pharmacokinetics is highly variable and difficult to accurately predict, especially in patients with acute hepatitis. It is possible for a patient with liver disease to have relatively normal or grossly abnormal lidocaine clearance, volumes of distribution, and half-life. An index of liver dysfunction can be gained by applying the Child-Pugh clinical classification system to the patient[23] (Table 7-2). Child-Pugh scores are discussed in detail in Chapter 3 but are briefly discussed here.

The Child-Pugh score consists of five laboratory tests or clinical symptoms: serum albumin, total bilirubin, prothrombin time, ascites, and hepatic encephalopathy. Each of these areas is given a score of 1 (normal) to 3 (severely abnormal; see Table 7-2), and the scores for the five areas are totaled. The Child-Pugh score for a patient with normal liver function is 5, whereas the score for a patient with grossly abnormal serum albumin, total bilirubin, and prothrombin time values in addition to severe ascites and hepatic encephalopathy is 15. A Child-Pugh score greater than 8 is grounds for a decrease in the initial daily drug dose for lidocaine ($t_{1/2}$ = 5 hours). As in any patient with or without liver dysfunction, initial doses are meant as starting points for dosage titration based on patient response and avoidance of adverse effects. Lidocaine serum concentrations and the presence of adverse drug effects should be monitored frequently in patients with liver cirrhosis.

Heart failure causes reduced lidocaine clearance because of decreased hepatic blood flow secondary to compromised cardiac output[5,12,21,24,25] (Table 7-3). Patients with cardio-

TABLE 7-1 Disease States and Conditions That Alter Lidocaine Pharmacokinetics

DISEASE STATE/ CONDITION	HALF-LIFE (h)	CENTRAL VOLUME OF DISTRIBUTION (Vc) (L/kg)	VOLUME OF DISTRIBUTION FOR ENTIRE BODY (V_{area}) (L/kg)	COMMENT
Adult, normal liver function	1.5 (range, 1–2)	0.5 (range, 0.4–0.6)	1.5 (range, 1–2)	Lidocaine has a high hepatic extraction ratio of ~70%, so liver blood flow is a primary determinant of clearance rate. Accumulation of serum lidocaine concentrations can occur with long-term (>24 h) infusions.
Adult, hepatic disease (liver cirrhosis or acute hepatitis)	5	0.6	2.6	Lidocaine is metabolized >95% by hepatic microsomal enzymes (primarily CYP3A), so loss of functional liver tissue, as well as reduced liver blood flow, decreases lidocaine clearance. Pharmacokinetic parameters are highly variable in liver disease patients. Volumes of distribution are larger due to decreased α_1-acid glycoprotein and albumin drug binding in the plasma.
Adult, heart failure	2	0.3	1	Decreased liver blood flow secondary to reduced cardiac output reduces lidocaine clearance. Volumes of distribution are smaller because of in-

TABLE 7-1 ***(continued)***

DISEASE STATE/ CONDITION	HALF-LIFE (h)	CENTRAL VOLUME OF DISTRIBUTION (Vc) (L/kg)	VOLUME OF DISTRIBUTION FOR ENTIRE BODY (V_{area}) (L/kg)	COMMENT
Adult, heart failure *(continued)*				creased α_1-acid glycoprotein drug binding in the plasma. Heart failure results in large and variable reductions in lidocaine clearance. Cardiac status must be monitored closely in heart failure patients, since lidocaine clearance changes with acute changes in cardiac output.
Adult, postmyocardial infarction (<12 h)	4	0.5	1.5	Myocardial infarction reduces cardiac output, resulting in variable reductions in lidocaine clearance. These patients are especially prone to accumulation of serum lidocaine concentrations during long-term (>24 h) infusions owing to secretion of α_1-acid glycoprotein.
Adult, obese (>30% over ideal body weight)	According to other disease states or conditions that affect lidocaine pharmacokinetics	According to other disease states or conditions that affect lidocaine pharmacokinetics	According to other disease states or conditions that affect lidocaine pharmacokinetics	Lidocaine doses should be based on ideal body weight for patients whose weight is >30% above IBW.

genic shock experience extreme declines in lidocaine clearance owing to severe decreases in cardiac output and liver blood flow. Central volume of distribution (Vc = 0.3 L/kg) and volume of distribution for the entire body (V_{area} = 1 L/kg) are decreased because heart failure patients have elevated AAG serum concentrations, which lead to increased lidocaine plasma protein binding and decreased lidocaine unbound fraction. In patients with heart failure, an average lidocaine half-life is 2 hours (range, 1 to 24 hours). Half-life ($t_{1/2}$) does not change as much as expected from the change in clearance (Cl), because the volume of distribution simultaneously decreases [$t_{1/2} = (0.693 \cdot \downarrow V_{area})/\downarrow Cl$]. Obviously, the effect that heart failure has on lidocaine pharmacokinetics is highly variable and difficult to accurately predict. It is possible for a patient with heart failure to have relatively normal or grossly abnormal lidocaine clearance and half-life. For heart failure patients, initial doses are meant as starting points for dosage titration based on patient response and avoidance of adverse effects. Lidocaine serum concentrations and the presence of adverse drug effects should be monitored frequently in patients with heart failure.

Patients with myocardial infarction may develop serious ventricular arrhythmias that require therapy with lidocaine. After a myocardial infarction, serum AAG concentrations increase up to 50% over a 12- to 72-hour time period.[8,10,11] As AAG serum concentrations increase, plasma protein binding of lidocaine decreases, and the unbound fraction of lidocaine decreases from about 30% to about 20%. Although lidocaine is considered a high hepatic extraction ratio drug with liver blood flow having the major influence on lidocaine clearance, a decline in the unbound fraction of lidocaine in the plasma decreases lidocaine clearance. The reduction in lidocaine clearance is continuous as long as AAG concentrations continue to rise. A result of this phenomenon is that lidocaine serum concentrations do not reach steady state during long-term (>24 hours) intravenous infusions of lidocaine in myocardial infarction patients, and results of pharmacokinetic studies in this patient population differ according to when the investigation took place in relation to the myocardial damage. When studied within 12 hours of myocardial infarction, patients had decreased lidocaine clearance due to decreased cardiac output and liver blood flow, relatively normal volumes of distribution (Vc = 0.5 L/kg, V_{area} = 1.5 L/kg), and a prolonged half-life of 4 hours.[25–27] When similar myocardial infarction patients are studied after

TABLE 7-2 Child-Pugh Scores for Patients With Liver Disease

TEST/SYMPTOM	SCORE 1 POINT	SCORE 2 POINTS	SCORE 3 POINTS
Total bilirubin (mg/dL)	<2.0	20–3.0	>3.0
Serum albumin (g/dL)	>3.5	2.8–3.5	<2.8
Prothrombin time (seconds prolonged over control)	<4	4–6	>6
Ascites	Absent	Slight	Moderate
Hepatic encephalopathy	None	Moderate	Severe

From Pugh RN, Murray-Lyon IM, Dawson JL, Pietroni MC, Williams R. Transection of the oesophagus for bleeding oesophageal varices. Br J Surg 1973;60:646–649.

TABLE 7-3 New York Heart Association Functional Classification of Heart Failure

CLASS	DESCRIPTION
I	Patients with cardiac disease but without limitations of physical activity. Ordinary physical activity does not cause undue fatigue, dyspnea, or palpitation.
II	Patients with cardiac disease that results in slight limitations of physical activity. Ordinary physical activity results in fatigue, palpitation, dyspnea, or angina.
III	Patients with cardiac disease that results in marked limitations of physical activity. Although patients are comfortable at rest, less than ordinary activity leads to symptoms.
IV	Patients with cardiac disease that results in an inability to carry on physical activity without discomfort. Symptoms of congestive heart failure are present even at rest. With any physical activity, increased discomfort is experienced.

From Johnson JA, Parker RB, Geraci SA. Heart failure. In: DiPiro JT, Talbert RL, Yee GC, Matzke GR, Wells BG, Posey LM, eds. Pharmacotherapy—a pathophysiologic approach. Stamford, CT: Appleton & Lange, 1999:153–181.

longer lidocaine infusions, the central volume of distribution and volume of distribution representing the entire body are smaller, because AAG serum concentrations have had an opportunity to increase and change lidocaine plasma protein binding.[8,10,11]

Although the volume of distribution representing the entire body (V_{area}) correlates most closely with total body weight, obese patients (>30% above ideal body weight) should have central volume of distribution and clearance estimates based on ideal body weight.[18] Lidocaine pharmacokinetic parameter estimates should be based on the concurrent disease states and conditions in the patient. If weight-based dosage recommendations are to be used, ideal body weight should be used to compute maintenance infusions (mg/kg per minute) and loading doses (mg/kg) for obese persons.

Patient age has an effect on lidocaine volumes of distribution and half-life.[24] For elderly patients over the age of 65, studies indicate that lidocaine clearance is unchanged, the volumes of distribution are slightly larger, and lidocaine half-life is longer (average half-life = 2.3 hours, range, 1.7 to 4.5 hours) compared with those of younger subjects. A confounding factor found in lidocaine pharmacokinetic studies conducted in older adults is the possible accidental inclusion of subjects that have subclinical or mild cases of the disease states associated with reduced lidocaine clearance (e.g., heart failure and liver disease). In addition, most patients with serious ventricular arrhythmias studied in all of the previously mentioned studies are older, and those results include any influence of age. Thus, in most cases elderly patients are treated with lidocaine according to their other disease states or conditions that influence lidocaine pharmacokinetics.

Lidocaine serum concentrations accumulate in patients receiving long-term (>24 hours) infusions, even if the patient did not have a myocardial infarction.[9,17] Accumulation of lidocaine in these patients is due to competition for hepatic metabolism between parent drug and metabolites. Because MEGX and GX metabolites are eliminated to some extent by the kidney, patients with renal failure should be monitored for lidocaine adverse effects due to metabolite accumulation, even though lidocaine serum concentrations are within the therapeutic range. Lidocaine is not appreciably removed by hemodialysis.

DRUG INTERACTIONS

Lidocaine has serious drug interactions with β-adrenergic receptor blockers and cimetidine, which decrease lidocaine clearance 30% or more.[28] Propranolol, metoprolol, and nadolol have been reported to reduce lidocaine clearance owing to the decrease in cardiac output caused by β-blocker agents. Decreased cardiac output results in reduced liver blood flow, which explains the decline in lidocaine clearance caused by these drugs. Cimetidine also decreases lidocaine clearance, but the mechanism of the interaction is different. Because cimetidine does not change liver blood flow, cimetidine is believed to decrease lidocaine clearance by inhibiting hepatic microsomal enzymes.[29,30]

Lidocaine clearance may be accelerated by concomitant use of phenobarbital or phenytoin.[28] Both of these agents are known to be hepatic drug-metabolizing enzyme inducers, and this is the probable mechanism of their drug interaction with lidocaine. It is important to remember that phenytoin has antiarrhythmic effects and is also classified as a type IB antiarrhythmic agent. Because of this, phenytoin and lidocaine may have additive pharmacologic effects that could result in a pharmacodynamic drug interaction.

INITIAL DOSAGE DETERMINATION METHODS

Pharmacokinetic Dosing Method

The goal of initial dosing of lidocaine is to compute the best dose possible for the patient, given the patient's set of disease states and conditions that influence lidocaine pharmacokinetics and the arrhythmia being treated. To do this, pharmacokinetic parameters are estimated using average parameters measured in other patients with similar disease states and condition profiles.

ESTIMATE OF HALF-LIFE AND ELIMINATION RATE CONSTANT

Lidocaine is predominantly metabolized by the liver. Unfortunately, there is no good way to estimate the elimination characteristics of liver-metabolized drugs using an endogenous marker of liver function in the same manner that serum creatinine and estimated creatinine clearance are used to estimate the elimination of agents that are renally eliminated. Because of this, a patient is categorized according to the disease states and conditions that are known to change lidocaine half-life, and the half-life previously measured in these studies is used as an estimate of the current patient's half-life (see Table 7-1). For example, if a patient has suffered an uncomplicated myocardial infarction, lidocaine half-life is assumed to be 4 hours. Alternatively, for a patient with moderate heart failure [New York Heart Association (NYHA) CHF class III], lidocaine half-life is assumed to be 2 hours, whereas a patient with severe liver disease (Child-Pugh score, 12) is assigned an estimated lidocaine half-life of 5 hours. To produce the most conservative lidocaine doses in patients with multiple concurrent disease states or conditions that affect lidocaine pharmacokinetics, the disease state or condition associated with the longest half-life should be used to compute doses. This approach prevents accidental overdosage as much as currently possible. Once the correct half-life is identified for the patient, it can be converted into the lidocaine elimination rate constant (k) using the following equation: $k = 0.693/t_{1/2}$.

ESTIMATE OF VOLUME OF DISTRIBUTION

As with the half-life estimate, lidocaine volume of distribution values are chosen according to the disease states and conditions that are present (see Table 7-1). The central volume of distribution (Vc) is used to compute loading doses because lidocaine has a rapid onset of action after administration, and the heart acts as if it is in the central compartment of the two-compartment model used to describe lidocaine pharmacokinetics. The central volume of distribution is assumed to be 0.6 L/kg for liver disease patients, 0.3 L/kg for heart failure and cardiogenic shock patients, and 0.5 L/kg for all other patients. The volume of distribution for the entire body after distribution is complete (V_{area}) is used to help compute lidocaine clearance and is assumed to be 2.6 L/kg for liver disease patients, 1 L/kg for heart failure and cardiogenic shock patients, and 1.5 L/kg for all other patients. For obese patients (>30% above ideal body weight), ideal body weight is used to compute lidocaine volume of distribution. Thus, for a not obese 80-kg patient without heart failure or liver disease, the estimated lidocaine central volume of distribution is 40 L: Vc = 0.5 L/kg · 80 kg = 40 L. For a 150-kg obese patient with an ideal body weight of 60 kg and normal cardiac and liver function, the estimated lidocaine volume of distribution is 30 L: V = 0.5 L/kg · 60 kg = 30 L.

SELECTION OF APPROPRIATE PHARMACOKINETIC MODEL AND EQUATIONS

When given by continuous intravenous infusion, lidocaine follows a two-compartment pharmacokinetic model (see Figures 7-1 through 7-3). A simple pharmacokinetic equation that computes the lidocaine steady-state serum concentration (Css in μg/mL = mg/L) is widely used and allows dosage calculation for a continuous infusion: Css = k_0/Cl or k_0 = Css · Cl, where k_0 is the dose of lidocaine in mg/h and Cl is lidocaine clearance in L/h. Clearance is computed using estimates of lidocaine elimination rate constant (k) and volume of distribution for the entire body after distribution is complete (V_{area}): Cl = kV_{area}. For example, if a patient has an estimated elimination rate constant of 0.173 h^{-1} and an estimated volume of distribution of 105 L, the estimated clearance would be 18.2 L/h: Cl = 0.173 h^{-1} · 105 L = 18.2 L/h.

The equation used to calculate an intravenous loading dose (LD in mg) is based on a two-compartment model: LD = (Css · Vc), where Css is the desired lidocaine steady-state concentration in μg/mL, which is equivalent to mg/L, and Vc is the lidocaine central volume of distribution. Intravenous lidocaine loading doses should be given as an intravenous bolus no faster than 25 to 50 mg/min.

STEADY-STATE CONCENTRATION SELECTION

The general accepted therapeutic range for lidocaine is 1.5 to 5 μg/mL. However, lidocaine therapy must be individualized for each patient to achieve optimal responses and minimal side effects.

Example 1 LK is a 50-year-old, 75-kg, 178-cm (70-in) male with ventricular tachycardia who requires therapy with intravenous lidocaine. He has normal liver and cardiac function. Suggest an initial intravenous lidocaine dosage regimen designed to achieve a steady-state lidocaine concentration of 3 μg/mL.

1. *Estimate the half-life and elimination rate constant according to the disease states and conditions of the patient.*

The expected lidocaine half-life ($t_{1/2}$) is 1.5 hours. The elimination rate constant is computed using the following formula: $k = 0.693/t_{1/2} = 0.693/1.5\ h = 0.462\ h^{-1}$.

2. *Estimate the volume of distribution and clearance.*

The patient is not obese, so the estimated lidocaine central volume of distribution and the volume of distribution for the entire body (V_{area}) is based on actual body weight: $Vc = 0.5\ L/kg \cdot 75\ kg = 38\ L$, $V_{area} = 1.5\ L/kg \cdot 75\ kg = 113\ L$. Estimated lidocaine clearance is computed by taking the product of V_{area} and the elimination rate constant: $Cl = kV_{area} = 0.462\ h^{-1} \cdot 113\ L = 52.2\ L/h$.

3. *Compute the dosage regimen.*

Therapy is started by administering an intravenous loading dose of lidocaine to the patient (note: μg/mL = mg/L, and this concentration unit was substituted for Css in the calculations so that unnecessary unit conversion was not required): $LD = Css \cdot Vc = 3\ mg/L \cdot 38\ L = 114\ mg$, rounded to 100 mg intravenously over 2 to 4 minutes. An additional dose of 50% of the loading dose can be given if arrhythmias recur 20 to 30 minutes after the initial loading dose.

A lidocaine continuous intravenous infusion is started immediately after the loading dose has been administered. The dosage equation for intravenous lidocaine is $k_0 = Css \cdot Cl = (3\ mg/L \cdot 52.2\ L/h)/(60\ min/h) = 2.6\ mg/min$, rounded to 2.5 mg/min.

A steady-state lidocaine serum concentration can be measured after steady-state is attained in 3 to 5 half-lives. Since lidocaine is expected to have a half-life of 1.5 hours in the patient, the lidocaine steady-state concentration can be obtained any time after the first 8 hours of dosing (5 half-lives $= 5 \cdot 1.5\ h = 7.5\ h$). Lidocaine serum concentrations should also be measured if the patient experiences a return of ventricular arrhythmia or if the patient develops potential signs or symptoms of lidocaine toxicity.

Example 2 OI is a 60-year-old, 85-kg, 185-cm (73-in) male with ventricular fibrillation who requires therapy with intravenous lidocaine. He has liver cirrhosis (Child-Pugh score, 11). Suggest an initial intravenous lidocaine dosage regimen designed to achieve a steady-state lidocaine concentration of 4 μg/mL.

1. *Estimate the half-life and elimination rate constant according to the disease states and conditions of the patient.*

The expected lidocaine half-life ($t_{1/2}$) is 5 hours. The elimination rate constant is computed using the following formula: $k = 0.693/t_{1/2} = 0.693/5\ h = 0.139\ h^{-1}$.

2. *Estimate the volume of distribution and clearance.*

The patient is not obese, so the estimated lidocaine central volume of distribution and the volume of distribution for the entire body (V_{area}) can be based on actual body weight: $Vc = 0.6\ L/kg \cdot 85\ kg = 51\ L$, $V_{area} = 2.6\ L/kg \cdot 85\ kg = 221\ L$. Estimated lidocaine clearance is computed by taking the product of V_{area} and the elimination rate constant: $Cl = kV_{area} = 0.139\ h^{-1} \cdot 221\ L = 31\ L/h$.

3. *Compute the dosage regimen.*

Therapy is started by administering an intravenous loading dose of lidocaine to the patient (note: μg/mL = mg/L, and this concentration unit was substituted for Css in the calculations to avoid unnecessary unit conversion): LD = Css · Vc = 4 mg/L · 51 L = 204 mg, rounded to 200 mg intravenously over 4 to 8 minutes (note: longer administration time due to larger dose). An additional dose of 50% of the loading dose can be given if arrhythmias recur 20 to 30 minutes after the initial loading dose.

A lidocaine continuous intravenous infusion is started immediately after the loading dose has been administered. The dosage equation for intravenous lidocaine is k_0 = Css · Cl = (4 mg/L · 31 L/h)/(60 min/h) = 2.1 mg/min, rounded to 2 mg/min.

A steady-state lidocaine serum concentration can be measured after steady-state is attained in 3 to 5 half-lives. Since lidocaine is expected to have a half-life of 5 hours in the patient, the lidocaine steady-state concentration can be obtained any time after the first day of dosing (5 half-lives = 5 · 5 h = 25 h). Lidocaine serum concentrations should also be measured if the patient experiences a return of ventricular arrhythmia or develops potential signs or symptoms of lidocaine toxicity.

Example 3 MN is a 64-year-old, 78-kg, 175-cm (69-in) male with ventricular tachycardia who requires therapy with intravenous lidocaine. He has moderate heart failure (NYHA CHF class III). Suggest an initial intravenous lidocaine dosage regimen designed to achieve a steady-state lidocaine concentration of 3 μg/mL.

1. *Estimate the half-life and elimination rate constant according to the disease states and conditions of the patient.*

The expected lidocaine half-life ($t_{1/2}$) is 2 hours. The elimination rate constant is computed using the following formula: k = 0.693/$t_{1/2}$ = 0.693/2 h = 0.347 h^{-1}.

2. *Estimate the volume of distribution and clearance.*

The patient is not obese, so the estimated lidocaine central volume of distribution and the volume of distribution for the entire body (V_{area}) can be based on actual body weight: Vc = 0.3 L/kg · 78 kg = 23 L, V_{area} = 1 L/kg · 78 kg = 78 L. Estimated lidocaine clearance is computed by taking the product of V_{area} and the elimination rate constant: Cl = kV_{area} = 0.347 h^{-1} · 78 L = 27 L/h.

3. *Compute the dosage regimen.*

Therapy is started by administering an intravenous loading dose of lidocaine to the patient (note: μg/mL = mg/L, and this concentration unit was substituted for Css in the calculations to avoid unnecessary unit conversion): LD = Css · Vc = 3 mg/L · 23 L = 69 mg, rounded to 75 mg intravenously over 2 to 3 minutes. An additional dose of 50% of the loading dose can be given if arrhythmias recur 20 to 30 minutes after the initial loading dose.

A lidocaine continuous intravenous infusion is started immediately after the loading dose has been administered. The dosage equation for intravenous lidocaine is k_0 = Css · Cl = (3 mg/L · 27 L/h)/(60 min/h) = 1.4 mg/min, rounded to 1.5 mg/min.

A steady-state lidocaine serum concentration can be measured after steady state is attained in 3 to 5 half-lives. Because lidocaine is expected to have a half-life of 2 hours in the patient, the lidocaine steady-state concentration can be obtained any time after the first 10 to 12 hours of dosing (5 half-lives = 5 · 2 h = 10 h). Lidocaine serum concentrations should also be measured if the patient experiences a return of ventricular arrhythmia or develops potential signs or symptoms of lidocaine toxicity.

Literature-Based Recommended Dosing

Because of the large amount of variability in lidocaine pharmacokinetics, even when concurrent disease states and conditions are identified, many clinicians believe that the use of standard lidocaine doses for various situations is warranted.[31] The original computation of these doses was based on the pharmacokinetic dosing method described in the previous section and subsequently modified based on clinical experience. In general, the lidocaine steady-state serum concentration expected from the lower end of the dosage range was 1.5 to 3 μg/mL and 3 to 5 μg/mL for the upper end of the dosage range. Suggested intravenous lidocaine continuous infusion maintenance doses are 1 to 2 mg/min for patients with liver disease or heart failure and 3 to 4 mg/min for all other patients. When more than one disease state or condition is present in a patient, choosing the lowest infusion rate results in the safest, most conservative dosage recommendation. With regard to loading doses, lidocaine is given intravenously at 1 to 1.5 mg/kg (not to exceed 25 to 50 mg/min) to all patients except those with heart failure. The suggested lidocaine intravenous loading dose for heart failure patients is 0.5 to 0.75 mg/kg (not to exceed 25 to 50 mg/min), although some clinicians advocate full loading doses of lidocaine in patients with heart failure. Ideal body weight is used to compute loading doses for obese patients (>30% over ideal body weight).

To illustrate the similarities and differences between this method of dosage calculation and the pharmacokinetic dosing method, the same examples used in the previous section are used here.

Example 1 LK is a 50-year-old, 75-kg, 178-cm (70-in) male with ventricular tachycardia who requires therapy with intravenous lidocaine. He has normal liver and cardiac function. Suggest an initial intravenous lidocaine dosage regimen designed to achieve a steady-state lidocaine concentration of 3 μg/mL.

1. *Choose a lidocaine dose based on the disease states and conditions of the patient.*

A lidocaine loading dose of 1 to 1.5 mg/kg and a maintenance infusion of 3 to 4 mg/min are suggested for a patient without heart failure or liver disease.

2. *Compute the dosage regimen.*

Because the desired concentration is in the lower end of the therapeutic range, a dose in the lower end of the suggested ranges is used. A lidocaine loading dose of 1 mg/kg is administered: LD = 1 mg/kg · 75 kg = 75 mg over 1.5 to 3 minutes. A lidocaine maintenance infusion of 3 mg/min will be administered after the loading dose is given. An additional dose of 50% of the loading dose can be given if arrhythmias recur 20 to 30 minutes after the initial loading dose.

A steady-state lidocaine serum concentration can be measured after steady state is attained in 3 to 5 half-lives. Because lidocaine is expected to have a half-life of 1.5 hours in the patient, the lidocaine steady-state concentration can be obtained any time after the first 8 hours of dosing (5 half-lives = 5 · 1.5 h = 7.5 h). Lidocaine serum concentrations should also be measured if the patient experiences a return of ventricular arrhythmia or develops potential signs or symptoms of lidocaine toxicity.

Example 2 OI is a 60-year-old, 85-kg, 185-cm (73-in) male with ventricular fibrillation who requires therapy with intravenous lidocaine. He has liver cirrhosis (Child-Pugh score, 11). Suggest an initial intravenous lidocaine dosage regimen designed to achieve a steady-state lidocaine concentration of 4 μg/mL.

1. *Choose a lidocaine dose based on the disease states and conditions of the patient.*

A lidocaine loading dose of 1 to 1.5 mg/kg and a maintenance infusion of 1 to 2 mg/min are suggested for a patient with liver disease.

2. *Compute the dosage regimen.*

Because the desired concentration is in the upper end of the therapeutic range, a dose in the upper end of the suggested ranges is used. A lidocaine loading dose of 1.5 mg/kg is administered: LD = 1.5 mg/kg · 85 kg = 128 mg, rounded to 150 mg over 3 to 6 minutes. A lidocaine maintenance infusion of 2 mg/min is administered after the loading dose is given. An additional dose of 50% of the loading dose can be given if arrhythmias recur 20 to 30 minutes after the initial loading dose.

A steady-state lidocaine serum concentration can be measured after steady state is attained in 3 to 5 half-lives. Because lidocaine is expected to have a half-life of 5 hours in the patient, the lidocaine steady-state concentration can be obtained any time after the first day of dosing (5 half-lives = 5 · 5 h = 25 h). Lidocaine serum concentrations should also be measured if the patient experiences a return of ventricular arrhythmia or develops potential signs or symptoms of lidocaine toxicity.

Example 3 MN is a 64-year-old, 78-kg, 175-cm (69-in) male with ventricular tachycardia who requires therapy with intravenous lidocaine. He has moderate heart failure (NYHA CHF class III). Suggest an initial lidocaine dosage regimen designed to achieve a steady-state lidocaine concentration of 3 μg/mL.

1. *Choose a lidocaine dose based on the disease states and conditions of the patient.*

A lidocaine loading dose of 0.5 to 0.75 mg/kg and a maintenance infusion of 1 to 2 mg/min are suggested for a patient with heart failure.

2. *Compute the dosage regimen.*

Because the desired concentration is in the lower end of the therapeutic range, a dose in the lower end of the suggested ranges is used. A lidocaine loading dose of 0.5 mg/kg is administered: LD = 0.5 mg/kg · 78 kg = 39 mg, rounded to 50 mg over 1 to 2 minutes. A lidocaine maintenance infusion of 1 mg/min is administered after the loading dose is given. An additional dose of 50% of the loading dose can be given if arrhythmias recur 20 to 30 minutes after the initial loading dose.

A steady-state lidocaine serum concentration can be measured after steady state is attained in 3 to 5 half-lives. Because lidocaine is expected to have a half-life of 2 hours in the patient, the lidocaine steady-state concentration can be obtained any time after the first 10 to 12 hours of dosing (5 half-lives = 5 · 2 h = 10 h). Lidocaine serum concentrations should also be measured if the patient experiences a return of ventricular arrhythmia or develops potential signs or symptoms of lidocaine toxicity.

USE OF LIDOCAINE SERUM CONCENTRATIONS TO ALTER DOSES

Because of the large amount of pharmacokinetic variability among patients, it is likely that doses computed using patient population characteristics will not always produce lidocaine serum concentrations that are expected or desirable. Because of pharmacokinetic variability, the narrow therapeutic index of lidocaine and the desire to prevent lidocaine adverse side effects, measurement of lidocaine serum concentrations can be a useful adjunct for patients to ensure that therapeutic, nontoxic levels are present. In addition to lidocaine serum concentrations, important patient parameters (e.g., ECG, clinical signs and symptoms of ventricular arrhythmia, potential lidocaine side effects) should be monitored to confirm that the patient is responding to treatment and not developing adverse drug reactions.

When lidocaine serum concentrations are measured in patients and a dosage change is necessary, clinicians should seek to use the simplest, most straightforward method available to determine a dose that will provide safe and effective treatment. In most cases, a simple dosage ratio can be used to change lidocaine doses, assuming that the drug follows *linear pharmacokinetics.* Although it has been clearly demonstrated in research studies that lidocaine serum concentrations accumulate in patients during long-term (>24 hours) infusions, in the clinical setting most patients' steady-state serum concentrations change proportionally with lidocaine dose for shorter infusion times. Thus, linear pharmacokinetics is assumed to be adequate for dosage adjustments in most patients.

Sometimes it is useful to compute lidocaine pharmacokinetic constants for a patient and to base dosage adjustments on these constants. In this case, it may be possible to calculate and use *pharmacokinetic parameters* to alter the lidocaine dose. In some situations, it may be necessary to compute lidocaine clearance for the patient during a continuous infusion before steady-state conditions occur and to use this pharmacokinetic parameter to calculate the best drug dose. Computerized methods that incorporate expected population pharmacokinetic characteristics (*Bayesian pharmacokinetics computer programs*) can be used in difficult cases in which serum concentrations are obtained at suboptimal times or the patient was not at steady state when serum concentrations were measured.

Linear Pharmacokinetics Method

Because lidocaine follows linear, dose-proportional pharmacokinetics in most patients during short-term (<24 hours) infusions, steady-state serum concentrations change in proportion to dose according to the following equation: $D_{new}/Css_{new} = D_{old}/Css_{old}$ or $D_{new} = (Css_{new}/Css_{old})D_{old}$, where D is the dose, Css is the steady-state concentration, old indicates the dose that produced the steady-state concentration that the patient is receiving, and new denotes the dose necessary to produce the desired steady-state concentration. The advantage of this method is that it is quick and simple. The disadvantages are that steady-state concentrations are required and that accumulation of serum lidocaine concentrations can occur with long-term (>24 hours) infusions. When steady-state serum concentrations are higher than expected during long-term lidocaine infusions, lidocaine accumulation pharmacokinetics is a possible explanation for the observation. Because of this, suggested dosage increases greater than 75% using this method should be scrutinized by the prescribing clinician and the risk-versus-benefit ratio assessed for the patient before initiating large dosage increases (>75% over current dose).

Example 1 LK is a 50-year-old, 75-kg, 178-cm (70-in) male with ventricular tachycardia who requires therapy with intravenous lidocaine. He has normal liver and cardiac function. His steady-state lidocaine concentration is 2.2 μg/mL at 2 mg/min. Compute a lidocaine dose that will provide a steady-state concentration of 4 μg/mL.

1. *Compute the new dose to achieve desired serum concentration.*

The patient is expected to achieve steady-state conditions after 8 hours (5 half-lives = 5 · 1.5 h = 7.5 h) of therapy.

With the use of linear pharmacokinetics, the new dose to attain the desired concentration should be proportional to the old dose that produced the measured concentration:

$$D_{new} = (Css_{new}/Css_{old})D_{old} = [(4\ \mu g/mL)/(2.2\ \mu g/mL)]\ 2\ mg/min$$
$$= 3.6\ mg/min,\ \text{rounded to } 3.5\ mg/min$$

The new suggested dose is 3.5 mg/min of intravenous lidocaine to be started immediately.

A steady-state lidocaine serum concentration can be measured after steady state is attained in 3 to 5 half-lives. Because lidocaine is expected to have a half-life of 1.5 hours in the patient, the lidocaine steady-state concentration can be obtained any time after the first 8 hours of dosing (5 half-lives = 5 · 1.5 h = 7.5 h). Lidocaine serum concentrations should also be measured if the patient experiences a return of ventricular arrhythmia or develops potential signs or symptoms of lidocaine toxicity.

Example 2 OI is a 60-year-old, 85-kg, 185-cm (73-in) male with ventricular fibrillation who requires therapy with intravenous lidocaine. He has liver cirrhosis (Child-Pugh score, 11). His steady-state lidocaine concentration is 6.4 μg/mL at 2 mg/min. Compute a lidocaine dose that will provide a steady-state concentration of 3 μg/mL.

1. *Compute a new dose to achieve the desired serum concentration.*

The patient is expected to achieve steady-state conditions after a day (5 half-lives = 5 · 5 h = 25 h) of therapy.

Using linear pharmacokinetics, the new dose to attain the desired concentration should be proportional to the old dose that produced the measured concentration:

$$D_{new} = (Css_{new}/Css_{old})D_{old} = [(3\ \mu g/mL)/(6.4\ \mu g/mL)]\ 2\ mg/min$$
$$= 0.9\ mg/min,\ \text{rounded to } 1\ mg/min$$

The new suggested dose is 1 mg/min of intravenous lidocaine. If the patient is experiencing adverse drug effects, the infusion can be held for 1 estimated half-life (5 hours) until the new dose is started.

A steady-state lidocaine serum concentration can be measured after steady state is attained in 3 to 5 half-lives. Because lidocaine is expected to have a half-life of 5 hours in the patient, the lidocaine steady-state concentration can be obtained any time after the first day of dosing (5 half-lives = 5 · 5 h = 25 h). Lidocaine serum concentrations should also be measured if the patient experiences a return of ventricular arrhythmia or develops potential signs or symptoms of lidocaine toxicity.

Example 3 MN is a 64-year-old, 78-kg, 175-cm (69-in) male with ventricular tachycardia who requires therapy with intravenous lidocaine. He has moderate heart failure (NYHA CHF class III). His steady-state lidocaine concentration is 2.2 μg/mL at 1 mg/min. Compute a lidocaine dose that will provide a steady-state concentration of 4 μg/mL.

1. *Compute a new dose to achieve the desired serum concentration.*

The patient is expected to achieve steady-state conditions after 10 to 12 hours (5 half-lives = 5 · 2 h = 10 h) of therapy.

Using linear pharmacokinetics, the new dose to attain the desired concentration should be proportional to the old dose that produced the measured concentration:

$$D_{new} = (Css_{new}/Css_{old})D_{old} = [(4\ \mu g/mL)/(2.2\ \mu g/mL)]\ 1\ mg/min$$
$$= 1.8\ mg/min,\ rounded\ to\ 2\ mg/min$$

The new suggested dose is 2 mg/min of intravenous lidocaine to begin immediately.

A steady-state lidocaine serum concentration can be measured after steady state is attained in 3 to 5 half-lives. Because lidocaine is expected to have a half-life of 2 hours in the patient, the lidocaine steady-state concentration can be obtained any time after the first 10 to 12 hours of dosing (5 half-lives = 5 · 2 h = 10 h). Lidocaine serum concentrations should also be measured if the patient experiences a return of ventricular arrhythmia or develops potential signs or symptoms of lidocaine toxicity.

Pharmacokinetic Parameter Method

The pharmacokinetic parameter method of adjusting drug doses was among the first techniques available for changing doses using serum concentrations. It allows the computation of a person's unique pharmacokinetic constants and uses them to calculate a dose that achieves desired lidocaine concentrations. The pharmacokinetic parameter method requires that steady state has been achieved and uses only a steady-state lidocaine concentration (Css in mg/L or μg/mL). During a continuous intravenous infusion, the following equation is used to compute lidocaine clearance (Cl in L/min): $Cl = k_0/Css$, where k_0 is the dose of lidocaine in mg/min. The clearance measured using this technique is the patient's unique lidocaine pharmacokinetic constant and can be used in the intravenous continuous infusion equation to compute the required dose (k_0 in mg/min) to achieve any desired steady-state serum concentration (Css in mg/L or μg/mL): $k_0 = Css \cdot Cl$, where Cl is lidocaine clearance in L/min. Because this method also assumes linear pharmacokinetics, lidocaine doses computed using the pharmacokinetic parameter method and using the linear pharmacokinetic method should be identical.

Example 1 LK is a 50-year-old, 75-kg, 178-cm (70-in) male with ventricular tachycardia who requires therapy with intravenous lidocaine. He has normal liver and cardiac function. His steady-state lidocaine concentration is 2.2 μg/mL at 2 mg/min. Compute a lidocaine dose that will provide a steady-state concentration of 4 μg/mL.

1. *Compute the pharmacokinetic parameters.*

The patient is expected to achieve steady-state conditions after the first 8 hours (5 half-lives = 1.5 · 5 h = 7.5 h) of therapy.

Lidocaine clearance can be computed using a steady-state lidocaine concentration: Cl = k_0/Css = (2 mg/min)/(2.2 mg/L) = 0.91 L/min. (Note: μg/mL = mg/L, and this concentration unit was substituted for Css in the calculations to avoid unnecessary unit conversion.)

2. *Compute the lidocaine dose.*

Lidocaine clearance is used to compute the new lidocaine infusion rate: k_0 = Css · Cl = 4 mg/L · 0.91 L/min = 36 mg/min, rounded to 3.5 mg/min.

The new lidocaine infusion rate is instituted immediately.

A steady-state lidocaine serum concentration can be measured after steady state is attained in 3 to 5 half-lives. Because lidocaine is expected to have a half-life of 1.5 hours in the patient, the lidocaine steady-state concentration can be obtained any time after the first 8 hours of dosing (5 half-lives = 5 · 1.5 h = 7.5 h). Lidocaine serum concentrations also should be measured if the patient experiences a return of ventricular arrhythmia or develops potential signs or symptoms of lidocaine toxicity.

Example 2 OI is a 60-year-old, 85-kg, 185-cm (73-in) male with ventricular fibrillation who requires therapy with intravenous lidocaine. He has liver cirrhosis (Child-Pugh score, 11). His steady-state lidocaine concentration is 6.4 μg/mL at 2 mg/min. Compute a lidocaine dose that will provide a steady-state concentration of 3 μg/mL.

1. *Compute the pharmacokinetic parameters.*

The patient is expected to achieve steady-state conditions after a day (5 half-lives = 5 · 5 h = 25 h) of therapy.

Lidocaine clearance can be computed using a steady-state lidocaine concentration: Cl = k_0/Css = (2 mg/min)/(6.4 mg/L) = 0.31 L/min. (Note: μg/mL = mg/L, and this concentration unit was substituted for Css in the calculations to avoid unnecessary unit conversion.)

2. *Compute the lidocaine dose.*

Lidocaine clearance is used to compute the new lidocaine infusion rate: k_0 = Css · Cl = 3 mg/L · 0.31 L/min = 0.9 mg/min, rounded to 1 mg/min.

The new suggested dose is 1 mg/min of intravenous lidocaine. If the patient is experiencing adverse drug effects, the infusion can be held for 1 estimated half-life (5 hours) until the new dose is started.

A steady-state lidocaine serum concentration can be measured after steady state is attained in 3 to 5 half-lives. Because lidocaine is expected to have a half-life of 5 hours in the patient, the lidocaine steady-state concentration can be obtained any time after the first day of dosing (5 half-lives = 5 · 5 h = 25 h). Lidocaine serum concentrations should also be measured if the patient experiences a return of ventricular arrhythmia or develops potential signs or symptoms of lidocaine toxicity.

Example 3 MN is a 64-year-old, 78-kg, 175-cm (69-in) male with ventricular tachycardia who requires therapy with intravenous lidocaine. He has moderate heart failure (NYHA CHF class III). His steady-state lidocaine concentration is 2.2 μg/mL at 1 mg/min. Compute a lidocaine dose that will provide a steady-state concentration of 4 μg/mL.

1. *Compute the pharmacokinetic parameters.*

The patient is expected to achieve steady-state conditions after 10 to 12 hours (5 half-lives = 5 · 2 h = 10 h) of therapy.

Lidocaine clearance can be computed using a steady-state lidocaine concentration: $Cl = k_0/Css$ = (1 mg/min)/(2.2 mg/L) = 0.45 L/min. (Note: μg/mL = mg/L, and this concentration unit was substituted for Css in the calculations to avoid unnecessary unit conversion.)

2. *Compute the lidocaine dosage.*

Lidocaine clearance is used to compute the new lidocaine infusion rate: $k_0 = Css \cdot Cl$ = 4 mg/L · 0.45 L/min = 1.8 mg/min, rounded to 2 mg/min.

The new suggested dose is 2 mg/min of intravenous lidocaine to begin immediately.

A steady-state lidocaine serum concentration can be measured after steady state is attained in 3 to 5 half-lives. Because lidocaine is expected to have a half-life of 2 hours in the patient, the lidocaine steady-state concentration can be obtained any time after the first 10 to 12 hours of dosing (5 half-lives = 5 · 2 h = 10 h). Lidocaine serum concentrations should also be measured if the patient experiences a return of ventricular arrhythmia or develops potential signs or symptoms of lidocaine toxicity.

BAYESIAN PHARMACOKINETICS COMPUTER PROGRAMS

Computer programs are available that can assist in the computation of pharmacokinetic parameters for patients. The most reliable computer programs use a nonlinear regression algorithm that incorporates components of Bayes' theorem. Nonlinear regression is a statistical technique that uses an iterative process to compute the best pharmacokinetic parameters for a concentration–time data set. Briefly, the patient's drug dosage schedule and serum concentrations are entered into the computer. The computer program has a pharmacokinetic equation preprogrammed for the drug and administration method (e.g., oral, intravenous bolus, intravenous infusion). Typically, a one-compartment model is used, although some programs allow the user to choose among several different equations. Using population estimates based on demographic information for the patient (e.g., age, weight, gender, liver function, cardiac status) supplied by the user, the computer program then computes estimated serum concentrations each time there are actual serum concentrations. Kinetic parameters are then changed by the computer program, and a new set of estimated serum concentrations are computed. The pharmacokinetic parameters that generated the estimated serum concentrations closest to the actual values are remembered by the computer program, and the process is repeated until the set of pharmacokinetic parameters that result in estimated serum concentrations that are statistically closest to the actual serum concentrations is generated. These pharmacokinetic parameters can then be used to compute improved dosing schedules for patients.

Bayes' theorem is used in the computer algorithm to balance the results of the computations between values based solely on the patient's serum drug concentrations and those based only on patient population parameters. Results from studies that compare various methods of dosage adjustment have consistently found that these types of computer dosing programs perform at least as well as experienced clinical pharmacokineticists and clinicians and better than inexperienced clinicians.

Some clinicians use Bayesian pharmacokinetics computer programs exclusively to alter drug doses based on serum concentrations. An advantage of this approach is that consistent dosage recommendations are made when several different practitioners are involved in therapeutic drug-monitoring programs. However, because simpler dosing methods work just as well for patients with stable pharmacokinetic parameters and steady-state drug concentrations, many clinicians reserve the use of computer programs for more difficult situations. Those situations include serum concentrations that are not at steady state, serum concentrations not obtained at the specific times needed to use simpler methods, and unstable pharmacokinetic parameters. Many Bayesian pharmacokinetics computer programs are available to users, and most provide answers similar to the one used in the following examples. The program used to solve problems in this book is DrugCalc, written by Dr. Dennis Mungall, and is available on his Internet web site (http://members.aol.com/thertch/index.htm).[32]

Example 1 OY is a 57-year-old, 79-kg, 173-cm (68-in) male with ventricular tachycardia who requires therapy with intravenous lidocaine. He has normal liver (bilirubin, 0.7 mg/dL; albumin, 4.0 g/dL) and cardiac function. He received a 100-mg loading dose of lidocaine at 0800 H, and a continuous intravenous infusion of lidocaine was started at 0810 H at 2 mg/min. His lidocaine serum concentration is 2.1 μg/mL at 1030 H. Compute a lidocaine infusion rate that will provide a steady-state concentration of 4 μg/mL.

1. *Enter the patient's demographic, drug dosing, and serum concentration–time data into the computer program.*

This patient is unlikely to be at steady state, so the linear pharmacokinetics method cannot be used. The DrugCalc program requires lidocaine infusion rates to be entered in terms of mg/h. A 2-mg/min infusion rate is equivalent to 120 mg/h (k_0 = 2 mg/min · 60 min/h = 120 mg/h).

2. *Compute the pharmacokinetic parameters for the patient using the Bayesian pharmacokinetics computer program.*

The pharmacokinetic parameters computed by the program are a volume of distribution for the entire body (V_{area}) of 100 L, a half-life of 1.6 hours, and a clearance of 43.6 L/h.

3. *Compute the dose required to achieve the desired lidocaine serum concentrations.*

The continuous intravenous infusion equation used by the program to compute doses indicates that a dose of 180 mg/h or 3 mg/min [k_0 = (180 mg/h)/(60 min/h) = 3 mg/min] will produce a steady-state lidocaine concentration of 4.1 μg/mL. This infusion rate is started immediately.

Example 2 SL is a 71-year-old, 82-kg, 178-cm (70-in) male with ventricular fibrillation who requires therapy with intravenous lidocaine. He has liver cirrhosis (Child-Pugh score, 12; bilirubin, 3.2 mg/dL; albumin, 2.5 g/dL) and normal cardiac function. He received a 150-mg loading dose of lidocaine at 1300 H, and a continuous intravenous infusion of lidocaine was started at 1305 H at 2 mg/min. The lidocaine serum concentration is 5.7 μg/mL at 2300 H. Compute a lidocaine infusion rate that will provide a steady-state concentration of 4 μg/mL.

1. *Enter the patient's demographic, drug dosing, and serum concentration–time data into the computer program.*

This patient is unlikely to be at steady state, so the linear pharmacokinetics method cannot be used. The DrugCalc program requires lidocaine infusion rates to be entered in terms of mg/h. A 2-mg/min infusion rate is equivalent to 120 mg/h (k_0 = 2 mg/min · 60 min/h = 120 mg/h).

2. *Compute the pharmacokinetic parameters for the patient using the Bayesian pharmacokinetics computer program.*

The pharmacokinetic parameters computed by the program are a volume of distribution for the entire body (V_{area}) of 142 L, a half-life of 6.5 hours, and a clearance of 15 L/h.

3. *Compute the dose required to achieve the desired lidocaine serum concentrations.*

The continuous intravenous infusion equation used by the program to compute doses indicates that a dose of 60 mg/h or 1 mg/min [k_0 = (60 mg/h)/(60 min/h) = 1 mg/min] will produce a steady-state lidocaine concentration of 4 μg/mL. This infusion rate can be started immediately, or if the patient is experiencing adverse drug effects, the infusion can be held for 1/2 to 1 half-life to allow lidocaine serum concentrations to decline and restarted at that time.

Example 3 TR is a 75-year-old, 85-kg, 173-cm (68-in) male with ventricular tachycardia who requires therapy with intravenous lidocaine. He has moderate heart failure

(NYHA CHF class III). He received a 75-mg loading dose of lidocaine at 0100 H, and a continuous intravenous infusion of lidocaine was started at 0115 H at 1 mg/min. The lidocaine serum concentration is 1.7 μg/mL at 0400 H. Compute a lidocaine infusion rate that will provide a steady-state concentration of 3 μg/mL.

1. *Enter the patient's demographic, drug dosing, and serum concentration–time data into the computer program.*

This patient is unlikely to be at steady state, so the linear pharmacokinetics method cannot be used. The DrugCalc program requires lidocaine infusion rates to be entered in terms of mg/h. A 1-mg/min infusion rate is equivalent to 60 mg/h (k_0 = 1 mg/min · 60 min/h = 60 mg/h).

2. *Compute the pharmacokinetic parameters for the patient using the Bayesian pharmacokinetics computer program.*

The pharmacokinetic parameters computed by the program are a volume of distribution for the entire body (V_{area}) of 74 L, a half-life of 1.8 hours, and a clearance of 29 L/h.

3. *Compute the dose required to achieve the desired lidocaine serum concentrations.*

The continuous intravenous infusion equation used by the program to compute doses indicates that a dose of 90 mg/h or 1.5 mg/min [k_0 = (90 mg/h)/(60 min/h) = 1.5 mg/min] will produce a steady-state lidocaine concentration of 3 μg/mL. This infusion rate should be started immediately.

USE OF LIDOCAINE BOOSTER DOSES TO IMMEDIATELY INCREASE SERUM CONCENTRATIONS

If a patient has a subtherapeutic lidocaine serum concentration and is experiencing ventricular arrhythmias in an acute situation, it is desirable to increase the lidocaine concentration as quickly as possible. In this setting, it is not acceptable to simply increase the maintenance dose and wait 3 to 5 half-lives for therapeutic serum concentrations to be established. A rational way to increase the serum concentrations rapidly is to administer a booster dose of lidocaine, a process also known as "reloading" the patient with lidocaine, which is computed using pharmacokinetic techniques. A modified loading dose equation is used to accomplish computation of the booster dose (BD), which takes into account the current lidocaine concentration in the patient: $BD = (C_{desired} - C_{actual})Vc$, where $C_{desired}$ is the desired lidocaine concentration, C_{actual} is the actual current lidocaine concentration for the patient, and Vc is the central volume of distribution for lidocaine. If the central volume of distribution for lidocaine is known for the patient, it can be used in the calculation. However, this value is not usually known and is typically assumed to equal the population average appropriate for the disease states and conditions present in the patient (see Table 7-1).

Concurrent with the administration of the booster dose, the maintenance dose of the lidocaine is usually increased. Clinicians need to recognize that a booster dose does not alter the time required to achieve steady-state conditions when a new lidocaine dosage rate is prescribed (see Figure 7-3). It still requires 3 to 5 half-lives to attain steady state when the dosage rate is changed. However, usually the difference between the postbooster dose lidocaine concentration and the ultimate steady-state concentration has been reduced by giving the extra dose of the drug.

Example 1 BN is a 57-year-old, 50-kg, 157-cm (62-in) female with ventricular tachycardia who is receiving therapy with intravenous lidocaine. She has normal liver function and does not have heart failure. After receiving an initial loading dose of lidocaine (75 mg) and a maintenance infusion of lidocaine of 2 mg/min for 2 hours, her arrhythmia reappears and a lidocaine concentration is measured at 1.2 μg/mL. Compute a booster dose of lidocaine to achieve a lidocaine concentration of 4 μg/mL.

1. *Estimate the volume of distribution according to the disease states and conditions of the patient.*

In the case of lidocaine, the population average central volume of distribution is 0.5 L/kg, which can be used to estimate the parameter for the patient. The patient is not obese, so her actual body weight is used in the computation: $V = 0.5\ L/kg \cdot 50\ kg = 25\ L$.

2. *Compute the booster dose.*

The booster dose is computed using the following equation: $BD = (C_{desired} - C_{actual})Vc = (4\ mg/L - 1.2\ mg/L)25\ L = 70\ mg$, rounded to 75 mg of lidocaine intravenously over 1.5 to 3 minutes. (Note: μg/mL = mg/L, and this concentration unit was substituted for C in the calculations to avoid unnecessary unit conversion.) If the maintenance dose was increased, it will take an additional 3 to 5 estimated half-lives for new steady-state conditions to be achieved. Lidocaine serum concentrations can be measured at this time. Lidocaine serum concentrations should also be measured if the patient experiences a return of ventricular arrhythmia or develops potential signs or symptoms of lidocaine toxicity.

PROBLEMS

The following problems are intended to emphasize the computation of initial and individualized doses using clinical pharmacokinetic techniques. Clinicians should always consult the patient's chart to confirm that current antiarrhythmic and other drug therapy are appropriate. In addition, all other medications that the patient is taking, including prescription and nonprescription drugs, should be noted and checked to ascertain whether a potential drug interaction with lidocaine exists.

1. VC is a 67-year-old, 72-kg, 185-cm (73-in) male with ventricular tachycardia who requires therapy with intravenous lidocaine. He has normal liver function and does not have heart failure. Suggest an initial oral lidocaine dosage regimen designed to achieve a steady-state lidocaine concentration of 3 μg/mL.

2. Patient VC (see problem 1) was prescribed intravenous lidocaine at 2 mg/min after receiving a loading dose. The current steady-state lidocaine concentration is 2.5 μg/mL. Compute a new lidocaine infusion rate that will provide a steady-state concentration of 4 μg/mL.

3. EM is a 56-year-old, 81-kg, 175-cm (69-in) male with ventricular tachycardia who requires therapy with intravenous lidocaine. He has cirrhosis (Child-Pugh score, 10) and does not have heart failure. Suggest an initial lidocaine dosage regimen designed to achieve a steady-state lidocaine concentration of 4 μg/mL.

4. Patient EM (see problem 3) was prescribed intravenous lidocaine at 2 mg/min. The current steady-state lidocaine concentration is 6.2 μg/mL. Compute a new intravenous lidocaine continuous infusion that will provide a steady-state concentration of 4 μg/mL.

5. OF is a 71-year-old, 60-kg, 157-cm (62-in) female with ventricular fibrillation who requires therapy with intravenous lidocaine. She has severe heart failure (NYHA CHF class IV) and normal liver function. Suggest an initial lidocaine dosage regimen designed to achieve a steady-state lidocaine concentration of 5 μg/mL.

6. Patient OF (see problem 5) was prescribed a lidocaine continuous infusion at 2 mg/min after receiving a loading dose. A steady-state lidocaine serum concentration was obtained and was 6.7 μg/mL. Compute a new intravenous lidocaine continuous infusion that will provide a steady-state concentration of 4 μg/mL.

7. FK is a 67-year-old, 130-kg, 183-cm (71-in) male with ventricular tachycardia who requires therapy with intravenous lidocaine. He has severe heart failure (NYHA CHF class IV) and normal liver function. Suggest an initial lidocaine dosage regimen designed to achieve a steady-state lidocaine concentration of 3 μg/mL.

8. Patient FK (see problem 9) was prescribed intravenous lidocaine. A lidocaine loading dose of 150 mg was given at 1230 H followed by a continuous infusion of 2 mg/min, starting at 1245 H. A lidocaine serum concentration was obtained at 1630 H and was 6.2 μg/mL. Compute a new lidocaine dose that will provide a steady-state concentration of 4 μg/mL.

9. GP is a 76-year-old, 90-kg, 183-cm (71-in) male who suffered a myocardial infarction. Three hours after his heart attack, he developed ventricular tachycardia and requires therapy with intravenous lidocaine. He has normal liver function and does not have heart failure. Suggest an initial intravenous lidocaine dosage regimen designed to achieve a steady-state lidocaine concentration of 4 μg/mL.

10. Patient GP (see problem 9) was prescribed intravenous lidocaine at 2 mg/min 15 minutes after receiving a 100-mg loading dose at 1520 H. At 1930 H, the lidocaine concentration is 1.9 μg/mL. Compute a new lidocaine infusion rate that will provide a steady-state concentration of 4 μg/mL.

11. CV is a 69-year-old, 90-kg, 185-cm (71-in) male with ventricular tachycardia who requires therapy with intravenous lidocaine. He has liver cirrhosis (Child-Pugh score, 11; total bilirubin, 2.7 mg/dL; albumin, 2.1 g/dL) and moderate heart failure (NYHA CHF class III). At 0200 H, he received 100 mg of intravenous lidocaine as a loading dose, and a maintenance intravenous infusion of 2 mg/min was started at 0215 H. Because the patient was experiencing mental status changes, the lidocaine infusion rate

was decreased to 1 mg/min at 0900 H. A lidocaine serum concentration was measured at 1000 H and was 5.4 μg/mL. Suggest a lidocaine continuous infusion rate that will achieve a steady-state concentration of 3 μg/mL.

12. FP is a 59-year-old, 90-kg, 163-cm (64-in) female with ventricular fibrillation who requires therapy with intravenous lidocaine. She has liver cirrhosis (Child-Pugh score, 9) and mild heart failure (NYHA CHF class II). At 1130 H, she received 100 mg of intravenous lidocaine as a loading dose, and a maintenance intravenous infusion of 3 mg/min was started at 1200 H. Because the patient was experiencing confusion, agitation, and dysarthria, the lidocaine infusion rate was decreased to 1 mg/min at 1500 H. At 2000 H, the patient began experiencing ventricular tachycardia, and an additional lidocaine booster dose of 100 mg was given while the continuous infusion was left unchanged. A lidocaine serum concentration was measured at 2200 H and was 4.3 μg/mL. Suggest a lidocaine continuous infusion rate that will achieve a steady-state concentration of 5 μg/mL.

ANSWERS TO PROBLEMS

1. The initial lidocaine dose for patient VC is calculated as follows.

Pharmacokinetic Dosing Method

1. *Estimate the half-life and elimination rate constant according to the disease states and conditions of the patient.*

The expected lidocaine half-life ($t_{1/2}$) is 1.5 hours. The elimination rate constant is computed using the following formula: $k = 0.693/t_{1/2} = 0.693/1.5\ h = 0.462\ h^{-1}$.

2. *Estimate the volume of distribution and clearance.*

The patient is not obese, so the estimated lidocaine central volume of distribution and the volume of distribution for the entire body (V_{area}) is based on the patient's actual body weight: $Vc = 0.5\ L/kg \cdot 72\ kg = 36\ L$, $V_{area} = 1.5\ L/kg \cdot 72\ kg = 108\ L$. Estimated lidocaine clearance is computed by taking the product of V_{area} and the elimination rate constant: $Cl = kV_{area} = 0.462\ h^{-1} \cdot 108\ L = 50\ L/h$.

3. *Compute the dosage regimen.*

Therapy is started by administering an intravenous loading dose of lidocaine to the patient (note: μg/mL = mg/L, and this concentration unit was substituted for Css in the calculations to avoid unnecessary unit conversion): $LD = Css \cdot Vc = 3\ mg/L \cdot 36\ L = 108\ mg$, rounded to 100 mg intravenously over 2 to 4 minutes. An additional dose of 50% of the loading dose can be given if arrhythmias recur 20 to 30 minutes after the initial loading dose.

A lidocaine continuous intravenous infusion is started immediately after the loading dose has been administered. The dosage equation for intravenous lidocaine is $k_0 = Css \cdot Cl = (3\ mg/L \cdot 50\ L/h)/(60\ min/h) = 2.5\ mg/min$.

A steady-state lidocaine serum concentration can be measured after steady-state is attained in 3 to 5 half-lives. Since lidocaine is expected to have a half-life of 1.5 hours in the patient, the lidocaine steady-state concentration can be obtained any time after the first 8 hours of dosing (5 half-lives = 5 · 1.5 h = 7.5 h). Lidocaine serum concentrations should also be measured if the patient experiences a return of ventricular arrhythmia or develops potential signs or symptoms of lidocaine toxicity.

Literature-Based Recommended Dosing

1. *Choose a lidocaine dose based on the disease states and conditions of the patient.*

A lidocaine loading dose of 1 to 1.5 mg/kg and a maintenance infusion of 3 to 4 mg/min are suggested for a patient without heart failure or liver disease.

2. *Compute the dosage regimen.*

Because the desired concentration is in the lower end of the therapeutic range, a dose in the lower end of the suggested ranges is used. A lidocaine loading dose of 1 mg/kg is administered: LD = 1 mg/kg · 72 kg = 72 mg, rounded to 75 mg over 1.5 to 3 minutes. A lidocaine maintenance infusion of 3 mg/min is administered after the loading dose is given. An additional dose of 50% of the loading dose can be given if arrhythmias recur 20 to 30 minutes after the initial loading dose.

A steady-state lidocaine serum concentration can be measured after steady state is attained in 3 to 5 half-lives. Since lidocaine is expected to have a half-life of 1.5 hours in the patient, the lidocaine steady-state concentration can be obtained any time after the first 8 hours of dosing (5 half-lives = 5 · 1.5 h = 7.5 h). Lidocaine serum concentrations should also be measured if the patient experiences a return of ventricular arrhythmia or develops potential signs or symptoms of lidocaine toxicity.

2. The revised lidocaine dose for patient VC is calculated as follows.

Linear Pharmacokinetics Method

1. *Compute a new dose to achieve the desired serum concentration.*

The patient is expected to achieve steady-state conditions after 8 hours (5 half-lives = 5 · 1.5 h = 7.5 h) of therapy.

With the use of linear pharmacokinetics, the new dose to attain the desired concentration should be proportional to the old dose that produced the measured concentration:

$$D_{new} = (Css_{new}/Css_{old})D_{old} = [(4\ \mu g/mL)/(2.5\ \mu g/mL)]\ 2\ mg/min$$
$$= 3.2\ mg/min,\ \text{rounded to}\ 3\ mg/min$$

The new suggested dose is 3 mg/min of intravenous lidocaine to be started immediately.

A steady-state lidocaine serum concentration can be measured after steady state is attained in 3 to 5 half-lives. Since lidocaine is expected to have a half-life of 1.5

hours in the patient, the lidocaine steady-state concentration can be obtained any time after the first 8 hours of dosing (5 half-lives = 5 · 1.5 h = 7.5 h). Lidocaine serum concentrations should also be measured if the patient experiences a return of ventricular arrhythmia or develops potential signs or symptoms of lidocaine toxicity.

Pharmacokinetic Parameter Method

1. *Compute the pharmacokinetic parameters.*

The patient is expected to achieve steady-state conditions after the first 8 hours (5 half-lives = 1.5 · 5 h = 7.5 h) of therapy.

Lidocaine clearance can be computed using a steady-state lidocaine concentration: $Cl = k_0/Css$ = (2 mg/min)/(2.5 mg/L) = 0.8 L/min. (Note: μg/mL = mg/L, and this concentration unit was substituted for Css in the calculations to avoid unnecessary unit conversion.)

2. *Compute the lidocaine dose.*

Lidocaine clearance is used to compute the new lidocaine infusion rate: k_0 = Css · Cl = 4 mg/L · 0.8 L/min = 3.2 mg/min, rounded to 3 mg/min.

The new lidocaine infusion rate should be instituted immediately.

A steady-state lidocaine serum concentration can be measured after steady state is attained in 3 to 5 half-lives. Since lidocaine is expected to have a half-life of 1.5 hours in the patient, the lidocaine steady-state concentration can be obtained any time after the first 8 hours of dosing (5 half-lives = 5 · 1.5 h = 7.5 h). Lidocaine serum concentrations should also be measured if the patient experiences a return of ventricular arrhythmia or develops potential signs or symptoms of lidocaine toxicity.

Computation of Booster Dose

1. *Use the central volume of distribution (Vc) to calculate the booster dose (if needed).*

The booster dose is computed using the following equation (Vc population average estimate used from problem 1): $BD = (C_{desired} - C_{actual})Vc$ = (4 mg/L − 2.5 mg/L)36 L = 54 mg, rounded to 50 mg of lidocaine intravenously over 1 to 2 minutes. (Note: μg/mL = mg/L, and this concentration unit was substituted for C in the calculations to avoid unnecessary unit conversion.) If the maintenance dose is increased, it will take an additional 3 to 5 estimated half-lives for new steady-state conditions to be achieved.

3. The initial lidocaine dose for patient EM is calculated as follows.

Pharmacokinetic Dosing Method

1. *Estimate the half-life and elimination rate constant according to the disease states and conditions of the patient.*

The expected lidocaine half-life ($t_{1/2}$) is 5 hours. The elimination rate constant is computed using the following formula: $k = 0.693/t_{1/2}$ = 0.693/5 h = 0.139 h^{-1}.

2. *Estimate the volume of distribution and clearance.*

The patient is not obese, so the estimated lidocaine central volume of distribution and the volume of distribution for the entire body (V_{area}) are based on the patient's actual body weight: Vc = 0.6 L/kg · 81 kg = 49 L, V_{area} = 2.6 L/kg · 81 kg = 211 L. Estimated lidocaine clearance is computed by taking the product of V_{area} and the elimination rate constant: Cl = kV_{area} = 0.139 h^{-1} · 211 L = 29.3 L/h.

3. *Compute the dosage regimen.*

Therapy is started by administering an intravenous loading dose of lidocaine to the patient (note: μg/mL = mg/L, and this concentration unit was substituted for Css in the calculations to avoid unnecessary unit conversion): LD = Css · Vc = 4 mg/L · 49 L = 196 mg, rounded to 200 mg intravenously over 4 to 8 minutes. An additional dose of 50% of the loading dose can be given if arrhythmias recur 20 to 30 minutes after the initial loading dose.

A lidocaine continuous intravenous infusion is started immediately after the loading dose has been administered. The dosage equation for intravenous lidocaine is k_0 = Css · Cl = (4 mg/L · 29.3 L/h)/(60 min/h) = 2 mg/min.

A steady-state lidocaine serum concentration can be measured after steady state is attained in 3 to 5 half-lives. Since lidocaine is expected to have a half-life of 5 hours in the patient, the lidocaine steady-state concentration can be obtained any time after the first day of dosing (5 half-lives = 5 · 5 h = 25 h). Lidocaine serum concentrations should also be measured if the patient experiences a return of ventricular arrhythmia or develops potential signs or symptoms of lidocaine toxicity.

Literature-Based Recommended Dosing

1. *Choose a lidocaine dose based on the disease states and conditions of the patient.*

A lidocaine loading dose of 1 to 1.5 mg/kg and a maintenance infusion of 1 to 2 mg/min are suggested for a patient with liver disease.

2. *Compute the dosage regimen.*

Because the desired concentration is in the upper end of the therapeutic range, doses in the upper end of the suggested ranges are used. A lidocaine loading dose of 1.5 mg/kg is administered: LD = 1.5 mg/kg · 81 kg = 122 mg, rounded to 100 mg over 2 to 4 minutes. A lidocaine maintenance infusion of 2 mg/min is administered after the loading dose is given. An additional dose of 50% of the loading dose can be given if arrhythmias recur 20 to 30 minutes after the initial loading dose.

A steady-state lidocaine serum concentration can be measured after steady state is attained in 3 to 5 half-lives. Since lidocaine is expected to have a half-life of 5 hours in the patient, the lidocaine steady-state concentration can be obtained any time after the first day of dosing (5 half-lives = 5 · 5 h = 25 h). Lidocaine serum concentrations should also be measured if the patient experiences a return of ventricular arrhythmia or develops potential signs or symptoms of lidocaine toxicity.

4. The revised lidocaine dose for patient EM is calculated as follows.

Linear Pharmacokinetics Method

1. *Compute a new dose to achieve the desired serum concentration.*

The patient is expected to achieve steady-state conditions after 1 day (5 half-lives = 5 · 5 h = 25 h) of therapy.

With the use of linear pharmacokinetics, the new dose to attain the desired concentration should be proportional to the old dose that produced the measured concentration:

$$D_{new} = (Css_{new}/Css_{old})D_{old} = [(4\ \mu g/mL)/(6.2\ \mu g/mL)]\ 2\ mg/min$$
$$= 1.3\ mg/min,\ rounded\ to\ 1.5\ mg/min$$

The new suggested dose is 1.5 mg/min of intravenous lidocaine to be started immediately. If the patient is experiencing lidocaine side effects, the lidocaine infusion can be held for approximately 1 half-life to allow concentrations to decline, and the new infusion can be started at that time.

A steady-state lidocaine serum concentration can be measured after steady state is attained in 3 to 5 half-lives. Since lidocaine is expected to have a half-life of 5 hours in the patient, the lidocaine steady-state concentration can be obtained any time after the first day of dosing (5 half-lives = 5 · 5 h = 25 h). Lidocaine serum concentrations should also be measured if the patient experiences a return of ventricular arrhythmia or develops potential signs or symptoms of lidocaine toxicity.

Pharmacokinetic Parameter Method

1. *Compute the pharmacokinetic parameters.*

The patient is expected to achieve steady-state conditions after the first day (5 half-lives = 5 · 5 h = 25 h) of therapy.

Lidocaine clearance can be computed using a steady-state lidocaine concentration: $Cl = k_0/Css$ = (2 mg/min)/(6.2 mg/L) = 0.32 L/min. (Note: μg/mL = mg/L, and this concentration unit was substituted for Css in the calculations to avoid unnecessary unit conversion.)

2. *Compute the lidocaine dose.*

Lidocaine clearance is used to compute the new lidocaine infusion rate: k_0 = Css · Cl = 4 mg/L · 0.32 L/min = 1.3 mg/min, rounded to 1.5 mg/min.

The new suggested dose is 1.5 mg/min of intravenous lidocaine to be started immediately. If the patient is experiencing lidocaine side effects, the lidocaine infusion can be held for approximately 1 half-life to allow concentrations to decline, and the new infusion can be started at that time.

A steady-state lidocaine serum concentration can be measured after steady state is attained in 3 to 5 half-lives. Since lidocaine is expected to have a half-life of 5 hours in the patient, the lidocaine steady-state concentration can be obtained any time after the first day of dosing (5 half-lives = 5 · 5 h = 25 h). Lidocaine serum concentrations should also be measured if the patient experiences a return of ventricular arrhythmia or develops potential signs or symptoms of lidocaine toxicity.

5. The initial lidocaine dose for patient OF is calculated as follows.

Pharmacokinetic Dosing Method

1. *Estimate the half-life and elimination rate constant according to the disease states and conditions of the patient.*

The expected lidocaine half-life ($t_{1/2}$) is 2 hours. The elimination rate constant is computed using the following formula: $k = 0.693/t_{1/2} = 0.693/2\ h = 0.347\ h^{-1}$.

2. *Estimate the volume of distribution and clearance.*

The patient is not obese, so the estimated lidocaine central volume of distribution and the volume of distribution for the entire body (V_{area}) are based on actual body weight: $Vc = 0.3\ L/kg \cdot 60\ kg = 18\ L$, $V_{area} = 1\ L/kg \cdot 60\ kg = 60\ L$. Estimated lidocaine clearance is computed by taking the product of V_{area} and the elimination rate constant: $Cl = kV_{area} = 0.347\ h^{-1} \cdot 60\ L = 20.8\ L/h$.

3. *Compute the dosage regimen.*

Therapy is started by administering an intravenous loading dose of lidocaine to the patient (Note: μg/mL = mg/L, and this concentration unit was substituted for Css in the calculations to avoid unnecessary unit conversion): LD = Css · Vc = 5 mg/L · 18 L = 90 mg, rounded to 100 mg intravenously over 2 to 4 minutes. An additional dose of 50% of the loading dose can be given if arrhythmias recur 20 to 30 minutes after the initial loading dose.

A lidocaine continuous intravenous infusion is started immediately after the loading dose has been administered. The dosage equation for intravenous lidocaine is k_0 = Css · Cl = (5 mg/L · 20.8 L/h)/(60 min/h) = 1.7 mg/min, rounded to 1.5 mg/min.

A steady-state lidocaine serum concentration can be measured after steady state is attained in 3 to 5 half-lives. Since lidocaine is expected to have a half-life of 2 hours in the patient, the lidocaine steady-state concentration can be obtained any time after the first 10 to 12 hours of dosing (5 half-lives = 5 · 2 h = 10 h). Lidocaine serum concentrations also should be measured if the patient experiences a return of ventricular arrhythmia or develops potential signs or symptoms of lidocaine toxicity.

Literature-Based Recommended Dosing

1. *Choose a lidocaine dose based on the disease states and conditions of the patient.*

A lidocaine loading dose of 0.5 to 0.75 mg/kg and a maintenance infusion of 1 to 2 mg/min are suggested for a patient with heart failure.

2. *Compute the dosage regimen.*

Because the desired concentration is in the upper end of the therapeutic range, doses in the upper end of the suggested ranges are used. A lidocaine loading dose of

0.75 mg/kg is administered: LD = 0.75 mg/kg · 60 kg = 45 mg, rounded to 50 mg over 1 to 2 minutes. A lidocaine maintenance infusion of 2 mg/min is administered after the loading dose is given. An additional dose of 50% of the loading dose can be given if arrhythmias recur 20 to 30 minutes after the initial loading dose.

A steady-state lidocaine serum concentration can be measured after steady state is attained in 3 to 5 half-lives. Since lidocaine is expected to have a half-life of 2 hours in the patient, the lidocaine steady-state concentration can be obtained any time after the first 10 to 12 hours of dosing (5 half-lives = 5 · 2 h = 10 h). Lidocaine serum concentrations also should be measured if the patient experiences a return of ventricular arrhythmia or develops potential signs or symptoms of lidocaine toxicity.

6. The revised lidocaine dose for patient OF is calculated as follows.

Linear Pharmacokinetics Method

1. *Compute a new dose to achieve the desired serum concentration.*

The patient is expected to achieve steady-state conditions after 10 to 12 hours (5 half-lives = 5 · 2 h = 10 h) of therapy.

With the use of linear pharmacokinetics, the new dose to attain the desired concentration should be proportional to the old dose that produced the measured concentration:

$$D_{new} = (Css_{new}/Css_{old})D_{old} = [(4\ \mu g/mL)/(6.7\ \mu g/mL)]\ 2\ mg/min = 1.2\ mg/min, \text{ rounded to } 1\ mg/min$$

The new suggested dose is 1 mg/min of intravenous lidocaine to be started immediately. If the patient is experiencing lidocaine side effects, the lidocaine infusion can be held for approximately 1 half-life to allow concentrations to decline, and the new infusion can be started at that time.

A steady-state lidocaine serum concentration can be measured after steady state is attained in 3 to 5 half-lives. Since lidocaine is expected to have a half-life of 2 hours in the patient, the lidocaine steady-state concentration can be obtained any time after the first 10 to 12 hours of dosing (5 half-lives = 5 · 2 h = 10 h). Lidocaine serum concentrations also should be measured if the patient experiences a return of ventricular arrhythmia or develops potential signs or symptoms of lidocaine toxicity.

Pharmacokinetic Parameter Method

1. *Compute the pharmacokinetic parameters.*

The patient is expected to achieve steady-state conditions after the first 10 to 12 hours (5 half-lives = 5 · 2 h = 10 h) of therapy.

Lidocaine clearance can be computed using a steady-state lidocaine concentration: $Cl = k_0/Css = (2\ mg/min)/(6.7\ mg/L) = 0.30\ L/min$. (Note: μg/mL = mg/L, and this concentration unit was substituted for Css in the calculations to avoid unnecessary unit conversion.)

2. *Compute the lidocaine dose.*

Lidocaine clearance is used to compute the new lidocaine infusion rate: k_0 = Css · Cl = 4 mg/L · 0.30 L/min = 1.2 mg/min, rounded to 1 mg/min.

The new suggested dose is 1 mg/min of intravenous lidocaine to be started immediately. If the patient is experiencing lidocaine side effects, the lidocaine infusion can be held for approximately 1 half-life to allow concentrations to decline, and the new infusion can be started at that time.

A steady-state lidocaine serum concentration can be measured after steady state is attained in 3 to 5 half-lives. Since lidocaine is expected to have a half-life of 2 hours in the patient, the lidocaine steady-state concentration can be obtained any time after the first 10 to 12 hours of dosing (5 half-lives = 5 · 2 h = 10 h). Lidocaine serum concentrations also should be measured if the patient experiences a return of ventricular arrhythmia or develops potential signs or symptoms of lidocaine toxicity.

7. The initial lidocaine dose for patient FK is calculated as follows.

Pharmacokinetic Dosing Method

1. *Estimate the half-life and elimination rate constant according to the disease states and conditions of the patient.*

The expected lidocaine half-life ($t_{1/2}$) is 2 hours. The elimination rate constant is computed using the following formula: $k = 0.693/t_{1/2} = 0.693/2\ h = 0.347\ h^{-1}$.

2. *Estimate the volume of distribution and clearance.*

The patient is obese (>30% over ideal body weight), so the estimated lidocaine central volume of distribution (Vc) and the volume of distribution for the entire body (V_{area}) are based on ideal body weight: IBW_{men} (in kg) = 50 kg + 2.3(Ht − 60 in) = 50 kg + 2.3(71 − 60) = 75 kg, Vc = 0.3 L/kg · 75 kg = 23 L, V_{area} = 1 L/kg · 75 kg = 75 L. Estimated lidocaine clearance is computed by taking the product of V_{area} and the elimination rate constant: $Cl = kV_{area} = 0.347\ h^{-1} \cdot 75\ L = 26\ L/h$.

3. *Compute the dosage regimen.*

Therapy is started by administering an intravenous loading dose of lidocaine to the patient (note: μg/mL = mg/L, and this concentration unit was substituted for Css in the calculations to avoid unnecessary unit conversion): LD = Css · Vc = 3 mg/L · 23 L = 69 mg, rounded to 75 mg intravenously over 1.5 to 3 minutes. An additional dose at 50% of the loading dose can be given if arrhythmias recur 20 to 30 minutes after the initial loading dose.

A lidocaine continuous intravenous infusion is started immediately after the loading dose has been administered. The dosage equation for intravenous lidocaine is k_0 = Css · Cl = (3 mg/L · 26 L/h)/(60 min/h) = 1.3 mg/min, rounded to 1.5 mg/min.

A steady-state lidocaine serum concentration can be measured after steady state is attained in 3 to 5 half-lives. Since lidocaine is expected to have a half-life of 2 hours in the patient, the lidocaine steady-state concentration can be obtained any time after the first 10 to 12 hours of dosing (5 half-lives = 5 · 2 h = 10 h). Lidocaine serum concentrations also should be measured if the patient experiences a return of ventricular arrhythmia or develops potential signs or symptoms of lidocaine toxicity.

Literature-Based Recommended Dosing

1. *Choose a lidocaine dose based on the disease states and conditions of the patient.*

A lidocaine loading dose of 0.5 to 0.75 mg/kg and a maintenance infusion of 1 to 2 mg/min are suggested for a patient with heart failure. The patient is obese (>30% over ideal body weight), so lidocaine doses are based on ideal body weight: IBW_{men} (in kg) = 50 kg + 2.3(Ht − 60 in) = 50 kg + 2.3(71 − 60) = 75 kg.

2. *Compute the dosage regimen.*

Because the desired concentration is in the lower end of the therapeutic range, doses in the lower end of the suggested ranges are used. A lidocaine loading dose of 0.5 mg/kg is administered: LD = 0.5 mg/kg · 75 kg = 38 mg, rounded to 50 mg over 1 to 2 minutes. A lidocaine maintenance infusion of 1 mg/min is administered after the loading dose is given. An additional dose at 50% of the loading dose can be given if arrhythmias recur 20 to 30 minutes after the initial loading dose.

A steady-state lidocaine serum concentration can be measured after steady state is attained in 3 to 5 half-lives. Since lidocaine is expected to have a half-life of 2 hours in the patient, the lidocaine steady-state concentration can be obtained any time after the first 10 to 12 hours of dosing (5 half-lives = 5 · 2 h = 10 h). Lidocaine serum concentrations should also be measured if the patient experiences a return of ventricular arrhythmia or develops potential signs or symptoms of lidocaine toxicity.

8. The revised lidocaine dose for patient FK is calculated as follows.

Bayesian Pharmacokinetics Computer Program Method

1. *Enter the patient's demographic, drug dosing, and serum concentration–time data into the computer program.*

This patient is unlikely to be at steady state, so the linear pharmacokinetics method cannot be used. The DrugCalc program requires lidocaine infusion rates to be entered in terms of mg/h. A 2-mg/min infusion rate is equivalent to 120 mg/h (k_0 = 2 mg/min · 60 min/h = 120 mg/h).

2. *Compute the pharmacokinetic parameters for the patient using the Bayesian pharmacokinetics computer program.*

The pharmacokinetic parameters computed by the program are a volume of distribution for the entire body (V_{area}) of 60 L, a half-life of 2.9 hours, and a clearance of 14.5 L/h.

3. *Compute a dose required to achieve the desired lidocaine serum concentrations.*

The continuous intravenous infusion equation used by the program to compute doses indicates that a dose of 60 mg/h or 1 mg/min [k_0 = (60 mg/h)/(60 min/h) = 1 mg/min] will produce a steady-state lidocaine concentration of 4 μg/mL. This infusion rate can be started immediately. If the patient is experiencing lidocaine side effects, the lidocaine infusion can be held for approximately 1 half-life to allow concentrations to decline, and the new infusion is started at that time.

9. The initial lidocaine dose for patient GP is calculated as follows.

Pharmacokinetic Dosing Method

1. *Estimate the half-life and elimination rate constant according to the disease states and conditions of the patient.*

The expected lidocaine half-life ($t_{1/2}$) is 4 hours. The elimination rate constant is computed using the following formula: $k = 0.693/t_{1/2} = 0.693/4\ h = 0.173\ h^{-1}$.

2. *Estimate the volume of distribution and clearance.*

The patient is not obese, so the estimated lidocaine central volume of distribution and the volume of distribution for the entire body (V_{area}) are based on actual body weight: $Vc = 0.5\ L/kg \cdot 90\ kg = 45\ L$, $V_{area} = 1.5\ L/kg \cdot 90\ kg = 135\ L$. Estimated lidocaine clearance is computed by taking the product of V_{area} and the elimination rate constant: $Cl = kV_{area} = 0.173\ h^{-1} \cdot 135\ L = 23.4\ L/h$.

3. *Compute the dosage regimen.*

Therapy is started by administering an intravenous loading dose of lidocaine to the patient (note: μg/mL = mg/L, and this concentration unit was substituted for Css in the calculations to avoid unnecessary unit conversion): $LD = Css \cdot Vc = 4\ mg/L \cdot 45\ L = 180\ mg$, rounded to 200 mg intravenously over 4 to 8 minutes. An additional dose at 50% of the loading dose can be given if arrhythmias recur 20 to 30 minutes after the initial loading dose.

A lidocaine continuous intravenous infusion is started immediately after the loading dose has been administered. The dosage equation for intravenous lidocaine is $k_0 = Css \cdot Cl = (4\ mg/L \cdot 23.4\ L/h)/(60\ min/h) = 1.6\ mg/min$, rounded to 1.5 mg/min.

A steady-state lidocaine serum concentration can be measured after steady state is attained in 3 to 5 half-lives. Since lidocaine is expected to have a half-life of 4 hours in the patient, the lidocaine steady-state concentration can be obtained any time after the first day of dosing (5 half-lives = $5 \cdot 4\ h = 20\ h$). Lidocaine serum concentrations should also be measured if the patient experiences a return of ventricular arrhythmia or develops potential signs or symptoms of lidocaine toxicity.

Literature-Based Recommended Dosing

1. *Choose a lidocaine dose based on the disease states and conditions of the patient.*

A lidocaine loading dose of 1 to 1.5 mg/kg and a maintenance infusion of 3 to 4 mg/min are suggested for a patient without heart failure or liver disease.

2. *Compute the dosage regimen.*

Because the desired concentration is in the upper end of the therapeutic range, a dose in the upper end of the suggested ranges is used. A lidocaine loading dose of 1.5 mg/kg is administered: $LD = 1.5\ mg/kg \cdot 90\ kg = 135\ mg$, rounded to 150 mg over 3 to 6 minutes. A lidocaine maintenance infusion of 3 mg/min is administered after the loading dose is given. An additional dose of 50% of the loading dose can be given if arrhythmias recur 20 to 30 minutes after the initial loading dose.

A steady-state lidocaine serum concentration can be measured after steady state is attained in 3 to 5 half-lives. Since lidocaine is expected to have a half-life of 4 hours in the patient, the lidocaine steady-state concentration can be obtained any time after the first day of dosing (5 half-lives = 5 · 4 h = 20 h). Lidocaine serum concentrations should also be measured if the patient experiences a return of ventricular arrhythmia or develops potential signs or symptoms of lidocaine toxicity.

10. The revised lidocaine dose for patient GP is calculated as follows.

Bayesian Pharmacokinetics Computer Program Method

1. *Enter the patient's demographic, drug dosing, and serum concentration–time data into the computer program.*

This patient is unlikely to be at steady state, so the linear pharmacokinetics method cannot be used. The DrugCalc program requires lidocaine infusion rates to be entered in terms of mg/h. A 2-mg/min infusion rate is equivalent to 120 mg/h (k_0 = 2 mg/min · 60 min/h = 120 mg/h).

2. *Compute the pharmacokinetic parameters for the patient using the Bayesian pharmacokinetics computer program.*

The pharmacokinetic parameters computed by the program are a volume of distribution for the entire body (V_{area}) of 118 L, a half-life of 1.4 hours, and a clearance of 57 L/h.

3. *Compute a dose required to achieve the desired lidocaine serum concentrations.*

The continuous intravenous infusion equation used by the program to compute doses indicates that 240 mg/h or 4 mg/min [k_0 = (240 mg/h)/(60 min/h) = 4 mg/min] will produce a steady-state lidocaine concentration of 4.2 μg/mL. This infusion rate should be started immediately.

Computation of Booster Dose

1. *Use the central volume of distribution (Vc) to calculate booster dose (if needed).*

The booster dose is computed using the following equation (Vc population average estimate used from problem 9): BD = ($C_{desired}$ − C_{actual})Vc = (4.2 mg/L − 1.9 mg/L)45 L = 104 mg, rounded to 100 mg of lidocaine intravenously over 2 to 4 minutes. (Note: μg/mL = mg/L, and this concentration unit was substituted for C in the calculations to avoid unnecessary unit conversion.) If the maintenance dose is increased, it will take an additional 3 to 5 estimated half-lives for new steady-state conditions to be achieved.

11. The revised lidocaine dose for patient CV is calculated as follows.

Bayesian Pharmacokinetics Computer Program Method

1. *Enter the patient's demographic, drug dosing, and serum concentration–time data into the computer program.*

This patient is unlikely to be at steady state, and multiple infusion rates have been prescribed, so the linear pharmacokinetics method cannot be used. In addition, the patient has two disease states that change lidocaine pharmacokinetics. The DrugCalc program requires lidocaine infusion rates to be entered in terms of mg/h. A 2-mg/min infusion rate is equivalent to 120 mg/h (k_0 = 2 mg/min · 60 min/h = 120 mg/h), and a 1-mg/min infusion rate is equivalent to 60 mg/h (k_0 = 1 mg/min · 60 min/h = 60 mg/h).

2. *Compute the pharmacokinetic parameters for the patient using the Bayesian pharmacokinetics computer program.*

The pharmacokinetic parameters computed by the program are a volume of distribution for the entire body (V_{area}) of 112 L, a half-life of 6 hours, and a clearance of 13 L/h.

3. *Compute the dose required to achieve the desired lidocaine serum concentrations.*

The continuous intravenous infusion equation used by the program to compute doses indicates that 39 mg/h or 0.7 mg/min [k_0 = (39 mg/h)/(60 min/h) = 0.7 mg/min] will produce a steady-state lidocaine concentration of 3 μg/mL. This infusion rate can be started immediately. If the patient is experiencing lidocaine side effects, the lidocaine infusion can be held for approximately 1 half-life to allow concentrations to decline, and the new infusion can be started at that time.

12. The revised lidocaine dose for patient FP is calculated as follows.

Bayesian Pharmacokinetics Computer Program Method

1. *Enter the patient's demographic, drug dosing, and serum concentration–time data into the computer program.*

This patient is unlikely to be at steady state, and multiple infusion rates and loading doses have been prescribed, so the linear pharmacokinetics method cannot be used. In addition, the patient has two disease states that change lidocaine pharmacokinetics. The DrugCalc program requires lidocaine infusion rates to be entered in terms of mg/h. A 3-mg/min infusion rate is equivalent to 180 mg/h (k_0 = 3 mg/min · 60 min/h = 180 mg/h), and a 1-mg/min infusion rate is equivalent to 60 mg/h (k_0 = 1 mg/min · 60 min/h = 60 mg/h).

2. *Compute the pharmacokinetic parameters for the patient using the Bayesian pharmacokinetics computer program.*

The pharmacokinetic parameters computed by the program are a volume of distribution for the entire body (V_{area}) of 136 L, a half-life of 5.6 hours, and a clearance of 17 L/h.

3. *Compute the dose required to achieve the desired lidocaine serum concentrations.*

The continuous intravenous infusion equation used by the program to compute doses indicates that 83 mg/h or 1.4 mg/min [k_0 = (83 mg/h)/(60 min/h) = 1.4 mg/min], rounded to 1.5 mg/min, will produce a steady-state lidocaine concentration of 5 μg/mL. This infusion rate can be started immediately.

REFERENCES

1. Bauman JL, Schoen MD. Arrhythmias. In: DiPiro JT, Talbert RL, Yee GC, Matzke GR, Wells BG, Posey LM, eds. Pharmacotherapy. Stamford, CT: Appleton & Lange, 1999:232–264.
2. Roden DM. Antiarrhythmic drugs. In: Hardman JG, Limbird LE, Molinoff PB, Ruddon RW, Gilman AG, eds. The pharmacological basis of therapeutics. New York: McGraw-Hill, 1996: 839–874.
3. Boyes RN, Scott DB, Jebson PJ, Godman MJ, Julian DG. Pharmacokinetics of lidocaine in man. Clin Pharmacol Ther 1971;12:105–116.
4. Wyman MG, Lalka D, Hammersmith L, Cannom DS, Goldreyer BN. Multiple bolus technique for lidocaine administration during the first hours of an acute myocardial infarction. Am J Cardiol 1978;41:313–317.
5. Halkin H, Meffin P, Melmon KL, Rowland M. Influence of congestive heart failure on blood vessels of lidocaine and its active monodeethylated metabolite. Clin Pharmacol Ther 1975;17: 669–676.
6. Strong JM, Mayfield DE, Atkinson AJ, Jr, Burris BC, Raymon F, Webster LT, Jr. Pharmacological activity, metabolism, and pharmacokinetics of glycinexylidide. Clin Pharmacol Ther 1975; 17:184–194.
7. Narang PK, Crouthamel WG, Carliner NH, Fisher ML. Lidocaine and its active metabolites. Clin Pharmacol Ther 1978;24:654–662.
8. Barchowsky A, Shand DG, Stargel WW, Wagner GS, Routledge PA. On the role of alpha 1-acid glycoprotein in lignocaine accumulation following myocardial infarction. Br J Clin Pharmacol 1982;13:411–415.
9. Bauer LA, Brown T, Gibaldi M, et al. Influence of long-term infusions on lidocaine kinetics. Clin Pharmacol Ther 1982;31:433–437.
10. Routledge PA, Stargel WW, Wagner GS, Shand DG. Increased alpha-1-acid glycoprotein and lidocaine disposition in myocardial infarction. Ann Intern Med 1980;93:701–704.
11. Routledge PA, Shand DG, Barchowsky A, Wagner G, Stargel WW. Relationship between alpha 1-acid glycoprotein and lidocaine disposition in myocardial infarction. Clin Pharmacol Ther 1981;30:154–157.
12. Thomson PD, Rowland M, Melmon KL. The influence of heart failure, liver disease, and renal failure on the disposition of lidocaine in man. Am Heart J 1971;82:417–421.
13. Scott DB, Jebson PJ, Vellani CW, Julian DG. Plasma-lignocaine levels after intravenous and intramuscular injection. Lancet 1970;1:41.
14. Routledge PA, Stargel WW, Kitchell BB, Barchowsky A, Shand DG. Sex-related differences in the plasma protein binding of lignocaine and diazepam. Br J Clin Pharmacol 1981;11:245–250.
15. Routledge PA, Barchowsky A, Bjornsson TD, Kitchell BB, Shand DG. Lidocaine plasma protein binding. Clin Pharmacol Ther 1980;27:347–351.
16. McNamara PJ, Slaughter RL, Pieper JA, Wyman MG, Lalka D. Factors influencing serum protein binding of lidocaine in humans. Anesth Analg 1981;60:395–400.
17. Suzuki T, Fujita S, Kawai R. Precursor-metabolite interaction in the metabolism of lidocaine. J Pharm Sci 1984;73:136–138.
18. Abernethy DR, Greenblatt DJ. Lidocaine disposition in obesity. Am J Cardiol 1984;53: 1183–1186.
19. Forrest JA, Finlayson ND, Adjepon-Yamoah KK, Prescott LF. Antipyrine, paracetamol, and lignocaine elimination in chronic liver disease. Br Med J 1977;1:1384–1387.
20. Huet PM, Lelorier J. Effects of smoking and chronic hepatitis B on lidocaine and indocyanine green kinetics. Clin Pharmacol Ther 1980;28:208–215.
21. Thomson PD, Melmon KL, Richardson JA, et al. Lidocaine pharmacokinetics in advanced heart failure, liver disease, and renal failure in humans. Ann Intern Med 1973;78:499–508.

22. Williams RL, Blaschke TF, Meffin PJ, Melmon KL, Rowland M. Influence of viral hepatitis on the disposition of two compounds with high hepatic clearance: lidocaine and indocyanine green. Clin Pharmacol Ther 1976;20:290–299.
23. Pugh RN, Murray-Lyon IM, Dawson JL, Pietroni MC, Williams R. Transection of the oesophagus for bleeding oesophageal varices. Br J Surg 1973;60:646–649.
24. Nation RL, Triggs EJ, Selig M. Lignocaine kinetics in cardiac patients and aged subjects. Br J Clin Pharmacol 1977;4:439–448.
25. Prescott LF, Adjepon-Yamoah KK, Talbot RG. Impaired lignocaine metabolism in patients with myocardial infarction and cardiac failure. Br Med J 1976;1:939–941.
26. Bax ND, Tucker GT, Woods HF. Lignocaine and indocyanine green kinetics in patients following myocardial infarction. Br J Clin Pharmacol 1980;10:353–361.
27. LeLorier J, Grenon D, Latour Y, et al. Pharmacokinetics of lidocaine after prolonged intravenous infusions in uncomplicated myocardial infarction. Ann Intern Med 1977;87:700–706.
28. Hansten PD, Horn JR. Drug interactions analysis and management. Vancouver, WA: Applied Therapeutics, 1998:527.
29. Bauer LA, Edwards WA, Randolph FP, Blouin RA. Cimetidine-induced decrease in lidocaine metabolism. Am Heart J 1984;108:413–415.
30. Bauer LA, McDonnell N, Horn JR, Zierler B, Opheim K, Strandness DE, Jr. Single and multiple doses of oral cimetidine do not change liver blood flow in humans. Clin Pharmacol Ther 1990;48:195–200.
31. Mutnick AH, Burke TG. Antiarrhythmics. In: Schumacher GE, ed. Therapeutic drug monitoring. Stamford, CT: Appleton & Lange, 1995:684.
32. Wandell M, Mungall D. Computer assisted drug interpretation and drug regimen optimization. Am Assoc Clin Chem 1984;6:1–11.
33. Johnson JA, Parker RB, Geraci SA. Heart failure. In: DiPiro JT, Talbert RL, Yee GC, Matzke GR, Wells BG, Posey LM, eds. Pharmacotherapy—a pathophysiologic approach. Stamford, CT: Appleton & Lange, 1999:153–181.

8

PROCAINAMIDE AND *N*-ACETYL PROCAINAMIDE

INTRODUCTION

Procainamide is an effective antiarrhythmic agent that is used intravenously and orally. Classified as a type IA antiarrhythmic agent, it can be used for the treatment of either supraventricular or ventricular arrhythmias.[1,2] It is a drug of choice for the treatment of stable monomorphic ventricular tachycardia in patients with a normal cardiac ejection fraction. Procainamide is a useful agent in the treatment of stable polymorphic ventricular fibrillation in patients with a normal baseline QT interval and normal ejection fraction. It can also be used to test shock-refractory ventricular fibrillation. For episodes of sustained ventricular tachycardia (>30 seconds, >150 beats/min) with serious signs or symptoms of hemodynamic instability (angina, pulmonary edema, hypotension, hemodynamic collapse), electrical cardioversion is the treatment of choice. However, for ventricular rates <150 beats/min in patients who are more hemodynamically stable, sustained monomorphic ventricular tachycardia may be successfully treated with antiarrhythmic (primary agents: procainamide or sotalol; secondary agents: amiodarone or lidocaine) therapy. The primary treatment for ventricular fibrillation is also direct-current cardioversion. Procainamide is the second-line antiarrhythmic agent for patients whose fibrillation does not convert using electrical shock and intravenous epinephrine or vasopressin. Given orally, procainamide is a widely used agent for long-term suppression of ventricular arrhythmias.

Procainamide is also effective in the long-term prevention of chronic supraventricular arrhythmias, such as supraventricular tachycardia, atrial flutter, and atrial fibrillation. After ventricular rate has been controlled, procainamide therapy can be used to chemically convert atrial fibrillation to normal sinus rhythm for a patient with a normal cardiac ejection fraction. Procainamide inhibits transmembrane sodium influx into the conduction system of the heart, thereby decreasing conduction velocity.[1,2] It also increases the duration of the action potential, increases threshold potential toward zero, and decreases the slope of phase 4 of the action potential. Automaticity is decreased during procainamide therapy. The net effect of these cellular changes is that procainamide causes increased refractoriness and decreased conduction in heart conduction tissue, which establishes a bidirectional block in reentrant pathways.

N-acetyl procainamide (NAPA) is an active metabolite of procainamide and has type III antiarrhythmic effects.[1,2] A common characteristic of type III antiarrhythmic agents (bretylium, amiodarone, sotalol) is prolongation of the duration of the action potential, resulting in an increased absolute refractory period.

THERAPEUTIC AND TOXIC CONCENTRATIONS

When given intravenously, the serum procainamide concentration–time curve follows a two-compartment model[3] (Figure 8-1). If an intravenous loading dose is followed by a continuous infusion, serum concentrations decline rapidly at first because of distribution of the loading dose from blood to tissues[3] (Figure 8-2). When oral dosage forms are given, absorption occurs more slowly than distribution, so a distribution phase is not seen[4–8] (Figure 8-3).

The generally accepted therapeutic range for procainamide is 4 to 10 μg/mL. Serum concentrations in the upper end of the therapeutic range (≥8 μg/mL) may result in minor side effects such as gastrointestinal disturbances (anorexia, nausea, vomiting, diarrhea), weakness, malaise, decreased mean arterial pressure (<20%), and a 10% to 30% prolongation of electrocardiogram (ECG) intervals (PR and QT intervals, QRS complex). Procainamide serum concentrations higher than 12 μg/mL can cause increased PR-interval, QT-interval, or QRS-complex widening (>30%) on the ECG; heart block; ventricular conduction disturbances; new ventricular arrhythmias; or cardiac arrest. Procainamide therapy is also associated with *torsades de pointes*.[1,2] Torsades de pointes ("twisting of the

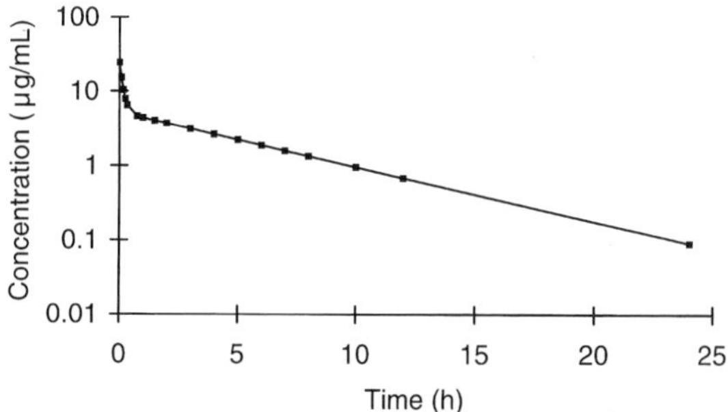

FIGURE 8-1 Procainamide serum concentrations initially drop rapidly after an intravenous bolus while the drug distributes from blood into the tissues during the distribution phase. During the distribution phase, the drug leaves the blood because of tissue distribution and elimination. After 20 to 30 minutes, an equilibrium is established because the blood and tissues, and serum concentrations drop more slowly, because elimination is the primary process for removing drug from the blood. This type of serum concentration–time profile is described by a two-compartment model.

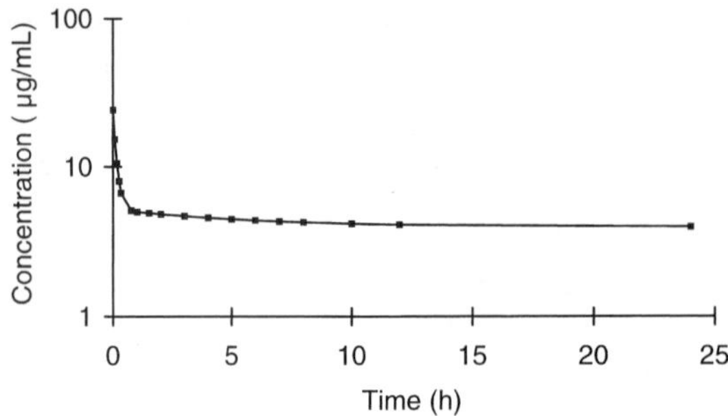

FIGURE 8-2 To maintain therapeutic procainamide concentrations, an intravenous loading dose (over 25 to 30 minutes) is followed by a continuous intravenous infusion of the drug. A distribution phase is still seen because of the administration of the loading dose. Note that the administration of a loading dose may not establish steady-state conditions immediately, and the infusion needs to run 3 to 5 half-lives until steady-state concentrations are attained.

points") is a form of polymorphic ventricular tachycardia preceded by QT-interval prolongation. It is characterized by polymorphic QRS complexes that change in amplitude and length, giving the appearance of oscillations around the ECG baseline. Torsades de pointes can develop into multiple episodes of nonsustained polymorphic ventricular tachycardia, syncope, ventricular fibrillation, or sudden cardiac death.

Nondose- or concentration-related side effects to procainamide include rash, agranulocytosis, and a systemic lupus-like syndrome. Symptoms of the lupus-like syndrome include rash, photosensitivity, arthralgias, pleuritis or pericarditis, hemolytic anemia or leukopenia, and a positive antinuclear antibody test. Patients who metabolize the drug more rapidly via *N*-acetyltransferase, known as "rapid acetylators," appear to have a lower incidence of this adverse effect or at least take more time and higher doses for it to appear. Although the lupus-like syndrome is usually not life-threatening, it does occur in 30% to 50% of patients taking procainamide for longer than 6 to 12 months and requires discontinuation of the drug. Most symptoms abate within several weeks to months, but

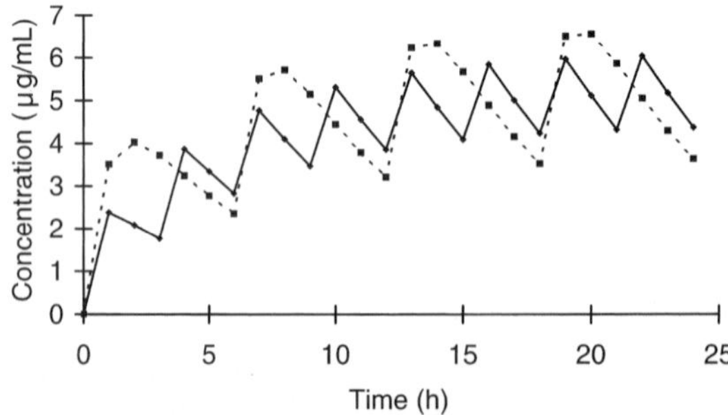

FIGURE 8-3 Serum concentration–time profile for rapid-release procainamide (*solid line;* given every 3 hours) and sustained-release procainamide (*dashed line;* given every 6 hours) oral dosage forms after multiple doses until steady state is achieved. The curves shown are typical for an adult with normal renal and hepatic function.

some patients require a year or more to recover completely. Intravenous procainamide doses must be given no faster than 25 to 50 mg/min because faster injection can cause profound hypotension.

An active procainamide metabolite, known as *N*-acetyl procainamide (NAPA) or acecainide, also possesses antiarrhythmic effects.[9–11] Based on limited clinical trials of NAPA, effective concentrations are 10 to 30 μg/mL. Concentration-dependent adverse effects for NAPA are similar to those given for procainamide. However, NAPA does not appear to cause a systemic lupus-like syndrome. NAPA is not commercially available in the United States and has been given orphan drug status by the US Food and Drug Administration with an indication for prevention of life-threatening ventricular arrhythmias in patients with documented procainamide-induced lupus. Some laboratories report the sum of procainamide and NAPA concentrations for a patient as the "total procainamide concentration," using the therapeutic range of 10 to 30 μg/mL. However, because procainamide and NAPA have different antiarrhythmic potencies, serum concentrations for each agent should be considered individually. Also, many feel that it is more important to maintain therapeutic procainamide concentrations in patients rather than to maintain NAPA or total procainamide levels in the suggested ranges. Clinicians should understand that all patients with "toxic" procainamide or NAPA serum concentrations in the listed ranges do not exhibit signs or symptoms of procainamide toxicity. Rather, procainamide and NAPA concentrations in the given ranges increase the likelihood that an adverse effect will occur.

For dose adjustment purposes, procainamide serum concentrations during oral administration are best measured as a predose or trough level at steady state after the patient has received a consistent dosage regimen for 3 to 5 drug half-lives. If the drug is given as a continuous intravenous infusion, procainamide serum concentrations can be measured at steady state after the patient has received a consistent infusion rate for 3 to 5 drug half-lives. Procainamide half-life varies from 2.5 to 5 hours in normal adults to 14 hours or more in adult patients with renal failure. Average NAPA half-lives are 6 hours for normal adults and 41 hours for adult patients with renal failure. If procainamide is given orally or intravenously on a stable schedule, steady-state serum concentrations for parent drug and metabolite are achieved in about 1 day ($5 \cdot 5$ h = 25 h for procainamide and $5 \cdot 6$ h = 30 h for NAPA). For a patient in renal failure, it takes 3 days for steady-state concentrations to occur for procainamide and 9 days for steady-state conditions to be established for NAPA ($5 \cdot 14$ h = 70 h or ~3 days for procainamide, $5 \cdot 41$ h = 205 h or ~9 days for NAPA).

CLINICAL MONITORING PARAMETERS

The electrocardiogram (ECG or EKG) should be monitored to determine the response to procainamide. The goal of therapy is suppression of arrhythmias and avoidance of adverse drug reactions. Electrophysiologic studies using programmed stimulation to replicate the ventricular arrhythmia or 24-hour ECG Holter monitoring can be performed in patients who are receiving various antiarrhythmic agents to determine effective antiarrhythmic drug therapy.[2]

Because many procainamide therapeutic and side effects are not correlated with its serum concentration, it is often not necessary to obtain serum procainamide concentrations in patients receiving appropriate doses who currently have no arrhythmia or adverse drug effects. However, procainamide serum concentrations should be obtained in patients who have a recurrence of tachyarrhythmias, are experiencing possible procainamide side effects, or are receiving procainamide doses not consistent with disease states and conditions known to alter procainamide pharmacokinetics (see Effects of Disease States and Conditions on Procainamide Pharmacokinetics and Dosing). Serum concentration monitoring can aid in the decision to increase or decrease the procainamide dose. For instance, if an arrhythmia reappears and the procainamide serum concentration is <10 μg/mL, increasing the procainamide dose is a therapeutic option. However, if the procainamide serum concentration is over 10 to 12 μg/mL, a dosage increase is less likely to be effective in suppressing the arrhythmia, and drug side effects are more likely to occur. Some patients have responded to procainamide serum concentrations as high as 20 μg/mL without experiencing severe adverse effects.[12] Similarly, if a possible concentration-related procainamide adverse drug reaction is noted in a patient and the procainamide serum concentration is <4 μg/mL, the observed problem may not be due to procainamide treatment, and other sources can be investigated. While receiving procainamide, patients should be monitored for the following adverse drug effects: anorexia, nausea, vomiting, diarrhea, weakness, malaise, decreased blood pressure, ECG changes (increased PR-interval, QT-interval, or QRS-complex widening >30%), heart block, ventricular conduction disturbances, new ventricular arrhythmias, rash, agranulocytosis, and the systemic lupus-like syndrome.

BASIC CLINICAL PHARMACOKINETIC PARAMETERS

Procainamide is eliminated by both hepatic metabolism (~50%) and renal elimination of unchanged drug (~50%).[9–11,13,14] Hepatic metabolism is mainly via *N*-acetyltransferase (NAT).[9–11] NAPA is the primary active metabolite resulting from procainamide metabolism by *N*-acetyltransferase. It exhibits a bimodal genetic polymorphism that results in "slow acetylator" and "rapid acetylator" phenotypes. If the patient has normal renal function, acetylator status can be estimated using the ratio of NAPA and procainamide (PA) steady-state concentrations: acetylator ratio = NAPA/PA.[15,16] If this ratio is 1.2 or greater, the patient is probably a rapid acetylator. If the ratio is 0.8 or less, the patient is probably a slow acetylator. The Caucasian and African-American populations appear to be about evenly split between slow and rapid acetylators. Eighty to 90% of the Japanese and Eskimo populations are rapid acetylators, whereas only 20% or less of Egyptians and certain Jewish populations are of the rapid phenotype. Obviously, ethnic background can play an important role in the procainamide dose required to achieve a therapeutic effect as well as in the potential for development of systemic lupus-like adverse effects. Metabolism of procainamide to other metabolites may be mediated by CYP2D6.[17] The ratio of procainamide renal clearance and creatinine clearance is 2 to 3, implying that net renal tubular secretion is taking place in the kidney.[13,14] The renal secretion probably takes place in the proximal tubule. Although some reports indicate that procainamide follows nonlinear pharmacokinetics, for the purposes of clinical drug dosing in patients, linear pharmacokinetic concepts and equations can be effectively used to compute doses and estimate serum concentrations.[18,19]

The average oral bioavailability of procainamide for both immediate-release and sustained-release dosage forms is 83%.[4–8] A lag time of 20 to 30 minutes occurs in some patients between oral dosage administration and the time that procainamide first appears in the serum. Plasma protein binding of procainamide in normal persons is only about 15%. The recommended dose of procainamide is based on the concurrent disease states and conditions in the patient that can influence procainamide pharmacokinetics. Procainamide pharmacokinetic parameters used to compute doses are given in the following section for specific patient profiles.

EFFECTS OF DISEASE STATES AND CONDITIONS ON PROCAINAMIDE PHARMACOKINETICS AND DOSING

In healthy adults without the disease states and conditions given later in this section and with normal liver and renal function, an average procainamide half-life is 3.3 hours (range, 2.5 to 4.6 hours) and a volume of distribution for the entire body is 2.7 L/kg (V = 2 to 3.8 L/kg; Table 8-1).[20–22] *N*-acetyltransferase is the enzyme responsible for conversion of procainamide to NAPA. The genetic polymorphism of *N*-acetyltransferase produces a bimodal frequency distribution for procainamide half-life and clearance, which divides the population into rapid and slow acetylators (Figure 8-4). The mean procainamide half-life in rapid acetylators is 2.7 hours, whereas in slow acetylators, it is 5.2 hours. Not all studies conducted with procainamide have separated results from rapid and slow acetylators when analyzing the pharmacokinetic data. Unfortunately, it is not practical to phenotype a patient as a slow or rapid metabolizer before administering the drug, so average population half-life and clearance are used for initial dosage computation. Disease states and conditions that change procainamide pharmacokinetics and dosage requirements may alter clearance and the volume of distribution. The elimination rate constant ($k = 0.693/t_{1/2}$, where $t_{1/2}$ is the half-life) and clearance ($Cl = kV$) can be computed from the aforementioned pharmacokinetic parameters.

Because about 50% of a procainamide dose is eliminated unchanged by the kidneys, renal dysfunction is the most important disease state that affects procainamide pharmacokinetics.[23–25] The procainamide clearance rate decreases as creatinine clearance decreases, but this relationship is not as helpful as it is with other drugs that are primarily renally eliminated. For example, digoxin, vancomycin, and the aminoglycoside antibiotics are eliminated mostly by glomerular filtration. Creatinine clearance is used as an estimate of glomerular filtration rate in patients because it is relatively easy to calculate or estimate. Because the major route of renal clearance for procainamide is by proximal tubular secretion, creatinine clearance is not as reliable a parameter to aid in the estimation of procainamide clearance. In patients with renal failure, the average procainamide half-life is 13.9 hours, and the volume of distribution is 1.7 L/kg.

Uncompensated heart failure reduces procainamide clearance because of decreased hepatic blood flow secondary to compromised cardiac output[22,23] (Table 8-2). Volume of distribution (V = 1.7 L/kg) is decreased in uncompensated heart failure patients as well. Because both clearance and volume of distribution simultaneously decrease, the increase in half-life is not as dramatic as might be expected, and in patients with uncompensated heart failure, an average procainamide half-life is 5.5 hours ($t_{1/2} = [0.693 \cdot \downarrow V]/\downarrow Cl$). The effect that uncompensated heart failure has on procainamide pharmacokinetics is highly variable and difficult to accurately predict. It is possible for patients with uncompensated heart failure to have relatively normal or grossly abnormal procainamide clearance and

TABLE 8-1 Disease States and Conditions That Alter Procainamide Pharmacokinetics

DISEASE STATE/ CONDITION	HALF-LIFE (h)	VOLUME OF DISTRIBUTION (L/kg)	COMMENTS
Adult, normal renal and liver function	3.3 (range, 2.6–4.6)	2.7 (range, 2–3.8)	Procainamide is eliminated ~50% unchanged in the urine and ~50% metabolized. *N*-acetyltransferase converts procainamide to an active metabolite (*N*-acetyl procainamide or NAPA). Genetically, some individuals are "rapid acetylators" and convert more procainamide to NAPA than do "slow acetylators." NAPA is 85% eliminated unchanged by the kidneys.
Adult, renal failure (creatinine clearance ≤10 mL/min)	13.9	1.7	Because 50% of procainamide and 85% of NAPA are eliminated unchanged by the kidneys, clearance of both agents is reduced in renal failure.
Adult, liver cirrhosis	N/A	N/A	Procainamide is metabolized ~50% by hepatic enzymes (primarily *N*-acetyltransferase). Clearance of procainamide is decreased in liver cirrhosis patients, but NAPA clearance does not substantially change. Pharmacokinetic parameters are highly variable in liver disease patients.

TABLE 8-1 ***(continued)***

DISEASE STATE/ CONDITION	HALF-LIFE (h)	VOLUME OF DISTRIBUTION (L/kg)	COMMENTS
Adult, uncompensated heart failure	5.5	1.6	Decreased liver blood flow secondary to reduced cardiac output reduces procainamide clearance. Heart failure results in variable reductions in procainamide clearance.
Adult, obese (>30% over ideal body weight)	According to other disease states and conditions that affect procainamide pharmacokinetics	According to other disease states and conditions that affect procainamide pharmacokinetics	Procainamide volume of distribution should be based on ideal body weight (IBW) for patients who weigh >30% over IBW, but clearance should be based on total body weight (TBW) (0.52 L/h/kg TBW for patients with normal renal function).

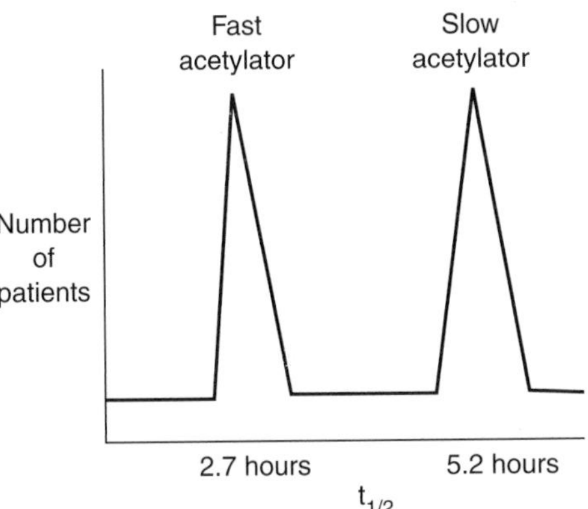

FIGURE 8-4 *N*-acetyltransferase converts procainamide to its active metabolite, *N*-acetyl procainamide (NAPA). Patients can be phenotyped into two groups according to their ability to metabolize procainamide to NAPA via acetylation of the parent drug: in fast acetylators procainamide is converted to NAPA rapidly and has a shorter half-life ($t_{1/2}$), whereas in slow acetylators procainamide is converted to NAPA more slowly and has a longer procainamide half-life. This leads to a bimodal distribution of procainamide half-life for adults with normal renal function.

TABLE 8-2 New York Heart Association (NYHA) Functional Classification for Heart Failure

CLASS	DESCRIPTION
I	Patients with cardiac disease but without limitations of physical activity. Ordinary physical activity does not cause undue fatigue, dyspnea, or palpitation.
II	Patients with cardiac disease that results in slight limitations of physical activity. Ordinary physical activity results in fatigue, palpitation, dyspnea, or angina.
III	Patients with cardiac disease that results in marked limitations of physical activity. Although patients are comfortable at rest, less than ordinary activity leads to symptoms.
IV	Patients with cardiac disease that results in an inability to carry on physical activity without discomfort. Symptoms of congestive heart failure are present even at rest. With any physical activity, increased discomfort is experienced.

From Johnson JA, Parker RB, Geraci SA. Heart failure. In: DiPiro JT, Talbert RL, Yee GC, Matzke GR, Wells BG, Posey LM, eds. Pharmacotherapy—a pathophysiologic approach. Stamford, CT: Appleton & Lange, 1999:153–181.

half-life. For these patients, initial doses are meant as starting points for dosage titration based on patient response and avoidance of adverse effects. Most clinicians reduce initial procainamide doses by 25% to 50% for patients with uncompensated heart failure (Table 8-3). Patients with compensated heart failure receiving appropriate treatment with good clinical response may have normal procainamide pharmacokinetics.[26] Procainamide serum concentrations and the presence of adverse drug effects should be monitored frequently in patients with heart failure.

Procainamide pharmacokinetics have not been adequately studied in patients with liver cirrhosis or hepatitis. However, most *N*-acetyltransferase responsible for the conversion of procainamide to NAPA is thought to reside in the liver. Because of this, most clinicians recommend a decrease in initial doses of procainamide in patients with liver disease.[27] An index of liver dysfunction can be gained by applying the Child-Pugh clinical classification system to the patient[28] (Table 8-4). Child-Pugh scores are completely discussed in Chapter 3 but are briefly discussed here. The Child-Pugh score consists of five laboratory tests or clinical symptoms: serum albumin, total bilirubin, prothrombin time, ascites, and hepatic encephalopathy. Each of these areas is given a score of 1 (normal) to 3 (severely abnormal; see Table 8-4), and the scores for the five areas are totaled. The Child-Pugh score of a patient with normal liver function is 5, whereas the score of a patient with grossly abnormal serum albumin, total bilirubin, and prothrombin time values in addition to severe ascites and hepatic encephalopathy is 15. A Child-Pugh score of 8 to 10 is grounds for a decrease of 25% in the initial daily drug dosage for procainamide, whereas a score of 11 or higher suggests the need for a decrease of 50% (see Table 8-3). As in any patient with or without liver dysfunction, initial doses are meant to be starting points for dosage titration based on patient response and avoidance of adverse effects. Procainamide serum concentrations and the presence of adverse drug effects should be monitored frequently in patients with cirrhosis or hepatitis.

Studies investigating the impact of obesity (>30% over ideal body weight) on procainamide pharmacokinetics have found that volume of distribution correlates best with ideal body weight, but clearance correlates best with total body weight.[29] The volume of

TABLE 8-3 Literature-Based Recommended Oral Procainamide Initial Dosage Ranges for Various Disease States and Conditions

DISEASE STATE/CONDITION	PROCAINAMIDE (ORAL TABLETS)	PROCAINAMIDE (CONTINUOUS INTRAVENOUS INFUSION)
Adult, normal renal function (creatinine clearance >50 mL/min)	50 mg/kg/d	2–6 mg/min
Adult, renal dysfunction	Creatinine clearance 10–50 mL/min: 25%–50% dosage decrease Creatinine clearance <10 mL/min: 50%–75% dosage decrease	Creatinine clearance 10–50 mL/min: 25%–50% dosage decrease Creatinine clearance <10 mL/min: 50%–75% dosage decrease
Adult, uncompensated heart failure	NYHA CHF class II: 25% dosage decrease NYHA CHF class III or IV: 50% dosage decrease	NYHA CHF class II: 25% dosage decrease NYHA CHF class III or IV: 50% dosage decrease
Adult, liver disease	Child-Pugh score 8–10: 25% dosage decrease Child-Pugh score >10: 50% dosage decrease	Child-Pugh score, 8–10: 25% dosage decrease Child-Pugh score >10: 50% dosage decrease
Adult, obese (>30% over ideal body weight)	Base dose on total body weight according to other disease states and conditions	Base dose on total body weight according to other disease states and conditions

CHF = congestive heart failure; NYHA = New York Heart Association.

TABLE 8-4 Child-Pugh Scores for Patients with Liver Disease

TEST/SYMPTOM	SCORE 1 POINT	SCORE 2 POINTS	SCORE 3 POINTS
Total bilirubin (mg/dL)	<2.0	2.0–3.0	>3.0
Serum albumin (g/dL)	>3.5	2.8–3.5	<2.8
Prothrombin time (seconds prolonged over control)	<4	4–6	>6
Ascites	Absent	Slight	Moderate
Hepatic encephalopathy	None	Moderate	Severe

From Pugh RN, Murray-Lyon IM, Dawson JL, Pietroni MC, Williams R. Transection of the oesophagus for bleeding oesophageal varices. Br J Surg 1973;60:646–649.

distribution for procainamide should be based on ideal body weight for obese persons according to the other disease states and conditions of the patient. Clearance should be based on total body weight (TBW) in obese patients (0.52 L/h per kg TBW for normal renal function).

Procainamide is significantly removed by hemodialysis but not by peritoneal dialysis.[30] Patients undergoing hemodialysis treatments may receive an additional dose of the usual amount of procainamide after the procedure is finished.

NAPA is primarily eliminated unchanged in the urine via glomerular filtration and renal tubular secretion.[13,14,20,25,31] When NAPA is given orally, 85% of the administered dose is recovered in the urine as unchanged drug. In patients with normal renal and liver function, NAPA has an average half-life of 6 hours.[10] NAPA half-life increases to 41 hours on average in patients with renal failure.[25,31] The volume of distribution of NAPA in healthy persons is 1.4 L/kg. NAPA is significantly removed by hemodialysis but not by peritoneal dialysis.[31] In most patients with renal dysfunction, the ratio of NAPA to procainamide steady-state concentration exceeds 1, even if the patient is a slow acetylator. This is because NAPA elimination is much more dependent on renal function, so NAPA concentrations accumulate more than procainamide concentrations do in patients with renal dysfunction. Thus, in patients with renal failure, NAPA may be the predominant antiarrhythmic agent in the serum.

DRUG INTERACTIONS

Procainamide has serious drug interactions with other drugs that are capable of inhibiting its renal tubular secretion.[32,33] Cimetidine, trimethoprim, and ofloxacin all compete for tubular secretion with procainamide and NAPA. When given with these other agents, procainamide renal clearance decreases by 30% to 50%, and NAPA renal clearance decreases by 10% to 30%. Amiodarone increases the steady-state concentrations of procainamide and NAPA by 57% and 32%, respectively.

INITIAL DOSAGE DETERMINATION METHODS

Pharmacokinetic Dosing Method

The goal of initial dosing of procainamide is to compute the best possible dose for the patient given the patient's disease states and conditions that influence procainamide pharmacokinetics and the arrhythmia being treated. To do this, pharmacokinetic parameters are estimated by means of average parameters measured in other patients with similar disease states and condition profiles.

ESTIMATE OF HALF-LIFE AND ELIMINATION RATE CONSTANT

Depending on the acetylator status of the patient, procainamide is metabolized by the liver and eliminated unchanged by the kidney almost equally in patients with normal hepatic and renal function. Unfortunately, there is no good way to estimate the elimination characteristics of liver-metabolized drugs using an endogenous marker of liver function in the same manner that serum creatinine and estimated creatinine clearance are used to estimate the elimination of agents that are renally eliminated by glomerular filtration. In addition, creatinine clearance does not accurately reflect the renal elimination of procainamide, because the mechanism of elimination includes active tubular secretion. Because of this, a patient is categorized according to the disease states and conditions that are known to change procainamide half-life, and the half-life previously measured in these studies is used as an estimate of the patient's half-life (see Table 8-1). For a patient with moderate to severe heart failure (New York Heart Association [NYHA] heart failure classes II to IV), procainamide half-life is assumed to be 5.5 hours, whereas a patient with renal failure is assigned an estimated half-life of 13.9 hours. To produce the most conservative procainamide doses in patients with multiple concurrent disease states or conditions that affect procainamide pharmacokinetics, the disease state or condition with the longest half-life should be used to compute doses. This approach prevents accidental overdosage as much as is currently possible. After the correct half-life is identified for the patient, it can be converted into the procainamide elimination rate constant (k) using the following equation: $k = 0.693/t_{1/2}$.

ESTIMATE OF VOLUME OF DISTRIBUTION

As with the half-life estimate, the procainamide volume of distribution is chosen according to the disease states and conditions that are present (see Table 8-1). The volume of distribution is used to help compute procainamide clearance and is assumed to be 1.7 L/kg for patients with renal failure, 1.6 L/kg for patients with uncompensated heart failure, and 2.7 L/kg for all other patients. For obese patients (>30% above ideal body weight), ideal body weight is used to compute procainamide volume of distribution. Thus, for a nonobese 80-kg patient without heart failure or liver disease, the estimated procainamide volume of distribution is 216 L: $V = 2.7\ L/kg \cdot 80\ kg = 216\ L$. For a 150-kg obese patient with an ideal body weight of 60 kg and normal cardiac and liver function, the estimated procainamide volume of distribution is 162 L: $V = 2.7\ L/kg \cdot 60\ kg = 162\ L$.

SELECTION OF APPROPRIATE PHARMACOKINETIC MODEL AND EQUATIONS

When given orally, procainamide follows a one-compartment pharmacokinetic model (see Figure 8-3). Because procainamide has such a short half-life, most patients receive oral procainamide therapy using sustained-release dosage forms. Procainamide sustained-release dosage forms provide good bioavailability (F = 0.83), supply a continuous release of procainamide into the gastrointestinal tract, and provide a smooth procainamide serum concentration–time curve that emulates an intravenous infusion when doses are given two to four times daily. In the United States, two sustained-release dosage forms have been approved that provide every-6-hour or every-12-hour dosing. Because of this, a very simple pharmacokinetic equation that computes the average procainamide steady-state serum concentration (Css in μg/mL = mg/L) is widely used and allows maintenance dosage calculation: $Css = [F(D/\tau)]/Cl$ or $D = (Css \cdot Cl \cdot \tau)/F$, where F is the bioavailability fraction of the oral dosage form (F = 0.83 for most oral procainamide sustained-release products), D is the dose of procainamide in mg, and τ is the dosage interval in hours. Cl is procainamide clearance in liters per hour (L/h) and is computed using estimates of procainamide elimination rate constant (k) and volume of distribution: Cl = kV. For example, for a patient with an estimated elimination rate constant of $0.210\ h^{-1}$ and an estimated volume of distribution of 189 L, the estimated clearance is 39.7 L/h: $Cl = 0.210\ h^{-1} \cdot 189\ L = 39.7\ L/h$.

When intravenous therapy is required, a similar pharmacokinetic equation that computes the procainamide steady-state serum concentration (Css in μg/mL = mg/L) is widely used and allows dosage calculation for a continuous infusion: Css = k_0/Cl or k_0 = Css · Cl, where k_0 is the dose of procainamide in mg/min, and Cl is procainamide clearance in L/min and is computed using estimates of procainamide elimination rate constant (k) and volume of distribution: Cl = kV.

The equation used to calculate an intravenous loading dose (LD in mg) is based on a simple one-compartment model: LD = Css · V, where Css is the desired procainamide steady-state concentration in μg/mL, which is equivalent to mg/L, and V is the procainamide volume of distribution. Intravenous procainamide loading doses should be infused no faster than 25 to 50 mg/min to prevent severe hypotension. Two methods are used to administer procainamide loading doses. One method administers 100 mg every 5 minutes to a maximum of 500 mg; a 10-minute waiting period to allow drug distribution to tissues is used if more than 500 mg is needed to abate the arrhythmia. The other method administers the loading dose as a short-term infusion at a rate of 20 mg/min over 25 to 30 minutes, not to exceed a total dose of 500 to 600 mg. Current advanced cardiac life-support guidelines recommend that loading doses do not exceed 17 mg/kg of procainamide.

SELECTION OF STEADY-STATE CONCENTRATION

The generally accepted therapeutic range for procainamide is 4 to 10 μg/mL. If procainamide + NAPA ("total procainamide") concentrations are used, the typical therapeutic range is 10 to 30 μg/mL; note that procainamide and NAPA are not equipotent antiarrhythmics. However, procainamide therapy must be individualized for each patient to achieve optimal responses and minimal side effects.

Example 1 LK is a 50-year-old, 75-kg, 178-cm (70-in) man with ventricular tachycardia who receives therapy with oral procainamide sustained-release tablets. He has normal liver and cardiac function. Suggest an initial oral procainamide dosage regimen designed to achieve a steady-state procainamide concentration of 4 μg/mL.

1. *Estimate the half-life and elimination rate constant according to the disease states and conditions of the patient.*

The expected procainamide half-life ($t_{1/2}$) in an individual with normal hepatic and renal function is 3.3 hours. The elimination rate constant is computed according to the following formula: k = 0.693/$t_{1/2}$ = 0.693/3.3 h = 0.210 h^{-1}.

2. *Estimate the volume of distribution and clearance.*

The patient is not obese, so the estimated procainamide volume of distribution is based on actual body weight: V = 2.7 L/kg · 75 kg = 203 L. Estimated procainamide clearance is computed by taking the product of the volume of distribution and the elimination rate constant: Cl = kV = 0.210 h^{-1} · 203 L = 42.6 L/h.

3. *Compute the dosage regimen.*

Oral sustained-release procainamide tablets are prescribed for this patient (F = 0.83). Because procainamide has a rapid clearance and short half-life in this patient, the initial dosage interval (τ) is set to 6 hours. (Note: μg/mL = mg/L, and this concentration unit was substituted for Css in the calculations to avoid unnecessary unit conversion.) The dosage equation for oral procainamide is D = (Css · Cl · τ)/F = (4 mg/L · 42.6 L/h · 6 h)/0.83 = 1231 mg, rounded to 1250 mg every 6 hours.

Steady-state procainamide and NAPA serum concentrations can be measured after steady state is attained in 3 to 5 half-lives. Because procainamide is expected to have a half-life of 3.3 hours and NAPA a half-life of 6 hours in the patient, the steady-state concentrations can be obtained any time after the first day of dosing (5 half-lives = 5 · 3.3 h = 16.5 h for procainamide; 5 half-lives = 5 · 6 h = 30 h for NAPA). Procainamide and NAPA serum concentrations also should be measured if the patient experiences a return of arrhythmia or develops potential signs or symptoms of procainamide toxicity.

Example 2 OI is a 60-year-old, 85-kg, 185-cm (73-in) man with atrial fibrillation who requires therapy with oral procainamide. He has renal failure and an estimated creatinine clearance = 9 mL/min. Suggest an initial extended-release procainamide dosage regimen designed to achieve a steady-state procainamide concentration of 4 μg/mL.

1. *Estimate the half-life and elimination rate constant according to the disease states and conditions of the patient.*

Patients with severe renal disease have highly variable procainamide pharmacokinetics and dosage requirements. Renal failure decreases procainamide renal clearance, and the expected procainamide half-life ($t_{1/2}$) is 13.9 hours. The elimination rate constant is computed using the following formula: $k = 0.693/t_{1/2} = 0.693/13.9\ h = 0.050\ h^{-1}$.

2. *Estimate the volume of distribution and clearance.*

The patient is not obese, so the estimated procainamide volume of distribution is based on actual body weight: V = 1.7 L/kg · 85 kg = 145 L. Estimated procainamide clearance is computed by taking the product of the volume of distribution and the elimination rate constant: $Cl = kV = 0.050\ h^{-1} \cdot 145\ L = 7.25\ L/h$.

3. *Compute the dosage regimen.*

Oral sustained-release procainamide tablets are prescribed to this patient (F = 0.83). The initial dosage interval (τ) is set to 12 hours. (Note: μg/mL = mg/L, and this concentration unit was substituted for Css in the calculations to avoid unnecessary unit conversion.) The dosage equation for oral procainamide is D = (Css · Cl · τ)/F = (4 mg/L · 7.25 L/h · 12 h)/0.83 = 419 mg, rounded to 500 mg every 12 hours.

Steady-state procainamide and NAPA serum concentrations can be measured after steady state is attained in 3 to 5 half-lives. Because procainamide is expected to have a half-life of 13.9 hours and NAPA a half-life of 41 hours in the patient, the steady-state concentrations can be obtained any time after 3 to 9 days of dosing (5 half-lives = 5 · 13.9 h = 69.5 h for procainamide; 5 half-lives = 5 · 41 h = 205 h for NAPA). Procainamide and NAPA serum concentrations should also be measured if the patient experiences a return of arrhythmia or develops potential signs or symptoms of procainamide toxicity.

To illustrate the differences and similarities between oral and intravenous procainamide dosage regimen design, the same cases are used to compute intravenous procainamide loading doses and continuous infusions.

Example 1 LK is a 50-year-old, 75-kg, 178-cm (70-in) male with ventricular tachycardia who requires therapy with intravenous procainamide. He has normal liver and cardiac function. Suggest an intravenous procainamide dosage regimen designed to achieve a steady-state procainamide concentration of 4 μg/mL.

1. *Estimate the half-life and elimination rate constant according to the disease states and conditions of the patient.*

The expected procainamide half-life ($t_{1/2}$) in an individual with normal hepatic and renal function is 3.3 hours. The elimination rate constant is computed using the following formula: $k = 0.693/t_{1/2} = 0.693/3.3\ h = 0.210\ h^{-1}$.

2. *Estimate the volume of distribution and clearance.*

The patient is not obese, so the estimated procainamide volume of distribution is based on actual body weight: V = 2.7 L/kg · 75 kg = 203 L. Estimated procainamide clearance is computed by taking the product of the volume of distribution and the elimination rate constant: $Cl = kV = 0.210\ h^{-1} \cdot 203\ L = 42.6\ L/h$.

3. *Compute the dosage regimen.*

Therapy is started by administering an intravenous loading dose of procainamide to the patient: LD = Css · V = 4 mg/L · 203 L = 812 mg, rounded to 800 mg intravenously. Initially, a maximum dose of 600 mg over 25 to 30 minutes is given, and the additional 200 mg is given, if needed, at 20 mg/min. (Note: μg/mL = mg/L, and this concentration unit was substituted for Css in the calculations to avoid unnecessary unit conversion.)

A procainamide continuous intravenous infusion is started immediately after the loading dose has been administered. The dosage equation for intravenous procainamide is k_0 = Css · Cl = (4 mg/L · 42.6 L/h)/(60 min/h) = 2.8 mg/min, rounded to 3 mg/min.

Steady-state procainamide and NAPA serum concentrations can be measured after steady state is attained in 3 to 5 half-lives. Because procainamide is expected to have a half-life of 3.3 hours and NAPA a half-life of 6 hours in the patient, the steady-state concentrations can be obtained any time after the first day of dosing (5 half-lives = 5 · 3.3 h = 16.5 h for procainamide; 5 half-lives = 5 · 6 h = 30 h for NAPA). Procainamide and NAPA serum concentrations also should be measured if the patient experiences a return of arrhythmia or develops potential signs or symptoms of procainamide toxicity.

Example 2 OI is a 60-year-old, 85-kg, 185-cm (73-in) male with atrial fibrillation who requires therapy with intravenous procainamide. He has renal failure with an estimated creatinine clearance of 9 mL/min. Suggest an initial intravenous procainamide dosage regimen designed to achieve a steady-state procainamide concentration of 4 μg/mL.

1. *Estimate the half-life and elimination rate constant according to the disease states and conditions of the patient.*

Patients with severe renal disease have highly variable procainamide pharmacokinetics and dosage requirements. Renal failure decreases procainamide renal clearance, and the expected procainamide half-life ($t_{1/2}$) is 13.9 hours. The elimination rate constant is computed using the following formula: $k = 0.693/t_{1/2} = 0.693/13.9\ h = 0.050\ h^{-1}$.

2. *Estimate the volume of distribution and clearance.*

The patient is not obese, so the estimated procainamide volume of distribution is based on actual body weight: V = 1.7 L/kg · 85 kg = 145 L. Estimated procainamide clearance is computed by taking the product of the volume of distribution and the elimination rate constant: Cl = kV = 0.050 h^{-1} · 145 L = 7.25 L/h.

3. *Compute the dosage regimen.*

Therapy is started by administering an intravenous loading dose of procainamide: LD = Css · V = 4 mg/L · 145 L = 580 mg, rounded to 600 mg intravenously over 25 to 30 minutes. (Note: μg/mL = mg/L, and this concentration unit was substituted for Css in the calculations to avoid unnecessary unit conversion.)

A procainamide continuous intravenous infusion is started immediately after the loading dose has been administered. The dosage equation for intravenous procainamide is k_0 = Css · Cl = (4 mg/L · 7.25 L/h)/(60 min/h) = 0.48 mg/min, rounded to 0.5 mg/min.

Steady-state procainamide and NAPA serum concentrations can be measured after steady state is attained in 3 to 5 half-lives. Because procainamide is expected to have a half-life of 13.9 hours and NAPA a half-life of 41 hours in the patient, the steady-state concentrations can be obtained any time after 3 to 9 days of dosing (5 half-lives = 5 · 13.9 h = 69.5 h for procainamide; 5 half-lives = 5 · 41 h = 205 h for NAPA). Procainamide and NAPA serum concentrations also should be measured if the patient experiences a return of arrhythmia or develops potential signs or symptoms of procainamide toxicity.

Literature-Based Recommended Dosing

Because of the wide variability in procainamide pharmacokinetics, even when concurrent disease states and conditions are identified, many clinicians believe that standard procainamide doses for various situations are warranted. The original computation of these doses was based on the pharmacokinetic dosing method described in the previous section, which was subsequently modified based on clinical experience. In general, the procainamide steady-state serum concentration expected from the lower end of the dosage range was 4 to 6 μg/mL and 6 to 10 μg/mL for the upper end of the dosage range. Suggested procainamide maintenance doses are given in Table 8-3. A 25% to 50% reduction in initial procainamide dose is suggested for patients with moderate to severe liver disease (Child-Pugh score, ≥8) or moderate to severe heart failure (NYHA class II or greater). A 25% to 75% decrease is indicated with renal dysfunction. When more than one disease state or condition is present in a patient, choice of the lowest daily dose results in the safest, most conservative dosage recommendation.

To illustrate the similarities and differences between the literature-based method and the pharmacokinetic dosing method of dosage calculation, the same examples used in the previous section are used here.

Example 1 LK is a 50-year-old, 75-kg, 178-cm (70-in) man with ventricular tachycardia who requires therapy with oral procainamide sustained-release tablets. He has normal liver and cardiac function. Suggest an initial oral procainamide dosage regimen designed to achieve a steady-state procainamide concentration of 4 μg/mL.

1. *Choose a procainamide dose based on the disease states and conditions of the patient.*

A procainamide maintenance dose of 50 mg/kg per day is suggested for a patient with no heart failure or liver disease who requires a procainamide steady-state serum concentration in the lower end of the therapeutic range. The suggested initial dose is 3750 mg/d (50 mg/kg/d · 75 kg = 3750 mg/d), rounded to 4000 mg/d or 1000 mg every 6 hours.

Steady-state procainamide and NAPA serum concentrations can be measured after steady state is attained in 3 to 5 half-lives. Because procainamide is expected to have a half-life of 3.3 hours and NAPA a half-life of 6 hours in the patient, the steady-state concentrations can be obtained any time after the first day of dosing (5 half-lives = 5 · 3.3 h = 16.5 h for procainamide; 5 half-lives = 5 · 6 h = 30 h for NAPA). Procainamide and NAPA serum concentrations also should be measured if the patient experiences a return of arrhythmia or develops potential signs or symptoms of procainamide toxicity.

Example 2 OI is a 60-year-old, 85-kg, 185-cm (73-in) man with atrial fibrillation who requires therapy with oral procainamide. He has renal failure with an estimated creatinine clearance of 9 mL/min. Suggest an initial extended-release procainamide dosage regimen designed to achieve a steady-state procainamide concentration of 4 μg/mL.

1. *Choose a procainamide dose based on the disease states and conditions of the patient.*

A procainamide maintenance dose of 12.5 mg/kg per day (50 mg/kg/d · 0.25 = 12.5 mg/kg/d) is suggested for a patient with renal failure who requires a procainamide steady-state serum concentration in the lower end of the therapeutic range. The suggested initial dose is 1063 mg/d (12.5 mg/kg/d · 85 kg = 1063 mg/d), rounded to 1000 mg/d or 500 mg every 12 hours.

Steady-state procainamide and NAPA serum concentrations can be measured after steady state is attained in 3 to 5 half-lives. Because procainamide is expected to have a half-life of 13.9 hours and NAPA a half-life of 41 hours in the patient, the steady-state concentrations can be obtained any time after 3 to 9 days of dosing (5 half-lives = 5 · 13.9 h = 69.5 h for procainamide; 5 half-lives = 5 · 41 h = 205 h for NAPA). Procainamide and NAPA serum concentrations also should be measured if the patient experiences a return of arrhythmia or develops potential signs or symptoms of procainamide toxicity.

To illustrate the differences and similarities between oral and intravenous procainamide dosage regimen design, the same cases are used here to compute intravenous procainamide loading doses and continuous infusions.

Example 1 LK is a 50-year-old, 75-kg, 178-cm (70-in) male with ventricular tachycardia who requires therapy with intravenous procainamide. He has normal liver and cardiac function. Suggest an intravenous procainamide dosage regimen designed to achieve a steady-state procainamide concentration of 4 μg/mL.

1. *Choose a procainamide dose based on the disease states and conditions of the patient.*

A procainamide maintenance dose of 2 to 4 mg/min is suggested for a patient with no heart failure or liver disease who requires a procainamide steady-state serum concentration in the lower end of the therapeutic range. The suggested initial continuous infusion is 3 mg/min. If needed, a loading dose of 500 mg infused over 25 to 30 minutes can also be given.

Steady-state procainamide and NAPA serum concentrations can be measured after steady state is attained in 3 to 5 half-lives. Because procainamide is expected to have a half-life of 3.3 hours and NAPA a half-life of 6 hours in the patient, the steady-state concentrations can be obtained any time after the first day of dosing (5 half-lives = 5 · 3.3 h = 16.5 h for procainamide; 5 half-lives = 5 · 6 h = 30 h for NAPA). Procainamide and NAPA serum concentrations also should be measured if the patient experiences a return of arrhythmia or develops potential signs or symptoms of procainamide toxicity.

Example 2 OI is a 60-year-old, 85-kg, 185-cm (73-in) male with atrial fibrillation who requires therapy with intravenous procainamide. He has renal failure with an estimated creatinine clearance of 9 mL/min. Suggest an initial intravenous procainamide dosage regimen designed to achieve a steady-state procainamide concentration of 4 μg/mL.

1. *Choose a procainamide dose based on the disease states and conditions of the patient.*

A procainamide maintenance dose of 1 to 2 mg/min is suggested for a patient with renal failure requiring a procainamide steady-state serum concentration in the lower end of the therapeutic range. The suggested initial dose is 1 mg/min. If needed, a loading dose of 500 mg infused over 25 to 30 minutes can also be given.

Steady-state procainamide and NAPA serum concentrations can be measured after steady state is attained in 3 to 5 half-lives. Because procainamide is expected to have a half-life of 13.9 hours and NAPA a half-life of 41 hours in the patient, the steady-state concentrations can be obtained any time after 3 to 9 days of dosing (5 half-lives = 5 · 13.9 h = 69.5 h for procainamide; 5 half-lives = 5 · 41 h = 205 h for NAPA). Procainamide and NAPA serum concentrations also should be measured if the patient experiences a return of arrhythmia or develops potential signs or symptoms of procainamide toxicity.

USE OF PROCAINAMIDE AND *N*-ACETYL PROCAINAMIDE SERUM CONCENTRATIONS TO ALTER DOSES

Because of the large amount of pharmacokinetic variability among patients, it is likely that doses computed using patient population characteristics will not always produce procainamide or NAPA serum concentrations that are expected or desirable. Because of pharmacokinetic variability, the narrow therapeutic index of procainamide, and the desire to prevent procainamide adverse side effects, measurement of procainamide and NAPA serum concentrations in patients can be a useful adjunct to ensure that therapeutic, nontoxic levels are present. In addition to procainamide serum concentrations, important patient parameters (e.g., ECG, clinical signs and symptoms of the arrhythmia, potential procainamide side effects) should be monitored to confirm that the patient is responding to treatment and not developing adverse drug reactions.

When procainamide and NAPA serum concentrations are measured and a dosage change is necessary, clinicians should seek the simplest, most straightforward method available to determine a dose that will provide safe and effective treatment. In most cases, a simple dosage ratio can be used to change procainamide doses, assuming the drug follows *linear pharmacokinetics.* Thus, assuming linear pharmacokinetics is adequate for dosage adjustments in most patients.

Sometimes it is useful to compute procainamide pharmacokinetic constants for a patient and base dosage adjustments on these parameters. In this case, it may be possible to calculate and use *pharmacokinetic parameters* to alter the procainamide dose. In some situations, it may be necessary to compute procainamide pharmacokinetic parameters as soon as possible before steady-state conditions occur and to use these parameters to calculate the best drug dose. Computerized methods that incorporate expected population pharmacokinetic characteristics (*Bayesian pharmacokinetics computer programs*) can be used in difficult cases in which the patient's serum concentrations are obtained at suboptimal times or in which the patient was not at steady state when serum concentrations were measured.

Linear Pharmacokinetics Method

Because procainamide follows linear, dose-proportional pharmacokinetics in most patients, steady-state procainamide and NAPA serum concentrations change in proportion to dose according to the following equation: $D_{new}/Css_{new} = D_{old}/Css_{old}$ or $D_{new} = (Css_{new}/Css_{old})D_{old}$, where D is the dose, Css is the steady-state concentration, old indicates the dose that produced the steady-state concentration that the patient is receiving, and new denotes the dose necessary to produce the desired steady-state concentration. The advantage of this method is that it is quick and simple. The disadvantage is that steady-state concentrations are required. Because nonlinear pharmacokinetics for procainamide has been observed in some patients, suggested dosage increases greater than 75% using this method should be scrutinized by the prescribing clinician and the risk-benefit for the patient assessed before initiating large dosage increases (>75% over current dose).

Example 1 LK is a 50-year-old, 75-kg, 178-cm (70-in) male with ventricular tachycardia who requires therapy with procainamide sustained-release tablets. He has normal liver and cardiac function. His steady-state procainamide and NAPA concentrations are 2.2 μg/mL and 1.5 μg/mL, respectively (total procainamide concentration = 3.7 μg/mL), at 1000 mg every 12 hours. Compute a procainamide dosage that will provide a steady-state concentration of 4 μg/mL.

1. *Compute a new dose to achieve the desired serum concentration.*

The patient is expected to achieve steady-state conditions after the first day (5 half-lives = 5 · 3.3 h = 17 h for procainamide; 5 half-lives = 5 · 6 h = 30 h for NAPA) of therapy.

Using linear pharmacokinetics, the new dose to attain the desired concentration should be proportional to the old dose that produced the measured concentration. (Note: Total daily dose = 1000 mg/dose · 2 doses/d = 2000 mg/d.)

$$D_{new} = (Css_{new}/Css_{old})D_{old} = [(4\ \mu g/mL)/(2.2\ \mu g/mL)]\ 2000\ mg/d$$
$$= 3636\ mg/d, \text{ rounded to } 4000\ mg/d \text{ or } 2000\ mg \text{ every } 12 \text{ hours}$$

The new suggested dosage is 2000 mg of oral procainamide every 12 hours to be started immediately.

The expected NAPA steady-state serum concentration increases in proportion to the procainamide dosage increase:

$$Css_{new} = (D_{new}/D_{old})Css_{old} = [(4000 \text{ mg/d})/(2000 \text{ mg/d})]\ 1.5\ \mu\text{g/mL} = 3\ \mu\text{g/mL}$$

A steady-state procainamide serum concentration can be measured after steady state is attained in 3 to 5 half-lives. Because procainamide is expected to have a half-life of 3.3 hours and NAPA a half-life of 6 hours in the patient, procainamide and NAPA steady-state concentrations can be obtained any time after the first day of dosing (5 half-lives = 5 · 3.3 h = 17 h for procainamide; 5 half-lives = 5 · 6 h = 30 h for NAPA). Procainamide and NAPA serum concentrations should also be measured if the patient experiences a return of arrhythmia or develops potential signs or symptoms of procainamide toxicity.

Example 2 OI is a 60-year-old, 85-kg, 185-cm (73-in) male with atrial fibrillation who requires therapy with oral procainamide sustained-release tablets. He has renal failure with an estimated creatinine clearance of 9 mL/min. His steady-state procainamide and NAPA concentrations are 13.1 μg/mL and 25.2 μg/mL, respectively (total procainamide concentration = 38.3 μg/mL), at 1000 mg every 12 hours. Compute a procainamide dose that will provide a steady-state concentration of 6 μg/mL.

1. *Compute a new dose to achieve the desired serum concentration.*

The patient is expected to achieve steady-state conditions after the ninth day (5 half-lives = 5 · 13.9 h = 70 h, or 3 days for procainamide; 5 half-lives = 5 · 41 h = 205 h, or 9 days for NAPA) of therapy.

With the use of linear pharmacokinetics, the new dose to attain the desired concentration should be proportional to the old dose that produced the measured concentration. (Note: Total daily dose = 1000 mg/dose · 2 doses/d = 2000 mg/d.)

$$D_{new} = (Css_{new}/Css_{old})D_{old} = [(6\ \mu\text{g/mL})/(13.1\ \mu\text{g/mL})]\ 2000 \text{ mg/d}$$
$$= 916 \text{ mg/d, rounded to 1000 mg/d or 500 mg every 12 hours}$$

The new suggested dosage is 500 mg of oral procainamide every 12 hours to be started immediately.

The expected NAPA steady-state serum concentration decreases in proportion to the procainamide dosage increase:

$$Css_{new} = (D_{new}/D_{old})Css_{old} = [(1000 \text{ mg/d})/(2000 \text{ mg/d})]\ 25.2\ \mu\text{g/mL} = 12.6\ \mu\text{g/mL}$$

A steady-state procainamide serum concentration can be measured after steady state is attained in 3 to 5 half-lives. Because procainamide is expected to have a half-life of 13.9 hours and NAPA a half-life of 41 hours in the patient, procainamide and NAPA steady-state concentrations can be obtained any time after the ninth day of dosing (5 half-lives = 5 · 13.9 h = 70 h for procainamide; 5 half-lives = 5 · 41 h = 205 h for NAPA). Procainamide and NAPA serum concentrations also should be measured if the patient experiences a return of arrhythmia or develops potential signs or symptoms of procainamide toxicity.

Example 3 MN is a 64-year-old, 78-kg, 175-cm (69-in) man with ventricular tachycardia who requires therapy with intravenous procainamide. He has moderate heart failure (NYHA CHF class III). His steady-state procainamide and NAPA concentrations are 4.5 μg/mL and 7.9 μg/mL, respectively (total procainamide concentration = 12.4 μg/mL), at 1 mg/min. Compute a procainamide dose that will provide a steady-state concentration of 8 μg/mL.

1. *Compute a new dose to achieve the desired serum concentration.*

The patient is expected to achieve steady-state conditions after the second day (5 half-lives = 5 · 5.5 h = 28 h for procainamide; 5 half-lives = 5 · 6 h = 30 h for NAPA, assuming normal renal function) of therapy.

With the use of linear pharmacokinetics, the new dose to attain the desired concentration should be proportional to the old dose that produced the measured concentration:

$$D_{new} = (Css_{new}/Css_{old})D_{old} = [(8\ \mu g/mL)/(4.5\ \mu g/mL)]\ 1\ mg/min$$
$$= 1.8\ mg/min,\ \text{rounded to}\ 2\ mg/min$$

The new suggested dose is 2 mg/min of intravenous procainamide to be started immediately.

The expected NAPA steady-state serum concentration increases in proportion to the procainamide dosage increase:

$$Css_{new} = (D_{new}/D_{old})Css_{old} = [(2\ mg/min)/(1\ mg/min)]\ 7.9\ \mu g/mL = 15.8\ \mu g/mL$$

A steady-state procainamide serum concentration can be measured after steady state is attained in 3 to 5 half-lives. Because procainamide is expected to have a half-life of 5.5 hours and NAPA a half-life of 6 hours in the patient, procainamide and NAPA steady-state concentrations can be obtained any time after the second day of dosing (5 half-lives = 5 · 5.5 h = 28 h for procainamide; 5 half-lives = 5 · 6 h = 30 h for NAPA). Procainamide and NAPA serum concentrations also should be measured if the patient experiences a return of arrhythmia or develops potential signs or symptoms of procainamide toxicity.

Pharmacokinetic Parameter Method

The pharmacokinetic parameter method of adjusting drug doses was among the first techniques available to change doses using serum concentrations. It allows the computation of an individual's unique pharmacokinetic constants and uses these to calculate a dose that achieves the desired procainamide concentrations. The pharmacokinetic parameter method requires that steady state has been achieved and uses only a steady-state procainamide concentration (Css). During a continuous intravenous infusion, the following equation is used to compute procainamide clearance (Cl): $Cl = k_0/Css$, where k_0 is the dose of procainamide in mg/min. If the patient is receiving oral procainamide therapy, procainamide clearance (Cl) can be calculated using the following formula: $Cl = [F(D/\tau)]/Css$, where F is the bioavailability fraction for the oral dosage form (F = 0.83 for most oral procainamide products), D is the dose of procainamide in mg, Css is the steady-state procainamide concentration, and τ is the dosage interval in hours. For both oral and intravenous procainamide routes of administration, the expected NAPA steady-state serum concentration increases in proportion to the procainamide dosage increase: $Css_{new} = (D_{new}/D_{old})Css_{old}$, where D is the dose, Css is the steady-state concentration, old is the dose that produced the steady-state concentration that the patient is currently receiving, and new is the dose necessary to produce the desired steady-state concentration. Because this method also assumes linear pharmacokinetics, procainamide doses computed using the pharmacokinetic parameter method and the linear pharmacokinetic method should be identical.

Example 1 LK is a 50-year-old, 75-kg, 178-cm (70-in) male with ventricular tachycardia who requires therapy with procainamide sustained-release tablets. He has normal liver and cardiac function. His steady-state procainamide and NAPA concentrations are 2.2 μg/mL and 1.5 μg/mL, respectively (total procainamide concentration = 3.7 μg/mL), at 1000 mg every 12 hours. Compute a procainamide dose that will provide a steady-state concentration of 4 μg/mL.

1. *Compute the pharmacokinetic parameters.*

The patient is expected to achieve steady-state conditions after the first day (5 half-lives = 5 · 3.3 h = 17 h for procainamide; 5 half-lives = 5 · 6 h = 30 h for NAPA) of therapy.

Procainamide clearance can be computed using a steady-state procainamide concentration: $Cl = [F(D/\tau)]/Css = [0.83\ (1000\ mg/12\ h)]/(2.2\ mg/L) = 31.4\ L/h$. (Note: μg/mL = mg/L, and this concentration unit was substituted for Css in the calculations to avoid unnecessary unit conversion.)

2. *Compute the procainamide dose.*

Procainamide clearance is used to compute the new dose: $D = (Css \cdot Cl \cdot \tau)/F = (4\ mg/L \cdot 31.4\ L/h \cdot 12\ h)/0.83 = 1816\ mg$, rounded to 2000 mg every 12 hours.

The expected NAPA steady-state serum concentration increases in proportion to the procainamide dosage increase:

$$Css_{new} = (D_{new}/D_{old})Css_{old} = [(4000\ mg/d)/(2000\ mg/d)]\ 1.5\ \mu g/mL = 3\ \mu g/mL$$

The new procainamide dose should be instituted immediately.

A steady-state procainamide serum concentration can be measured after steady state is attained in 3 to 5 half-lives. Because procainamide is expected to have a half-life of 3.3 hours and NAPA a half-life of 6 hours in the patient, procainamide and NAPA steady-state concentrations can be obtained any time after the first day of dosing (5 half-lives = 5 · 3.3 h = 17 h for procainamide; 5 half-lives = 5 · 6 h = 30 h for NAPA). Procainamide and NAPA serum concentrations also should be measured if the patient experiences a return of arrhythmia or develops potential signs or symptoms of procainamide toxicity.

Example 2 OI is a 60-year-old, 85-kg, 185-cm (73-in) male with atrial fibrillation who requires therapy with oral procainamide sustained-release tablets. He has renal failure with an estimated creatinine clearance of 9 mL/min. His steady-state procainamide and NAPA concentrations are 13.1 μg/mL and 25.2 μg/mL, respectively (total procainamide concentration = 38.3 μg/mL), at 1000 mg every 12 hours. Compute a procainamide dose that will provide a steady-state concentration of 6 μg/mL.

1. *Compute the pharmacokinetic parameters.*

The patient is expected to achieve steady-state conditions after the ninth day (5 half-lives = 5 · 13.9 h = 70 h, or 3 days for procainamide; 5 half-lives = 5 · 41 h = 205 h, or 9 days for NAPA) of therapy.

Procainamide clearance can be computed using a steady-state procainamide concentration: $Cl = [F(D/\tau)]/Css = [0.83\ (1000\ mg/12\ h)]/(13.1\ mg/L) = 5.28\ L/h$. (Note: μg/mL = mg/L, and this concentration unit was substituted for Css in the calculations to avoid unnecessary unit conversion.)

2. *Compute the procainamide dose.*

Procainamide clearance is used to compute the new dose: $D = (Css \cdot Cl \cdot \tau)/F = (6\ mg/L \cdot 5.28\ L/h \cdot 12\ h)/0.83 = 458\ mg$, rounded to 500 mg every 12 hours.

The expected NAPA steady-state serum concentration changes in proportion to the procainamide dosage change:

$$Css_{new} = (D_{new}/D_{old})Css_{old} = [(1000\ mg/d)/(2000\ mg/d)]\ 25.2\ \mu g/mL = 12.6\ \mu g/mL$$

If the patient is experiencing side effects, the new dosage regimen can be held for 1 estimated half-life. Otherwise, the new procainamide dose is instituted immediately.

A steady-state procainamide serum concentration can be measured after steady state is attained in 3 to 5 half-lives. Because procainamide is expected to have a half-life of 13.9 hours and NAPA a half-life of 41 hours in the patient, procainamide and NAPA steady-state concentrations can be obtained any time after the ninth day of dosing (5 half-lives = 5 · 13.9 h = 70 h for procainamide; 5 half-lives = 5 · 41 h = 205 h for NAPA). Procainamide and NAPA serum concentrations also should be measured if the patient experiences a return of arrhythmia or develops potential signs or symptoms of procainamide toxicity.

Example 3 MN is a 64-year-old, 78-kg, 175-cm (69-in) male with ventricular tachycardia who requires therapy with intravenous procainamide. He has moderate heart failure (NYHA CHF class III). His steady-state procainamide and NAPA concentrations are 4.5 μg/mL and 7.9 μg/mL, respectively (total procainamide concentration = 12.4 μg/mL), at 1 mg/min. Compute a procainamide dose that will provide a steady-state concentration of 8 μg/mL.

1. *Compute the pharmacokinetic parameters.*

The patient is expected to achieve steady-state conditions after the second day (5 half-lives = 5 · 5.5 h = 28 h for procainamide; 5 half-lives = 5 · 6 h = 30 h for NAPA, assuming normal renal function) of therapy.

Procainamide clearance can be computed using a steady-state procainamide concentration: $Cl = k_0/Css = (1\ mg/min)/(4.5\ mg/L) = 0.22\ L/min$. (Note: μg/mL = mg/L, and this concentration unit was substituted for Css in calculations to avoid unnecessary unit conversion.)

2. *Compute the procainamide dose.*

Procainamide clearance is used to compute the new dose: k_0 = Css · Cl = 8 mg/L · 0.22 L/min = 1.8 mg/min, rounded to 2 mg/min. (Note: μg/mL = mg/L, and this concentration unit was substituted for Css in the calculations to avoid unnecessary unit conversion.)

The expected NAPA steady-state serum concentration increases in proportion to the procainamide dosage increase:

$$Css_{new} = (D_{new}/D_{old})Css_{old} = [(2\ mg/min)/(1\ mg/min)]\ 7.9\ \mu g/mL = 15.8\ \mu g/mL$$

The new procainamide dose is instituted immediately.

A steady-state procainamide serum concentration can be measured after steady state is attained in 3 to 5 half-lives. Because procainamide is expected to have a half-life of 5.5 hours and NAPA a half-life of 6 hours in the patient, procainamide and NAPA steady-state concentrations can be obtained any time after the second day of dosing (5 half-lives = 5 · 5.5 h = 28 h for procainamide; 5 half-lives = 5 · 6 h = 30 h for NAPA). Procainamide and NAPA serum concentrations also should be measured if the patient experiences a return of arrhythmia or develops potential signs or symptoms of procainamide toxicity.

CHIOU METHOD

For some patients, it is desirable to individualize procainamide infusion rates as rapidly as possible before steady state is achieved.[34] Examples of these cases include patients with renal dysfunction, heart failure, or hepatic cirrhosis, in whom procainamide pharmacokinetic parameters are variable and procainamide half-lives are long. In this situation, two procainamide serum concentrations obtained at least 4 to 6 hours apart during a continuous infusion can be used to compute procainamide clearance and dosing rates. In addition to this requirement, the only way procainamide can be entering the patient's body must be by intravenous infusion. Thus, the last dose of sustained-release procainamide must have been administered no less than 12 to 16 hours before this technique is used; otherwise, some residual oral procainamide is still absorbed from the gastrointestinal tract and causes computation errors.

The following equation is used to compute procainamide clearance (Cl) using the procainamide concentrations:

$$Cl = \frac{2\ k_0}{C_1 + C_2} + \frac{2V(C_1 - C_2)}{(C_1 + C_2)\ (t_2 - t_1)}$$

where k_0 is the infusion rate of procainamide, V is procainamide volume of distribution (chosen according to disease states and conditions of the patient; see Table 8-1), C_1 and C_2 are the first and second procainamide serum concentrations, and t_1 and t_2 are the times that C_1 and C_2 were obtained. After procainamide clearance (Cl) is determined, it can be used to adjust the procainamide infusion rate (k_0) according to the following relationship: k_0 = Css · Cl.

Example 1 JB is a 50-year-old, 60-kg, 170-cm (67-in) male with heart failure (NYHA CHF class III) started on a 5-mg/min procainamide infusion after being administered an intravenous loading dose. The procainamide concentration was 10.6 μg/mL at 1000 H and 14.3 μg/mL at 1400 H. What procainamide infusion rate is needed to achieve a Css of 8 μg/mL?

1. *Compute the procainamide clearance and dose.*

$$Cl = \frac{2\ k_0}{C_1 + C_2} + \frac{2V(C_1 - C_2)}{(C_1 + C_2)\ (t_2 - t_1)}$$

$$Cl = \frac{2(5\ mg/min)}{10.6\ mg/L + 14.3\ mg/L} + \frac{2(1.6\ L/kg \cdot 60\ kg)(10.6\ mg/L - 14.3\ mg/L)}{(10.6\ mg/L + 14.3\ mg/L)\ 240\ min} = 0.28\ L/min$$

Note: μg/mL = mg/L, and this concentration unit was substituted for concentrations to avoid unnecessary unit conversion. In addition, the time difference between t_2 and t_1, in minutes, was determined and placed directly in the calculation.

$$k_0 = Css \cdot Cl = 8\ mg/L \cdot 0.28\ L/min = 2.2\ mg/min\ \text{of procainamide}$$

Example 2 YU is a 64-year-old, 80-kg, 175-cm (69-in) male who was started on a 3-mg/min procainamide infusion after being administered an intravenous loading dose at 0900 H. The procainamide concentration was 10.3 μg/mL at 1000 H and 7.1 μg/mL at 1600 H. What procainamide infusion rate is needed to achieve a Css of 10 μg/mL?

1. *Compute the procainamide clearance and dose.*

$$Cl = \frac{2\ k_0}{C_1 + C_2} + \frac{2V(C_1 - C_2)}{(C_1 + C_2)\ (t_2 - t_1)}$$

$$Cl = \frac{2(3\ mg/min)}{10.3\ mg/L + 7.1\ mg/L} + \frac{2(2.7\ L/kg \cdot 80\ kg)(10.3\ mg/L - 7.1\ mg/L)}{(10.3\ mg/L + 7.1\ mg/L)\ 360\ min} = 0.57\ L/min$$

Note: μg/mL = mg/L, and this concentration unit was substituted for concentrations to avoid unnecessary unit conversion. In addition, the time difference between t_2 and t_1, in minutes, was determined and placed directly in the calculation.

$$k_0 = Css \cdot Cl = 10\ mg/L \cdot 0.57\ L/min = 5.7\ mg/min\ \text{of procainamide}$$

BAYESIAN PHARMACOKINETICS COMPUTER PROGRAMS

Computer programs are available that can assist in the computation of pharmacokinetic parameters for patients. The most reliable computer programs use a nonlinear regression algorithm, which incorporates components of Bayes' theorem. Nonlinear regression is a statistical technique that uses an iterative process to compute the best pharmacokinetic parameters for a concentration–time data set. Briefly, the patient's drug dosage schedule and serum concentrations are entered into the computer. The computer program has a pharmacokinetic equation preprogrammed for the drug and administration method (e.g., oral, intravenous bolus, intravenous infusion). Typically, a one-compartment model is used, although some programs allow the user to choose among several different equations. Using population estimates based on demographic information for the patient (e.g., age, weight, gender, liver function, cardiac status) supplied by the user, the computer program then computes estimated serum concentrations each time there are actual serum concentrations. Kinetic parameters are then changed by the computer program, and a new set of estimated serum concentrations are computed. The pharmacokinetic parameters that generated the estimated serum concentrations closest to the actual values are remembered by the computer program, and the process is repeated until the set of pharmacokinetic parameters that result in estimated serum concentrations that are statistically closest to the actual serum concentrations are generated. These pharmacokinetic parameters can then be used to compute improved dosing schedules for patients. Bayes' theorem is used in the computer algorithm to balance the results of the computations between values based solely on the patient's serum drug concentrations and those based only on patient population parameters. Results from studies that compare various methods of dosage adjustment have consistently found that these types of computer dosing programs perform at least as well as experienced clinical pharmacokineticists and clinicians and better than inexperienced clinicians.

Some clinicians use Bayesian pharmacokinetics computer programs exclusively to alter drug doses based on serum concentrations. An advantage of this approach is that consistent dosage recommendations are made when several different practitioners are involved in therapeutic drug-monitoring programs. However, since simpler dosing methods work just as well for patients with stable pharmacokinetic parameters and steady-state drug concentrations, many clinicians reserve the use of computer programs for more difficult situations. Such situations include serum concentrations that are not at steady state, serum concentrations not obtained at the specific times needed for simpler methods, and unstable pharmacokinetic parameters. Many Bayesian pharmacokinetics computer programs are available to users, and most provide answers similar to the one used in the following examples. The program used to solve problems in this book is DrugCalc, written by Dr. Dennis Mungall, and is available on his Internet web site (http://members.aol.com/thertch/index.htm).[35]

Example 1 OY is a 57-year-old, 79-kg, 173-cm (68-in) male with ventricular tachycardia who requires therapy with oral procainamide. He has normal liver (bilirubin = 0.7 mg/dL, albumin = 4.0 g/dL), renal (serum creatinine = 1.0 mg/dL), and cardiac function. He started taking procainamide sustained-release tablets 500 mg four times daily at 0700, 1200, 1800, and 2200 H. His procainamide serum concentration is 2.1 μg/mL at 2130 H before the third dose is given on the first day of therapy. Compute a procainamide dose that will provide a steady-state concentration of 6 μg/mL.

1. *Enter the patient's demographic, drug dosing, and serum concentration–time data into the computer program.*

This patient is unlikely to be at steady state, so the linear pharmacokinetics method cannot be used.

2. *Compute the pharmacokinetic parameters for the patient using the Bayesian pharmacokinetics computer program.*

The pharmacokinetic parameters computed by the program are a volume of distribution of 152 L, a half-life of 3.1 hours, and a clearance of 33.9 L/h.

3. *Compute the dose required to achieve the desired procainamide serum concentrations.*

The oral one-compartment model equation used by the program to compute doses indicates that 2000 mg of procainamide every 6 hours will produce a steady-state trough concentration of 6.1 μg/mL. This dose is to be started immediately.

Example 2 SL is a 71-year-old, 82-kg, 178-cm (70-in) male with atrial fibrillation who requires therapy with oral procainamide. He has cirrhosis (Child-Pugh score, 12; bilirubin, 3.2 mg/dL; albumin, 2.5 g/dL) and normal cardiac function. He began procainamide sustained-release tablets 500 mg every 12 hours at 0700 H. On the second day of therapy before the morning dose is administered, the procainamide serum concentration is 4.5 μg/mL at 0700 H. Compute a procainamide dose that will provide a steady-state concentration of 5 μg/mL.

1. *Enter the patient's demographic, drug dosing, and serum concentration–time data into the computer program.*

This patient is unlikely to be at steady state, so the linear pharmacokinetics method cannot be used.

2. *Compute the pharmacokinetic parameters for the patient using the Bayesian pharmacokinetics computer program.*

The pharmacokinetic parameters computed by the program are a volume of distribution of 110 L, a half-life of 15.5 hours, and a clearance of 4.93 L/h.

3. *Compute the dose required to achieve the desired procainamide serum concentrations.*

The oral one-compartment model equation used by the program to compute doses indicates that 250 mg of procainamide sustained-release tablets every 8 hours will produce a steady-state trough concentration of 5.5 μg/mL. This dose should be started immediately.

Example 3 TR is a 75-year-old, 85-kg, 173-cm (68-in) male with atrial flutter who requires therapy with procainamide sustained-release tablets. He has moderate heart failure (NYHA CHF class III). Yesterday, he was prescribed procainamide 500 mg four times daily and received the first two doses at 0800 H and 1200 H. Because he felt that his arrhythmia had returned, he phoned his physician, who advised him to increase the dose to 1000 mg (1800 H and 2200 H). His procainamide serum concentration is 10.7 μg/mL at 1000 H, 2 hours after the morning dose (at 0800 H, 1000 mg procainamide). Compute a procainamide sustained-release tablet dose that will provide a steady-state trough concentration of 6 μg/mL.

1. *Enter the patient's demographic, drug dosing, and serum concentration–time data into the computer program.*

This patient is unlikely to be at steady state, so the linear pharmacokinetics method cannot be used.

2. *Compute the pharmacokinetic parameters for the patient using the Bayesian pharmacokinetics computer program.*

The pharmacokinetic parameters computed by the program are a volume of distribution of 114 L, a half-life of 7.3 hours, and a clearance of 10.8 L/h.

3. *Compute the dose required to achieve the desired procainamide serum concentrations.*

The oral one-compartment model equation used by the program to compute doses indicates that 500 mg of procainamide immediate-release tablets taken every 6 hours will produce a steady-state trough concentration of 5.9 μg/mL. This dose should be started immediately.

USE OF PROCAINAMIDE BOOSTER DOSES TO IMMEDIATELY INCREASE SERUM CONCENTRATIONS

If a patient has a subtherapeutic procainamide serum concentration in an acute situation, it may be desirable to increase the procainamide concentration as quickly as possible. In this setting, it is not acceptable to simply increase the maintenance dose and wait 3 to 5 half-lives for therapeutic serum concentrations to be established in the patient. A rational way to increase the serum concentrations rapidly is to administer a booster dose of procainamide—a process also known as "reloading" the patient with procainamide—computed using pharmacokinetic techniques. A modified loading dose equation is used to accomplish computation of the booster dose (BD), which takes into account the current procainamide concentration in the patient: $BD = (C_{desired} - C_{actual})V$, where $C_{desired}$ is the desired procainamide concentration, C_{actual} is the actual current procainamide concentration for the patient, and V is the volume of distribution for procainamide. If the volume of distribution for procainamide is known for the patient, it can be used in the calculation. However, this value is not usually known and is assumed to equal the population average for the disease states and conditions of the patient (see Table 8-1).

Concurrent with the administration of the booster dose, the maintenance dose of procainamide is usually increased. Clinicians need to recognize that a booster dose does not alter the time required to achieve steady-state conditions when a new procainamide dosage rate is prescribed. It still requires 3 to 5 half-lives to attain steady state when the dosage rate is changed. However, usually the difference between the postbooster dose procainamide concentration and the ultimate steady-state concentration has been reduced by giving the extra dose of drug.

Example 1 BN is a 42-year-old, 50-kg, 157-cm (62-in) woman with atrial flutter who is receiving therapy with intravenous procainamide. She has normal liver and cardiac function. After receiving an initial loading dose of procainamide (300 mg) and a maintenance infusion of procainamide of 4 mg/min for 16 hours, her procainamide concentration is measured at 2.1 μg/mL, and her atrial rate continues to be rapid. Compute a booster dose of procainamide to achieve a procainamide concentration of 6 μg/mL.

1. *Estimate the volume of distribution according to the disease states and conditions of the patient.*

In the case of procainamide, the population average volume of distribution is 2.7 L/kg and will be used to estimate the parameter for the patient. The patient is not obese, so her actual body weight is used in the computation: $V = 2.7\ L/kg \cdot 50\ kg = 135\ L$.

2. *Compute the booster dose.*

The booster dose is computed according to the following equation: $BD = (C_{desired} - C_{actual})V = (6\ mg/L - 2.1\ mg/L)135\ L = 527\ mg$, rounded to 500 mg of procainamide infused over 25 to 30 minutes. (Note: μg/mL = mg/L, and this concentration unit was substituted for Css in the calculations to avoid unnecessary unit conversion.) If the maintenance dose is increased, it will take an additional 3 to 5 estimated half-lives for new steady-state conditions to be achieved. Procainamide serum concentrations can be measured at this time.

CONVERSION OF PROCAINAMIDE DOSES FROM INTRAVENOUS TO ORAL ROUTE OF ADMINISTRATION

Occasionally, there is a need to convert the route of administration of a patient stabilized on procainamide therapy from the oral route to an equivalent continuous infusion, or vice versa. In general, oral procainamide dosage forms, including most sustained-release tablets and capsules, have a bioavailability of 0.83. Assuming that equal procainamide serum concentrations are desired, this makes conversion between the intravenous [$k_0 = Css \cdot Cl$] and oral [$D = (Css \cdot Cl \cdot \tau)/F$] routes of administration simple, because equivalent doses of drug are prescribed: $k_0 = FD_{po}/(60 \text{ min/h} \cdot \tau)$ or $D_{po} = (k_0 \cdot \tau \cdot 60 \text{ min/h})/F$, where k_0 is the equivalent intravenous infusion rate for the procainamide in mg/min, D_{po} is the equivalent dose of oral procainamide in mg, τ is the dosage interval in hours, and F is the bioavailability fraction of oral procainamide.

Example 1 JH is receiving oral sustained-release procainamide 1000 mg every 6 hours. She is responding well to therapy, has no adverse drug effects, and has steady-state procainamide and NAPA concentrations of 8.3 μg/mL and 14.7 μg/mL, respectively. Suggest an equivalent dose of procainamide given as an intravenous infusion.

1. *Calculate the equivalent intravenous dose of procainamide.*

The equivalent intravenous procainamide dose would be $k_0 = FD_{po}/(60 \text{ min/h} \cdot \tau) = (0.83 \cdot 1000 \text{ mg})/(60 \text{ min/h} \cdot 6 \text{ h}) = 2.3$ mg/min of procainamide as a continuous intravenous infusion.

Example 2 LK is receiving a continuous infusion of procainamide 5 mg/min. He is responding well to therapy, has no adverse drug effects, and has steady-state procainamide and NAPA concentrations of 6.2 μg/mL and 4.3 μg/mL, respectively. Suggest an equivalent dose of sustained-release oral procainamide.

1. *Calculate the equivalent oral dose of procainamide.*

The equivalent oral sustained-release procainamide dose using a 12-hour dosage interval would be $D_{po} = (k_0 \cdot \tau \cdot 60 \text{ min/h})/F = (5 \text{ mg/min} \cdot 12 \text{ h} \cdot 60 \text{ min/h})/0.83 = 4337$ mg, rounded to 4000 mg. The patient is prescribed procainamide sustained-release tablets 4000 mg orally every 12 hours.

PROBLEMS

The following problems are intended to emphasize the computation of initial and individualized doses using clinical pharmacokinetic techniques. Clinicians should always consult the patient's chart to confirm that current antiarrhythmic and other drug therapy is appropriate. In addition, all other medications that the patient is taking, including prescription and nonprescription drugs, should be noted and checked to ascertain whether a potential drug interaction with procainamide exists.

1. NJ is a 67-year-old, 72-kg, 185-cm (73-in) male with ventricular tachycardia who requires therapy with oral procainamide. He has normal renal and liver function and does not have uncompensated heart failure. Suggest an initial oral procainamide dosage regimen designed to achieve a steady-state procainamide concentration of 4 μg/mL.

2. Patient NJ (see problem 1) was prescribed procainamide sustained-release tablets 1000 mg orally every 6 hours. His steady-state procainamide and NAPA concentrations are 4.2 μg/mL and 2.5 μg/mL, respectively (total procainamide concentration = 6.7 μg/mL). Compute a new oral procainamide dose that will provide a procainamide steady-state concentration of 6 μg/mL.

3. GF is a 56-year-old, 81-kg, 175-cm (69-in) male with ventricular tachycardia who requires therapy with oral procainamide. He has renal failure (estimated creatinine clearance = 10 mL/min) and normal liver function. Suggest an initial procainamide dosage regimen designed to achieve a steady-state procainamide concentration of 4 μg/mL.

4. Patient GF (see problem 3) was prescribed procainamide sustained-release tablets 1000 mg orally every 12 hours. His steady-state procainamide and NAPA concentrations are 9.5 μg/mL and 32.5 μg/mL, respectively (total procainamide concentration = 42 μg/mL). Compute a new oral procainamide dose that will provide a procainamide steady-state concentration of 6 μg/mL.

5. YU is a 71-year-old, 60-kg, 157-cm (62-in) female with paroxysmal atrial tachycardia who requires therapy with oral procainamide. She has severe uncompensated heart failure (NYHA CHF class IV) and normal liver function. Suggest an initial procainamide dosage regimen designed to achieve a steady-state procainamide concentration of 5 μg/mL.

6. Patient YU (see problem 5) was prescribed procainamide sustained-release tablets 1000 mg orally every 12 hours. The procainamide and NAPA concentrations obtained just before the third dose of this regimen were 11.4 μg/mL and 10.1 μg/mL, respectively (total procainamide concentration = 21.5 μg/mL). Assuming that the procainamide concentration was zero before the first dose, compute a new oral procainamide dose that will provide a steady-state concentration of 8 μg/mL.

7. WE is a 54-year-old, 55-kg, 165-cm (65-in) female with atrial fibrillation who requires therapy with oral procainamide. She has severe cirrhosis (Child-Pugh score, 13). Suggest an initial oral procainamide dosage regimen designed to achieve a steady-state procainamide concentration of 5 μg/mL.

8. Patient WE (see problem 7) was prescribed procainamide sustained-release tablets 1000 mg orally every 12 hours. The procainamide and NAPA concentrations obtained just before the third dose of this regimen were 9.5 μg/mL and 7.2 μg/mL,

respectively (total procainamide concentration = 16.7 μg/mL). Assuming that the procainamide concentration was zero before the first dose, compute a new oral procainamide dose that will provide a steady-state concentration of 7 μg/mL.

9. IO is a 62-year-old, 130-kg, 180-cm (71-in) male with atrial flutter who requires therapy with oral procainamide. He has normal liver and renal function. Suggest an initial procainamide sustained-release dosage regimen designed to achieve a steady-state procainamide concentration of 4 μg/mL.

10. Patient IO (see problem 9) was prescribed procainamide sustained-release tablets 2000 mg orally every 12 hours. After the first dose, the patient's arrhythmia returned, and his clinician advised a dosage increase to 3000 mg every 12 hours. Procainamide and NAPA serum concentrations were obtained just before the third dose (i.e., after one 2000-mg and one 3000-mg dose) and the procainamide concentration was 2.8 μg/mL. Assuming that the procainamide concentration was zero before the first dose, compute a new oral procainamide dose that will provide a steady-state procainamide concentration of 4 μg/mL.

11. LG is a 53-year-old, 69-kg, 178-cm (70-in) male with atrial flutter who requires therapy with intravenous procainamide. He has normal liver and cardiac function. Suggest an initial procainamide dosage regimen designed to achieve a steady-state procainamide concentration of 4 μg/mL.

12. Patient LG (see problem 11) was prescribed intravenous procainamide 3 mg/min. The procainamide and NAPA concentrations obtained after 24 hours of this regimen were 4.5 μg/mL and 2.5 μg/mL, respectively (total procainamide concentration = 7 μg/mL). Compute a new intravenous procainamide infusion and a procainamide booster dose that will provide a steady-state concentration of 8 μg/mL.

13. CV is a 69-year-old, 90-kg, 185-cm (73-in) male with ventricular tachycardia who requires therapy with intravenous procainamide. He has cirrhosis (Child-Pugh score, 11) and normal cardiac function. Suggest an initial intravenous procainamide dosage regimen designed to achieve a steady-state procainamide concentration of 5 μg/mL.

14. Patient CV (see problem 13) was prescribed intravenous procainamide 3 mg/min and administered a loading dose of procainamide 500 mg over 30 minutes before continuous infusion was begun. Procainamide serum concentration obtained after 12 hours of the infusion was 11.2 μg/mL. Compute a new intravenous procainamide infusion that will provide a steady-state concentration of 6 μg/mL.

15. PE is a 61-year-old, 67-kg, 168-cm (66-in) female with atrial fibrillation who requires therapy with intravenous procainamide. She has severe heart failure (NYHA CHF class IV) and normal liver function. Suggest an initial intravenous procainamide dosage regimen designed to achieve a steady-state procainamide concentration of 4 μg/mL.

16. Patient PE (see problem 15) was prescribed intravenous procainamide 4 mg/min and administered a loading dose of procainamide 500 mg over 30 minutes before continuous infusion was begun. Procainamide serum concentrations were obtained 4 hours and 8 hours after the infusion began and were 4.3 μg/mL and 8.8 μg/mL, respectively. Compute a new intravenous procainamide infusion that will provide a steady-state concentration of 6 μg/mL.

ANSWERS TO PROBLEMS

1. The initial procainamide dose for patient NJ is calculated as follows.

Pharmacokinetic Dosing Method

1. *Estimate the half-life and elimination rate constant according to the disease states and conditions of the patient.*

The expected procainamide half-life ($t_{1/2}$) is 3.3 hours. The elimination rate constant is computed using the following formula: $k = 0.693/t_{1/2} = 0.693/3.3\ h = 0.210\ h^{-1}$.

2. *Estimate the volume of distribution and clearance.*

The patient is not obese, so the estimated procainamide volume of distribution is based on actual body weight: V = 2.7 L/kg · 72 kg = 194 L. Estimated procainamide clearance is computed by taking the product of the volume of distribution and the elimination rate constant: $Cl = kV = 0.210\ h^{-1} \cdot 194\ L = 40.7\ L/h$.

3. *Compute the dosage regimen.*

Oral sustained-release procainamide tablets are prescribed to this patient (F = 0.83). Because the patient has a rapid procainamide clearance and half-life, the initial dosage interval (τ) is set to 6 hours. (Note: μg/mL = mg/L, and this concentration unit was substituted for Css in the calculations to avoid unnecessary unit conversion.) The dosage equation for oral procainamide is D = (Css · Cl · τ)/F = (4 mg/L · 40.7 L/h · 6 h)/0.83 = 1177 mg, rounded to 1000 mg every 6 hours.

Steady-state procainamide and NAPA serum concentrations can be measured after steady state is attained in 3 to 5 half-lives. Because procainamide is expected to have a half-life of 3.3 hours and NAPA a half-life of 6 hours for the patient, the steady-state concentrations can be obtained any time after the first day of dosing (5 half-lives = 5 · 3.3 h = 16.5 h for procainamide; 5 half-lives = 5 · 6 h = 30 h for NAPA). Procainamide and NAPA serum concentrations also should be measured if the patient experiences a return of arrhythmia or develops potential signs or symptoms of procainamide toxicity.

Literature-Based Recommended Dosing

1. *Choose the procainamide dose based on the disease states and conditions of the patient.*

A procainamide dose of 50 mg/kg per day is suggested by Table 8-3 for an adult with normal renal and hepatic function.

2. *Compute the dosage regimen.*

Oral sustained-release procainamide tablets are prescribed to this patient every 6 hours: D = procainamide dose · Wt = 50 mg/kg/d · 72 kg = 3600 mg/d, rounded to

4000 mg/d or 1000 mg every 6 hours. This dose is identical to that suggested by the pharmacokinetic dosing method.

Steady-state procainamide and NAPA serum concentrations can be measured after steady state is attained in 3 to 5 half-lives. Because procainamide is expected to have a half-life of 3.3 hours and NAPA a half-life of 6 hours in the patient, the steady-state concentrations can be obtained any time after the first day of dosing (5 half-lives = 5 · 3.3 h = 16.5 h for procainamide; 5 half-lives = 5 · 6 h = 30 h for NAPA). Procainamide and NAPA serum concentrations should also be measured if the patient experiences a return of arrhythmia or develops potential signs or symptoms of procainamide toxicity.

2. The revised procainamide dose for patient NJ is calculated as follows.

Linear Pharmacokinetics Method

1. *Compute a new dose to achieve the desired serum concentration.*

The patient is expected to achieve steady-state conditions after the second day (5 half-lives = 5 · 3.3 h = 17 h for procainamide; 5 half-lives = 5 · 6 h = 30 h for NAPA) of therapy.

With linear pharmacokinetics, the new dose to attain the desired concentration should be proportional to the old dose that produced the measured concentration. (Note: Total daily dose = 1000 mg/dose · 4 doses/d = 4000 mg/d.)

$$D_{new} = (Css_{new}/Css_{old})D_{old} = [(6\ \mu g/mL)/(4.2\ \mu g/mL)]\ 4000\ mg/d$$
$$= 5714\ mg/d, \text{ rounded to } 6000\ mg/d \text{ or } 1500\ mg \text{ every } 6 \text{ hours}$$

The new suggested dose is 1500 mg every 6 hours of oral procainamide to be started immediately.

The expected NAPA steady-state serum concentration changes in proportion to the procainamide dosage alteration:

$$Css_{new} = (D_{new}/D_{old})Css_{old} = [(6000\ mg/d)/(4000\ mg/d)]\ 2.5\ \mu g/mL = 3.8\ \mu g/mL$$

A steady-state procainamide serum concentration can be measured after steady state is attained in 3 to 5 half-lives. Because procainamide is expected to have a half-life of 3.3 hours and NAPA a half-life of 6 hours in the patient, procainamide and NAPA steady-state concentrations can be obtained any time after the second day of dosing (5 half-lives = 5 · 3.3 h = 17 h for procainamide; 5 half-lives = 5 · 6 h = 30 h for NAPA). Procainamide and NAPA serum concentrations also should be measured if the patient experiences a return of arrhythmia or develops potential signs or symptoms of procainamide toxicity.

Pharmacokinetic Parameter Method

1. *Compute the pharmacokinetic parameters.*

The patient is expected to achieve steady-state conditions after the second day (5 half-lives = 5 · 3.3 h = 17 h for procainamide; 5 half-lives = 5 · 6 h = 30 h for NAPA) of therapy.

Procainamide clearance can be computed using a steady-state procainamide concentration: $Cl = [F(D/\tau)]/Css = [0.83\ (1000\ mg/6\ h)]/(4.2\ mg/L) = 32.9\ L/h$. (Note: μg/mL = mg/L, and this concentration unit was substituted for Css in the calculations to avoid unnecessary unit conversion.)

2. *Compute the procainamide dose.*

Procainamide clearance is used to compute the new dose: $D = (Css \cdot Cl \cdot \tau)/F = (6\ mg/L \cdot 32.9\ L/h \cdot 6\ h)/0.83 = 1427\ mg$, rounded to 1500 mg every 6 hours.

The expected NAPA steady-state serum concentration changes in proportion to the procainamide dosage alteration:

$$Css_{new} = (D_{new}/D_{old})Css_{old} = [(6000\ mg/d)/(4000\ mg/d)]\ 2.5\ \mu g/mL = 3.8\ \mu g/mL$$

The new procainamide dose is instituted immediately.

A steady-state procainamide serum concentration can be measured after steady state is attained in 3 to 5 half-lives. Because procainamide is expected to have a half-life of 3.3 hours and NAPA a half-life of 6 hours in the patient, procainamide and NAPA steady-state concentrations can be obtained any time after the second day of dosing (5 half-lives = $5 \cdot 3.3\ h = 17\ h$ for procainamide; 5 half-lives = $5 \cdot 6\ h = 30\ h$ for NAPA). Procainamide and NAPA serum concentrations also should be measured if the patient experiences a return of arrhythmia or develops potential signs or symptoms of procainamide toxicity.

3. The initial procainamide dose for patient GF is calculated as follows.

Pharmacokinetic Dosing Method

1. *Estimate the half-life and elimination rate constant according to the disease states and conditions of the patient.*

The expected procainamide half-life ($t_{1/2}$) is 13.9 hours. The elimination rate constant is computed using the following formula: $k = 0.693/t_{1/2} = 0.693/13.9\ h = 0.050\ h^{-1}$.

2. *Estimate the volume of distribution and clearance.*

The patient is not obese, so the estimated procainamide volume of distribution is based on actual body weight: $V = 1.7\ L/kg \cdot 81\ kg = 138\ L$. Estimated procainamide clearance is computed by taking the product of the volume of distribution and the elimination rate constant: $Cl = kV = 0.050\ h^{-1} \cdot 138\ L = 6.9\ L/h$.

3. *Compute the dosage regimen.*

Oral sustained-release procainamide tablets are prescribed to this patient (F = 0.83). Because procainamide has a slow clearance and a long half-life in this patient, the initial dosage interval (τ) is set to 12 hours. (Note: μg/mL = mg/L, and this concentration unit was substituted for Css in the calculations to avoid unnecessary unit conversion.) The dosage equation for oral procainamide is $D = (Css \cdot Cl \cdot \tau)/F = (4\ mg/L \cdot 6.9\ L/h \cdot 12\ h)/0.83 = 399\ mg$, rounded to 500 mg every 12 hours.

Steady-state procainamide and NAPA serum concentrations can be measured after steady state is attained in 3 to 5 half-lives. Because procainamide is expected to have a half-life of 13.9 hours and NAPA a half-life of 41 hours in the patient, the steady-state concentration can be obtained any time after the ninth day of dosing (5 half-lives = 5 · 13.9 h = 70 h for procainamide; 5 half-lives = 5 · 41 h = 205 h for NAPA). Procainamide and NAPA serum concentrations also should be measured if the patient experiences a return of arrhythmia or develops potential signs or symptoms of procainamide toxicity.

Literature-Based Recommended Dosing

1. *Choose the procainamide dose based on the disease states and conditions of the patient.*

A procainamide dose of 12.5 mg/kg per day (50 mg/kg per day normal dose, reduced by 75%) is suggested by Table 8-3 for an adult with severe renal failure.

2. *Compute the dosage regimen.*

Oral sustained-release procainamide tablets are prescribed for this patient every 12 hours: D = procainamide dose · Wt = 12.5 mg/kg/d · 81 kg = 1013 mg/d, rounded to 1000 mg/d or 500 mg every 12 hours. This dose is identical to that suggested by the pharmacokinetic dosing method.

Steady-state procainamide and NAPA serum concentrations can be measured after steady state is attained in 3 to 5 half-lives. Because procainamide is expected to have a half-life of 13.9 hours and NAPA a half-life of 41 hours in the patient, the steady-state concentrations can be obtained any time after the ninth day of dosing (5 half-lives = 5 · 13.9 h = 70 h for procainamide; 5 half-lives = 5 · 41 h = 205 h for NAPA). Procainamide and NAPA serum concentrations also should be measured if the patient experiences a return of arrhythmia or develops potential signs or symptoms of procainamide toxicity.

4. The revised procainamide dose for patient GF is calculated as follows.

Linear Pharmacokinetics Method

1. *Compute a new dose to achieve the desired serum concentration.*

The patient is expected to achieve steady-state conditions after the ninth day of dosing (5 half-lives = 5 · 13.9 h = 70 h for procainamide; 5 half-lives = 5 · 41 h = 205 h for NAPA).

With the use of linear pharmacokinetics, the new dose to attain the desired concentration should be proportional to the old dose that produced the measured concentration. (Note: Total daily dose = 1000 mg/dose · 2 doses/d = 2000 mg/d.)

$$D_{new} = (Css_{new}/Css_{old})D_{old} = [(6\ \mu g/mL)/(9.5\ \mu g/mL)]\ 2000\ mg/d$$
$$= 1263\ mg/d, \text{ rounded to } 1500\ mg/d \text{ or } 750\ mg \text{ every } 12\ hours$$

The new suggested dose is 750 mg oral procainamide every 12 hours to be started immediately if no adverse effects are present. If side effects are observed, the new dosage regimen can be held for 1 procainamide half-life before being instituted.

The expected NAPA steady-state serum concentration changes in proportion to the procainamide dosage alteration:

$$Css_{new} = (D_{new}/D_{old})Css_{old} = [(1500\ mg/d)/(2000\ mg/d)]\ 32.5\ \mu g/mL = 24.4\ \mu g/mL$$

Steady-state procainamide and NAPA serum concentrations can be measured after steady state is attained in 3 to 5 half-lives. Because procainamide is expected to have a half-life of 13.9 hours and NAPA a half-life of 41 hours in the patient, the steady-state concentrations can be obtained any time after the ninth day of dosing (5 half-lives = 5 · 13.9 h = 70 h for procainamide; 5 half-lives = 5 · 41 h = 205 h for NAPA). Procainamide and NAPA serum concentrations also should be measured if the patient experiences a return of arrhythmia or develops potential signs or symptoms of procainamide toxicity.

Pharmacokinetic Parameter Method

1. *Compute the pharmacokinetic parameters.*

The patient is expected to achieve steady-state conditions after the ninth day of dosing (5 half-lives = 5 · 13.9 h = 70 h for procainamide; 5 half-lives = 5 · 41 h = 205 h for NAPA).

Procainamide clearance can be computed using a steady-state procainamide concentration: $Cl = [F(D/\tau)]/Css = [0.83\ (1000\ mg/12\ h)]/(9.5\ mg/L) = 7.3\ L/h$. (Note: μg/mL = mg/L, and this concentration unit was substituted for Css in the calculations to avoid unnecessary unit conversion.)

2. *Compute the procainamide dose.*

Procainamide clearance is used to compute the new dose: $D = (Css \cdot Cl \cdot \tau)/F = (6\ mg/L \cdot 7.3\ L/h \cdot 12\ h)/0.83 = 633\ mg$, rounded to 750 mg every 12 hours.

The expected NAPA steady-state serum concentration changes in proportion to the procainamide dosage alteration:

$$Css_{new} = (D_{new}/D_{old})Css_{old} = [(1500\ mg/d)/(2000\ mg/d)]\ 32.5\ \mu g/mL = 24.4\ \mu g/mL$$

The new suggested dose is 750 mg oral procainamide every 12 hours to be started immediately if no adverse effects are present. If side effects are observed, the new dosage regimen can be held for 1 procainamide half-life before being instituted.

Steady-state procainamide and NAPA serum concentrations can be measured after steady state is attained in 3 to 5 half-lives. Because procainamide is expected to have a half-life of 13.9 hours and NAPA a half-life of 41 hours in the patient, the steady-state concentrations can be obtained any time after the ninth day of dosing (5 half-lives = 5 · 13.9 h = 70 h for procainamide; 5 half-lives = 5 · 41 h = 205 h for NAPA). Procainamide and NAPA serum concentrations also should be measured if the patient experiences a return of arrhythmia or develops potential signs or symptoms of procainamide toxicity.

5. The initial procainamide dose for patient YU is calculated as follows.

1. *Estimate the half-life and elimination rate constant according to the disease states and conditions of the patient.*

Patients with severe uncompensated heart failure have highly variable procainamide pharmacokinetics and dosage requirements. Patients with heart failure have decreased cardiac output, which leads to decreased liver blood flow, and the expected procainamide half-life ($t_{1/2}$) is 5.5 hours. The elimination rate constant is computed using the following formula: $k = 0.693/t_{1/2} = 0.693/5.5\ h = 0.126\ h^{-1}$.

2. *Estimate the volume of distribution and clearance.*

The patient is not obese, so the estimated procainamide volume of distribution is based on actual body weight: V = 1.6 L/kg · 60 kg = 96 L. Estimated procainamide clearance is computed by taking the product of the volume of distribution and the elimination rate constant: $Cl = kV = 0.126\ h^{-1} \cdot 96\ L = 12.1\ L/h$.

3. *Compute the dosage regimen.*

Oral sustained-release procainamide tablets are prescribed to this patient (F = 0.83). The initial dosage interval (τ) is set to 12 hours. (Note: μg/mL = mg/L, and this concentration unit was substituted for Css in the calculations to avoid unnecessary unit conversion.) The dosage equation for oral procainamide is D = (Css · Cl · τ)/F = (5 mg/L · 12.1 L/h · 12 h)/0.83 = 875 mg, rounded to 750 mg every 12 hours.

Steady-state procainamide and NAPA serum concentrations can be measured after steady state is attained in 3 to 5 half-lives. Because procainamide is expected to have a half-life of 5.5 hours and NAPA a half-life of 6 hours in the patient (assuming that heart failure has no effect on NAPA pharmacokinetics), the steady-state concentrations can be obtained any time after the second day of dosing (5 half-lives = 5 · 5.5 h = 27.5 h for procainamide; 5 half-lives = 5 · 6 h = 30 h for NAPA). Procainamide and NAPA serum concentrations also should be measured if the patient experiences a return of arrhythmia or develops potential signs or symptoms of procainamide toxicity. Procainamide pharmacokinetic parameters can change as the patient's cardiac status changes. If heart failure improves, cardiac output will increase, resulting in increased liver blood flow and procainamide clearance. Alternatively, if heart failure worsens, cardiac output decreases further, resulting in decreased liver blood flow and procainamide clearance. Thus, patients with heart failure who are receiving procainamide therapy must be monitored very carefully.

Literature-Based Recommended Dosing

1. *Choose a procainamide dose based on the disease states and conditions of the patient.*

A procainamide dose of 25 mg/kg per day (50 mg/kg per day normal dose, reduced by 50%) is suggested by Table 8-3 for an adult with severe uncompensated heart failure.

2. *Compute the dosage regimen.*

Oral sustained-release procainamide tablets are prescribed for this patient every 12 hours: D = procainamide dose · Wt = 25 mg/kg/d · 60 kg = 1500 mg/d, 750 mg every 12 hours. This dose is identical to that suggested by the pharmacokinetic dosing method.

Steady-state procainamide and NAPA serum concentrations can be measured after steady state is attained in 3 to 5 half-lives. Because procainamide is expected to have a half-life of 5.5 hours and NAPA a half-life of 6 hours in the patient (assuming that heart failure has no effect on NAPA pharmacokinetics), the steady-state concentrations can be obtained any time after the second day of dosing (5 half-lives = 5 · 5.5 h = 27.5 h for procainamide; 5 half-lives = 5 · 6 h = 30 h for NAPA). Procainamide and NAPA serum concentrations also should be measured if the patient experiences a return of arrhythmia or develops potential signs or symptoms of procainamide toxicity. Procainamide pharmacokinetic parameters can change as the patient's cardiac status changes. If heart failure improves, cardiac output increases, resulting in increased liver blood flow and procainamide clearance. Alternatively, if heart failure worsens, cardiac output decreases further, resulting in decreased liver blood flow and procainamide clearance. Thus, patients with heart failure who are receiving procainamide therapy must be monitored very carefully.

6. The revised procainamide dose for patient YU is calculated as follows.

The patient has severe heart failure and is expected to achieve steady-state conditions after the second day (5 half-lives = 5 · 5.5 h = 27.5 h) of therapy. Because the procainamide serum concentration was obtained on the third day of therapy, it is unlikely that steady state has been attained, so the linear pharmacokinetics and pharmacokinetic parameter methods cannot be used.

Bayesian Pharmacokinetics Computer Program Method

1. *Enter the patient's demographic, drug dosing, and serum concentration–time data into the computer program.*

2. *Compute the pharmacokinetic parameters for the patient using the Bayesian pharmacokinetics computer program.*

The pharmacokinetic parameters computed by the program are a volume of distribution of 75 L, a half-life of 13.8 hours, and a clearance of 3.8 L/h.

3. *Compute the dose required to achieve the desired procainamide serum concentrations.*

The one-compartment model first-order absorption equations used by the program to compute doses indicate that 500 mg every 12 hours will produce a steady-state procainamide concentration of 8 μg/mL.

7. The initial procainamide dose for patient WE is calculated as follows.

Pharmacokinetic Dosing Method

Detailed pharmacokinetic studies have not been done in patients with severe liver disease, so this method cannot be used.

Literature-Based Recommended Dosing

1. *Choose a procainamide dose based on the disease states and conditions of the patient.*

A procainamide dose of 25 mg/kg per day (50 mg/kg per day normal dose, reduced by 50%) is suggested by Table 8-4 for an adult with severe liver disease.

2. *Compute the dosage regimen.*

Oral sustained-release procainamide tablets are prescribed for this patient every 12 hours: D = procainamide dose · Wt = 25 mg/kg/d · 55 kg = 1375 mg/d, rounded to 1500 mg or 750 mg every 12 hours.

Steady-state procainamide and NAPA serum concentrations can be measured after steady state is attained in 3 to 5 half-lives. Procainamide and NAPA serum concentrations also should be measured if the patient experiences a return of arrhythmia or develops potential signs or symptoms of procainamide toxicity. Procainamide pharmacokinetic parameters can change as the patient's hepatic status changes. Thus, patients with cirrhosis who are receiving procainamide therapy must be monitored very carefully.

8. The revised procainamide dose for patient WE is calculated as follows.

The patient has abnormal hepatic function and is expected to have a prolonged half-life. Because the procainamide serum concentration was obtained before the third dose, it is unlikely that the serum concentration was obtained at steady state, so the linear pharmacokinetics and pharmacokinetic parameter methods cannot be used.

Bayesian Pharmacokinetics Computer Program Method

1. *Enter the patient's demographic, drug dosing, and serum concentration–time data into the computer program.*

2. *Compute the pharmacokinetic parameters for the patient using the Bayesian pharmacokinetics computer program.*

The pharmacokinetic parameters computed by the program are a volume of distribution of 91 L, a half-life of 14 hours, and a clearance of 4.5 L/h.

3. *Compute the dose required to achieve the desired procainamide serum concentrations.*

The one-compartment model first-order absorption equations used by the program to compute doses indicate that 500 mg of procainamide every 12 hours will produce a steady-state procainamide concentration of 6.7 μg/mL.

9. The initial procainamide dose for patient IO is calculated as follows.

Pharmacokinetic Dosing Method

1. *Estimate the half-life and elimination rate constant according to the disease states and conditions of the patient.*

For an obese person, a clearance value based on total body weight (TBW) is used to compute procainamide doses.

2. *Estimate the volume of distribution and clearance.*

The patient is obese [IBW_{male} (in kg) = 50 kg + 2.3(Ht – 60 in) = 50 kg + 2.3(71 – 60) = 75 kg, patient >30% over ideal body weight], so the estimated procainamide clearance is based on total body weight and the population clearance value for obese persons: Cl = 0.52 L/h/kg · 130 kg = 67.6 L/h.

3. *Compute the dosage regimen.*

Oral sustained-release procainamide tablets are prescribed for this patient (F = 0.83). The initial dosage interval (τ) is set to 12 hours. (Note: μg/mL = mg/L, and this concentration unit was substituted for Css in the calculations to avoid unnecessary unit conversion.) The dosage equation for oral procainamide is D = (Css · Cl · τ)/F = (4 mg/L · 67.6 L/h · 12 h)/0.83 = 3909 mg, rounded to 4000 mg or 2000 mg every 12 hours.

A steady-state trough procainamide serum concentration can be measured after steady state is attained in 3 to 5 half-lives. Because procainamide is expected to have a half-life of 3.3 hours in the patient, the procainamide steady-state concentration can be obtained any time after the first day of dosing (5 half-lives = 5 · 3.3 h = 17 h). Procainamide serum concentrations also should be measured if the patient experiences an exacerbation of arrhythmia or develops potential signs or symptoms of procainamide toxicity.

Literature-Based Recommended Dosing

1. *Choose a procainamide dose based on the disease states and conditions of the patient.*

Procainamide 50 mg/kg per day is suggested by Table 8-4 for an adult with normal renal and hepatic function. Because the patient is obese [IBW_{men} (in kg) = 50 kg + 2.3(Ht − 60 in) = 50 kg + 2.3(71 − 60) = 75 kg, patient >30% over ideal body weight], total body weight is used to compute doses.

2. *Compute the dosage regimen.*

Oral sustained-release procainamide tablets are prescribed for this patient. The initial dosage interval is set to 12 hours: D = procainamide dose · Wt = 50 mg/kg/d · 130 kg = 6500 mg, rounded to 6000 mg or 3000 mg every 12 hours. (Note: Dose is rounded down to prevent possible overdosage.)

A steady-state trough procainamide serum concentration can be measured after steady state is attained in 3 to 5 half-lives. Because procainamide is expected to have a half-life of 3.3 hours in the patient, the procainamide steady-state concentration can be obtained any time after the first day of dosing (5 half-lives = 5 · 3.3 h = 17 h). Procainamide serum concentrations also should be measured if the patient experiences an exacerbation of arrhythmia or develops potential signs or symptoms of procainamide toxicity. Procainamide pharmacokinetic parameters can change as the patient's cardiac status changes.

10. The revised procainamide dose for patient IO is calculated as follows.

The patient has mild heart failure and is expected to achieve steady-state conditions after the first day (5 half-lives = 5 · 5.5 h = 27.5 h) of therapy. Because the procainamide serum concentration was obtained on the second day of therapy but two different doses were given on day 1, it is unlikely that the serum concentration was obtained at steady state. Therefore, neither the linear pharmacokinetics nor the pharmacokinetic parameter methods can be used.

Bayesian Pharmacokinetics Computer Program Method

1. *Enter the patient's demographic, drug dosing, and serum concentration–time data into the computer program.*

2. *Compute the pharmacokinetic parameters for the patient using the Bayesian pharmacokinetics computer program.*

The pharmacokinetic parameters computed by the program are a volume of distribution of 235 L, a half-life of 5.1 hours, and a clearance of 31.8 L/h.

3. *Compute the dose required to achieve the desired procainamide serum concentrations.*

The one-compartment model first-order absorption equations used by the program to compute doses indicate that 4000 mg procainamide every 12 hours will produce a steady-state procainamide concentration of 4.4 μg/mL.

A steady-state trough procainamide serum concentration can be measured after steady state is attained in 3 to 5 half-lives. Because procainamide is expected to have a half-life of 5.1 hours in the patient, the procainamide steady-state concentration can be obtained any time after the first day of dosing (5 half-lives = 5 · 5.1 h = 25.5 h). Procainamide serum concentrations also should be measured if the patient experiences an exacerbation of arrhythmia or develops potential signs or symptoms of procainamide toxicity.

11. The initial procainamide dose for patient LG is calculated as follows.

Pharmacokinetic Dosing Method

1. *Estimate the half-life and elimination rate constant according to the disease states and conditions of the patient.*

The expected procainamide half-life ($t_{1/2}$) is 3.3 hours. The elimination rate constant is computed using the following formula: $k = 0.693/t_{1/2} = 0.693/3.3\ h = 0.210\ h^{-1}$.

2. *Estimate the volume of distribution and clearance.*

The patient is not obese, so the estimated procainamide volume of distribution is based on actual body weight: V = 2.7 L/kg · 69 kg = 186 L. Estimated procainamide clearance is computed by taking the product of the volume of distribution and the elimination rate constant: $Cl = kV = 0.210\ h^{-1} \cdot 186\ L = 39.1\ L/h$.

3. *Compute the dosage regimen.*

Therapy is started by administering an intravenous loading dose of procainamide: LD = Css · V = 4 mg/L · 186 L = 744 mg, rounded to 750 mg. A maximum dose of 600 mg given intravenously over 25 to 30 minutes should be given and response assessed before giving the remainder of the computed loading dose. (Note: μg/mL =

mg/L, and this concentration unit was substituted for Css in the calculations to avoid unnecessary unit conversion.)

A procainamide continuous intravenous infusion is started immediately after the loading dose has been administered. The dosage equation for intravenous procainamide is k_0 = Css · Cl = (4 mg/L · 39.1 L/h)/(60 min/h) = 2.6 mg/min, rounded to 3 mg/min.

A steady-state procainamide serum concentration can be measured after steady state is attained in 3 to 5 half-lives. Because procainamide is expected to have a half-life of 3.3 hours in the patient, the procainamide steady-state concentration can be obtained any time after the first day of dosing (5 half-lives = 5 · 3.3 h = 16.5 h). Procainamide serum concentrations also should be measured if the patient experiences an exacerbation of arrhythmia or develops potential signs or symptoms of procainamide toxicity.

Literature-Based Recommended Dosing

1. *Choose a procainamide dose based on the disease states and conditions of the patient.*

A procainamide loading dose of 500 mg over 25 to 30 minutes is administered followed by a continuous infusion. A procainamide dose of 2 to 6 mg/min is suggested by Table 8-4 for an adult with normal hepatic and renal function. A dose of 3 mg/min is expected to attain a steady-state procainamide concentration in the lower end of the therapeutic range.

A procainamide serum concentration can be measured after steady state is attained in 3 to 5 half-lives. Because procainamide is expected to have a half-life of 3.3 hours in the patient, the procainamide steady-state concentration can be obtained any time after the first day of dosing (5 half-lives = 5 · 3.3 h = 16.5 h). Procainamide serum concentrations also should be measured if the patient experiences an exacerbation of arrhythmia or develops potential signs or symptoms of procainamide toxicity.

12. The revised procainamide dose for patient LG is calculated as follows.

Linear Pharmacokinetics Method

1. *Compute a new dose to achieve the desired serum concentration.*

The patient is expected to achieve steady-state conditions after the first day (5 half-lives = 5 · 3.3 h = 16.5 h) of therapy.

With the use of linear pharmacokinetics, the new infusion rate to attain the desired concentration should be proportional to the old infusion rate that produced the measured concentration:

$$D_{new} = (Css_{new}/Css_{old})D_{old} = [(8\ \mu g/mL)/(4.5\ \mu g/mL)]\ 3\ mg/min$$
$$= 5.3\ mg/min,\ rounded\ to\ 5\ mg/min$$

The new suggested infusion rate is 5 mg/min of procainamide.

The expected NAPA steady-state serum concentration changes in proportion to the procainamide dosage alteration:

$$Css_{new} = (D_{new}/D_{old})Css_{old} = [(5 \text{ mg/min})/(3 \text{ mg/min})] \ 2.5 \ \mu g/mL = 4.2 \ \mu g/mL$$

A booster dose of procainamide is computed using an estimated volume of distribution for the patient (2.7 L/kg · 69 kg = 186 L): BD = $(C_{desired} - C_{actual})V$ = (8 mg/L − 4.5 mg/L) 186 L = 651 mg, rounded to 600 mg of procainamide over 25 to 30 minutes. The booster dose is given to the patient before the infusion rate is increased to the new value.

A steady-state trough procainamide serum concentration can be measured after steady state is attained in 3 to 5 half-lives. Because procainamide is expected to have a half-life of 3.3 hours in the patient, the procainamide steady-state concentration can be obtained any time after the first day of dosing (5 half-lives = 5 · 3.3 h = 16.5 h). Procainamide serum concentrations also should be measured if the patient experiences an exacerbation of arrhythmia or develops potential signs or symptoms of procainamide toxicity.

Pharmacokinetic Parameter Method

1. *Compute the pharmacokinetic parameters.*

The patient is expected to achieve steady-state conditions after the first day (5 half-lives = 5 · 3.3 h = 16.5 h) of therapy.

Procainamide clearance can be computed using a steady-state procainamide concentration: Cl = k_0/Css = (3 mg/min)/(4.5 mg/L) = 0.67 L/min. (Note: μg/mL = mg/L, and this concentration unit was substituted for Css in the calculations to avoid unnecessary unit conversion.)

2. *Compute the procainamide dose.*

Procainamide clearance is used to compute the new procainamide infusion rate: k_0 = Css · Cl = 8 mg/L · 0.67 L/min = 5.4 mg/min, rounded to 5 mg/min.

The new suggested infusion rate is 5 mg/min of procainamide.

The expected NAPA steady-state serum concentration changes in proportion to the procainamide dosage alteration:

$$Css_{new} = (D_{new}/D_{old})Css_{old} = [(5 \text{ mg/min})/(3 \text{ mg/min})] \ 2.5 \ \mu g/mL = 4.2 \ \mu g/mL$$

A booster dose of procainamide is computed using an estimated volume of distribution for the patient (2.7 L/kg · 69 kg = 186 L): BD = $(C_{desired} - C_{actual})V$ = (8 mg/L − 4.5 mg/L) 186 L = 651 mg, rounded to 600 mg of procainamide over 25 to 30 minutes. The booster dose should be given to the patient before the infusion rate is increased to the new value.

A steady-state trough procainamide serum concentration can be measured after steady state is attained in 3 to 5 half-lives. Because procainamide is expected to have a half-life of 3.3 hours in the patient, the procainamide steady-state concentration can be obtained any time after the first day of dosing (5 half-lives = 5 · 3.3 h = 16.5 h).

Procainamide serum concentrations also should be measured if the patient experiences an exacerbation of arrhythmia or develops potential signs or symptoms of procainamide toxicity.

13. The initial procainamide dose for patient CV is calculated as follows.

Pharmacokinetic Dosing Method

Detailed pharmacokinetic studies have not been done in patients with severe liver disease, so this method cannot be used.

Literature-Based Recommended Dosing

1. *Choose a procainamide dose based on the disease states and conditions of the patient.*

A procainamide loading dose of 500 mg over 25 to 30 minutes is administered followed by a continuous infusion. A procainamide dose of 1 to 3 mg/min (2 to 6 mg/min normal dose, reduced by 50%) is suggested by Table 8-3 for an adult with severe liver disease. A dose in the lower end of this range should result in a procainamide steady-state concentration in the lower end of the therapeutic range. A dose of 1 mg/min is prescribed for the patient.

Steady-state procainamide and NAPA serum concentrations can be measured after steady state is attained in 3 to 5 half-lives. Procainamide and NAPA serum concentrations also should be measured if the patient experiences a return of arrhythmia or develops potential signs or symptoms of procainamide toxicity. Procainamide pharmacokinetic parameters can change as the patient's hepatic status changes. Thus, patients with liver failure who are receiving procainamide therapy must be monitored very carefully.

14. The revised procainamide dose for patient CV is calculated as follows.

The patient has cirrhosis and may not have achieved steady-state conditions after 12 hours of therapy. Because of this, it is unlikely that the serum concentration was obtained at steady state, even though a loading dose was given. Therefore, the linear pharmacokinetics and pharmacokinetic parameter methods cannot be used.

Bayesian Pharmacokinetics Computer Program Method

1. *Enter the patient's demographic, drug dosing, and serum concentration–time data into the computer program.*

Note: DrugCalc requires procainamide infusion rates to be entered in terms of mg/h (3 mg/min · 60 min/h = 180 mg/h).

2. *Compute the pharmacokinetic parameters for the patient using the Bayesian pharmacokinetics computer program.*

The pharmacokinetic parameters computed by the program are a volume of distribution of 139 L, a half-life of 8.2 hours, and a clearance of 11.8 L/h.

3. *Compute the dose required to achieve the desired procainamide serum concentrations.*

The one-compartment model infusion equations used by the program to compute doses indicate that a procainamide infusion of 71 mg/h or 1.2 mg/min [(71 mg/h)/(60 min/h) = 1.2 mg/min] will produce a steady-state procainamide concentration of 6 μg/mL. This dose should be started immediately if no adverse effects were noted. However, if the patient is experiencing drug side effects, the new infusion rate should be started after holding the infusion for 8 hours (~1 half-life) to allow procainamide serum concentrations to decrease by half.

15. The initial procainamide dose for patient PE is calculated as follows.

Pharmacokinetic Dosing Method

1. *Estimate the half-life and elimination rate constant according to the disease states and conditions of the patient.*

Patients with severe heart failure have highly variable procainamide pharmacokinetics and dosage requirements. Heart failure patients have decreased cardiac output, which leads to decreased liver blood flow, and the expected procainamide half-life ($t_{1/2}$) is 5.5 hours. The elimination rate constant is computed using the following formula: $k = 0.693/t_{1/2} = 0.693/5.5\ h = 0.126\ h^{-1}$.

2. *Estimate the volume of distribution and clearance.*

The patient is not obese, so the estimated procainamide volume of distribution is based on actual body weight: V = 1.6 L/kg · 67 kg = 107 L. Estimated procainamide clearance is computed by taking the product of the volume of distribution and the elimination rate constant: $Cl = kV = 0.126\ h^{-1} \cdot 107\ L = 13.5\ L/h$.

3. *Compute the dosage regimen.*

Therapy is started by administering an intravenous loading dose of procainamide to the patient: LD = Css · V = 4 mg/L · 107 L = 428 mg, rounded to 400 mg. A loading dose of 400 mg given intravenously over 25 to 30 minutes is given. (Note: μg/mL = mg/L, and this concentration unit was substituted for Css in the calculations to avoid unnecessary unit conversion.)

A procainamide continuous intravenous infusion is started immediately after the loading dose has been administered. The dosage equation for intravenous procainamide is $k_0 = Css \cdot Cl = (4\ mg/L \cdot 13.5\ L/h)/(60\ min/h) = 0.9\ mg/min$, rounded to 1 mg/min.

A steady-state procainamide serum concentration can be measured after steady state is attained in 3 to 5 half-lives. Because procainamide is expected to have a half-life of 5.5 hours in the patient, the procainamide steady-state concentration can be obtained any time after the second day of dosing (5 half-lives = 5 · 5.5 h = 27.5 h). Procainamide serum concentrations also should be measured if the patient experiences an exacerbation of arrhythmia or develops potential signs or symptoms of procainamide toxicity. Procainamide pharmacokinetic parameters can change as the patient's cardiac status changes. If heart failure improves, cardiac output will increase, resulting in increased liver blood flow and procainamide clearance. Alternatively, if heart failure worsens, cardiac output will decrease further, resulting in decreased liver blood flow and procainamide clearance. Thus, patients with heart failure who are receiving procainamide therapy must be monitored very carefully.

Literature-Based Recommended Dosing

1. *Choose a procainamide dose based on the disease states and conditions of the patient.*

A procainamide loading dose of 500 mg over 25 to 30 minutes is administered followed by a continuous infusion. A procainamide dose of 1 to 3 mg/min (2 to 6 mg/min normal dose, reduced by 50%) is suggested by Table 8-4 for an adult with severe heart failure. A dose in the lower end of this range should result in a procainamide steady-state concentration in the lower end of the therapeutic range. A dose of 1 mg/min is prescribed for the patient.

A steady-state procainamide serum concentration can be measured after steady state is attained in 3 to 5 half-lives. Because procainamide is expected to have a half-life of 5.5 hours in the patient, the procainamide steady-state concentration can be obtained any time after the second day of dosing (5 half-lives = 5 · 5.5 h = 27.5 h). Procainamide serum concentrations also should be measured if the patient experiences an exacerbation of arrhythmia or develops potential signs or symptoms of procainamide toxicity. Procainamide pharmacokinetic parameters can change as the patient's cardiac status changes. If heart failure improves, cardiac output increases, resulting in increased liver blood flow and procainamide clearance. Alternatively, if heart failure worsens, cardiac output will decrease further, resulting in decreased liver blood flow and procainamide clearance. Thus, patients with heart failure who are receiving procainamide therapy must be monitored very carefully.

16. The revised procainamide dose for patient PE is calculated as follows.

The patient has severe heart failure and is expected to achieve steady-state conditions after the second day (5 half-lives = 5 · 5.5 h = 27.5 h) of therapy. Because the procainamide serum concentrations were obtained after 4 hours and 8 hours of therapy, it is unlikely that the serum concentrations were obtained at steady state, even though a loading dose was given. Therefore, the linear pharmacokinetics method and the pharmacokinetic parameter method cannot be used.

Chiou Method

1. *Compute the procainamide clearance.*

$$Cl = \frac{2\,k_0}{C_1 + C_2} + \frac{2V(C_1 - C_2)}{(C_1 + C_2)\,(t_2 - t_1)}$$

$$Cl = \frac{2(4\text{ mg/min})}{4.3\text{ mg/L} + 8.8\text{ mg/L}} + \frac{2(1.6\text{ L/kg} \cdot 67\text{ kg})(4.3\text{ mg/L} - 8.8\text{ mg/L})}{(4.3\text{ mg/L} + 8.8\text{ mg/L})\ 240\text{ min}} = 0.30\text{ L/min}$$

Note: μg/mL = mg/L, and this concentration unit was substituted for concentrations to avoid unnecessary unit conversion. In addition, the time difference between t_2 and t_1, in minutes, was determined and placed directly in the calculation.

$$k_0 = Css \cdot Cl = 6 \text{ mg/L} \cdot 0.30 \text{ L/min} = 1.8 \text{ mg/min of procainamide}$$

Bayesian Pharmacokinetics Computer Program Method

1. *Enter the patient's demographic, drug dosing, and serum concentration–time data into the computer program.*

In this case, the patient is not at steady state, so the linear pharmacokinetics method cannot be used. DrugCalc requires procainamide continuous infusions to be entered in terms of mg/h (4 mg/min · 60 min/h = 240 mg/h).

2. *Compute the pharmacokinetic parameters for the patient using the Bayesian pharmacokinetics computer program.*

The pharmacokinetic parameters computed by the program are a volume of distribution of 246 L, a half-life of 13.9 hours, and a clearance of 12.3 L/h or 0.21 L/min [(12.3 L/h)/(60 min/h) = 0.21 L/h].

3. *Compute the dose required to achieve the desired procainamide serum concentrations.*

The one-compartment model infusion equations used by the program to compute doses indicate that a procainamide infusion of 74 mg/h or 1.2 mg/min ([74 mg/h] /60 min/h = 1.2 mg/min) will produce a steady-state procainamide concentration of 6 μg/mL.

REFERENCES

1. Roden DM. Antiarrhythmic drugs. In: Hardman JG, Limbird LE, Molinoff PB, Ruddon RW, Gilman AG, eds. The pharmacological basis of therapeutics. New York: McGraw-Hill, 1996: 839–874.
2. Bauman JL, Schoen MD. Arrhythmias. In: DiPiro JT, Talbert RL, Yee GC, Matzke GR, Wells BG, Posey LM, eds. Pharmacotherapy. Stamford, CT: Appleton & Lange, 1999:232–264.
3. Lima JJ, Conti DR, Goldfarb AL, Golden LH, Jusko WJ. Pharmacokinetic approach to intravenous procainamide therapy. Eur J Clin Pharmacol 1978;13:303–308.
4. Giardina EG, Fenster PE, Bigger JT, Jr, Mayersohn M, Perrier D, Marcus FI. Efficacy, plasma concentrations and adverse effects of a new sustained release procainamide preparation. Am J Cardiol 1980;46:855–862.
5. Manion CV, Lalka D, Baer DT, Meyer MB. Absorption kinetics of procainamide in humans. J Pharm Sci 1977;66:981–984.
6. Graffner C, Johnsson G, Sjogren J. Pharmacokinetics of procainamide intravenously and orally as conventional and slow-release tablets. Clin Pharmacol Ther 1975;17:414–423.
7. Smith TC, Kinkel AW. Plasma levels of procainamide after administration of conventional and sustained-release preparations. Curr Ther Res 1980;27:217–228.
8. Koup JR, Abel RB, Smithers JA, Eldon MA, de Vries TM. Effect of age, gender, and race on steady state procainamide pharmacokinetics after administration of Procanbid sustained-release tablets. Ther Drug Monit 1998;20:73–77.

9. Gibson TP, Matusik J, Matusik E, Nelson HA, Wilkinson J, Briggs WA. Acetylation of procainamide in man and its relationship to isonicotinic acid hydrazide acetylation phenotype. Clin Pharmacol Ther 1975;17:395–399.
10. Dutcher JS, Strong JM, Lucas SV, Lee WK, Atkinson AJ, Jr. Procainamide and *N*-acetylprocainamide kinetics investigated simultaneously with stable isotope methodology. Clin Pharmacol Ther 1977;22:447–457.
11. Lima JJ, Conti DR, Goldfarb AL, Tilstone WJ, Golden LH, Jusko WJ. Clinical pharmacokinetics of procainamide infusions in relation to acetylator phenotype. J Pharmacokinet Biopharm 1979;7:69–85.
12. Myerburg RJ, Kessler KM, Kiem I, et al. Relationship between plasma levels of procainamide, suppression of premature ventricular complexes and prevention of recurrent ventricular tachycardia. Circulation 1981;64:280–290.
13. Galeazzi RL, Sheiner LB, Lockwood T, Benet LZ. The renal elimination of procainamide. Clin Pharmacol Ther 1976;19:55–62.
14. Reidenberg MM, Camacho M, Kluger J, Drayer DE. Aging and renal clearance of procainamide and acetylprocainamide. Clin Pharmacol Ther 1980;28:732–735.
15. Lima JJ, Jusko WJ. Determination of procainamide acetylator status. Clin Pharmacol Ther 1978;23:25–29.
16. Reidenberg MM, Drayer DE, Levy M, Warner H. Polymorphic acetylation procainamide in man. Clin Pharmacol Ther 1975;17:722–730.
17. Lessard E, Fortin A, Belanger PM, Beaune P, Hamelin BA, Turgeon J. Role of CYP2D6 in the *N*-hydroxylation of procainamide. Pharmacogenetics 1997;7:381–390.
18. Tilstone WJ, Lawson DH. Capacity-limited elimination of procainamide in man. Res Commun Chem Pathol Pharmacol 1978;21:343–346.
19. Coyle JD, Boudoulas H, Mackichan JJ, Lima JJ. Concentration-dependent clearance of procainamide in normal subjects. Biopharm Drug Dispos 1985;6:159–165.
20. Giardina EG, Dreyfuss J, Bigger JT, Jr, Shaw JM, Schreiber EC. Metabolism of procainamide in normal and cardiac subjects. Clin Pharmacol Ther 1976;19:339–351.
21. Koch-Weser J. Pharmacokinetic of procainamide in man. Ann N Y Acad Sci 1971;179: 370–382.
22. Koch-Weser J, Klein SW. Procainamide dosage schedules, plasma concentrations, and clinical effects. JAMA 1971;215:1454–1460.
23. Bauer LA, Black D, Gensler A, Sprinkle J. Influence of age, renal function and heart failure on procainamide clearance and *N*-acetylprocainamide serum concentrations. Int J Clin Pharmacol Ther Toxicol 1989;27:213–216.
24. Gibson TP, Lowenthal DT, Nelson HA, Briggs WA. Elimination of procainamide in end stage renal failure. Clin Pharmacol Ther 1975;17:321–329.
25. Gibson TP, Atkinson AJ, Jr, Matusik E, Nelson LD, Briggs WA. Kinetics of procainamide and *N*-acetylprocainamide in renal failure. Kidney Int 1977;12:422–429.
26. Tisdale JE, Rudis MI, Padhi ID, et al. Disposition of procainamide in patients with chronic congestive heart failure receiving medical therapy. J Clin Pharmacol 1996;36:35–41.
27. Mutnick AH, Burke TG. Antiarrhythmics. In: Schumacher GE, ed. Therapeutic drug monitoring. Stamford, CT: Appleton & Lange, 1995:295–343.
28. Pugh RN, Murray-Lyon IM, Dawson JL, Pietroni MC, Williams R. Transection of the oesophagus for bleeding oesophageal varices. Br J Surg 1973;60:646–649.
29. Christoff PB, Conti DR, Naylor C, Jusko WJ. Procainamide disposition in obesity. Drug Intell Clin Pharm 1983;17:516–522.
30. Atkinson AJ, Jr, Krumlovsky FA, Huang CM, del Greco F. Hemodialysis for severe procainamide toxicity: clinical and pharmacokinetic observations. Clin Pharmacol Ther 1976;20: 585–592.

31. Gibson TP, Matusik EJ, Briggs WA. *N*-Acetylprocainamide levels in patients with end-stage renal failure. Clin Pharmacol Ther 1976;19:206–212.

32. Hansten PD, Horn JR. Drug interactions analysis and management. Vancouver, WA: Applied Therapeutics, 1998:527.

33. Bauer LA, Black D, Gensler A. Procainamide-cimetidine drug interaction in elderly male patients. J Am Geriatr Soc 1990;38:467–469.

34. Chiou WL, Gadalla MA, Peng GW. Method for the rapid estimation of the total body drug clearance and adjustment of dosage regimens in patients during a constant-rate intravenous infusion. J Pharmacokinet Biopharm 1978;6:135–151.

35. Wandell M, Mungall D. Computer assisted drug interpretation and drug regimen optimization. Am Assoc Clin Chem 1984;6:1–11.

36. Johnson JA, Parker RB, Geraci SA. Heart failure. In: DiPiro JT, Talbert RL, Yee GC, Matzke GR, Wells BG, Posey LM, eds. Pharmacotherapy—a pathophysiologic approach. Stamford, CT: Appleton & Lange, 1999:153–181.

9

QUINIDINE

INTRODUCTION

Quinidine was one of the first agents used for its antiarrhythmic effects. It is classified as a type IA antiarrhythmic agent and can be used for the management of supraventricular or ventricular arrhythmias.[1,2] After the ventricular rate has been controlled, quinidine therapy can be used to chemically convert atrial fibrillation to normal sinus rhythm. Because of its side-effect profile, quinidine is considered by many clinicians to be a second-line choice of antiarrhythmic agent. Quinidine inhibits transmembrane sodium influx into the conduction system of the heart and decreases conduction velocity.[1,2] It also increases the duration of the action potential, increases threshold potential toward zero, and decreases the slope of phase 4 of the action potential. Automaticity is decreased during quinidine therapy. The net effect of these cellular changes is that quinidine increases refractoriness and decreases conduction in heart conduction tissue, and these effects establish a bidirectional block in reentrant pathways.

THERAPEUTIC AND TOXIC CONCENTRATIONS

When quinidine is given intravenously, the quinidine serum concentration–time curve follows a two-compartment model.[3–6] However, because of marked hypotension and tachycardia when the drug is given intravenously to some patients, the oral route of administration is far more common. When oral quinidine is given as a rapidly absorbed dosage form, such as quinidine sulfate tablets, a similar distribution phase is observed with a duration of 20 to 30 minutes.[3,4,7,8] If extended-release oral dosage forms are given, absorption occurs more slowly than distribution, so a distribution phase does not occur (Figure 9-1).[9–13]

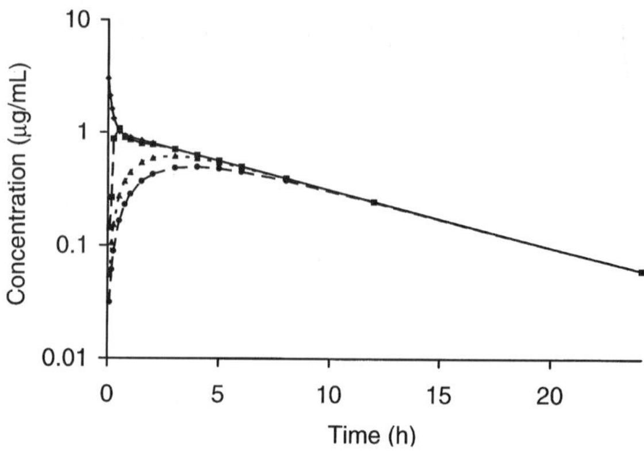

FIGURE 9-1 Quinidine serum concentrations after an intravenous dose (*diamonds*) and three different oral tablets (doses normalized to provide 200 mg of quinidine base systemically). After an intravenous dose, quinidine serum concentrations decline according to a two-compartment model, which demonstrates a distribution phase that lasts for 20 to 30 minutes after injection. Immediate-release quinidine tablets (*squares*) are rapidly absorbed and show a distinct distribution phase. Extended-release quinidine gluconate (*triangles*) and quinidine sulfate (*circles*) have slower absorption profiles, so the drug has an opportunity to distribute to tissues while absorption is occurring. Because of this, no distribution phase is observed for these dosage forms.

The generally accepted therapeutic range for quinidine is 2 to 6 μg/mL. Quinidine serum concentrations above the therapeutic range can cause increased QT-interval or QRS-complex widening (>35% to 50%) on an electrocardiogram (ECG), cinchonism, hypotension, high-degree atrioventricular block, and ventricular arrhythmias. Cinchonism is a collection of symptoms that includes tinnitus, blurred vision, light-headedness, tremor, giddiness, and altered hearing, which decreases in severity with lower quinidine concentrations. Gastrointestinal adverse effects such as anorexia, nausea, vomiting, and diarrhea, the most common side effects of quinidine therapy, can occur after both oral and intravenous quinidine administration but are not strongly correlated with specific serum levels. Quinidine therapy also is associated with syncope and torsades de pointes. Quinidine syncope occurs when ventricular tachycardia, ventricular fibrillation, or a prolongation of QT intervals occurs in a non–dose dependent manner. Torsades de pointes ("twisting of the points") is a form of polymorphic ventricular tachycardia preceded by prolongation of the QT interval. It is characterized by polymorphic QRS complexes that change in amplitude and length, giving the appearance of oscillations around the ECG baseline. Torsades de pointes can develop into multiple episodes of nonsustained polymorphic ventricular tachycardia, syncope, ventricular fibrillation, or sudden cardiac death. Hypersensitivity reactions to quinidine include rash, drug fever, thrombocytopenia, hemolytic anemia, asthma, respiratory depression, a systemic lupus-like syndrome, hepatitis, and anaphylactic shock.

Quinidine metabolites (3-hydroxyquinidine, 2′-quinidinone, quinidine-*N*-oxide, *O*-desmethylquinidine) all have antiarrhythmic effects in animal models.[14–17] Of these compounds, 3-hydroxyquinidine is the most potent (60% to 80% compared with the parent drug) and achieves high enough serum concentrations in humans that its antiarrhythmic effects probably contribute to the clinical effects observed during quinidine treatment. Dihydroquinidine is an impurity contained in commercially available quinidine products that also has antiarrhythmic effects.[18–20] Most products contain less than 10% of the labeled quinidine amount as dihydroquinidine. Clinicians should understand that not all patients with "toxic" quinidine serum concentrations in the listed ranges have signs or symptoms of quinidine toxicity. Rather, quinidine concentrations in the given ranges increase the likelihood that an adverse effect will occur.

For dose adjustment, quinidine serum concentrations are best measured as a predose or trough level at steady state after the patient has received a consistent dosage regimen for 3 to 5 drug half-lives. Quinidine half-life varies from 6 to 8 hours for healthy adults to 9 to 10 hours or more among adults with liver failure. If quinidine is given orally or intravenously on a stable schedule, steady-state serum concentrations are achieved in about 2 days ($5 \cdot 8\ h = 40\ h$).

CLINICAL MONITORING PARAMETERS

The ECG or EKG should be monitored to determine the response to quinidine. The goal of therapy is suppression of arrhythmia and avoidance of adverse drug reactions. Electrophysiologic studies with programmed stimulation to replicate the ventricular arrhythmia or 24-hour ECG monitoring with a Holter monitor can be performed while a patient receives a variety of antiarrhythmic agents to determine effective antiarrhythmic drug therapy.[1]

Because many therapeutic and side effects of quinidine are not correlated with its serum concentration, it is often not necessary to measure quinidine serum concentrations for patients receiving appropriate doses who currently have no arrhythmia or adverse drug effects. However, quinidine serum concentrations should be obtained for patients who have recurrence of tachyarrhythmia, are experiencing possible side effects of quinidine, or are receiving quinidine doses not consistent with disease states and conditions known to alter quinidine pharmacokinetics (see Effects of Disease States and Conditions on Quinidine Pharmacokinetics and Dosing). Serum concentration monitoring can aid in the decision to increase or decrease the quinidine dose. For example, if arrhythmia reappears and the quinidine serum concentration is <6 μg/mL, increasing the quinidine dose is a therapeutic option. However, if the quinidine serum concentration is >6 μg/mL, it is unlikely a dosage increase will be effective in suppressing the arrhythmia, and there is increased likelihood that drug side effects may occur. Similarly, if a patient has a possible concentration-related adverse reaction to quinidine and the quinidine serum concentration is <2 μg/mL, it is possible that the observed problem may not be caused by quinidine treatment, and other sources can be investigated. While receiving quinidine, patients should be monitored for the following adverse drug effects: anorexia, nausea, vomiting, diarrhea, cinchonism, syncope, increased QT-interval or QRS-complex widening (>35% to 50%) on an ECG, hypotension, high-degree atrioventricular block, ventricular arrhythmias, and hypersensitivity reactions (rash, drug fever, thrombocytopenia, hemolytic anemia, asthma, respiratory depression, lupus-like syndrome, hepatitis, and anaphylactic shock).

BASIC CLINICAL PHARMACOKINETIC PARAMETERS

Quinidine is almost completely eliminated by means of hepatic metabolism (~80%).[4,7] Hepatic metabolism is mainly through the cytochrome P450 3A (CYP3A) enzyme system. 3-Hydroxyquinidine is the primary active metabolite of quinidine metabolism, and dihydroquinidine is an active compound that is found as an impurity in most quinidine dosage forms. The hepatic extraction ratio of quinidine is about 30%, so quinidine is typically classified as an intermediate extraction ratio drug. Because of this, it is expected that liver blood flow, unbound fraction of drug in the blood, and intrinsic clearance will all be important factors influencing the clearance of quinidine. After oral administration, quinidine is subject to moderate first-pass metabolism by CYP3A contained in the liver and intestinal wall. Approximately 20% of a quinidine dose is eliminated unchanged in the urine. Although there have been some reports that quinidine follows nonlinear pharmacokinetics, for the purpose of clinical drug dosing, linear pharmacokinetic concepts and equations can be effectively used to compute doses and estimate serum concentrations.[21]

Three different salt forms of quinidine are available. Quinidine sulfate contains 83% quinidine base, quinidine gluconate contains 62% quinidine base, and quinidine polygalacturonate contains 60% quinidine base. The gluconate salt is available for intravenous injection and oral use. Quinidine sulfate and polygalacturonate are available only for oral use. The oral bioavailability of all three quinidine-based drugs is moderate and generally equals 70%, reflecting first-pass metabolism in the intestinal wall and liver.[3,7] Although quinidine injection can be given intramuscularly, this route of administration may cause erratic absorption and serum concentrations.[6]

Plasma protein binding of quinidine in healthy persons is about 80% to 90%.[22–24] The drug binds to both albumin and α_1-acid glycoprotein (AAG). AAG is classified as an acute-phase reactant protein that is present in small amounts in all persons but is secreted in large amounts in response to stresses and disease states such as trauma, heart failure, and myocardial infarction. Among patients with these disease states, quinidine binding to AAG can be even larger, resulting in an unbound fraction as low as 8%.

The recommended dose of quinidine is based on the concurrent disease states and conditions that can influence quinidine pharmacokinetics. Quinidine pharmacokinetic parameters used to compute doses are given in the following section for specific patient profiles.

EFFECTS OF DISEASE STATES AND CONDITIONS ON QUINIDINE PHARMACOKINETICS AND DOSING

Healthy adults without the disease states and conditions discussed later and with normal liver function have an average quinidine half-life of 7 hours (range, 6 to 8 hours) and a volume of distribution for the entire body of 2.4 L/kg (V = 2 to 3 L/kg; Table 9-1).[3–6,9,25–27] Disease states and conditions that change quinidine pharmacokinetics and dosage requirements may alter clearance and volume of distribution. The elimination rate constant ($k = 0.693/t_{1/2}$, where $t_{1/2}$ is the half-life) and clearance ($Cl = kV$) can be computed from the aforementioned pharmacokinetic parameters.

Patients with cirrhosis of the liver have increased quinidine clearance and volume of distribution, which result in a prolonged average quinidine half-life of 9 hours.[28,29] Clear-

TABLE 9-1 Disease States and Conditions That Alter Quinidine Pharmacokinetics

DISEASE STATE/ CONDITION	HALF-LIFE (h)	VOLUME OF DISTRIBUTION (L/kg)	COMMENTS
Adult, normal liver function	7 (range, 6–8)	2.4 (range, 2–3)	Quinidine has a moderate hepatic extraction ratio of ~30%, so liver blood flow, unbound fraction of drug in the blood, and intrinsic clearance are all important factors in clearance rate. Approximately 20% of quinidine is eliminated unchanged in urine.
Adult, liver cirrhosis	9	3.8	Quinidine is metabolized ~80% by hepatic microsomal enzymes (primarily CYP3A). Clearance of total drug is increased in patients with cirrhosis, but intrinsic clearance is decreased. Pharmacokinetic parameters are highly variable among patients with liver disease. Volume of distribution is larger owing to decreased α_1-acid glycoprotein and albumin production by liver, which decreases drug binding in the plasma.
Adult, heart failure	7	1.7	Decreased liver blood flow associated with reduced cardiac output reduces quinidine clearance. Volume of distribution is smaller owing to increased α_1-acid glycoprotein drug binding in the plasma. Heart failure causes large and variable reductions in

(continues)

TABLE 9-1 Disease States and Conditions That Alter Quinidine Pharmacokinetics *(continued)*

DISEASE STATE/ CONDITION	HALF-LIFE (h)	VOLUME OF DISTRIBUTION (L/kg)	COMMENTS
Adult, heart failure *(continued)*			quinidine clearance. Cardiac status must be monitored closely for patients with heart failure because quinidine clearance changes with acute changes in cardiac output.
Adult, obese (>30% over ideal body weight)	According to other disease states or conditions that affect quinidine pharmacokinetics	According to other disease states or conditions that affect quinidine pharmacokinetics	Quinidine doses should be based on ideal body weight for patients who weigh >30% over ideal body weight.

ance and volume of distribution are larger among patients with liver disease because albumin and AAG concentrations are lower among these patients. The result is reduced quinidine plasma protein binding (average V = 3.8 L/kg). The increased unbound fraction in the plasma allows more quinidine to enter the liver parenchyma, where hepatic drug-metabolizing enzymes are present. The result is increased drug clearance. A decrease in plasma protein binding also leads to higher unbound levels for a given total quinidine serum concentration. For example, a total quinidine serum concentration of 3 μg/mL would yield an unbound concentration of 0.3 μg/mL in a patient with normal plasma protein binding (3 μg/mL · 0.1 unbound fraction = 0.3 μg/mL) but an unbound concentration of 0.6 μg/mL in a patient with cirrhosis with decreased plasma protein binding (3 μg/mL · 0.2 unbound fraction = 0.6 μg/mL). The importance of this difference in unbound concentrations has not been assessed for patients with cirrhosis, but clinicians should bear it in mind when monitoring quinidine levels because only total serum concentrations are available from laboratories.

The exact effect of liver disease on quinidine pharmacokinetics is highly variable and difficult to predict accurately. It is possible for a patient with liver disease to have relatively normal or grossly abnormal quinidine clearance, volume of distribution, and half-life. An index of liver dysfunction can be gained by applying the Child-Pugh clinical classification system (Table 9-2).[30] Child-Pugh scores are discussed in Chapter 3 but are discussed briefly here. The Child-Pugh score consists of five laboratory tests or clinical symptoms: serum albumin, total bilirubin, prothrombin time, ascites, and hepatic encephalopathy. Each of these areas is given a score of 1 (normal) to 3 (severely abnormal; see Table 9-2), and the scores for the five areas are totaled. The Child-Pugh score for a patient with normal liver function is 5. The score for a patient with grossly abnormal serum albumin, total bilirubin, and prothrombin time values in addition to severe ascites and hepatic encephalopathy is 15. A Child-Pugh score greater than 8 is grounds for a de-

TABLE 9-2 Child-Pugh Scores for Patients with Liver Disease

TEST/SYMPTOM	SCORE 1 POINT	SCORE 2 POINTS	SCORE 3 POINTS
Total bilirubin (mg/dL)	<2.0	2.0–3.0	>3.0
Serum albumin (g/dL)	>3.5	2.8–3.5	<2.8
Prothrombin time (seconds prolonged over control)	<4	4–6	>6
Ascites	Absent	Slight	Moderate
Hepatic encephalopathy	None	Moderate	Severe

From Pugh RN, Murray-Lyon IM, Dawson JL, Pietroni MC, Williams R. Transection of the oesophagus for bleeding oesophageal varices. Br J Surg 1973;60:646–649.

crease of 25% to 50% in the initial daily drug dose of quinidine. As for any patient with or without liver dysfunction, initial doses are meant as starting points for dosage titration based on patient response and avoidance of adverse effects. Quinidine serum concentrations and the presence of adverse drug effects should be monitored frequently for patients with cirrhosis of the liver.

Heart failure reduces quinidine clearance because of decreased hepatic blood flow due to compromised cardiac output (Table 9-3).[7,8,31,32] Volume of distribution (V = 1.7 L/kg) is decreased because patients with heart failure have elevated AAG serum concentrations. The increase in AAG concentration causes increased quinidine plasma protein binding and a decrease in the unbound fraction of quinidine. Because clearance and volume of distribution decrease simultaneously, patients with heart failure have an average quinidine half-life of 7 hours, which is similar to that of a healthy person [$t_{1/2} = (0.693 \cdot \downarrow V)/\downarrow Cl$]. Increased plasma protein binding also leads to lower unbound levels of a given total quinidine serum concentration. For example, a total quinidine serum concentration of 3

TABLE 9-3 New York Heart Association Functional Classification for Heart Failure

CLASS	DESCRIPTION
I	Patients with cardiac disease but without limitations of physical activity. Ordinary physical activity does not cause undue fatigue, dyspnea, or palpitation.
II	Patients with cardiac disease that results in slight limitations of physical activity. Ordinary physical activity results in fatigue, palpitation, dyspnea, or angina.
III	Patients with cardiac disease that results in marked limitations of physical activity. Although patients are comfortable at rest, less than ordinary activity leads to symptoms.
IV	Patients with cardiac disease that results in an inability to carry on physical activity without discomfort. Symptoms of congestive heart failure are present even at rest. With any physical activity, increased discomfort is experienced.

From Johnson JA, Parker RB, Geraci SA. Heart failure. In: DiPiro JT, Talbert RL, Yee GC, Matzke GR, Wells BG, Posey LM, eds. Pharmacotherapy: a pathophysiologic approach. Stamford, CT: Appleton & Lange, 1999:153–181.

μg/mL would yield an unbound concentration of 0.3 μg/mL for a patient with normal plasma protein binding (3 μg/mL · 0.1 unbound fraction = 0.3 μg/mL) but an unbound concentration of 0.15 μg/mL in a patient with heart failure with increased plasma protein binding (3 μg/mL · 0.05 unbound fraction = 0.15 μg/mL). The clinical significance of this difference in unbound concentration has not been assessed for patients with heart failure. The effect of heart failure on quinidine pharmacokinetics is highly variable and difficult to predict accurately. It is possible for a patient with heart failure to have relatively normal or grossly abnormal quinidine clearance and half-life. For patients with heart failure, initial doses are meant as starting points for dosage titration based on patient response and avoidance of adverse effects. Quinidine serum concentrations and the presence of adverse drug effects should be monitored frequently for patients with heart failure.

Patients with myocardial infarction may have serious arrhythmias that necessitate therapy with quinidine. After a myocardial infarction, serum AAG concentrations increase as high as 50% over 12 to 72 hours. As AAG serum concentrations increase, plasma protein binding of quinidine increases, and the unbound fraction of quinidine decreases. Because quinidine is considered to have a moderate hepatic extraction ratio, a decline in the unbound fraction of quinidine in the plasma decreases quinidine clearance.

Patient age has an effect on quinidine clearance and half-life.[15,33] Among patients older than 65 years, studies indicate that quinidine clearance is reduced, the volume of distribution is unchanged, and half-life is longer (average half-life, 10 hours) compared with those of younger persons. A confounding factor found in pharmacokinetic studies of quinidine conducted with older adults is the possible accidental inclusion of subjects who have subclinical or mild cases of the conditions associated with reduced quinidine clearance, such as heart failure and liver disease. Most patients with serious arrhythmias who participated in the previously mentioned investigations were older, and those results include any influence of age. Thus in most cases, elderly patients are treated with quinidine according to the other diseases or conditions present that influence quinidine pharmacokinetics.

Because detailed studies have not been conducted with obese patients, ideal body weight (IBW) should be used to compute initial doses of quinidine to avoid accidental overdose among overweight persons (>30% greater than IBW). Because only 20% of a quinidine dose is eliminated unchanged by the kidney, dosage adjustments for patients with renal failure usually are not needed.[14,32] Quinidine is not appreciably removed with hemodialysis or peritoneal dialysis.[34,35]

DRUG INTERACTIONS

Quinidine has serious drug interactions with other drugs that are capable of inhibiting the CYP3A enzyme system.[36] Because this isozyme is present in the intestinal wall and liver, quinidine serum concentrations may increase owing to decreased clearance, decreased first-pass metabolism, or a combination of both. Erythromycin, ketoconazole, and verapamil have been reported to increase quinidine serum concentration or area under the concentration–time curve (AUC) by >30% to 50%. Other macrolide antibiotics, such as clarithromycin, or azole antifungals, such as fluconazole, miconazole, and itraconazole, that inhibit CYP3A probably cause similar drug interactions with quinidine. Cimetidine and amiodarone also have been reported to cause increases in quinidine concentrations or AUC of a similar magnitude. Drugs that induce CYP3A (phenytoin, phenobarbital, rifampin, rifabutin) decrease quinidine serum concentrations by increasing quinidine clearance and first-pass metabolism. It is important to remember that phenytoin has antiarrhythmic effects and is classified as a type IB antiarrhythmic agent. Because of this, phenytoin and quinidine may have additive pharmacologic effects that can cause a pharmacodynamic drug interaction.

Although it is not a substrate for the enzyme, quinidine is a potent inhibitor of the CYP2D6 enzyme system.[36–39] As little as 50 mg of quinidine can effectively turn an extensive metabolizer into a poor metabolizer of this isozyme. Because poor metabolizers of CYP2D6 substrates have little to none of this enzyme in the liver, administration of quinidine does not cause a drug interaction among these persons. Quinidine can decrease 30% or more the clearance of β-adrenergic receptor blockers eliminated by CYP2D6. Propranolol, metoprolol, and timolol have decreased clearance owing to quinidine coadministration. Tricyclic antidepressants (nortriptyline, imipramine, desipramine), haloperidol, and dextromethorphan also have increased serum concentrations when given with quinidine. Codeine is a prodrug with no analgesic effect that relies on conversion to morphine by the CYP2D6 enzyme system to decrease pain. When quinidine is given concomitantly with codeine, conversion from codeine to morphine does not take place, and patients do not experience analgesia. A similar drug interaction may occur with dihydrocodeine and hydrocodone. Although it may not be reported in the literature for a specific compound, clinicians should consider that a drug interaction is possible between quinidine and any CYP2D6 substrate.

Quinidine increases digoxin serum concentrations 30% to 50% by decreasing digoxin renal and nonrenal clearance and the volume of distribution of digoxin.[36] The probable mechanisms of this drug interaction are inhibition of elimination of digoxin renal and hepatic p-glycoprotein (PGP) and tissue binding displacement of digoxin by quinidine. Antacids can increase urinary pH. The increase in pH increases renal tubular reabsorption of un-ionized quinidine and decreases quinidine renal clearance. Administration of kaolin-pectin results in physical adsorption of quinidine in the gastrointestinal tract and decreases oral absorption of quinidine. The pharmacologic effects of warfarin and neuromuscular blockers have been enhanced when these drugs were given with quinidine.

INITIAL DOSAGE DETERMINATION METHODS

Pharmacokinetic Dosing Method

The goal of initial dosing of quinidine is to compute the best dose possible for the patient given the diseases and conditions that influence quinidine pharmacokinetics and the arrhythmia for which the patient is being treated. Pharmacokinetic parameters for the patient are estimated with average parameters measured for other patients with similar disease state and condition profiles.

ESTIMATE OF HALF-LIFE AND ELIMINATION RATE CONSTANT

Quinidine is predominately metabolized by the liver. There is no good way to estimate the elimination characteristics of liver-metabolized drugs with an endogenous marker of liver function in the same manner that serum creatinine and estimated creatinine clearance are used to estimate the elimination of agents that are eliminated by the kidney. Because of this, a patient is categorized according to the diseases and conditions known to change the half-life of quinidine. The half-life previously measured in these studies is used as an estimate of the current patient's half-life (see Table 9-1). For a patient with moderate heart failure (New York Heart Association [NYHA] congestive heart failure class III), the half-life of quinidine would be assumed to be 7 hours. A patient with severe liver disease (Child-Pugh score, 12) would be assigned an estimated half-life of 9 hours. To produce the most conservative quinidine doses for patients with several concurrent diseases or conditions that affect quinidine pharmacokinetics, the disease or condition with the longest half-life should be used to compute doses. This approach avoids accidental overdosage as much as currently possible. Once the correct half-life is identified for the patient, it can be converted into the quinidine elimination rate constant (k) with the following equation: $k = 0.693/t_{1/2}$.

ESTIMATE OF VOLUME OF DISTRIBUTION

As with the half-life estimate, the quinidine volume of distribution is chosen according to the disease states and conditions present (see Table 9-1). The volume of distribution is used to help compute quinidine clearance and is assumed to equal 3.8 L/kg for patients with liver disease, 1.7 L/kg for patients with heart failure, and 2.4 L/kg for all other patients. For obese patients (>30% above IBW), IBW is used to compute quinidine volume of distribution. Thus for a nonobese 80-kg patient without heart failure or liver disease, the estimated volume of distribution of quinidine is 192 L: $V = 2.4\ L/kg \cdot 80\ kg = 192\ L$. For a 150-kg obese patient with an ideal body weight of 60 kg and normal cardiac and liver function, the estimated volume of distribution of quinidine is 144 L: $V = 2.4\ L/kg \cdot 60\ kg = 144\ L$.

SELECTION OF APPROPRIATE PHARMACOKINETIC MODEL AND EQUATIONS

When given orally, quinidine follows a one- or two-compartment pharmacokinetic model (see Figure 9-1). When oral therapy is required, most clinicians use a sustained-release dosage form that has good bioavailability (F = 0.7), supplies a continuous release of quinidine into the gastrointestinal tract, and provides a smooth quinidine serum concentration–time curve that emulates intravenous infusion when given every 8 to 12 hours. Because of this, a very simple pharmacokinetic equation that computes the average steady-state serum concentration of quinidine (Css in μg/mL = mg/L) is widely used and allows maintenance dosage calculation: $Css = [F \cdot S\ (D/\tau)]/Cl$ or $D = (Css \cdot Cl \cdot \tau)/(F \cdot S)$, where F is the bioavailability fraction for the oral dosage form (F = 0.7 for most oral quinidine products); S is the fraction of the quinidine salt form that is active quinidine (S = 0.83 for sulfate, immediate-release tablets of 100, 200, 300 mg and extended-release tablets of 300 mg; S = 0.62 for gluconate, extended-release tablets of 324 mg; S = 0.60 for polygalacturonate, immediate-release tablets of 275 mg); D is the dose of quinidine salt in milligrams; and τ is the dosage interval in hours. Cl is quinidine clearance in L/h and is computed with estimates of quinidine elimination rate constant (k) and volume of distribution: Cl = kV. For example, for a patient with an estimated elimination rate constant of $0.099\ h^{-1}$ and an estimated volume of distribution of 168 L, the estimated clearance would equal 16.6 L/h: $Cl = 0.099\ h^{-1} \cdot 168\ L = 16.6\ L/h$.

SELECTION OF STEADY-STATE CONCENTRATION

The generally accepted therapeutic range of quinidine is 2 to 6 μg/mL. However, quinidine therapy must be individualized for each patient to achieve optimal responses and minimal side effects.

Example 1 LK is a 50-year-old, 75-kg (height, 178 cm) man with ventricular tachycardia who needs therapy with oral quinidine gluconate. He has normal liver and cardiac function. Suggest an initial oral quinidine dosage regimen designed to achieve a steady-state quinidine concentration of 3 μg/mL.

1. *Estimate the half-life and elimination rate constant according to disease states and conditions present in the patient.*

The expected quinidine half-life ($t_{1/2}$) is 7 hours. The elimination rate constant is computed with the following formula: $k = 0.693/t_{1/2} = 0.693/7\ h = 0.099\ h^{-1}$.

2. *Estimate the volume of distribution and clearance.*

The patient is not obese, so the estimated volume of distribution of quinidine is based on actual body weight: V = 2.4 L/kg · 75 kg = 180 L. Estimated quinidine clearance is computed by multiplying V and the elimination rate constant: $Cl = kV = 0.099\ h^{-1} \cdot 180\ L = 17.8\ L/h$.

3. *Compute the dosage regimen.*

Oral extended-release quinidine gluconate tablets will be prescribed to this patient (F = 0.7, S = 0.62). The initial dosage interval (τ) is set to 8 hours. (Note: μg/mL = mg/L, and this concentration unit was substituted for Css in the calculations to avoid unit conversion.) The dosage equation for oral quinidine is $D = (Css \cdot Cl \cdot \tau)/(F \cdot S) = (3\ mg/L \cdot 17.8\ L/h \cdot 8\ h)/(0.7 \cdot 0.62) = 984\ mg$, rounded to 972 mg every 8 hours.

Steady-state serum concentration of quinidine can be measured after steady state is attained in 3 to 5 half-lives. Because the drug is expected to have a half-life of 7 hours in this patient, the quinidine steady-state concentration can be obtained any time after the second day of dosing (5 half-lives = 5 · 7 h = 35 h). Serum concentration of quinidine should be measured if the patient has a return of arrhythmia or has signs or symptoms of quinidine toxicity.

Example 2 OI is a 60-year-old, 85-kg (height, 185 cm) man with atrial fibrillation who needs therapy with oral quinidine sulfate. He has cirrhosis of the liver (Child-Pugh score, 11). Suggest an initial extended-release quinidine sulfate dosage regimen designed to achieve a steady-state quinidine concentration of 2 μg/mL.

1. *Estimate the half-life and elimination rate constant according to disease states and conditions present in the patient.*

The expected quinidine half-life ($t_{1/2}$) is 9 hours. The elimination rate constant is computed with the following formula: $k = 0.693/t_{1/2} = 0.693/9\ h = 0.077\ h^{-1}$.

2. *Estimate the volume of distribution and clearance.*

The patient is not obese, so the estimated quinidine volume of distribution is based on actual body weight: V = 3.8 L/kg · 85 kg = 323 L. Estimated quinidine clearance is computed by multiplying V and the elimination rate constant: Cl = kV = 0.077 h^{-1} · 323 L = 24.9 L/h.

3. *Compute the dosage regimen.*

Oral extended-release quinidine sulfate tablets will be prescribed to this patient (F = 0.7, S = 0.83). The initial dosage interval (τ) will be set to 8 hours. (Note: μg/mL = mg/L, and this concentration unit was substituted for Css in the calculations to avoid unit conversion.) The dosage equation for oral quinidine is D = (Css · Cl · τ)/(F · S) = (2 mg/L · 24.9 L/h · 8 h)/(0.7 · 0.83) = 686 mg, rounded to 600 mg every 8 hours.

Steady-state serum concentration of quinidine can be measured after steady state is attained in 3 to 5 half-lives. Because the drug is expected to have a half-life of 9 hours in this patient, the quinidine steady-state concentration can be obtained any time after the second day of dosing (5 half-lives = 5 · 9 h = 45 h). Serum concentration of quinidine should be measured if the patient has a return of arrhythmia or if the patient has signs or symptoms of quinidine toxicity.

Example 3 MN is a 64-year-old, 78-kg (height, 175 cm) man with ventricular tachycardia who needs therapy with oral quinidine. He has moderate heart failure (NYHA class III). Suggest an initial extended-release quinidine gluconate dosage regimen designed to achieve a steady-state quinidine concentration of 3 μg/mL.

1. *Estimate the half-life and elimination rate constant according to disease states and conditions present in the patient.*

The expected quinidine half-life ($t_{1/2}$) is 7 hours. The elimination rate constant is computed with the following formula: k = 0.693/$t_{1/2}$ = 0.693/7 h = 0.099 h^{-1}.

2. *Estimate the volume of distribution and clearance.*

The patient is not obese, so the estimated quinidine volume of distribution is based on actual body weight: V = 1.7 L/kg · 78 kg = 133 L. Estimated quinidine clearance is computed by taking the product of V and the elimination rate constant: Cl = kV = 0.099 h^{-1} · 133 L = 13.2 L/h.

3. *Compute the dosage regimen.*

Oral extended-release quinidine gluconate tablets will be prescribed to this patient (F = 0.7, S = 0.62). The initial dosage interval (τ) will be set to 8 hours. (Note: μg/mL = mg/L, and this concentration unit was substituted for Css in the calculations to avoid unit conversion.) The dosage equation for oral quinidine is D = (Css · Cl · τ)/(F · S) = (3 mg/L · 13.2 L/h · 8 h)/(0.7 · 0.62) = 730 mg, rounded to 648 mg every 8 hours.

Steady-state serum concentration of quinidine can be measured after steady state is attained in 3 to 5 half-lives. Because the drug is expected to have a half-life of 7 hours in this patient, the quinidine steady-state concentration can be obtained any time after the second day of dosing (5 half-lives = 5 · 7 h = 35 h). Serum concentration of quinidine should be measured if the patient has a return of arrhythmia or if the patient has signs or symptoms of quinidine toxicity.

Literature-Based Recommended Dosing

Because of the large amount of variability in quinidine pharmacokinetics, even when concurrent disease states and conditions are identified, many clinicians believe that the use of standard quinidine doses for various situations is warranted. The original computation of these doses was based on the pharmacokinetic dosing method described in the previous section and subsequently modified on the basis of clinical experience. In general, the quinidine steady-state serum concentration expected from the lower end of the dosage range was 2 to 4 μg/mL and 4 to 6 μg/mL for the upper end of the dosage range. Suggested oral quinidine maintenance doses are given in Table 9-4. A 25% to 50% reduction in initial quinidine dose is suggested for patients with moderate to severe liver disease (Child-Pugh score, ≥8) or moderate-severe heart failure (NYHA class II or greater). When a patient has more than one disease or condition, choosing the lowest daily dose results in the safest, most conservative dosage recommendation.

To illustrate the similarities and differences between this method of dosage calculation and the pharmacokinetic dosing method, the examples from the previous section are repeated.

Example 1 LK is a 50-year-old, 75-kg (height, 178 cm) man with ventricular tachycardia who needs therapy with oral quinidine gluconate. He has normal liver and cardiac function. Suggest an initial oral quinidine dosage regimen designed to achieve a steady-state quinidine concentration of 3 μg/mL.

1. *Choose the quinidine dose based on disease states and conditions present in the patient.*

A quinidine gluconate maintenance dose of 628 mg every 12 hours (1256 mg/d) is suggested for a patient without heart failure or liver disease who needs a quinidine steady-state serum concentration in the lower end of the therapeutic range.

Steady-state serum concentration of quinidine can be measured after steady state is attained in 3 to 5 half-lives. Because the drug is expected to have a half-life of 7 hours in this patient, the quinidine steady-state concentration can be obtained any time after the second day of dosing (5 half-lives = 5 · 7 h = 35 h). Serum concentration of quinidine

TABLE 9-4 Literature-Based Recommended Oral Quinidine Initial Dosage Ranges for Various Disease States and Conditions

DISEASE STATE/ CONDITION	QUINIDINE SULFATE, IMMEDIATE-RELEASE TABLETS	QUINIDINE SULFATE, EXTENDED-RELEASE TABLETS	QUINIDINE GLUCONATE, EXTENDED-RELEASE TABLETS	QUINIDINE POLYGALACTURONATE, TABLETS
Adult, normal liver function	200–300 mg every 6–8 h	600 mg every 8–12 h	324–648 mg every 8–12 h	275–413 mg every 6–8 h
Adult, liver cirrhosis or heart failure	100–200 mg every 6–8 h	300 mg every 8–12 h	324 mg every 8–12 hours	138–275 mg every 6–8 h

should be measured if the patient has a return of arrhythmia or if the patient has signs or symptoms of quinidine toxicity.

Example 2 OI is a 60-year-old, 85-kg (height, 185 cm) man with atrial fibrillation who needs therapy with oral quinidine sulfate. He has liver cirrhosis (Child-Pugh score, 11). Suggest an initial immediate-release quinidine sulfate dosage regimen designed to achieve a steady-state quinidine concentration of 2 μg/mL.

1. *Choose the quinidine dose based on disease states and conditions present in the patient.*

A quinidine sulfate maintenance dose of 100 mg every 6 hours (400 mg/d) is suggested for a patient with liver disease who needs a quinidine steady-state serum concentration in the lower end of the therapeutic range.

Steady-state serum concentration of quinidine can be measured after steady state is attained in 3 to 5 half-lives. Because the drug is expected to have a half-life of 9 hours in this patient, the quinidine steady-state concentration can be obtained any time after the second day of dosing (5 half-lives = $5 \cdot 9$ h = 45 h). Serum concentration of quinidine should be measured if the patient has a return of arrhythmia or if the patient has signs or symptoms of quinidine toxicity.

Example 3 MN is a 64-year-old, 78-kg (height, 175 cm) man with ventricular tachycardia who needs therapy with oral quinidine. He has moderate heart failure (NYHA class III). Suggest an initial extended-release quinidine gluconate dosage regimen designed to achieve a steady-state quinidine concentration of 3 μg/mL.

1. *Choose the quinidine dose based on disease states and conditions present in the patient.*

A quinidine gluconate maintenance dose of 324 mg every 12 hours (648 mg/d) is suggested for a patient with heart failure who needs a quinidine steady-state serum concentration in the lower end of the therapeutic range.

Steady-state serum concentration of quinidine can be measured after steady state is attained in 3 to 5 half-lives. Because the drug is expected to have a half-life of 7 hours in this patient, the quinidine steady-state concentration can be obtained any time after the second day of dosing (5 half-lives = $5 \cdot 7$ h = 35 h). Serum concentration of quinidine should be measured if the patient has a return of arrhythmia or if the patient has signs or symptoms of quinidine toxicity.

USE OF QUINIDINE SERUM CONCENTRATIONS TO ALTER DOSES

Because of the large amount of pharmacokinetic variability among patients, it is likely that doses computed with patient population characteristics will not always produce quinidine serum concentrations that are expected or desirable. Because of pharmacokinetic variability, the narrow therapeutic index of quinidine, and the desire to avoid the adverse side effects of quinidine, measurement of quinidine serum concentrations can be a useful adjunct for patients to ensure that therapeutic, nontoxic levels are present. In addition to quinidine serum concentrations, important patient variables, such as ECG findings, clinical signs and symptoms of arrhythmia, and potential quinidine side effects, should be followed to confirm that the patient is responding to treatment and not developing adverse drug reactions.

When quinidine serum concentrations are measured for patients and a dosage change is necessary, clinicians should seek to use the simplest, most straightforward method available to determine a dose that will provide safe and effective treatment. In most cases, a simple dosage ratio can be used to change quinidine doses if the drug follows *linear pharmacokinetics*. Thus assuming linear pharmacokinetics is adequate for dosage adjustments for most patients.

Sometimes it is useful to compute quinidine pharmacokinetic constants for a patient and to base dosage adjustments on these parameters. In this case, it may be possible to calculate and use *pharmacokinetic parameters* to alter the quinidine dose. In some situations, it may be necessary to compute quinidine pharmacokinetic parameters as soon as possible for the patient before steady-state conditions occur and to use these parameters to calculate the best drug dose. Computerized methods that incorporate expected population pharmacokinetic characteristics (*Bayesian pharmacokinetics computer programs*) can be used in difficult situations in which serum concentrations are obtained at suboptimal times or the patient was not at steady state when serum concentrations were measured.

Linear Pharmacokinetics Method

Because quinidine follows linear, dose-proportional pharmacokinetics in most patients, steady-state serum concentrations change in proportion to dose according to the following equation: $D_{new}/Css_{new} = D_{old}/Css_{old}$ or $D_{new} = (Css_{new}/Css_{old})D_{old}$, where D is the dose, Css is the steady-state concentration, old indicates the dose that produced the steady-state concentration that the patient is currently receiving, and new denotes the dose necessary to produce the desired steady-state concentration. The advantages of this method are that it is quick and simple. The disadvantage is that steady-state concentrations are required. Because nonlinear pharmacokinetics of quinidine have been observed in some patients, suggested dosage increases >75% with this method should be scrutinized by the prescribing clinician. The risk versus benefit for the patient should be assessed before large dosage increases are initiated (>75% over current dose).

Example 1 LK is a 50-year-old, 75-kg (height, 178 cm) man with ventricular tachycardia who needs therapy with quinidine gluconate. He has normal liver and cardiac function. The current steady-state quinidine concentration is 2.2 μg/mL at a dose of 324 mg every 8 hours. Compute a quinidine dose that will provide a steady-state concentration of 4 μg/mL.

1. *Compute the new dose to achieve desired serum concentration.*

The patient is expected to achieve steady-state conditions after the second day (5 half-lives = 5 · 7 h = 35 h) of therapy.

With linear pharmacokinetics, the new dose to attain the desired concentration should be proportional to the old dose that produced the measured concentration. (Note: Total daily dose = 324 mg/dose · 3 doses/d = 972 mg/d.)

$$D_{new} = (Css_{new}/Css_{old})D_{old} = [(4\ \mu g/mL)/(2.2\ \mu g/mL)]\ 972\ mg/d$$
$$= 1767\ mg/d,\ \text{rounded to 1944 mg/d or 648 mg every 8 hours}$$

The new suggested dose is 648 mg every 8 hours of oral quinidine gluconate to be started immediately.

Steady-state serum concentration of quinidine can be measured after steady state is attained in 3 to 5 half-lives. Because the drug is expected to have a half-life of 7 hours in this patient, the quinidine steady-state concentration can be obtained any time after the second day of dosing (5 half-lives = 5 · 7 h = 35 h). Serum concentration of quinidine should be measured if the patient has a return of arrhythmia or if the patient has signs or symptoms of quinidine toxicity.

Example 2 OI is a 60-year-old, 85-kg (height, 185 cm) man with atrial fibrillation who needs therapy with oral quinidine sulfate extended-release tablets. He has cirrhosis of the liver (Child-Pugh score, 11). The current steady-state quinidine concentration is 7.4 μg/mL at a dose of 600 mg every 12 hours. Compute a quinidine dose that will provide a steady-state concentration of 3 μg/mL.

1. *Compute a new dose to achieve the desired serum concentration.*

The patient is expected to achieve steady-state conditions after 2 days (5 half-lives = 5 · 9 h = 45 h) of therapy.

With linear pharmacokinetics, the new dose to attain the desired concentration should be proportional to the old dose that produced the measured concentration. (Note: Total daily dose = 600 mg/dose · 2 doses/d = 1200 mg/d.)

$$D_{new} = (Css_{new}/Css_{old})D_{old} = [(3\ \mu g/mL)/(7.4\ \mu g/mL)]\ 1200\ mg/d$$
$$= 486\ mg/d,\ \text{rounded to}\ 600\ mg/d$$

The new suggested dose is 300 mg every 12 hours of quinidine sulfate extended-release tablets. If the patient is experiencing adverse drug effects, the new dosage regimen can be held for 1 or 2 estimated half-lives ($t_{1/2}$ = 9 h).

Steady-state serum concentration of quinidine can be measured after steady state is attained in 3 to 5 half-lives. Because the drug is expected to have a half-life of 9 hours in this patient, the quinidine steady-state concentration can be obtained any time after the second day of dosing (5 half-lives = 5 · 9 h = 45 h). Serum concentration of quinidine should be measured if the patient has a return of arrhythmia or if the patient has signs or symptoms of quinidine toxicity.

Example 3 MN is a 64-year-old, 78-kg (height, 175 cm) man with ventricular tachycardia who needs therapy with oral quinidine sulfate immediate-release tablets. He has moderate heart failure (NYHA class III). The current steady-state quinidine concentration is 2.2 μg/mL at a dose of 100 mg every 6 hours. Compute a quinidine dose that will provide a steady-state concentration of 4 μg/mL.

1. *Compute a new dose to achieve the desired serum concentration.*

The patient is expected to achieve steady-state conditions after 2 days (5 half-lives = 5 · 7 h = 35 h) of therapy.

With linear pharmacokinetics, the new dose to attain the desired concentration should be proportional to the old dose that produced the measured concentration. (Note: Total daily dose = 100 mg/dose · 4 doses/d = 400 mg/d.)

$$D_{new} = (Css_{new}/Css_{old})D_{old} = [(4\ \mu g/mL)/(2.2\ \mu g/mL)]\ 400\ mg/d$$
$$= 727\ mg/d, \text{ rounded to } 800\ mg/d \text{ or } 200\ mg \text{ every 6 hours}$$

The new suggested dose is 200 mg every 6 hours of quinidine sulfate immediate-release tablets to begin immediately.

Steady-state quinidine serum concentration can be measured after steady state is attained in 3 to 5 half-lives. Because the drug is expected to have a half-life of 7 hours in this patient, the quinidine steady-state concentration can be obtained any time after the second day of dosing (5 half-lives = 5 · 9 h = 45 h). Serum concentration of quinidine should be measured if the patient has a return of arrhythmia or if the patient has signs or symptoms of quinidine toxicity.

Pharmacokinetic Parameter Method

The pharmacokinetic parameter method of adjusting drug doses was among the first techniques available to change doses using serum concentrations. A patient's unique pharmacokinetic constants are computed and used to calculate a dose that achieves desired quinidine concentrations. Use of the pharmacokinetic parameter method requires that steady state has been achieved, and only a steady-state quinidine concentration (Css) is used. If the patient is receiving oral quinidine therapy, quinidine clearance (Cl) can be calculated with the following formula: $Cl = [F \cdot S\ (D/\tau)]/Css$, where F is the bioavailability fraction of the oral dosage form (F = 0.7 for most oral quinidine products), S is the fraction of the quinidine salt form that is active quinidine (S = 0.83 for quinidine sulfate, S = 0.62 for quinidine gluconate, S = 0.60 for quinidine polygalacturonate), D is the dose of quinidine salt in milligrams, Css is the steady-state quinidine concentration, and τ is the dosage interval in hours. Because linear pharmacokinetics are assumed, quinidine doses computed with the pharmacokinetic parameter method and the linear pharmacokinetic method should be identical.

Example 1 LK is a 50-year-old, 75-kg (height, 178 cm) man with ventricular tachycardia who needs therapy with quinidine gluconate. He has normal liver and cardiac function. The current steady-state quinidine concentration is 2.2 μg/mL at a dose of 324 mg every 8 hours. Compute a quinidine dose that will provide a steady-state concentration of 4 μg/mL.

1. *Compute the pharmacokinetic parameters.*

The patient is expected to achieve steady-state conditions after the second day (5 half-lives = 5 · 7 h = 35 h) of therapy.

Quinidine clearance can be computed with a steady-state quinidine concentration: $Cl = [F \cdot S\ (D/\tau)]/Css = [0.7 \cdot 0.62\ (324\ mg/8\ h)]/(2.2\ mg/L) = 7.99\ L/h$. (Note: μg/mL = mg/L, and this concentration unit was substituted for Css in the calculations to avoid unit conversion.)

2. *Compute the quinidine dose.*

Quinidine clearance is used to compute the new dose: D = (Css · Cl · τ)/(F · S) = (4 mg/L · 7.99 L/h · 8 h)/(0.7 · 0.62) = 589 mg, rounded to 648 mg every 8 hours.

The new quinidine dose is instituted immediately.

Steady-state serum concentration of quinidine can be measured after steady state is attained in 3 to 5 half-lives. Because the drug is expected to have a half-life of 7 hours in this patient, the quinidine steady-state concentration can be obtained any time after the second day of dosing (5 half-lives = 5 · 7 h = 35 h). Serum concentration of quinidine should be measured if the patient has a return of arrhythmia or if the patient has signs or symptoms of quinidine toxicity.

Example 2 OI is a 60-year-old, 85-kg (height, 185 cm) man with atrial fibrillation who needs therapy with oral quinidine sulfate extended-release tablets. He has cirrhosis of the liver (Child-Pugh score, 11). The current steady-state quinidine concentration is 7.4 μg/mL at a dose of 600 mg every 12 hours. Compute a quinidine dose that will provide a steady-state concentration of 3 μg/mL.

1. *Compute the pharmacokinetic parameters.*

The patient is expected to achieve steady-state conditions after the second day (5 half-lives = 5 · 9 h = 45 h) of therapy.

Quinidine clearance can be computed with a steady-state quinidine concentration: Cl = [F · S (D/τ)]/Css = [0.7 · 0.83 (600 mg/12 h)]/(7.4 mg/L) = 3.93 L/h. (Note: μg/mL = mg/L, and this concentration unit was substituted for Css in the calculations to avoid unit conversion.)

2. *Compute the quinidine dose.*

Quinidine clearance is used to compute the new dose: D = (Css · Cl · τ)/(F · S) = (3 mg/L · 3.93 L/h · 12 h)/(0.7 · 0.83) = 244 mg, rounded to 300 mg every 12 hours.

The new quinidine dose is instituted immediately.

Steady-state serum concentration of quinidine can be measured after steady state is attained in 3 to 5 half-lives. Because the drug is expected to have a half-life of 9 hours in this patient, the quinidine steady-state concentration can be obtained any time after the second day of dosing (5 half-lives = 5 · 9 h = 45 h). Serum concentration of quinidine should be measured if the patient has a return of arrhythmia or if the patient has signs or symptoms of quinidine toxicity.

Example 3 MN is a 64-year-old, 78-kg (height, 175 cm) man with ventricular tachycardia who needs therapy with oral quinidine sulfate immediate-release tablets. He has moderate heart failure (NYHA class III). The current steady-state quinidine concentration is 2.2 μg/mL at a dose of 100 mg every 6 hours. Compute a quinidine dose that will provide a steady-state concentration of 4 μg/mL.

1. *Compute the pharmacokinetic parameters.*

The patient is expected to achieve steady-state conditions after the second day (5 half-lives = 5 · 7 h = 35 h) of therapy.

Quinidine clearance can be computed with a steady-state quinidine concentration: Cl = [F · S (D/τ)]/Css = [0.7 · 0.83 (100 mg/6 h)]/(2.2 mg/L) = 4.40 L/h. (Note: μg/mL = mg/L, and this concentration unit was substituted for Css in the calculations to avoid unit conversion.)

2. *Compute the quinidine dose.*

Quinidine clearance is used to compute the new dose: D = (Css · Cl · τ)/(F · S) = (4 mg/L · 4.40 L/h · 6 h)/(0.7 · 0.83) = 182 mg, rounded to 200 mg every 6 hours.

The new quinidine dose is instituted immediately.

Steady-state serum concentration of quinidine can be measured after steady state is attained in 3 to 5 half-lives. Because the drug is expected to have a half-life of 7 hours in this patient, the quinidine steady-state concentration can be obtained any time after the second day of dosing (5 half-lives = 5 · 7 h = 35 h). Serum concentration of quinidine should be measured if the patient has a return of arrhythmia or if the patient has signs or symptoms of quinidine toxicity.

BAYESIAN PHARMACOKINETICS COMPUTER PROGRAMS

Computer programs are available that can assist in the computation of pharmacokinetic parameters for patients. The most reliable computer programs entail a nonlinear regression algorithm that incorporates components of Bayes' theorem. Nonlinear regression is a statistical technique in which an iterative process is used to compute the best pharmacokinetic parameters for a concentration–time data set. Briefly, the patient's drug dosage schedule and serum concentrations are entered into the computer. The computer program has a pharmacokinetic equation preprogrammed for the drug and administration method (e.g., oral, intravenous bolus, intravenous infusion). A one-compartment model typically is used, although some programs allow the user to choose among several equations. With population estimates based on demographic information for the patient (e.g., age, weight, sex, liver function, cardiac status) supplied by the user, the computer program computes estimated serum concentrations at each time there are actual serum concentrations. Kinetic parameters are then changed by the computer program, and a new set of estimated serum concentrations are computed. The pharmacokinetic parameters that generate the estimated serum concentrations closest to the actual values are remembered by the computer program, and the process is repeated until the set of pharmacokinetic parameters that result in estimated serum concentrations statistically closest to the actual serum concentrations are generated. These pharmacokinetic parameters can then be used to compute improved dosing schedules for patients. Bayes' theorem is used in the computer algorithm to balance the results of the computations between values based solely on the patient's serum drug concentrations and those based only on patient population parameters. Results of studies in which various methods of dosage adjustment have been compared have consistently shown that these types of computer dosing programs perform at least as well as experienced clinical pharmacokineticists and clinicians and better than inexperienced clinicians.

Some clinicians use Bayesian pharmacokinetics computer programs exclusively to alter drug doses on the basis of serum concentrations. An advantage of this approach is that consistent dosage recommendations are made when several different practitioners are involved in therapeutic drug monitoring programs. However, because simpler dosing methods work just as well for patients with stable pharmacokinetic parameters and steady-state drug concentrations, many clinicians reserve the use of computer programs for more difficult situations. Those situations include serum concentrations that are not at steady state, serum concentrations not obtained at the specific times needed to use simpler methods, and unstable pharmacokinetic parameters. Many Bayesian pharmacokinetics computer programs are available, and most should provide answers similar to those in the following examples. The program used to solve problems in this book is DrugCalc, written by Dr. Dennis Mungall. It is available on the Internet at http://members.aol.com/thertch/index.htm.[40]

Example 1 OY is a 57-year-old, 79-kg (height, 173 cm) man with ventricular tachycardia who needs therapy with oral quinidine gluconate. He has normal liver (bilirubin, 0.7 mg/dL; albumin, 4.0 g/dL) and cardiac function. He starts taking quinidine gluconate 648 mg every 12 hours at 0800 H. The quinidine serum concentration is 2.1 μg/mL at 0730 H before the morning dose is given on the second day of therapy. Compute a quinidine gluconate dose that will provide a steady-state concentration of 4 μg/mL.

1. *Enter the patient's demographic, drug dosing, and serum concentration–time data into the computer program.*

In this case, it is unlikely that the patient is at steady state, so the linear pharmacokinetics method cannot be used. The DrugCalc program requires that quinidine salt doses be entered in terms of quinidine base. A 648-mg dose of quinidine gluconate is equivalent to 400 mg of quinidine base (400 mg quinidine base = 648 mg quinidine gluconate · 0.62).

2. *Compute the pharmacokinetic parameters for the patient using the Bayesian pharmacokinetics computer program.*

The pharmacokinetic parameters computed with the program are a volume of distribution of 181 L, a half-life of 15.2 hours, and a clearance of 8.21 L/h.

3. *Compute the dose required to achieve desired quinidine serum concentrations.*

The oral one-compartment model equation used in the program to compute doses indicates that 972 mg of quinidine gluconate every 12 hours will produce a steady-state trough concentration of 4.7 μg/mL. (Note: DrugCalc uses salt form A and sustained-action options for quinidine gluconate.) This dose is started immediately.

Example 2 SL is a 71-year-old, 82-kg (height, 178 cm) man with atrial fibrillation who needs therapy with oral quinidine. He has cirrhosis of the liver (Child-Pugh score, 12; bilirubin, 3.2 mg/dL; albumin, 2.5 g/dL) and normal cardiac function. He begins taking quinidine sulfate extended-release tablets 600 mg every 12 hours at 0700 H. On the second day of therapy before the morning dose, the quinidine serum concentration is 4.5 μg/mL at 0700 H. Compute a quinidine sulfate dose that will provide a steady-state concentration of 4 μg/mL.

1. *Enter the patient's demographic, drug dosing, and serum concentration–time data into the computer program.*

In this case, it is unlikely that the patient is at steady state, so the linear pharmacokinetics method cannot be used. The DrugCalc program requires that quinidine salt doses be entered in terms of quinidine base. A 600-mg dose of quinidine sulfate is equivalent to 500 mg of quinidine base (500 mg quinidine base = 600 mg quinidine sulfate · 0.83).

2. *Compute the pharmacokinetic parameters for the patient using the Bayesian pharmacokinetics computer program.*

The pharmacokinetic parameters computed with the program are a volume of distribution of 161 L, a half-life of 21.4 hours, and a clearance of 5.24 L/h.

3. *Compute the dose needed to achieve the desired quinidine serum concentrations.*

The oral one-compartment model equation used in the program to compute doses indicates that 300 mg of quinidine sulfate extended-release tablets every 12 hours will produce a steady-state trough concentration of 4.1 μg/mL. (Note: DrugCalc uses salt form B and sustained-action options for quinidine sulfate extended-release tablets.) This dose is started immediately.

Example 3 TR is a 75-year-old, 85-kg (height, 173 cm) man with atrial flutter who needs therapy with quinidine sulfate immediate-release tablets. He has moderate heart failure (NYHA class III). Yesterday he was given a prescription for quinidine sulfate 200 mg four times daily and took the first two doses at 0800 H and 1200 H. Because he believes arrhythmia may have returned, the patient phones his physician, who advises the patient to increase the dose to 400 mg (1800 H and 2200 H). The quinidine serum concentration is 4.7 μg/mL at 1000 H, 2 hours after the morning dose (0800 H, 400 mg quinidine sulfate). Compute a quinidine sulfate dose that will provide a steady-state trough concentration of 4 μg/mL.

1. *Enter the patient's demographic, drug dosing, and serum concentration–time data into the computer program.*

In this case, it is unlikely that the patient is at steady state, so the linear pharmacokinetics method cannot be used. The DrugCalc program requires that quinidine salt doses be entered in terms of quinidine base. A 200-mg dose of quinidine sulfate is equivalent to 165 mg of quinidine base, and 400 mg of quinidine sulfate is equivalent to 330 mg of quinidine base (165 mg quinidine base = 200 mg quinidine sulfate · 0.83, 330 mg quinidine base = 400 mg quinidine sulfate · 0.83).

2. *Compute the pharmacokinetic parameters for the patient using the Bayesian pharmacokinetics computer program.*

The pharmacokinetic parameters computed with the program are a volume of distribution of 126 L, a half-life of 11.6 hours, and a clearance of 7.53 L/h.

3. *Compute the dose required to achieve the desired quinidine serum concentrations.*

The oral one-compartment model equation used in the program to compute doses indicates that 300 mg of quinidine sulfate immediate-release tablets every 6 hours will produce a steady-state trough concentration of 4.2 μg/mL. (Note: DrugCalc uses salt form B and oral options for quinidine sulfate immediate-release tablets.) This dose is started immediately.

CONVERSION OF QUINIDINE DOSES FROM ONE SALT FORM TO ANOTHER

Occasionally there is a need to convert stabilized quinidine therapy from one salt form to an equivalent amount of quinidine base in another salt form. In general, oral quinidine dosage forms, including most sustained-release tablets, have a bioavailability of 0.7. If equal quinidine serum concentrations are desired, this makes conversion between the two salt forms simple because equivalent doses of drug are prescribed: $D_{new} = (D_{old} \cdot S_{old})/S_{new}$, where D_{new} is the equivalent quinidine base dose for the new quinidine salt dosage form in milligrams per day, D_{old} is the dose of oral quinidine salt old dosage form in milligrams per day, and S_{old} and S_{new} are the fractions of the old and new quinidine salt dosage forms that are active quinidine.

Example 1 JH is taking oral extended-release quinidine sulfate 600 mg every 12 hours. She is responding well to therapy, has no adverse drug effects, and has a steady-state quinidine concentration of 4.7 μg/mL. Suggest an equivalent dose of extended-release quinidine gluconate to be taken every 8 hours by this patient.

1. *Calculate the equivalent oral dose of quinidine.*

The patient is receiving 600 mg every 12 hours or 1200 mg/d (600 mg/dose · 2 doses/d = 1200 mg/d) of quinidine sulfate. The equivalent quinidine gluconate dose is $D_{new} = (D_{old} \cdot S_{old})/S_{new}$ = (1200 mg/d · 0.83)/0.62 = 1606 mg/d, rounded to 1620 mg/d of quinidine gluconate, or 648 mg at 0700 H, 324 mg at 1500 H, and 648 mg at 2300 H.

Example 2 LK is taking oral extended-release quinidine gluconate 648 mg every 12 hours. He is responding well to therapy, has no adverse drug effects, and has a steady-state quinidine concentration of 3.3 μg/mL. Suggest an equivalent dose of immediate-release oral quinidine sulfate for this patient.

1. *Calculate the equivalent oral dose of quinidine.*

The patient is taking 648 mg every 12 hours or 1296 mg/d (648 mg/dose · 2 doses/d = 1296 mg/d) of quinidine gluconate. The equivalent quinidine sulfate dose is $D_{new} = (D_{old} \cdot S_{old})/S_{new}$ = (1296 mg/d · 0.62)/0.83 = 968 mg/d, rounded to 800 mg/d of quinidine sulfate or 200 mg every 6 hours.

PROBLEMS

The following problems are intended to emphasize the computation of initial and individualized doses by means of clinical pharmacokinetic techniques. Clinicians should always consult the patient's chart to confirm that current antiarrhythmic and other drug therapy is appropriate. All other medications that the patient is taking, including prescription and nonprescription drugs, should be recorded and checked to ascertain whether risk exists for a drug interaction with quinidine.

1. VC is a 67-year-old, 72-kg (height, 185 cm) man with ventricular tachycardia who needs therapy with oral quinidine. He has normal liver function and does not have heart failure. Suggest an initial extended-release quinidine gluconate dosage regimen designed to achieve a steady-state quinidine concentration of 3 μg/mL.

2. Patient VC (see problem 1) is given a prescription for oral quinidine gluconate 648 mg every 12 hours. The current steady-state quinidine concentration is 2.5 μg/mL. Compute a new quinidine gluconate dose that will provide a steady-state concentration of 4 μg/mL.

3. EM is a 56-year-old, 81-kg (height, 175 cm) man with ventricular tachycardia who needs therapy with oral quinidine. He has cirrhosis of the liver (Child-Pugh score, 10) and does not have heart failure. Suggest an initial quinidine gluconate extended-release tablet dosage regimen designed to achieve a steady-state quinidine concentration of 2 μg/mL.

4. Patient EM (see problem 3) is given a prescription for oral quinidine gluconate extended-release tablets 648 mg every 8 hours. The current steady-state quinidine concentration is 5.1 μg/mL, and the patient is experiencing symptoms that could be adverse effects of quinidine therapy. Compute a new quinidine gluconate dose that will provide a steady-state concentration of 3 μg/mL.

5. OF is a 71-year-old, 60-kg (height, 157 cm) woman with paroxysmal atrial tachycardia who needs therapy with oral quinidine. She has severe heart failure (NYHA class IV) and normal liver function. Suggest an initial quinidine sulfate extended-release dosage regimen designed to achieve a steady-state quinidine concentration of 4 μg/mL.

6. Patient OF (see problem 5) is given a prescription for quinidine sulfate extended-release tablets 600 mg orally every 12 hours. A steady-state quinidine serum concentration of 6.7 μg/mL is obtained. Compute a new quinidine sulfate dose that will provide a steady-state concentration of 4 μg/mL.

7. FK is a 67-year-old, 130-kg (height, 180 cm) man with ventricular tachycardia who needs therapy with oral quinidine. He has severe heart failure (NYHA class IV) and normal liver function. Suggest an initial quinidine sulfate immediate-release dosage regimen designed to achieve a steady-state quinidine concentration of 3 μg/mL.

8. Patient FK (see problem 7) is given a prescription for oral quinidine. Immediate-release quinidine sulfate tablets 300 mg every 8 hours are prescribed to start at 0700 H. A quinidine serum concentration of 1.7 μg/mL is obtained just before the third dose at 2300 H. Compute a new dose that will provide a steady-state concentration of 4 μg/mL.

9. CV is a 69-year-old, 90-kg (height, 185 cm) man with ventricular tachycardia who needs therapy with quinidine. He has cirrhosis of the liver (Child-Pugh score, 11; total bilirubin, 2.7 mg/dL; albumin, 2.1 g/dL) and moderate heart failure (NYHA class

III). At 0200 H, he receives 500 mg of intravenous quinidine gluconate over 2 hours as a loading dose. At 0800 H, quinidine gluconate 648 mg orally every 12 hours is started. A quinidine serum concentration is measured before the third dose at 0800 H the next day and is 5.4 μg/mL. Suggest an oral quinidine gluconate dosage regimen that will achieve a steady-state trough concentration of 4 μg/mL.

10. FP is a 59-year-old, 90-kg (height, 162 cm) woman with atrial fibrillation who needs therapy with oral quinidine. She has cirrhosis of the liver (Child-Pugh score, 9) and has mild heart failure (NYHA class II). She receives 600 mg of sustained-release quinidine sulfate every 12 hours at 0600 H and 1800 H for 9 doses. Because the patient has anorexia, nausea, vomiting, and a 40% widening of the QRS complex, the quinidine doses are held after the ninth dose. A quinidine serum concentration is measured at 0800 H the next morning and is 7.1 μg/mL. Suggest a quinidine sulfate immediate-release tablet dose that will achieve a steady-state trough concentration of 4 μg/mL.

ANSWERS TO PROBLEMS

1. The initial quinidine dose for patient VC is calculated as follows.

Pharmacokinetic Dosing Method

1. *Estimate the half-life and elimination rate constant according to disease states and conditions present in the patient.*

The expected quinidine half-life ($t_{1/2}$) is 7 hours. The elimination rate constant is computed with the following formula: $k = 0.693/t_{1/2} = 0.693/7\ h = 0.099\ h^{-1}$.

2. *Estimate the volume of distribution and clearance.*

The patient is not obese, so the estimated volume of distribution of quinidine is based on actual body weight: $V = 2.4\ L/kg \cdot 72\ kg = 173\ L$. Estimated quinidine clearance is computed by multiplying V and the elimination rate constant: $Cl = kV = 0.099\ h^{-1} \cdot 173\ L = 17.1\ L/h$.

3. *Compute the dosage regimen.*

Oral extended-release quinidine gluconate tablets are prescribed to this patient ($F = 0.7$, $S = 0.62$). The initial dosage interval (τ) is set to 8 hours. (Note: μg/mL = mg/L, and this concentration unit was substituted for Css in the calculations to avoid unit conversion.) The dosage equation for oral quinidine is $D = (Css \cdot Cl \cdot \tau)/(F \cdot S) = (3\ mg/L \cdot 17.1\ L/h \cdot 8\ h)/(0.7 \cdot 0.62) = 945\ mg$, rounded to 972 mg every 8 hours.

Steady-state serum concentration of quinidine can be measured after steady state is attained in 3 to 5 half-lives. Because the drug is expected to have a half-life of 7 hours in this patient, the quinidine steady-state concentration can be obtained any time after the second day of dosing (5 half-lives = $5 \cdot 7\ h = 35\ h$). Serum concentration of quinidine should be measured if the patient has a return of arrhythmia or if the patient has signs or symptoms of quinidine toxicity.

Literature-Based Recommended Dosing

1. *Choose the quinidine dose based on disease states and conditions present in the patient.*

A quinidine gluconate maintenance dose of 648 mg every 12 hours (1296 mg/d) is suggested for a patient without heart failure or liver disease who needs a quinidine steady-state serum concentration in the lower end of the therapeutic range.

Steady-state serum concentration of quinidine can be measured after steady state is attained in 3 to 5 half-lives. Because the drug is expected to have a half-life of 7 hours in this patient, the quinidine steady-state concentration can be obtained any time after the second day of dosing (5 half-lives = 5 · 7 h = 35 h). Serum concentration of quinidine should be measured if the patient has a return of arrhythmia or if the patient has signs or symptoms of quinidine toxicity.

2. The revised quinidine dose for patient VC is calculated as follows.

Linear Pharmacokinetics Method

1. *Compute the new dose to achieve the desired serum concentration.*

The patient is expected to achieve steady-state conditions after 2 days (5 half-lives = 5 · 7 h = 35 h) of therapy.

Using linear pharmacokinetics, the new dose to attain the desired concentration should be proportional to the old dose that produced the measured concentration. (Note: Total daily dose is 1296 mg/d = 648 mg/d · 2 doses/d.)

$$D_{new} = (Css_{new}/Css_{old})D_{old} = [(4\ \mu g/mL)/(2.5\ \mu g/mL)]\ 1296\ mg/d$$
$$= 2074\ mg/d, \text{ rounded to } 1944\ mg/d \text{ or } 648\ mg \text{ every } 8 \text{ hours}$$

The new suggested dose is 648 mg every 8 hours of quinidine gluconate to be started immediately.

Steady-state serum concentration of quinidine can be measured after steady state is attained in 3 to 5 half-lives. Because the drug is expected to have a half-life of 7 hours in this patient, the quinidine steady-state concentration can be obtained any time after 2 days of dosing (5 half-lives = 5 · 7 h = 35 h). Serum concentration of quinidine should be measured if the patient has a return of arrhythmia or if the patient has signs or symptoms of quinidine toxicity.

Pharmacokinetic Parameter Method

1. *Compute the pharmacokinetic parameters.*

The patient is expected to achieve steady-state conditions after the second day (5 half-lives = 5 · 7 h = 35 h) of therapy.

Quinidine clearance can be computed with a steady-state quinidine concentration: $Cl = [F \cdot S\ (D/\tau)]/Css = [0.7 \cdot 0.62\ (648\ mg/12\ h)]/(2.5\ mg/L) = 9.37\ L/h$. (Note: μg/mL = mg/L, and this concentration unit was substituted for Css in the calculations to avoid unit conversion.)

2. *Compute the quinidine dose.*

Quinidine clearance is used to compute the new dose: D = (Css · Cl · τ)/(F · S) = (4 mg/L · 9.37 L/h · 8 h)/(0.7 · 0.62) = 691 mg, rounded to 648 mg every 8 hours.

The new quinidine dose is instituted immediately.

Steady-state quinidine serum concentration can be measured after steady state is attained in 3 to 5 half-lives. Because the drug is expected to have a half-life of 7 hours in this patient, the quinidine steady-state concentration can be obtained any time after the second day of dosing (5 half-lives = 5 · 7 h = 35 h). Serum concentration of quinidine should be measured if the patient has a return of arrhythmia or if the patient has signs or symptoms of quinidine toxicity.

3. The initial quinidine dose for patient EM is calculated as follows.

Pharmacokinetic Dosing Method

1. *Estimate the half-life and elimination rate constant according to disease states and conditions present in the patient.*

The expected quinidine half-life ($t_{1/2}$) is 9 hours. The elimination rate constant is computed with the following formula: $k = 0.693/t_{1/2} = 0.693/9\ h = 0.077\ h^{-1}$.

2. *Estimate the volume of distribution and clearance.*

The patient is not obese, so the estimated quinidine volume of distribution is based on actual body weight: V = 3.8 L/kg · 81 kg = 308 L. Estimated quinidine clearance is computed by multiplying V and the elimination rate constant: Cl = kV = $0.077\ h^{-1}$ · 308 L = 23.7 L/h.

3. *Compute the dosage regimen.*

Oral extended-release quinidine gluconate tablets are prescribed to this patient (F = 0.7, S = 0.62). The initial dosage interval (τ) is set to 8 hours. (Note: μg/mL = mg/L, and this concentration unit was substituted for Css in the calculations to avoid unit conversion.) The dosage equation for oral quinidine is D = (Css · Cl · τ)/(F · S) = (2 mg/L · 23.7 L/h · 8 h)/(0.7 · 0.62) = 873 mg, rounded to 972 mg every 8 hours.

Steady-state serum concentration of quinidine can be measured after steady state is attained in 3 to 5 half-lives. Because the drug is expected to have a half-life of 9 hours in this patient, the quinidine steady-state concentration can be obtained any time after the second day of dosing (5 half-lives = 5 · 9 h = 45 h). Serum concentration of quinidine should be measured if the patient has a return of arrhythmia or if the patient has signs or symptoms of quinidine toxicity.

Literature-Based Recommended Dosing

1. *Choose the quinidine dose based on disease states and conditions present in the patient.*

A quinidine gluconate maintenance dose of 324 mg every 12 hours (648 mg/d) is suggested for a patient with liver disease who needs a quinidine steady-state serum concentration in the lower end of the therapeutic range.

Steady-state serum concentration of quinidine can be measured after steady state is attained in 3 to 5 half-lives. Because the drug is expected to have a half-life of 9 hours in this patient, the quinidine steady-state concentration can be obtained any time after the second day of dosing (5 half-lives = 5 · 9 h = 45 h). Serum concentration of quinidine should be measured if the patient has a return of arrhythmia or if the patient has signs or symptoms of quinidine toxicity.

4. The revised quinidine dose for patient EM is calculated as follows.

Linear Pharmacokinetics Method

1. *Compute the new dose to achieve the desired serum concentration.*

The patient is expected to achieve steady-state conditions after 2 days (5 half-lives = 5 · 9 h = 45 h) of therapy.

With linear pharmacokinetics, the new dose to attain the desired concentration should be proportional to the old dose that produced the measured concentration. (Note: Total daily dose is 1944 mg/d = 648 mg/d · 3 doses/d.)

$$D_{new} = (Css_{new}/Css_{old})D_{old} = [(3\ \mu g/mL)/(5.1\ \mu g/mL)]\ 1944\ mg/d$$
$$= 1144\ mg/d, \text{ rounded to } 1296\ mg/d \text{ or } 648\ mg \text{ every } 12 \text{ hours}$$

The new suggested dose is 648 mg every 12 hours of quinidine gluconate to be started in 1 or 2 half-lives (9 to 18 hours) to allow time for possible side effects to subside.

Steady-state serum concentration of quinidine can be measured after steady state is attained in 3 to 5 half-lives. Because the drug is expected to have a half-life of 9 hours in this patient, the quinidine steady-state concentration can be obtained any time after 2 days of dosing (5 half-lives = 5 · 9 h = 45 h). Serum concentration of quinidine should be measured if the patient has a return of arrhythmia or if the patient has signs or symptoms of quinidine toxicity.

Pharmacokinetic Parameter Method

1. *Compute the pharmacokinetic parameters.*

The patient is expected to achieve steady-state conditions after the second day (5 half-lives = 5 · 9 h = 45 h) of therapy.

Quinidine clearance can be computed with a steady-state quinidine concentration: $Cl = [F \cdot S\ (D/\tau)]/Css = [0.7 \cdot 0.62\ (648\ mg/8\ h)]/(5.1\ mg/L) = 6.89\ L/h$. (Note: μg/mL = mg/L, and this concentration unit was substituted for Css in the calculations to avoid unit conversion.)

2. *Compute the quinidine dose.*

Quinidine clearance is used to compute the new dose: $D = (Css \cdot Cl \cdot \tau)/(F \cdot S) = (3\ mg/L \cdot 6.89\ L/h \cdot 12\ h)/(0.7 \cdot 0.62) = 572\ mg$, rounded to 648 mg every 12 hours.

The new suggested dose is 648 mg every 12 hours of quinidine gluconate to be started in 1 or 2 half-lives (9 to 18 hours) to allow time for possible side effects to subside.

Steady-state serum concentration of quinidine can be measured after steady state is attained in 3 to 5 half-lives. Because the drug is expected to have a half-life of 9 hours in this patient, the quinidine steady-state concentration can be obtained any time after the 2 days of dosing (5 half-lives = 5 · 9 h = 45 h). Serum concentration of quinidine should be measured if the patient has a return of arrhythmia or if the patient has signs or symptoms of quinidine toxicity.

5. The initial quinidine dose for patient OF is calculated as follows.

Pharmacokinetic Dosing Method

1. *Estimate the half-life and elimination rate constant according to disease states and conditions present in the patient.*

The expected quinidine half-life ($t_{1/2}$) is 7 hours. The elimination rate constant is computed with the following formula: $k = 0.693/t_{1/2} = 0.693/7\ h = 0.099\ h^{-1}$.

2. *Estimate the volume of distribution and clearance.*

The patient is not obese, so the estimated quinidine volume of distribution is based on actual body weight: V = 1.7 L/kg · 60 kg = 102 L. Estimated quinidine clearance is computed by multiplying V and the elimination rate constant: Cl = kV = $0.099\ h^{-1} \cdot 102\ L = 10.1\ L/h$.

3. *Compute the dosage regimen.*

Oral extended-release quinidine sulfate tablets are prescribed to this patient (F = 0.7, S = 0.83). The initial dose interval (τ) is set to 12 hours. (Note: μg/mL = mg/L, and this concentration unit was substituted for Css in the calculations to avoid unit conversion.) The dosage equation for oral quinidine is D = (Css · Cl · τ)/(F · S) = (4 mg/L · 10.1 L/h · 12 h)/(0.7 · 0.83) = 834 mg, rounded to 900 mg every 12 hours.

Steady-state serum concentration of quinidine can be measured after steady state is attained in 3 to 5 half-lives. Because the drug is expected to have a half-life of 7 hours in this patient, the quinidine steady-state concentration can be obtained any time after the second day of dosing (5 half-lives = 5 · 7 h = 35 h). Serum concentration of quinidine should be measured if the patient has a return of arrhythmia or if the patient has signs or symptoms of quinidine toxicity.

Literature-Based Recommended Dosing

1. *Choose a quinidine dose based on disease states and conditions present in the patient.*

A quinidine sulfate maintenance dose of 300 mg every 8 hours (900 mg/d) is suggested for a patient with heart failure who needs a quinidine steady-state serum concentration in the upper end of the therapeutic range.

Steady-state serum concentration of quinidine can be measured after steady state is attained in 3 to 5 half-lives. Because the drug is expected to have a half-life of 7 hours in this patient, the quinidine steady-state concentration can be obtained any time after the second day of dosing (5 half-lives = 5 · 7 h = 35 h). Serum concentration of quinidine should be measured if the patient has a return of arrhythmia or if the patient has signs or symptoms of quinidine toxicity.

6. The revised quinidine dose for patient OF is calculated as follows.

Linear Pharmacokinetics Method

1. *Compute the new dose to achieve the desired serum concentration.*

The patient is expected to achieve steady-state conditions after 2 days (5 half-lives = 5 · 7 h = 35 h) of therapy.

With linear pharmacokinetics, the new dose to attain the desired concentration should be proportional to the old dose that produced the measured concentration. (Note: Total daily dose is 1200 mg/d = 600 mg/dose · 2 doses/d.)

$$D_{new} = (Css_{new}/Css_{old})D_{old} = [(4\ \mu g/mL)/(6.7\ \mu g/mL)]\ 1200\ mg/d$$
$$= 716\ mg/d,\ \text{rounded to 600 mg/d or 300 mg every 12 hours}$$

The new suggested dose is 300 mg every 12 hours of quinidine sulfate extended-release tablets to be started in 1 or 2 half-lives (7 to 14 hours) to allow time for serum concentrations to decline.

Steady-state serum concentration of quinidine can be measured after steady state is attained in 3 to 5 half-lives. Because the drug is expected to have a half-life of 7 hours in this patient, the quinidine steady-state concentration can be obtained any time after 2 days of dosing (5 half-lives = 5 · 7 h = 35 h). Serum concentration of quinidine should be measured if the patient has a return of arrhythmia or if the patient has signs or symptoms of quinidine toxicity.

Pharmacokinetic Parameter Method

1. *Compute the pharmacokinetic parameters.*

The patient is expected to achieve steady-state conditions after the second day (5 half-lives = 5 · 7 h = 35 h) of therapy.

Quinidine clearance can be computed with a steady-state quinidine concentration: $Cl = [F \cdot S\ (D/\tau)]/Css = [0.7 \cdot 0.83\ (600\ mg/12\ h)]/(6.7\ mg/L) = 4.34\ L/h$. (Note: μg/mL = mg/L, and this concentration unit was substituted for Css in the calculations to avoid unit conversion.)

2. *Compute the quinidine dose.*

Quinidine clearance is used to compute the new dose: $D = (Css \cdot Cl \cdot \tau)/(F \cdot S) = (4\ mg/L \cdot 4.34\ L/h \cdot 12\ h)/(0.7 \cdot 0.83) = 359\ mg$, rounded to 300 mg every 12 hours.

The new suggested dose is 300 mg every 12 hours of quinidine sulfate extended-release tablets to be started in 1 or 2 half-lives (7 to 14 hours) to allow time for possible side effects to subside.

Steady-state serum concentration of quinidine can be measured after steady state is attained in 3 to 5 half-lives. Because the drug is expected to have a half-life of 7 hours in this patient, the quinidine steady-state concentration can be obtained any time after 2 days of dosing (5 half-lives = 5 · 7 h = 35 h). Serum concentration of quinidine should be measured if the patient has a return of arrhythmia or if the patient has signs or symptoms of quinidine toxicity.

7. The initial quinidine dose for patient FK is calculated as follows.

Pharmacokinetic Dosing Method

1. *Estimate the half-life and elimination rate constant according to disease states and conditions present in the patient.*

The expected quinidine half-life ($t_{1/2}$) is 7 hours. The elimination rate constant is computed with the following formula: $k = 0.693/t_{1/2} = 0.693/7\ h = 0.099\ h^{-1}$.

2. *Estimate the volume of distribution and clearance.*

The patient is obese (>30% over ideal body weight), so the estimated quinidine volume of distribution is based on ideal body weight in kilograms: IBW_{males} = 50 kg + 2.3(Ht – 60) = 50 kg + 2.3(71 – 60) = 75 kg, where Ht is height in inches (height in centimeters divided by 2.54). The computation for V is then V = 1.7 L/kg · 75 kg = 128 L. Estimated quinidine clearance is computed by multiplying V and the elimination rate constant: Cl = kV = 0.099 h^{-1} · 128 L = 12.7 L/h.

3. *Compute the dosage regimen.*

Oral immediate-release quinidine sulfate tablets are prescribed to this patient (F = 0.7, S = 0.83). The initial dosage interval (τ) is set to 6 hours. (Note: μg/mL = mg/L, and this concentration unit was substituted for Css in the calculations to avoid unit conversion.) The dosage equation for oral quinidine is D = (Css · Cl · τ)/(F · S) = (3 mg/L · 12.7 L/h · 6 h)/(0.7 · 0.83) = 393 mg, rounded to 400 mg every 6 hours.

Steady-state serum concentration of quinidine can be measured after steady state is attained in 3 to 5 half-lives. Because the drug is expected to have a half-life of 7 hours in this patient, the quinidine steady-state concentration can be obtained any time after the second day of dosing (5 half-lives = 5 · 7 h = 35 h). Serum concentration of quinidine should be measured if the patient has a return of arrhythmia or if the patient has signs or symptoms of quinidine toxicity.

Literature-Based Recommended Dosing

1. *Choose a quinidine dose based on disease states and conditions present in the patient.*

A quinidine sulfate maintenance dose of 100 mg every 6 hours (400 mg/d) is suggested for a patient with heart failure who needs a quinidine steady-state serum concentration in the lower end of the therapeutic range.

Steady-state serum concentration of quinidine can be measured after steady state is attained in 3 to 5 half-lives. Because the drug is expected to have a half-life of 7 hours in this patient, the quinidine steady-state concentration can be obtained any time after the second day of dosing (5 half-lives = 5 · 7 h = 35 h). Serum concentration of quinidine should be measured if the patient has a return of arrhythmia or if the patient has signs or symptoms of quinidine toxicity.

8. The revised quinidine dose for patient FK is calculated as follows.

Bayesian Pharmacokinetics Computer Program Method

1. *Enter the patient's demographic, drug dosing, and serum concentration–time data into the computer program.*

In this case, it is unlikely that the patient is at steady state, so the linear pharmacokinetics method cannot be used. The DrugCalc program requires quinidine salt doses be entered in terms of quinidine base. A 300-mg dose of quinidine sulfate is equivalent to 250 mg of quinidine base (250 mg quinidine base = 300 mg quinidine sulfate · 0.83).

2. *Compute the pharmacokinetic parameters for the patient using the Bayesian pharmacokinetics computer program.*

The pharmacokinetic parameters computed with the program are a volume of distribution of 171 L, a half-life of 16.1 hours, and a clearance of 7.36 L/h.

3. *Compute the dose required to achieve the desired quinidine serum concentrations.*

The oral one-compartment model equation used in the program to compute doses indicates that 300 mg of quinidine sulfate immediate-release tablets every 6 hours will produce a steady-state trough concentration of 4.7 μg/mL. (Note: DrugCalc uses salt form B and oral options for quinidine sulfate immediate-release tablets.) This dose is started immediately.

9. The revised quinidine dose for patient CV is calculated as follows.

Bayesian Pharmacokinetics Computer Program Method

1. *Enter the patient's demographic, drug dosing, and serum concentration–time data into the computer program.*

In this case, it is unlikely that the patient is at steady state, so the linear pharmacokinetics method cannot be used. The DrugCalc program requires quinidine salt doses be entered in terms of quinidine base. A 500-mg dose of quinidine gluconate is equivalent to 300 mg of quinidine base, and a 648-mg dose of quinidine gluconate is equal to 400 mg of quinidine base (300 mg quinidine base = 500 mg quinidine gluconate · 0.62, 400 mg quinidine base = 648 mg quinidine gluconate · 0.62).

2. *Compute the pharmacokinetic parameters for the patient using the Bayesian pharmacokinetics computer program.*

The pharmacokinetic parameters computed with the program are a volume of distribution of 130 L, a half-life of 23.6 hours, and a clearance of 3.83 L/h.

3. *Compute the dose required to achieve the desired quinidine serum concentrations.*

The oral one-compartment model equation used in the program to compute doses indicates that 324 mg of quinidine gluconate extended-release tablets every 12 hours will produce a steady-state trough concentration of 4.2 μg/mL. (Note: DrugCalc uses salt form B and sustained-release options for quinidine gluconate extended-release tablets.) This dose can be held for 1 half-life (1 day) if adverse drug effects occur, or it can be started immediately.

10. The revised quinidine dose for patient FP is calculated as follows.

Bayesian Pharmacokinetics Computer Program Method

1. *Enter the patient's demographic, drug dosing, and serum concentration–time data into the computer program.*

In this case, it is unlikely that the patient is at steady state, so the linear pharmacokinetics method cannot be used. The DrugCalc program requires quinidine salt doses be entered in terms of quinidine base. A 600-mg dose of quinidine sulfate is equivalent to 500 mg of quinidine base (500 mg quinidine base = 600 mg quinidine sulfate · 0.83).

2. *Compute the pharmacokinetic parameters for the patient using the Bayesian pharmacokinetics computer program.*

The pharmacokinetic parameters computed with the program are a volume of distribution of 238 L, a half-life of 51.3 hours, and a clearance of 3.21 L/h.

3. *Compute the dose required to achieve the desired quinidine serum concentrations.*

The oral one-compartment model equation used in the program to compute doses indicates that 200 mg of quinidine sulfate immediate-release tablets every 12 hours will produce a steady-state trough concentration of 3.6 μg/mL. (Note: DrugCalc uses salt form B and oral options for quinidine sulfate immediate-release tablets.) This dose can be held for 1 half-life (2 days) if adverse drug effects continue to occur, or it can be started immediately.

REFERENCES

1. Bauman JL, Schoen MD. Arrhythmias. In: DiPiro JT, Talbert RL, Yee GC, Matzke GR, Wells BG, Posey LM, eds. Pharmacotherapy: a pathophysiologic approach. Stamford, CT: Appleton & Lange, 1999:232–264.
2. Roden DM. Antiarrhythmic drugs. In: Hardman JG, Limbird LE, Molinoff PB, Ruddon RW, Gilman AG, eds. The pharmacological basis of therapeutics. New York: McGraw-Hill, 1996: 839–874.
3. Ueda CT, Williamson BJ, Dzindzio BS. Absolute quinidine bioavailability. Clin Pharmacol Ther 1976;20:260–265.
4. Ueda CT, Hirschfeld DS, Scheinman MM, Rowland M, Williamson BJ, Dzindzio BS. Disposition kinetics of quinidine. Clin Pharmacol Ther 1976;19:30–36.
5. Woo E, Greenblatt DJ. A reevaluation of intravenous quinidine. Am Heart J 1978;96:829–832.
6. Greenblatt DJ, Pfeifer HJ, Ochs HR, et al. Pharmacokinetics of quinidine in humans after intravenous, intramuscular and oral administration. J Pharmacol Exp Ther 1977;202:365–378.
7. Ueda CT, Dzindzio BS. Quinidine kinetics in congestive heart failure. Clin Pharmacol Ther 1978;23:158–164.
8. Ueda CT, Dzindzio BS. Bioavailability of quinidine in congestive heart failure. Br J Clin Pharmacol 1981;11:571–577.

9. Covinsky JO, Russo J Jr, Kelly KL, Cashman J, Amick EN, Mason WD. Relative bioavailability of quinidine gluconate and quinidine sulfate in healthy volunteers. J Clin Pharmacol 1979;19: 261–269.
10. Gibson DL, Smith GH, Koup JR, Stewart DK. Relative bioavailability of a standard and a sustained-release quinidine tablet. Clin Pharm 1982;1:366–368.
11. McGilveray IJ, Midha KK, Rowe M, Beaudoin N, Charette C. Bioavailability of 11 quinidine formulations and pharmacokinetic variation in humans. J Pharm Sci 1981;70:524–529.
12. Ochs HR, Greenblatt DJ, Woo E, Franke K, Pfeifer HJ, Smith TW. Single and multiple dose pharmacokinetics of oral quinidine sulfate and gluconate. Am J Cardiol 1978;41:770–777.
13. Woo E, Greenblatt DJ, Ochs HR. Short- and long-acting oral quinidine preparations: clinical implications of pharmacokinetic differences. Angiology 1978;29:243–250.
14. Drayer DE, Lowenthal DT, Restivo KM, Schwartz A, Cook CE, Reidenberg MM. Steady-state serum levels of quinidine and active metabolites in cardiac patients with varying degrees of renal function. Clin Pharmacol Ther 1978;24:31–39.
15. Drayer DE, Hughes M, Lorenzo B, Reidenberg MM. Prevalence of high (3S)-3-hydroxyquinidine/quinidine ratios in serum, and clearance of quinidine in cardiac patients with age. Clin Pharmacol Ther 1980;27:72–75.
16. Holford NH, Coates PE, Guentert TW, Riegelman S, Sheiner LB. The effect of quinidine and its metabolites on the electrocardiogram and systolic time intervals: concentration-effect relationships. Br J Clin Pharmacol 1981;11:187–195.
17. Rakhit A, Holford NH, Guentert TW, Maloney K, Riegelman S. Pharmacokinetics of quinidine and three of its metabolites in man. J Pharmacokinet Biopharm 1984;12:1–21.
18. Ueda CT, Dzindzio BS. Pharmacokinetics of dihydroquinidine in congestive heart failure patients after intravenous quinidine administration. Eur J Clin Pharmacol 1979;16:101–105.
19. Ueda CT, Williamson BJ, Dzindzio BS. Disposition kinetics of dihydroquinidine following quinidine administration. Res Commun Chem Pathol Pharmacol 1976;14:215–225.
20. Narang PK, Crouthamel WG. Dihydroquinidine contamination of quinidine raw materials and dosage forms: rapid estimation by high-performance liquid chromatography. J Pharm Sci 1979; 68:917–919.
21. Russo J, Jr, Russo ME, Smith RA, Pershing LK. Assessment of quinidine gluconate for nonlinear kinetics following chronic dosing. J Clin Pharmacol 1982;22:264–270.
22. Chen BH, Taylor EH, Ackerman BH, Olsen K, Pappas AA. Effect of pH on free quinidine [letter]. Drug Intell Clin Pharm 1988;22:826.
23. Mihaly GW, Cheng MS, Klein MB. Difference in the binding of quinine and quinidine to plasma proteins. Br J Clin Pharmacol 1987;24:769–774.
24. Woo E, Greenblatt DJ. Pharmacokinetic and clinical implications of quinidine protein binding. J Pharm Sci 1979;68:466–470.
25. Carliner NH, Crouthamel WG, Fisher ML, et al. Quinidine therapy in hospitalized patients with ventricular arrhythmias. Am Heart J 1979;98:708–715.
26. Conrad KA, Molk BL, Chidsey CA. Pharmacokinetic studies of quinidine in patients with arrhythmias. Circulation 1977;55:1–7.
27. Guentert TW, Holford NH, Coates PE, Upton RA, Riegelman S. Quinidine pharmacokinetics in man: choice of a disposition model and absolute bioavailability studies. J Pharmacokinet Biopharm 1979;7:315–330.
28. Kessler KM, Humphries WC, Jr, Black M, Spann JF. Quinidine pharmacokinetics in patients with cirrhosis or receiving propranolol. Am Heart J 1978;96:627–635.
29. Powell JR, Okada R, Conrad KA, Guentert TW, Riegelman S. Altered quinidine disposition in a patient with chronic active hepatitis. Postgrad Med J 1982;58:82–84.
30. Pugh RN, Murray-Lyon IM, Dawson JL, Pietroni MC, Williams R. Transection of the oesophagus for bleeding oesophageal varices. Br J Surg 1973;60:646–649.

31. Crouthamel WG. The effect of congestive heart failure on quinidine pharmacokinetics. Am Heart J 1975;90:335–339.
32. Kessler KM, Lowenthal DT, Warner H, Gibson T, Briggs W, Reidenberg MM. Quinidine elimination in patients with congestive heart failure or poor renal function. N Engl J Med 1974;290: 706–709.
33. Ochs HR, Greenblatt DJ, Woo E, Smith TW. Reduced quinidine clearance in elderly persons. Am J Cardiol 1978;42:481–485.
34. Hall K, Meatherall B, Krahn J, Penner B, Rabson JL. Clearance of quinidine during peritoneal dialysis. Am Heart J 1982;104:646–647.
35. Chin TW, Pancorbo S, Comty C. Quinidine pharmacokinetics in continuous ambulatory peritoneal dialysis. Clin Exp Dial Apheresis 1981;5:391–397.
36. Hansten PD, Horn JR. Drug interactions analysis and management. Vancouver, WA: Applied Therapeutics, 1998:527.
37. Muralidharan G, Cooper JK, Hawes EM, Korchinski ED, Midha KK. Quinidine inhibits the 7-hydroxylation of chlorpromazine in extensive metabolisers of debrisoquine. Eur J Clin Pharmacol 1996;50:121–128.
38. von Moltke LL, Greenblatt DJ, Cotreau-Bibbo MM, Duan SX, Harmatz JS, Shader RI. Inhibition of desipramine hydroxylation in vitro by serotonin-reuptake-inhibitor antidepressants, and by quinidine and ketoconazole: a model system to predict drug interactions in vivo. J Pharmacol Exp Ther 1994;268:1278–1283.
39. von Moltke LL, Greenblatt DJ, Duan SX, Daily JP, Harmatz JS, Shader RI. Inhibition of desipramine hydroxylation (cytochrome P450-2D6) in vitro by quinidine and by viral protease inhibitors: relation to drug interactions in vivo. J Pharm Sci 1998;87:1184–1189.
40. Wandell M, Mungall D. Computer assisted drug interpretation and drug regimen optimization. Am Assoc Clin Chem 1984;6:1–11.

Part IV

ANTICONVULSANTS

10

PHENYTOIN

INTRODUCTION

Phenytoin is a hydantoin compound related to barbiturates. It is used for the treatment of patients with seizure disorders. Phenytoin is an effective anticonvulsant for the long-term management of tonic-clonic (grand mal) or partial seizures and the short-term management of generalized status epilepticus (Table 10-1).[1] After generalized status epilepticus has been controlled with intravenous benzodiazepine therapy and supportive measures have been instituted, phenytoin therapy usually is instituted immediately with the administration of intravenous phenytoin or fosphenytoin. Orally administered phenytoin is used in long-term therapy to provide prophylaxis against tonic-clonic or partial seizures. Phenytoin also is a type 1B antiarrhythmic agent that is particularly useful in the management of digitalis-induced arrhythmia. It is also used in the management of trigeminal neuralgia.

The antiseizure activity of phenytoin is related to its ability to inhibit the repetitive firing of action potentials caused by prolonged depolarization of neurons.[2,3] Phenytoin also stops the spread of abnormal discharges from epileptic foci and decreases the spread of seizure activity through the brain. Posttetanic potentiation at synaptic junctions is blocked, and the blockage alters synaptic transmission. At the cellular level, the mechanism of action of phenytoin appears related to its ability to prolong inactivation of voltage-activated sodium ion channels and to reduce the ability of neurons to fire at high frequencies.

THERAPEUTIC AND TOXIC CONCENTRATIONS

The usual therapeutic range for total (unbound + bound) phenytoin serum concentrations when the drug is used in the management of seizures is 10 to 20 μg/mL. Because it is highly bound (~90%) to albumin, phenytoin is prone to plasma protein binding displace-

TABLE 10-1 International Classification of Epileptic Seizures

MAJOR CLASS	SUBSET OF CLASS	DRUG THERAPY FOR SELECTED SEIZURE TYPE
Partial seizures (beginning locally)	1. Simple partial seizures (without impaired consciousness) a. With motor symptoms b. With somatosensory or special sensory symptoms c. With autonomic symptoms d. With psychological symptoms	Carbamazepine Phenytoin Valproic acid Phenobarbital Primidone
	2. Complex partial seizures (with impaired consciousness) a. Simple partial onset followed by impaired consciousness b. Impaired consciousness at onset	Carbamazepine Phenytoin Valproic acid Phenobarbital Primidone
	3. Partial seizures evolving into secondary generalized seizures	Carbamazepine Phenytoin Valproic acid Phenobarbital Primidone
Generalized seizures (convulsive or nonconvulsive)	1. Absence seizures (typical or atypical; also known as petit mal seizures)	Valproic acid Ethosuximide
	2. Tonic-clonic seizures (also known as grand mal seizures)	Carbamazepine Phenytoin Valproic acid Phenobarbital Primidone

Adapted from Brodie MJ, Dichter MA. Antiepileptic drugs. N Engl J Med 1996;334:168–175.

ment. Because of this displacement, unbound, or free, phenytoin concentrations are widely available. Although clinical data support the therapeutic range for total phenytoin concentrations, the suggested therapeutic range for unbound phenytoin concentrations is based on the usual unbound fraction (10%) of phenytoin among persons with normal plasma protein binding. Thus the generally accepted therapeutic range of unbound phenytoin concentrations is 1 to 2 μg/mL, which is simply 10% of the lower and upper limits for the total concentration range.

When the concentration is in the upper end of the therapeutic range (>15 μg/mL), some patients have minor central nervous system depression side effects, such as drowsiness or fatigue.[2,3] At total phenytoin concentrations >20 μg/mL, nystagmus may occur and can be especially prominent during lateral gaze. When total concentrations exceed 30 μg/mL, ataxia, slurred speech, and incoordination similar to those of ethanol intoxication can occur. If total phenytoin concentrations are >40 μg/mL, mental status changes, including decreased mentation, severe confusion or lethargy, and coma, are possible. Drug-induced seizure activity can occur at concentrations >50 to 60 μg/mL. Because phenytoin follows nonlinear or saturable metabolism pharmacokinetics, it is possible to attain excessive drug concentrations much easier than for other compounds that follow linear pharmacokinetics. Clinicians should understand that not all patients with high phenytoin serum concentrations in the aforementioned ranges have signs or symptoms of phenytoin toxicity. Rather, phenytoin concentrations in the ranges given increase the likelihood of an adverse drug effect.

CLINICAL USEFULNESS OF UNBOUND PHENYTOIN CONCENTRATIONS

Unbound phenytoin concentrations are an extremely useful monitoring tool when used correctly. The relation between total concentration (C), unbound, or free, concentration (C_f), and unbound, or free, fraction (f_B) is $C_f = f_B C$. For routine therapeutic drug monitoring, total phenytoin serum concentrations still are used to gauge therapy with the anticonvulsant. For most patients without known or identifiable abnormalities in plasma protein binding, the unbound fraction of phenytoin is normal (~10%) and measurement of unbound drug concentration is unnecessary. At present, it is 50% to 100% more expensive to measure unbound drug concentration than it is to measure total concentration. It also takes longer for a laboratory to perform the measurements and return the results to clinicians, and the means to obtain the measurements are not available at all laboratories. Monitoring of unbound phenytoin serum concentration generally should be restricted to patients with known reasons to have altered plasma protein binding of the drug. Exceptions to this approach are patients with an augmented or excessive pharmacologic response in relation to total phenytoin concentration. For example, a possible explanation for a satisfactory anticonvulsant response to a low total phenytoin concentration may be abnormal plasma protein binding (20%) of unknown causation. Although the total concentration is low (5 μg/mL), a therapeutic unbound concentration is present ($C_f = f_B C = 0.2 \cdot 5$ μg/mL = 1 μg/mL). If a patient has a phenytoin-related adverse drug reaction possibly due to phenytoin and the total phenytoin concentration is within the therapeutic range, an explanation may be abnormal protein binding (20%) of unknown causation. Although the total concentration appears appropriate (15 μg/mL), a toxic unbound concentration is present ($C_f = f_B C = 0.2 \cdot 15$ μg/mL = 3 μg/mL).

Unbound phenytoin serum concentrations should be measured for patients with factors known to alter plasma protein binding of phenytoin. These factors fall into three broad categories: (1) lack of binding protein when there are insufficient plasma concentrations of albumin, (2) displacement of phenytoin from albumin binding sites by endogenous compounds, and (3) displacement of phenytoin from albumin binding sites by exogenous compounds (Table 10-2).[4–22]

Low albumin concentrations, known as hypoalbuminemia, can be found among patients with liver disease or nephrotic syndrome, pregnant women, patients with cystic fibrosis, burn patients, trauma patients, malnourished persons, and the elderly. Albumin concentrations <3 g/dL are associated with high unbound fractions of phenytoin in the plasma. Pa-

TABLE 10-2 Diseases and Conditions That Alter Phenytoin Plasma Protein Binding

INSUFFICIENT ALBUMIN CONCENTRATION (HYPOALBUMINEMIA)	DISPLACEMENT BY ENDOGENOUS COMPOUNDS	DISPLACEMENT BY EXOGENOUS COMPOUNDS
Liver disease Nephrotic syndrome Pregnancy Cystic fibrosis Burns Trauma Malnourishment Elderly	Hyperbilirubinemia Jaundice Liver disease Renal dysfunction	Drug interactions Warfarin Valproic acid >2 g/d aspirin Nonsteroidal antiinflammatory drugs with high albumin binding capacity

tients with albumin concentrations of 2.5 to 3 g/dL typically have unbound fractions of phenytoin of 15% to 20%. Patients with albumin concentrations between 2.0 and 2.5 g/dL often have unbound fractions of phenytoin >20%. Albumin is manufactured by the liver, so patients with hepatic disease may have difficulty synthesizing the protein. Patients with nephrotic syndrome waste albumin by eliminating it in the urine. Malnourished patients can be so nutritionally deprived that albumin production is impeded. Malnourishment is the cause of hypoalbuminemia among some elderly patients, although there is a general decrease in albumin concentrations among older persons. While recovering from their injuries, burn and trauma patients can become hypermetabolic, and albumin concentration can decrease if insufficient caloric intake is supplied during this phase of disease. Albumin concentration can decrease during pregnancy as maternal reserves are shifted to the developing fetus. The decrease is especially prevalent during the third trimester.

Displacement of phenytoin from plasma protein binding sites by endogenous substances can occur among patients with hepatic or renal dysfunction. The mechanism is competition for albumin plasma protein binding sites between the endogenous substances and phenytoin. Bilirubin, a by-product of heme metabolism, is broken down by the liver, so patients with hepatic disease can have excessive bilirubin concentrations. Total bilirubin concentrations >2 mg/dL are associated with abnormal plasma protein binding of phenytoin. Patients with end-stage renal disease (creatinine clearance, <10 to 15 mL/min) and uremia (blood urea nitrogen concentration, >80 to 100 mg/dL) accumulate unidentified compounds in the blood that displace phenytoin from plasma protein binding sites. Abnormal phenytoin binding persists in these patients even when dialysis is instituted.

Displacement from plasma protein binding of phenytoin can be caused by exogenously administered compounds such as drugs. In this case, the mechanism is competition for albumin binding sites between phenytoin and other agents. Other drugs that are highly bound to albumin and cause drug interactions with phenytoin due to displacement of plasma protein binding include warfarin, valproic acid, aspirin (>2 g/d), and some highly bound nonsteroidal antiinflammatory agents.

Once the free fraction (f_B) has been determined for a patient with altered plasma protein binding of phenytoin ($f_B = C_f/C$, where C is the total concentration and C_f is the unbound concentration), it is often not necessary to measure additional concentrations of unbound drug. If the situation that caused altered plasma protein binding is stable, such as albumin or bilirubin concentration, hepatic or renal function, or other drug doses, total phenytoin concentration can be converted to the concurrent unbound value and used for therapeutic drug monitoring. For example, a patient with end-stage renal failure is receiving phenytoin as well as valproic acid and warfarin. The concurrently measured total and unbound phenytoin concentrations are 5 μg/mL and 1.5 μg/mL, respectively, yielding an unbound fraction of 30% [$f_B = C_f/C = (1.5\ \mu g/mL)/(5\ \mu g/mL) = 0.30$]. The next day, the total phenytoin concentration is 6 μg/mL. The estimated unbound concentration is 1.8 μg/mL: $C_f = f_B C = 0.30 \cdot 6\ \mu g/mL = 1.8\ \mu g/mL$. Of course, if the disease status or drug therapy changes, a new unbound fraction of phenytoin is present and must be measured with an unbound and total phenytoin concentration.

When unbound phenytoin concentrations are unavailable, several methods have been suggested to estimate the value or a surrogate measure of the value. The most common surrogate is estimation of the equivalent total phenytoin concentration that would provide the same unbound phenytoin concentration if the patient had a normal unbound fraction value of 10%. These calculations adjust the total phenytoin concentration so that it can be compared to the usual phenytoin therapeutic range of 10 to 20 μg/mL. The adjusted concentration can then be used to determine if dosage changes are warranted. The equation for hypoalbuminemia is $C_{Normal\ Binding} = C/(X \cdot Alb + 0.1)$, where $C_{Normal\ Binding}$ is the normalized total phenytoin concentration in micrograms per milliliter, C is the actual measured phenytoin concentration in micrograms per milliliter, X is a constant equal to 0.2 if protein binding measurements are conducted at 37°C or 0.25 if conducted at 25°C, and Alb is the albumin concentration in grams per deciliter.[23,24] If the patient has end-stage renal disease (creatinine clearance, <10 to 15 mL/min), the same equation is used with a different constant value (X = 0.1).[23] (Note: In most *experimental* laboratories protein binding is determined at normal body temperature [37°C]; in most *clinical* laboratories protein binding is determined at room temperature [25°C].) Because it is assumed that the normal unbound fraction of phenytoin is 10%, the estimated unbound concentration of phenytoin (C_{fEST}) is computed with the following formula: $(C_{fEST}) = 0.1\ C_{Normal\ Binding}$. A different approach is used in the equations for patients with concurrent valproic acid administration. In this case, the unbound phenytoin concentration (C_{fEST}) is estimated with simultaneously measured total concentrations of phenytoin (PHT in micrograms per milliliter) and valproic acid (VPA in micrograms per milliliter): $C_{fEST} = (0.095 + 0.001 \cdot VPA)PHT$.[25,26] This value is compared with the usual therapeutic range of unbound phenytoin concentrations (1 to 2 μg/mL) and used for dosage adjustment. These equations provide only estimates of the respective concentrations. Actual unbound concentrations of phenytoin should be measured whenever possible in the care of patients with suspected abnormal plasma protein binding of phenytoin.

Example 1 JM has epilepsy and is being treated with phenytoin. He has hypoalbuminemia (albumin level, 2.2 g/dL) and normal renal function (creatinine clearance, 90 mL/min). The total phenytoin concentration is 7.5 μg/mL. With the assumption that any unbound concentrations are measured at 25°C, compute an estimated normalized phenytoin concentration for this patient.

1. *Choose the appropriate equation to estimate normalized total phenytoin concentration at the appropriate temperature.*

$$C_{Normal\ Binding} = C/(0.25 \cdot Alb + 0.1) = (7.5\ \mu g/mL)/(0.25 \cdot 2.2\ g/dL + 0.1) = 11.5\ \mu g/mL$$

$$C_{fEST} = 0.1\ C_{Normal\ Binding} = 0.1 \cdot 11.5\ \mu g/mL = 1.2\ \mu g/mL$$

The estimated normalized total phenytoin concentration is expected to provide an unbound concentration equivalent to a total phenytoin concentration of 11.5 μg/mL for a patient with normal drug protein binding (C_{fEST} = 1.2 μg/mL). Because the estimated total value is within the therapeutic range of 10 to 20 μg/mL, it is likely that the patient has an unbound phenytoin concentration within the therapeutic range. If possible, this estimate should be confirmed by measuring the actual unbound concentration of phenytoin.

Example 2 LM has epilepsy and is being treated with phenytoin. He has hypoalbuminemia (albumin level, 2.2 g/dL) and poor renal function (creatinine clearance, 10 mL/min). The total phenytoin concentration is 7.5 μg/mL. Compute an estimated normalized phenytoin concentration for this patient.

1. *Choose the appropriate equation to estimate the normalized total phenytoin concentration.*

$$C_{\text{Normal Binding}} = C/(0.1 \cdot \text{Alb} + 0.1) = (7.5\ \mu\text{g/mL})/(0.1 \cdot 2.2\ \text{g/dL} + 0.1) = 23.4\ \mu\text{g/mL}$$

$$C_{fEST} = 0.1\ C_{\text{Normal Binding}} = 0.1 \cdot 23.4\ \mu\text{g/mL} = 2.3\ \mu\text{g/mL}$$

The estimated normalized total phenytoin concentration is expected to provide an unbound concentration equivalent to a total phenytoin concentration of 23.4 μg/mL for a patient with normal drug protein binding (C_{fEST} = 2.3 μg/mL). Because the estimated total value is above the therapeutic range of 10 to 20 μg/mL, it is likely that the patient has an unbound phenytoin concentration above the therapeutic range. If possible, this estimate should be confirmed by measuring the actual unbound concentration of phenytoin.

Example 3 PM has epilepsy and is being treated with phenytoin and valproic acid. He has a normal albumin concentration (4.2 g/dL) and normal renal function (creatinine clearance, 90 mL/min). The steady-state total phenytoin and valproic acid concentrations are 7.5 μg/mL and 100 μg/mL, respectively. Compute an estimated unbound phenytoin concentration for this patient.

1. *Choose the appropriate equation to estimate the unbound phenytoin concentration.*

$$C_{fEST} = (0.095 + 0.001 \cdot \text{VPA})\text{PHT} = (0.095 + 0.001 \cdot 100\ \mu\text{g/mL})\ 7.5\ \mu\text{g/mL} = 1.5\ \mu\text{g/mL}$$

The estimated unbound concentration of phenytoin is expected to be within the therapeutic range for unbound concentrations. If possible, this estimate should be confirmed by measuring the actual unbound concentration of phenytoin.

CLINICAL MONITORING PARAMETERS

The goal of therapy with anticonvulsants is to reduce seizure frequency and maximize quality of life with a minimum of adverse drug effects.[3] Although it is desirable to abolish all seizure episodes, it may not be possible to accomplish this for many patients. Patients should be observed for concentration-related side effects (drowsiness, fatigue, nystagmus, ataxia, slurred speech, lack of coordination, changes in mental status, decreased mentation, confusion, lethargy, and coma) and for adverse reactions associated with long-term use (behavioral changes, cerebellar syndrome, connective tissue changes, coarse facies, skin thickening, folate deficiency, gingival hyperplasia, lymphadenopathy, hirsutism, osteomalacia). Idiosyncratic side effects include skin rash, Stevens-Johnson syndrome, bone marrow suppression, systemic lupus-like reactions, and hepatitis.

Serum concentrations of phenytoin should be measured for most patients. Because epilepsy is an episodic disease, patients do not have seizures on a continuous basis. Thus during dosage titration, it is difficult to determine whether the patient is responding to drug therapy or simply is not having abnormal central nervous system discharges. Phenytoin serum concentrations are valuable in avoiding adverse drug effects. Patients are more likely to accept drug therapy if adverse reactions are held to the absolute minimum. Because phenytoin follows nonlinear or saturable pharmacokinetics, it is fairly easy to reach toxic concentrations with modest changes in drug dose.

BASIC CLINICAL PHARMACOKINETIC PARAMETERS

Phenytoin is eliminated primarily by means of hepatic metabolism (>95%). Hepatic metabolism occurs mainly through the CYP2C9 enzyme system; a smaller amount is metabolized by CYP2C19. About 5% of a phenytoin dose is recovered in the urine as unchanged drug. Phenytoin follows Michaelis-Menten or saturable pharmacokinetics.[27,28] This is the type of nonlinear pharmacokinetics that occurs when the number of drug molecules overwhelms or saturates the ability of the enzyme to metabolize the drug. When this happens, steady-state drug serum concentrations increase in a disproportionate manner after a dosage increase (Figure 10-1). In this case, the rate of drug removal is described by the classic Michaelis-Menten relation used for all enzyme systems: Rate of metabolism = $(V_{max} \cdot C)/(K_m + C)$, where V_{max} is the maximum rate of metabolism in mil-

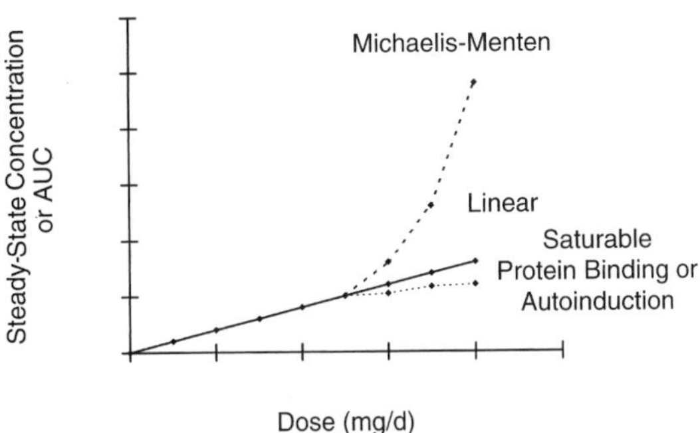

FIGURE 10-1 If a drug follows linear pharmacokinetics, steady-state concentration (Css) or the area under the concentration-time curve (AUC) increases in proportion to the dose. The result is a straight line on the plot. Nonlinear pharmacokinetics occurs when the Css or AUC versus dose plot produces something other than a straight line. If a drug, such as phenytoin or aspirin, follows Michaelis-Menten pharmacokinetics, as steady-state drug concentration approaches the Michaelis-Menten constant (K_m), serum concentrations increase more than expected owing to dose increases. If a drug, such as valproic acid or disopyramide, follows nonlinear protein binding, total steady-state drug concentrations increase less than expected as dose increases.

ligrams per day, C is the phenytoin concentration in milligrams per liter, and K_m is the substrate concentration in milligrams per liter and the rate of metabolism is $V_{max}/2$.

The clinical implication of Michaelis-Menten pharmacokinetics is that the clearance of phenytoin is not a constant, as it is with linear pharmacokinetics, but is concentration- or dose-dependent. As the dose or concentration of phenytoin increases, the clearance rate (Cl) decreases as the enzyme approaches saturable conditions: $Cl = V_{max}/(K_m + C)$. This is the reason concentrations increase disproportionately after a phenytoin dosage increase. For example, phenytoin follows saturable pharmacokinetics with average Michaelis-Menten constants of V_{max} = 500 mg/d and K_m = 4 mg/L. The therapeutic range of phenytoin is 10 to 20 μg/mL. As the steady-state concentration of phenytoin increases from 10 μg/mL to 20 μg/mL, clearance decreases from 36 L/d to 21 L/d: $Cl = V_{max}/(K_m + C)$; Cl = (500 mg/d)/(4 mg/L + 10 mg/L) = 36 L/d; Cl = (500 mg/d)/(4 mg/L + 20 mg/L) = 21 L/d. (Note: μg/mL = mg/L, and this substitution is made to avoid unit conversion.) There is so much interpatient variability in Michaelis-Menten pharmacokinetic parameters for phenytoin (typically V_{max} = 100 to 1000 mg/d and K_m = 1 to 15 μg/mL) that dosing the drug is extremely difficult.

Phenytoin volume of distribution (V = 0.7 L/kg) is unaffected by saturable metabolism and is still determined by the physiologic volume of blood (V_B) and tissues (V_T) as well as the unbound fraction of drug in the blood (f_B) and tissues (f_T): $V = V_B + (f_B/f_T)V_T$. Also, half-life ($t_{1/2}$) still is related to clearance and volume of distribution with the same equation used for linear pharmacokinetics: $t_{1/2} = (0.693 \cdot V)/Cl$. However, because clearance is dose- or concentration-dependent, half-life also changes with changes in phenytoin dosage or concentration. As doses or concentrations increase for a drug that follows Michaelis-Menten pharmacokinetics, clearance decreases and half-life becomes longer for the drug: $\uparrow t_{1/2} = (0.693 \cdot V)/\downarrow Cl$. According to the previous example for clearance and volume of distribution for a person weighing 70 kg (V = 0.7 L/kg · 70 kg ≈50 L), half-life changes from 1 d ($t_{1/2}$ = [0.693 · V]/Cl = [0.693 · 50 L]/[36 L/d] = 1 d) to 1.7 d ($t_{1/2}$ = [0.693 · 50 L]/[21 L/d] = 1.7 d) as the serum concentration of phenytoin increases from 10 μg/mL to 20 μg/mL. The clinical implication of this finding is that the time to steady state (3 to 5 half-lives) is longer as the dose or concentration of phenytoin increases. On average, the time to steady-state serum concentration is approximately 5 days at a dosage rate of 300 mg/d and 15 days at a dosage rate of 400 mg/d.[27]

Under steady-state conditions, the rate of drug administration equals the rate of drug removal.[29] Therefore the Michaelis-Menten equation can be used to compute the maintenance dose (MD in mg/d) needed to achieve a target steady-state serum concentration of phenytoin (Css in μg/mL or mg/L):

$$MD = \frac{V_{max} \cdot Css}{K_m + Css}$$

Or, solved for Css:

$$Css = \frac{K_m \cdot MD}{V_{max} - MD}$$

When phenytoin steady-state concentration is much less than the K_m value for a patient, this equation simplifies to MD = (V_{max}/K_m)Css or, because V_{max}/K_m is a constant, MD = Cl · Css. Therefore, when K_m >> Css, phenytoin follows linear pharmacokinetics.

When phenytoin steady-state concentration is much greater than the K_m value for a patient, the rate of metabolism becomes a constant equal to V_{max}. Under these conditions, only a fixed amount of phenytoin is metabolized per day because the enzyme system is completely saturated and cannot increase its metabolic capacity. This situation is also known as *zero-order pharmacokinetics. First-order pharmacokinetics* is another name for linear pharmacokinetics.

For parenteral use, phenytoin is available in two different dosage forms. Phenytoin sodium, the sodium salt of phenytoin, contains 92% phenytoin by weight. Although it is a salt of phenytoin, the drug is still relatively insoluble in water. To facilitate dissolution, ethanol and propylene glycol are added to the vehicle, and the pH of the solution is adjusted to between 10 and 12. Intramuscular injections of phenytoin sodium are extremely painful.[30] Some of the drug probably precipitates in the muscle injection site, and this causes prolonged absorption of the drug over several days. When phenytoin is given intravenously, the injection rate should not exceed 50 mg/min to avoid hypotension. Even at lower infusion rates, profound hypotension can occur in patients with unstable blood pressure or shock. Phenytoin sodium injection can be given by means of slow intravenous push of undiluted drug, or the drug can be added to normal saline solution at a concentration of 10 mg/mL or less and infused at <50 mg/min. When added to normal saline solution, the drug should be given as soon as possible after being mixed to avoid precipitation, and a 0.22-µm in-line filter should be used to remove any drug crystals before they reach the patient.

To avoid many of the problems associated with phenytoin sodium injection, a water-soluble phosphate ester prodrug of phenytoin, fosphenytoin, has been developed. Conversion of fosphenytoin to phenytoin is rapid; the half-life of fosphenytoin is approximately 15 minutes. To avoid confusion, fosphenytoin is prescribed in terms of phenytoin sodium equivalents (PE). Thus 100 mg PE of fosphenytoin is equivalent to 100 mg phenytoin sodium. Hypotension during intravenous administration of fosphenytoin is much less of a problem than during administration of phenytoin sodium. The maximal intravenous infusion rate is 150 mg PE per minute. Transient pruritis and paresthesia are associated with this route of administration. Intramuscular absorption is rapid; peak concentration is reached about 30 minutes after injection, and bioavailability with this route of administration is 100%. Fosphenytoin, however, is much more expensive than phenytoin sodium injection, so this has limited its widespread use. Most clinicians use fosphenytoin only for patients who need intramuscular phenytoin or for patients with unstable or low blood pressure that necessitates intravenous phenytoin therapy.

For oral use, capsules contain phenytoin sodium (92% phenytoin by weight), and tablets and suspension contain phenytoin acid. Phenytoin sodium capsules are labeled as *extended phenytoin sodium capsules* or *prompt phenytoin sodium capsules.* Extended phenytoin sodium capsules release phenytoin slowly from the gastrointestinal tract into the systemic circulation. The extended-release characteristics of this dosage form are produced by slow dissolution of the drug in gastric juices and are not the result of extended-release dosage form technology. Prompt phenytoin sodium capsules are absorbed fairly quickly from the gastrointestinal tract because they contain microcrystalline phenytoin sodium, which dissolves more quickly in gastric juices than does the extended form. Because of the sustained-release properties, extended phenytoin sodium capsules can be taken once or twice daily. Prompt phenytoin sodium capsules must be taken several times daily. Phenytoin sodium capsules are available in 100-mg and 30-mg strengths.

Phenytoin tablets (50 mg, chewable) and suspension (125 mg/5 mL and 30 mg/5 mL) for oral use are available as the acid form of the drug. Both the tablet and suspension dosage forms are absorbed more rapidly than extended phenytoin sodium capsules, and once-daily dosing with these may not be possible for some patients. The suspensions are thick, and it is difficult to disperse the drug evenly throughout the liquid. If the container is not shaken well before a dose is dispensed, the drug can flocculate into the bottom of the bottle. When this occurs, phenytoin concentration near the top of the bottle is less than average, and doses given when the bottle is two thirds or more full contain less phenytoin. Phenytoin concentration near the bottom of the bottle is greater than average, and doses given when the bottle is one third or less full contain more phenytoin. This problem can be avoided to a large extent if the dispensing pharmacist shakes the bottle for several minutes before giving it to the patient.

For most drugs, the 8% difference in dose between dosage forms containing phenytoin (suspension and tablets, 100 mg = 100 mg phenytoin) and phenytoin sodium (capsules and injection, 100 mg = 92 mg phenytoin) is trivial and easily ignored. However, because phenytoin follows nonlinear pharmacokinetics, an 8% difference in dose can cause substantial changes in the serum concentration of phenytoin. For example, if a patient is stabilized on a dose of intravenous phenytoin sodium 300 mg/d (300 mg/d phenytoin sodium × 0.92 = 276 mg phenytoin) with a steady-state concentration of 17 μg/mL, switching to phenytoin suspension 300 mg/d can cause steady-state phenytoin concentration to exceed 20 μg/mL (15% to 30% increase or more) and produce toxicity. If a different patient is stabilized on a dose of phenytoin suspension 300 mg/d with a steady-state concentration of 12 μg/mL, switching to intravenous phenytoin sodium 300 mg/d (300 mg/d phenytoin sodium × 0.92 = 276 mg phenytoin) can cause steady-state phenytoin concentrations less than 10 μg/mL (15% to 30% decrease or more) and result in loss of efficacy. Phenytoin doses usually are not fine-tuned to the point of directly accounting for the difference in phenytoin content (276 mg of phenytoin suspension would not be prescribed for a patient receiving 300 mg of phenytoin sodium injection). Rather, clinicians are aware that when phenytoin dosage forms are changed, phenytoin content may change. They anticipate that the drug concentration may increase or decrease because of this. Most clinicians recheck phenytoin serum concentrations after a change in dosage form is instituted.

The oral bioavailability of phenytoin approximates 100% for capsule, tablet, and suspension dosage forms.[31–34] At larger amounts, there is some dose dependency on absorption characteristics.[35] Single oral doses of 800 mg or more produce longer times for maximal concentrations to occur (T_{max}) and decreased bioavailability. Because larger oral doses also produce a higher incidence of gastrointestinal side effects (primarily nausea and vomiting due to local irritation), it is prudent to break maintenance doses larger than 800 mg/d into multiple doses. If oral phenytoin loading doses are given, a common total dose is 1000 mg given as 400 mg, 300 mg, and 300 mg separated by 2- to 6-hour intervals. Enteral feedings given by nasogastric tube interfere with phenytoin absorption.[36–39] Possible mechanisms include decreased gastrointestinal transit time, which reduces absorption contact time, binding of phenytoin to proteins contained in the feedings, and adherence of phenytoin to the lumen of the feeding tube. The solution to this problem is to stop the feedings, when possible, for 1 to 2 hours before and after phenytoin administration and to increase the oral phenytoin dose. It is not unusual for phenytoin oral dosage requirements to double or triple while a patient receives concurrent nasogastric feedings (e.g., usual dose of 300 to 400 mg/d increasing to 600 to 1200 mg/d during nasogastric feeding). Intravenous or intramuscular phenytoin or fosphenytoin doses also can be substituted while nasogastric feedings are being administered. Although poorly documented, phenytoin oral malabsorption can occur among patients with severe diarrhea, malabsorption syndromes, or gastric resection.

The typical recommended loading dose of phenytoin is 15 to 20 mg/kg or about 1000 mg for most adult patients. Usual initial maintenance doses are 5 to 10 mg/kg per day for children (6 months to 16 years of age) and 4 to 6 mg/kg per day for adults. For adults, the most prescribed dose is 300 to 400 mg/d of phenytoin. Because of an increased incidence of adverse effects among patients older than 65 years, many clinicians prescribe a maximum of 200 mg/d as an initial dose for these patients.[40,41]

EFFECT OF ALTERED PLASMA PROTEIN BINDING ON THE PHARMACOKINETICS OF PHENYTOIN

The pharmacokinetic alterations that occur with altered plasma protein binding cause complex changes in total and unbound steady-state concentrations of phenytoin and drug response. As discussed (in Chapter 3), hepatic drug metabolism is described with the following equation:

$$Cl_H = \frac{LBF \cdot (f_B \cdot Cl'_{int})}{LBF + (f_B \cdot Cl'_{int})}$$

where LBF is liver blood flow, f_B is the fraction of unbound drug in the blood, and Cl'_{int} is intrinsic clearance. For drugs such as phenytoin that have a low hepatic extraction ratio (≤30%), the numeric value of liver blood flow is much greater than the product of unbound fraction of drug in the blood and the intrinsic clearance of the compound ($LBF >> f_B \cdot Cl'_{int}$), and the sum in the denominator of the hepatic clearance equation is almost equal to liver blood flow [$LBF \approx LBF + (f_B \cdot Cl'_{int})$]. When this substitution is made into the hepatic clearance equation, hepatic clearance equals the product of free fraction in the blood and the intrinsic clearance of the drug for a drug with a low hepatic extraction ratio, as follows:

$$Cl_H = \frac{LBF \cdot (f_B \cdot Cl'_{int})}{LBF} = f_B \cdot Cl'_{int}$$

A graphic technique is used to illustrate the differences that may occur in steady-state drug concentration and pharmacologic effects among patients with altered plasma protein binding of phenytoin (Figure 10-2A). In the example, it is assumed that phenytoin is being given to a patient as a continuous intravenous infusion and that all physiologic, pharmacokinetic, and drug effect parameters (*y*-axis) are initially stable. However, the same changes occur for average total and unbound steady-state concentrations when the drug is given on a continuous dosage schedule (every 8, 12, and 24 hours and so on) or orally. On the *x*-axis, an arrow indicates that plasma protein binding of phenytoin decreases and that the unbound fraction increases in the patient; an assumption made for this illustration is that any changes in the parameters are instantaneous. An increase in a parameter is denoted as an uptick in the line, and a decrease in the parameter is shown as a downtick in the line.

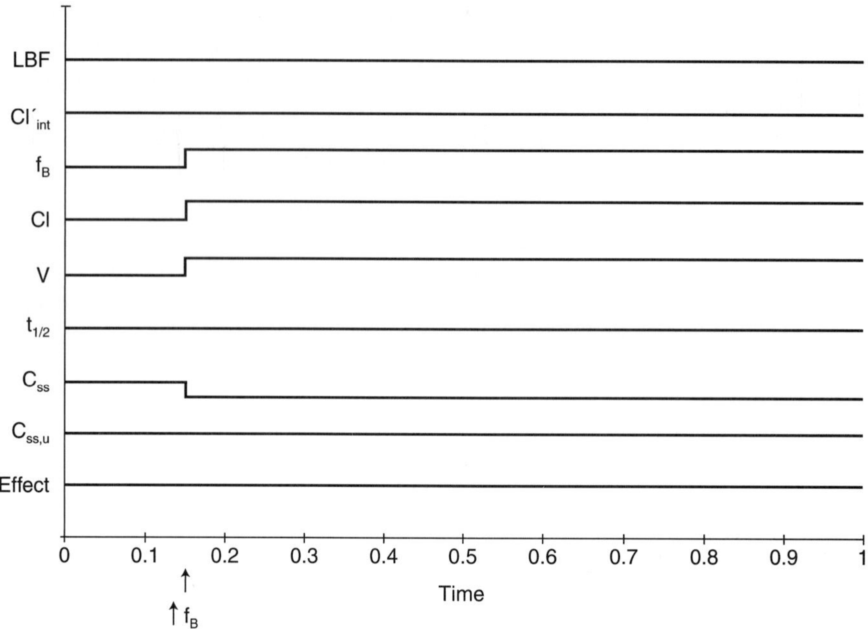

FIGURE 10-2 (A) Schematic of physiologic (*LBF*, liver blood flow; Cl'_{int}, intrinsic or unbound clearance; f_B, unbound fraction of drug in blood/plasma), pharmacokinetic (*Cl*, clearance; *V*, volume of distribution; $t_{1/2}$, half-life; C_{ss}, total steady-state drug concentration; $C_{ss,u}$, unbound steady-state drug concentration), and pharmacodynamic (*Effect*, pharmacodynamic effect) changes that occur with decreased protein binding of phenytoin (*arrow,* $\uparrow f_B$).

For a drug with a low hepatic extraction ratio, drug interactions that displace plasma protein binding cause major pharmacokinetic alterations but are not clinically significant because the pharmacologic effect of the drug does not change (see Figure 10-2A). Because the clearance of the drug depends on the fraction of unbound drug in the blood and intrinsic clearance for an agent with a low hepatic extraction ratio, a decrease in plasma protein binding and an increase in unbound fraction increase clearance ($\uparrow Cl = \uparrow f_B Cl'_{int}$) and volume of distribution ($\uparrow V = V_B + [\uparrow f_B/f_T]V_T$). Because half-life depends on clearance and volume of distribution, it is likely that because both parameters increase, half-life does not change substantially ($t_{1/2} = [0.693 \cdot \uparrow V]/\uparrow Cl$). However, it is possible that if either clearance or volume of distribution changes disproportionately, half-life also changes. The total steady-state concentration declines because of the increase in clearance ($\downarrow Css = k_0/\uparrow Cl$, where k_0 is the infusion rate of drug). The unbound steady-state concentration remains unaltered because the free fraction of drug in the blood is higher than it was before the increase in unbound fraction ($Css_u = \uparrow f_B \downarrow Css$). The pharmacologic effect of the drug does not change, because the free concentration of drug in the blood is unchanged. This outcome can be unexpected for the decrease in plasma protein binding, especially because the total steady-state concentration of the drug decreases. Clinicians need to be aware of situations such as this because the total drug concentration (Bound + Unbound) can be misleading and cause an unwarranted increase in drug dosage. Unbound concentrations of drugs should be used to persuade clinicians that an increase in drug dosage is not needed despite a decrease in total concentrations caused by this interaction.

EFFECTS OF DISEASES AND CONDITIONS ON PHARMACOKINETICS AND DOSING

Adults without the diseases and conditions discussed later and who have normal liver and renal function and normal plasma protein binding (~90%) have an average phenytoin V_{max} of 7 mg/kg per day (range, 1.5 to 14 mg/kg per day) and K_m of 4 μg/mL (range, 1 to 15 μg/mL).[28] Michaelis-Menten parameters for children 6 months to 6 years of age are V_{max} of 12 mg/kg per day and K_m of 6 μg/mL. For children 7 to 16 years of age, V_{max} is 9 mg/kg per day and K_m is 6 μg/mL.[42–47] The most difficult and frustrating aspect of phenytoin dosage determination is the 10- to 15-fold variation in Michaelis-Menten pharmacokinetic parameters that produces huge variability in dose requirements. An individualized dosage regimen must be determined to accomplish therapeutic goals. Unfortunately, measurement of V_{max} and K_m for phenytoin is difficult. Because of this, the effects of diseases and conditions on these parameters are largely unknown. By necessity, phenytoin is discussed in qualitative terms.

Patients with cirrhosis of the liver or acute hepatitis have reduced phenytoin clearance because of destruction of liver parenchyma. This loss of functional hepatic cells decreases the amount of CYP2C9 and CYP2C19 available to metabolize the drug and decreases V_{max}. The volume of distribution is larger because of reduced plasma protein binding. Protein binding is reduced, and unbound fraction is increased due to hypoalbuminemia or hyperbilirubinemia, especially albumin ≤3 g/dL or total bilirubin ≥2 mg/dL). However, the effects of liver disease on phenytoin pharmacokinetics are highly variable and difficult to predict accurately. It is possible for a patient with liver disease to have relatively normal or grossly abnormal phenytoin clearance and volume of distribution. For example, a patient with liver disease who has relatively normal albumin and bilirubin concentrations can have a normal volume of distribution of phenytoin. An index of liver dysfunction can be gained by applying the Child-Pugh clinical classification system (Table 10-3).[48] Child-Pugh scores are discussed in detail in Chapter 3, but are discussed briefly here.

The Child-Pugh score is based on five laboratory test results or clinical symptoms: serum albumin level, total bilirubin level, prothrombin time, presence of ascites, and presence of hepatic encephalopathy. Each of these areas is given a score of 1 (normal) to 3 (severely abnormal), and the scores for the five areas are added. The Child-Pugh score for a patient with normal liver function is 5, and the score for a patient with grossly abnormal serum albumin, total bilirubin, and prothrombin time values in addition to severe ascites and hepatic encephalopathy is 15. A Child-Pugh score greater than 8 is grounds for a decrease of 25% to 50% in the initial daily dose of phenytoin. As for any patient with or without liver dysfunction, initial doses are meant as starting points for dosage titration based on patient response and avoidance of adverse effects. Serum concentrations of phenytoin and the presence of adverse drug effects should be assessed frequently for patients with cirrhosis of the liver.

TABLE 10-3 Child-Pugh Scores for Patients with Liver Disease

TEST/SYMPTOM	SCORE 1 POINT	SCORE 2 POINTS	SCORE 3 POINTS
Total bilirubin (mg/dL)	<2.0	2.0–3.0	>3.0
Serum albumin (g/dL)	>3.5	2.8–3.5	<2.8
Prothrombin time (seconds prolonged over control)	<4	4–6	>6
Ascites	Absent	Slight	Moderate
Hepatic encephalopathy	None	Moderate	Severe

Adapted from Pugh RN, Murray-Lyon IM, Dawson JL, Pietroni MC, Williams R. Transection of the oesophagus for bleeding oesophageal varices. Br J Surg 1973;60:646–9.

Patients who have sustained trauma or burns have an increased ability to metabolize phenytoin that begins 3 to 7 days after the injury.[49,50] At that time, these patients become hypermetabolic to repair damaged tissue, and the V_{max} for phenytoin increases owing to this general increase in metabolic rate. If caloric needs are not met during this phase of recovery for trauma patients, many become hypoalbuminemic, and plasma protein binding of phenytoin decreases. The result is an increase in unbound fraction. Phenytoin dosage requirements increase while trauma patients are in the hypermetabolic phase, and monitoring of unbound concentration is indicated when patients have low albumin concentrations, especially albumin levels ≤3 g/dL.

Pregnant women taking phenytoin have increased dosage requirements, particularly during the third trimester (27 weeks and later).[4,5,51–55] There are several reasons for this change, including malabsorption of drug resulting in decreased bioavailability, increased metabolism of phenytoin, and decreased protein binding due to low albumin concentrations. Aggressive monitoring of drug serum concentration, including measurement of unbound phenytoin concentrations if the patient is hypoalbuminemic, is necessary to avoid seizures and harm to the unborn fetus. An additional concern in the administration of phenytoin to pregnant patients is the development of fetal hydantoin syndrome.

Elderly individuals older than 65 years have a decreased capacity to metabolize phenytoin, possibly because age-related losses of liver parenchyma decrease the amount of CYP2C9 and CYP2C19.[40,41] Older patients also may have hypoalbuminemia with resulting decreases in plasma protein binding and increases in unbound fraction.[21,22] Many elderly patients also seem to have an increased propensity for central nervous system side effects of phenytoin. Because of these pharmacokinetic and pharmacodynamic changes, clinicians tend to prescribe lower initial doses of phenytoin to older patients (~200 mg/d).

Patients with end-stage renal disease and creatinine clearance <10 to 15 mL/min have an unidentified substance in their blood that displaces phenytoin from its plasma protein binding sites.[14–18,20] This unknown compound is not removed with dialysis.[19] These patients also tend to have hypoalbuminemia, which increases the unbound fraction of phenytoin even further. Monitoring of the unbound serum concentration of phenytoin is helpful in determining dosage requirements for patients with renal failure. Other patients prone to hypoalbuminemia are those with nephrotic syndrome, cystic fibrosis, or malnutrition. High bilirubin concentrations can be found among patients with biliary tract obstruction or hemolysis. Monitoring of the unbound concentration of phenytoin should be considered in the care of these patients, especially when albumin concentrations are ≤3 g/dL or total bilirubin concentration is ≥2 mg/dL.

DRUG INTERACTIONS

Because it is so highly metabolized in the liver by CYP2C9 and CYP2C19, phenytoin is prone to drug interactions that inhibit hepatic microsomal enzymes.[56] Cimetidine, valproic acid, amiodarone, choramphenicol, isoniazid, disulfiram, and omeprazole have been reported to inhibit phenytoin metabolism and increase the serum concentration of phenytoin. Phenytoin also is a broad-based hepatic enzyme inducer that affects most cytochrome P450 systems. Drugs with narrow therapeutic ranges that can have their metabolism increased by concurrent phenytoin administration include carbamazepine, phenobarbital, cyclosporine, tacrolimus, and warfarin. When phenytoin therapy is added to the medication regimen for a patient, a comprehensive review for drug interactions should be conducted. Valproic acid, aspirin (>2 g/d), some highly protein-bound nonsteroidal antiinflammatory drugs, and warfarin can displace phenytoin from plasma protein binding sites. This necessitates monitoring of unbound phenytoin concentration.

The drug interaction between valproic acid and phenytoin deserves special examination because of its complexity and because these two agents are regularly used together for the management of seizures.[6–9] The drug interaction involves displacement of plasma protein binding and inhibition of intrinsic clearance of phenytoin by valproic acid. What makes this interaction so difficult to detect and understand is that these two changes do not occur simultaneously, so the impression left by the drug interaction depends on when it is observed. For example, a patient is stabilized on phenytoin therapy (Figure 10-2B), but because adequate control of seizures has not been attained, valproic acid is added to the regimen. As valproic acid accumulates, the first interaction observed is phenytoin plasma protein binding displacement as the two drugs compete for binding sites on albumin. The result of this portion of the drug interaction is an increase in unbound fraction of phenytoin and a decrease in total serum concentration of phenytoin, but the unbound serum concentration of phenytoin remains the same. As valproic acid serum concentrations achieve steady-state conditions, the higher concentrations of the drug bathe the hepatic microsomal enzyme system and inhibit intrinsic clearance of phenytoin. This portion of the interaction decreases intrinsic clearance and hepatic clearance of phenytoin, so both unbound and total concentrations of phenytoin increase. When phenytoin concentrations finally equilibrate and reach steady state under the new plasma protein binding and intrinsic clearance conditions imposed by concurrent valproic acid therapy, the total concentration of phenytoin often is at about the same level as before the drug interaction occurred, but unbound phenytoin concentrations are much higher. If only total phenytoin concentrations are measured at this point in time, clinicians will be under the impression that total concentrations did not change and that no drug interaction occurred. However, if unbound phenytoin concentrations are simultaneously measured, it will be found that these concentrations have increased and that the unbound fraction of phenytoin is twice or more (≥20%) the baseline amount. In this situation, the patient may have unbound phenytoin concentrations that are toxic, and a decrease in phenytoin dosage may be in order.

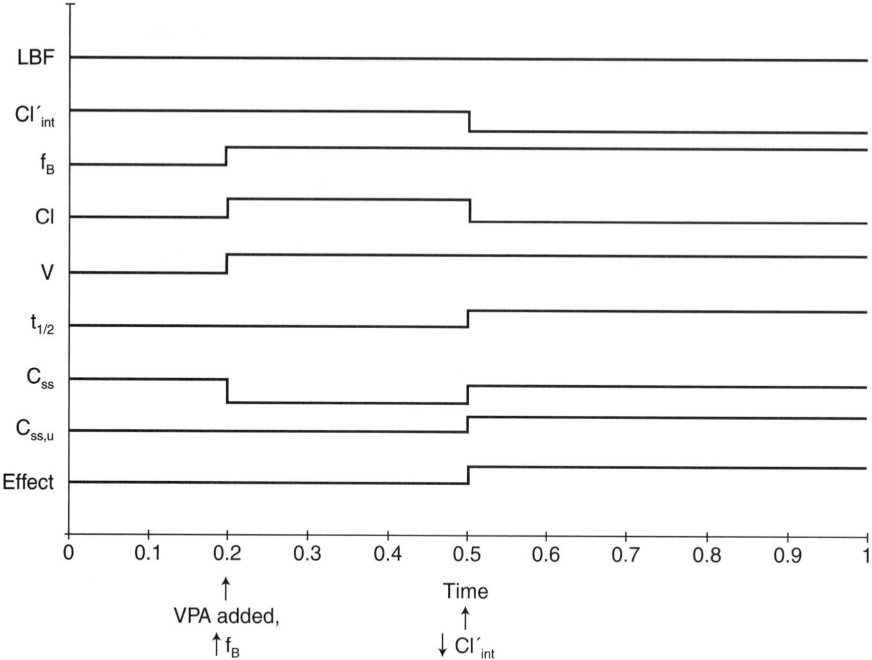

FIGURE 10-2 (B) Schematic of the effect of initiating valproic acid (*VPA*) treatment of a patient who is stabilized with phenytoin therapy (see Figure 10-2**A** for definitions of symbols). Valproic acid initially decreases plasma protein binding of phenytoin by means of competitive displacement for binding sites on albumin (*arrow*, $\uparrow f_B$). As valproic acid concentrations increase, the hepatic enzyme inhibition component of the drug interaction comes into play (*arrow*, $\downarrow Cl'_{int}$). The net result is a total phenytoin concentration largely unchanged from baseline but an increased unbound concentration of phenytoin and an enhanced pharmacologic effect.

INITIAL DOSAGE DETERMINATION METHODS

Pharmacokinetic Dosing Method

The goal of initial dosing with phenytoin is to compute the best dose possible for the patient given the diseases and conditions that influence phenytoin pharmacokinetics. The optimal way to reach this goal is to use average parameters measured for other patients with similar diseases and conditions as estimates of pharmacokinetic constants for the patient currently being treated with the drug. Because of the difficulty in computing Michaelis-Menten parameters, accurate estimates of V_{max} and K_m are not available for many important patient populations. Even if average population Michaelis-Menten constants are available, the 10- to 15-fold variation in these parameters means that initial doses derived from these parameters will not be successful in meeting the goals for all patients. Monitoring of the serum concentration of phenytoin, including measurement of unbound concentration if altered plasma protein binding is suspected, is an important component of therapy with this drug. If the patient has serious hepatic dysfunction

(Child-Pugh score, ≥8), maintenance doses computed with this method should be decreased 25% to 50% depending on the aggressiveness of therapy needed.

ESTIMATE OF MICHAELIS-MENTEN PARAMETERS

Otherwise healthy adults with normal liver and renal function and normal plasma protein binding have an average phenytoin V_{max} of 7 mg/kg per day and K_m of 4 μg/mL. Michaelis-Menten parameters for children 6 months to 6 years of age are a V_{max} of 12 mg/kg per day and a K_m of 6 μg/mL. For children 7 to 16 years of age, V_{max} is 9 mg/kg per day and K_m is 6 μg/mL. These are the only parameters needed to estimate a maintenance dosage of phenytoin.

ESTIMATE OF VOLUME OF DISTRIBUTION

The volume of distribution for patients with normal phenytoin plasma protein binding is estimated to be 0.7 L/kg for adults. For obese persons 30% or more above their ideal body weight, the volume of distribution can be estimated with the following equation: V = 0.7 L/kg [IBW + 1.33(TBW − IBW)], where IBW is ideal body weight in kilograms; $IBW_{females}$ = 45 + 2.3(Ht − 60) or IBW_{males} = 50 + 2.3(Ht − 60), where Ht is height in inches (height in centimeters divided by 2.54) and TBW is total body weight in kilograms.[57] This parameter is used to estimate the loading dose (LD in mg) of phenytoin, if one is indicated: LD = Css · V, where Css is the desired total phenytoin concentration in milligrams per liter (Note: mg/L = μg/mL, and this change was directly made to avoid unit conversion) and V is volume of distribution in liters. For example, the volume of distribution for a 70-kg patient who is not obese is 49 L (V = 0.7 L/kg · 70 kg = 49 L). The loading dose to achieve a total phenytoin concentration of 15 μg/mL is 750 mg: LD = Css · V = 15 mg/L · 49 L = 735 mg, rounded to 750 mg. (Note: mg/L = μg/mL, and this change was directly made to avoid unit conversion.) For an obese person with a total body weight of 150 kg and an ideal body weight of 70 kg, the volume of distribution is 123 L: V = 0.7 L/kg [IBW + 1.33(TBW − IBW)] = 0.7 L/kg [70 kg + 1.33(150 kg − 70 kg)] = 123 L.

SELECTION OF APPROPRIATE PHARMACOKINETIC MODEL AND EQUATIONS

When given by means of short-term intravenous infusion or orally, phenytoin follows a one-compartment pharmacokinetic model. When oral therapy is required, most clinicians use an extended phenytoin capsule dosage form that has good bioavailability (F = 1), supplies a continuous release of phenytoin into the gastrointestinal tract, and provides a smooth phenytoin serum concentration–time curve that emulates that of intravenous infusion after once- or twice-daily dosing. Because of this, the Michaelis-Menten pharmacokinetic equation used to compute the average phenytoin steady-state serum concentration (Css in μg/mL = mg/L) is widely used and allows calculation of maintenance dosage, as follows:

$$MD = \frac{V_{max} \cdot Css}{S(K_m + Css)}$$

Or, solved for Css:

$$Css = \frac{K_m \cdot (S \cdot MD)}{V_{max} - (S \cdot MD)}$$

where V_{max} is the maximum rate of metabolism in milligrams per day, S is the fraction of phenytoin salt that is active phenytoin (0.92 for phenytoin sodium injection and capsules; 0.92 for fosphenytoin because doses are prescribed as a phenytoin sodium equivalent, or PE; 1.0 for phenytoin acid suspensions and tablets), MD is the maintenance dose of the phenytoin salt contained in the dosage form in milligrams per day, Css is the phenytoin concentration in milligrams per liter (equivalent to micrograms per milliliter), and K_m is the substrate concentration in milligrams per liter (equivalent to micrograms per milliliter) when the rate of metabolism is $V_{max}/2$.

The equation used to calculate loading doses (LD in mg) is based on a simple one-compartment model: $LD = (Css \cdot V)/S$, where Css is the desired phenytoin steady-state concentration in micrograms per milliliter, which is equivalent to milligrams per liter, V is the volume of distribution of phenytoin, and S is the fraction of phenytoin salt that is active (0.92 for phenytoin sodium injection and capsules; 0.92 for fosphenytoin because doses are prescribed as a phenytoin sodium equivalent, or PE; 1.0 for phenytoin acid suspensions and tablets). Intravenous phenytoin sodium doses should be short-term infusions administered at no more than 50 mg/min. Intravenous administration of fosphenytoin should be a short-term infusion given at no more than 150 mg/min PE.

SELECTION OF STEADY-STATE CONCENTRATION

The generally accepted therapeutic ranges for total and unbound concentrations of phenytoin are 10 to 20 μg/mL and 1 to 2 μg/mL, respectively, for the management of seizures. The unbound concentration is the portion of phenytoin in equilibrium with the central nervous system and most accurately reflects drug concentration at the site of action. Thus for patients with altered phenytoin plasma protein binding, it is more important to have the unbound concentration within therapeutic range than it is total concentration. To establish that the unbound fraction (f_B) is altered for a patient, total and unbound concentrations of phenytoin should be measured simultaneously from the same blood sample: $f_B = C/C_f$, where C is the total phenytoin concentration in micrograms per milliliter and C_f is the unbound, or free, phenytoin concentration in micrograms per milliliter. As long as the disease or condition that caused altered phenytoin plasma protein binding is stable, a previously measured unbound fraction can be used to convert newly measured total phenytoin concentrations to the unbound equivalent ($C_f = f_BC$). Phenytoin therapy must be individualized to achieve optimal responses and minimal side effects.

Example 1 TD is a 50-year-old, 75-kg (height, 178 cm) man who has simple partial seizures. He needs therapy with oral phenytoin. He has normal liver and renal function. Suggest an initial phenytoin dosage regimen designed to achieve a steady-state phenytoin concentration of 12 μg/mL.

1. *Estimate the Michaelis-Menten constants according to disease states and conditions present in the patient.*

The V_{max} for an adult who is not obese and has normal liver and renal function is 7 mg/kg per day. For a 75-kg patient, V_{max} is 525 mg/d: $V_{max} = 7 \text{ mg/kg/d} \cdot 75 \text{ kg} = 525$ mg/d. For this patient, K_m is 4 mg/L.

2. *Compute the dosage regimen.*

Oral extended phenytoin sodium capsules are prescribed to this patient (F = 1, S = 0.92). The initial dosage interval (τ) is set to 24 hours. (Note: μg/mL = mg/L, and this concentration unit was substituted for Css in the calculations to avoid unit conversion.) The dosage equation for phenytoin is

$$MD = \frac{V_{max} \cdot Css}{S(K_m + Css)} = \frac{525 \text{ mg/d} \cdot 12 \text{ mg/L}}{0.92(4 \text{ mg/L} + 12 \text{ mg/L})} = 428 \text{ mg/d, rounded to } 400 \text{ mg/d}$$

A steady-state minimum total serum concentration of phenytoin should be measured after steady state is attained in 7 to 14 days. Serum concentration of phenytoin also should be measured if the patient has an exacerbation of epilepsy or if the patient has signs or symptoms of phenytoin toxicity.

Example 2 UO is a 10-year-old, 40-kg boy who has simple partial seizures. He needs therapy with oral phenytoin. He has normal liver and renal function. Suggest an initial phenytoin dosage regimen designed to achieve a steady-state phenytoin concentration of 12 μg/mL.

1. *Estimate the Michaelis-Menten constants according to disease states and conditions present in the patient.*

The V_{max} for a 7- to 16-year-old patient with normal liver and renal function is 9 mg/kg per day. For a 40-kg patient, V_{max} is 360 mg/d: V_{max} = 9 mg/kg/d · 40 kg = 360 mg/d. For this patient, K_m is 6 mg/L.

2. *Compute the dosage regimen.*

Oral phenytoin suspension is prescribed to this patient (F = 1, S = 1). The initial dosage interval (τ) is set to 12 hours. (Note: μg/mL = mg/L, and this concentration unit was substituted for Css in the calculations to avoid unit conversion.) The dosage equation for phenytoin is

$$MD = \frac{V_{max} \cdot Css}{S(K_m + Css)} = \frac{360 \text{ mg/d} \cdot 12 \text{ mg/L}}{1.0(6 \text{ mg/L} + 12 \text{ mg/L})} = 240 \text{ mg/d, rounded to } 250 \text{ mg/d}$$

Phenytoin suspension 125 mg every 12 hours is prescribed to this patient. A steady-state minimum total serum concentration of phenytoin should be measured after steady state is attained in 7 to 14 days. Serum concentration of phenytoin also should be measured if the patient has an exacerbation of epilepsy or if the patient has signs or symptoms of phenytoin toxicity.

To illustrate the differences and similarities between oral and intravenous phenytoin dosage regimens, the same cases are used to compute intravenous phenytoin or fosphenytoin loading and maintenance doses.

Example 3 TD is a 50-year-old, 75-kg (height, 178 cm) man who has simple partial seizures. He needs therapy with intravenous phenytoin sodium. He has normal liver and renal function. Suggest an initial phenytoin dosage regimen designed to achieve a steady-state phenytoin concentration of 12 μg/mL.

1. *Estimate the Michaelis-Menten and volume of distribution constants according to disease states and conditions present in the patient.*

The V_{max} for an adult who is not obese and has normal liver and renal function is 7 mg/kg per day. For a 75-kg patient, V_{max} is 525 mg/d: V_{max} = 7 mg/kg/d · 75 kg = 525 mg/d. For this patient, K_m is 4 mg/L. The volume of distribution for this patient is 53 L: V = 0.7 L/kg · 75 kg = 53 L.

2. *Compute the dosage regimen.*

Intravenous phenytoin sodium is prescribed to this patient (F = 1, S = 0.92). If a loading dose is needed, it is computed with the following equation: LD = (V · Css)/S = (53 L · 12 mg/L)/0.92 = 691 mg, rounded to 700 mg given at a maximal rate of 50 mg/min. (Note: μg/mL = mg/L, and this concentration unit was substituted for Css in the calculations to avoid unit conversion.)

For the maintenance dose, the initial dosage interval (τ) is set to 12 hours. The dosage equation for phenytoin is

$$MD = \frac{V_{max} \cdot Css}{S(K_m + Css)} = \frac{525 \text{ mg/d} \cdot 12 \text{ mg/L}}{0.92(4 \text{ mg/L} + 12 \text{ mg/L})} = 428 \text{ mg/d, rounded to 400 mg/d}$$

The patient is given a prescription for a 200-mg phenytoin sodium injection every 12 hours at an infusion rate no greater than 50 mg/min. A steady-state minimum total phenytoin serum concentration should be measured after steady state is attained in 7 to 14 days. Phenytoin serum concentrations also should be measured if the patient has an exacerbation of epilepsy or if the patient has signs or symptoms of phenytoin toxicity.

Example 4 UO is a 10-year-old, 40-kg boy who has simple partial seizures. He needs therapy with intravenous fosphenytoin. He has normal liver and renal function. Suggest an initial phenytoin dosage regimen designed to achieve a steady-state phenytoin concentration of 12 μg/mL.

1. *Estimate the Michaelis-Menten and volume of distribution constants according to disease states and conditions present in the patient.*

The V_{max} for a 7- to 16-year-old patient with normal liver and renal function is 9 mg/kg per day. For a 40-kg patient, V_{max} is 360 mg/d: V_{max} = 9 mg/kg/d · 40 kg = 360 mg/d. For this patient, K_m is 6 mg/L. The volume of distribution for this patient is 28 L: V = 0.7 L/kg · 40 kg = 28 L.

2. *Compute the dosage regimen.*

Intravenous fosphenytoin is prescribed in phenytoin sodium equivalents, or PE (F = 1, S = 0.92). If a loading dose is needed, it is computed with the following equation: LD = (V · Css)/S = (28 L · 12 mg/L)/0.92 = 365 mg, rounded to 350 mg given at a maximal rate of 150 mg/min PE. (Note: μg/mL = mg/L, and this concentration unit was substituted for Css in the calculations to avoid unit conversion.) The dosage equation for phenytoin is

$$MD = \frac{V_{max} \cdot Css}{S(K_m + Css)} = \frac{360 \text{ mg/d} \cdot 12 \text{ mg/L}}{0.92(6 \text{ mg/L} + 12 \text{ mg/L})} = 261 \text{ mg/d, rounded to 250 mg/d}$$

Intravenous fosphenytoin 125 mg PE every 12 hours given at no more than 150 mg/min PE is prescribed. A steady-state minimum total serum concentration of phenytoin is measured after steady state is attained in 7 to 14 days. Serum concentrations of phenytoin also should be measured if the patient has an exacerbation of epilepsy or if the patient has signs or symptoms of phenytoin toxicity.

Literature-Based Recommended Dosing

Because of the large variability in phenytoin pharmacokinetics, even when concurrent diseases and conditions are identified, many clinicians believe that the use of standard phenytoin doses for various situations is warranted. The original computation of these doses was based on the pharmacokinetic dosing methods described earlier and was modified according to clinical experience. In general, the expected steady-state serum concentration of phenytoin used to compute these doses is 10 to 15 μg/mL. Suggested phenytoin maintenance doses are 4 to 6 mg/kg per day for adults and 5 to 10 mg/kg per day for children 6 months to 16 years of age. Phenytoin loading doses are 15 to 20 mg/kg. For obese patients (>30% over ideal body weight), adjusted body weight (ABW) in kilograms should be used to compute loading doses, as follows: ABW = IBW + 1.33(TBW − IBW), where IBW is ideal body weight in kilograms; $IBW_{females} = 45 + 2.3(Ht - 60)$ or $IBW_{males} = 50 + 2.3(Ht - 60)$, where Ht is height in inches (centimeters divided by 2.54) and TBW is total body weight in kilograms.[57] Although clearance probably increases among patients with obesity, precise information regarding the best weight factor is lacking for computation of the maintenance dose, so most clinicians use ideal body weight to calculate this dose. If the patient has serious hepatic dysfunction (Child-Pugh score, ≥8), maintenance doses prescribed with this method should be decreased 25% to 50% depending on the aggressiveness of therapy needed. Doses of phenytoin, phenytoin sodium, or fosphenytoin (in PE) are computed with these dosage rates because doses are rounded to clinically acceptable amounts.

To illustrate the similarities and differences between this method of dosage calculation and the pharmacokinetic dosing method, the previous examples are used.

Example 1 TD is a 50-year-old, 75-kg (height, 178 cm) man who has simple partial seizures. He needs therapy with oral phenytoin. He has normal liver and renal function. Suggest an initial phenytoin dosage regimen designed to achieve a steady-state phenytoin concentration of 12 μg/mL.

1. *Estimate the phenytoin dose according to disease states and conditions present in the patient.*

The suggested initial dosage for extended phenytoin sodium capsules to be taken by an adult is 4 to 6 mg/kg per day. At a rate of 5 mg/kg per day, the initial dose is 400 mg/d: 5 mg/kg/d · 75 kg = 375 mg/d, rounded to 400 mg/d. Using a dosage interval of 24 hours, the prescribed dose is 400 mg of extended phenytoin sodium capsules daily.

Steady-state minimum total phenytoin serum concentration should be measured after steady state is attained in 7 to 14 days. Phenytoin serum concentrations also should be measured if the patient experiences an exacerbation of epilepsy or if the patient has signs or symptoms of phenytoin toxicity.

Example 2 UO is a 10-year-old, 40-kg boy who has simple partial seizures. He needs therapy with oral phenytoin. He has normal liver and renal function. Suggest an initial phenytoin dosage regimen designed to achieve a steady-state phenytoin concentration of 12 μg/mL.

1. *Estimate the phenytoin dose according to disease states and conditions present in the patient.*

The suggested initial dosage rate for phenytoin suspension to be administered to an older child is 5 to 10 mg/kg per day. At a rate of 6 mg/kg per day, the initial dose is 250 mg/d: 6 mg/kg/d · 40 kg = 240 mg/d, rounded to 250 mg/d. With a dosage interval of 12 hours, the prescribed dosage is 125 mg of phenytoin suspension every 12 hours.

Steady-state minimum total serum concentration of phenytoin should be measured after steady state is attained in 7 to 14 days. Phenytoin serum concentrations also should be measured if the patient has an exacerbation of epilepsy or if the patient has signs or symptoms of phenytoin toxicity.

To illustrate the differences and similarities between the designs of oral and intravenous phenytoin dosage regimens, the cases presented earlier are used to compute intravenous phenytoin or fosphenytoin loading and maintenance doses.

Example 3 TD is a 50-year-old, 75-kg (height, 178 cm) man who has simple partial seizures. He needs therapy with intravenous phenytoin sodium. He has normal liver and renal function. Suggest an initial phenytoin dosage regimen designed to achieve a steady-state phenytoin concentration of 12 μg/mL.

1. *Estimate the phenytoin dose according to disease states and conditions present in the patient.*

The suggested initial dosage of phenytoin sodium injection for an adult patient is 4 to 6 mg/kg per day. At a rate of 5 mg/kg per day, the initial dose is 400 mg/d: 5 mg/kg/d · 75 kg = 375 mg/d, rounded to 400 mg/d. With a dosage interval of 12 hours, the prescribed dose is 200 mg of phenytoin sodium injection every 12 hours. If loading-dose administration is necessary, the suggested amount is 15 to 20 mg/kg. At 15 mg/kg, the suggested loading dose is 1250 mg of phenytoin sodium injection given no faster than 50 mg/min: 15 mg/kg · 75 kg = 1125 mg, rounded to 1250 mg.

Steady-state minimum total serum concentration of phenytoin should be measured after steady state is attained in 7 to 14 days. Phenytoin serum concentrations also should be measured if the patient has an exacerbation of epilepsy or if the patient has signs or symptoms of phenytoin toxicity.

Example 4 UO is a 10-year-old, 40-kg boy who has simple partial seizures. He needs therapy with intravenous fosphenytoin. He has normal liver and renal function. Suggest an initial phenytoin dosage regimen designed to achieve a steady-state phenytoin concentration of 12 μg/mL.

1. *Estimate the phenytoin dose according to disease states and conditions present in the patient.*

The suggested initial dosage of fosphenytoin injection for an older child is 5 to 10 mg/kg per day PE. At a rate of 6 mg/kg per day, the initial dose is 250 mg/d PE: 6

mg/kg/d · 40 kg = 240 mg/d, rounded to 250 mg/d. With a dosage interval of 12 hours, the prescribed dose is 125 mg of fosphenytoin injection every 12 hours. If loading-dose administration is necessary, the suggested amount is 15 to 20 mg/kg PE. At 15 mg/kg, the suggested loading dose is 600 mg PE of fosphenytoin injection given no faster than 150 mg/min PE: 15 mg/kg · 40 kg = 600 mg.

Steady-state minimum total serum concentration of phenytoin should be measured after steady state is attained in 7 to 14 days. Phenytoin serum concentrations also should be measured if the patient has an exacerbation of epilepsy or if the patient has signs or symptoms of phenytoin toxicity.

USE OF PHENYTOIN SERUM CONCENTRATIONS TO ALTER DOSES

Because of the large pharmacokinetic variability among patients, it is likely that doses computed according to patient population characteristics will not always produce phenytoin serum concentrations that are expected or desirable. Because of pharmacokinetic variability, the Michaelis-Menten pharmacokinetics followed by the drug, the narrow therapeutic index of phenytoin, and the desire to avoid adverse side effects of phenytoin, measurement of phenytoin serum concentrations is conducted for almost all patients to ensure that therapeutic, nontoxic levels are present. In addition to phenytoin serum concentrations, important patient characteristics, such as seizure frequency and risk of side effects of phenytoin, should be followed to confirm that the patient is responding to treatment and not having an adverse drug reaction.

When serum concentrations of phenytoin are measured, and a dosage change is necessary, clinicians should use the simplest, most straightforward method available to determine a dose that will provide safe and effective treatment. A variety of methods are used to estimate new maintenance doses or Michaelis-Menten parameters when one steady-state phenytoin serum concentration is available.

Sometimes it is useful to compute phenytoin pharmacokinetic constants for a patient and base dosage adjustments on these. If two or more steady-state serum concentrations of phenytoin are available from two to more daily dosage rates, it may be possible to calculate and use pharmacokinetic parameters to alter the phenytoin dose. Finally, computerized methods that incorporate expected population pharmacokinetic characteristics (Bayesian pharmacokinetics computer programs) can be used in difficult cases in which serum concentrations are obtained at suboptimal times or the patient was not at steady state when serum concentrations were measured. To compare the results obtained with the different methods, the same cases are used to compute adjusted doses of phenytoin.

Single Total Phenytoin Steady-State Serum Concentration Methods

EMPIRIC DOSING METHOD

With the knowledge of population Michaelis-Menten pharmacokinetic parameters, it is possible to suggest empiric dosage increases for phenytoin when one steady-state serum concentration is available (Table 10-4).[58] The lower end of the suggested dosage range for each category tends to produce more conservative increases in steady-state concentration. The upper end of the suggested dosage range tends to produce more aggressive increases.

TABLE 10-4 Empiric Phenytoin Dosage Increases Based on a Single Total Steady-State Concentration

MEASURED PHENYTOIN TOTAL SERUM CONCENTRATION (μg/mL)	SUGGESTED DOSAGE INCREASE*
<7	100 mg/d or more
7–12	50–100 mg/d
>12	30–50 mg/d

* Higher dosage used if more aggressive therapy desired, lower dosage used if less aggressive therapy desired. Adapted from Mauro LS, Mauro VF, Bachmann KA, Higgins JT. Accuracy of two equations in determining normalized phenytoin concentrations. DICP 1989;23:64–8.

Whenever possible, clinicians should avoid using more than one strength of solid dosage form (e.g., 30- and 100-mg extended phenytoin capsules) to treat a patient. An effective way to increase the phenytoin dose for a patient who needs an increase in dose of 50 mg/d when using the 100-mg extended phenytoin sodium capsule dosage form is to increase the dose 100 mg every other day. For example, if a dosage increase of 50 mg/d is desired for a patient taking 300 mg/d of extended phenytoin sodium capsules, a dosage increase of 300 mg/d alternating with 400 mg/d is possible if the patient can comply with a more complex dosage schedule. Dosage aids such as calendars, prefilled dosage cassettes, or memory aiding schemes (400 mg/d on even days, 300 mg/d on odd days) are useful in different patient situations. Alternate daily dosages are possible because of the extended-release characteristics of extended phenytoin capsules and the long half-life of phenytoin.

Example 1 TD is a 50-year-old, 75-kg (height, 178 cm) man who has simple partial seizures. He needs therapy with oral phenytoin. He has normal liver and renal function. The patient is given a prescription for 400 mg/d of extended phenytoin sodium capsules for 1 month. Steady-state total concentration of phenytoin is 6.2 μg/mL. The patient is found to be compliant with the dosage regimen. Suggest an initial phenytoin dosage regimen designed to achieve a steady-state phenytoin concentration in the therapeutic range.

1. *Use Table 10-4 to suggest the new phenytoin dosage.*

Table 10-4 suggests a dosage increase of ≥100 mg/d for this patient. The dose is increased to 500 mg/d.

Steady-state minimum total serum concentration of phenytoin should be measured after steady state is attained in 7 to 14 days. Serum concentration of phenytoin also should be measured if the patient has an exacerbation of epilepsy or if the patient has signs or symptoms of phenytoin toxicity.

Example 2 GF is a 35-year-old, 55-kg (height, 157 cm) woman who has tonic-clonic seizures. She needs therapy with oral phenytoin. She has normal liver and renal function. The patient is given a prescription for 300 mg/d of extended phenytoin sodium capsules for 1 month. Steady-state total concentration of phenytoin is 10.7 μg/mL. The patient is found to be compliant with the dosage regimen. Suggest an initial phenytoin dosage regimen designed to achieve a steady-state phenytoin concentration in the middle of the therapeutic range.

1. *Use Table 10-4 to suggest the new phenytoin dose.*

The table suggests a dosage increase of 50 to 100 mg/d for this patient. The dose is increased to 300 mg/d alternating with 400 mg/d.

Steady-state minimum total serum concentration of phenytoin should be measured after steady state is attained in 7 to 14 days. Serum concentration of phenytoin also should be measured if the patient has an exacerbation of epilepsy or if the patient has signs or symptoms of phenytoin toxicity.

PSEUDOLINEAR PHARMACOKINETICS METHOD

A simple, easy way to approximate new total serum concentrations after a dosage adjustment of phenytoin is to temporarily assume linear pharmacokinetics, then to add 15% to 33% for a dosage increase or to subtract 15% to 33% for a dosage decrease to account for Michaelis-Menten pharmacokinetics: $Css_{new} = (D_{new}/D_{old})Css_{old}$, where Css_{new} is the expected steady-state concentration of the new phenytoin dose in micrograms per milliliter, Css_{old} is the measured steady-state concentration of the old phenytoin dose in micrograms per milliliter, D_{new} is the new phenytoin dose to be prescribed in milligrams per day, and D_{old} is the currently prescribed phenytoin dose in milligrams per day.[59]

Example 3 TD is a 50-year-old, 75-kg (height, 178 cm) man who has simple partial seizures. He needs therapy with oral phenytoin. He has normal liver and renal function. The patient is given a prescription for 400 mg/d of extended phenytoin sodium capsules for 1 month. Steady-state total concentration of phenytoin is 6.2 μg/mL. The patient is found to be compliant with the dosage regimen. Suggest an initial phenytoin dosage regimen designed to achieve a steady-state phenytoin concentration in the therapeutic range.

1. *Use pseudolinear pharmacokinetics to predict a new concentration for a dosage increase, then compute the 15% to 33% factor to account for Michaelis-Menten pharmacokinetics.*

Because the patient is receiving extended phenytoin sodium capsules, a convenient dosage change is 100 mg/d, and an increase to 500 mg/d is suggested. According to pseudolinear pharmacokinetics, the resulting total steady-state serum concentration of phenytoin is $Css_{new} = (D_{new}/D_{old})Css_{old} = [(500 \text{ mg/d})/(400 \text{ mg/d})]\ 6.2\ \mu g/mL = 7.8\ \mu g/mL$. Because of Michaelis-Menten pharmacokinetics, the serum concentration is expected to increase 15%, or 1.15 times, to 33%, or 1.33 times, greater than that predicted with linear pharmacokinetics: $Css = 7.8\ \mu g/mL \cdot 1.15 = 9.0\ \mu g/mL$, and $Css = 7.8\ \mu g/mL \cdot 1.33 = 10.4\ \mu g/mL$. Thus a dosage increase of 100 mg/d is expected to yield a total steady-state serum concentration of phenytoin between 9 and 10 μg/mL.

Steady-state minimum total serum concentration of phenytoin should be measured after steady state is attained in 7 to 14 days. Serum concentration of phenytoin also should be measured if the patient has an exacerbation of epilepsy or if the patient has signs or symptoms of phenytoin toxicity.

Example 4 GF is a 35-year-old, 55-kg (hieight, 157 cm) woman who has tonic-clonic seizures. She needs therapy with oral phenytoin. She has normal liver and renal function. The patient is given a prescription for 300 mg/d of extended phenytoin sodium capsules for 1 month. Steady-state total concentration of phenytoin is 10.7 μg/mL. The patient is found to be compliant with the dosage regimen. Suggest an initial phenytoin dosage regimen designed to achieve a steady-state phenytoin concentration in the middle of the therapeutic range.

1. *Use pseudolinear pharmacokinetics to predict a new concentration for a dosage increase, then compute the 15% to 33% factor to account for Michaelis-Menten pharmacokinetics.*

Because the patient is receiving extended phenytoin sodium capsules, a convenient dosage change is 100 mg/d, and an increase to 400 mg/d is suggested. According to pseudolinear pharmacokinetics, the resulting total steady-state serum concentration of phenytoin is $Css_{new} = (D_{new}/D_{old})Css_{old}$ = [(400 mg/d)/(300 mg/d)] 10.7 μg/mL = 14.3 μg/mL. Because of Michaelis-Menten pharmacokinetics, the serum concentration is expected to increase 15%, or 1.15 times, to 33%, or 1.33 times, greater than that predicted with linear pharmacokinetics: Css = 14.3 μg/mL · 1.15 = 16.4 μg/mL, and Css = 14.3 μg/mL · 1.33 = 19.0 μg/mL. Thus a dosage increase of 100 mg/d is expected to yield a total steady-state serum concentration of phenytoin between 16 and 19 μg/mL.

Steady-state minimum total serum concentration of phenytoin should be measured after steady state is attained in 7 to 14 days. Serum concentration of phenytoin also should be measured if the patient has an exacerbation of epilepsy or if the patient has signs or symptoms of phenytoin toxicity.

GRAVES-CLOYD METHOD

With this dosage-adjustment method, a steady-state serum concentration of phenytoin is used to compute the patient's own phenytoin clearance rate (D_{old}/Css_{old}, where D_{old} is the administered phenytoin dose in milligrams per day and Css_{old} is the resulting measured total steady-state concentration of phenytoin in micrograms per milliliter) at the dosage being given. The measured concentration and desired concentration (Css_{new} in μg/mL) then are used to estimate a new dose (D_{new} in mg/d) for the patient[60]: $D_{new} = (D_{old}/Css_{old}) \cdot Css_{new}^{0.199} \cdot Css_{old}^{0.804}$.

Example 5 TD is a 50-year-old, 75-kg (height, 178 cm) man who has simple partial seizures. He needs therapy with oral phenytoin. He has normal liver and renal function. The patient is given a prescription for 400 mg/d of extended phenytoin sodium capsules for 1 month. Steady-state phenytoin total concentration is 6.2 μg/mL. The patient is found to be compliant with the dosage regimen. Suggest an initial phenytoin dosage regimen designed to achieve a steady-state phenytoin concentration in the therapeutic range.

1. *Use the Graves-Cloyd method to estimate a new phenytoin dose for the desired steady-state concentration.*

Phenytoin sodium 400 mg contains 368 mg of phenytoin (400 mg · 0.92 = 368 mg). A new total steady-state serum concentration of phenytoin of 10 μg/mL is chosen for the patient: $D_{new} = (D_{old}/Css_{old}) \cdot Css_{new}^{0.199} \cdot Css_{old}^{0.804}$ = [(368 mg/d)/(6.2 mg/L)] · (10 mg/L)$^{0.199}$ · (6.2 mg/L)$^{0.804}$ = 407 mg/d. This is equivalent to 442 mg/d of phenytoin sodium (407 mg/0.92 = 442 mg), rounded to 450 mg/d, or 400 mg/d on even days alternating with 500 mg/d on odd days.

Steady-state minimum total serum concentration of phenytoin should be measured after steady state is attained in 7 to 14 days. Serum concentration of phenytoin also should be measured if the patient has an exacerbation of epilepsy or if the patient has signs or symptoms of phenytoin toxicity.

Example 6 GF is a 35-year-old, 55-kg (height, 157 cm) woman who has tonic-clonic seizures. She needs therapy with oral phenytoin. She has normal liver and renal function. The patient is given a prescription for 300 mg/d of extended phenytoin sodium capsules for 1 month. Steady-state total concentration of phenytoin is 10.7 μg/mL. The patient is found to be compliant with the dosage regimen. Suggest an initial phenytoin dosage regimen designed to achieve a steady-state phenytoin concentration of 18 μg/mL.

1. *Use the Graves-Cloyd method to estimate a new phenytoin dose for the desired steady-state concentration.*

Phenytoin sodium 300 mg contains 276 mg of phenytoin (300 mg · 0.92 = 276 mg). A new total steady-state serum concentration of phenytoin of 18 μg/mL is chosen for the patient: $D_{new} = (D_{old}/Css_{old}) \cdot Css_{new}^{0.199} \cdot Css_{old}^{0.804}$ = [(276 mg/d)/(10.7 mg/L)] · (18 mg/L)$^{0.199}$ · (10.7 mg/L)$^{0.804}$ = 308 mg/d. This is equivalent to 335 mg/d of phenytoin sodium (308 mg/0.92 = 335 mg), rounded to 350 mg/d, or 300 mg/d on odd days alternating with 400 mg/d on even days.

Steady-state minimum total phenytoin serum concentration should be measured after steady state is attained in 7 to 14 days. Serum concentration of phenytoin also should be measured if the patient has an exacerbation of epilepsy or if the patient has signs or symptoms of phenytoin toxicity.

VOZEH-SHEINER OR ORBIT GRAPH METHOD

A graphic method of adjusting phenytoin dosage entails population Michaelis-Menten information, Bayes' theorem, and a single steady-state total concentration.[61] With this method a series of orbs encompassing 50%, 75%, 85%, and so on, of the population parameter combinations for V_{max} and K_m are used on the plot suggested by Mullen[62] for use with multiple steady-state dosage pairs (Figure 10-3). The use of the population parameter orbs allows use of the plot with one phenytoin steady-state concentration-dose pair.

The graph is divided into two sectors. On the left side of the *x*-axis, a steady-state total phenytoin concentration is plotted. On the *y*-axis, the phenytoin dosage rate in milligrams per kilogram per day of phenytoin (S = 0.92 for phenytoin sodium and fosphenytoin PE dosage forms) is plotted. A straight line is drawn between these two points and is extended into the right sector and through the orbs contained in the right sector. If the line intersects more than one orb, the innermost orb is selected, and the midpoint of the line contained within that orb is found and marked with a point. The midpoint within the orb and the desired steady-state total concentration of phenytoin (on the left portion of the *x*-axis) are connected with a straight line. The intersection of this line with the *y*-axis is the new phenytoin dose needed to achieve the new phenytoin concentration. If necessary, the phenytoin dose is converted to phenytoin sodium or fosphenytoin amounts. If a line parallel to the *y*-axis is drawn down to the *x*-axis from the midpoint of the line contained within the orb, an estimate of K_m in micrograms per milliliter is obtained. Similarly, if a line parallel to the *x*-axis is drawn to the left to the *y*-axis from the midpoint of the line

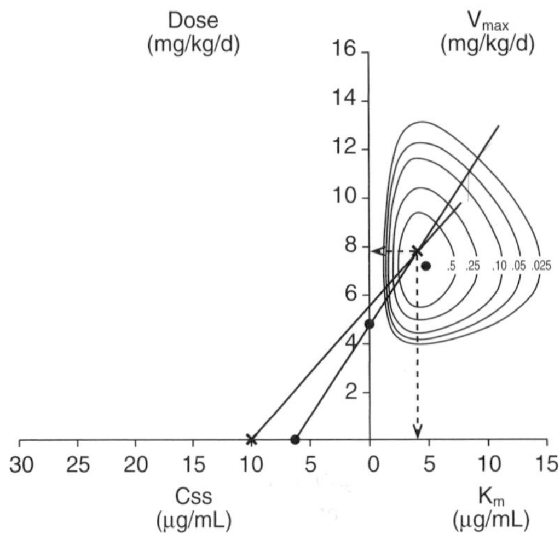

FIGURE 10-3 Vozeh-Sheiner or orbit graph in which Bayesian feedback is used to estimate Michaelis-Menten parameters and phenytoin dose with one steady-state concentration-dose pair (data from example 7). The orbs represent 50%, 75%, 85%, and so on, of the population parameter combinations for V_{max} and K_m. The drug dose is converted into an amount of phenytoin in milligrams per kilogram per day and plotted on the *y*-axis (*circle,* 4.9 mg/kg per day). The concurrent steady-state serum concentration of phenytoin is plotted on the left portion of the *x*-axis (*circle,* 6.2 µg/mL), and the two points are joined with a straight line across the orbs. If the line intersects more than one orb, the innermost orb is selected, and the midpoint of the line contained within that orb is found and marked (*x* within orbs). The new desired steady-state concentration is identified on the left portion of the *x*-axis (*X* on *x*-axis, 10 µg/mL), and the two *x* marks are connected with a straight line. The required phenytoin dose is identified at the intersection of the drawn line and the *y*-axis (5.5 mg/kg per day). If necessary, the dose is converted to phenytoin sodium or fosphenytoin amounts. Estimates of V_{max} (7.9 mg/kg per day) and K_m (4 µg/mL) are obtained by means of extrapolating parallel lines to the *y*- and *x*-axes, respectively.

contained within the orb, an estimate of V_{max} in milligrams per kilogram per day is obtained.

Example 7 TD is a 50-year-old, 75-kg (height, 178 cm) man who has simple partial seizures. He needs therapy with oral phenytoin. He has normal liver and renal function. The patient is given a prescription for 400 mg/d of extended phenytoin sodium capsules for 1 month. Steady-state total concentration of phenytoin is 6.2 µg/mL. The patient is found to be compliant with the dosage regimen. Suggest an initial phenytoin dosage regimen designed to achieve a steady-state phenytoin concentration in the therapeutic range.

1. *Use the Vozeh-Sheiner method to estimate a new phenytoin dose for the desired steady-state concentration.*

A new total phenytoin steady-state serum concentration of 10 µg/mL is chosen for the patient. With the orbit graph, the serum concentration-dose information is plotted. The phenytoin dose is 0.92 · phenytoin sodium dose = 0.92 · 400 mg/d = 368 mg/d; (368 mg/d)/(75 kg) = 4.9 mg/kg/d (see Figure 10-3). According to the graph, a dose of

5.5 mg/kg per day of phenytoin is needed to achieve a steady-state concentration of 10 μg/mL. This is an extended phenytoin sodium capsule dose of 450 mg/d, administered by means of alternating 400 mg/d on even days and 500 mg/d on odd days: (5.5 mg/kg/d · 75 kg)/0.92 = 448 mg/d, rounded to 450 mg/d.

Steady-state minimum total serum concentration of phenytoin should be measured after steady state is attained in 7 to 14 days. Serum concentration of phenytoin also should be measured if the patient has an exacerbation of epilepsy or if the patient has signs or symptoms of phenytoin toxicity.

Example 8 GF is a 35-year-old, 55-kg (height, 157 cm) woman who has tonic-clonic seizures. She needs therapy with oral phenytoin. She has normal liver and renal function. The patient is given a prescription for 300 mg/d of extended phenytoin sodium capsules for 1 month. Steady-state total concentration of phenytoin is 10.7 μg/mL. The patient is found to be compliant with the dosage regimen. Suggest an initial phenytoin dosage regimen designed to achieve a steady-state phenytoin concentration of 18 μg/mL.

1. *Use the Vozeh-Sheiner method to estimate a new phenytoin dose for the desired steady-state concentration.*

A new total steady-state serum concentration of phenytoin of 18 μg/mL is chosen for the patient. The serum concentration–dose information is plotted on an orbit graph (Note: phenytoin dose = 0.92 · phenytoin sodium dose = 0.92 · 300 mg/d = 276 mg/d: (276 mg/d)/(55 kg) = 5.0 mg/kg/d; Figure 10-4). According to the graph, a dose of 5.7 mg/kg per day of phenytoin is required to achieve a steady-state concentration of 18 μg/mL. This equals an extended phenytoin sodium capsule dose of 350 mg/d, administered by alternating 300 mg/d on even days and 400 mg/d on odd days: (5.7 mg/kg/d · 55 kg)/0.92 = 341 mg/d, rounded to 350 mg/d.

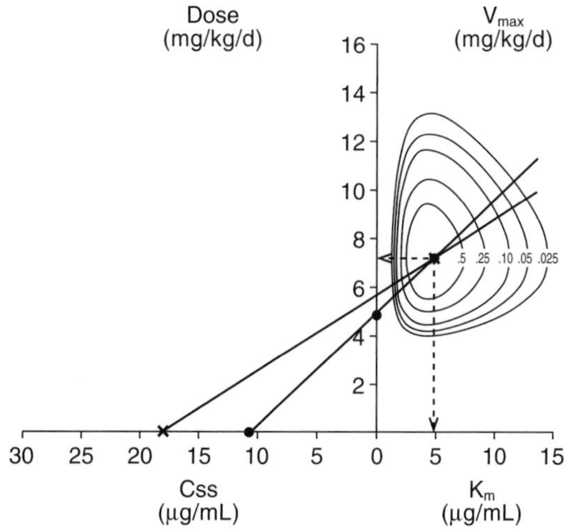

FIGURE 10-4 Vozeh-Sheiner or orbit graph in which Bayesian feedback is used to estimate Michaelis-Menten parameters and phenytoin dose with one steady-state concentration-dose pair. The graph shows the solution for example 8.

Steady-state minimum total serum concentration of phenytoin should be measured after steady state is attained in 7 to 14 days. Serum concentration of phenytoin also should be measured if the patient has an exacerbation of epilepsy or if the patient has signs or symptoms of phenytoin toxicity.

Methods for Two or More Phenytoin Steady-State Serum Concentrations at Two or More Dosage Levels

To use each of the dosage schemes in this section, at least two steady-state serum concentrations of phenytoin at different dosage rates are needed. This requirement can be difficult to achieve.

EMPIRIC DOSING METHOD

With a knowledge of population Michaelis-Menten pharmacokinetic parameters, it is possible to suggest empiric dosage increases for phenytoin when there are two or more steady-state serum concentrations at two or more dosage levels.[59] For instance, if a patient has a steady-state phenytoin concentration of 11.2 μg/mL with 300 mg/d of phenytoin sodium and 25.3 μg/mL with 400 mg/d of phenytoin sodium, it is obvious that a dose of 350 mg/d of phenytoin sodium will probably produce a steady-state phenytoin serum concentration in the middle to upper end of the therapeutic range. Similarly, if a patient has a steady-state phenytoin concentration of 11.2 μg/mL with 300 mg/d of phenytoin sodium and 15.0 μg/mL with 400 mg/d of phenytoin sodium, it is apparent that a dose of 450 mg/d of phenytoin sodium will probably produce a steady-state phenytoin serum concentration in the upper end of the therapeutic range. In the latter situation, Table 10-4 can be useful for suggesting dosage increases.

Example 1 TD is a 50-year-old, 75-kg (height, 178 cm) man who has simple partial seizures. He needs therapy with oral phenytoin. He has normal liver and renal function. The patient is given a prescription for 400 mg/d of extended phenytoin sodium capsules for 1 month. Steady-state total concentration of phenytoin is 6.2 μg/mL. The dosage is increased to 500 mg/d of extended phenytoin sodium capsules for another month, and steady-state total concentration of phenytoin is 22.0 μg/mL. The patient has some lateral-gaze nystagmus with the new dosage. The patient is found to be compliant with the dosage regimen. Suggest a new phenytoin dosage regimen designed to achieve a steady-state phenytoin concentration in the middle to upper end of the therapeutic range.

1. *Empirically suggest the new phenytoin dose.*

The next logical dose to prescribe is phenytoin sodium 450 mg/d to be taken by the patient as 400 mg/d on even days and 500 mg/d on odd days.

Steady-state minimum total serum concentration of phenytoin should be measured after steady state is attained in 7 to 14 days. Serum concentration of phenytoin also should be measured if the patient has an exacerbation of epilepsy or if the patient has signs or symptoms of phenytoin toxicity.

Example 2 GF is a 35-year-old, 55-kg (height, 157 cm) woman who has tonic-clonic seizures. She needs therapy with oral phenytoin. She has normal liver and renal function. The patient is given a prescription for 300 mg/d of extended phenytoin sodium capsules for 1 month. Steady-state total concentration of phenytoin is 10.7 μg/mL. The dose is increased to 350 mg/d of extended phenytoin sodium capsules for an additional month, and the resulting steady-state concentration is 15.8 μg/mL. The patient is found to be compliant with the dosage regimen. Suggest a new phenytoin dosage increase designed to achieve a steady-state phenytoin concentration in the upper end of the therapeutic range.

1. *Empirically suggest the new phenytoin dose.*

The next logical dose to prescribe is phenytoin sodium 400 mg/d (see Table 10-4).

Steady-state minimum total serum concentration of phenytoin should be measured after steady state is attained in 7 to 14 days. Serum concentration of phenytoin also should be measured if the patient has an exacerbation of epilepsy or if the patient has signs or symptoms of phenytoin toxicity.

MULLEN METHOD

In the Mullen method, a concentration-dose plot is used as that described for the Vozeh-Sheiner or orbit graph method, but the population orbs denoting the Bayesian distribution of V_{max} and K_m parameters are omitted.[62,63] As before, the graph is divided into two sectors. The left side of the *x*-axis is steady-state total concentration of phenytoin. The *y*-axis is phenytoin dosage rate in milligrams per kilogram per day of phenytoin (S = 0.92 for phenytoin sodium and fosphenytoin PE dosage forms). A straight line is drawn between these two points and extended into the right sector. This process is repeated for all steady-state concentration-dose pairs that are available. The intersection of these lines in the right sector provides the Michaelis-Menten constant values for the patient. If a line parallel to the *y*-axis is drawn down to the *x*-axis from the intersection point, K_m in micrograms per milliliter is obtained. Similarly, if a line parallel to the *x*-axis is drawn to the left to the *y*-axis from the intersection point, an estimate of V_{max} in milligrams per kilogram per day is obtained. To compute the new phenytoin dose, the intersection point and the desired steady-state total concentration of phenytoin (left portion of the *x*-axis) are connected with a straight line. The intersection of this line with the *y*-axis is the new phenytoin dose needed to achieve the new phenytoin concentration. If needed, the phenytoin dose is converted to phenytoin sodium or fosphenytoin amounts.

Example 3 TD is a 50-year-old, 75-kg (height, 178 cm) man who has simple partial seizures. He needs therapy with oral phenytoin. He has normal liver and renal function. The patient is given a prescription for 400 mg/d of extended phenytoin sodium capsules for 1 month. Steady-state total concentration of phenytoin is 6.2 μg/mL. The dosage is increased to 500 mg/d of extended phenytoin sodium capsules for another month, and steady-state total concentration of phenytoin is 22.0 μg/mL. The patient has lateral-gaze nystagmus with the new dosage. The patient is found to be compliant with the dosage regimen. Suggest a new phenytoin dosage regimen designed to achieve a steady-state phenytoin concentration in the therapeutic range.

1. *Use the Mullen method to estimate a new phenytoin dose for the desired steady-state concentration.*

The serum concentration–dose information is plotted on the graph (Note: phenytoin dose = 0.92 · phenytoin sodium dose = 0.92 · 400 mg/d = 368 mg/d, (368 mg/d)/75 kg =

4.9 mg/kg/d; phenytoin dose = 0.92 · phenytoin sodium dose = 0.92 · 500 mg/d = 460 mg/d, (460 mg/d)/75 kg = 6.1 mg/kg/d; Figure 10-5). According to the graph, a dose of 5.5 mg/kg per day of phenytoin is needed to achieve a steady-state concentration of 11.5 μg/mL. This equals an extended phenytoin sodium capsule dose of 450 mg/d, administered by means of alternating 400 mg/d on even days and 500 mg/d on odd days: (5.5 mg/kg/d · 75 kg)/0.92 = 448 mg/d, rounded to 450 mg/d. V_{max} = 6.8 mg/kg per day and K_m = 2.2 μg/mL for this patient.

Steady-state minimum total serum concentration of phenytoin should be measured after steady state is attained in 7 to 14 days. Serum concentration of phenytoin also should be measured if the patient has an exacerbation of epilepsy or if the patient has signs or symptoms of phenytoin toxicity.

Example 4 GF is a 35-year-old, 55-kg (height, 157 cm) woman who has tonic-clonic seizures. She needs therapy with oral phenytoin. She has normal liver and renal function. The patient is given a prescription for 300 mg/d of extended phenytoin sodium capsules for 1 month. Steady-state total concentration of phenytoin is 10.7 μg/mL. The dose is increased to 350 mg/d of extended phenytoin sodium capsules for an additional month, and the resulting steady-state concentration is 15.8 μg/mL. The patient is found to be compliant with the dosage regimen. Suggest a new phenytoin dosage increase de-

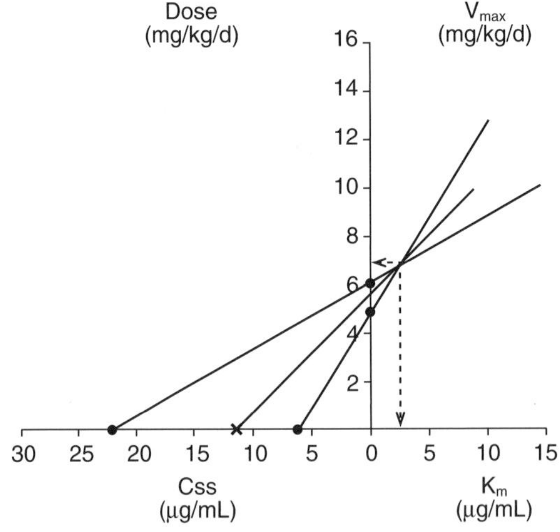

FIGURE 10-5 Mullen graph used to compute Michaelis-Menten parameters and phenytoin dose with two or more steady-state concentration-dose pairs (data from example 3). The first dose and concentration are plotted as *circles* on the *y*- (4.9 mg/kg per day) and *x*-axes (6.2 μg/mL) and joined with a straight line. This process is repeated for the second concentration-dose pair (6.1 mg/kg per day, 22 μg/mL) and any others that are available. The intersection of the lines in the right sector of the graph is used to compute a new dose by means of drawing a straight line between the intersection and the new desired steady-state concentration on the left portion of the *x*-axis (*X* on *x*-axis, 11.5 μg/mL). The required dose is the intersection of this new line with the *y*-axis (5.5 mg/kg per day). Estimates of V_{max} (6.8 mg/kg per day) and K_m (2.2 μg/mL) are obtained by means of extrapolating parallel lines to the *y*- and *x*-axes, respectively.

signed to achieve a steady-state phenytoin concentration in the upper end of the therapeutic range.

1. *Use the Mullen method to estimate a new phenytoin dose for the desired steady-state concentration.*

The serum concentration–dose information is plotted on the graph (Note: phenytoin dose = 0.92 · phenytoin sodium dose = 0.92 · 300 mg/d = 276 mg/d, (276 mg/d)/55 kg = 5 mg/kg/d; phenytoin dose = 0.92 · phenytoin sodium dose = 0.92 · 350 mg/d = 322 mg/d, (322 mg/d)/55 kg = 5.9 mg/kg/d; Figure 10-6). According to the graph, a dose of 6.7 mg/kg per day of phenytoin is needed to achieve a steady-state concentration of 22 μg/mL. This equals an extended phenytoin sodium capsule dose of 400 mg/d: (6.7 mg/kg/d · 55 kg)/0.92 = 401 mg/d, rounded to 400 mg/d. V_{max} = 9.4 mg/kg per day and K_m = 9.5 μg/mL for this patient.

Steady-state minimum total serum concentration of phenytoin should be measured after steady state is attained in 7 to 14 days. Serum concentration of phenytoin also should be measured if the patient has an exacerbation of epilepsy or if the patient has signs or symptoms of phenytoin toxicity.

LUDDEN METHOD

The Ludden method involves arrangement of the Michaelis-Menten equation so that two or more maintenance doses (MD in milligrams per day of phenytoin) and steady-state concentrations (Css in milligrams per liter or micrograms per milliliter) can be used to obtain graphic solutions for V_{max} and K_m: MD = $-K_m$(MD/Css) + V_{max}.[29] When maintenance dose is plotted on the *y*-axis and MD/Css is plotted on the *x*-axis of cartesian graph paper, a straight line with a *y*-intercept of V_{max} and a slope of $-K_m$ is found. If three or more concentration-dose pairs are available, it is best to plot the data so the best straight

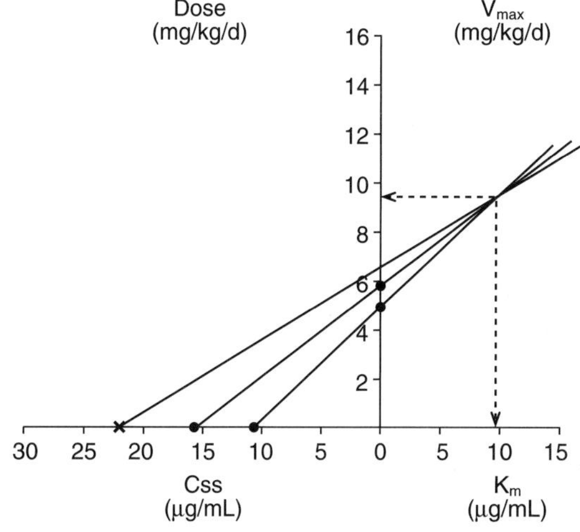

FIGURE 10-6 Mullen graph used to estimate Michaelis-Menten parameters and phenytoin dose with two or more steady-state concentration-dose pairs. The graph shows the solution for example 4.

line can be drawn through the points. However, if only two concentration-dose pairs are available, a direct mathematical solution can be used. The slope for a simple linear equation is the quotient of the change in the *y*-axis value (Δy) and the change in the *x*-axis value (Δx): slope = $\Delta y/\Delta x$. Applying this to rearrangement of the Michaelis-Menten equation gives $-K_m = (MD_1 - MD_2)/[(MD_1/Css_1) - (MD_2/Css_2)]$, where the subscript 1 indicates the higher dose and 2 indicates the lower dose. Once the Michaelis-Menten equation is rearranged, V_{max} can be found: $V_{max} = MD + K_m(MD/Css)$. The Michaelis-Menten equation can be used to compute steady-state concentrations for a given dose and vice versa.

Example 5 TD is a 50-year-old, 75-kg (height, 178 cm) man who has simple partial seizures. He needs therapy with oral phenytoin. He has normal liver and renal function. The patient is given a prescription for 400 mg/d of extended phenytoin sodium capsules for 1 month. Steady-state total concentration of phenytoin is 6.2 μg/mL. The dosage is increased to 500 mg/d of extended phenytoin sodium capsules for another month, and the steady-state total concentration of phenytoin is 22.0 μg/mL. The patient has lateral-gaze nystagmus with the new dosage. The patient is found to be compliant with the dosage regimen. Suggest a new phenytoin dosage regimen designed to achieve a steady-state phenytoin concentration in the therapeutic range.

1. *Use the Ludden method to estimate V_{max} and K_m.*

Serum concentration–dose information is plotted on the graph (Note: phenytoin dose = 0.92 · phenytoin sodium dose = 0.92 · 400 mg/d = 368 mg/d; phenytoin dose = 0.92 · phenytoin sodium dose = 0.92 · 500 mg/d = 460 mg/d; Figure 10-7). According to the graph, V_{max} is 510 mg/d and K_m is 2.4 mg/L.

Because only two steady-state concentration-dose pairs are available, a direct mathematical solution can be found: $-K_m = (MD_1 - MD_2)/[(MD_1/Css_1) - (MD_2/Css_2)]$ = (460

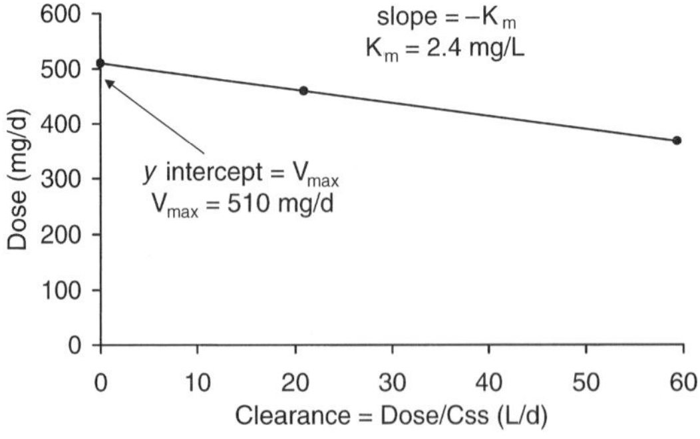

FIGURE 10-7 Ludden graph used to compute Michaelis-Menten parameters and phenytoin dose with two or more steady-state concentration-dose pairs (data from example 5). Dose is plotted on the *y*-axis and clearance (*Dose/Css*) on the *x*-axis for each data pair. The best straight line is drawn through the points. Slope equals $-K_m$, and V_{max} is the *y* intercept. These values are used to compute the required maintenance dose (MD) for any desired steady-state serum concentration: $MD = (V_{max} \cdot Css)/[S(K_m + Css)]$.

mg/d – 368 mg/d)/{[(460 mg/d)/(22 mg/L)] – [(368 mg/d)/(6.2 mg/L)]} = –2.4 mg/L, K_m = 2.4 mg/L; V_{max} = MD + [K_m(MD/Css)] = 368 mg/d + {2.4[(368 mg/d)/(6.2 mg/L)]} = 510 mg/d.

2. *Use the Michaelis-Menten equation to compute a new phenytoin dose for the desired steady-state concentration.*

According to the Michaelis-Menten equation, a dose of 450 mg of phenytoin sodium is needed to achieve a steady-state concentration of 10.4 µg/mL:

$$Css = \frac{K_m \cdot (S \cdot MD)}{V_{max} - (S \cdot MD)} = \frac{2.4\ mg/L \cdot (0.92 \cdot 450\ mg/d)}{510\ mg/d - (0.92 \cdot 450\ mg/d)} = 10.4\ mg/L$$

This dose is administered by means of alternating 400 mg/d on even days and 500 mg/d on odd days.

Steady-state minimum total serum concentration of phenytoin should be measured after steady state is attained in 7 to 14 days. Serum concentration of phenytoin also should be measured if the patient has an exacerbation of epilepsy or if the patient has signs or symptoms of phenytoin toxicity.

Example 6 GF is a 35-year-old, 55-kg (height, 157 cm) woman who has tonic-clonic seizures. She needs therapy with oral phenytoin. She has normal liver and renal function. The patient is given a prescription for 300 mg/d of extended phenytoin sodium capsules for 1 month. Steady-state total concentration of phenytoin is 10.7 µg/mL. The dose is increased to 350 mg/d of extended phenytoin sodium capsules for an additional month. The resulting steady-state concentration is 15.8 µg/mL. The patient is found to be compliant with the dosage regimen. Suggest a new phenytoin dosage regimen increase designed to achieve a steady-state phenytoin concentration in the upper end of the therapeutic range.

1. *Use the Ludden method to estimate V_{max} and K_m.*

The serum concentration–dose information is plotted on the graph (Note: phenytoin dose = 0.92 · phenytoin sodium dose = 0.92 · 300 mg/d = 276 mg/d; phenytoin dose = 0.92 · phenytoin sodium dose = 0.92 · 350 mg/d = 322 mg/d; Figure 10-8). According to the graph, V_{max} is 495 mg/d and K_m is 8.5 mg/L.

Because only two steady-state concentration-dose pairs are available, a direct mathematical solution can also be conducted: $-K_m = (MD_1 - MD_2)/[(MD_1/Css_1) - (MD_2/Css_2)]$ = (322 mg/d – 276 mg/d)/{[(322 mg/d)/(15.8 mg/L)] – [(276 mg/d)/(10.7 mg/L)]} = –8.5 mg/L, K_m = 8.5 mg/L; V_{max} = MD + [K_m(MD/Css)] = 322 mg/d + {8.5 mg/L [(322 mg/d)/(15.8 mg/L)]} = 495 mg/d.

2. *Use the Michaelis-Menten equation to compute a new phenytoin dose for the desired steady-state concentration.*

According to the Michaelis-Menten equation, a dose of 400 mg of phenytoin sodium is needed to achieve a steady-state concentration of 24.6 µg/mL:

$$Css = \frac{K_m \cdot (S \cdot MD)}{V_{max} - (S \cdot MD)} = \frac{8.5\ mg/L \cdot (0.92 \cdot 400\ mg/d)}{495\ mg/d - (0.92 \cdot 400\ mg/d)} = 24.6\ mg/L$$

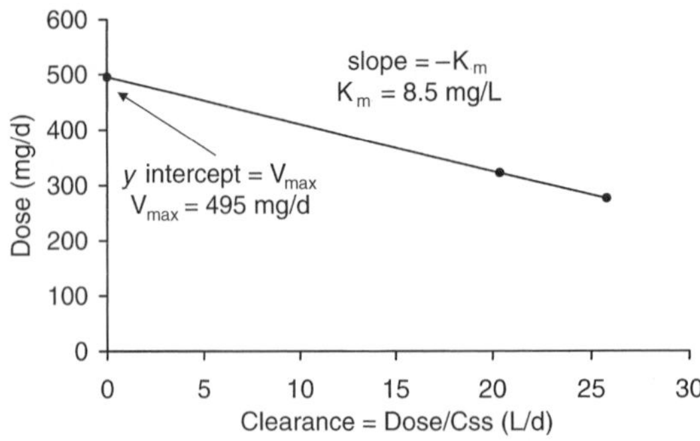

FIGURE 10-8 Ludden graph used to compute Michaelis-Menten parameters and phenytoin dose with two or more steady-state concentration-dose pairs. The graph shows the solution for example 6.

A steady-state minimum serum concentration of phenytoin should be measured after steady state is attained in 7 to 14 days. Serum concentration of phenytoin also should be measured if the patient has an exacerbation of epilepsy or if the patient has signs or symptoms of phenytoin toxicity.

BAYESIAN PHARMACOKINETICS COMPUTER PROGRAMS

Computer programs are available that can assist in the computation of pharmacokinetic parameters for patients. In the most reliable computer programs, a nonlinear regression algorithm incorporates components of Bayes' theorem. Nonlinear regression is a statistical technique in which an iterative process is used to compute the best pharmacokinetic parameters for a concentration–time data set. Briefly, the patient's drug dosage schedule and serum concentrations are entered into a computer. The computer program contains a pharmacokinetic equation for the drug and administration method (e.g., oral, intravenous bolus, intravenous infusion). A one-compartment model typically is used, although some programs allow the user to choose among several equations. With population estimates based on demographic information for the patient (e.g., age, weight, sex, liver function, cardiac status) supplied by the user, the computer program is used to compute estimated serum concentrations at each time there are actual serum concentrations. Kinetic parameters are changed by means of the computer program, and a new set of estimated serum concentrations are computed. The pharmacokinetic parameters that generated the estimated serum concentrations closest to the actual values are stored in the computer memory, and the process is repeated until the set of pharmacokinetic parameters that provide estimated serum concentrations statistically closest to the actual serum concentrations are generated. These pharmacokinetic parameters can be used to compute improved dosing schedules for patients. Bayes' theorem is used in the computer algorithm to balance the results of the computations between values based solely on the patient's serum drug concentrations and those based only on patient population parameters. Results of studies that compare various methods of dosage adjustment have consistently shown that these types of computer dosing programs perform at least as well as experienced clinical pharmacokineticists and clinicians and better than inexperienced clinicians.

Some clinicians use Bayesian pharmacokinetics computer programs exclusively to alter drug doses based on serum concentration. An advantage of this approach is that consistent dosage recommendations are made when several different practitioners are involved in therapeutic drug-monitoring programs. However, because simpler dosing methods work just as well for patients with stable pharmacokinetic parameters and steady-state drug concentrations, many clinicians reserve the use of computer programs for more difficult situations. Those situations include serum concentrations that are not at steady state, serum concentrations not obtained at the specific times needed to use simpler methods, and unstable pharmacokinetic parameters. There are distinct advantages over other methods used to adjust phenytoin dose on the basis of one steady-state serum concentration. Many Bayesian pharmacokinetics computer programs are available, and most should provide answers similar to the ones used in the following examples. The program used to solve problems in this book is DrugCalc, written by Dr. Dennis Mungall, and is available on his Internet web site (http://members.aol.com/thertch/index.htm).[64]

Example 1 TD is a 50-year-old, 75-kg (height, 178 cm) man who has simple partial seizures. He needs therapy with oral phenytoin. He has normal liver and renal function (total bilirubin, 0.5 mg/dL; albumin, 4.0 g/dL; serum creatinine, 0.9 mg/dL). The patient is given a prescription for 400 mg/d of extended phenytoin sodium capsules for 1 month. Steady-state total concentration of phenytoin is 6.2 μg/mL. The patient is found to be compliant with the dosage regimen. Suggest an initial phenytoin dosage regimen designed to achieve a steady-state phenytoin concentration in the therapeutic range.

1. *Enter the patient's demographic, drug dosing, and serum concentration–time data into the computer program.*

DrugCalc requires that doses be entered as phenytoin. A 400-mg dose of phenytoin sodium contains 368 mg of phenytoin (400 mg phenytoin sodium · 0.92 = 368 mg phenytoin). Extended phenytoin sodium capsules are entered as a slow-release dosage form.

2. *Compute the pharmacokinetic parameters for the patient with the Bayesian pharmacokinetics computer program.*

The pharmacokinetic parameters computed with the program are a volume of distribution of 53 L, a V_{max} of 506 mg/d, and a K_m of 4.3 mg/L.

3. *Compute the dose required to achieve the desired phenytoin serum concentrations.*

The one-compartment model Michaelis-Menten equations used in the program to compute doses indicate that a dose of 414 mg/d of phenytoin produces a total steady-state concentration of 12.1 μg/mL. This is equivalent to 450 mg/d of phenytoin sodium: [(414 mg/d phenytoin)/0.92] = 450 mg/d phenytoin sodium. Extended phenytoin sodium capsules are prescribed as 400 mg/d on even days alternating with 500 mg/d on odd days.

Steady-state minimum total serum concentration of phenytoin should be measured after steady state is attained in 7 to 14 days. Serum concentration of phenytoin also should be measured if the patient has an exacerbation of epilepsy or if the patient has signs or symptoms of phenytoin toxicity.

Example 2 GF is a 35-year-old, 55-kg (height, 157 cm) woman who has tonic-clonic seizures. She needs therapy with oral phenytoin. She has normal liver and renal function (total bilirubin, 0.6 mg/dL; albumin, 4.6 g/dL; serum creatinine, 0.6 mg/dL). The patient is given a prescription for 300 mg/d of extended phenytoin sodium capsules for 1 month. Steady-state total concentration of phenytoin is 10.7 μg/mL. The patient is found to be compliant with the dosage regimen. Suggest an initial phenytoin dosage regimen designed to achieve a steady-state phenytoin concentration of 18 μg/mL.

1. *Enter the patient's demographic, drug dosing, and serum concentration–time data into the computer program.*

DrugCalc requires that doses be entered as phenytoin. A 300-mg dose of phenytoin sodium contains 276 mg of phenytoin (300 mg phenytoin sodium · 0.92 = 276 mg phenytoin). Extended phenytoin sodium capsules are entered as a slow-release dosage form.

2. *Compute the pharmacokinetic parameters for the patient with the Bayesian pharmacokinetics computer program.*

The pharmacokinetic parameters computed with the program are a volume of distribution of 34 L, a V_{max} of 354 mg/d, and a K_m of 5.8 mg/L.

3. *Compute the dose required to achieve the desired phenytoin serum concentrations.*

The one-compartment model Michaelis-Menten equations used in the program to compute doses indicate that a dose of 304 mg/d of phenytoin produces a total steady-state concentration of 19.6 μg/mL. This is equivalent to 330 mg/d of phenytoin sodium: [(304 mg/d phenytoin)/0.92] = 330 mg/d phenytoin sodium. Extended phenytoin sodium capsules are prescribed as 330 mg/d (three 100-mg capsules + one 30-mg capsule).

Steady-state minimum total serum concentration of phenytoin should be measured after steady state is attained in 7 to 14 days. Serum concentration of phenytoin also should be measured if the patient has an exacerbation of epilepsy or if the patient has signs or symptoms of phenytoin toxicity.

Example 3 TY is a 27-year-old, 60-kg (height, 168 cm) woman who has complex partial seizures. She needs therapy with oral phenytoin. She has normal liver and renal function (total bilirubin, 0.8 mg/dL; albumin, 5.1 g/dL; serum creatinine, 0.4 mg/dL). The patient is given a prescription for 300 mg/d of extended phenytoin sodium capsules for 1 month. Steady-state total concentration of phenytoin is 8.7 μg/mL. The dosage is increased to 400 mg/d of extended phenytoin sodium capsules for an additional month, and the resulting steady-state concentration is 13.2 μg/mL. The patient is found to be compliant with the dosage regimen. Suggest a new phenytoin dosage increase designed to achieve a steady-state phenytoin concentration in the upper end of the therapeutic range.

1. *Enter the patient's demographic, drug dosing, and serum concentration–time data into the computer program.*

DrugCalc requires that doses be entered as phenytoin. A 300-mg dose of phenytoin sodium contains 276 mg of phenytoin (300 mg phenytoin sodium · 0.92 = 276 mg phenytoin), and a 400 mg dose of phenytoin sodium contains 368 mg of phenytoin (400 mg phenytoin sodium · 0.92 = 368 mg phenytoin). Extended phenytoin sodium capsules are entered as a slow-release dosage form.

2. *Compute the pharmacokinetic parameters for the patient with the Bayesian pharmacokinetics computer program.*

The pharmacokinetic parameters computed with the program are a volume of distribution of 43 L, a V_{max} of 586 mg/d, and a K_m of 13.2 mg/L.

3. *Compute the dose required to achieve the desired phenytoin serum concentrations.*

The one-compartment model Michaelis-Menten equations used in the program to compute doses indicate that a dose of 396 mg/d of phenytoin produces a total steady-state concentration of 20.4 μg/mL. This is equivalent to 430 mg/d of phenytoin sodium: [(396 mg/d phenytoin)/0.92] = 430 mg/d phenytoin sodium. Extended phenytoin sodium capsules are prescribed as 430 mg/d (four 100-mg capsules + one 30-mg capsule).

Steady-state minimum total serum concentration of phenytoin should be measured after steady state is attained in 7 to 14 days. Serum concentration of phenytoin also should be measured if the patient has an exacerbation of epilepsy or if the patient has signs or symptoms of phenytoin toxicity.

USE OF PHENYTOIN BOOSTER DOSES FOR IMMEDIATE INCREASES IN SERUM CONCENTRATION

If a patient has a subtherapeutic phenytoin serum concentration in an acute situation, it may be desirable to increase the phenytoin concentration as quickly as possible. In this setting, it is not acceptable simply to increase the maintenance dose and wait for therapeutic steady-state serum concentrations to be established. A rational way to increase serum concentration rapidly is to administer a booster dose of phenytoin, a process also known as "reloading" the patient with phenytoin. The dose is computed with pharmacokinetic techniques. The modified loading dose equation used to compute the booster dose (BD) takes into account the current phenytoin concentration in the patient: $BD = [(C_{desired} - C_{actual})V]/S$, where $C_{desired}$ is the desired phenytoin concentration, C_{actual} is the actual current phenytoin concentration for the patient, S is the fraction of phenytoin salt that is active phenytoin (0.92 for phenytoin sodium injection and capsules; 0.92 for fosphenytoin because doses are prescribed as a phenytoin sodium equivalent, or PE; 1.0 for phenytoin acid suspensions and tablets), and V is the volume of distribution of phenytoin. If the volume of distribution of phenytoin is known for the patient, it can be used in the calculation. However, this value is not usually known and is assumed to be the population average of 0.7 L/kg. For persons 30% or more above ideal body weight, the volume of distribution can be estimated with the following equation: $V = 0.7\ L/kg\ [IBW + 1.33(TBW - IBW)]$, where IBW is ideal body weight in kilograms: $IBW_{females} = 45 + 2.3(Ht - 60)$ or $IBW_{males} = 50 + 2.3(Ht - 60)$; Ht is height in inches (height in centimeters divided by 2.54); and TBW is total body weight in kilograms.

With administration of the booster dose, the maintenance dose of phenytoin usually is increased. Clinicians need to recognize that administration of a booster dose does not alter the time needed to achieve steady-state conditions when a new phenytoin dosage rate is prescribed. A sufficient time period still is needed to attain steady state when the dosage rate is changed. However, the difference between phenytoin concentration after the booster dose and the ultimate steady-state concentration usually decreases with the extra dose of drug.

Example 1 BN is a 22-year-old, 85-kg (height, 188 cm) man who has complex partial seizures, and he is receiving therapy with intravenous phenytoin sodium. He has normal liver and renal function. After an initial loading dose of phenytoin sodium (1000 mg) and a maintenance dose of 300 mg/d of phenytoin sodium for 5 days, the phenytoin concentration is 5.6 μg/mL immediately after seizure activity is observed. Compute a booster dose of phenytoin to achieve a phenytoin concentration of 15 μg/mL.

1. *Estimate the volume of distribution according to disease states and conditions present in the patient.*

In the case of phenytoin, the population average volume of distribution is 0.7 L/kg. This value is used to estimate the parameter for the patient. The patient is not obese, so actual body weight is used in the computation: $V = 0.7\ L/kg \cdot 85\ kg = 60\ L$.

2. *Compute the booster dose.*

The booster dose is computed with the following equation: $BD = [(C_{desired} - C_{actual})V]/S = [(15\ mg/L - 5.6\ mg/L)\ 60\ L]/0.92 = 613\ mg$, rounded to 600 mg of phenytoin sodium infused no faster than 50 mg/min. (Note: μg/mL = mg/L, and this concentration unit was substituted for Css in the calculations to avoid unit conversion.) If the maintenance dose is increased, it will take additional time for new steady-state conditions to be achieved. Serum concentration of phenytoin should be measured at this time.

PROBLEMS

The following problems are intended to emphasize the computation of initial and individualized doses using clinical pharmacokinetic techniques. Clinicians always should consult the patient's chart to confirm that current anticonvulsant therapy is appropriate. All other medications that the patient is taking, including prescription and nonprescription drugs, should be recorded and checked to ascertain the risk of drug interaction with phenytoin.

1. DF is a 23-year-old, 85-kg (height, 185 cm) man who has tonic-clonic seizures. He needs therapy with oral phenytoin. He has normal liver and renal function (bilirubin, 1.0 mg/dL; albumin, 4.9 g/dL; serum creatinine, 0.7 mg/dL). Suggest an initial extended phenytoin sodium capsule dosage regimen designed to achieve a steady-state phenytoin concentration of 10 μg/mL.

2. Patient DF (see problem 1) is given a prescription for extended phenytoin sodium capsules 500 mg/d orally. The current steady-state phenytoin concentration is 23.5 μg/mL. Compute a new oral phenytoin dose that will provide a steady-state concentration of 15 μg/mL.

3. TR is a 56-year-old, 70-kg (height, 175 cm) man who has complex partial seizures. He needs therapy with oral phenytoin. He has normal liver and renal function (bilirubin, 0.8 mg/dL; albumin, 4.4 g/dL; serum creatinine, 0.9 mg/dL). Suggest an initial

phenytoin suspension dosage regimen designed to achieve a steady-state phenytoin concentration of 15 μg/mL.

4. Patient TR (see problem 3) is given a prescription for phenytoin suspension 200 mg orally every 12 hours. The current steady-state phenytoin concentration is 8 μg/mL. Compute a new oral phenytoin dose that will provide a steady-state concentration of 15 μg/mL.

5. PL is a 64-year-old, 60-kg (height, 157 cm) woman who has simple partial seizures. She needs therapy with intravenous fosphenytoin. She has normal liver and renal function (bilirubin, 0.8 mg/dL; albumin, 3.6 g/dL; serum creatinine, 1.2 mg/dL). Suggest an initial intravenous fosphenytoin regimen designed to achieve a steady-state phenytoin concentration of 12 μg/mL.

6. Patient PL (see problem 5) is prescribed intravenous fosphenytoin injection 200 mg/d PE. The serum concentration of phenytoin just before the fourth dose of this regimen is 4.1 μg/mL. Assuming the phenytoin concentration was zero before the first dose, compute a new intravenous fosphenytoin injection that will provide a steady-state concentration of 12 μg/mL.

7. MN is a 24-year-old, 55-kg (height, 165 cm) woman who has complex partial seizures. She needs therapy with intravenous phenytoin sodium. She has normal liver and renal function (bilirubin, 0.8 mg/dL; albumin, 3.6 g/dL; serum creatinine, 1.2 mg/dL). Suggest an initial intravenous dosage regimen of phenytoin sodium designed to achieve a steady-state phenytoin concentration of 12 μg/mL.

8. Patient MN (see problem 7) is prescribed intravenous phenytoin sodium injection 300 mg/d. Serum concentration of phenytoin at steady state is 6.4 μg/mL. The dose is increased to intravenous phenytoin sodium injection 400 mg/d and the measured steady-state concentration is 10.7 μg/mL. Compute a new intravenous injection dosage of phenytoin sodium that will provide a steady-state concentration of 15 μg/mL.

9. SA is a 62-year-old, 130-kg (height, 180 cm) man who has complex partial seizures. He needs therapy with oral phenytoin. He has normal liver and renal function (bilirubin, 0.6 mg/dL; albumin, 3.9 g/dL; serum creatinine, 1.0 mg/dL). Suggest an initial dosage regimen of extended phenytoin sodium capsules designed to achieve a steady-state concentration of 10 μg/mL.

10. Patient SA (see problem 9) is given a prescription for extended phenytoin sodium capsules 200 mg orally every 12 hours. Phenytoin serum concentration at steady state is 6.2 μg/mL. The dose is increased to extended phenytoin sodium capsules 300 mg orally every 12 hours, and the measured steady-state concentration is 25.7 μg/mL. Compute a new oral phenytoin dose that will provide a steady-state concentration of 15 μg/mL.

11. VG has epilepsy and is being treated with phenytoin. He has hypoalbuminemia (albumin, 2.4 g/dL) and normal renal function (creatinine clearance, 90 mL/min). Total phenytoin concentration is 8.9 μg/mL. Assuming that the clinical laboratory measures unbound concentration at 25°C, compute an estimated normalized phenytoin concentration for this patient.

12. DE has epilepsy and is being treated with phenytoin. He has hypoalbuminemia (albumin, 2.0 g/dL) and poor renal function (creatinine clearance, 10 mL/min). Total phenytoin concentration is 8.1 μg/mL. Compute an estimated normalized phenytoin concentration for this patient.

13. KL has epilepsy and is being treated with phenytoin and valproic acid. Albumin concentration (albumin, 4.0 g/dL) and renal function (creatinine clearance, 95 mL/min) are normal. Steady-state total concentrations of phenytoin and valproic acid are 6 μg/mL and 90 μg/mL, respectively. Compute an estimated unbound phenytoin concentration for this patient.

ANSWERS TO PROBLEMS

1. The initial phenytoin dose for patient DF is calculated as follows.

Pharmacokinetic Dosing Method

1. *Estimate the Michaelis-Menten constants according to disease states and conditions present in the patient.*

The V_{max} for an adult patient who is not obese and has normal liver and renal function is 7 mg/kg per day. For an 85-kg patient, V_{max} = 595 mg/d: V_{max} = 7 mg/kg/d · 85 kg = 595 mg/d. For this patient, K_m = 4 mg/L.

2. *Compute the dosage regimen.*

Oral phenytoin sodium capsules are prescribed to this patient (F = 1, S = 0.92). The initial dosage interval (τ) is set to 24 hours. (Note: μg/mL = mg/L, and this concentration unit was substituted for Css in the calculations to avoid unit conversion.) The dosage equation for phenytoin is

$$MD = \frac{V_{max} \cdot Css}{S(K_m + Css)} = \frac{595\ \text{mg/d} \cdot 10\ \text{mg/L}}{0.92\ (4\ \text{mg/L} + 10\ \text{mg/L})} = 462\ \text{mg/d, rounded to } 500\ \text{mg/d}$$

Steady-state minimum total serum concentration of phenytoin should be measured after steady state is attained in 7 to 14 days. Serum concentration of phenytoin also should be measured if the patient has an exacerbation of epilepsy or if the patient has signs or symptoms of phenytoin toxicity.

Literature-Based Recommended Dosing

1. *Estimate the phenytoin dose according to disease states and conditions present in the patient.*

The suggested initial dosage rate for extended phenytoin sodium capsules administered to an adult patient is 4 to 6 mg/kg per day. At a rate of 5 mg/kg per day, the initial dose is 400 mg/d: 5 mg/kg/d · 85 kg = 425 mg/d, rounded to 400 mg/d. With a dosage interval of 24 hours, the prescribed dose is 400 mg of extended phenytoin sodium capsules daily.

Steady-state minimum total serum concentration of phenytoin should be measured after steady state is attained in 7 to 14 days. Serum concentration of phenytoin also should be measured if the patient has an exacerbation of epilepsy or if the patient has signs or symptoms of phenytoin toxicity.

2. The revised phenytoin dose for patient DF is calculated as follows.

Empiric Dosing Method

1. *Suggest a new phenytoin dose.*

Because the patient is receiving extended phenytoin sodium capsules, a convenient dosage change is 100 mg/d, and a decrease to 400 mg/d is suggested.

Steady-state minimum total serum concentration of phenytoin should be measured after steady state is attained in 7 to 14 days. Serum concentration of phenytoin also should be measured if the patient has an exacerbation of epilepsy or if the patient has signs or symptoms of phenytoin toxicity.

Pseudolinear Pharmacokinetics Method

1. *Use pseudolinear pharmacokinetics to predict a new concentration for a dosage decrease, then compute the 15% to 33% factor to account for Michaelis-Menten pharmacokinetics.*

Because the patient is receiving extended phenytoin sodium capsules, a convenient dosage change is 100 mg/d, and a decrease to 400 mg/d is suggested. According to pseudolinear pharmacokinetics, the resulting total steady-state phenytoin serum concentration is $Css_{new} = (D_{new}/D_{old})Css_{old}$ = [(400 mg/d)/(500 mg/d)] 23.5 μg/mL = 18.8 μg/mL. Because of Michaelis-Menten pharmacokinetics, the serum concentration is expected to decrease 15%, or 0.85 times, to 33%, or 0.67 times, greater than that predicted by linear pharmacokinetics: Css = 18.8 μg/mL · 0.85 = 16 μg/mL, and Css = 18.8 μg/mL · 0.67 = 12.6 μg/mL. Thus a dosage decrease of 100 mg/d is expected to yield a total steady-state serum concentration of phenytoin of 12 to 16 μg/mL.

Steady-state minimum total serum concentration of phenytoin should be measured after steady state is attained in 7 to 14 days. Serum concentration of phenytoin also should be measured if the patient has an exacerbation of epilepsy or if the patient has signs or symptoms of phenytoin toxicity.

Graves-Cloyd Method

1. *Use the Graves-Cloyd method to estimate a new phenytoin dose for the desired steady-state concentration.*

A new total steady-state serum concentration of phenytoin of 15 μg/mL is chosen for the patient (460 mg phenytoin = 500 mg phenytoin sodium · 0.92): $D_{new} = (D_{old}/Css_{old}) \cdot Css_{new}^{0.199} \cdot Css_{old}^{0.804}$ = [(460 mg/d)/(23.5 mg/L)] · $(15\ \text{mg/L})^{0.199}$ · $(23.5\ \text{mg/L})^{0.804}$ = 425 mg/d of phenytoin acid, which equals 462 mg of phenytoin sodium (462 mg phenytoin sodium = 425 mg phenytoin/0.92). This dose is rounded to 450 mg/d, or 400 mg/d on even days alternating with 500 mg/d on odd days.

Steady-state minimum total serum concentration of phenytoin should be measured after steady state is attained in 7 to 14 days. Serum concentration of phenytoin also should be measured if the patient has an exacerbation of epilepsy or if the patient has signs or symptoms of phenytoin toxicity.

Vozeh-Sheiner Method

1. *Use the Vozeh-Sheiner method to estimate a new phenytoin dose for the desired steady-state concentration.*

A new total steady-state serum concentration of phenytoin of 15 μg/mL is chosen for the patient. The serum concentration–dose information is plotted on the orbit graph (Note: phenytoin dose = 0.92 · phenytoin sodium dose = 0.92 · 500 mg/d = 460 mg/d; (460 mg/d)/85 kg = 5.4 mg/kg/d; Figure 10-9). According to the graph, a dose of 4.9 mg/kg per day of phenytoin is needed to achieve a steady-state concentration of 15 μg/mL. This is an extended phenytoin sodium capsule dose of 450 mg/d, administered by means of alternating 400 mg/d on even days and 500 mg/d on odd days: (4.9 mg/kg/d · 85 kg)/0.92 = 453 mg/d, rounded to 450 mg/d.

Steady-state minimum total serum concentration of phenytoin should be measured after steady state is attained in 7 to 14 days. Serum concentration of phenytoin also should be measured if the patient has an exacerbation of epilepsy or if the patient has signs or symptoms of phenytoin toxicity.

3. The initial phenytoin dose for patient TR is calculated as follows.

Pharmacokinetic Dosing Method

1. *Estimate the Michaelis-Menten constants according to disease states and conditions present in the patient.*

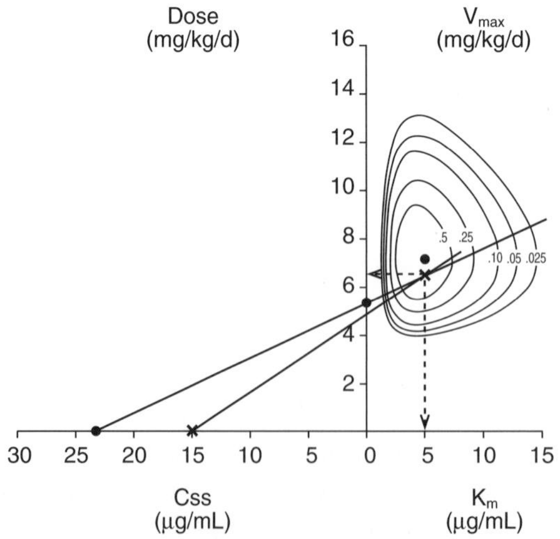

FIGURE 10-9 Solution to problem 2 obtained with Vozeh-Sheiner or orbit graph.

The V_{max} for an adult who is not obese and has normal hepatic and renal function is 7 mg/kg per day. For a 70-kg patient, V_{max} = 490 mg/d: V_{max} = 7 mg/kg/d · 70 kg = 490 mg/d. For this patient, K_m = 4 mg/L.

2. *Compute the dosage regimen.*

Oral phenytoin suspension is prescribed to this patient (F = 1, S = 1). The initial dosage interval (τ) is set to 12 hours. (Note: μg/mL = mg/L, and this concentration unit was substituted for Css in the calculations to avoid unit conversion.) The dosage equation for phenytoin is

$$MD = \frac{V_{max} \cdot Css}{S(K_m + Css)} = \frac{490 \text{ mg/d} \cdot 15 \text{ mg/L}}{1\ (4 \text{ mg/L} + 15 \text{ mg/L})} = 387 \text{ mg/d, rounded to } 400 \text{ mg/d}$$

A dosage of phenytoin suspension 200 mg every 12 hours is prescribed. A steady-state minimum total serum concentration of phenytoin should be measured after steady state is attained in 7 to 14 days. Serum concentration of phenytoin also should be measured if the patient has an exacerbation of epilepsy or if the patient has signs or symptoms of phenytoin toxicity.

Literature-Based Recommended Dosing

1. *Estimate the phenytoin dose according to disease states and conditions present in the patient.*

The suggested initial dosage rate for extended phenytoin sodium capsules taken by an adult patient is 4 to 6 mg/kg per day. Using a rate of 5 mg/kg per day, the initial dose is 400 mg/d: 5 mg/kg/d · 70 kg = 350 mg/d, rounded to 400 mg/d. With a dosage interval of 12 hours, the prescribed dose is 200 mg of phenytoin suspension every 12 hours.

Steady-state minimum total serum concentration of phenytoin should be measured after steady state is attained in 7 to 14 days. Serum concentration of phenytoin also should be measured if the patient has an exacerbation of epilepsy or if the patient has signs or symptoms of phenytoin toxicity.

4. The revised phenytoin dose of patient TR is calculated as follows.

Empiric Dosing Method

1. *Suggest a new phenytoin dose.*

Because the patient is receiving phenytoin suspension, a convenient dosage change would be 100 mg/d, and an increase to 500 mg/d or 250 mg every 12 hours is suggested (see Table 10-4).

Steady-state minimum total serum concentration of phenytoin should be measured after steady state is attained in 7 to 14 days. Serum concentration of phenytoin also should be measured if the patient has an exacerbation of epilepsy or if the patient has signs or symptoms of phenytoin toxicity.

Pseudolinear Pharmacokinetics Method

1. *Use pseudolinear pharmacokinetics to predict a new concentration for a dosage increase, then compute the 15% to 33% factor to account for Michaelis-Menten pharmacokinetics.*

Because the patient is receiving phenytoin suspension, a convenient dosage change would be 100 mg/d, and an increase to 500 mg/d is suggested. According to pseudolinear pharmacokinetics, the resulting total steady-state serum concentration of phenytoin is $Css_{new} = (D_{new}/D_{old})Css_{old}$ = [(500 mg/d)/(400 mg/d)] 8 μg/mL = 10 μg/mL. Because of Michaelis-Menten pharmacokinetics, the serum concentration is expected to increase 15%, or 1.15 times, to 33%, or 1.33 times, greater than that predicted with linear pharmacokinetics: Css = 10 μg/mL · 1.15 = 11.5 μg/mL, and Css = 10 μg/mL · 1.33 = 13.3 μg/mL. Thus a dosage increase of 100 mg/d is expected to yield a total steady-state serum concentration of phenytoin of 11 to 13 μg/mL.

Steady-state minimum total serum concentration of phenytoin should be measured after steady state is attained in 7 to 14 days. Serum concentration of phenytoin also should be measured if the patient has an exacerbation of epilepsy or if the patient has signs or symptoms of phenytoin toxicity.

Graves-Cloyd Method

1. *Use the Graves-Cloyd method to estimate a new phenytoin dose for the desired steady-state concentration.*

A new total steady-state serum concentration of phenytoin of 15 μg/mL is chosen for the patient: $D_{new} = (D_{old}/Css_{old}) \cdot Css_{new}^{0.199} \cdot Css_{old}^{0.804}$ = [(400 mg/d)/(8 mg/L)] · $(15\ \text{mg/L})^{0.199} \cdot (8\ \text{mg/L})^{0.804}$ = 456 mg/d, rounded to 450 mg/d, or 225 mg every 12 hours.

Steady-state minimum total serum concentration of phenytoin should be measured after steady state is attained in 7 to 14 days. Serum concentration of phenytoin also should be measured if the patient has an exacerbation of epilepsy or if the patient has signs or symptoms of phenytoin toxicity.

Vozeh-Sheiner Method

1. *Use the Vozeh-Sheiner method to estimate a new phenytoin dose for the desired steady-state concentration.*

A new total steady-state serum concentration of phenytoin of 15 μg/mL is chosen for the patient. The serum concentration–dose information is plotted on the orbit graph (Note: (400 mg/d)/70 kg = 5.7 mg/kg/d; Figure 10-10). According to the graph, a dose of 6.6 mg/kg per day of phenytoin is needed to achieve a steady-state concentration of 15 μg/mL. This equals a phenytoin suspension dose of 450 mg/d administered as 225 mg every 12 hours: 6.6 mg/kg/d · 70 kg = 462 mg/d, rounded to 450 mg/d.

Steady-state minimum total serum concentration of phenytoin should be measured after steady state is attained in 7 to 14 days. Serum concentration of phenytoin also

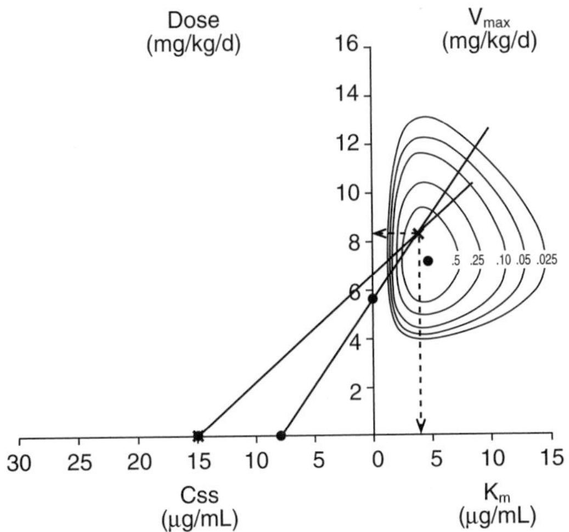

FIGURE 10-10 Solution to problem 4 obtained with Vozeh-Sheiner or orbit graph.

should be measured if the patient has an exacerbation of epilepsy or if the patient has signs or symptoms of phenytoin toxicity.

5. The initial phenytoin dose for patient PL is calculated as follows.

Pharmacokinetic Dosing Method

1. *Estimate the Michaelis-Menten constants and volume of distribution according to disease states and conditions present in the patient.*

The V_{max} for an adult who is not obese and has normal hepatic and renal function is 7 mg/kg per day. For a 60-kg patient, V_{max} = 420 mg/d: V_{max} = 7 mg/kg/d · 60 kg = 420 mg/d. For this patient, K_m = 4 mg/L. The volume of distribution for this patient is 42 L: V = 0.7 L/kg · 60 kg = 42 L.

2. *Compute the dosage regimen.*

Fosphenytoin is given to this patient, and it is prescribed in phenytoin sodium equivalents, or PE (F = 1, S = 0.92). The initial dosage interval (τ) is set to 12 hours. (Note: μg/mL = mg/L, and this concentration unit was substituted for Css in the calculations to avoid unit conversion.) The dosage equation for phenytoin is

$$MD = \frac{V_{max} \cdot Css}{S(K_m + Css)} = \frac{420 \text{ mg/d} \cdot 12 \text{ mg/L}}{0.92\ (4 \text{ mg/L} + 12 \text{ mg/L})} = 342 \text{ mg/d, rounded to } 350 \text{ mg}$$

$$LD = (V \cdot Css)/S = (42 \text{ L} \cdot 12 \text{ mg/L})/0.92 = 548 \text{ mg, rounded to } 550 \text{ mg}$$

The maintenance dose is given as 175 mg every 12 hours. Infusion rates of maintenance and loading doses should not exceed 150 mg/min PE. A steady-state minimum total serum concentration of phenytoin should be measured after steady state is attained in 7 to 14 days. Serum concentration of phenytoin also should be measured if the patient has an exacerbation of epilepsy or if the patient has signs or symptoms of phenytoin toxicity.

Literature-Based Recommended Dosing

1. *Estimate the phenytoin dose according to disease states and conditions present in the patient.*

The suggested initial dosage rate of fosphenytoin injection for an adult patient is 4 to 6 mg/kg per day PE. At a rate of 5 mg/kg per day, the initial dose is 300 mg/d or 150 mg every 12 hours: 5 mg/kg/d · 60 kg = 300 mg/d. The suggested loading doses of fosphenytoin is 15 to 20 mg/kg PE. With the dose of 18 mg/kg PE, the loading dose is 1000 mg PE: 18 mg/kg PE · 60 kg = 1080 mg PE, rounded to 1000 mg PE. Infusion rates of maintenance and loading dose should not exceed 150 mg/min PE.

Steady-state minimum total serum concentration of phenytoin should be measured after steady state is attained in 7 to 14 days. Serum concentration of phenytoin also should be measured if the patient has an exacerbation of epilepsy or if the patient has signs or symptoms of phenytoin toxicity.

6. The revised phenytoin dose of patient PL is calculated as follows.

Bayesian Pharmacokinetics Computer Program Method

Because the patient has only received three doses of fosphenytoin, it is unlikely the measured serum concentration is a steady-state concentration. Thus methods that require a single steady-state serum concentration should not be used.

1. *Enter the patient's demographic, drug dosing, and serum concentration–time data into the computer program.*

DrugCalc requires that doses be entered as phenytoin. A 200 mg/d PE dose of fosphenytoin contains 184 mg of phenytoin (200 mg PE fosphenytoin · 0.92 = 184 mg phenytoin). This dose is entered into the program along with a dose length time of 1.

2. *Compute the pharmacokinetic parameters for the patient using the Bayesian pharmacokinetics computer program.*

The pharmacokinetic parameters computed with the program are a volume of distribution of 47 L, a V_{max} of 299 mg/d, and a K_m of 6.0 mg/L.

3. *Compute the dose required to achieve the desired phenytoin serum concentrations.*

The one-compartment model Michaelis-Menten equations used in the program to compute doses indicate that a dose of 200 mg/d of phenytoin produces a total steady-state concentration of 12 μg/mL. This is equivalent to 217 mg/d of phenytoin sodium [(200 mg/d phenytoin)/0.92 = 217 mg/d PE fosphenytoin], and this dose is rounded to 200 mg/d PE. Fosphenytoin is prescribed as 200 mg/d PE at an infusion rate no greater than 150 mg/min PE.

Steady-state minimum total serum concentration of phenytoin should be measured after steady state is attained in 7 to 14 days. Serum concentration of phenytoin also

should be measured if the patient has an exacerbation of epilepsy or if the patient has signs or symptoms of phenytoin toxicity.

7. The initial phenytoin dose for patient MN is calculated as follows.

Pharmacokinetic Dosing Method

1. *Estimate the Michaelis-Menten constants and volume of distribution according to disease states and conditions present in the patient.*

The V_{max} for an adult who is not obese and has normal hepatic and renal function is 7 mg/kg per day. For a 55-kg patient, V_{max} = 385 mg/d: V_{max} = 7 mg/kg/d · 55 kg = 385 mg/d. For this patient, K_m = 4 mg/L. The volume of distribution for this patient is 39 L: V = 0.7 L/kg · 55 kg = 39 L.

2. *Compute the dosage regimen.*

Phenytoin sodium injection is given to this patient (F = 1, S = 0.92). The initial dosage interval (τ) is set to 12 hours. (Note: μg/mL = mg/L, and this concentration unit was substituted for Css in the calculations to avoid unit conversion.) The dosage equation for phenytoin is

$$MD = \frac{V_{max} \cdot Css}{S(K_m + Css)} = \frac{385 \text{ mg/d} \cdot 12 \text{ mg/L}}{0.92\ (4 \text{ mg/L} + 12 \text{ mg/L})} = 314 \text{ mg/d, rounded to 300 mg/d}$$

$$LD = (V \cdot Css)/S = (39 \text{ L} \cdot 12 \text{ mg/L})/0.92 = 509 \text{ mg, rounded to 500 mg}$$

The maintenance dose is given as 150 mg every 12 hours. Infusion rates of maintenance and loading doses should not exceed 50 mg/min. A steady-state minimum total serum concentration of phenytoin should be measured after steady state is attained in 7 to 14 days. Serum concentration of phenytoin also should be measured if the patient has an exacerbation of epilepsy or if the patient has signs or symptoms of phenytoin toxicity.

Literature-Based Recommended Dosing

1. *Estimate the phenytoin dose according to disease states and conditions present in the patient.*

The suggested initial dosage rate of phenytoin sodium injection for an adult patient is 4 to 6 mg/kg per day PE. At a rate of 5 mg/kg per day, the initial dose is 300 mg/d, or 150 mg every 12 hours: 5 mg/kg/d · 55 kg = 275 mg/d, rounded to 300 mg/d. The suggested loading dose of phenytoin sodium injection is 15 to 20 mg/kg. At a dose of 18 mg/kg, the loading dose is 1000 mg: 18 mg/kg · 55 kg = 990 mg PE, rounded to 1000 mg PE. Infusion rates of maintenance and loading doses should not exceed 50 mg/min.

Steady-state minimum total serum concentration of phenytoin should be measured after steady state is attained in 7 to 14 days. Serum concentration of phenytoin also should be measured if the patient has an exacerbation of epilepsy or if the patient has signs or symptoms of phenytoin toxicity.

8. The revised phenytoin dose of patient MN is calculated as follows.

Empiric Dosing Method

1. *Empirically suggest new phenytoin dose.*

The next logical dose to prescribe is phenytoin sodium 500 mg/d (see Table 10-4).

Steady-state minimum total serum concentration of phenytoin should be measured after steady state is attained in 7 to 14 days. Serum concentration of phenytoin also should be measured if the patient has an exacerbation of epilepsy or if the patient has signs or symptoms of phenytoin toxicity.

Mullen Method

1. *Use the Mullen method to estimate a new phenytoin dose for the desired steady-state concentration.*

Serum concentration–dose information is plotted on the graph (Note: phenytoin dose = 0.92 · phenytoin sodium dose = 0.92 · 300 mg/d = 276 mg/d, [(276 mg/d)/55 kg] = 5 mg/kg/d; phenytoin dose = 0.92 · phenytoin sodium dose = 0.92 · 400 mg/d = 368 mg/d, [(368 mg/d)/55 kg] = 6.7 mg/kg/d; Figure 10-11). According to the graph, a dose of 7.7 mg/kg per day of phenytoin is needed to achieve a steady-state concentration of 15 μg/mL. This is a phenytoin sodium injection dose of 450 mg/d, or 225 mg every 12 hours: (7.7 mg/kg/d · 55 kg)/0.92 = 460 mg/d, rounded to 450 mg/d. The dose is given as 225 mg every 12 hours. V_{max} = 13.4 mg/kg per day, and K_m = 10.6 μg/mL for this patient.

Steady-state minimum total serum concentration of phenytoin should be measured after steady state is attained in 7 to 14 days. Serum concentration of phenytoin also should be measured if the patient has an exacerbation of epilepsy or if the patient has signs or symptoms of phenytoin toxicity.

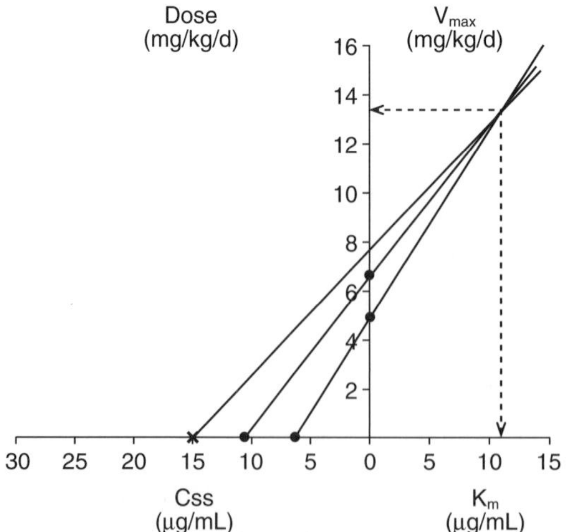

FIGURE 10-11 Solution to problem 8 obtained with Mullen graph.

Ludden Method

1. *Use the Ludden method to estimate V_{max} and K_m.*

The serum concentration–dose information is plotted on the graph (Note: phenytoin dose = 0.92 · phenytoin sodium dose = 0.92 · 300 mg/d = 276 mg/d, (276 mg/d)/55 kg = 5 mg/kg/d; phenytoin dose = 0.92 · phenytoin sodium dose = 0.92 · 400 mg/d = 368 mg/d, (368 mg/d)/55 kg = 6.7 mg/kg/d; Figure 10-12). According to the graph, V_{max} = 729 mg/d and K_m = 10.5 mg/L.

Because only two steady-state concentration-dose pairs are available, a direct mathematical solution can be attained: $-K_m = (MD_1 - MD_2)/[(MD_1/Css_2) - (MD_2/Css_2)]$ = [(368 mg/d) – (276 mg/d)]/{[(368 mg/d)/(10.7 mg/L)] – [(276 mg/d)/(6.4 mg/L)]} = –10.5 mg/L, K_m = 10.5 mg/L; $V_{max} = MD + K_m(MD/Css)$ = 368 mg/d + 10.5 mg/L [(368 mg/d)/(10.7 mg/L)] = 729 mg/d.

2. *Use the Michaelis-Menten equation to compute a new phenytoin dose for the desired steady-state concentration.*

According to the Michaelis-Menten equation, a dose of 450 mg of phenytoin sodium is needed to achieve a steady-state concentration of 10.4 μg/mL:

$$MD = \frac{V_{max} \cdot Css}{S(K_m + Css)} = \frac{729 \text{ mg/d} \cdot 15 \text{ mg/L}}{0.92\ (10.5 \text{ mg/L} + 15 \text{ mg/L})} = 466 \text{ mg/d, rounded to } 450 \text{ mg/d}$$

This dose is administered by means of giving 225 mg every 12 hours.

Steady-state minimum total serum concentration of phenytoin should be measured after steady state is attained in 7 to 14 days. Serum concentration of phenytoin also should be measured if the patient has an exacerbation of epilepsy or if the patient has signs or symptoms of phenytoin toxicity.

Bayesian Pharmacokinetics Computer Program Method

1. *Enter the patient's demographic, drug dosing, and serum concentration–time data into the computer program.*

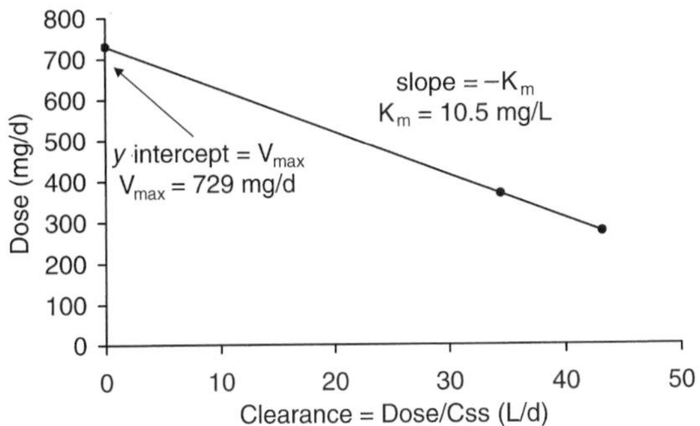

FIGURE 10-12 Solution to problem 8 obtained with Ludden graph.

DrugCalc requires that doses be entered as phenytoin (phenytoin dose = 0.92 · phenytoin sodium dose = 0.92 · 300 mg/d = 276 mg/d; phenytoin dose = 0.92 · phenytoin sodium dose = 0.92 · 400 mg/d = 368 mg/d). These doses are entered into the program with a dose length time of 1.

2. *Compute the pharmacokinetic parameters for the patient using the Bayesian pharmacokinetics computer program.*

The pharmacokinetic parameters computed with the program are a volume of distribution of 49 L, a V_{max} of 633 mg/d, and a K_m of 10.8 mg/L.

3. *Compute the dose required to achieve the desired phenytoin serum concentrations.*

The one-compartment model Michaelis-Menten equations used in the program to compute doses indicates that a dose of 414 mg/d of phenytoin produces a total steady-state concentration of 20.3 μg/mL. This is equivalent to 450 mg/d of phenytoin sodium [(414 mg/d phenytoin)/0.92 = 450 mg/d phenytoin sodium], and this dose is given as 225 mg every 12 hours.

Steady-state minimum total serum concentration of phenytoin should be measured after steady state is attained in 7 to 14 days. Serum concentration of phenytoin also should be measured if the patient has an exacerbation of epilepsy or if the patient has signs or symptoms of phenytoin toxicity.

9. The initial phenytoin dose for patient SA is calculated as follows.

Pharmacokinetic Dosing Method

1. *Estimate the Michaelis-Menten constants and volume of distribution according to disease states and conditions present in the patient.*

The V_{max} for an adult with normal hepatic and renal function is 7 mg/kg per day. In the care of obese persons, it is unclear whether to use ideal body weight (IBW) or total body weight (TBW) to calculate the maintenance dose. Most clinicians use ideal body weight because it produces the most conservative dosage recommendation: $IBW_{males} = 50 + 2.3(Ht - 60) = 50 + 2.3(71 - 60) = 75$ kg, where Ht is height in inches (height in centimeters divided by 2.54). For a 75-kg patient, V_{max} = 525 mg/d: V_{max} = 7 mg/kg/d · 75 kg = 525 mg/d. For this patient, K_m = 4 mg/L.

2. *Compute the dosage regimen.*

Extended phenytoin sodium capsules are given to this patient (F = 1, S = 0.92). The initial dosage interval (τ) is set to 24 hours. (Note: μg/mL = mg/L, and this concentration unit was substituted for Css in the calculations to avoid unit conversion.) The dosage equation for phenytoin is

$$MD = \frac{V_{max} \cdot Css}{S(K_m + Css)} = \frac{525 \text{ mg/d} \cdot 10 \text{ mg/L}}{0.92\ (4 \text{ mg/L} + 10 \text{ mg/L})} = 408 \text{ mg/d, rounded to } 400 \text{ mg/d}$$

The maintenance dose is given as 400 mg/d. A steady-state minimum total serum concentration of phenytoin should be measured after steady state is attained in 7 to 14 days. Serum concentration of phenytoin also should be measured if the patient has an exacerbation of epilepsy or if the patient has signs or symptoms of phenytoin toxicity.

Literature-Based Recommended Dosing

1. *Estimate the phenytoin dose according to disease states and conditions present in the patient.*

The suggested initial dosage rate for phenytoin sodium injection for an adult patient is 4 to 6 mg/kg per day. For obese persons, it is unclear whether to use ideal body weight (IBW) or total body weight (TBW) for dose calculation. Most clinicians use ideal body weight because it produces the most conservative dosage recommendation: $IBW_{males} = 50 + 2.3(Ht - 60) = 50 + 2.3(71 - 60) = 75$ kg, where 71 is height in inches (180 cm). At a rate of 5 mg/kg per day, the initial dose is 400 mg/d, or 200 mg every 12 hours: 5 mg/kg/d · 75 kg = 375 mg/d, rounded to 400 mg/d.

Steady-state minimum total serum concentration of phenytoin should be measured after steady state is attained in 7 to 14 days. Serum concentration of phenytoin also should be measured if the patient has an exacerbation of epilepsy or if the patient has signs or symptoms of phenytoin toxicity.

10. The revised phenytoin dose of patient SA is calculated as follows.

Empiric Dosing Method

1. *Empirically suggest a new phenytoin dose.*

The next logical dose to prescribe is phenytoin sodium 200 mg every morning plus 300 mg every evening.

Steady-state minimum total serum concentration of phenytoin should be measured after steady state is attained in 7 to 14 days. Serum concentration of phenytoin also should be measured if the patient has an exacerbation of epilepsy or if the patient has signs or symptoms of phenytoin toxicity.

Mullen Method

1. *Use the Mullen method to estimate a new phenytoin dose for the desired steady-state concentration.*

The serum concentration–dose information is plotted on the graph (Note: phenytoin dose = 0.92 · phenytoin sodium dose = 0.92 · 600 mg/d = 552 mg/d, (552 mg/d)/75 kg IBW = 7.4 mg/kg/d; phenytoin dose = 0.92 · phenytoin sodium dose = 0.92 · 400 mg/d = 368 mg/d, (368 mg/d)/75 kg IBW = 4.9 mg/kg/d; Figure 10-13). According to the graph, a dose of 6.7 mg/kg per day of phenytoin is needed to achieve a steady-state concentration of 15 μg/mL. This is an extended phenytoin sodium capsule dose of 500 mg/d, or 200 mg every morning plus 300 mg every evening: (6.7 mg/kg/d · 75 kg)/0.92 = 546 mg/d, rounded to 500 mg/d. V_{max} = 8.8 mg/kg per day, and K_m = 5 μg/mL for this patient.

Steady-state minimum total serum concentration of phenytoin should be measured after steady state is attained in 7 to 14 days. Serum concentration of phenytoin also

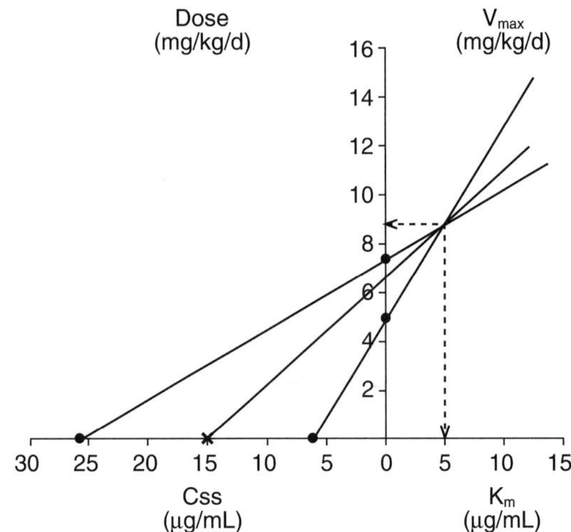

FIGURE 10-13 Solution to problem 10 obtained with Mullen graph.

should be measured if the patient has an exacerbation of epilepsy or if the patient has signs or symptoms of phenytoin toxicity.

Ludden Method

1. *Use the Ludden method to estimate V_{max} and K_m.*

Serum concentration–dose information is plotted on the graph (Note: phenytoin dose = 0.92 · phenytoin sodium dose = 0.92 · 600 mg/d = 552 mg/d, (552 mg/d)/75 kg IBW = 7.4 mg/kg/d; phenytoin dose = 0.92 · phenytoin sodium dose = 0.92 · 400 mg/d = 368 mg/d, (368 mg/d)/75 kg IBW = 4.9 mg/kg/d; Figure 10-14). According to the graph, V_{max} = 659 mg/d, and K_m = 4.9 mg/L.

Because only two steady-state concentration-dose pairs are available, a direct mathematical solution can be obtained: $-K_m = (MD_1 - MD_2)/[(MD_1/Css_1) - (MD_2/Css_2)]$ = [(552 mg/d) – (368 mg/d)]/{[(552 mg/d)/(25.7 mg/L)] – (368 mg/d)/(6.2 mg/L)]} = –4.9 mg/L, K_m = 4.9 mg/L; $V_{max} = MD + K_m(MD/Css)$ = 368 mg/d + 4.9 mg/L [(368 mg/d)/(6.2 mg/L)] = 659 mg/d.

2. *Use the Michaelis-Menten equation to compute a new phenytoin dose for the desired steady-state concentration.*

According to the Michaelis-Menten equation, a dose of 500 mg of phenytoin sodium is needed to achieve a steady-state concentration equal to 15 µg/mL:

$$MD = \frac{V_{max} \cdot Css}{S(K_m + Css)} = \frac{659\ \text{mg/d} \cdot 15\ \text{mg/L}}{0.92\ (4.9\ \text{mg/L} + 15\ \text{mg/L})} = 540\ \text{mg/d, rounded to 500 mg/d}$$

This dose is administered by means of giving 200 mg every morning plus 300 mg every evening.

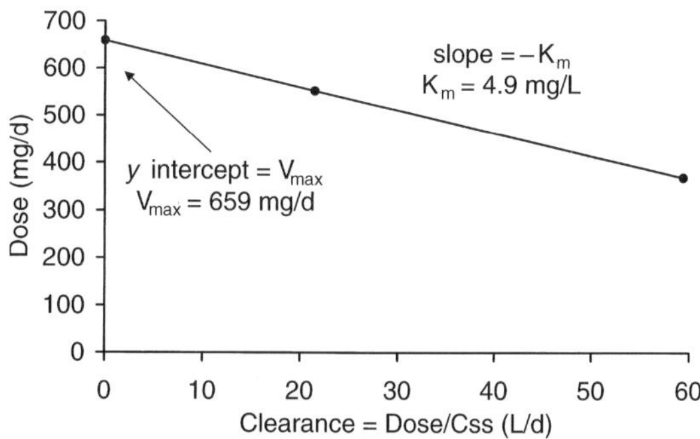

FIGURE 10-14 Solution to problem 10 obtained with Ludden graph.

Steady-state minimum total serum concentration of phenytoin should be measured after steady state is attained in 7 to 14 days. Serum concentration of phenytoin also should be measured if the patient has an exacerbation of epilepsy or if the patient has signs or symptoms of phenytoin toxicity.

Bayesian Pharmacokinetics Computer Program Method

1. *Enter the patient's demographic, drug dosing, and serum concentration–time data into the computer program.*

DrugCalc requires that doses be entered as phenytoin (phenytoin dose = 0.92 · phenytoin sodium dose = 0.92 · 600 mg/d = 552 mg/d; phenytoin dose = 0.92 · phenytoin sodium dose = 0.92 · 400 mg/d = 368 mg/d).

2. *Compute the pharmacokinetic parameters for the patient using the Bayesian pharmacokinetics computer program.*

The pharmacokinetic parameters computed with the program are a volume of distribution of 90 L, a V_{max} of 510 mg/d, and a K_m equal to 4.3 mg/L.

3. *Compute the dose required to achieve desired phenytoin serum concentrations.*

The one-compartment model Michaelis-Menten equations used in the program to compute doses indicate that a dose of 440 mg/d of phenytoin produces a total steady-state concentration of 15 μg/mL. This is equivalent to 478 mg/d of phenytoin sodium [(440 mg/d phenytoin)/0.92 = 478 mg/d phenytoin sodium]. This dose is rounded to 500 mg/d given as 200 mg in the morning plus 300 mg in the evening.

Steady-state minimum total serum concentration of phenytoin should be measured after steady state is attained in 7 to 14 days. Serum concentration of phenytoin also should be measured if the patient has an exacerbation of epilepsy or if the patient has signs or symptoms of phenytoin toxicity.

11. Solution for patient VG.

1. *Choose an appropriate equation to estimate normalized total phenytoin concentration at the appropriate temperature.*

$$C_{Normal\ Binding} = C/(0.25 \cdot Alb + 0.1) = (8.9\ \mu g/mL)/(0.25 \cdot 2.4\ g/dL + 0.1) = 12.7\ \mu g/mL$$

$$C_{fEST} = 0.1\ C_{Normal\ Binding} = 0.1 \cdot 12.7\ \mu g/mL = 1.3\ \mu g/mL$$

The estimated normalized total phenytoin concentration is expected to provide an unbound concentration equivalent to a total phenytoin concentration of 12.7 μg/mL for a patient with normal drug protein binding (C_{fEST} = 1.3 μg/mL). Because the estimated total value is within the therapeutic range of 10 to 20 μg/mL, it is likely that the patient has an unbound phenytoin concentration within the therapeutic range. If possible, this should be confirmed by means of measurement of the actual unbound concentration of phenytoin.

12. Solution for patient DE.

1. *Choose an appropriate equation to estimate normalized total phenytoin concentration.*

$$C_{Normal\ Binding} = C/(0.1 \cdot Alb + 0.1) = (8.1\ \mu g/mL)/(0.1 \cdot 2.0\ g/dL + 0.1) = 27\ \mu g/mL$$

$$C_{fEST} = 0.1\ C_{Normal\ Binding} = 0.1 \cdot 27\ \mu g/mL = 2.7\ \mu g/mL$$

The estimated normalized total phenytoin concentration is expected to provide an unbound concentration equivalent to a total phenytoin concentration of 27 μg/mL for a patient with normal drug protein binding (C_{fEST} = 2.7 μg/mL). Because the estimated total value is larger than the therapeutic range of 10 to 20 μg/mL, it is likely that the patient has an unbound phenytoin concentration greater than the therapeutic range. If possible, this should be confirmed by means of measurement of the actual unbound concentration of phenytoin.

13. Solution for patient KL.

1. *Choose an appropriate equation to estimate unbound concentration of phenytoin.*

$$C_{fEST} = (0.095 + 0.001 \cdot VPA)PHT = (0.095 + 0.001 \cdot 90\ \mu g/mL)\ 6\ \mu g/mL = 1.1\ \mu g/mL$$

The estimated unbound concentration of phenytoin is expected to be within the therapeutic range for unbound concentrations. If possible, this should be confirmed by means of measurement of the actual unbound concentration of phenytoin.

REFERENCES

1. Brodie MJ, Dichter MA. Antiepileptic drugs. N Engl J Med 1996;334:168–75.
2. McNamara JO. Drugs effective in the therapy of the epilepsies. In: Hardman JG, Limbird LE, Molinoff PB, Ruddon RW, Gilman AG, eds. The pharmacological basis of therapeutics. New York: McGraw-Hill, 1996:461–86.
3. Graves NM, Garnett WR. Epilepsy. In: DiPiro JT, Talbert RL, Yee GC, Matzke GR, Wells BG, Posey LM, eds. Pharmacotherapy: a pathophysiologic approach. Stamford, CT: Appleton & Lange, 1999:952–75.
4. Chen SS, Perucca E, Lee JN, Richens A. Serum protein binding and free concentration of phenytoin and phenobarbitone in pregnancy. Br J Clin Pharmacol 1982;13:547–52.

5. Knott C, Williams CP, Reynolds F. Phenytoin kinetics during pregnancy and the puerperium. Br J Obstet Gynaecol 1986;93:1030–7.
6. Perucca E, Hebdige S, Frigo GM, Gatti G, Lecchini S, Crema A. Interaction between phenytoin and valproic acid: plasma protein binding and metabolic effects. Clin Pharmacol Ther 1980;28: 779–89.
7. Pisani FD, Di Perri RG. Intravenous valproate: effects on plasma and saliva phenytoin levels. Neurology 1981;31:467–70.
8. Riva R, Albani F, Contin M, et al. Time-dependent interaction between phenytoin and valproic acid. Neurology 1985;35:510–5.
9. Frigo GM, Lecchini S, Gatti G, Perucca E, Crema A. Modification of phenytoin clearance by valproic acid in normal subjects. Br J Clin Pharmacol 1979;8:553–6.
10. Paxton JW. Effects of aspirin on salivary and serum phenytoin kinetics in healthy subjects. Clin Pharmacol Ther 1980;27:170–8.
11. Leonard RF, Knott PJ, Rankin GO, Robinson DS, Melnick DE. Phenytoin-salicylate interaction. Clin Pharmacol Ther 1981;29:56–60.
12. Fraser DG, Ludden TM, Evens RP, Sutherland EWd. Displacement of phenytoin from plasma binding sites by salicylate. Clin Pharmacol Ther 1980;27:165–9.
13. Olanow CW, Finn AL, Prussak C. The effects of salicylate on the pharmacokinetics of phenytoin. Neurology 1981;31:341–2.
14. Mabuchi H, Nakahashi H. A major inhibitor of phenytoin binding to serum protein in uremia. Nephron 1988;48:310–4.
15. Dasgupta A, Malik S. Fast atom bombardment mass spectrometric determination of the molecular weight range of uremic compounds that displace phenytoin from protein binding: absence of midmolecular uremic toxins. Am J Nephrol 1994;14:162-8.
16. Odar-Cederlof I, Borga O. Kinetics of diphenylhydantoin in uraemic patients: consequences of decreased plasma protein binding. Eur J Clin Pharmacol 1974;7:31–7.
17. Odar-Cederlof I, Borga O. Impaired plasma protein binding of phenytoin in uremia and displacement effect of salicylic acid. Clin Pharmacol Ther 1976;20:36–47.
18. Odar-Cederlof I. Plasma protein binding of phenytoin and warfarin in patients undergoing renal transplantation. Clin Pharmacokinet 1977;2:147–153.
19. Dodson WE, Loney LC. Hemodialysis reduces the unbound phenytoin in plasma. J Pediatr 1982;101:465–8.
20. Kinniburgh DW, Boyd ND. Isolation of peptides from uremic plasma that inhibit phenytoin binding to normal plasma proteins. Clin Pharmacol Ther 1981;30:276–80.
21. Peterson GM, McLean S, Aldous S, Von Witt RJ, Millingen KS. Plasma protein binding of phenytoin in 100 epileptic patients. Br J Clin Pharmacol 1982;14:298–300.
22. Patterson M, Heazelwood R, Smithurst B, Eadie MJ. Plasma protein binding of phenytoin in the aged: in vivo studies. Br J Clin Pharmacol 1982;13:423–5.
23. Winter ME, Tozer TN. Phenytoin. In: Evans WE, Schentag JJ, Jusko WJ, eds. Applied pharmacokinetics. Vancouver, WA: Applied Therapeutics, 1992;25:1–44.
24. Anderson GD, Pak C, Doane KW, et al. Revised Winter-Tozer equation for normalized phenytoin concentrations in trauma and elderly patients with hypoalbuminemia. Ann Pharmacother 1997;31:279–84.
25. Haidukewych D, Rodin EA, Zielinski JJ. Derivation and evaluation of an equation for prediction of free phenytoin concentration in patients co-medicated with valproic acid. Ther Drug Monit 1989;11:134–9.
26. Kerrick JM, Wolff DL, Graves NM. Predicting unbound phenytoin concentrations in patients receiving valproic acid: a comparison of two prediction methods. Ann Pharmacother 1995; 29:470–4.
27. Allen JP, Ludden TM, Burrow SR, Clementi WA, Stavchansky SA. Phenytoin cumulation kinetics. Clin Pharmacol Ther 1979;26:445–8.

28. Grasela TH, Sheiner LB, Rambeck B, et al. Steady-state pharmacokinetics of phenytoin from routinely collected patient data. Clin Pharmacokinet 1983;8:355–64.
29. Ludden TM, Allen JP, Valutsky WA, et al. Individualization of phenytoin dosage regimens. Clin Pharmacol Ther 1977;21:287–93.
30. Perrier D, Rapp R, Young B, et al. Maintenance of therapeutic phenytoin plasma levels via intramuscular administration. Ann Intern Med 1976;85:318–21.
31. Jusko WJ, Koup JR, Alvan G. Nonlinear assessment of phenytoin bioavailability. J Pharmacokinet Biopharm 1976;4:327–36.
32. Gugler R, Manion CV, Azarnoff DL. Phenytoin: pharmacokinetics and bioavailability. Clin Pharmacol Ther 1976;19:135–42.
33. Smith TC, Kinkel A. Absorption and metabolism of phenytoin from tablets and capsules. Clin Pharmacol Ther 1976;20:738–42.
34. Chakrabarti S, Belpaire F, Moerman E. Effect of formulation on dissolution and bioavailability of phenytoin tablets. Pharmazie 1980;35:627–9.
35. Jung D, Powell JR, Walson P, Perrier D. Effect of dose on phenytoin absorption. Clin Pharmacol Ther 1980;28:479–85.
36. Fleisher D, Sheth N, Kou JH. Phenytoin interaction with enteral feedings administered through nasogastric tubes. JPEN J Parenter Enteral Nutr 1990;14:513–6.
37. Cacek AT, DeVito JM, Koonce JR. In vitro evaluation of nasogastric administration methods for phenytoin. Am J Hosp Pharm 1986;43:689–92.
38. Bauer LA. Interference of oral phenytoin absorption by continuous nasogastric feedings. Neurology 1982;32:570–2.
39. Ozuna J, Friel P. Effect of enteral tube feeding on serum phenytoin levels. J Neurosurg Nurs 1984;16:289–91.
40. Bach B, Molholm Hansen J, Kampmann JP, Rasmussen SN, Skovsted L. Disposition of antipyrine and phenytoin correlated with age and liver volume in man. Clin Pharmacokinet 1981; 6:389–96.
41. Bauer LA, Blouin RA. Age and phenytoin kinetics in adult epileptics. Clin Pharmacol Ther 1982;31:301–4.
42. Blain PG, Mucklow JC, Bacon CJ, Rawlins MD. Pharmacokinetics of phenytoin in children. Br J Clin Pharmacol 1981;12:659–61.
43. Chiba K, Ishizaki T, Miura H, Minagawa K. Apparent Michaelis-Menten kinetic parameters of phenytoin in pediatric patients. Pediatr Pharmacol 1980;1:171–80.
44. Chiba K, Ishizaki T, Miura H, Minagawa K. Michaelis-Menten pharmacokinetics of diphenylhydantoin and application in the pediatric age patient. J Pediatr 1980;96:479–84.
45. Dodson WE. Nonlinear kinetics of phenytoin in children. Neurology 1982;32:42–8.
46. Leff RD, Fischer LJ, Roberts RJ. Phenytoin metabolism in infants following intravenous and oral administration. Dev Pharmacol Ther 1986;9:217–23.
47. Bauer LA, Blouin RA. Phenytoin Michaelis-Menten pharmacokinetics in Caucasian paediatric patients. Clin Pharmacokinet 1983;8:545–9.
48. Pugh RN, Murray-Lyon IM, Dawson JL, Pietroni MC, Williams R. Transection of the oesophagus for bleeding oesophageal varices. Br J Surg 1973;60:646–9.
49. Bauer LA, Edwards WA, Dellinger EP, Raisys VA, Brennan C. Importance of unbound phenytoin serum levels in head trauma patients. J Trauma 1983;23:1058–60.
50. Boucher BA, Rodman JH, Jaresko GS, Rasmussen SN, Watridge CB, Fabian TC. Phenytoin pharmacokinetics in critically ill trauma patients. Clin Pharmacol Ther 1988;44:675–83.
51. Chiba K, Ishizaki T, Tabuchi T, Wagatsuma T, Nakazawa Y. Antipyrine disposition in relation to lowered anticonvulsant plasma level during pregnancy. Obstet Gynecol 1982;60:620–6.
52. Dickinson RG, Hooper WD, Wood B, Lander CM, Eadie MJ. The effect of pregnancy in humans on the pharmacokinetics of stable isotope labelled phenytoin. Br J Clin Pharmacol 1989;28:17–27.

53. Lander CM, Smith MT, Chalk JB, et al. Bioavailability and pharmacokinetics of phenytoin during pregnancy. Eur J Clin Pharmacol 1984;27:105–10.
54. Kochenour NK, Emery MG, Sawchuk RJ. Phenytoin metabolism in pregnancy. Obstet Gynecol 1980;56:577–82.
55. Landon MJ, Kirkley M. Metabolism of diphenylhydantoin (phenytoin) during pregnancy. Br J Obstet Gynaecol 1979;86:125–32.
56. Hansten PD, Horn JR. Drug interactions analysis and management. Vancouver, WA: Applied Therapeutics, 1999:480.
57. Abernethy DR, Greenblatt DJ. Phenytoin disposition in obesity: determination of loading dose. Arch Neurol 1985;42:468–71.
58. Mauro LS, Mauro VF, Bachmann KA, Higgins JT. Accuracy of two equations in determining normalized phenytoin concentrations. DICP 1989;23:64–8.
59. Bauer LA. Clinical pharmacokinetics and pharmacodynamics. In: DiPiro JT, Talbert RL, Yee GC, Matzke GR, Wells BG, Posey LM, eds. Pharmacotherapy: a pathophysiologic approach. Stamford, CT: Appleton & Lange, 1999:21–43.
60. Graves N, Cloyd J, Leppik I. Phenytoin dosage predictions using population clearances. Ann Pharmacother 1982;16:473–8.
61. Vozeh S, Muir KT, Sheiner LB, Follath F. Predicting individual phenytoin dosage. J Pharmacokinet Biopharm 1981;9:131–46.
62. Mullen PW. Optimal phenytoin therapy: a new technique for individualizing dosage. Clin Pharmacol Ther 1978;23:228–32.
63. Mullen PW, Foster RW. Comparative evaluation of six techniques for determining the Michaelis-Menten parameters relating phenytoin dose and steady-state serum concentrations. J Pharm Pharmacol 1979;31:100–4.
64. Wandell M, Mungall D. Computer assisted drug interpretation and drug regimen optimization. Am Assoc Clin Chem 1984;6:1–11.

11

CARBAMAZEPINE

INTRODUCTION

Carbamazepine is an iminostilbene derivative related to the tricyclic antidepressants that is used in the treatment of tonic-clonic (grand mal), partial, or secondarily generalized seizures (Table 11-1).[1,2] Although methods have been suggested to manage acute seizures with carbamazepine, lack of an intravenous dosage form has limited use of this drug in this area. Thus carbamazepine is used primarily as a prophylactic agent in long-term therapy for epilepsy. Carbamazepine also is a useful agent for managing trigeminal neuralgia and bipolar affective disorders.[2]

The antiseizure activity of carbamazepine is related to its ability to decrease transmission in the nucleus ventralis anterior section of the thalamus, an area of the brain thought to be involved with the generalization and propagation of epileptic discharges.[1,2] Although the exact cellular mechanism of action is unclear, inhibition of voltage-gated sodium channels appears to be involved. Carbamazepine also depresses posttetanic potentiation and may prevent increases in cyclic adenosine monophosphate (cAMP).

THERAPEUTIC AND TOXIC CONCENTRATIONS

The accepted therapeutic range for carbamazepine is 4 to 12 μg/mL when the drug is used for the management of seizures. Plasma protein binding of carbamazepine is quite variable among individuals because it is bound to both albumin and α_1-acid glycoprotein (AAG). Among patients with normal concentrations of these proteins, plasma protein binding is 75% to 80%, which produces a free fraction of drug of 20% to 25%.[3–5] AAG is classified as an acute-phase reactant protein present in lower amounts in all persons. It is

TABLE 11-1 International Classification of Epileptic Seizures

MAJOR CLASS	SUBSET OF CLASS	DRUG THERAPY FOR SELECTED SEIZURE TYPE
Partial seizures (beginning locally)	1. Simple partial seizures (without impaired consciousness) a. With motor symptoms b. With somatosensory or special sensory symptoms c. With autonomic symptoms d. With psychological symptoms	Carbamazepine Phenytoin Valproic acid Phenobarbital Primidone
	2. Complex partial seizures (with impaired consciousness) a. Simple partial onset followed by impaired consciousness b. Impaired consciousness at onset	Carbamazepine Phenytoin Valproic acid Phenobarbital Primidone
	3. Partial seizures evolving into secondary generalized seizures	Carbamazepine Phenytoin Valproic acid Phenobarbital Primidone
Generalized seizures (convulsive or nonconvulsive)	1. Absence seizures (typical or atypical; also known as petit mal seizures)	Valproic acid Ethosuximide
	2. Tonic-clonic seizures (also known as grand mal seizures)	Carbamazepine Phenytoin Valproic acid Phenobarbital Primidone

Adapted from Brodie MJ, Dichter MA. Antiepileptic drugs. N Engl J Med 1996;334:168–175.

secreted in large amounts in response to stresses and diseases such as trauma, heart failure, and myocardial infarction. Among patients with these conditions, carbamazepine binding to AAG can be even larger. The result can be an unbound fraction as low as 10% to 15%.

Little prospective research has been done to establish the therapeutic range for unbound serum concentrations of carbamazepine or the clinical situations in which measurement of the unbound serum concentration is useful. As an initial guide, 25% of the total therapeutic range of carbamazepine has been used to establish a preliminary desirable range of 1 to 3 μg/mL for unbound serum concentration of carbamazepine. Although carbamazepine is highly plasma protein bound, it is difficult to displace this agent to the extent that a clinically important change in protein binding takes place. In general, a doubling in unbound fraction in the plasma is needed to produce such an alteration. In comparison, phenytoin is 90% protein bound under usual circumstances, and the result is an unbound fraction in the plasma of 10%. It is relatively easy to change the protein binding of phenytoin from 90% to 80% in a variety of diseases or conditions. Doing so increases the unbound fraction in the plasma from 10% to 20%. It is difficult, however, to change the protein binding of carbamazepine from 80% to 60% to achieve the same doubling of unbound fraction in the plasma (20% to 40%). As a result, measurement of unbound serum concentration of carbamazepine currently is limited to the care of (1) patients who have total concentrations within the therapeutic range but have the adverse effects that usually occur at higher concentrations and (2) patients who have total concentrations below the therapeutic range but have a therapeutic response that usually occurs at higher concentrations.

Carbamazepine-10,11-epoxide is an active metabolite of carbamazepine that contributes to both the therapeutic and toxic effects of the drug. It can be measured in serum samples at a small number of epilepsy centers.[6–12] The concentration of the epoxide often is related to the presence or absence of other inhibitors or inducers of hepatic drug-metabolizing enzymes. Epoxide concentrations tend to be higher among patients taking enzyme inducers and lower among patients taking enzyme inhibitors. Among persons undergoing long-term treatment, the average percentage of parent drug that is epoxide is about 12% for carbamazepine monotherapy, 14% when carbamazepine is taken with phenobarbital, 18% when carbamazepine is taken with phenytoin, and about 25% when carbamazepine is taken with both phenytoin and phenobarbital. The therapeutic range of carbamazepine-10,11-epoxide is not known, although a suggested range of 0.4 to 4 μg/mL is used at several research centers.

When the dose of carbamazepine is in the upper end of the therapeutic range (>8 μg/mL), some patients begin to experience concentration-related adverse effects, including nausea, vomiting, lethargy, dizziness, drowsiness, headache, blurred vision, diplopia, unsteadiness, ataxia, and incoordination. Because carbamazepine induces its own hepatic metabolism, these adverse effects also can occur early during dosage titration periods soon after dosage increases are made. To improve patient acceptance, it is important to initiate and titrate carbamazepine doses at a slow rate to minimize side effects. Clinicians should understand that not all patients with "toxic" carbamazepine serum concentrations in the listed ranges have signs or symptoms of carbamazepine toxicity. Rather, carbamazepine concentrations in the ranges given increase the likelihood that an adverse drug effect will occur.

CLINICAL MONITORING PARAMETERS

The goal of therapy with anticonvulsants is to reduce seizure frequency and maximize quality of life with a minimum of adverse drug effects. Although it is desirable to abolish all seizure episodes, it may not be possible to accomplish this for many patients. Patients should be observed for concentration-related side effects (nausea, vomiting, lethargy, dizziness, drowsiness, headache, blurred vision, diplopia, unsteadiness, ataxia, incoordination). Because carbamazepine has antidiuretic effects associated with reduced levels of antidiuretic hormone, some patients may have hyponatremia during long-term therapy with carbamazepine, and serum sodium concentrations can be measured periodically.

Hematologic adverse effects can be divided into two types. The first is leukopenia, which occurs among many patients and requires no therapeutic intervention. The typical clinical situation is that a patient with a previously normal leukocyte count has a transient decrease in this index. In some patients, a decreased, stable leukocyte count of 3000 cells/mm^2 or fewer may persist and does not appear to cause any deleterious effects. The second hematologic effect is severe and usually necessitates discontinuation of the drug. Thrombocytopenia, leukopenia (trend downward in leukocyte count with <2500 cells/mm^2 or absolute neutrophil count <1000 cells/mm^2), and anemia are in this category. In rare instances, aplastic anemia and agranulocytosis have been reported during carbamazepine treatment. Drug-induced hepatitis due to carbamazepine therapy also has been reported. The severe hematologic and hepatic adverse effects tend to occur early in treatment. Because of this, many clinicians obtain a complete blood cell count and liver function tests monthly for the first 3 to 6 months after a patient begins carbamazepine treatment. These tests are performed every 3 to 6 months for the first year. Other idiosyncratic side effects include skin rash, Stevens-Johnson syndrome, and systemic lupus-like reactions.

Serum concentrations of carbamazepine should be measured for most patients. Because epilepsy is an episodic disease, patients do not have seizures on a continuous basis. During dosage titration, it is difficult to determine whether a patient is responding to drug therapy or simply is not having any abnormal central nervous system discharges. Knowledge of serum concentration of carbamazepine is a valuable tool for avoiding adverse drug effects. Patients are more likely to accept drug therapy if adverse reactions are held to the absolute minimum. Because carbamazepine induces its own hepatic metabolism, it is fairly easy to attain toxic concentrations with modest increases in drug doses before maximal enzyme induction has occurred.

BASIC CLINICAL PHARMACOKINETIC PARAMETERS

More than 99% of carbamazepine is eliminated by means of hepatic metabolism, mainly by the CYP3A4 enzyme system.[13,14] Altogether, 33 metabolites have been identified, carbamazepine-10,11-epoxide being the major species. The epoxide metabolite is active and probably contributes to both the therapeutic and toxic side effects that occur during therapy. Carbamazepine is a potent inducer of hepatic drug-metabolizing enzymes and induces its own metabolism, a process known as *autoinduction* (Figure 11-1).[15–19] As a result, patients cannot initially be given the dose of carbamazepine that will ultimately result in a safe and effective outcome. At first, patients are given one-fourth to one-third the desired maintenance dose. This exposes hepatic drug-metabolizing enzymes to carbamazepine and begins the induction process. The dose is increased a similar amount every 2 to 3 weeks until the total desired daily dose is given. This gradual exposure to carbamazepine allows induction of liver enzymes and an increase in carbamazepine clearance over a 6- to 12-week period. Therapeutic effect and steady-state serum concentration of carbamazepine can be assessed 2 to 3 weeks after the final dosage increase. Autoinduction continues to occur among patients whose condition is stabilized with a carbamazepine dose but who need a dosage increase. It appears that 2 to 3 weeks also is needed under chronic dosing conditions for maximal autoinduction to occur after a

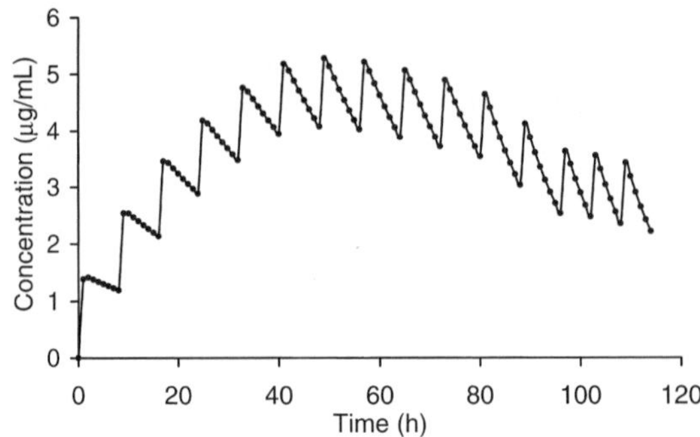

FIGURE 11-1 Carbamazepine induces its own metabolism through the CYP3A4 hepatic microsomal enzyme system. This process is known as *autoinduction.* When dosing is initiated, serum concentrations increase according to baseline clearance and half-life. After a few doses of carbamazepine, enough autoinduction has occurred that clearance increases, half-life decreases, and drug accumulation slows. With additional exposure of liver tissue to carbamazepine, clearance continues to increase, and half-life continues to shorten. As a result of these pharmacokinetic changes, carbamazepine concentration declines and ultimately stabilizes in accord with the new clearance and half-life values. Maximal autoinduction usually occurs 2 to 3 weeks after dosing begins. Because of the autoinduction phenomenon, the ultimate desired maintenance dose cannot be started with the first dose. Additional autoinduction occurs with subsequent increases in dose.

dosage increase. The effects of autoinduction are reversible even when dose administration is discontinued for as few as 6 days.[20]

An injectable form of carbamazepine is not available. For oral use, the drug is available as immediate-release tablets (chewable 100 mg, regular 200 mg), sustained-release tablets (100, 200, 400 mg), sustained-release capsule (300 mg), and suspension (100 mg/5 mL). The rapid-release dosage forms are erratically absorbed from the gastrointestinal tract. The result is a peak concentration 2 to 24 hours after a single dose of tablets (average, 6 hours). Multiple-dose studies have shown that after maximal autoinduction has taken place, peak concentration occurs about 3 hours after tablet administration. Peak concentration after multiple doses of sustained-release dosage forms occurs 3 to 12 hours after administration. Rectal administration of an extemporaneously compounded carbamazepine retention enema produced serum concentrations similar to that produced by a comparable immediate-release tablet.[21,22]

The absolute oral bioavailability of carbamazepine is not known because no intravenous form of the drug is available for comparison. According to the best estimates available, carbamazepine bioavailability is good and averages about 85% to 90%. The relative bioavailability of other dosage forms (chewable tablet, suspension, and sustained-release tablets and capsule) compared with that of the immediate-release tablet approaches 100%. If a patient is receiving a stable dose of carbamazepine in one dosage form, the same total daily dose of another dosage form can typically be substituted without adjustment. However, some bioequivalence problems have been reported for generic carbamazepine products.[23–25]

Usual initial maintenance doses are 10 to 20 mg/kg per day for children younger than 6 years, 200 mg/d for children 6 to 12 years of age, and 400 mg/d for adults. Twice-daily dosing is used until autoinduction takes place. Dosage increases to allow for autoinduction are made every 2 to 3 weeks depending on response and adverse effects. Most adults need 800 to 1200 mg/d of carbamazepine. Older children need 400 to 800 mg/d. Although minor side effects occur, single loading doses of 8 mg/kg have been given to adults as suspension or immediate-release tablets to achieve therapeutic concentrations within 2 to 4 hours after administration.[26]

EFFECTS OF DISEASES AND CONDITIONS ON PHARMACOKINETICS AND DOSING

After single doses of carbamazepine, the oral clearance (Cl/F) is 11 to 26 mL/h per kilogram, and the half-life is 35 hours for adults.[27–29] During multiple dosing after maximal autoinduction has taken place, oral clearance is 50 to 100 mL/h per kilogram, and half-life is 5 to 27 hours. Among children 6 to 12 years of age, oral clearance and half-life are 50 to 200 mL/h per kilogram and 3 to 15 hours during long-term dosing, respectively. Clearance rates can be higher and half-lives shorter among patients receiving other hepatic drug-metabolizing enzyme inducers, such as phenytoin, phenobarbital, or rifampin.[30–32] The apparent volume of distribution of carbamazepine calculated using immediate-release tablets (V/F) is 1 to 2 L/kg.

Patients with cirrhosis of the liver or acute hepatitis have impaired carbamazepine clearance because of destruction of liver parenchyma. This loss of functional hepatic cells decreases the amount of CYP3A4 available to metabolize the drug and decreases clearance. The volume of distribution may be larger because of a reduction in plasma protein binding. Protein binding may be decreased and unbound fraction increased because of hypoalbuminemia or hyperbilirubinemia (especially albumin ≤3 g/dL or total bilirubin ≥2 mg/dL). However, the effects of liver disease on carbamazepine pharmacokinetics are highly variable and difficult to predict accurately. It is possible for a patient with liver disease to have relatively normal or grossly abnormal carbamazepine clearance and volume of distribution. For example, a patient with liver disease who has relatively normal albumin and bilirubin concentrations can have a normal volume of distribution of carbamazepine. An index of liver dysfunction can be gained by applying the Child-Pugh clinical classification system (Table 11-2).[33] Child-Pugh scores are discussed in detail in Chapter 3 but are briefly discussed here.

The Child-Pugh score consists of five laboratory findings or clinical symptoms: serum albumin, total bilirubin, prothrombin time, ascites, and hepatic encephalopathy. Each of these areas is given a score of 1 (normal) to 3 (severely abnormal; see Table 11-2), and the scores for the five areas are summed. The Child-Pugh score for a patient with normal liver function is 5, and the score for a patient with grossly abnormal serum albumin, total bilirubin, and prothrombin time values in addition to severe ascites and hepatic encephalopathy is 15. A Child-Pugh score greater than 8 is grounds for a decrease of 25% to 50% in the initial daily dose of carbamazepine. As for any patient with or without liver dysfunction, initial doses are meant as starting points for dosage titration based on patient response and avoidance of adverse effects. Serum concentration of carbamazepine and the presence of adverse drug effects should be assessed frequently for patients with cirrhosis of the liver.

TABLE 11-2 Child-Pugh Scores for Patients with Liver Disease

TEST/SYMPTOM	SCORE 1 POINT	SCORE 2 POINTS	SCORE 3 POINTS
Total bilirubin (mg/dL)	<2.0	2.0–3.0	> 3.0
Serum albumin (g/dL)	>3.5	2.8–3.5	<2.8
Prothrombin time (seconds prolonged over control)	<4	4–6	>6
Ascites	Absent	Slight	Moderate
Hepatic encephalopathy	None	Moderate	Severe

Adapted from Pugh RN, Murray-Lyon IM, Dawson JL, Pietroni MC, Williams R. Transection of the oesophagus for bleeding oesophageal varices. Br J Surg 1973;60:646–649.

Elderly patients have lower oral clearance rates of carbamazepine than do younger adults, so lower initial doses (100 mg/d) may be used to treat older persons. During the third trimester of pregnancy, oral clearance of carbamazepine may decrease and necessitate dosage adjustment. Doses of carbamazepine do not have to be adjusted for patients with renal failure, and the drug is not removed during dialysis.[34,35] The concentration of carbamazepine in breast milk is about 60% of concurrent serum concentration.

DRUG INTERACTIONS

Carbamazepine is a potent inducer of hepatic drug-metabolizing enzyme systems.[36] The CYP1A2, CYP2C9, and CYP3A4 enzyme systems are induced by carbamazepine, and drug substrates for other enzyme systems also have known drug interactions with carbamazepine. Other antiepileptic drugs that have increased clearance rates and decreased steady-state concentrations in the presence of carbamazepine-related enzyme induction include felbamate, lamotrigine, phenytoin, primidone, tiagabine, topiramate, and valproic acid. Carbamazepine therapy also increases the clearance and decreases steady-state concentration of many other drugs, including oral contraceptives, calcium channel blockers, tricyclic antidepressants, cyclosporine, tacrolimus, theophylline, and warfarin. As a rule, when carbamazepine is added to a patient's drug regimen, loss of therapeutic effect of one of the other drugs the patient is taking must be considered as a possible drug interaction with carbamazepine.

Carbamazepine is a substrate for CYP3A4, and other drugs can affect carbamazepine clearance and steady-state serum concentration.[36] Phenytoin and phenobarbital can increase carbamazepine clearance and decrease steady-state serum concentration of carbamazepine. Cimetidine, macrolide antibiotics, azole antifungals, fluoxetine, fluvoxamine, nefazodone, cyclosporine, diltiazem, verapamil, indinavir, and ritonavir are examples of drugs that decrease the clearance of carbamazepine and increase the steady-state concentration. Administration of single doses of carbamazepine with grapefruit juice increases about 40% both the area under the serum concentration–time curve (AUC) and the maximal serum concentration (C_{max}) of carbamazepine.

INITIAL DOSAGE DETERMINATION METHODS

Because of the large amount of variability in the pharmacokinetics of carbamazepine, even when concurrent diseases and conditions are identified, most clinicians believe that the use of standard carbamazepine doses for various situations is warranted. The original computation of these doses was based on pharmacokinetic dosing methods. It later was modified on the basis of clinical experience. In general, the expected steady-state serum concentration of carbamazepine used to compute these doses was 6 to 8 μg/mL. Usual initial maintenance doses are 10 to 20 mg/kg per day for children younger than 6 years, 200 mg/d for children 6 to 12 years of age, and 400 mg/d for adults. Twice-daily dosing is used until autoinduction takes place. Dosage increases to allow for autoinduction are made every 2 to 3 weeks depending on response and adverse effects. Most adults need 800 to 1200 mg/d of carbamazepine. Older children need 400 to 800 mg/d. Immediate-release dosage forms are usually given three or four times daily, while sustained-release dosage forms are prescribed twice daily. If the patient has significant hepatic dysfunction (Child-Pugh score, ≥8), maintenance doses prescribed with this method should be decreased by 25% to 50% depending on the aggressiveness of therapy.

Example 1 KL is a 51-year-old, 75-kg (height, 178 cm) man who has simple partial seizures. He needs therapy with oral carbamazepine. He has normal liver function. Suggest an initial carbamazepine dosage regimen designed to achieve a steady-state carbamazepine concentration of 6 to 8 μg/mL.

1. *Estimate carbamazepine dose according to disease states and conditions present in the patient.*

The suggested initial dosage rate for immediate-release carbamazepine tablets in the treatment of an adult patient is 200 mg twice a day (400 mg/d). This dose is titrated upward in 200-mg increments every 2 to 3 weeks while the patient is observed for adverse and therapeutic effects. The goals of therapy are maximal suppression of seizures, avoidance of side effects, and a target drug range of 800 to 1200 mg/d.

Steady-state minimum total serum concentration of carbamazepine should be measured after steady state is achieved in 2 to 3 weeks at the highest dosage rate attained. Serum concentration of carbamazepine also should be measured if the patient has an exacerbation of epilepsy or if the patient has signs or symptoms of carbamazepine toxicity.

Example 2 UO is a 10-year-old, 40-kg boy who has simple partial seizures. He needs therapy with oral carbamazepine. He has normal liver function. Suggest an initial carbamazepine dosage regimen designed to achieve a steady-state carbamazepine concentration of 6 to 8 μg/mL.

1. *Estimate carbamazepine dose according to disease states and conditions present in the patient.*

The suggested initial dosage of immediate-release carbamazepine tablets for a child in this age range is 100 mg twice a day (200 mg/d). This dose is titrated upward in 100-mg increments every 2 to 3 weeks while the patient is observed for adverse and therapeutic effects. The goals of therapy are maximal suppression of seizures, avoidance of side effects, and a target drug range of 400 to 800 mg/d.

Steady-state minimum total serum concentration of carbamazepine should be measured after steady state is achieved in 2 to 3 weeks at the highest dosage rate attained. Serum concentration of carbamazepine also should be measured if the patient has an exacerbation of epilepsy or if the patient has signs or symptoms of carbamazepine toxicity.

USE OF SERUM CONCENTRATION OF CARBAMAZEPINE TO ALTER DOSES

Because of the great pharmacokinetic variability among patients, it is likely that doses computed with patient population characteristics will not always produce serum concentrations of carbamazepine that are expected or desirable. Because of pharmacokinetic variability, the autoinduction pharmacokinetics of the drug, the narrow therapeutic index of carbamazepine, and the desire to avoid adverse side effects, serum concentration of carbamazepine is measured for almost all patients to ensure that therapeutic, nontoxic levels are present. In addition to serum concentration of carbamazepine, important patient parameters such as seizure frequency and presence of side effects should be followed to confirm that the patient is responding to treatment and not having an adverse drug reaction. When serum concentration of carbamazepine is measured and a dosage change is found necessary, clinicians should use the simplest, most straightforward method available to choose a dose that will provide safe and effective treatment.

Pseudolinear Pharmacokinetics Method

A simple, easy way to approximate new total serum concentrations after a dosage adjustment of carbamazepine is to temporarily assume linear pharmacokinetics, then to subtract 10% to 20% for a dosage increase or add 10% to 20% for a dosage decrease to account for autoinduction pharmacokinetics: $Css_{new} = (D_{new}/D_{old})Css_{old}$, where Css_{new} is the expected steady-state concentration from the new carbamazepine dose in micrograms per milliliter, Css_{old} is the measured steady-state concentration from the old carbamazepine dose in micrograms per milliliter, D_{new} is the new carbamazepine dose to be prescribed in milligrams per day, and D_{old} is the currently prescribed carbamazepine dose in milligrams per day.

Example 1 KL is a 51-year-old, 75-kg (height, 178 cm) man who has simple partial seizures. He needs therapy with oral carbamazepine. He has normal liver function. After dosage titration, the patient is given a prescription for 200 mg in the morning, 200 mg in the afternoon, and 400 mg at bedtime (800 mg/d) of carbamazepine tablets for 1 month. Steady-state total concentration of carbamazepine is 3.8 μg/mL. The patient is found to be compliant with the dosage regimen. Suggest a carbamazepine dosage regimen designed to achieve a steady-state carbamazepine concentration in the therapeutic range.

1. *Use pseudolinear pharmacokinetics to predict a new concentration for a dosage increase, then compute the 10% to 20% factor to account for autoinduction pharmacokinetics.*

Because the patient is receiving carbamazepine tablets, a convenient dosage change would be 200 mg/d, and an increase to 1000 mg/d (400 mg in the morning and at bedtime,

200 mg in the afternoon) is suggested. According to pseudolinear pharmacokinetics, the resulting total steady-state serum concentration of carbamazepine is $Css_{new} = (D_{new}/D_{old})Css_{old}$ = [(1000 mg/d)/(800 mg/d)] 3.8 μg/mL = 4.8 μg/mL. Because of autoinduction pharmacokinetics, the serum concentration is expected to increase 10% less, or 0.90 times, to 20%, or 0.80 times, less than that predicted with linear pharmacokinetics: Css = 4.8 μg/mL · 0.90 = 4.3 μg/mL, and Css = 4.8 μg/mL · 0.80 = 3.8 μg/mL. Thus a dosage increase of 200 mg/d is expected to yield a total steady-state serum concentration of carbamazepine of 3.8 to 4.3 μg/mL.

Steady-state minimum total serum concentration of carbamazepine should be measured after steady state is attained in 2 to 3 weeks. Serum concentration of carbamazepine also should be measured if the patient has an exacerbation of epilepsy or if the patient has signs or symptoms of carbamazepine toxicity.

Example 2 UO is a 10-year-old, 40-kg boy who has simple partial seizures. He needs therapy with oral carbamazepine. He has normal liver function. After dosage titration, the patient is given a prescription for 200 mg three times a day (600 mg/d) of carbamazepine tablets for 1 month. Steady-state carbamazepine total concentration is 5.1 μg/mL. The patient is found to be compliant with the dosage regimen. Suggest a carbamazepine dosage regimen designed to achieve a steady-state concentration of carbamazepine in the middle of the therapeutic range.

1. *Use pseudolinear pharmacokinetics to predict a new concentration for a dosage increase, then compute the 10% to 20% factor to account for autoinduction pharmacokinetics.*

Because the patient is receiving carbamazepine tablets, a convenient dosage change would be 200 mg/d, and an increase to 800 mg/d (300 mg in the morning and at bedtime, 200 mg in the afternoon) is suggested. According to pseudolinear pharmacokinetics, the resulting total steady-state serum concentration of carbamazepine is $Css_{new} = (D_{new}/D_{old})Css_{old}$ = [(800 mg/d)/(600 mg/d)] 5.1 μg/mL = 6.8 μg/mL. Because of autoinduction pharmacokinetics, the serum concentration is expected to increase 10% less, or 0.90 times, to 20%, or 0.80 times, less than that predicted with linear pharmacokinetics: Css = 6.8 μg/mL · 0.90 = 6.1 μg/mL, and Css = 6.8 μg/mL · 0.80 = 5.4 μg/mL. Thus a dosage increase of 200 mg/d is expected to yield a total steady-state serum concentration of carbamazepine of 5.4 to 6.1 μg/mL.

Steady-state minimum total serum concentration of carbamazepine should be measured after steady state is attained in 2 to 3 weeks. Serum concentration of carbamazepine also should be measured if the patient has an exacerbation of epilepsy or if the patient has signs or symptoms of carbamazepine toxicity.

BAYESIAN PHARMACOKINETICS COMPUTER PROGRAMS

Computer programs can be used to calculate pharmacokinetic parameters for patients.[37] In the most reliable computer programs, a nonlinear regression algorithm incorporates components of Bayes' theorem. Nonlinear regression is a statistical technique in which an iterative process is used to compute the best pharmacokinetic parameters for a concentration–time data set. Unfortunately, these types of computer programs have not been able to give acceptable solutions unless four or more carbamazepine concentrations are available. This is because of the complexity of the autoinduction pharmacokinetics that carbamazepine follows under long-term dosing conditions. Because of the large number of concentrations needed, this dosage adjustment approach cannot be recommended.

PROBLEMS

The following problems are intended to emphasize the computation of initial and individualized doses with clinical pharmacokinetic techniques. Clinicians should always consult the patient's chart to confirm that current anticonvulsant therapy is appropriate. All other medications that the patient is taking, including prescription and nonprescription drugs, should be recorded and checked to ascertain the risk of drug interaction with carbamazepine.

1. TY is a 47-year-old, 85-kg (height, 185 cm) man who has tonic-clonic seizures. He needs therapy with oral carbamazepine. He has normal liver function. Suggest an initial carbamazepine dosage regimen designed to achieve a steady-state carbamazepine concentration of 6 to 8 μg/mL.

2. Patient TY (see problem 1) is given a prescription for 400 mg every 12 hours of sustained-release carbamazepine tablets for 1 month after dosage titration. Steady-state carbamazepine total concentration is 4.5 μg/mL. The patient is found to be compliant with the dosage regimen. Suggest a carbamazepine dosage regimen designed to achieve a steady-state carbamazepine concentration in the middle portion of the therapeutic range.

3. IU is a 9-year-old, 35-kg girl who has simple partial seizures. She needs therapy with oral carbamazepine. She has normal liver function. Suggest an initial carbamazepine dosage regimen designed to achieve a steady-state carbamazepine concentration of 6 to 8 μg/mL.

4. Patient IU (see problem 3) is given a prescription for 150 mg three times a day (450 mg/d) of carbamazepine suspension for 1 month after dosage titration. Steady-state total concentration of carbamazepine is 4.9 μg/mL. The patient is found to be compliant with the dosage regimen. Suggest a carbamazepine dosage regimen designed to achieve a steady-state carbamazepine concentration in the middle of the therapeutic range.

5. LK is a 4-year-old, 22-kg boy with complex partial seizures. He needs therapy with carbamazepine suspension. He has normal liver function. Suggest an initial carbamazepine dosage regimen designed to achieve a steady-state carbamazepine concentration of 6 to 8 μg/mL.

6. Patient LK (see problem 5) is given a prescription for 100 mg three times a day (300 mg/d) of carbamazepine suspension for 1 month after dosage titration. Steady-state carbamazepine total concentration is 6.1 μg/mL. The patient is found to be compliant

with the dosage regimen. Suggest a carbamazepine dosage regimen designed to achieve a steady-state carbamazepine concentration in the upper end of the therapeutic range.

ANSWERS TO PROBLEMS

1. Solution to problem 1.

1. *Estimate carbamazepine dose according to disease states and conditions present in the patient.*

The suggested initial dose of immediate-release carbamazepine tablets in the care of an adult patient is 200 mg twice a day (400 mg/d). This dose is titrated upward in 200-mg increments every 2 to 3 weeks while the patient is observed for adverse and therapeutic effects. The goals of therapy are maximal suppression of seizures, avoidance of side effects, and a target drug range of 800 to 1200 mg/d.

Steady-state minimum total serum concentration of carbamazepine should be measured after steady state is achieved in 2 to 3 weeks at the highest dosage rate attained. Serum concentration of carbamazepine also should be measured if the patient has an exacerbation of epilepsy or if the patient has signs or symptoms of carbamazepine toxicity.

2. Solution to problem 2.

1. *Use pseudolinear pharmacokinetics to predict a new concentration for a dosage increase, then compute the 10% to 20% factor to account for autoinduction pharmacokinetics.*

Because the patient is receiving sustained-release carbamazepine tablets, a convenient dosage change is 400 mg/d, and an increase to 1200 mg/d (600 mg every 12 hours) is suggested. According to pseudolinear pharmacokinetics, the resulting total steady-state serum concentration of carbamazepine is $Css_{new} = (D_{new}/D_{old})Css_{old}$ = [(1200 mg/d)/(800 mg/d)] 4.5 μg/mL = 6.8 μg/mL. Because of autoinduction pharmacokinetics, the serum concentration is expected to increase 10% less, or 0.90 times, to 20%, or 0.80 times, less than that predicted with linear pharmacokinetics: Css = 6.8 μg/mL · 0.90 = 6.1 μg/mL, and Css = 6.8 μg/mL · 0.80 = 5.4 μg/mL. Thus a dosage increase of 400 mg/d is expected to yield a total steady-state serum concentration of carbamazepine of 5.4 to 6.1 μg/mL.

Steady-state minimum total serum concentration of carbamazepine should be measured after steady state is attained in 2 to 3 weeks. Serum concentration of carbamazepine also should be measured if the patient has an exacerbation of epilepsy or if the patient has signs or symptoms of carbamazepine toxicity.

3. Solution to problem 3.

1. *Estimate carbamazepine dose according to disease states and conditions present in the patient.*

The suggested initial dosage rate for carbamazepine suspension in a child in this age range is 100 mg twice daily (200 mg/d). This dose would be titrated upward in 100-mg increments every 2 to 3 weeks while monitoring for adverse and therapeutic effects. The goals of therapy are maximal suppression of seizures, avoidance of side effects, and a target drug range of 400 to 800 mg/d.

Steady-state minimum total serum concentration of carbamazepine should be measured after steady state is achieved in 2 to 3 weeks at the highest dosage rate attained. Serum concentration of carbamazepine also should be measured if the patient has an exacerbation of epilepsy or if the patient has signs or symptoms of carbamazepine toxicity.

4. Solution to problem 4.

1. *Use pseudolinear pharmacokinetics to predict a new concentration for a dosage increase, then compute the 10% to 20% factor to account for autoinduction pharmacokinetics.*

Because the patient is receiving carbamazepine suspension, a convenient dosage change is 150 mg/d, and an increase to 600 mg/d (200 mg three times daily) is suggested. According to pseudolinear pharmacokinetics, the resulting total steady-state serum concentration of carbamazepine is $Css_{new} = (D_{new}/D_{old})Css_{old}$ = [(600 mg/d)/(450 mg/d)] 4.9 μg/mL = 6.5 μg/mL. Because of autoinduction pharmacokinetics, the serum concentration is expected to increase 10% less, or 0.90 times, to 20%, or 0.80 times, less than that predicted with linear pharmacokinetics: Css = 6.5 μg/mL · 0.90 = 5.9 μg/mL, and Css = 6.5 μg/mL · 0.80 = 5.2 μg/mL. Thus a dosage increase of 150 mg/d is expected to yield a total steady-state serum concentration of carbamazepine of 5.2 to 5.9 μg/mL.

Steady-state minimum total serum concentration of carbamazepine should be measured after steady state is attained in 2 to 3 weeks. Serum concentration of carbamazepine also should be measured if the patient has an exacerbation of epilepsy or if the patient has signs or symptoms of carbamazepine toxicity.

5. Solution to problem 5.

1. *Estimate carbamazepine dose according to disease states and conditions present in the patient.*

The suggested initial dose of carbamazepine suspension in the care of a child in this age range is 10 to 20 mg/kg per day. At a dose of 15 mg/kg per day, the target maintenance dose is 300 mg/d (15 mg/kg/d · 22 kg = 330 mg/d, rounded to 300 mg/d). The starting dose is one-fourth to one-third the target maintenance dose, or 100 mg/d given as 50 mg twice a day. This dose is titrated upward in 100-mg/d increments every 2 to 3 weeks while the patient is observed for adverse and therapeutic effects. The goals of therapy are maximal suppression of seizures, avoidance of side effects, and a target drug range of 300 mg/d given as 100 mg three times a day.

Steady-state minimum total serum concentration of carbamazepine should be measured after steady state is achieved in 2 to 3 weeks at the highest dosage rate attained. Serum concentration of carbamazepine also should be measured if the patient has an exacerbation of epilepsy or if the patient has signs or symptoms of carbamazepine toxicity.

6. Solution to problem 6.

1. *Use pseudolinear pharmacokinetics to predict a new concentration for a dosage increase, then compute the 10% to 20% factor to account for autoinduction pharmacokinetics.*

Because the patient is receiving carbamazepine suspension, a convenient dosage change is 150 mg/d, and an increase to 450 mg/d (150 mg three times daily) is suggested. According to pseudolinear pharmacokinetics, the resulting total steady-state serum concentration of carbamazepine is $Css_{new} = (D_{new}/D_{old})Css_{old}$ = [(450 mg/d)/(300 mg/d)] 6.1 μg/mL = 9.2 μg/mL. Because of autoinduction pharmacokinetics, the serum concentration is expected to increase 10% less, or 0.90 times, to 20%, or 0.80 times, less than that predicted with linear pharmacokinetics: Css = 9.2 μg/mL · 0.90 = 8.3 μg/mL, and Css = 9.2 μg/mL · 0.80 = 7.4 μg/mL. Thus a dosage increase of 150 mg/d is expected to yield a total steady-state serum concentration of carbamazepine of 7.4 to 8.3 μg/mL.

Steady-state minimum total serum concentration of carbamazepine should be measured after steady state is attained in 2 to 3 weeks. Serum concentration of carbamazepine also should be measured if the patient has an exacerbation of epilepsy or if the patient has signs or symptoms of carbamazepine toxicity.

REFERENCES

1. Graves NM, Garnett WR. Epilepsy. In: DiPiro JT, Talbert RL, Yee GC, Matzke GR, Wells BG, Posey LM, eds. Pharmacotherapy: a pathophysiologic approach. Stamford, CT: Appleton & Lange, 1999:952–75.
2. McNamara JO. Drugs effective in the therapy of the epilepsies. In: Hardman JG, Limbird LE, Molinoff PB, Ruddon RW, Gilman AG, eds. The pharmacological basis of therapeutics. New York: McGraw-Hill, 1996:461–86.
3. Hooper WD, Dubetz DK, Bochner F, et al. Plasma protein binding of carbamazepine. Clin Pharmacol Ther 1975;17:433–40.
4. Lawless LM, DeMonaco HJ, Muido LR. Protein binding of carbamazepine in epileptic patients. Neurology 1982;32:415–8.
5. Paxton JW, Donald RA. Concentrations and kinetics of carbamazepine in whole saliva, parotid saliva, serum ultrafiltrate, and serum. Clin Pharmacol Ther 1980;28:695–702.
6. Rane A, Hojer B, Wilson JT. Kinetics of carbamazepine and its 10,11-epoxide metabolite in children. Clin Pharmacol Ther 1976;19:276–83.
7. McKauge L, Tyrer JH, Eadie MJ. Factors influencing simultaneous concentrations of carbamazepine and its epoxide in plasma. Ther Drug Monit 1981;3:63–70.
8. Brodie MJ, Forrest G, Rapeport WG. Carbamazepine-10,11-epoxide concentrations in epileptics on carbamazepine alone and in combination with other anticonvulsants. Br J Clin Pharmacol 1983;16:747–9.
9. Eichelbaum M, Bertilsson L, Lund L, Palmer L, Sjoqvist F. Plasma levels of carbamazepine and carbamazepine-10,11-epoxide during treatment of epilepsy. Eur J Clin Pharmacol 1976;9:417–21.

10. MacKichan JJ, Duffner PK, Cohen ME. Salivary concentrations and plasma protein binding of carbamazepine and carbamazepine-10,11-epoxide in epileptic patients. Br J Clin Pharmacol 1981;12:31–7.
11. Hundt HK, Aucamp AK, Muller FO, Potgieter MA. Carbamazepine and its major metabolites in plasma: a summary of eight years of therapeutic drug monitoring. Ther Drug Monit 1983;5:427–35.
12. Elyas AA, Patsalos PN, Agbato OA, Brett EM, Lascelles PT. Factors influencing simultaneous concentrations of total and free carbamazepine and carbamazepine-10,11-epoxide in serum of children with epilepsy. Ther Drug Monit 1986;8:288–92.
13. Bertilsson L, Tybring G, Widen J, Chang M, Tomson T. Carbamazepine treatment induces the CYP3A4 catalysed sulphoxidation of omeprazole, but has no or less effect on hydroxylation via CYP2C19. Br J Clin Pharmacol 1997;44:186–9.
14. Kerr BM, Thummel KE, Wurden CJ, et al. Human liver carbamazepine metabolism: role of CYP3A4 and CYP2C8 in 10,11-epoxide formation. Biochem Pharmacol 1994;47:1969–79.
15. Perucca E, Bittencourt P, Richens A. Effect of dose increments on serum carbamazepine concentration in epileptic patients. Clin Pharmacokinet 1980;5:576–82.
16. McNamara PJ, Colburn WA, Gibaldi M. Time course of carbamazepine self-induction. J Pharmacokinet Biopharm 1979;7:63–68.
17. Eichelbaum M, Kothe KW, Hoffmann F, von Unruh GE. Use of stable labelled carbamazepine to study its kinetics during chronic carbamazepine treatment. Eur J Clin Pharmacol 1982;23:241–4.
18. Pitlick WH, Levy RH, Tropin AS, Green JR. Pharmacokinetic model to describe self-induced decreases in steady-state concentrations of carbamazepine. J Pharm Sci 1976;65:462–3.
19. Bertilsson L, Hojer B, Tybring G, Osterloh J, Rane A. Autoinduction of carbamazepine metabolism in children examined by a stable isotope technique. Clin Pharmacol Ther 1980;27:83–8.
20. Schaffler L, Bourgeois BF, Luders HO. Rapid reversibility of autoinduction of carbamazepine metabolism after temporary discontinuation. Epilepsia 1994;35:195–8.
21. Neuvonen PJ, Tokola O. Bioavailability of rectally administered carbamazepine mixture. Br J Clin Pharmacol 1987;24:839–41.
22. Graves NM, Kriel RL, Jones-Saete C, Cloyd JC. Relative bioavailability of rectally administered carbamazepine suspension in humans. Epilepsia 1985;26:429–33.
23. Hartley R, Aleksandrowicz J, Ng PC, McLain B, Bowmer CJ, Forsythe WI. Breakthrough seizures with generic carbamazepine: a consequence of poorer bioavailability? Br J Clin Pract 1990;44:270–3.
24. Meyer MC, Straughn AB, Mhatre RM, Shah VP, Williams RL, Lesko LJ. The relative bioavailability and in vivo–in vitro correlations for four marketed carbamazepine tablets. Pharm Res 1998;15:1787–91.
25. Olling M, Mensinga TT, Barends DM, Groen C, Lake OA, Meulenbelt J. Bioavailability of carbamazepine from four different products and the occurrence of side effects. Biopharm Drug Dispos 1999;20:19–28.
26. Cohen H, Howland MA, Luciano DJ, et al. Feasibility and pharmacokinetics of carbamazepine oral loading doses. Am J Health Syst Pharm 1998;55:1134–40.
27. Cotter LM, Eadie MJ, Hooper WD, Lander CM, Smith GA, Tyrer JH. The pharmacokinetics of carbamazepine. Eur J Clin Pharmacol 1977;12:451–6.
28. Levy RH, Pitlick WH, Troupin AS, Green JR, Neal JM. Pharmacokinetics of carbamazepine in normal man. Clin Pharmacol Ther 1975;17:657–68.
29. Rawlins MD, Collste P, Bertilsson L, Palmer L. Distribution and elimination kinetics of carbamazepine in man. Eur J Clin Pharmacol 1975;8:91–6.
30. Monaco F, Riccio A, Benna P, et al. Further observations on carbamazepine plasma levels in epileptic patients: relationships with therapeutic and side effects. Neurology 1976;26:936–73.

31. Battino D, Bossi L, Croci D, et al. Carbamazepine plasma levels in children and adults: influence of age, dose, and associated therapy. Ther Drug Monit 1980;2:315–22.
32. Eichelbaum M, Kothe KW, Hoffman F, von Unruh GE. Kinetics and metabolism of carbamazepine during combined antiepileptic drug therapy. Clin Pharmacol Ther 1979;26:366–71.
33. Pugh RN, Murray-Lyon IM, Dawson JL, Pietroni MC, Williams R. Transection of the oesophagus for bleeding oesophageal varices. Br J Surg 1973;60:646–9.
34. Lee CS, Wang LH, Marbury TC, Bruni J, Perchalski RJ. Hemodialysis clearance and total body elimination of carbamazepine during chronic hemodialysis. Clin Toxicol 1980;17:429–38.
35. Kandrotas RJ, Oles KS, Gal P, Love JM. Carbamazepine clearance in hemodialysis and hemoperfusion. DICP 1989;23:137–40.
36. Hansten PD, Horn JR. Drug interactions analysis and management. Vancouver, WA: Applied Therapeutics, 1999:480.
37. Wandell M, Mungall D. Computer assisted drug interpretation and drug regimen optimization. Am Assoc Clin Chem 1984;6:1–11.

12

VALPROIC ACID

INTRODUCTION

Valproic acid is chemically related to free fatty acids and is used in the management of generalized, partial, and absence (petit mal) seizures.[1] As such, it has the widest spectrum of activity of the other currently available antiepileptic drugs (Table 12-1). Now available in intravenous as well as oral form, valproic acid can be used for immediate management and long-term prophylaxis of seizures. Valproic acid also is a useful agent in the management of bipolar affective disorders. Although the precise mechanism of action of valproic acid is unknown, the antiepileptic effect is thought to be due to its ability to increase the concentration of the neuroinhibitor γ-aminobutyric acid (GABA), to potentiate the postsynaptic response to GABA, or to exert a direct effect on cellular membranes.[2]

THERAPEUTIC AND TOXIC CONCENTRATIONS

The generally accepted therapeutic range for total steady-state concentration of valproic acid is 50 to 100 μg/mL, although some clinicians suggest drug concentrations as high as 175 μg/mL with appropriate monitoring of serum concentration and possible adverse effects. Valproic acid is highly protein bound to albumin with typical values of 90% to 95%.[3,4] Plasma protein binding of valproic acid can be saturated within the therapeutic range. The result is less protein binding and higher unbound fraction of drug at higher concentrations. The concentration-dependent protein binding of valproic acid causes the drug to follow nonlinear pharmacokinetics (Figure 12-1). This type of nonlinear pharmacokinetics is fundamentally different from that observed during phenytoin administration. The hepatic metabolism of phenytoin becomes saturated, and Michaelis-Menten pharma-

TABLE 12-1 International Classification of Epileptic Seizures

MAJOR CLASS	SUBSET OF CLASS	DRUG THERAPY FOR SELECTED SEIZURE TYPE
Partial seizures (beginning locally)	1. Simple partial seizures (without impaired consciousness) a. With motor symptoms b. With somatosensory or special sensory symptoms c. With autonomic symptoms d. With psychological symptoms	Carbamazepine Phenytoin Valproic acid Phenobarbital Primidone
	2. Complex partial seizures (with impaired consciousness) a. Simple partial onset followed by impaired consciousness b. Impaired consciousness at onset	Carbamazepine Phenytoin Valproic acid Phenobarbital Primidone
	3. Partial seizures evolving into secondary generalized seizures	Carbamazepine Phenytoin Valproic acid Phenobarbital Primidone
Generalized seizures (convulsive or nonconvulsive)	1. Absence seizures (typical or atypical; also known as petit mal seizures)	Valproic acid Ethosuximide
	2. Tonic-clonic seizures (also known as grand mal seizures)	Phenytoin Carbamazepine Valproic acid Phenobarbital Primidone

Adapted from Brodie MJ, Dichter MA. Antiepileptic drugs. N Engl J Med 1996;334:168–75.

cokinetics occurs. As a result, when phenytoin doses are increased, total and unbound steady-state concentrations increase more than a proportional amount (e.g., when the dose is doubled, serum concentration may increase threefold to fivefold or more). In the case of valproic acid, when the dose is increased, total steady-state concentration of the drug increases less than expected, but unbound steady-state concentration increases in a proportional manner (e.g., when the dose is doubled, total serum concentration increases 1.6 to 1.9 times, but unbound steady-state serum concentration doubles; Figure 12-2). The pharmacokinetic rationale for these changes is explained fully in Basic Clinical Pharmacokinetic Parameters (see later chapter section).

Insufficient prospective research has been done to establish the therapeutic range for unbound steady-state serum concentration of valproic acid. As an initial guide, 5% of the lower end and 10% of the upper end of the total concentration therapeutic range is used to

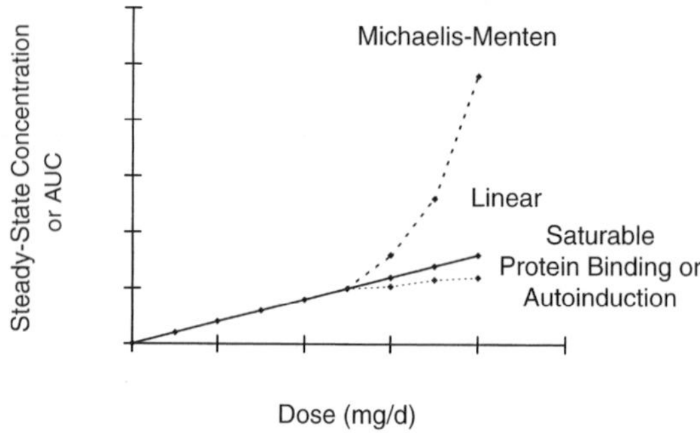

FIGURE 12-1 If a drug follows linear pharmacokinetics, steady-state concentration (Css) or the area under the concentration-time curve (AUC) increases in proportion to the dose. The result is a straight line on the plot. Nonlinear pharmacokinetics occurs when the Css or AUC versus dose plot produces other than a straight line. If a drug (e.g., phenytoin, aspirin) follows Michaelis-Menten pharmacokinetics, as steady-state drug concentration approaches the Michaelis-Menten constant (K_m), serum concentration increases more than expected due to dose increases. If a drug (e.g., valproic acid, disopyramide) follows nonlinear protein binding, total steady-state drug concentration increases less than expected as dose increases.

construct the preliminary unbound steady-state concentration therapeutic range for valproic acid of 2.5 to 10 μg/mL. The percentage used in each case is the average unbound fraction of drug at the appropriate concentration.

More information is available that identifies the clinical situations in which measurement of unbound serum concentration of valproic acid is useful. As is the case with phenytoin, measurement of unbound valproic acid serum concentration should be considered in the treatment of patients with factors known to alter plasma protein binding of valproic acid.[4–8] These factors fall into three broad categories: (1) lack of binding protein

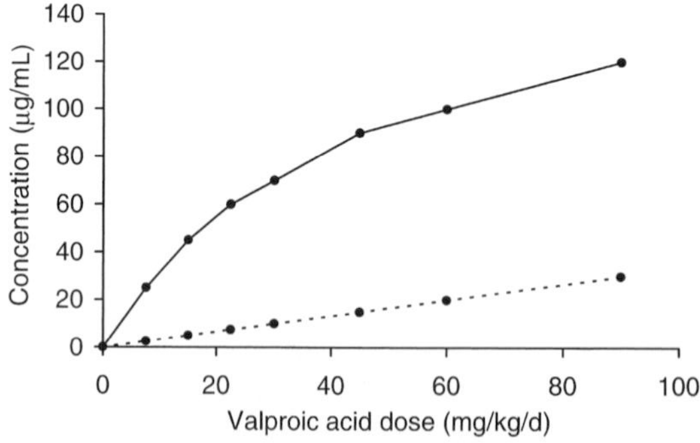

FIGURE 12-2 Although total valproic acid concentration increases in a nonlinear manner with dosage increases (*solid line*), unbound, or free, valproic acid concentration increases in a linear fashion with dosage increases (*dashed line*). Valproic acid is a low-extraction ratio drug, and the unbound serum concentration is only a function of intrinsic clearance (Cl'_{int}): $Css_u = (D/\tau)/Cl'_{int}$, where D is valproic acid dose in milligrams, τ is the dosage interval in hours, and Css_u is the unbound steady-state concentration of valproic acid.

when plasma concentration of albumin is insufficient, (2) displacement of valproic acid from albumin binding sites by endogenous compounds, and (3) displacement of valproic acid from albumin binding sites by exogenous compounds (Table 12-2).

Low albumin concentration, known as hypoalbuminemia, occurs among patients with liver disease or the nephrotic syndrome, pregnant women, patients with cystic fibrosis, burn patients, trauma patients, persons with malnutrition, and the elderly. Albumin concentration less than 3 g/dL is associated with a high unbound fraction of valproic acid in the plasma. Albumin is manufactured by the liver, so patients with hepatic disease may have difficulty synthesizing the protein. Patients with nephrotic syndrome waste albumin by eliminating it in the urine. Some patients can be so nutritionally deprived that albumin production is impeded. Malnutrition is the cause of hypoalbuminemia among some elderly patients, although there is a general decrease in albumin concentration among older patients. However, the unbound fraction of valproic acid is higher among elderly patients even if albumin concentration is within the normal range. While recovering from their injuries, burn and trauma patients can become hypermetabolic, and albumin concentration can decrease if enough calories are not supplied during this phase of disease. Albumin concentration may decline during pregnancy as maternal reserves are shifted to the developing fetus; the decline is especially prevalent during the third trimester.

Displacement of valproic acid from plasma protein binding sites by endogenous substances can occur among patients with hepatic or renal dysfunction. The mechanism is competition for albumin plasma protein binding sites between the endogenous substances and valproic acid. Bilirubin (a by-product of heme metabolism) is broken down by the liver, so patients with hepatic disease can have an excessive bilirubin concentration. Total bilirubin concentration in excess of 2 mg/dL is associated with abnormal plasma protein binding of valproic acid. Patients with end-stage renal disease (creatinine clearance <10 to 15 mL/min) and uremia (blood urea nitrogen concentration >80 to 100 mg/dL) accumulate unidentified compounds in the blood that displace valproic acid from plasma protein binding sites. Abnormal valproic acid binding persists in these patients even when dialysis is instituted.

Displacement of plasma protein binding of valproic acid also can be caused by exogenously administered compounds such as drugs. In this case, the mechanism is competition for albumin binding sites between valproic acid and other agents. Other drugs that

TABLE 12-2 Diseases and Conditions That Alter Plasma Protein Binding of Valproic Acid

INSUFFICIENT ALBUMIN CONCENTRATION (HYPOALBUMINEMIA)	DISPLACEMENT BY ENDOGENOUS COMPOUNDS	DISPLACEMENT BY EXOGENOUS COMPOUNDS
Liver disease	Hyperbilirubinemia	Drug interactions
Nephrotic syndrome	Jaundice	Warfarin
Pregnancy	Liver disease	Phenytoin
Cystic fibrosis	Renal dysfunction	Aspirin (>2 g/d)
Burns		Nonsteroidal antiinflammatory drugs with high albumin binding
Trauma		
Malnourishment		
Elderly		

are highly bound to albumin and cause drug interactions due to displacement of plasma protein binding with valproic acid include warfarin, phenytoin, aspirin (>2 g/d), and some highly bound nonsteroidal antiinflammatory agents.

When the serum concentration is in the upper end of the therapeutic range (>75 μg/mL), some patients experience the concentration-dependent adverse effects of valproic acid therapy, including ataxia, sedation, lethargy, and fatigue. For many patients, these side effects dissipate with continued dosing, and slow dosage titration may help minimize these adverse reactions among newly treated patients. Other concentration-related side effects of valproic acid therapy include tremor at concentrations greater than 100 μg/mL and stupor or coma at concentrations greater than 175 μg/mL. Thrombocytopenia associated with valproic acid therapy usually can be limited with a decrease in dosage.

CLINICAL MONITORING PARAMETERS

The goals of therapy with anticonvulsants are to reduce seizure frequency and maximize quality of life with a minimum of adverse drug effects. Although it is desirable to abolish all seizure episodes, it may not be possible to accomplish this for many patients. Patients should be observed for concentration-related side effects (ataxia, sedation, lethargy, fatigue, tremor, stupor, coma, thrombocytopenia) and for gastrointestinal upset associated with local irritation of the gastric mucosa (nausea, vomiting, anorexia).[9] Elevated results of liver function tests, increased serum ammonia level, alopecia, and weight gain can occur during long-term valproic acid treatment. Serious, but rare, idiosyncratic side effects include hepatotoxicity, pancreatitis, pitting edema, systemic lupus-like reactions, and leukopenia with bone marrow changes.

Serum concentration of valproic acid should be measured for most patients. Because epilepsy is an episodic disease, patients do not have seizures on a continuous basis. During dosage titration it is difficult to determine whether the patient is responding to drug therapy or simply is not having abnormal central nervous system discharges. Knowledge of serum concentration of valproic acid is valuable to avoid adverse drug effects. Patients are more likely to accept drug therapy if adverse reactions are held to the absolute minimum.

BASIC CLINICAL PHARMACOKINETIC PARAMETERS

More than 95% of valproic acid is eliminated by means of hepatic metabolism. Hepatic metabolism occurs through glucuronidation, beta oxidation, and alpha hydroxylation. More than 10 metabolites of valproic acid have been identified. The 4-en metabolite of valproic acid may be associated with the propensity of the drug to cause hepatotoxicity. About 1% to 5% of a valproic acid dose is recovered in the urine as unchanged drug. Valproic acid follows nonlinear pharmacokinetics due to saturable, or concentration-dependent, plasma protein binding. This type of nonlinear pharmacokinetics occurs when the number of drug molecules overwhelms or saturates the ability of albumin to bind the drug in the plasma. When this occurs, total steady-state serum concentration of the drug increases in a disproportionate manner after a dosage increase, but unbound steady-state serum concentration increases in a proportionate manner (see Figure 12-2). Valproic acid is eliminated almost completely by means of hepatic metabolism, and it has a low hepatic extraction ratio. In this case the hepatic clearance rate is described with the classic relation used to describe hepatic clearance: $Cl_H = [LBF \cdot (f_B Cl'_{int})]/(LBF + f_B Cl'_{int})$, where LBF is liver blood flow, f_B is the unbound fraction of drug in the blood, and Cl'_{int} is the intrinsic ability of the enzyme system to metabolize the drug. Because valproic acid has a low hepatic extraction ratio, this expression for hepatic clearance simplifies to $Cl_H = f_B Cl'_{int}$.

The clinical implication of concentration-dependent plasma protein binding pharmacokinetics is that the clearance of valproic acid is not a constant as it is with linear pharmacokinetics but is concentration- or dose-dependent. As the dose or concentration of valproic acid increases, the clearance rate (Cl) increases because more unbound drug is available to hepatic enzymes for metabolism: $\uparrow Cl_H = \uparrow f_B Cl'_{int}$. This is why total steady-state concentration increases disproportionately after the dosage of valproic acid is increased: $\uparrow Css = [F(\Uparrow D/\tau)]/\uparrow Cl_H$, where F is the bioavailability of valproic acid, D is the dose of valproic acid, τ is the dosage interval, and Cl_H is hepatic clearance. When the dose of valproic acid is increased, the unbound fraction increases and causes an increase in hepatic clearance. Because dose and hepatic clearance increase simultaneously, total valproic acid concentration increases, but by a smaller than expected amount. For example, valproic acid follows concentration-dependent plasma protein binding pharmacokinetics with an average unbound fraction of 5% in the lower end of the therapeutic range (50 μg/mL) and 10% in the upper end of the therapeutic range (100 μg/mL). When the dose is increased and steady-state concentration of valproic acid increases from 50 μg/mL to 100 μg/mL, the unbound fraction increases by a factor of 2, from 5% to 10%, and hepatic clearance of total drug doubles within the therapeutic range: $2Cl_H = 2f_B Cl'_{int}$. Unfortunately, there is so much interpatient variability in concentration-dependent plasma protein binding parameters for valproic acid that predicting changes in unbound fraction and hepatic clearance is extremely difficult. However, because unbound steady-state concentrations are influenced only by intrinsic clearance, unbound concentration increases in proportion to dose: $Css_u = [F(D/\tau)]/Cl'_{int}$.

The volume of distribution of valproic acid (V = 0.15 to 0.2 L/kg) is affected by concentration-dependent plasma protein binding and is determined by the physiologic volume of blood (V_B) and tissues (V_T) as well as the unbound fraction of drug in the blood (f_B) and tissues (f_T): $V = V_B + [(f_B/f_T)V_T]$. As valproic acid concentrations increase, unbound fraction of drug in the blood increases, which causes an increase in the volume of distribution for the drug: $\uparrow V = V_B + [(\uparrow f_B/f_T)V_T]$. Half-life ($t_{1/2}$) is related to clearance and volume of distribution with the same equation as for linear pharmacokinetics: $t_{1/2} = (0.693 \cdot V)/Cl$. However, because clearance and volume of distribution are functions of dose- or concentration-dependent plasma protein binding for valproic acid, half-life changes with changes in drug dosage or concentration. As doses or concentrations increase for a drug that follows concentration-dependent plasma protein binding pharmacokinetics, clearance and volume of distribution increase simultaneously, and changes in half-life vary depending on the relative changes in clearance and volume of distribution: $\leftrightarrow t_{1/2} = (0.693 \cdot \uparrow V)/\uparrow Cl$. With the average clearance and volume of distribution for an adult (V = 0.15 L/kg, Cl = 10 mL/h/kg or 0.010 L/h/kg), half-life remains 10 h ($t_{1/2} = [0.693 \cdot V]/Cl = [0.693 \cdot 0.15\ L/kg]/[0.010\ L/h/kg] = 10\ h$). Clearance and volume of distribution increase to 0.30 L/kg and 0.020 L/h per kilogram because of decreased protein binding ($t_{1/2}$ = [0.693 · 0.30 L]/[0.020 L/h/kg] = 10 h) as serum concentration of valproic acid increases from 50 μg/mL to 100 μg/mL. The clinical implication of this finding is that the time to steady state (3 to 5 $t_{1/2}$) may vary as the dose or concentration of valproic acid increases. On average, the half-life of valproic acid is 10 to 18 hours among adults with total concentrations in the therapeutic range.

Valproic acid is available as three different entities, and all of them are prescribed as valproic acid equivalents: valproic acid, sodium valproate (the sodium salt of valproic acid), and divalproex sodium (a stable coordination compound consisting of a 1:1 ratio of valproic acid and sodium valproate). For parenteral use, valproic acid is available as a 100 mg/mL solution. When given intravenously, it should be diluted in at least 50 mL of intravenous solution and given over 1 hour (infusion rates should not exceed 20 mg/min). For oral use, a syrup (50 mg/mL), soft capsule (250 mg), enteric coated capsules (125, 250, and 500 mg), and sprinkle capsule (125 mg, used to sprinkle into foods) are available. The enteric coated capsules are not sustained-release products but only delay the absorption of drug after ingestion. As a result, there are fewer instances of gastrointestinal side effects with the enteric coated product. The oral bioavailability of valproic acid is good for all dosage forms and approximates 100%. Because of this, the same total daily dose of valproic acid can be used whether or not intravenous or oral valproic acid is administered. For example, if a patient's condition is stabilized with an oral valproic acid product and it is necessary to switch to intravenous administration, the same total daily dose of injectable valproic acid can be given.

The typical maintenance dosage of valproic acid is 15 mg/kg per day, resulting in 1000 mg or 500 mg twice a day for most adults. However, because age and coadministration of other antiepileptic drugs that are enzyme inducers, such as carbamazepine, phenytoin, and phenobarbital, affect the pharmacokinetics of valproic acid, many clinicians recommend administration of 7.5 mg/kg per day for adults or 10 mg/kg per day for children younger than 12 years receiving monotherapy and 15 mg/kg per day for adults or 20 mg/kg per day for children younger than 12 years receiving other drugs that are enzyme inducers.[10]

EFFECTS OF DISEASES AND CONDITIONS ON PHARMACOKINETICS AND DOSING

For valproic acid, oral clearance (Cl/F) is 7 to 12 mL/h per kilogram, and half-life is 12 to 18 hours for adults.[11] Among children 6 to 12 years of age, oral clearance and half-life are 10 to 20 mL/h per kilogram and 6 to 8 hours.[12] Clearance rates can be higher and half-lives shorter among patients receiving other hepatic drug-metabolizing enzyme inducers (phenytoin, phenobarbital, carbamazepine). Among adults receiving other antiepileptic drugs that are enzyme inducers, valproic acid clearance is 15 to 18 mL/h per kilogram, and half-life ranges from 4 to 12 hours. Similarly, if children receive therapy with other antiepileptic drugs that are enzyme inducers, clearance is 20 to 30 mL/h per kilogram, and half-life is 4 to 6 hours.[13,14] The volume of distribution (V/F) of valproic acid is 0.15 to 0.2 L/kg.[11,15]

Patients with cirrhosis of the liver or acute hepatitis have reduced valproic acid clearance because of destruction of the liver parenchyma.[16] This loss of functional hepatic cells decreases the amount of enzymes available to metabolize the drug and decreases clearance. Valproic acid clearance among patients with liver disease is 3 to 4 mL/h per kilogram. The volume of distribution may be larger because of reduced plasma protein binding (free fraction ≈ 29%). Protein binding may be reduced and unbound fraction may be increased owing to hypoalbuminemia or hyperbilirubinemia (especially albumin ≤3 g/dL or total bilirubin ≥2 mg/dL). The average half-life of valproic acid among patients with liver disease is 25 hours. However, the effects of liver disease on valproic acid pharmacokinetics are highly variable and difficult to predict accurately. It is possible for a patient with liver disease to have relatively normal or grossly abnormal valproic acid clearance and volume of distribution. For example, a patient with liver disease who has relatively normal albumin and bilirubin concentrations can have a normal volume of distribution of valproic acid. An index of liver dysfunction can be gained by applying the Child-Pugh clinical classification system (Table 12-3).[17] Child-Pugh scores are discussed in detail in Chapter 3 but are discussed briefly here.

The Child-Pugh score consists of five laboratory values or clinical symptoms: serum albumin, total bilirubin, prothrombin time, ascites, and hepatic encephalopathy. Each of these areas is given a score of 1 (normal) to 3 (severely abnormal; see Table 12-3), and the scores for the five areas are summed. The Child-Pugh score for a patient with normal liver function is 5. The score for a patient with grossly abnormal serum albumin, total bilirubin, and prothrombin time values in addition to severe ascites and hepatic encephalopathy is 15. A Child-Pugh score greater than 8 is grounds for a decrease of 25% to 50% in the initial daily dose of valproic acid. As for any patient with or without liver dysfunction, initial doses are meant as starting points for dosage titration based on patient response and avoidance of adverse effects. Serum concentration of valproic acid and the presence of adverse drug effects should be monitored frequently for patients with liver cirrhosis.

Elderly patients have lower oral clearance rates of valproic acid and higher unbound fractions than do younger adults, so lower initial doses may be used to treat older persons.[4] During the third trimester of pregnancy, oral clearance of valproic acid may de-

TABLE 12-3 Child-Pugh Scores for Patients with Liver Disease

TEST/SYMPTOM	SCORE 1 POINT	SCORE 2 POINTS	SCORE 3 POINTS
Total bilirubin (mg/dL)	<2.0	2.0–3.0	>3.0
Serum albumin (g/dL)	>3.5	2.8–3.5	<2.8
Prothrombin time (seconds prolonged over control)	<4	4–6	>6
Ascites	Absent	Slight	Moderate
Hepatic encephalopathy	None	Moderate	Severe

Adapted from Pugh RN, Murray-Lyon IM, Dawson JL, Pietroni MC, Williams R. Transection of the oesophagus for bleeding oesophageal varices. Br J Surg 1973;60:646–9.

crease and necessitate dosage adjustment.[18] Serum concentration of valproic acid has some diurnal variation in its value, so the time at which steady-state serum concentration is measured should be recorded if several are being compared.[4,19] Doses of valproic acid do not have to be adjusted for patients with renal failure, and the drug is not removed by dialysis.[20] The concentration of valproic acid in breast milk is about 10% of concurrent serum concentration.

DRUG INTERACTIONS

Valproic acid is a potent inhibitor of hepatic drug-metabolizing enzyme systems and glucuronidation.[21–23] Other antiepileptic drugs that have their clearance rates decreased and steady-state concentrations increased by valproic acid–related enzyme inhibition include clonazepam, carbamazepine, phenytoin, primidone, lamotrigine, and ethosuximide. Valproic acid therapy also decreases the clearance and increases steady-state concentration of other drugs, including zidovudine, amitriptyline, and nortriptyline. As a rule, when valproic acid is added to a patient's drug regimen, an adverse effect due to one of the other drugs must be considered as a possible drug interaction with valproic acid.

Additionally, other drugs can affect valproic acid clearance and steady-state serum concentrations.[21] Phenytoin, lamotrigine, rifampin, and carbamazepine can increase valproic acid clearance and decrease steady-state serum concentration of valproic acid. Cimetidine, chlorpromazine, and felbamate are examples of drugs that decrease valproic acid clearance and increase valproic acid steady-state concentrations.

Because valproic acid is highly protein bound, plasma protein binding drug interactions can occur with other drugs that are highly bound to albumin.[21] Aspirin, warfarin, and phenytoin all have plasma protein binding drug interactions with valproic acid, and these drugs have higher unbound fractions when given concurrently with valproic acid. The drug interaction between valproic acid and phenytoin deserves special examination because of its complexity and because these two agents are regularly used together for the management of seizures.[24–27] The drug interaction involves the plasma protein binding displacement and intrinsic clearance inhibition of phenytoin by valproic acid. What makes this interaction so difficult to detect and understand is that these two changes do not occur simultaneously, so the impression left by the drug interaction depends on when it is observed. For example, a patient's condition is stabilized with phenytoin therapy (Figure 12-3), but because adequate control of seizures has not been attained, valproic acid is added to the regimen. As valproic acid accumulates, the first interaction is plasma protein binding displacement of phenytoin as the two drugs compete for binding sites on albumin. The result of this portion of the drug interaction is an increase in unbound fraction of phenytoin and a decrease in total serum concentration of phenytoin, but the unbound phenytoin serum concentration remains the same. As valproic acid serum concentrations reach steady state, the higher concentrations of drug bathe the hepatic microsomal enzyme system and inhibit intrinsic clearance of phenytoin. This portion of the interaction decreases intrinsic clearance and hepatic clearance of phenytoin, so both unbound and total phenytoin concentrations increase. When phenytoin concentrations finally equilibrate and reach steady state under the new plasma protein binding and intrinsic clearance conditions imposed by concurrent valproic acid therapy, the total concentration of phenytoin often is about the same as before the drug interaction occurred, but

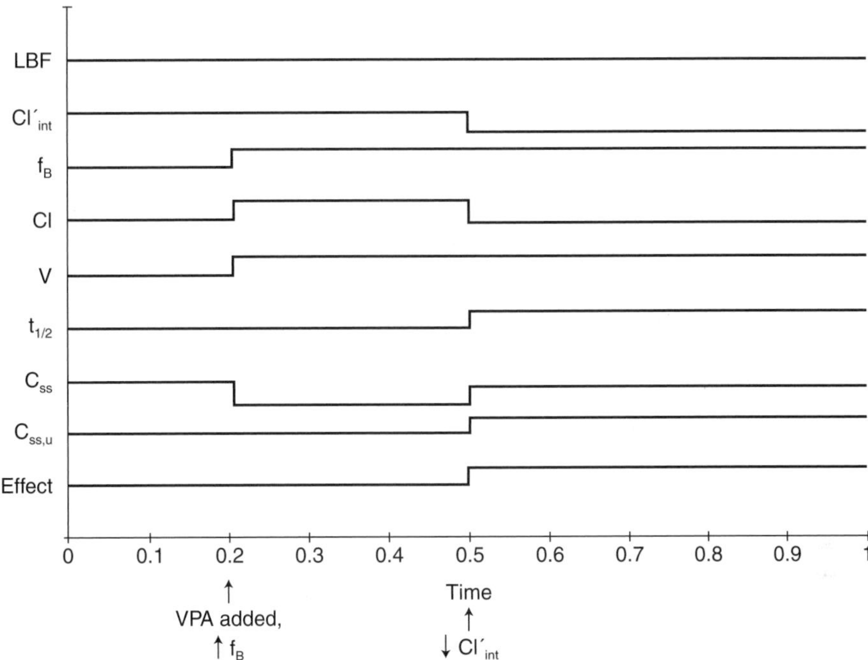

FIGURE 12-3 Schematic of physiologic (*LBF*, liver blood flow; Cl'_{int}, intrinsic or unbound clearance; f_B, unbound fraction of drug in blood/plasma), pharmacokinetic (*Cl*, clearance; *V*, volume of distribution; $t_{1/2}$, half-life; C_{ss}, total steady-state drug concentration; $C_{ss,u}$, unbound steady-state drug concentration), and pharmacodynamic (*Effect*, pharmacodynamic effect) parameters during valproic acid (*VPA*) treatment of a patient whose condition has been stabilized with phenytoin therapy. Valproic acid initially decreases phenytoin plasma protein binding by means of competitive displacement for binding sites on albumin ($\uparrow f_B$). As valproic acid concentration increases, the hepatic enzyme inhibition component of the drug interaction comes into play ($\downarrow Cl'_{int}$). The net result is that total phenytoin concentration is largely unchanged from baseline, but unbound phenytoin concentration and the pharmacologic effect increase.

unbound phenytoin concentration is much higher. If only total phenytoin concentration is measured at this point, clinicians will be under the impression that total concentration did not change and that no drug interaction occurred. However, simultaneous measurement of unbound phenytoin concentration shows that this concentration has increased and that the unbound fraction of phenytoin is twice or more (≥20%) the baseline amount. In this situation, the patient may have an unbound concentration of phenytoin that is toxic, and a decrease in phenytoin dosage may be in order.

INITIAL DOSAGE DETERMINATION METHODS

Pharmacokinetic Dosing Method

The goal of initial dosing of valproic acid is to compute the best dose possible for the patient given the diseases and conditions that influence valproic acid pharmacokinetics and the epileptic disorder for which the patient is being treated. To do this, pharmacokinetic parameters for the patient are estimated with average parameters measured for other patients with similar disease and condition profiles.

ESTIMATE OF CLEARANCE

Valproic acid is predominately metabolized by liver. Unfortunately, there is no good way to estimate the elimination characteristics of liver-metabolized drugs with an endogenous marker of liver function in the same manner that serum creatinine and estimated creatinine clearance are used to estimate the elimination of agents removed by the kidneys. Because of this, a patient is categorized according to the diseases and conditions known to change valproic acid clearance, and the clearance previously measured in these studies is used as an estimate of the current patient's clearance. For example, for a 70-kg adult with cirrhosis of the liver or acute hepatitis, valproic acid clearance is assumed to be 3 to 4 mL/h per kilogram: 70 kg · 3.5 mL/h/kg = 245 mL/h or 0.245 L/h. To produce the most conservative valproic acid doses for patients with several concurrent diseases or conditions that affect valproic acid pharmacokinetics, the disease or condition with the smallest clearance should be used to compute doses. This approach avoids accidental overdosage as much as is currently possible.

ESTIMATE OF VOLUME OF DISTRIBUTION

The volume of distribution of valproic acid is assumed to be 0.15 L/kg for adults and 0.2 L/kg for children younger than 12 years. For an 80-kg adult, the estimated valproic volume of distribution is 12 L: V = 0.15 L/kg · 80 kg = 12 L. Patients with cirrhosis or renal failure may have larger volumes of distribution because of decreased plasma protein binding.

ESTIMATE OF HALF-LIFE AND ELIMINATION RATE CONSTANT

Once the correct clearance and volume of distribution estimates are identified for the patient, they can be converted into the valproic acid half-life ($t_{1/2}$) and elimination rate constant (k) estimates with the following equations: $t_{1/2} = (0.693 \cdot V)/Cl$, $k = 0.693/t_{1/2} = Cl/V$.

SELECTION OF APPROPRIATE PHARMACOKINETIC MODEL AND EQUATIONS

When given by intravenous infusion or orally, valproic acid follows a one-compartment pharmacokinetic model. When oral therapy is required, valproic acid has good bioavailability (F = 1), and dosing every 8 to 12 hours provides a relatively smooth serum concentration–time curve that emulates intravenous infusion. Because of this, a simple pharmacokinetic equation for determining average steady-state serum concentration of valproic acid (Css in μg/mL or mg/L) is widely used and allows calculation of a maintenance dosage: $Css = [F(D/\tau)]/Cl$, or $D = (Css \cdot Cl \cdot \tau)/F$, where F is the bioavailability fraction for the oral dosage form (F = 1 for oral valproic acid products), D is the dose of valproic acid in milligrams, τ is the dosage interval in hours, and Cl is clearance in liters per hour. When intravenous therapy is required, the same pharmacokinetic equation is widely used: $Css = (D/\tau)/Cl$, or $D = Css \cdot Cl \cdot \tau$, where D is the dose of valproic acid in milligrams, τ is the dosage interval in hours, and Cl is clearance in liters per hour.

The equation used to calculate an intravenous loading dose (LD) in milligrams is based on a simple one-compartment model: $LD = Css \cdot V$, where Css is the desired steady-state concentration of valproic acid in micrograms per milliliter, which is equivalent to milligrams per liter, and V is the volume of distribution in liters. Intravenous dosage of valproic acid should be by means of infusion that lasts at least 60 minutes (≤20 mg/min).

Example 1 KL is a 51-year-old, 75-kg (height, 178 cm) man who has tonic-clonic seizures. He needs therapy with oral valproic acid. He has normal liver function and takes no medications that induce hepatic enzymes. Suggest an initial valproic acid dosage regimen designed to achieve a steady-state valproic acid concentration of 50 μg/mL.

1. *Estimate clearance and volume of distribution according to disease states and conditions present in the patient.*

The clearance rate for an adult patient not taking other drugs that induce hepatic drug metabolism is 7 to 12 mL/h per kilogram. For a value of 10 mL/h per kilogram, the estimated clearance is 0.75 L/h: Cl = 75 kg · 10 mL/h/kg = 750 mL/h, or 0.75 L/h. At 0.15 L/kg, the estimated volume of distribution is 11 L: 75 kg · 0.15 L/kg = 11 L.

2. *Estimate half-life and elimination rate constant.*

Once the correct clearance and volume of distribution estimates are identified for the patient, they can be converted into the valproic acid half-life ($t_{1/2}$) and elimination rate constant (k) estimates with the following equations: $t_{1/2} = (0.693 \cdot V)/Cl = (0.693 \cdot 11\ L)/(0.75\ L/h) = 10\ h$; $k = 0.693/t_{1/2} = 0.693/10\ h = 0.069\ h^{-1}$.

3. *Compute the dosage regimen.*

Oral enteric coated divalproex sodium tablets are prescribed to this patient (F = 1). (Note: μg/mL = mg/L, and this concentration unit was substituted for Css in the calculations to avoid unit conversion.) The dosage equation for oral valproic acid is $D = (Css \cdot Cl \cdot \tau)/F = (50\ mg/L \cdot 0.75\ L/h \cdot 12\ h)/1 = 450\ mg$, rounded to 500 mg every 12 hours.

Steady-state minimum serum concentration of valproic acid should be measured after steady state is attained in 3 to 5 half-lives. Because the drug is expected to have a half-life of 10 hours in this patient, the steady-state concentration of valproic acid can be measured any time after the second day of dosing (5 half-lives = 5 · 10 h = 50 h). Serum concentration of valproic acid should be measured if the patient has an exacerbation of epilepsy or if the patient has signs or symptoms of valproic acid toxicity.

Example 2 UO is a 10-year-old, 40-kg boy who has absence seizures. He needs therapy with oral valproic acid. He has normal liver function and takes carbamazepine. Suggest an initial valproic acid dosage regimen designed to achieve a steady-state valproic acid concentration of 50 μg/mL.

1. *Estimate clearance and volume of distribution according to disease states and conditions present in the patient.*

The clearance rate for a child who takes other drugs that induce hepatic drug metabolism is 20 to 30 mL/h per kilogram. With a value of 25 mL/h per kilogram, the estimated clearance is 1 L/h: Cl = 40 kg · 25 mL/h/kg = 1000 mL/h or 1 L/h. At 0.2 L/kg, the estimated volume of distribution is 8 L: 40 kg · 0.2 L/kg = 8 L.

2. *Estimate half-life and elimination rate constant.*

Once the correct clearance and volume of distribution estimates are identified for the patient, they can be converted into the valproic acid half-life ($t_{1/2}$) and elimination rate constant (k) estimates with the following equations: $t_{1/2} = (0.693 \cdot V)/Cl = (0.693 \cdot 8\ L)/(1\ L/h) = 6\ h$; $k = 0.693/t_{1/2} = 0.693/6\ h = 0.116\ h^{-1}$.

3. *Compute the dosage regimen.*

Oral valproic acid syrup is prescribed to this patient (F = 1). (Note: μg/mL = mg/L, and this concentration unit was substituted for Css in the calculations to avoid unit conversion.) The dosage equation for oral valproic acid is $D = (Css \cdot Cl \cdot \tau)/F = (50\ mg/L \cdot 1\ L/h \cdot 8\ h)/1 = 400\ mg$, or 400 mg every 8 h.

Steady-state minimum serum concentration of valproic acid should be measured after steady state is attained in 3 to 5 half-lives. Because the drug is expected to have a half-life of 6 hours in this patient, the steady-state concentration of valproic acid can be measured any time after the first day of dosing (5 half-lives = 5 · 6 h = 30 h). Serum concentration of valproic acid should be measured if the patient has an exacerbation of epilepsy or if the patient has signs or symptoms of valproic acid toxicity.

Example 3 HU is a 25-year-old, 85-kg (height, 188 cm) man who has tonic-clonic seizures. He needs therapy with intravenous valproic acid. He has normal liver function and takes no medications that induce hepatic enzymes. Suggest an initial valproic acid dosage regimen designed to achieve a steady-state valproic acid concentration of 75 μg/mL.

1. *Estimate clearance and volume of distribution according to disease states and conditions present in the patient.*

The clearance rate for an adult patient not taking other drugs that induce hepatic drug metabolism is 7 to 12 mL/h per kilogram. With a value of 10 mL/h per kilogram, the estimated clearance is 0.85 L/h: $Cl = 85\ kg \cdot 10\ mL/h/kg = 850\ mL/h$, or 0.85 L/h. At 0.15 L/kg, the estimated volume of distribution is 13 L: $85\ kg \cdot 0.15\ L/kg = 13\ L$.

2. *Estimate half-life and elimination rate constant.*

Once the correct clearance and volume of distribution estimates are identified for the patient, they can be converted into the valproic acid half-life ($t_{1/2}$) and elimination rate constant (k) estimates with the following equations: $t_{1/2} = (0.693 \cdot V)/Cl = (0.693 \cdot 13\ L)/(0.85\ L/h) = 11\ h$; $k = 0.693/t_{1/2} = 0.693/11\ h = 0.063\ h^{-1}$.

3. *Compute the dosage regimen.*

Valproic acid injection is prescribed to this patient (F = 1). (Note: μg/mL = mg/L, and this concentration unit was substituted for Css in the calculations to avoid unit conversion.) The maintenance dosage equation for valproic acid is $D = (Css \cdot Cl \cdot \tau)/F = (75\ mg/L \cdot 0.85\ L/h \cdot 8\ h)/1 = 510\ mg$, rounded to 500 mg every 8 hours. The loading dose equation for valproic acid is $LD = Css \cdot V = 75\ mg/L \cdot 13\ L = 975\ mg$, rounded to 1000 mg. Intravenous doses should be given over 1 hour (≤20 mg/min).

Steady-state minimum serum concentration of valproic acid should be measured after steady state is attained in 3 to 5 half-lives. Because the drug is expected to have a half-life of 11 hours in this patient, the steady-state concentration of valproic acid can be measured any time after the second day of dosing (5 half-lives = 5 · 11 h = 55 h). Serum concentration of valproic acid should be measured if the patient has an exacerbation of epilepsy or if the patient has signs or symptoms of valproic acid toxicity.

Literature-Based Recommended Dosing

Because of the large variability in valproic acid pharmacokinetics, even when concurrent diseases and conditions are identified, most clinicians believe that the use of standard valproic acid doses for various situations is warranted. The original computation of these doses was based on pharmacokinetic dosing methods and modified on the basis of clinical experience. In general, the expected steady-state serum concentration of valproic acid used to compute these doses was 50 μg/mL. The usual initial maintenance dose for pediatric patients is 10 mg/kg per day if the child is not taking a hepatic enzyme inducer (phenytoin, phenobarbital, carbamazepine, rifampin) or 20 mg/kg per day if the child is taking a hepatic enzyme inducer. For adults, the initial maintenance dose is 7.5 mg/kg per day if the patient is not taking hepatic enzyme inducers or 15 mg/kg per day if a hepatic enzyme inducer is concurrently administered. Two or three divided daily doses are initially used for these total doses. To avoid gastrointestinal side effects, doses more than 1500 mg at one time should be avoided. Dosage increases of 5 to 10 mg/kg per day are made every 1 to 2 weeks depending on response and adverse effects. Most adults need 1500 to 3000 mg/d of valproic acid. If the patient has significant hepatic dysfunction (Child-Pugh score ≥8), maintenance doses prescribed with this method should be decreased 25% to 50% depending on the aggressiveness of therapy. To illustrate the similarities and differences between this method of dosage calculation and the pharmacokinetic dosing method, the previous examples are used.

Example 4 KL is a 51-year-old, 75-kg (height, 178 cm) man who has tonic-clonic seizures. He needs therapy with oral valproic acid. He has normal liver function and takes no medications that induce hepatic enzymes. Suggest an initial valproic dosage regimen for this patient.

1. *Estimate the valproic acid dose according to disease states and conditions present in the patient.*

Oral enteric coated divalproex sodium tablets are prescribed to this patient. The suggested initial maintenance dosage of valproic acid for an adult patient not taking enzyme inducers is 7.5 mg/kg per day: 75 kg · 7.5 mg/kg/d = 563 mg/d, rounded to 500 mg/d or 250 mg every 12 hours. This dose is titrated upward in increments of 5 to 10 mg/kg per day every 1 to 2 weeks while the patient is observed for adverse and therapeutic effects. The goals of therapy are maximal suppression of seizures and avoidance of side effects.

Steady-state minimum total serum concentration of valproic acid should be measured after steady state is attained in 1 to 2 weeks. Serum concentration of valproic acid also should be measured if the patient has an exacerbation of epilepsy or if the patient has signs or symptoms of valproic acid toxicity.

Example 5 UO is a 10-year-old, 40-kg boy who has absence seizures. He needs therapy with oral valproic acid. He has normal liver function and currently takes carbamazepine. Suggest an initial valproic acid dosage regimen for this patient.

1. *Estimate the valproic acid dose according to disease states and conditions present in the patient.*

Oral valproic acid syrup is prescribed to this patient. The suggested initial maintenance dosage of valproic acid for a child taking enzyme inducers is 20 mg/kg per day: 40 kg · 20 mg/kg/d = 800 mg/d, rounded to 750 mg/d or 250 mg every 8 hours. This dose is titrated upward in increments of 5 to 10 mg/kg per day every 1 to 2 weeks while the patient is observed for adverse and therapeutic effects. The goals of therapy are maximal suppression of seizures and avoidance of side effects.

Steady-state minimum total serum concentration of valproic acid should be measured after steady state is attained in 1 to 2 weeks. Serum concentration of valproic acid also should be measured if the patient has an exacerbation of epilepsy or if the patient has signs or symptoms of valproic acid toxicity.

Example 6 HU is a 25-year-old, 85-kg (height, 188 cm) man who has tonic-clonic seizures. He needs therapy with intravenous valproic acid. He has normal liver function and takes no medications that induce hepatic enzymes. Suggest an initial valproic acid dosage regimen for this patient.

1. *Estimate the valproic acid dose according to disease states and conditions present in the patient.*

Intravenous valproic acid injection is prescribed to this patient. The suggested initial maintenance dosage for an adult patient not taking enzyme inducers is 7.5 mg/kg per day: 85 kg · 7.5 mg/kg/d = 638 mg/d, rounded to 750 mg/d, or 250 mg every 8 hours. This dose is titrated upward in increments of 5 to 10 mg/kg per day every 1 to 2 weeks while the patient is observed for adverse and therapeutic effects. If needed, a loading dose of 7.5 mg/kg can be given as the first dose: 85 kg · 7.5 mg/kg = 638 mg, rounded to 750 mg. Intravenous doses should be administered over 1 hour (≤20 mg/min). The goals of therapy are maximal suppression of seizures and avoidance of side effects.

Steady-state minimum total serum concentration of valproic acid should be measured after steady state is attained in 1 to 2 weeks. Serum concentration of valproic acid also should be measured if the patient has an exacerbation of epilepsy or if the patient has signs or symptoms of valproic acid toxicity.

USE OF SERUM CONCENTRATION OF VALPROIC ACID TO ALTER DOSES

Because of the large pharmacokinetic variability among patients, it is likely that doses computed with patient population characteristics will not always produce serum concentrations of valproic acid that are expected or desirable. Because of pharmacokinetic variability, the nonlinear pharmacokinetics followed by the drug owing to concentration-dependent plasma protein binding, the narrow therapeutic index of valproic acid, and the desire to avoid adverse side effects of valproic acid, serum concentration of valproic acid is measured for most patients to ensure that therapeutic, nontoxic levels are present. In addition to valproic acid serum concentration, important patient parameters, such as seizure frequency and risk of side effects of valproic acid, should be followed to confirm that the patient is responding to treatment and not having an adverse drug reaction. When serum concentration of valproic acid is measured, and a dosage change is necessary, clinicians should use the simplest, most straightforward method available to determine a dose that will provide safe and effective treatment.

Pseudolinear Pharmacokinetics Method

A simple, easy way to approximate new total serum concentrations after adjustment of the dosage of valproic acid is temporarily to assume linear pharmacokinetics, then subtract 10% to 20% for a dosage increase or add 10% to 20% for a dosage decrease to account for nonlinear, concentration-dependent plasma protein binding pharmacokinetics: $D_{new} = (Css_{new}/Css_{old})D_{old}$, where Css_{new} is the expected steady-state concentration of the new valproic acid dose in micrograms per milliliter, Css_{old} is the measured steady-state concentration of the old valproic acid dose in micrograms per milliliter, D_{new} is the new valproic acid dose to be prescribed in milligrams per day, and D_{old} is the currently prescribed dosage of valproic acid in milligrams per day. Unbound steady-state concentration increases or decreases in a linear manner with dose.

Example 7 KL is a 51-year-old, 75-kg (height, 178 cm) man who has tonic-clonic seizures. He needs therapy with oral valproic acid. The patient is given a prescription for 500 mg every 12 hours of enteric coated divalproex sodium tablets (1000 mg/d) for 1 month. Steady-state total concentration of valproic acid is 38 μg/mL. The patient is found to be compliant with the dosage regimen. Suggest a valproic acid dosage regimen designed to achieve a steady-state valproic acid concentration of 80 μg/mL.

1. *Use pseudolinear pharmacokinetics to predict a new concentration for a dosage increase, then compute the 10% to 20% factor to account for nonlinear, concentration-dependent plasma protein binding pharmacokinetics.*

According to pseudolinear pharmacokinetics, the resulting total steady-state serum concentration of valproic acid is $D_{new} = (Css_{new}/Css_{old})D_{old}$ = [(80 μg/mL)/(38 μg/mL)] 1000 mg/d = 2105 mg/d, rounded to 2000 mg/d, or 1000 mg every 12 hours. Because of nonlinear, concentration-dependent protein binding pharmacokinetics, the total steady-state serum concentration is expected to be 10% less, or 0.90 times, to 20% less, or 0.80 times, than that predicted with linear pharmacokinetics: Css = 80 μg/mL · 0.90 = 72 μg/mL, and Css = 80 μg/mL · 0.80 = 64 μg/mL. Thus a dosage of 2000 mg/d is expected to yield a total steady-state serum concentration of valproic acid of 64 to 72 μg/mL.

Steady-state minimum total serum concentration of valproic acid should be measured after steady state is attained in 1 to 2 weeks. Serum concentration of valproic acid also should be measured if the patient has an exacerbation of epilepsy or if the patient has signs or symptoms of valproic acid toxicity.

Example 8 UO is a 10-year-old, 40-kg boy who has absence seizures. He needs therapy with oral valproic acid. He has normal liver function. The patient is given a prescription for 400 mg three times daily (1200 mg/d) of valproic acid syrup for 1 month. Steady-state total concentration of valproic acid is 130 μg/mL. The patient is found to be compliant with the dosage regimen. Suggest a valproic acid dosage regimen designed to achieve a steady-state valproic acid concentration of 75 μg/mL.

1. *Use pseudolinear pharmacokinetics to predict a new concentration for a dosage decrease, then compute the 10% to 20% factor to account for nonlinear, concentration-dependent plasma protein binding pharmacokinetics.*

According to pseudolinear pharmacokinetics, the resulting total steady-state serum concentration of valproic acid is $D_{new} = (Css_{new}/Css_{old})D_{old}$ = [(75 μg/mL)/(130 μg/mL)] 1200 mg/d = 692 mg/d, rounded to 750 mg/d, or 250 mg every 8 hours. Because of nonlinear, concentration-dependent protein binding pharmacokinetics, the total steady-state serum concentration is expected to be 10% greater, or 1.10 times, to 20% greater, or 1.20 times, than that predicted with linear pharmacokinetics: Css = 75 μg/mL · 1.10 = 83 μg/mL, and Css = 75 μg/mL · 1.20 = 90 μg/mL. Thus a dosage of 750 mg/d is expected to yield a total steady-state serum concentration of valproic acid of 83 to 90 μg/mL.

Steady-state minimum total serum concentration of valproic acid should be measured after steady state is attained in 1 to 2 weeks. Serum concentration of valproic acid also should be measured if the patient has an exacerbation of epilepsy or if the patient has signs or symptoms of valproic acid toxicity.

Pharmacokinetic Parameter Method

The pharmacokinetic parameter method of adjusting drug doses was among the first techniques for changing doses using serum concentrations. It allows computation of patients' unique pharmacokinetic constants and calculation of a dose that achieves desired valproic acid concentrations. The pharmacokinetic parameter method requires that steady state has been achieved, and only a steady-state concentration (Css) of valproic acid is used. During intravenous dosing, the following equation is used to compute valproic acid clearance (Cl): $Cl = (D/\tau)/Css$, where D is the dose of valproic acid in milligrams, Css is the steady-state concentration of valproic acid in milligrams per liter, and τ is the dosage interval in hours. If the patient is receiving oral valproic acid therapy, valproic acid clearance (Cl) can be calculated with the following formula: $Cl = [F(D/\tau)]/Css$, where F is the bioavailability fraction for the oral dosage form (F = 1 for oral valproic acid products), D is the dose of valproic acid in milligrams, Css is the steady-state concentration of valproic acid in milligrams per liter, and τ is the dosage interval in hours.

Serum concentration of valproic acid sometimes is measured before and after an intravenous dose is administered. In a one-compartment model, volume of distribution (V) is calculated with the following equation: $V = D/(C_{postdose} - C_{predose})$, where D is the dose of valproic acid in milligrams, $C_{postdose}$ is the concentration after the loading dose in milligrams per liter, and $C_{predose}$ is the concentration in milligrams per liter before the loading dose is administered. ($C_{predose}$ should be measured within 30 minutes of administration; $C_{postdose}$ should be measured 30 to 60 minutes after the end of infusion to avoid any distribution phase.) If the predose concentration is also the steady-state concentration, valproic acid clearance also can be computed. If both clearance (Cl) and volume of distribution (V) have been measured with these techniques, the half-life $[t_{1/2} = (0.693 \cdot V)/Cl]$ and elimination rate constant ($k = 0.693/t_{1/2} = Cl/V$) can be computed. The clearance, volume of distribution, elimination rate constant, and half-life measured with these techniques are the patient's unique pharmacokinetic constants for valproic acid and can be used in one-compartment model equations to compute the dose required to achieve any desired serum concentration. Because linear pharmacokinetics also are assumed, valproic acid doses computed with the pharmacokinetic parameter method and the pseudolinear pharmacokinetic method should be identical. To account for nonlinear, concentration-dependent plasma protein binding pharmacokinetics, 10% to 20% for a dosage increase can be subtracted or 10% to 20% for a dosage decrease can be added to the expected steady-state serum concentration. To illustrate the similarities and differences between this method of dosage calculation and the pharmacokinetic parameter method, the previous examples are used.

Example 9 KL is a 51-year-old, 75-kg (height, 178 cm) man who has tonic-clonic seizures. He needs therapy with oral valproic acid. The patient is given a prescription for 500 mg every 12 hours of enteric coated divalproex sodium tablets (1000 mg/d) for 1 month. Steady-state total concentration of valproic acid is 38 μg/mL. The patient is found to be compliant with the dosage regimen. Suggest a valproic acid dosage regimen designed to achieve a steady-state valproic acid concentration of 80 μg/mL.

1. *Compute the pharmacokinetic parameters.*

The patient is expected to achieve steady-state conditions after 2 to 3 days of therapy. Valproic acid clearance can be computed with steady-state valproic acid concentration: $Cl = [F(D/\tau)]/Css = [1(500\ mg/12\ h)]/(38\ mg/L) = 1.1\ L/h$. (Note: μg/mL = mg/L, and this concentration unit was substituted for Css in the calculations to avoid unit conversion.)

2. *Compute the valproic acid dose.*

Valproic acid clearance is used to compute the new dose: $D = (Css \cdot Cl \cdot \tau)/F = (80\ mg/L \cdot 1.1\ L/h \cdot 12\ h)/1 = 1056\ mg$, rounded to 1000 mg every 12 hours.

Because of nonlinear, concentration-dependent protein binding pharmacokinetics, the total steady-state serum concentration is expected to be 10% less, or 0.90 times, to 20% less, or 0.80 times, than that predicted with linear pharmacokinetics: $Css = 80\ \mu g/mL \cdot 0.90 = 72\ \mu g/mL$, and $Css = 80\ \mu g/mL \cdot 0.80 = 64\ \mu g/mL$. Thus a dosage of 2000 mg/d is expected to yield a total steady-state serum concentration of valproic acid of 64 to 72 μg/mL.

Steady-state minimum total serum concentration of valproic acid should be measured after steady state is attained in 1 to 2 weeks. Serum concentration of valproic acid also should be measured if the patient has an exacerbation of epilepsy or if the patient has signs or symptoms of valproic acid toxicity.

Example 10 UO is a 10-year-old, 40-kg boy who has absence seizures. He needs therapy with oral valproic acid. He has normal liver function. The patient is given a prescription for 400 mg three times daily (1200 mg/d) of valproic acid syrup for 1 month. Steady-state total concentration of valproic acid is 130 μg/mL. The patient is found to be compliant with the dosage regimen. Suggest a valproic acid dosage regimen designed to achieve a steady-state valproic acid concentration of 75 μg/mL.

1. *Compute the pharmacokinetic parameters.*

The patient is expected to achieve steady-state conditions after 2 to 3 days of therapy. Valproic acid clearance can be computed with steady-state valproic acid concentration: $Cl = [F(D/\tau)]/Css = [1(400\ mg/8\ h)]/(130\ mg/L) = 0.38\ L/h$. (Note: μg/mL = mg/L, and this concentration unit was substituted for Css in the calculations to avoid unit conversion.)

2. *Compute the valproic acid dose.*

Valproic acid clearance is used to compute the new dose: $D = (Css \cdot Cl \cdot \tau)/F = (75\ mg/L \cdot 0.38\ L/h \cdot 8\ h)/1 = 228\ mg$, rounded to 250 mg every 8 hours.

Because of nonlinear, concentration-dependent protein binding pharmacokinetics, the total steady-state serum concentration is expected to be 10% more, or 1.10 times, to 20% more, or 1.20 times, than that predicted with linear pharmacokinetics: $Css = 75\ \mu g/mL \cdot 1.10 = 83\ \mu g/mL$, and $Css = 75\ \mu g/mL \cdot 1.20 = 90\ \mu g/mL$. Thus a dosage of 750 mg/d is expected to yield a total steady-state serum concentration of valproic acid of 83 to 90 μg/mL.

Steady-state minimum total serum concentration of valproic acid should be measured after steady state is attained in 1 to 2 weeks. Serum concentration of valproic acid also should be measured if the patient has an exacerbation of epilepsy or if the patient has signs or symptoms of valproic acid toxicity.

Example 11 PP is a 59-year-old, 65-kg (height, 173 cm) man who has tonic-clonic seizures. He is receiving valproic acid injection 500 mg every 8 hours. The current steady-state concentration of valproic acid (obtained 30 min before administration of a booster dose) is 40 μg/mL. Compute a maintenance dose of valproic acid that will provide a steady-state concentration of 75 μg/mL. In an attempt to boost valproic acid concentration as soon as possible, an additional, single booster dose of 500 mg valproic acid over 60 minutes is given before the maintenance dosage is increased. The total serum concentration of valproic acid 30 minutes after the additional dose is 105 μg/mL.

1. *Compute the pharmacokinetic parameters.*

The patient is expected to achieve steady-state conditions after 2 to 3 days of therapy. Valproic acid clearance can be computed with steady-state valproic acid concentration: $Cl = [F(D/\tau)]/Css = [1(500\ mg/8\ h)]/(40\ mg/L) = 1.6\ L/h$. (Note: μg/mL = mg/L, and this concentration unit was substituted for Css in the calculations to avoid unit conversion.)

Volume of distribution of valproic acid can be computed with the concentrations before and after the bolus dose is administered: $V = D/(C_{postdose} - C_{predose}) = 500\ mg/(105\ mg/L - 40\ mg/L) = 8\ L$. (Note: μg/mL = mg/L, and this concentration unit was substituted for Css in the calculations to avoid unit conversion.)

Valproic acid half-life ($t_{1/2}$) and elimination rate constant (k) can be computed as follows: $t_{1/2} = (0.693 \cdot V)/Cl = (0.693 \cdot 8\ L)/(1.6\ L/h) = 3.5\ h$; $k = Cl/V = (1.6\ L/h)/(8\ L) = 0.20\ h^{-1}$.

2. *Compute the valproic acid dose.*

Valproic acid clearance is used to compute the new maintenance dose of valproic acid: $D = (Css \cdot Cl \cdot \tau) = (75\ mg/L \cdot 1.6\ L/h \cdot 8\ h) = 960\ mg$, rounded to 1000 mg every 8 hours.

Because of nonlinear, concentration-dependent protein binding pharmacokinetics, the total steady-state serum concentration is expected to be 10% less, or 0.90 times, to 20% less, or 0.80 times, than that predicted with linear pharmacokinetics: Css = 75 μg/mL · 0.90 = 68 μg/mL, and Css = 75 μg/mL · 0.80 = 60 μg/mL. Thus a dosage of 3000 mg/d is expected to yield a total steady-state serum concentration of valproic acid of 60 to 68 μg/mL. The new valproic acid maintenance dose is instituted one dosage interval after the additional booster dose is given.

Serum concentration of valproic acid should be measured after steady state is attained in 3 to 5 half-lives. Because the drug has a half-life of 3.5 hours in this patient, the steady-state concentration of valproic acid can be measured after 1 day of continuous dosing (5 half-lives = 5 · 3.5 h = 17.5 h). Serum concentration of valproic acid should be measured if the patient has an exacerbation of epilepsy or if the patient has signs or symptoms of valproic acid toxicity.

BAYESIAN PHARMACOKINETICS COMPUTER PROGRAMS

Computer programs can assist in calculation of pharmacokinetic parameters for patients. In the most reliable computer programs a nonlinear regression algorithm incorporates components of Bayes' theorem.[28] Nonlinear regression is a statistical technique in which an iterative process is used to compute the best pharmacokinetic parameters for a concentration–time data set. Briefly, the patient's drug dosage schedule and serum concentrations are entered into the computer. The computer program has a pharmacokinetic equation programmed for the drug and administration method (e.g., oral, intravenous bolus, intravenous infusion). A one-compartment model typically is used, although some programs allow the user to choose among several different equations. With population estimates based on demographic information for the patient, such as age, weight, sex, liver function, and cardiac status, the user runs the computer program to estimate serum concentration for each time at which actual serum concentration is known. Kinetic parameters are then changed with the computer program, and a new set of estimated serum concentrations are computed. The pharmacokinetic parameters that generate the estimated serum concentration closest to the actual value are stored in the computer program, and the process is repeated until the set of pharmacokinetic parameters that give estimated serum concentrations statistically closest to actual serum concentrations are generated. These pharmacokinetic parameters can then be used to compute improved dosing schedules for patients. Bayes' theorem is used in the computer algorithm to balance the results of the computations between values based solely on the patient's serum drug concentrations and those based only on patient population parameters. Results of studies in which the various methods of dosage adjustment have been compared show that these types of computer dosing programs perform at least as well as experienced clinical pharmacokineticists and clinicians and better than inexperienced clinicians.

Some clinicians use Bayesian pharmacokinetics computer programs exclusively to alter drug doses on the basis of serum concentration. An advantage of this approach is that consistent dosage recommendations are made when several practitioners are involved in therapeutic drug monitoring programs. However, because simpler dosing methods work just as well for patients with stable pharmacokinetic parameters and steady-state drug concentrations, many clinicians reserve the use of computer programs for more difficult situations. Those situations include serum concentrations that are not at steady state, serum concentrations not obtained at the specific times needed to use simpler methods, and unstable pharmacokinetic parameters. Many Bayesian pharmacokinetics computer programs are available, and most should provide answers similar to the one used in the following examples. The program used to solve problems in this book is DrugCalc, written by Dr. Dennis Mungall. It is available on his Internet web site (http://members.aol.com/thertch/index.htm).[28]

Example 12 LK is a 50-year-old, 75-kg (height, 178 cm) man who has complex partial seizures. He is receiving 500 mg every 8 hours of oral enteric coated valproic acid tablets. He has normal liver function (bilirubin, 0.7 mg/dL; albumin, 4.0 g/dL) and takes 1200 mg/d of carbamazepine. The current steady-state concentration of valproic acid is 31 μg/mL. Compute a valproic acid dose that will provide a steady-state concentration of 70 μg/mL.

1. *Enter the patient's demographic, drug dosing, and serum concentration–time data into the computer program.*

2. *Compute the pharmacokinetic parameters for the patient with a Bayesian pharmacokinetics computer program.*

The pharmacokinetic parameters computed with the program are a volume of distribution of 8.6 L, a half-life of 5.2 hours, and a clearance of 1.13 L/h.

3. *Compute the dose required to achieve the desired serum concentration of valproic acid.*

The one-compartment model, first-order absorption equations used in the program to compute doses indicate that a dose of 1000 mg every 8 hours will produce a steady-state valproic acid concentration of 68 μg/mL.

Example 13 HJ is a 62-year-old, 87-kg (height, 185 cm) man who has tonic-clonic seizures. He is given a new prescription for 500 mg of oral valproic acid capsules every 12 hours. He has cirrhosis of the liver (Child-Pugh score, 12; bilirubin, 3.2 mg/dL; albumin, 2.5 g/dL). The minimum valproic acid concentration before the seventh dose is 72 μg/mL. The patient is having minor adverse effects (sedation, lethargy, fatigue). Compute a valproic acid dose that will provide a total steady-state concentration of 50 μg/mL.

1. *Enter the patient's demographic, drug dosing, and serum concentration–time data into the computer program.*

In this case, it is unlikely that the patient is at steady state, so the linear pharmacokinetics method cannot be used.

2. *Compute the pharmacokinetic parameters for the patient with a Bayesian pharmacokinetics computer program.*

The pharmacokinetic parameters computed with the program are a volume of distribution of 12.5 L, a half-life of 19 hours, and a clearance of 0.46 L/h.

3. *Compute the dose required to achieve the desired serum concentration of valproic acid.*

The one-compartment model, first-order absorption equations used in the program to compute doses indicate that a dose of 750 mg every 24 hours produces a steady-state concentration of 46 μg/mL.

Example 14 JB is a 50-year-old, 60-kg (height, 170 cm) man who has tonic-clonic seizures. Valproic acid 500 mg every 8 hours intravenously is administered after an intravenous loading dose of 750 mg valproic acid beginning at 0800 H and lasting 60 minutes. The valproic acid concentration is 30 μg/mL before the third maintenance dose. What valproic acid dose is needed to achieve a steady-state concentration of 75 μg/mL?

1. *Enter the patient's demographic, drug dosing, and serum concentration–time data into the computer program.*

In this case, it is unlikely that the patient is at steady state, so the linear pharmacokinetics method cannot be used. Valproic acid doses are input as intravenous bolus doses.

2. *Compute the pharmacokinetic parameters for the patient with a Bayesian pharmacokinetics computer program.*

The pharmacokinetic parameters computed with the program are a volume of distribution of 8.9 L, a half-life of 15 hours, and clearance of 0.42 L/h.

3. *Compute the dose required to achieve the desired serum concentration of valproic acid.*

The one-compartment model, intravenous bolus equations used in the program to compute doses indicate that a dose of valproic acid 300 mg every 8 hours produces a steady-state concentration of 75 μg/mL.

PROBLEMS

The following problems are intended to emphasize computation of initial and individualized doses with clinical pharmacokinetic techniques. Clinicians always should consult the patient's chart to confirm that current anticonvulsant therapy is appropriate. All other medications that the patient is taking, including prescription and nonprescription drugs, should be recorded and checked to ascertain the risk of drug interaction with valproic acid.

1. CD is a 42-year-old, 85-kg (height, 185 cm) man who has tonic-clonic seizures. He needs therapy with oral valproic acid. He has normal liver function. Suggest an initial valproic acid dosage regimen designed to achieve a steady-state valproic acid concentration of 50 μg/mL.

2. Patient CD (see problem 1) is given a prescription for 750 mg every 12 hours of enteric coated divalproex sodium tablets for 1 month. Steady-state total concentration of valproic acid is 40 μg/mL. This patient is found to be compliant with the dosage regimen. Suggest a valproic acid dosage regimen designed to achieve a steady-state valproic acid concentration of 75 μg/mL.

3. BP is a 9-year-old, 35-kg (height, 137 cm) girl who has absence seizures. She needs therapy with oral valproic acid. She has normal liver function. Suggest an initial valproic acid dosage regimen designed to achieve a steady-state valproic acid concentration of 75 μg/mL.

4. Patient BP (see problem 3) is given a prescription for 150 mg three times a day (450 mg/d) of valproic acid syrup for 2 weeks. Steady-state total concentration of valproic

acid is 55 μg/mL. The patient is found to be compliant with the dosage regimen. Suggest a valproic acid dosage regimen designed to achieve a steady-state valproic acid concentration of 90 μg/mL.

5. PH is a 4-year-old, 22-kg (height, 102 cm) boy who has tonic-clonic seizures. He needs therapy with valproic acid syrup. He has normal liver function and also is being treated with carbamazepine. Suggest an initial valproic acid dosage regimen designed to achieve a steady-state valproic acid concentration of 50 μg/mL.

6. Patient PH (see problem 5) is given a prescription for 100 mg three times a day (300 mg/d) of valproic acid syrup for 1 week. Steady-state total concentration of valproic acid is 40 μg/mL. The patient is found to be compliant with the dosage regimen. Suggest a valproic acid dosage regimen designed to achieve a steady-state valproic acid concentration of 60 μg/mL.

7. FL is a 29-year-old, 75-kg (height, 180 cm) man who has tonic-clonic seizures. He needs therapy with oral valproic acid. He has normal liver function and is also undergoing phenytoin therapy. Suggest an initial valproic acid dosage regimen designed to achieve a steady-state valproic acid concentration of 50 μg/mL.

8. Patient FL (see problem 7) is given a prescription for 750 mg every 8 hours of enteric coated divalproex sodium tablets for 2 weeks. Steady-state total concentration of valproic acid is 55 μg/mL. The patient is found to be compliant with the dosage regimen. Suggest a valproic acid dosage regimen designed to achieve a steady-state valproic acid concentration of 90 μg/mL.

9. WE is a 55-year-old, 68-kg (height, 173 cm) man who has complex partial seizures. He is receiving 500 mg every 8 hours of oral enteric coated divalproex sodium tablets. He has normal liver function (bilirubin, 0.7 mg/dL; albumin, 4.0 g/dL) and also takes 800 mg/d of carbamazepine. Total valproic acid concentration is 22 μg/mL before the fourth dose. Compute a valproic acid dose that will provide a steady-state concentration of 50 μg/mL.

10. YF is a 5-year-old, 20-kg (height, 107 cm) girl who has tonic-clonic seizures. She is given a new prescription of 250 mg every 12 hours of oral valproic acid capsules. She has normal liver function and is receiving no enzyme inducers. Minimum valproic acid concentration before the third dose is 42 μg/mL. Compute a valproic acid dose that will provide a total steady-state concentration of 75 μg/mL.

ANSWERS TO PROBLEMS

1. Solution to problem 1.

Pharmacokinetic Dosing Method

1. *Estimate clearance and volume of distribution according to disease states and conditions present in the patient.*

The clearance rate for an adult patient not taking other drugs that induce hepatic drug metabolism is 7 to 12 mL/h per kilogram. At a value of 10 mL/h per kilogram the estimated clearance is 0.85 L/h: Cl = 85 kg · 10 mL/h/kg = 850 mL/h or 0.85 L/h. At 0.15 L/kg, the estimated volume of distribution is 13 L: 85 kg · 0.15 L/kg = 13 L.

2. *Estimate half-life and elimination rate constant.*

Once the correct clearance and volume of distribution estimates are identified for the patient, they can be converted into the valproic acid half-life ($t_{1/2}$) and elimination rate constant (k) estimates with the following equations: $t_{1/2} = (0.693 \cdot V)/Cl = (0.693 \cdot 13\ L)/(0.85\ L/h) = 11\ h$; $k = 0.693/t_{1/2} = 0.693/11\ h = 0.063\ h^{-1}$.

3. *Compute the dosage regimen.*

Oral enteric coated divalproex sodium tablets are prescribed to this patient (F = 1). (Note: μg/mL = mg/L, and this concentration unit was substituted for Css in the calculations to avoid unit conversion.) The dosage equation for oral valproic acid is $D = (Css \cdot Cl \cdot \tau)/F = (50\ mg/L \cdot 0.85\ L/h \cdot 12\ h)/1 = 510\ mg$, rounded to 500 mg every 12 hours.

Steady-state minimum serum concentration of valproic acid should be measured after steady state is attained in 3 to 5 half-lives. Because the drug is expected to have a half-life of 11 hours in this patient, steady-state concentration of valproic acid can be measured any time after the second day of dosing (5 half-lives = 5 · 11 h = 55 h). Serum concentration of valproic acid should be measured if the patient has an exacerbation of epilepsy or if the patient has signs or symptoms of valproic acid toxicity.

Literature-Based Recommended Dosing

1. *Estimate the valproic acid dose according to disease states and conditions present in the patient.*

Oral enteric coated divalproex sodium tablets are prescribed to this patient. The suggested initial maintenance dosage of valproic acid for an adult patient not taking enzyme inducers is 7.5 mg/kg per day: 85 kg · 7.5 mg/kg/d = 638 mg/d, rounded to 750 mg, or 250 mg every 8 hours. This dose is titrated upward in increments of 5 to 10 mg/kg per day every 1 to 2 weeks while the patient is observed for adverse and therapeutic effects. The goals of therapy are maximal suppression of seizures and avoidance of side effects.

Steady-state minimum total serum concentration of valproic acid should be measured after steady state is attained in 1 to 2 weeks. Serum concentration of valproic acid also should be measured if the patient has an exacerbation of epilepsy or if the patient has signs or symptoms of valproic acid toxicity.

2. Solution to problem 2.

Pseudolinear Pharmacokinetics Method

1. *Use pseudolinear pharmacokinetics to predict a new concentration for a dosage increase, then compute the 10% to 20% factor to account for nonlinear, concentration-dependent plasma protein binding pharmacokinetics.*

According to pseudolinear pharmacokinetics, the resulting total steady-state serum concentration of valproic acid is $D_{new} = (Css_{new}/Css_{old})D_{old}$ = [(75 μg/mL)/(40 μg/mL)] 1500 mg/d = 2813 mg/d, rounded to 3000 mg/d, or 1000 mg every 8 hours. Because of nonlinear, concentration-dependent protein binding pharmacokinetics, the total steady-state serum concentration is expected to be 10% less, or 0.90 times, to 20% less, or 0.80 times, than that predicted with linear pharmacokinetics: Css = 75 μg/mL · 0.90 = 68 μg/mL, and Css = 75 μg/mL · 0.80 = 60 μg/mL. Thus a dosage of 3000 mg/d is expected to yield a total steady-state serum concentration of valproic acid of 60 to 68 μg/mL.

Steady-state minimum total serum concentration of valproic acid should be measured after steady state is attained in 1 to 2 weeks. Serum concentration of valproic acid also should be measured if the patient has an exacerbation of their epilepsy or if the patient has signs or symptoms of valproic acid toxicity.

Pharmacokinetic Parameter Method

1. *Compute the pharmacokinetic parameters.*

The patient is expected to achieve steady-state conditions after 2 to 3 days of therapy. Valproic acid clearance can be computed with steady-state valproic acid concentration: $Cl = [F(D/\tau)]/Css$ = [1(750 mg/12 h)]/(40 mg/L) = 1.6 L/h. (Note: μg/mL = mg/L, and this concentration unit was substituted for Css in the calculations to avoid unit conversion.)

2. *Compute the valproic acid dose.*

Valproic acid clearance is used to compute the new dose: $D = (Css \cdot Cl \cdot \tau)/F$ = (75 mg/L · 1.6 L/h · 8 h)/1 = 960 mg, rounded to 1000 mg every 8 hours. (Note: dosage interval was changed to every 8 hours to avoid large single doses and gastrointestinal upset.)

Because of nonlinear, concentration-dependent protein binding pharmacokinetics, total steady-state serum concentration is expected to be 10% less, or 0.90 times, to 20% less, or 0.80 times, than that predicted with linear pharmacokinetics: Css = 75 μg/mL · 0.90 = 68 μg/mL, and Css = 75 μg/mL · 0.80 = 60 μg/mL. Thus a dose of 2000 mg/d is expected to yield a total steady-state serum concentration of valproic acid of 60 to 68 μg/mL.

Steady-state minimum total serum concentration of valproic acid should be measured after steady state is attained in 1 to 2 weeks. Serum concentration of valproic acid also should be measured if the patient has an exacerbation of epilepsy or if the patient has signs or symptoms of valproic acid toxicity.

Bayesian Pharmacokinetics Computer Program Method

1. *Enter the patient's demographic, drug dosing, and serum concentration–time data into the computer program.*

2. *Compute the pharmacokinetic parameters for the patient with a Bayesian pharmacokinetics computer program.*

The pharmacokinetic parameters computed with the program are a volume of distribution of 10.7 L, a half-life of 8.1 hours, and a clearance of 0.91 L/h.

3. *Compute the dose required to achieve the desired serum concentration of valproic acid.*

The one-compartment model, first-order absorption equations used by the program to compute doses indicate that a dose of 750 mg every 8 hours will produce a steady-state valproic acid concentration of 78 μg/mL.

3. Solution to problem 3.

Pharmacokinetic Dosing Method

1. *Estimate clearance and volume of distribution according to disease states and conditions present in the patient.*

The clearance rate for a pediatric patient not taking other drugs that induce hepatic drug metabolism is 10 to 20 mL/h per kilogram. At a value of 15 mL/h per kilogram, the estimated clearance is 0.53 L/h: Cl = 35 kg · 15 mL/h/kg = 525 mL/h, or 0.53 L/h. At 0.2 L/kg, the estimated volume of distribution is 7 L: 35 kg · 0.2 L/kg = 7 L.

2. *Estimate half-life and elimination rate constant.*

Once the correct clearance and volume of distribution estimates are identified for the patient, they can be converted into the valproic acid half-life ($t_{1/2}$) and elimination rate constant (k) estimates with the following equations: $t_{1/2} = (0.693 \cdot V)/Cl = (0.693 \cdot 7\ L)/(0.53\ L/h) = 9\ h$; $k = 0.693/t_{1/2} = 0.693/9\ h = 0.077\ h^{-1}$.

3. *Compute the dosage regimen.*

Oral valproic acid syrup is prescribed to this patient (F = 1). (Note: μg/mL = mg/L, and this concentration unit was substituted for Css in the calculations to avoid unit conversion.) The dosage equation for oral valproic acid is $D = (Css \cdot Cl \cdot \tau)/F = (75\ mg/L \cdot 0.53\ L/h \cdot 8\ h)/1 = 318\ mg$, rounded to 300 mg every 8 hours.

Steady-state minimum serum concentration of valproic acid should be measured after steady state is attained in 3 to 5 half-lives. Because the drug is expected to have a half-life of 9 hours in this patient, steady-state concentration of valproic acid can be measured any time after the second day of dosing (5 half-lives = 5 · 9 h = 45 h). Serum concentration of valproic acid should be measured if the patient has an exacerbation of seizures or if the patient has signs or symptoms of valproic acid toxicity.

Literature-Based Recommended Dosing

1. *Estimate the valproic acid dose according to disease states and conditions present in the patient.*

Oral valproic acid syrup is prescribed to this patient. The suggested initial maintenance dosage of valproic acid for a pediatric patient not taking enzyme inducers is 10 mg/kg per day: 35 kg · 10 mg/kg/d = 350 mg/d, rounded to 400 mg, or 200 mg every 12 hours. This dose is titrated upward in increments of 5 to 10 mg/kg per day every 1 to

2 weeks while the patient is observed for adverse and therapeutic effects. The goals of therapy are maximal suppression of seizures and avoidance of side effects.

Steady-state minimum total serum concentration of valproic acid should be measured after steady state is attained in 1 to 2 weeks. Serum concentration of valproic acid also should be measured if the patient has an exacerbation of epilepsy or if the patient has signs or symptoms of valproic acid toxicity.

4. Solution to problem 4.

Pseudolinear Pharmacokinetics Method

1. *Use pseudolinear pharmacokinetics to predict a new concentration for a dosage increase, then compute the 10% to 20% factor to account for nonlinear, concentration-dependent plasma protein binding pharmacokinetics.*

According to pseudolinear pharmacokinetics, the resulting total steady-state serum concentration of valproic acid is $D_{new} = (Css_{new}/Css_{old})D_{old}$ = [(90 μg/mL)/(55 μg/mL)] 450 mg/d = 736 mg/d, rounded to 750 mg/d, or 250 mg every 8 hours. Because of nonlinear, concentration-dependent protein binding pharmacokinetics, the total steady-state serum concentration is expected to be 10% less, or 0.90 times, to 20% less, or 0.80 times, than that predicted with linear pharmacokinetics: Css = 90 μg/mL · 0.90 = 81 μg/mL, and Css = 90 μg/mL · 0.80 = 72 μg/mL. Thus a dosage of 750 mg/d is expected to yield a total steady-state serum concentration of valproic acid of 72 to 81 μg/mL.

Steady-state minimum total serum concentration of valproic acid should be measured after steady state is attained in 1 to 2 weeks. Serum concentration of valproic acid also should be measured if the patient has an exacerbation of epilepsy or if the patient has signs or symptoms of valproic acid toxicity.

Pharmacokinetic Parameter Method

1. *Compute the pharmacokinetic parameters.*

The patient is expected to achieve steady-state conditions after 2 to 3 days of therapy. Valproic acid clearance can be computed with a steady-state valproic acid concentration: Cl = [F(D/τ)]/Css = [1(150 mg/8 h)]/(55 mg/L) = 0.34 L/h. (Note: μg/mL = mg/L, and this concentration unit was substituted for Css in the calculations to avoid unit conversion.)

2. *Compute the valproic acid dose.*

Valproic acid clearance is used to compute the new dose: D = (Css · Cl · τ)/F = (90 mg/L · 0.34 L/h · 8 h)/1 = 245 mg, rounded to 250 mg every 8 hours.

Because of nonlinear, concentration-dependent protein binding pharmacokinetics, total steady-state serum concentration is expected to be 10% less, or 0.90 times, to 20% less, or 0.80 times, than that predicted with linear pharmacokinetics: Css = 90 μg/mL · 0.90 = 81 μg/mL, and Css = 90 μg/mL · 0.80 = 72 μg/mL. Thus a dosage of 750 mg/d is expected to yield a total steady-state serum concentration of valproic acid of 72 to 81 μg/mL.

Steady-state minimum total serum concentration of valproic acid should be measured after steady state is attained in 1 to 2 weeks. Serum concentration of valproic acid also should be measured if the patient has an exacerbation of epilepsy or if the patient has signs or symptoms of valproic acid toxicity.

Bayesian Pharmacokinetics Computer Program Method

1. *Enter the patient's demographic, drug dosing, and serum concentration–time data into the computer program.*

2. *Compute the pharmacokinetic parameters for the patient with a Bayesian pharmacokinetics computer program.*

The pharmacokinetic parameters computed with the program are a volume of distribution of 2 L, a half-life of 6.4 hours, and a clearance of 0.21 L/h.

3. *Compute the dose required to achieve the desired serum concentration of valproic acid.*

The one-compartment model, first-order absorption equations used in the program to compute doses indicate that a dose of 250 mg every 8 hours produces a steady-state valproic acid concentration of 100 μg/mL.

5. Solution to problem 5.

Pharmacokinetic Dosing Method

1. *Estimate clearance and volume of distribution according to disease states and conditions present in the patient.*

The clearance rate for a pediatric patient who takes other drugs that induce hepatic drug metabolism is 20 to 30 mL/h per kilogram. At a value of 25 mL/h per kilogram the estimated clearance is 0.55 L/h: $Cl = 22\ kg \cdot 25\ mL/h/kg = 550\ mL/h$, or 0.55 L/h. At 0.2 L/kg, the estimated volume of distribution is 4.4 L: $22\ kg \cdot 0.2\ L/kg = 4.4\ L$.

2. *Estimate half-life and elimination rate constant.*

Once the correct clearance and volume of distribution estimates are identified for the patient, they can be converted into the valproic acid half-life ($t_{1/2}$) and elimination rate constant (k) estimates with the following equations: $t_{1/2} = (0.693 \cdot V)/Cl = (0.693 \cdot 4.4\ L)/(0.55\ L/h) = 5.5\ h$; $k = 0.693/t_{1/2} = 0.693/5.5\ h = 0.126\ h^{-1}$.

3. *Compute the dosage regimen.*

Oral valproic acid syrup is prescribed to this patient (F = 1). (Note: μg/mL = mg/L, and this concentration unit was substituted for Css in the calculations to avoid unit conversion.) The dosage equation for oral valproic acid is $D = (Css \cdot Cl \cdot \tau)/F = (50\ mg/L \cdot 0.55\ L/h \cdot 8\ h)/1 = 220\ mg$, rounded to 250 mg every 8 hours.

Steady-state minimum serum concentration of valproic acid should be measured after steady state is attained in 3 to 5 half-lives. Because the drug is expected to have a half-life of 5.5 hours in this patient, steady-state concentration of valproic acid can be measured any time after the first day of dosing (5 half-lives = 5 · 5.5 h = 28 h). Serum concentration of valproic acid should be measured if the patient has an exacerbation of seizures or if the patient has signs or symptoms of valproic acid toxicity.

Literature-Based Recommended Dosing

1. *Estimate the valproic acid dose according to disease states and conditions present in the patient.*

Oral valproic acid syrup is prescribed to this patient. The suggested initial maintenance dosage of valproic acid for a pediatric patient taking enzyme inducers is 20 mg/kg per day: 22 kg · 20 mg/kg/d = 440 mg/d, rounded to 400 mg, or 200 mg every 12 hours. This dose is titrated upward in increments of 5 to 10 mg/kg per day every 1 to 2 weeks while the patient is observed for adverse and therapeutic effects. The goals of therapy are maximal suppression of seizures and avoidance of side effects.

Steady-state minimum total serum concentration of valproic acid should be measured after steady state is attained in 1 to 2 weeks. Serum concentration of valproic acid also should be measured if the patient has an exacerbation of epilepsy or if the patient has signs or symptoms of valproic acid toxicity.

6. Solution to problem 6.

Pseudolinear Pharmacokinetics Method

1. *Use pseudolinear pharmacokinetics to predict a new concentration for a dosage increase, then compute the 10% to 20% factor to account for nonlinear, concentration-dependent plasma protein binding pharmacokinetics.*

According to pseudolinear pharmacokinetics, the resulting total steady-state serum concentration of valproic acid is $D_{new} = (Css_{new}/Css_{old})D_{old}$ = [(60 μg/mL)/(40 μg/mL)] 300 mg/d = 450 mg/d, 150 mg every 8 hours. Because of nonlinear, concentration-dependent protein binding pharmacokinetics, the total steady-state serum concentration is expected to be 10% less, or 0.90 times, to 20% less, or 0.80 times, than that predicted with linear pharmacokinetics: Css = 60 μg/mL · 0.90 = 54 μg/mL, and Css = 60 μg/mL · 0.80 = 48 μg/mL. Thus a dosage of 450 mg/d is expected to yield a total steady-state serum concentration of valproic acid of 48 to 54 μg/mL.

Steady-state minimum total serum concentration of valproic acid should be measured after steady state is attained in 1 to 2 weeks. Serum concentration of valproic acid also should be measured if the patient has an exacerbation of epilepsy or if the patient has signs or symptoms of valproic acid toxicity.

Pharmacokinetic Parameter Method

1. *Compute the pharmacokinetic parameters.*

The patient is expected to achieve steady-state conditions after 2 to 3 days of therapy. Valproic acid clearance can be computed with steady-state valproic acid concentration: $Cl = [F(D/\tau)]/Css$ = [1(100 mg/8 h)]/(40 mg/L) = 0.31 L/h. (Note: μg/mL = mg/L, and this concentration unit was substituted for Css in the calculations to avoid unit conversion.)

2. *Compute the valproic acid dose.*

Valproic acid clearance is used to compute the new dose: D = (Css · Cl · τ)/F = (60 mg/L · 0.31 L/h · 8 h)/1 = 149 mg, rounded to 150 mg every 8 hours.

Because of nonlinear, concentration-dependent protein binding pharmacokinetics, total steady-state serum concentration is expected to be 10% less, or 0.90 times, to 20% less, or 0.80 times, than that predicted with linear pharmacokinetics: Css = 60 μg/mL · 0.90 = 54 μg/mL, and Css = 60 μg/mL · 0.80 = 48 μg/mL. Thus a dosage of 450 mg/d is expected to yield a total steady-state serum concentration of valproic acid of 48 to 54 μg/mL.

Steady-state minimum total serum concentration of valproic acid should be measured after steady state is attained in 1 to 2 weeks. Serum concentration of valproic acid also should be measured if the patient has an exacerbation of epilepsy or if the patient has signs or symptoms of valproic acid toxicity.

Bayesian Pharmacokinetics Computer Program Method

1. *Enter the patient's demographic, drug dosing, and serum concentration–time data into the computer program.*

2. *Compute the pharmacokinetic parameters for the patient with a Bayesian pharmacokinetics computer program.*

The pharmacokinetic parameters computed with the program are a volume of distribution of 2.9 L, a half-life of 8.9 hours, and a clearance of 0.23 L/h.

3. *Compute the dose required to achieve the desired serum concentration of valproic acid.*

The one-compartment model, first-order absorption equations used in the program to compute doses indicate that a dose of 150 mg every 8 hours produces a steady-state concentration of valproic acid of 64 μg/mL.

7. Solution to problem 7.

Pharmacokinetic Dosing Method

1. *Estimate clearance and volume of distribution according to disease states and conditions present in the patient.*

The clearance rate for an adult patient taking other drugs that induce hepatic drug metabolism is 15 to 18 mL/h per kilogram. At a value of 16 mL/h per kilogram, the estimated clearance would equal 1.2 L/h: Cl = 75 kg · 16 mL/h/kg = 1200 mL/h or 1.2 L/h. At 0.15 L/kg, the estimated volume of distribution would be 11 L: 75 kg · 0.15 L/kg = 11 L.

2. *Estimate half-life and elimination rate constant.*

Once the correct clearance and volume of distribution estimates are identified for the patient, they can be converted into valproic acid half-life ($t_{1/2}$) and elimination rate constant (k) estimates with the following equations: $t_{1/2} = (0.693 \cdot V)/Cl = (0.693 \cdot 11\ L)/(1.2\ L/h) = 6\ h$; $k = 0.693/t_{1/2} = 0.693/6\ h = 0.116\ h^{-1}$.

3. *Compute the dosage regimen.*

Oral enteric coated divalproex sodium tablets are prescribed to this patient (F = 1). (Note: μg/mL = mg/L, and this concentration unit was substituted for Css in the calculations to avoid unit conversion.) The dosage equation for oral valproic acid is $D = (Css \cdot Cl \cdot \tau)/F = (50 \text{ mg/L} \cdot 1.2 \text{ L/h} \cdot 8 \text{ h})/1 = 480$ mg, rounded to 500 mg every 8 hours.

Steady-state minimum serum concentration of valproic acid should be measured after steady state is attained in 3 to 5 half-lives. Because the drug is expected to have a half-life of 6 hours in this patient, steady-state concentration of valproic acid can be measured any time after the second day of dosing (5 half-lives = 5 · 6 h = 30 h). Serum concentration of valproic acid should be measured if the patient has an exacerbation of epilepsy or if the patient has signs or symptoms of valproic acid toxicity.

Literature-Based Recommended Dosing

1. *Estimate the valproic acid dose according to disease states and conditions present in the patient.*

Oral enteric coated divalproex sodium tablets are prescribed to this patient. The suggested initial maintenance dosage of valproic acid for an adult patient taking enzyme inducers is 15 mg/kg per day: 75 kg · 15 mg/kg/d = 1125 mg/d, rounded to 1000 mg, or 500 mg every 12 hours. This dose is titrated upward in increments of 5 to 10 mg/kg per day every 1 to 2 weeks while the patient is observed for adverse and therapeutic effects. The goals of therapy are maximal suppression of seizures and avoidance of side effects.

Steady-state minimum total serum concentration of valproic acid should be measured after steady state is attained in 1 to 2 weeks. Serum concentration of valproic acid should be measured if the patient has an exacerbation of epilepsy or if the patient has signs or symptoms of valproic acid toxicity.

8. Solution to problem 8.

Pseudolinear Pharmacokinetics Method

1. *Use pseudolinear pharmacokinetics to predict a new concentration for a dosage increase, then compute the 10% to 20% factor to account for nonlinear, concentration-dependent plasma protein binding pharmacokinetics.*

According to pseudolinear pharmacokinetics, the resulting total steady-state serum concentration of valproic acid is $D_{new} = (Css_{new}/Css_{old})D_{old} = [(90 \text{ μg/mL})/(55 \text{ μg/mL})]\ 2250$ mg/d = 3682 mg/d, rounded to 3750 mg/d, or 1250 mg every 8 hours. Because of nonlinear, concentration-dependent protein binding pharmacokinetics, the total steady-state serum concentration is expected to be 10% less, or 0.90 times, to 20% less, or 0.80 times, than that predicted with linear pharmacokinetics: Css = 90 μg/mL · 0.90 = 81 μg/mL, and Css = 90 μg/mL · 0.80 = 72 μg/mL. Thus a dosage of 3750 mg/d is expected to yield a total steady-state serum concentration of valproic acid of 72 to 81 μg/mL.

Steady-state minimum total serum concentration of valproic acid should be measured after steady state is attained in 1 to 2 weeks. Serum concentration of valproic acid also should be measured if the patient has an exacerbation of epilepsy or if the patient has signs or symptoms of valproic acid toxicity.

Pharmacokinetic Parameter Method

1. *Compute the pharmacokinetic parameters.*

The patient is expected to achieve steady-state conditions after 2 to 3 days of therapy. Valproic acid clearance can be computed with steady-state valproic acid concentration: Cl = [F(D/τ)]/Css = [1(750 mg/8 h)]/(55 mg/L) = 1.7 L/h. (Note: μg/mL = mg/L, and this concentration unit was substituted for Css in the calculations to avoid unit conversion.)

2. *Compute the valproic acid dose.*

Valproic acid clearance is used to compute the new dose: D = (Css · Cl · τ)/F = (90 mg/L · 1.7 L/h · 8 h)/1 = 1224 mg, rounded to 1250 mg every 8 hours.

Because of nonlinear, concentration-dependent protein binding pharmacokinetics, total steady-state serum concentration is expected to be 10% less, or 0.90 times, to 20% less, or 0.80 times, than that predicted with linear pharmacokinetics: Css = 90 μg/mL · 0.90 = 81 μg/mL, and Css = 90 μg/mL · 0.80 = 72 μg/mL. Thus a dosage of 3750 mg/d is expected to yield a total steady-state serum concentration of valproic acid of 72 to 81 μg/mL.

Steady-state minimum total serum concentration of valproic acid should be measured after steady state is attained in 1 to 2 weeks. Serum concentration of valproic acid also should be measured if the patient has an exacerbation of epilepsy or if the patient has signs or symptoms of valproic acid toxicity.

Bayesian Pharmacokinetics Computer Program Method

1. *Enter the patient's demographic, drug dosing, and serum concentration–time data into the computer program.*

2. *Compute the pharmacokinetic parameters for the patient with a Bayesian pharmacokinetics computer program.*

The pharmacokinetic parameters computed with the program are a volume of distribution of 9 L, a half-life of 6.1 hours, and a clearance of 1 L/h.

3. *Compute the dose required to achieve the desired serum concentration of valproic acid.*

The one-compartment model, first-order absorption equations used in the program to compute doses indicate that a dose of 1000 mg every 8 hours produces a steady-state concentration of valproic acid of 82 μg/mL.

9. Solution to problem 9.

Bayesian Pharmacokinetics Computer Program Method

1. *Enter the patient's demographic, drug dosing, and serum concentration–time data into the computer program.*

2. *Compute the pharmacokinetic parameters for the patient with a Bayesian pharmacokinetics computer program.*

The pharmacokinetic parameters computed with the program are a volume of distribution of 6.8 L, a half-life of 3.9 hours, and a clearance of 1.2 L/h.

3. *Compute the dose required to achieve the desired serum concentration of valproic acid.*

The one-compartment model, first-order absorption equations used in the program to compute doses indicate that a dose of 1000 mg every 8 hours produces a steady-state concentration of valproic acid of 50 μg/mL.

10. Solution to problem 10.

Bayesian Pharmacokinetics Computer Program Method

1. *Enter the patient's demographic, drug dosing, and serum concentration–time data into the computer program.*

2. *Compute the pharmacokinetic parameters for the patient with a Bayesian pharmacokinetics computer program.*

The pharmacokinetic parameters computed with the program are a volume of distribution of 4.3 L, a half-life of 9.2 hours, and a clearance of 0.32 L/h.

3. *Compute the dose required to achieve the desired serum concentration of valproic acid.*

The one-compartment model, first-order absorption equations used in the program to compute doses indicate that a dose of 250 mg every 8 hours produces a steady-state valproic acid concentration of 70 μg/mL. (Note: dosage interval was decreased to avoid excessive doses and gastrointestinal side effects.)

REFERENCES

1. Brodie MJ, Dichter MA. Antiepileptic drugs. N Engl J Med 1996;334:168–75.
2. McNamara JO. Drugs effective in the therapy of the epilepsies. In: Hardman JG, Limbird LE, Molinoff PB, Ruddon RW, Gilman AG, eds. The pharmacological basis of therapeutics. New York: McGraw-Hill, 1996:461–86.
3. Kodama Y, Koike Y, Kimoto H, et al. Binding parameters of valproic acid to serum protein in healthy adults at steady state. Ther Drug Monit 1992;14:55–60.
4. Bauer LA, Davis R, Wilensky A, Raisys V, Levy RH. Valproic acid clearance: unbound fraction and diurnal variation in young and elderly adults. Clin Pharmacol Ther 1985;37:697–700.
5. Urien S, Albengres E, Tillement JP. Serum protein binding of valproic acid in healthy subjects and in patients with liver disease. Int J Clin Pharmacol Ther Toxicol 1981;19:319–25.
6. Brewster D, Muir NC. Valproate plasma protein binding in the uremic condition. Clin Pharmacol Ther 1980;27:76–82.
7. Bruni J, Wang LH, Marbury TC, Lee CS, Wilder BJ. Protein binding of valproic acid in uremic patients. Neurology 1980;30:557–9.
8. Gugler R, Mueller G. Plasma protein binding of valproic acid in healthy subjects and in patients with renal disease. Br J Clin Pharmacol 1978;5:441–6.

9. Graves NM, Garnett WR. Epilepsy. In: DiPiro JT, Talbert RL, Yee GC, Matzke GR, Wells BG, Posey LM, eds. Pharmacotherapy: a pathophysiologic approach. Stamford, CT: Appleton & Lange, 1999:952–75.
10. Garnett WR. Antiepileptics. In: Schumacher GE, ed. Therapeutic drug monitoring. Stamford, CT: Appleton & Lange, 1995:345–95.
11. Zaccara G, Messori A, Moroni F. Clinical pharmacokinetics of valproic acid—1988. Clin Pharmacokinet 1988;15:367–89.
12. Hall K, Otten N, Johnston B, Irvine-Meek J, Leroux M, Seshia S. A multivariable analysis of factors governing the steady-state pharmacokinetics of valproic acid in 52 young epileptics. J Clin Pharmacol 1985;25:261–8.
13. Cloyd JC, Kriel RL, Fischer JH. Valproic acid pharmacokinetics in children, II: discontinuation of concomitant antiepileptic drug therapy. Neurology 1985;35:1623–7.
14. Chiba K, Suganuma T, Ishizaki T, et al. Comparison of steady-state pharmacokinetics of valproic acid in children between monotherapy and multiple antiepileptic drug treatment. J Pediatr 1985;106:653–8.
15. Gugler R, von Unruh GE. Clinical pharmacokinetics of valproic acid. Clin Pharmacokinet 1980;5:67–83.
16. Klotz U, Rapp T, Muller WA. Disposition of valproic acid in patients with liver disease. Eur J Clin Pharmacol 1978;13:55–60.
17. Pugh RN, Murray-Lyon IM, Dawson JL, Pietroni MC, Williams R. Transection of the oesophagus for bleeding oesophageal varices. Br J Surg 1973;60:646–9.
18. Omtzigt JG, Nau H, Los FJ, Pijpers L, Lindhout D. The disposition of valproate and its metabolites in the late first trimester and early second trimester of pregnancy in maternal serum, urine, and amniotic fluid: effect of dose, co-medication, and the presence of spina bifida. Eur J Clin Pharmacol 1992;43:381–8.
19. Bauer LA, Davis R, Wilensky A, Raisys V, Levy RH. Diurnal variation in valproic acid clearance. Clin Pharmacol Ther 1984;35:505–9.
20. Kandrotas RJ, Love JM, Gal P, Oles KS. The effect of hemodialysis and hemoperfusion on serum valproic acid concentration. Neurology 1990;40:1456–8.
21. Hansten PD, Horn JR. Drug interactions analysis and management. Vancouver, WA: Applied Therapeutics, 1999:480.
22. Bauer LA, Harris C, Wilensky AJ, Raisys VA, Levy RH. Ethosuximide kinetics: possible interaction with valproic acid. Clin Pharmacol Ther 1982;31:741–5.
23. Trapnell CB, Klecker RW, Jamis-Dow C, Collins JM. Glucuronidation of 3′-azido-3′-deoxythymidine (zidovudine) by human liver microsomes: relevance to clinical pharmacokinetic interactions with atovaquone, fluconazole, methadone, and valproic acid. Antimicrob Agents Chemother 1998;42:1592–6.
24. Pisani FD, Di Perri RG. Intravenous valproate: effects on plasma and saliva phenytoin levels. Neurology 1981;31:467–70.
25. Perucca E, Hebdige S, Frigo GM, Gatti G, Lecchini S, Crema A. Interaction between phenytoin and valproic acid: plasma protein binding and metabolic effects. Clin Pharmacol Ther 1980;28:779–89.
26. Riva R, Albani F, Contin M, et al. Time-dependent interaction between phenytoin and valproic acid. Neurology 1985;35:510–5.
27. Frigo GM, Lecchini S, Gatti G, Perucca E, Crema A. Modification of phenytoin clearance by valproic acid in normal subjects. Br J Clin Pharmacol 1979;8:553–6.
28. Wandell M, Mungall D. Computer assisted drug interpretation and drug regimen optimization. Am Assoc Clin Chem 1984;6:1–11.

13

PHENOBARBITAL/PRIMIDONE

INTRODUCTION

Phenobarbital is a barbiturate, and primidone is a deoxybarbiturate. These agents are effective in the management of generalized tonic-clonic and partial seizures (Table 13-1).[1] Phenobarbital is available as a separate agent but is also an active metabolite produced through hepatic metabolism during primidone treatment. Because of this, and because they share a similar antiseizure spectrum, these two drugs are considered together in this chapter. The probable mechanism of action of phenobarbital is elevation of seizure threshold by interacting with γ-aminobutyric $acid_A$ ($GABA_A$) postsynaptic receptors. This interaction potentiates synaptic inhibition.[2,3] Although the exact mechanism of action of the antiepileptic effect of primidone is not known, a portion of the antiseizure activity is produced by the active metabolites phenobarbital and phenylethylmalonamide (PEMA).[2,3]

THERAPEUTIC AND TOXIC CONCENTRATIONS

The therapeutic ranges for phenobarbital and primidone are defined by most laboratories as 15 to 40 μg/mL and 5 to 12 μg/mL, respectively. When primidone is given, sufficient doses usually are administered to produce therapeutic concentrations of both phenobarbital and primidone. At present, concentrations of the other possible active metabolite of primidone, PEMA, are not routinely measured. Although results of animal experiments indicate that primidone has inherent antiseizure activity, some clinicians believe that phenobarbital is the predominate species responsible for the therapeutic effect of primidone in humans.[4] Because phenobarbital and PEMA are produced through hepatic metabolism

TABLE 13-1 International Classification of Epileptic Seizures

MAJOR CLASS	SUBSET OF CLASS	DRUG THERAPY FOR SELECTED SEIZURE TYPE
Partial seizures (beginning locally)	1. Simple partial seizures (without impaired consciousness) a. With motor symptoms b. With somatosensory or special sensory symptoms c. With autonomic symptoms d. With psychological symptoms	Carbamazepine Phenytoin Valproic acid Phenobarbital Primidone
	2. Complex partial seizures (with impaired consciousness) a. Simple partial onset followed by impaired consciousness b. Impaired consciousness at onset	Carbamazepine Phenytoin Valproic acid Phenobarbital Primidone
	3. Partial seizures evolving into secondary generalized seizures	Carbamazepine Phenytoin Valproic acid Phenobarbital Primidone
Generalized seizures (convulsive or nonconvulsive)	1. Absence seizures (typical or atypical; also known as petit mal seizures)	Valproic acid Ethosuximide
	2. Tonic-clonic seizures (also known as grand mal seizures)	Phenytoin Carbamazepine Valproic acid Phenobarbital Primidone

Adapted from Brodie MJ, Dichter MA. Antiepileptic drugs. N Engl J Med 1996;334:168–75.

of primidone, it is difficult to study the antiepileptic activity of primidone alone in patients.

The most common concentration-related adverse effects of phenobarbital involve the central nervous system. They include ataxia, headache, unsteadiness, sedation, confusion, and lethargy.[2,5] Other concentration-related side effects are nausea and, in children, irritability and hyperactivity. At phenobarbital concentrations greater than 60 μg/mL, stupor and coma can occur. During long-term treatment with phenobarbital, changes in behavior, porphyria, decreased cognitive function, and osteomalacia can occur. For primidone, concentration-related side effects include nausea, vomiting, diplopia, dizziness, sedation, unsteadiness, and ataxia.[2,5] Slow dosage titration, administration of smaller doses, and more frequent dosing of the drug usually produce relief of these side effects. Long-term treatment with primidone is associated with behavioral changes, decreased cognitive function, and disorders of the connective tissue. Some of the adverse effects that occur during treatment with primidone may be caused by phenobarbital. Idiosyncratic side effects independent of concentration of both drugs include skin rash and blood dyscrasia.

CLINICAL MONITORING PARAMETERS

The goals of therapy with anticonvulsants are to reduce seizure frequency and maximize quality of life with a minimum of adverse drug effects. Although it is desirable to abolish all seizure episodes, it may not be possible to accomplish this for many patients. Patients should be observed for concentration-related side effects (diplopia, ataxia, dizziness, headache, unsteadiness, sedation, confusion, lethargy) and gastrointestinal upset (nausea, vomiting) when receiving these drugs. Serious but rare idiosyncratic side effects include connective tissue disorders, blood dyscrasia, and skin rash.

Serum concentrations of phenobarbital, or of primidone plus phenobarbital for those receiving primidone therapy, should be measured for most patients. Because epilepsy is an episodic disease, patients do not have seizures on a continuous basis. Thus, during dosage titration it is difficult to determine whether a patient is responding to drug therapy or simply is not having abnormal central nervous system discharges at that time. Measurement of serum concentration is a valuable tool to avoid adverse drug effects. Patients are more likely to accept drug therapy if adverse reactions are held to the absolute minimum.

BASIC CLINICAL PHARMACOKINETIC PARAMETERS

Phenobarbital is eliminated primarily (65% to 70%) through hepatic metabolism to inactive metabolites.[6] About 30% to 35% of a phenobarbital dose is recovered as unchanged drug in the urine. Renal excretion of unchanged phenobarbital is pH dependent; alkaline urine increases renal clearance. Phenobarbital is about 50% bound to plasma proteins. The absolute bioavailability of oral phenobarbital in humans approaches 100%.[7] Phenobarbital is available in tablet (15, 16, 30, 60, and 100 mg), capsule (16 mg), elixir (15 and 20 mg/5 mL), and injectable (30, 60, 65, and 130 mg/mL for intravenous or intramuscular use) forms. The typical maintenance dose of phenobarbital is 2.5 to 5 mg/kg per day for neonates, 3 to 4.5 mg/kg per day for children younger than 10 years, and 1.5 to 2 mg/kg per day for older patients.[2,5] For the immediate management of status epilepticus, intravenous phenobarbital doses of 15 to 20 mg/kg are used.

Primidone is eliminated through hepatic metabolism (40% to 60%) and renal excretion of unchanged drug (40% to 60%).[8] In adults, approximately 15% to 20% of a primidone dose is converted by the liver into phenobarbital. PEMA is another active metabolite of primidone.[8,9] When treatment with primidone is begun, PEMA can be detected after the first dose, but phenobarbital concentration may not be measurable for 5 to 7 days (Figure 13-1). Primidone does not bind substantially to plasma proteins in humans. Because an intravenous form of the drug is not commercially available, the absolute bioavailability of primidone in humans is not known. Primidone is available as tablets (50 and 250 mg) and oral suspension (250 mg/5 mL). The usual maintenance dose of primidone is 12 to 20 mg/kg per day for neonates, 12 to 23 mg/kg per day for children younger than 15 years, and 10 to 25 mg/kg per day for older patients.

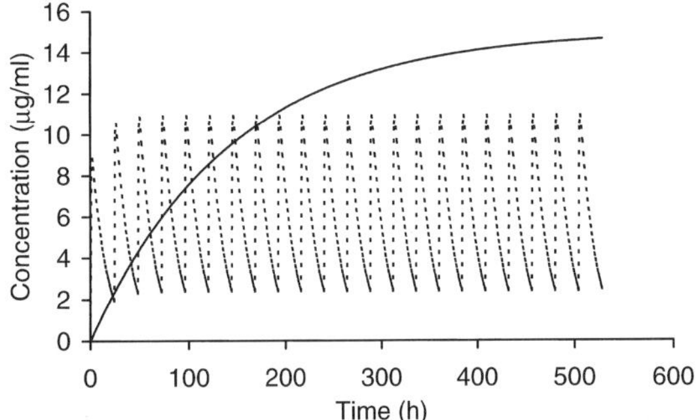

FIGURE 13-1 Primidone and phenobarbital concentrations after administration of primidone. Primidone concentration fluctuates over the dosage interval with a half-life of 8 to 15 hours, but phenobarbital accumulates slowly with an average half-life of 100 hours in adults as primidone is converted to phenobarbital. Because of this, primidone concentration achieves steady state long before phenobarbital concentration reaches steady state. To measure steady-state serum concentrations of both drugs, one must wait at least 3 to 4 weeks after a change in primidone dosage.

EFFECTS OF DISEASES AND CONDITIONS ON PHARMACOKINETICS AND DOSING

The clearance rate (Cl) of phenobarbital for children 12 years and older and for adults is 4 mL/h per kilogram. For children younger than 12 years, it is 8 mL/h per kilogram.[5,7,10] The volume of distribution (V) is 0.7 L/kg, and the half-life averages 120 hours in neonates (0 to 4 weeks of age), 60 hours in infants and children (2 months and older), and 100 hours in adults. Although results of only limited studies involving patients with hepatic disease are available, a 50% increase in half-life occurs among adults with cirrhosis of the liver or acute viral hepatitis.[11] These findings suggest that patients with cirrhosis of the liver or acute hepatitis may have reduced phenobarbital clearance because of destruction of liver parenchyma. This loss of functional hepatic cells reduces the amount of enzymes available to metabolize the drug and decreases clearance. An index of liver dysfunction can be gained by applying the Child-Pugh clinical classification system (Table 13-2).[12] Child-Pugh scores are discussed in detail in Chapter 3, but are discussed briefly here.

The Child-Pugh score consists of five laboratory tests or clinical symptoms: serum albumin, total bilirubin, prothrombin time, ascites, and hepatic encephalopathy. Each of these areas is given a score of 1 (normal) to 3 (severely abnormal; see Table 13-2), and the scores for the five areas are summed. The Child-Pugh score for a patient with normal liver function is 5, and the score for a patient with grossly abnormal serum albumin, total bilirubin, and prothrombin time values in addition to severe ascites and hepatic encephalopathy is 15. A Child-Pugh score greater than 8 is grounds for a decrease of 25% to 50% in the initial daily dose of phenobarbital. As for any patient with or without liver dysfunction, initial doses are meant as starting points for dosage titration based on patient response and avoidance of adverse effects. Serum concentration of phenobarbital and the presence of adverse drug effects should be monitored frequently in the care of patients with cirrhosis of the liver. Because phenobarbital is also eliminated by the kidney, patients with renal dysfunction (creatinine clearance, <30 mL/min) receiving phenobarbital

TABLE 13-2 Child-Pugh Scores for Patients with Liver Disease

TEST/SYMPTOM	SCORE 1 POINT	SCORE 2 POINTS	SCORE 3 POINTS
Total bilirubin (mg/dL)	<2.0	2.0–3.0	>3.0
Serum albumin (g/dL)	>3.5	2.8–3.5	<2.8
Prothrombin time (seconds prolonged over control)	<4	4–6	>6
Ascites	Absent	Slight	Moderate
Hepatic encephalopathy	None	Moderate	Severe

Adapted from Pugh RN, Murray-Lyon IM, Dawson JL, Pietroni MC, Williams R. Transection of the oesophagus for bleeding oesophageal varices. Br J Surg 1973;60:646–9.

should be closely observed. Phenobarbital is significantly removed (~30% of total body amount) during hemodialysis, and supplemental doses may have to be given after a dialysis session. Phenobarbital enters the breast milk, so nursing infants should be monitored for possible adverse drug reactions.[13]

The clearance rate (Cl/F) of primidone for patients 12 years and older taking primidone alone is 35 mL/h per kilogram.[14] However, the clearance rate of primidone increases to 50 mL/h per kilogram for older patients if they are receiving concurrent therapy with phenytoin or carbamazepine.[14] Among children, primidone clearance averages 125 mL/h per kilogram.[15] The volume of distribution (V/F) is 0.7 L/kg, and the half-life averages 8 hours in adults taking phenytoin or carbamazepine and children younger than 12 years and 15 hours among adults taking primidone alone.[5,14,15] No results of studies involving patients with hepatic or renal disease are available. However, because almost equal amounts of primidone are eliminated by the liver and kidney, patients with renal or hepatic dysfunction receiving primidone should be closely observed. A Child-Pugh score greater than 8 or creatinine clearance less than 30 mL/min is grounds for a decrease of 25% to 50% in the initial daily dose of primidone. As in the care of any patient with or without liver dysfunction, initial doses are meant as starting points for dosage titration based on patient response and avoidance of adverse effects. Serum concentrations of primidone and phenobarbital and the presence of adverse drug effects should be monitored frequently for patients with liver or kidney disease taking primidone. Primidone is significantly removed (~30% of total body amount) during hemodialysis, and supplemental doses may have to be given after a dialysis session.

DRUG INTERACTIONS

Phenobarbital is a potent inducer of hepatic drug metabolism for the CYP1A2, CYP2C9, and CYP3A4 enzyme systems.[16] Because phenobarbital also is a metabolite produced during primidone therapy, primidone has similar drug interaction potential. Because phenobarbital is such a broad-based hepatic enzyme inducer, patients should be observed closely for drug interactions whenever either of these agents is added to a therapeutic regimen. A brief list of compounds the metabolism and clearance of which are increased by concurrent phenobarbital treatment includes carbamazepine, lamotrigine, valproic acid, cyclosporine, nifedipine, diltiazem, verapamil, oral contraceptives, tricyclic antidepressants, quinidine, theophylline, and warfarin. Other anticonvulsants that decrease the metabolism and clearance of phenobarbital are felbamate and valproic acid. Phenytoin also may have an interaction with phenobarbital in which the agents change the metabolism and clearance of each other. The result of this drug interaction is quite variable; it can be an increase, decrease, or no change in the steady-state concentration of both drugs. Primidone metabolism and clearance are increased by carbamazepine and phenytoin treatment, whereas valproic acid therapy decreases primidone metabolism and clearance.

INITIAL DOSAGE DETERMINATION METHODS

Pharmacokinetic Dosing Method

The goal of initial dosing of phenobarbital or primidone is to compute the best dose possible for the patient given the diseases and conditions that influence the pharmacokinetics of the drugs and the epileptic disorder for which the patient is being treated. To do this, pharmacokinetic parameters for the patient are estimated with average parameters measured for other patients with similar disease and condition profiles.

ESTIMATE OF CLEARANCE

Phenobarbital is predominately metabolized by the liver, and primidone is about 50% eliminated by the liver. There is no good way to estimate the elimination characteristics of liver-metabolized drugs with an endogenous marker of liver function in the same manner that serum creatinine and estimated creatinine clearance are used to estimate the elimination of agents eliminated by the kidney. Because of this, a patient is categorized according to the diseases and conditions known to change drug clearance, and the clearance previously measured in these studies is used as an estimate of the current patient's clearance. For example, for a 70-kg adult, phenobarbital clearance is assumed to be 4 mL/h per kilogram: 70 kg · 4 mL/h/kg = 280 mL/h, or 0.28 L/h. To produce the most conservative phenobarbital or primidone doses for patients with several concurrent diseases or conditions that affect pharmacokinetics, the disease or condition with the smallest clearance should be used to compute doses. This approach avoids accidental overdosage as much as currently possible.

ESTIMATE OF VOLUME OF DISTRIBUTION

The volume of distribution of both drugs is assumed to be 0.7 L/kg for adults and children. Thus, for a 70-kg adult, the estimated volume of distribution is 49 L: V = 0.7 L/kg · 70 kg = 49 L.

ESTIMATE OF HALF-LIFE AND ELIMINATION RATE CONSTANT

Once the correct clearance and volume of distribution estimates are identified for a patient, they can be converted into the half-life ($t_{1/2}$) and elimination rate constant (k) estimates with the following equations: $t_{1/2} = (0.693 \cdot V)/Cl$; $k = 0.693/t_{1/2} = Cl/V$.

SELECTION OF APPROPRIATE PHARMACOKINETIC MODEL AND EQUATIONS

Primidone and phenobarbital follow a one-compartment pharmacokinetic model. When oral therapy with either drug or intramuscular treatment with phenobarbital is required, both anticonvulsants have good bioavailability (assume F = 1), and one dose of phenobarbital a day or several doses of primidone a day provide a relatively smooth serum concentration–time curve that emulates that of intravenous infusion. A simple pharmacokinetic equation for computing the average steady-state serum concentration of phenobarbital or primidone (Css in μg/mL = mg/L) is widely used and allows calculation of a maintenance dosage: $Css = [F(D/\tau)]/Cl$, or $D = (Css \cdot Cl \cdot \tau)/F$, where F is the bioavailability fraction for the oral dosage form (F = 1 for both drugs), D is the dose of the anticonvulsant in milligrams, Cl is anticonvulsant clearance in liters per hour, and τ is the dosage interval in hours.

When intravenous therapy with phenobarbital is required, a similar pharmacokinetic equation is widely used: $Css = (D/\tau)/Cl$, or $D = Css \cdot Cl \cdot \tau$, where D is the dose of phenobarbital in milligrams, τ is the dosage interval in hours, Cl is phenobarbital clearance in liters per hour. The equation used to calculate an intravenous loading dose of phenobarbital (LD in milligrams) is based on a simple one-compartment model: $LD = Css \cdot V$, where Css is the desired phenobarbital steady-state concentration in micrograms per milliliter, which is equivalent to milligrams per liter, and V is the volume of distribution of phenobarbital. Intravenous phenobarbital doses should administered no faster than 100 mg/min.

Example 1 GO is a 50-year-old, 75-kg (height, 178 cm) man who has tonic-clonic seizures. He needs therapy with oral phenobarbital. He has normal liver and renal function. Suggest an initial phenobarbital dosage regimen designed to achieve a steady-state concentration of 20 μg/mL.

1. *Estimate clearance and volume of distribution according to disease states and conditions present in the patient.*

The clearance rate for an older patient is 4 mL/h per kilogram. With this value, the estimated clearance is 0.3 L/h: Cl = 75 kg · 4 mL/h/kg = 300 mL/h, or 0.3 L/h. The estimated volume of distribution is 53 L: 75 kg · 0.7 L/kg = 53 L.

2. *Estimate half-life and elimination rate constant.*

Once the correct clearance and volume of distribution estimates are identified for the patient, they can be converted into phenobarbital half-life ($t_{1/2}$) and elimination rate constant (k) estimates with the following equations: $t_{1/2} = (0.693 \cdot V)/Cl = (0.693 \cdot 53\ L)/(0.3\ L/h) = 122\ h$; $k = Cl/V = (0.3\ L/h)/53\ L = 0.0057\ h^{-1}$.

3. *Compute the dosage regimen.*

Oral phenobarbital tablets are prescribed to this patient (F = 1). (Note: μg/mL = mg/L, and this concentration unit was substituted for Css in the calculations to avoid unit conversion.) The dosage equation for oral phenobarbital is $D = (Css \cdot Cl \cdot \tau)/F = (20\ mg/L \cdot 0.3\ L/h \cdot 24\ h)/1 = 144\ mg$, rounded to 120 every 24 hours.

Steady-state minimum phenobarbital serum concentration should be measured after steady state is attained in 3 to 5 half-lives. Because the drug is expected to have a half-life of 122 hours in this patient, steady-state concentration of phenobarbital can be measured any time after 4 weeks of dosing (5 half-lives = 5 · 122 h = 610 h, or 25 d). Serum concentration of phenobarbital should be measured if the patient has an exacerbation of epilepsy or if the patient has signs or symptoms of phenobarbital toxicity.

Example 2 GO is a 50-year-old, 75-kg (height, 178 cm) man who has tonic-clonic seizures. He needs therapy with intravenous phenobarbital. He has normal liver and renal function. Suggest an initial phenobarbital dosage regimen designed to achieve a steady-state concentration of 20 μg/mL.

1. *Estimate clearance and volume of distribution according to disease states and conditions present in the patient.*

The clearance rate for an older patient is 4 mL/h per kilogram. With this value, the estimated clearance is 0.3 L/h: Cl = 75 kg · 4 mL/h/kg = 300 mL/h, or 0.3 L/h. The estimated volume of distribution is 53 L: 75 kg · 0.7 L/kg = 53 L.

2. *Estimate half-life and elimination rate constant.*

Once the correct clearance and volume of distribution estimates are identified for the patient, they can be converted into phenobarbital half-life ($t_{1/2}$) and elimination rate constant (k) estimates with the following equations: $t_{1/2}$ = (0.693 · V)/Cl = (0.693 · 53 L)/(0.3 L/h) = 122 h; k = Cl/V = (0.3 L/h)/53 L = 0.0057 h^{-1}.

3. *Compute the dosage regimen.*

Intravenous phenobarbital is prescribed to this patient. (Note: μg/mL = mg/L, and this concentration unit was substituted for Css in the calculations to avoid unit conversion.) The dosage equation for intravenous phenobarbital is D = Css · Cl · τ = 20 mg/L · 0.3 L/h · 24 h = 144 mg, rounded to 120 every 24 hours. If needed, an intravenous loading dose can be computed for the patient: LD = Css · V = 20 mg/L · 53 L = 1060 mg, rounded to 1000 mg. Intravenous loading doses should be administered no faster than 100 mg/min.

Steady-state minimum phenobarbital serum concentration should be measured after steady state is attained in 3 to 5 half-lives. Because the drug is expected to have a half-life of 122 hours in this patient, steady-state concentration of phenobarbital can be measured any time after 4 weeks of dosing (5 half-lives = 5 · 122 h = 610 h, or 25 d). Serum concentration of phenobarbital should be measured if the patient has an exacerbation of epilepsy or if the patient has signs or symptoms of phenobarbital toxicity.

Example 3 BI is a 23-year-old, 65-kg (height, 167 cm) man who has complex partial seizures. He needs therapy with oral primidone. He has normal liver and renal function and takes carbamazepine. Suggest an initial primidone dosage regimen designed to achieve a steady-state primidone concentration of 6 μg/mL.

1. *Estimate clearance and volume of distribution according to disease states and conditions present in the patient.*

The clearance rate of primidone for an adult patient taking carbamazepine is 50 mL/h per kilogram. At this value, the estimated clearance is 3.25 L/h: Cl = 65 kg · 50 mL/h/kg = 3250 mL/h, or 3.25 L/h. The estimated volume of distribution is 46 L: 65 kg · 0.7 L/kg = 46 L.

2. *Estimate half-life and elimination rate constant.*

Once the correct clearance and volume of distribution estimates are identified for the patient, they can be converted into primidone half-life ($t_{1/2}$) and elimination rate constant (k) estimates with the following equations: $t_{1/2} = (0.693 \cdot V)/Cl = (0.693 \cdot 46\ L)/(3.25\ L/h) = 10\ h$; $k = Cl/V = (3.25\ L/h)/46\ L = 0.071\ h^{-1}$.

3. *Compute the dosage regimen.*

Oral primidone tablets are prescribed to this patient (F = 1). (Note: μg/mL = mg/L, and this concentration unit was substituted for Css in the calculations to avoid unit conversion.) The dosage equation for oral primidone is $D = (Css \cdot Cl \cdot \tau)/F = (6\ mg/L \cdot 3.25\ L/h \cdot 12\ h)/1 = 234\ mg$, rounded to 250 mg every 12 hours. To avoid side effects, the starting dose is 50% of this anticipated maintenance dose (125 mg every 12 hours) and is titrated to the full dose over 1 to 2 weeks.

Steady-state minimum serum concentrations of primidone and phenobarbital should be measured after steady state of both agents is attained in 3 to 5 half-lives. Because phenobarbital is expected to have a half-life of 100 hours or more in this patient, steady-state concentration can be measured any time after 3 to 4 weeks of dosing at the full primidone maintenance dose (5 phenobarbital half-lives = $5 \cdot 100\ h = 500\ h$, or 21 d). Serum concentrations of primidone and phenobarbital should be measured if the patient has an exacerbation of epilepsy or if the patient has signs or symptoms of primidone toxicity.

Literature-Based Recommended Dosing

Because of the large amount of variability in phenobarbital and primidone pharmacokinetics, even when concurrent disease states and conditions are identified, most clinicians believe that the use of standard drug doses for various situations is warranted. The original computation of these doses was based on pharmacokinetic dosing methods and modified according to clinical experience. In general, the expected steady-state serum concentration used to compute these doses was in the lower end of the therapeutic range for each drug (Table 13-3). Phenobarbital usually is administered once or twice a day. Primidone is given 2 to 4 times a day. To avoid side effects, primidone doses are started at 25% to 50% of the ultimate desired maintenance dose, and dosage is increased every 1 to 2 weeks depending on response and presence of adverse effects. If the patient has serious

TABLE 13-3 Literature-Based Initial Doses of Phenobarbital and Primidone

PATIENT PROFILE	PHENOBARBITAL DOSE (mg/kg/d)	PRIMIDONE DOSE (mg/kg/d)
Neonate	2.5–5	12–20
Child	3–4.5	12–23
Adult	1.5–2	10–25

Intravenous loading doses for phenobarbital are 15 to 20 mg/kg for status epilepticus.

hepatic dysfunction (Child-Pugh score, ≥8) or renal disease (creatinine clearance, <30 mL/min), maintenance doses prescribed with this method should be decreased 25% to 50% depending on the aggressiveness of therapy. To illustrate the similarities and differences between this method of dosage calculation and the pharmacokinetic dosing method, the previous examples are used.

Example 4 GO is a 50-year-old, 75-kg (height, 178 cm) man who has tonic-clonic seizures. He needs therapy with oral phenobarbital. He has normal liver and renal function. Suggest an initial phenobarbital dosage regimen designed to achieve a steady-state concentration of 20 μg/mL.

1. *Estimate the phenobarbital dose according to disease states and conditions present in the patient.*

Oral phenobarbital tablets are prescribed to this patient. The suggested initial maintenance dosage of phenobarbital in the care of an adult patient is 1.5 to 2 mg/kg per day. At 1.5 mg/kg per day, the dose is 75 kg · 1.5 mg/kg/d = 113 mg/d, rounded to 120 mg/d.

Minimum phenobarbital serum concentrations should be measured after steady state is attained in 3 to 5 half-lives. Because phenobarbital is expected to have a half-life of 100 hours or more in this patient, steady-state concentration can be obtained any time after 3 to 4 weeks of dosing (5 phenobarbital half-lives = 5 · 100 h = 500 h, or 21 d). Serum concentration of phenobarbital also should be measured if the patient has an exacerbation of epilepsy or if the patient has signs or symptoms of phenobarbital toxicity.

Example 5 GO is a 50-year-old, 75-kg (height, 178 cm) man who has tonic-clonic seizures. He needs therapy with intravenous phenobarbital. He has normal liver and renal function. Suggest an initial phenobarbital dosage regimen designed to achieve a steady-state concentration of 8 to 20 μg/mL.

1. *Estimate the phenobarbital dose according to disease states and conditions present in the patient.*

Intravenous phenobarbital is prescribed to this patient. The suggested initial maintenance dosage of phenobarbital in the care of an adult patient is 1.5 to 2 mg/kg per day. At 1.5 mg/kg per day, the maintenance dose is 75 kg · 1.5 mg/kg/d = 113 mg/d, rounded to 120 mg/d. If needed, the loading dose range is 15 to 20 mg/kg. At 15 mg/kg, the loading dose is 75 kg · 15 mg/kg = 1125 mg, rounded to 1000 mg.

Steady-state minimum phenobarbital serum concentration should be measured after steady state is attained in 3 to 4 weeks. Phenobarbital serum concentration should also be measured if the patient experiences an exacerbation of their epilepsy or if the patient develops potential signs or symptoms of phenobarbital toxicity.

Example 6 BI is a 23-year-old, 65-kg (height, 167 cm) man who has complex partial seizures. He needs therapy with oral primidone. He has normal liver and renal function and takes carbamazepine. Suggest an initial primidone dosage regimen designed to achieve a steady-state primidone concentration of 6 μg/mL.

1. *Estimate the primidone dose according to disease states and conditions present in the patient.*

Oral primidone tablets are prescribed to this patient. The suggested initial maintenance dosage of primidone in the care of an adult patient is 10 to 25 mg/kg per day. Because the patient is taking carbamazepine, which is known to induce primidone metabolism, a dose of 15 mg/kg per day is used to compute the initial dose: 65 kg · 15 mg/kg/d = 975 mg/d, rounded to 1000 mg/d and given as 250 mg every 6 hours. To avoid side effects, the starting dose is 50% of this anticipated maintenance dose (125 mg every 6 hours) and is titrated to the full dose over 1 to 2 weeks according to response and adverse effects.

Steady-state minimum primidone and phenobarbital serum concentrations should be measured after steady state of both agents is attained in 3 to 5 half-lives. Because phenobarbital is expected to have a half-life of 100 hours or more in this patient, steady-state concentration can be measured any time after 3 to 4 weeks of dosing at the full maintenance dose of primidone (5 phenobarbital half-lives = 5 · 100 h = 500 h, or 21 d). Serum concentrations of primidone and phenobarbital should be measured if the patient has an exacerbation of epilepsy or if the patient has signs or symptoms of primidone toxicity.

USE OF SERUM CONCENTRATIONS OF PHENOBARBITAL AND PRIMIDONE TO ALTER DOSES

Because of the large amount of pharmacokinetic variability among patients, it is likely that doses computed with patient population characteristics will not always produce serum concentration of phenobarbital or primidone that is expected or desirable. Because of pharmacokinetic variability, the narrow therapeutic index of phenobarbital and primidone, and the desire to avoid adverse side effects, measurement of serum concentrations of these anticonvulsants is conducted for most patients to ensure that therapeutic, nontoxic levels are present. In addition to serum concentration of phenobarbital or primidone, important patient parameters, such as seizure frequency and side effects, should be followed to confirm that the patient is responding to treatment and not having adverse drug reactions. When serum concentration of phenobarbital or primidone is measured, and a dosage change is necessary, clinicians should seek to use the simplest, most straightforward method available to determine a dose that will provide safe and effective treatment.

Linear Pharmacokinetics Method

Because phenobarbital and primidone follow linear, dose-proportional pharmacokinetics, steady-state serum concentration changes in proportion to dose according to the following equation: $D_{new}/Css_{new} = D_{old}/Css_{old}$ or $D_{new} = (Css_{new}/Css_{old})D_{old}$, where D is the dose, Css is steady-state concentration, old indicates the dose that produced the steady-state concentration that the patient is currently receiving, and new denotes the dose necessary to produce the desired steady-state concentration. The advantages of this method are that it is quick and simple. The disadvantages are that steady-state concentrations are required, and primidone may undergo induction of its hepatic clearance at higher doses as phenobarbital concentrations increase. This method works for phenobarbital regardless of route of administration. When primidone is administered to the patient, phenobarbital is produced as an active metabolite. The phenobarbital concentration changes in a linear manner. The phenobarbital concentration resulting from a change in primidone dosage can be estimated with a rearrangement of the foregoing equation: $Css_{new} = (D_{new}/D_{old}) Css_{old}$, where D is the primidone dose, Css is the steady-state concentration of phenobarbital, old indicates the primidone dose that produced the steady-state phenobarbital concentration that the patient is currently receiving, and new denotes the primidone dose necessary to produce the desired steady-state phenobarbital concentration.

Example 7 LK is a 13-year-old, 47-kg (height, 155 cm) girl who has complex partial seizures. She needs therapy with oral primidone. After dosage titration, the patient is given a prescription for 250 mg every 8 hours of primidone tablets (750 mg/d) for 1 month. Steady-state concentrations of primidone and phenobarbital are 3 μg/mL and 15 μg/mL, respectively. The patient is found to be compliant with the dosage regimen. Suggest a primidone dosage regimen designed to achieve a steady-state primidone concentration of 6 μg/mL.

1. *Compute a new dose to achieve the desired serum concentration.*

According to linear pharmacokinetics, the primidone dose necessary to cause the change in steady-state concentration is $D_{new} = (Css_{new}/Css_{old})D_{old} = [(6\ \mu g/mL)/(3\ \mu g/mL)]\ 750\ mg/d = 1500\ mg/d$, or 500 mg every 8 hours. The dosage regimen is titrated to this value over 1 to 2 weeks to avoid adverse effects. According to linear pharmacokinetics, the resulting steady-state phenobarbital serum concentration is $Css_{new} = (D_{new}/D_{old})Css_{old} = [(1500\ mg/d)/(750\ mg/d)]\ 15\ \mu g/mL = 30\ \mu g/mL$.

Steady-state minimum serum concentrations of primidone and phenobarbital should be measured after steady state is attained in 3 to 4 weeks. Serum concentrations of primidone and phenobarbital also should be measured if the patient has an exacerbation of epilepsy or if the patient has signs or symptoms of primidone toxicity.

Example 8 HI is a 42-year-old, 75-kg (height, 178 cm) man who has tonic-clonic seizures. He needs therapy with oral phenobarbital. After dosage titration, the patient is given a prescription for 120 mg/d of phenobarbital tablets for 1 month. Steady-state phenobarbital concentration is 20 μg/mL. The patient is found to be compliant with the dosage regimen. Suggest a phenobarbital dosage regimen designed to achieve a steady-state phenobarbital concentration of 30 μg/mL.

1. *Compute a new dose to achieve the desired serum concentration.*

According to linear pharmacokinetics, the resulting steady-state serum concentration of phenobarbital is $D_{new} = (Css_{new}/Css_{old})D_{old} = [(30\ \mu g/mL)/(20\ \mu g/mL)]\ 120\ mg/d = 180\ mg/d$.

Steady-state minimum serum concentration of phenobarbital should be measured after steady state is attained in 3 to 4 weeks. Serum concentration of phenobarbital also should be measured if the patient has an exacerbation of epilepsy or if the patient has signs or symptoms of phenobarbital toxicity.

Pharmacokinetic Parameter Method

The pharmacokinetic parameter method of adjusting drug doses was among the first techniques used to change doses with serum concentration. It allows computation of a patient's unique pharmacokinetic constants. The constants are used to calculate a dose that achieves the desired concentration of phenobarbital or primidone. For patients receiving oral phenobarbital, the pharmacokinetic parameter method necessitates that steady state has been achieved, and only a steady-state concentration (Css) of phenobarbital is used. Phenobarbital clearance (Cl) can be calculated with the following formula: $Cl = [F(D/\tau)]/Css$, where F is the bioavailability fraction for the oral dosage form (F = 1 for oral phenobarbital products), D is the dose of phenobarbital in milligrams, Css is the steady-state phenobarbital concentration in milligrams per liter, and τ is the dosage interval in hours. Phenobarbital clearance during intravenous therapy can be computed with the equivalent formula: $Cl = (D/\tau)/Css$, where D is the dose of phenobarbital in milligrams, Css is the steady-state concentration of phenobarbital in milligrams per liter, and τ is the dosage interval in hours.

If the patient is receiving oral primidone, primidone clearance (Cl) is computed with the same equation: $Cl = [F(D/\tau)]/Css$, where F is the bioavailability fraction of the oral dosage form (F = 1 for oral primidone products), D is the dose of primidone in milligrams, Css is the steady-state primidone concentration in milligrams per liter, and τ is the dosage interval in hours. As with the linear pharmacokinetics method discussed previously, phenobarbital concentration during primidone treatment can be easily calculated. The phenobarbital concentration resulting from a change in primidone dosage can be estimated with the following equation: $Css_{new} = (D_{new}/D_{old})Css_{old}$, where D is the primidone dose, Css is the steady-state phenobarbital concentration, old indicates the primidone dose that produced the steady-state phenobarbital concentration that the patient is currently receiving, and new denotes the primidone dose necessary to produce the desired steady-state phenobarbital concentration. To illustrate the similarities and differences between this method of dosage calculation and the pharmacokinetic parameter method, the previous examples are used.

Example 9 LK is a 13-year-old, 47-kg (height, 155 cm) girl who has complex partial seizures. She needs therapy with oral primidone. After dosage titration, the patient is given a prescription for 250 mg every 8 hours of primidone tablets (750 mg/d) for 1 month. Steady-state concentrations of primidone and phenobarbital are 3 μg/mL and 15 μg/mL, respectively. The patient is found to be compliant with the dosage regimen. Suggest a primidone dosage regimen designed to achieve a steady-state primidone concentration of 6 μg/mL.

1. *Compute pharmacokinetic parameters.*

The patient is expected to achieve steady-state conditions of both primidone and phenobarbital after 3 to 4 weeks of therapy. Primidone clearance can be computed with steady-state primidone concentration: $Cl = [F(D/\tau)]/Css = [1(250 \text{ mg}/8 \text{ h})]/(3 \text{ mg/L}) = 10 \text{ L/h}$. (Note: μg/mL = mg/L, and this concentration unit was substituted for Css in the calculations to avoid unit conversion.)

2. *Compute primidone dose and resulting phenobarbital concentration.*

Primidone clearance is used to compute the new dose: $D = (Css \cdot Cl \cdot \tau)/F = (6 \text{ mg/L} \cdot 10 \text{ L/h} \cdot 8 \text{ h})/1 = 480 \text{ mg}$, rounded to 500 mg every 8 hours. According to linear pharmacokinetics, the resulting steady-state phenobarbital serum concentration is $Css_{new} = (D_{new}/D_{old})Css_{old} = [(1500 \text{ mg/d})/(750 \text{ mg/d})]\ 15\ \mu\text{g/mL} = 30\ \mu\text{g/mL}$.

Steady-state minimum serum concentrations of primidone and phenobarbital should be measured after steady-state is attained in 3 to 4 weeks. Serum concentrations of primidone and phenobarbital also should be measured if the patient has an exacerbation of epilepsy or if the patient has signs or symptoms of primidone toxicity.

Example 10 HI is a 42-year-old, 75-kg (height, 178 cm) man who has tonic-clonic seizures. He needs therapy with oral phenobarbital. After dosage titration, the patient is given a prescription for 120 mg/d of phenobarbital tablets for 1 month. Steady-state phenobarbital concentration is 20 μg/mL. The patient is found to be compliant with the dosage regimen. Suggest a phenobarbital dosage regimen designed to achieve a steady-state phenobarbital concentration of 30 μg/mL.

1. *Compute pharmacokinetic parameters.*

The patient is expected to achieve steady-state conditions after 3 to 4 weeks of therapy. Phenobarbital clearance can be computed with steady-state phenobarbital concentration: $Cl = [F(D/\tau)]/Css = [1(120\ mg/24\ h)]/(20\ mg/L) = 0.25\ L/h$. (Note: μg/mL = mg/L, and this concentration unit was substituted for Css in the calculations to avoid unit conversion.)

2. *Compute the phenobarbital dose.*

Phenobarbital clearance is used to compute the new dose: $D = (Css \cdot Cl \cdot \tau)/F = (30\ mg/L \cdot 0.25\ L/h \cdot 24\ h)/1 = 180$ mg every 24 hours.

Steady-state minimum serum concentration of phenobarbital should be measured after steady state is attained in 3 to 4 weeks. Serum concentration of phenobarbital also should be measured if the patient has an exacerbation of epilepsy or if the patient has signs or symptoms of phenobarbital toxicity.

BAYESIAN PHARMACOKINETICS COMPUTER PROGRAMS

Computer programs can assist in the computation of pharmacokinetic parameters for patients. In the most reliable computer programs a nonlinear regression algorithm incorporates components of Bayes' theorem. Nonlinear regression is a statistical technique in which an iterative process is used to compute the best pharmacokinetic parameters for a concentration–time data set. The patient's drug dosage schedule and serum concentrations are entered into the computer. The computer program has a pharmacokinetic equation programmed for the drug and administration method, such as oral, intravenous bolus, intravenous infusion. A one-compartment model typically is used, although some programs allow the user to choose among several equations. With population estimates based on demographic information for the patient, such as age, weight, sex, liver function, and cardiac status, supplied by the user, the program computes estimated serum concentration for each actual serum concentration. Kinetic parameters are changed by the computer program, and a new set of estimated serum concentrations are computed. The pharmacokinetic parameters that generated the estimated serum concentrations closest to the actual values are stored in the computer memory, and the process is repeated until the set of pharmacokinetic parameters that give estimated serum concentrations statistically closest to the actual serum concentrations are generated. These pharmacokinetic parameters can be used to compute improved dosing schedules for patients. Bayes' theorem is used in the computer algorithm to balance the results of the computations between values based solely on the patient's serum drug concentrations and those based only on patient population parameters. Results of studies in which various methods of dosage adjustment have been compared have consistently shown these types of computer dosing programs perform at least as well as experienced clinical pharmacokineticists and clinicians and better than inexperienced clinicians.

Some clinicians use Bayesian pharmacokinetics computer programs exclusively to alter drug doses based on serum concentrations. An advantage of this approach is that consistent dosage recommendations are made when several practitioners are involved in therapeutic drug-monitoring programs. However, because simpler dosing methods work just as well for patients with stable pharmacokinetic parameters and steady-state drug concentrations, many clinicians reserve the use of computer programs for more difficult situations. Those situations include serum concentrations that are not at steady state, serum concentrations not obtained at the specific times needed to use simpler methods, and unstable pharmacokinetic parameters. Many Bayesian pharmacokinetics computer programs are available, and most provide answers similar to the ones in the following examples. The program used to solve problems in this book is DrugCalc, written by Dr. Dennis Mungall, and is available on his Internet web site (http://members.aol.com/thertch/index.htm).[17] Currently, this program is available only for phenobarbital.

Example 11 HI is a 42-year-old, 75-kg (height, 178 cm) man who has tonic-clonic seizures. He needs therapy with oral phenobarbital. After dosage titration, the patient is given a prescription for 120 mg/d of phenobarbital tablets for 1 month. Steady-state phenobarbital concentration is 20 μg/mL. The patient is found to be compliant with the dosage regimen. Suggest a phenobarbital dosage regimen designed to achieve steady-state phenobarbital concentration of 30 μg/mL.

1. *Enter the patient's demographic, drug dosing, and serum concentration–time data into the computer program.*

2. *Compute pharmacokinetic parameters for the patient with a Bayesian pharmacokinetics computer program.*

The pharmacokinetic parameters computed with the program are a volume of distribution of 51 L, a half-life of 185 hours, and a clearance of 0.19 L/h.

3. *Compute the dose required to achieve the desired serum concentration of phenobarbital.*

The one-compartment model, first-order absorption equations used in the program to compute doses indicate that a dose of 180 mg every 24 hours produces a steady-state phenobarbital concentration of 36 μg/mL.

Example 12 JB is an 8-year-old, 35-kg (height, 127 cm) boy who has absence seizures. Phenobarbital elixir 100 mg every 24 hours has been started. The phenobarbital concentration is 12 μg/mL before the tenth maintenance dose. What phenobarbital dose is needed to achieve a Css of 25 μg/mL?

1. *Enter the patient's demographic, drug dosing, and serum concentration–time data into the computer program.*

In this case, it is unlikely that the patient is at steady state, so the linear pharmacokinetics method cannot be used.

2. *Compute pharmacokinetic parameters for the patient with a Bayesian pharmacokinetics computer program.*

The pharmacokinetic parameters computed with the program are a volume of distribution of 26 L, a half-life of 82 hours, and clearance of 0.22 L/h.

3. *Compute the dose required to achieve the desired serum concentration of phenobarbital.*

The one-compartment model, oral equations used in the program to compute doses indicate that a dose of phenobarbital 175 mg every 24 hours produces a steady-state concentration of 26 μg/mL.

PROBLEMS

The following problems are intended to emphasize the computation of initial and individualized doses with clinical pharmacokinetic techniques. Clinicians always should consult the patient's chart to confirm that current anticonvulsant therapy is appropriate. All other medications that the patient is taking, including prescription and nonprescription drugs, should be recorded and checked to ascertain the risk of drug interaction with phenobarbital or primidone.

1. FH is a 37-year-old, 85-kg (height, 185 cm) man who has tonic-clonic seizures. He needs therapy with oral phenobarbital. He has normal liver and renal function. Suggest an initial phenobarbital dosage regimen designed to achieve a steady-state phenobarbital concentration of 15 μg/mL.

2. Patient FH (see problem 1) is given a prescription for 90 mg every 24 hours of phenobarbital tablets for 1 month. Steady-state phenobarbital concentration is 12 μg/mL. The patient is found to be compliant with the dosage regimen. Suggest a phenobarbital dosage regimen designed to achieve a steady-state phenobarbital concentration of 20 μg/mL.

3. AS is a 9-year-old, 35-kg (height, 137 cm) girl who has complex partial seizures. She needs therapy with oral phenobarbital. She has normal liver and renal function. Suggest an initial phenobarbital dosage regimen designed to achieve a steady-state phenobarbital concentration of 20 μg/mL.

4. Patient AS (see problem 3) is given a prescription for 30 mg twice a day (60 mg/d) of phenobarbital elixir for 3 weeks. Steady-state phenobarbital concentration is 8.3 μg/mL. The patient is found to be compliant with the dosage regimen. Suggest a phenobarbital dosage regimen designed to achieve a steady-state phenobarbital concentration of 15 μg/mL.

5. FL is a 29-year-old, 75-kg (height, 180 cm) man who has tonic-clonic seizures. He needs therapy with oral primidone. He has normal liver function and also is receiving phenytoin therapy. Suggest an initial primidone dosage regimen designed to achieve a steady-state primidone concentration of 5 μg/mL.

6. Patient FL (see problem 5) is given a prescription for 500 mg every 12 hours of primidone tablets for 4 weeks. Steady-state total concentrations of primidone and phenobarbital are 4.3 μg/mL and 11.6 μg/mL, respectively. The patient is found to be compliant with the dosage regimen. Suggest a primidone dosage regimen designed to achieve a steady-state primidone concentration of 6 μg/mL and estimate the resulting phenobarbital concentration.

7. PH is a 4-year-old, 22-kg (height, 102 cm) boy who has tonic-clonic seizures. He needs therapy with primidone suspension. He has normal liver and renal function and also is treated with carbamazepine. Suggest an initial primidone dosage regimen designed to achieve a steady-state primidone concentration of 5 μg/mL.

8. Patient PH (see problem 7) is given a prescription for 75 mg three times daily (225 mg/d) of primidone suspension for 3 weeks. Steady-state concentrations of primidone and phenobarbital are 5.5 μg/mL and 18 μg/mL, respectively. The patient is found to be compliant with the dosage regimen. Suggest a primidone dosage regimen designed to achieve a steady-state primidone concentration of 8 μg/mL and estimate the resulting phenobarbital concentration.

9. PU is a 55-year-old, 68-kg (height, 173 cm) man who has complex partial seizures. He is receiving 90 mg/d of phenobarbital. He has normal liver and renal (bilirubin, 0.7 mg/dL; albumin, 4.0 g/dL; serum creatinine, 1.1 mg/dL) function and takes 800 mg/d of carbamazepine. The phenobarbital concentration is 14 μg/mL before the eighth dose. Compute a phenobarbital dose that will provide a steady-state concentration of 25 μg/mL.

10. LH is a 25-year-old, 60-kg (height, 160 cm) woman who has tonic-clonic seizures. She is given a new prescription of 120 mg/d of phenobarbital tablets. She has normal liver and renal function and also is being treated with phenytoin. The minimum phenobarbital concentration before the tenth dose is 10 μg/mL. Compute a phenobarbital dose that will provide a steady-state concentration of 30 μg/mL.

ANSWERS TO PROBLEMS

1. Answer to problem 1.

Pharmacokinetic Dosing Method

1. *Estimate clearance and volume of distribution according to disease states and conditions present in the patient.*

The clearance rate for an older patient is 4 mL/h per kilogram. At this value, estimated clearance is 0.34 L/h: Cl = 85 kg · 4 mL/h/kg = 340 mL/h, or 0.34 L/h. The estimated volume of distribution is 60 L: 85 kg · 0.7 L/kg = 60 L.

2. *Estimate half-life and elimination rate constant.*

Once the correct clearance and volume of distribution estimates are identified for the patient, they can be converted into phenobarbital half-life ($t_{1/2}$) and elimination rate constant (k) estimates with the following equations: $t_{1/2} = (0.693 \cdot V)/Cl = (0.693 \cdot 60\ L)/(0.34\ L/h) = 122\ h$; $k = Cl/V = (0.34\ L/h)/60\ L = 0.0057\ h^{-1}$.

3. *Compute the dosage regimen.*

Oral phenobarbital tablets are prescribed to this patient (F = 1). (Note: μg/mL = mg/L, and this concentration unit was substituted for Css in the calculations to avoid unit conversion.) The dosage equation for oral phenobarbital is $D = (Css \cdot Cl \cdot \tau)/F = (15\ mg/L \cdot 0.34\ L/h \cdot 24\ h)/1 = 122\ mg$, rounded to 120 every 24 hours.

Steady-state minimum serum concentration of phenobarbital should be measured after steady state is attained in 3 to 5 half-lives. Because the drug is expected to have a half-life of 122 hours in this patient, steady-state concentration of phenobarbital can be measured any time after 4 weeks of dosing (5 half-lives = 5 · 122 h = 610 h, or 25 d). Serum concentration of phenobarbital should be measured if the patient has an exacerbation of epilepsy or if the patient has signs or symptoms of phenobarbital toxicity.

Literature-Based Recommended Dosing

1. *Estimate the phenobarbital dose according to disease states and conditions present in the patient.*

Oral phenobarbital tablets are prescribed to this patient. The suggested initial maintenance dosage of phenobarbital for an adult patient is 1.5 to 2 mg/kg per day. At 1.5 mg/kg per day, the dose is 85 kg · 1.5 mg/kg/d = 128 mg/d, rounded to 120 mg/d.

Minimum serum concentration of phenobarbital should be measured after steady state is attained in 3 to 5 half-lives. Because phenobarbital is expected to have a half-life of 100 hours or more in this patient, steady-state concentration can be measured any time after 3 to 4 weeks of dosing (5 phenobarbital half-lives = 5 · 100 h = 500 h, or 21 d). Serum concentration of phenobarbital should be measured if the patient has an exacerbation of epilepsy or if the patient has signs or symptoms of phenobarbital toxicity.

2. Answer to problem 2.

Linear Pharmacokinetics Method

1. *Compute a new dose to achieve the desired serum concentration.*

According to linear pharmacokinetics, the resulting steady-state serum concentration of phenobarbital is $D_{new} = (Css_{new}/Css_{old})D_{old} = [(20\ \mu g/mL)/(12\ \mu g/mL)]\ 90\ mg/d = 150\ mg/d$.

Steady-state minimum serum concentration of phenobarbital should be measured after steady state is attained in 3 to 4 weeks. Serum concentration of phenobarbital also should be measured if the patient has an exacerbation of epilepsy or if the patient has signs or symptoms of phenobarbital toxicity.

Pharmacokinetic Parameter Method

1. *Compute pharmacokinetic parameters.*

The patient is expected to achieve steady-state conditions after 3 to 4 weeks of therapy. Phenobarbital clearance can be computed with steady-state phenobarbital concentration: $Cl = [F(D/\tau)]/Css = [1(90 \text{ mg}/24 \text{ h})]/(12 \text{ mg/L}) = 0.31 \text{ L/h}$. (Note: μg/mL = mg/L, and this concentration unit was substituted for Css in the calculations to avoid unit conversion.)

2. *Compute the phenobarbital dose.*

Phenobarbital clearance is used to compute the new dose: $D = (Css \cdot Cl \cdot \tau)/F = (20 \text{ mg/L} \cdot 0.31 \text{ L/h} \cdot 24 \text{ h})/1 = 149 \text{ mg}$, rounded to 150 mg every 24 hours.

Steady-state minimum serum concentration of phenobarbital should be measured after steady state is attained in 3 to 4 weeks. Serum concentration of phenobarbital also should be measured if the patient has an exacerbation of epilepsy or if the patient has signs or symptoms of phenobarbital toxicity.

3. Answer to problem 3.

Pharmacokinetic Dosing Method

1. *Estimate clearance and volume of distribution according to disease states and conditions present in the patient.*

The clearance rate for a pediatric patient is 8 mL/h per kilogram. At this value, estimated clearance is 0.28 L/h: $Cl = 35 \text{ kg} \cdot 8 \text{ mL/h/kg} = 280 \text{ mL/h}$, or 0.28 L/h. The estimated volume of distribution is 25 L: $35 \text{ kg} \cdot 0.7 \text{ L/kg} = 25 \text{ L}$.

2. *Estimate half-life and elimination rate constant.*

Once the correct clearance and volume of distribution estimates are identified for the patient, they can be converted into phenobarbital half-life ($t_{1/2}$) and elimination rate constant (k) estimates with the following equations: $t_{1/2} = (0.693 \cdot V)/Cl = (0.693 \cdot 25 \text{ L})/(0.28 \text{ L/h}) = 62 \text{ h}$; $k = Cl/V = (0.28 \text{ L/h})/25 \text{ L} = 0.011 \text{ h}^{-1}$.

3. *Compute the dosage regimen.*

Oral phenobarbital elixir is prescribed to this patient (F = 1). (Note: μg/mL = mg/L, and this concentration unit was substituted for Css in the calculations to avoid unit conversion.) The dosage equation for oral phenobarbital is $D = (Css \cdot Cl \cdot \tau)/F = (20 \text{ mg/L} \cdot 0.28 \text{ L/h} \cdot 24 \text{ h})/1 = 134 \text{ mg}$, rounded to 120 every 24 hours.

Steady-state minimum serum concentration of phenobarbital should be measured after steady state is attained in 3 to 5 half-lives. Because the drug is expected to have a half-life of 62 hours in this patient, steady-state concentration of phenobarbital can be measured any time after 2 weeks of dosing (5 half-lives = $5 \cdot 62 \text{ h} = 310 \text{ h}$, or 13 d).

Serum concentration of phenobarbital should be measured if the patient has an exacerbation of epilepsy or if the patient has signs or symptoms of phenobarbital toxicity.

Literature-Based Recommended Dosing

1. *Estimate the phenobarbital dose according to disease states and conditions present in the patient.*

Oral phenobarbital elixir is prescribed to this patient. The suggested initial maintenance dosage rate for phenobarbital in a pediatric patient is 3 to 4.5 mg/kg per day. At 3 mg/kg per day, the dosage is 35 kg · 3 mg/kg/d = 105 mg/d, rounded to 100 mg/d.

Mimimum serum concentration of phenobarbital should be measured after steady state is attained in 3 to 5 half-lives. Because phenobarbital is expected to have a half-life of 60 hours in this patient, steady-state concentration can be measured any time after 2 weeks of dosing (5 phenobarbital half-lives = 5 · 60 h = 300 h, or 13 d). Serum concentration of phenobarbital should be measured if the patient has an exacerbation of epilepsy or if the patient has signs or symptoms of phenobarbital toxicity.

4. Answer to problem 4.

Linear Pharmacokinetics Method

1. *Compute a new dose to achieve the desired serum concentration.*

According to linear pharmacokinetics, the resulting steady-state phenobarbital serum concentration is $D_{new} = (Css_{new}/Css_{old})D_{old}$ = [(15 μg/mL)/(8.3 μg/mL)] 60 mg/d = 108 mg/d, rounded to 100 mg every 24 hours.

Steady-state minimum serum concentration of phenobarbital should be measured after steady state is attained in 2 weeks. Serum concentration of phenobarbital also should be measured if the patient has an exacerbation of epilepsy or if the patient has signs or symptoms of phenobarbital toxicity.

Pharmacokinetic Parameter Method

1. *Compute pharmacokinetic parameters.*

The patient is expected to achieve steady-state conditions after 2 weeks of therapy. Phenobarbital clearance can be computed with steady-state phenobarbital concentration: $Cl = [F(D/\tau)]/Css$ = [1(30 mg/12 h)]/(8.3 mg/L) = 0.30 L/h. (Note: μg/mL = mg/L, and this concentration unit was substituted for Css in the calculations to avoid unit conversion.)

2. *Compute the phenobarbital dose.*

Phenobarbital clearance is used to compute the new dose: $D = (Css \cdot Cl \cdot \tau)/F$ = (15 mg/L · 0.30 L/h · 12 h)/1 = 54 mg, rounded to 60 mg every 12 hours.

Steady-state minimum serum concentration of phenobarbital should be measured after steady state is attained in 2 weeks. Serum concentration of phenobarbital also should be measured if the patient has an exacerbation of epilepsy or if the patient has signs or symptoms of phenobarbital toxicity.

5. Answer to problem 5.

Pharmacokinetic Dosing Method

1. *Estimate clearance and volume of distribution according to disease states and conditions present in the patient.*

The primidone clearance rate for an adult patient taking phenytoin is 50 mL/h per kilogram. At this value, the estimated clearance is 3.75 L/h: Cl = 75 kg · 50 mL/h/kg = 3750 mL/h, or 3.75 L/h. The estimated volume of distribution is 53 L: 75 kg · 0.7 L/kg = 53 L.

2. *Estimate half-life and elimination rate constant.*

Once the correct clearance and volume of distribution estimates are identified for the patient, they can be converted into primidone half-life ($t_{1/2}$) and elimination rate constant (k) estimates with the following equations: $t_{1/2}$ = (0.693 · V)/Cl = (0.693 · 53 L)/(3.75 L/h) = 10 h; k = Cl/V = (3.75 L/h)/53 L = 0.071 h^{-1}.

3. *Compute the dosage regimen.*

Oral primidone tablets are prescribed to this patient (F = 1). (Note: μg/mL = mg/L, and this concentration unit was substituted for Css in the calculations to avoid unit conversion.) The dosage equation for oral primidone is D = (Css · Cl · τ)/F = (5 mg/L · 3.75 L/h · 12 h)/1 = 225 mg, rounded to 250 mg every 12 hours. To avoid side effects, the starting dose is 50% of this anticipated maintenance dose (125 mg every 12 hours) and is titrated to the full dose over 1 to 2 weeks.

Steady-state minimum serum concentrations of primidone and phenobarbital should be measured after steady state of both agents is attained in 3 to 5 half-lives. Because phenobarbital is expected to have a half-life of 100 hours or more in this patient, steady-state concentrations can be measured any time after 3 to 4 weeks of dosing at the full primidone maintenance dose (5 phenobarbital half-lives = 5 · 100 h = 500 h, or 21 d). Serum concentrations of primidone and phenobarbital should be measured if the patient has an exacerbation of epilepsy or if the patient has signs or symptoms of primidone toxicity.

Literature-Based Recommended Dosing

1. *Estimate the primidone dose according to disease states and conditions present in the patient.*

Oral primidone tablets are prescribed to this patient. The suggested initial maintenance dosage of primidone for an adult patient is 10 to 25 mg/kg per day. Because the patient is taking phenytoin, which is known to induce primidone metabolism, a dose of 15 mg/kg per day is used to compute the initial dose: 75 kg · 15 mg/kg/d = 1125 mg/d, rounded to 1000 mg/d and given as 250 mg every 6 hours. To avoid side effects, the starting dose is 50% of this anticipated maintenance dose (125 mg every 6 hours) and is titrated to the full dose over 1 to 2 weeks according to response and adverse effects.

Steady-state minimum serum concentrations of primidone and phenobarbital should be measured after steady state of both agents is attained in 3 to 5 half-lives. Because phenobarbital is expected to have a half-life of 100 hours or more in this patient, steady-state concentrations can be measured any time after 3 to 4 weeks of dosing at the full primidone maintenance dose (5 phenobarbital half-lives = 5 · 100 h = 500 h, or 21 d). Serum concentrations of primidone and phenobarbital should be measured if the patient has an exacerbation of epilepsy or if the patient has signs or symptoms of primidone toxicity.

6. Answer to problem 6.

Linear Pharmacokinetics Method

1. *Compute a new dose to achieve the desired serum concentration.*

According to linear pharmacokinetics, the primidone dose necessary to change steady-state concentration is $D_{new} = (Css_{new}/Css_{old})D_{old}$ = [(6 μg/mL)/(4.3 μg/mL)] 1000 mg/d = 1395 mg/d, rounded to 1500 mg/d, or 500 mg every 8 hours. The dosage regimen is titrated to this value over 1 to 2 weeks to avoid adverse effects. According to linear pharmacokinetics, the resulting steady-state serum concentration of phenobarbital is $Css_{new} = (D_{new}/D_{old})\ Css_{old}$ = [(1500 mg/d)/(1000 mg/d)] 11.6 μg/mL = 17.4 μg/mL.

Steady-state minimum serum concentrations of primidone and phenobarbital should be measured after steady state is attained in 3 to 4 weeks. Serum concentrations of primidone and phenobarbital also should be measured if the patient has an exacerbation of epilepsy or if the patient has signs or symptoms of primidone toxicity.

Pharmacokinetic Parameter Method

1. *Compute pharmacokinetic parameters.*

The patient is expected to achieve steady-state conditions of both primidone and phenobarbital after 3 to 4 weeks of therapy. Primidone clearance can be computed with steady-state primidone concentration: $Cl = [F(D/\tau)]/Css$ = [1(500 mg/12 h)]/(4.3 mg/L) = 9.7 L/h. (Note: μg/mL = mg/L, and this concentration unit was substituted for Css in the calculations to avoid unit conversion.)

2. *Compute primidone dose and resulting phenobarbital concentration.*

Primidone clearance is used to compute the new dose: $D = (Css \cdot Cl \cdot \tau)/F$ = (6 mg/L · 9.7 L/h · 8 h)/1 = 466 mg, rounded to 500 mg every 8 hours. According to linear pharmacokinetics, the resulting steady-state serum concentration of phenobarbital is $Css_{new} = (D_{new}/D_{old})Css_{old}$ = [(1500 mg/d)/(1000 mg/d)] 11.6 μg/mL = 17.4 μg/mL.

Steady-state minimum serum concentrations of primidone and phenobarbital should be measured after steady state is attained in 3 to 4 weeks. Serum concentrations of primidone and phenobarbital also should be measured if the patient has an exacerbation of epilepsy or if the patient has signs or symptoms of primidone toxicity.

7. Solution to problem 7.

Pharmacokinetic Dosing Method

1. *Estimate clearance and volume of distribution according to disease states and conditions present in the patient.*

The clearance rate for a pediatric patient is 125 mL/h per kilogram. At this value, the estimated clearance is 2.75 L/h: Cl = 22 kg · 125 mL/h/kg = 2750 mL/h, or 2.75 L/h. The estimated volume of distribution is 15 L: 22 kg · 0.7 L/kg = 15 L.

2. *Estimate half-life and elimination rate constant.*

Once the correct clearance and volume of distribution estimates are identified for the patient, they can be converted into primidone half-life ($t_{1/2}$) and elimination rate constant (k) estimates with the following equations: $t_{1/2}$ = (0.693 · V)/Cl = (0.693 · 15 L)/(2.75 L/h) = 4 h; k = Cl/V = (2.75 L/h)/15 L = 0.183 h^{-1}.

3. *Compute the dosage regimen.*

Oral primidone suspension is prescribed to this patient (F = 1). (Note: μg/mL = mg/L, and this concentration unit was substituted for Css in the calculations to avoid unit conversion.) The dosage equation for oral primidone is D = (Css · Cl · τ)/F = (5 mg/L · 2.75 L/h · 6 h)/1 = 82.5 mg, rounded to 100 mg every 6 hours. To avoid side effects, the starting dose is 50% of this anticipated maintenance dose (50 mg every 6 hours) and is titrated to the full dose over 1 to 2 weeks.

Steady-state minimum serum concentrations of primidone and phenobarbital should be measured after steady state of both agents is attained in 3 to 5 half-lives. Because phenobarbital is expected to have a half-life of 60 hours or more in this patient, steady-state concentrations can be measured any time after 2 weeks of dosing at the full primidone maintenance dose (5 phenobarbital half-lives = 5 · 60 h = 300 h, or 13 d). Serum concentrations of primidone and phenobarbital should be measured if the patient has an exacerbation of epilepsy or if the patient has signs or symptoms of primidone toxicity.

Literature-Based Recommended Dosing

1. *Estimate the primidone dose according to disease states and conditions present in the patient.*

Oral primidone suspension is prescribed to this patient. The suggested initial maintenance dosage of primidone for a pediatric patient is 12 to 23 mg/kg per day. Because the patient is taking phenytoin, which is known to induce primidone metabolism, a dose of 15 mg/kg per day is used to compute the initial dose: 22 kg · 15 mg/kg/d = 330 mg/d, rounded to 300 mg/d and given as 100 mg every 8 hours. To avoid side effects, the starting dose is 50% of this anticipated maintenance dose (50 mg every 8 hours) and is titrated to the full dose over 1 to 2 weeks according to response and adverse effects.

Steady-state minimum serum concentrations of primidone and phenobarbital should be measured after steady state of both agents is attained in 3 to 5 half-lives. Because phenobarbital is expected to have a half-life of 60 hours or more in this patient, steady-state concentrations can be measured any time after 2 weeks of dosing at the full primidone maintenance dose (5 phenobarbital half-lives = 5 · 60 h = 300 h, or 13 d). Serum concentrations of primidone and phenobarbital should be measured if the patient has an exacerbation of epilepsy or if the patient has signs or symptoms of primidone toxicity.

8. Answer to problem 8.

Linear Pharmacokinetics Method

1. *Compute a new dose to achieve the desired serum concentration.*

According to linear pharmacokinetics, the primidone dose necessary to change steady-state concentration is $D_{new} = (Css_{new}/Css_{old})D_{old}$ = [(8 μg/mL)/(5.5 μg/mL)] 225 mg/d = 327 mg/d, rounded to 300 mg/d, or 100 mg every 8 hours. The dosage regimen is titrated to this value over 1 to 2 weeks to avoid adverse effects. According to linear pharmacokinetics, the resulting steady-state serum concentration of phenobarbital is $Css_{new} = (D_{new}/D_{old})Css_{old}$ = [(300 mg/d)/(225 mg/d)] 18 μg/mL = 24 μg/mL.

Steady-state minimum serum concentrations of primidone and phenobarbital should be measured after steady state is attained in 2 weeks. Serum concentrations of primidone and phenobarbital also should be measured if the patient has an exacerbation of epilepsy or if the patient has signs or symptoms of primidone toxicity.

Pharmacokinetic Parameter Method

1. *Compute pharmacokinetic parameters.*

The patient is expected to achieve steady-state conditions of both primidone and phenobarbital after 2 weeks of therapy. Primidone clearance can be computed with steady-state primidone concentration: $Cl = [F(D/\tau)]/Css$ = [1(75 mg/8 h)]/(5.5 mg/L) = 1.7 L/h. (Note: μg/mL = mg/L, and this concentration unit was substituted for Css in the calculations to avoid unit conversion.)

2. *Compute primidone dose and resulting phenobarbital concentration.*

Primidone clearance is used to compute the new dose: $D = (Css \cdot Cl \cdot \tau)/F$ = (8 mg/L · 1.7 L/h · 8 h)/1 = 109 mg, rounded to 100 mg every 8 hours. According to linear pharmacokinetics, the resulting steady-state serum concentration of phenobarbital is $Css_{new} = (D_{new}/D_{old})Css_{old}$ = [(300 mg/d)/(225 mg/d)] 18 μg/mL = 24 μg/mL.

Steady-state minimum serum concentrations of primidone and phenobarbital should be measured after steady state is attained in 2 weeks. Serum concentrations of primidone and phenobarbital also should be measured if the patient has an exacerbation of epilepsy or if the patient has signs or symptoms of primidone toxicity.

9. Solution to problem 9.

1. *Enter the patient's demographic, drug dosing, and serum concentration–time data into the computer program.*

After less than 4 weeks of phenobarbital therapy, it is unlikely the patient is at steady state.

2. *Compute pharmacokinetic parameters for the patient with a Bayesian pharmacokinetics computer program.*

The pharmacokinetic parameters computed with the program are a volume of distribution of 36 L, a half-life of 217 hours, and a clearance of 0.11 L/h.

3. *Compute the dose required to achieve the desired serum concentration of phenobarbital.*

The one-compartment model, first-order absorption equations used in the program to compute doses indicate that a dose of 60 mg every 24 hours produces a steady-state phenobarbital concentration of 21 μg/mL.

10. Solution to problem 10.

1. *Enter the patient's demographic, drug dosing, and serum concentration–time data into the computer program.*

After less than 4 weeks of phenobarbital therapy, it is unlikely the patient is at steady state.

2. *Compute pharmacokinetic parameters for the patient with a Bayesian pharmacokinetics computer program.*

The pharmacokinetic parameters computed with the program are a volume of distribution of 44 L, a half-life of 97 hours, and a clearance of 0.31 L/h.

3. *Compute the dose required to achieve the desired serum concentration of phenobarbital.*

The one-compartment model, first-order absorption equations used in the program to compute doses indicate that a dose of 240 mg every 24 hours produces a steady-state phenobarbital concentration of 29 μg/mL.

REFERENCES

1. Brodie MJ, Dichter MA. Antiepileptic drugs. N Engl J Med 1996;334:168–75.
2. Graves NM, Garnett WR. Epilepsy. In: DiPiro JT, Talbert RL, Yee GC, Matzke GR, Wells BG, Posey LM, eds. Pharmacotherapy: a pathophysiologic approach. Stamford, CT: Appleton & Lange, 1999:952–75.
3. McNamara JO. Drugs effective in the therapy of the epilepsies. In: Hardman JG, Limbird LE, Molinoff PB, Ruddon RW, Gilman AG, eds. The pharmacological basis of therapeutics. New York: McGraw-Hill, 1996:461–86.
4. Smith DB. Primidone: clinical use. In: Levy R, Mattson R, Meldrum B, eds. Antiepileptic drugs. New York: Raven Press, 1989:423–38.

5. Garnett WR. Antiepileptics. In: Schumacher GE, ed. Therapeutic drug monitoring. Stamford, CT: Appleton & Lange, 1995:345–95.
6. Browne TR, Evans JE, Szabo GK, Evans BA, Greenblatt DJ. Studies with stable isotopes: II. phenobarbital pharmacokinetics during monotherapy. J Clin Pharmacol 1985;25:51–8.
7. Nelson E, Powell JR, Conrad K, et al. Phenobarbital pharmacokinetics and bioavailability in adults. J Clin Pharmacol 1982;22:141–8.
8. Streete JM, Berry DJ, Pettit LI, Newberry JE. Phenylethylmalonamide serum levels in patients treated with primidone and the effects of other antiepileptic drugs. Ther Drug Monit 1986;8:161–5.
9. Baumel IP, Gallagher BB, Mattson RH. Phenylethylmalonamide (PEMA): an important metabolite of primidone. Arch Neurol 1972;27:34–41.
10. Heimann G, Gladtke E. Pharmacokinetics of phenobarbital in childhood. Eur J Clin Pharmacol 1977;12:305–10.
11. Alvin J, McHorse T, Hoyumpa A, Bush MT, Schenker S. The effect of liver disease in man on the disposition of phenobarbital. J Pharmacol Exp Ther 1975;192:224–35.
12. Pugh RN, Murray-Lyon IM, Dawson JL, Pietroni MC, Williams R. Transection of the oesophagus for bleeding oesophageal varices. Br J Surg 1973;60:646–9.
13. Rust RS, Dodson WE. Phenobarbital: absorption, distribution, and excretion. In: Levy RH, Mattson R, Meldrum B, eds. Antiepileptic drugs. New York: Raven Press, 1989:293–304.
14. Cloyd JC, Miller KW, Leppik IE. Primidone kinetics: effects of concurrent drugs and duration of therapy. Clin Pharmacol Ther 1981;29:402–7.
15. Kauffman RE, Habersang R, Lansky L. Kinetics of primidone metabolism and excretion in children. Clin Pharmacol Ther 1977;22:200–5.
16. Hansten PD, Horn JR. Drug interactions analysis and management. Vancouver, WA: Applied Therapeutics, 1999:480.
17. Wandell M, Mungall D. Computer assisted drug interpretation and drug regimen optimization. Am Assoc Clin Chem 1984;6:1–11.

14

ETHOSUXIMIDE

INTRODUCTION

Ethosuximide is a succinimide compound effective in the management of absence (petit mal) seizures (Table 14-1).[1] It is the product of an intense research effort into structure activity to find a specific agent to suppress absence seizures that had a relatively low side-effect profile. Although the exact mechanism of action is not known, the antiepileptic effect of ethosuximide is thought to be its ability to decrease low-threshold calcium currents in thalamic neurons.[2] The thalamus has a key role in the production of 3-Hz spike-wave rhythms that are a hallmark of absence seizures. Ethosuximide may inhibit the sodium-potassium ATPase system and NADPH-linked aldehyde reductase.[3]

THERAPEUTIC AND TOXIC CONCENTRATIONS

The therapeutic range of ethosuximide is defined by most laboratories as 40 to 100 μg/mL, although some clinicians suggest drug concentrations as high as 150 μg/mL with appropriate monitoring of serum concentrations and possible side effects.[4] The most common adverse effects of ethosuximide are gastric distress, nausea, vomiting, and anorexia, but these gastrointestinal problems appear to be caused by local irritation of gastric mucosa. In general, administration of smaller doses and more frequent dosing of the drug produce relief from these side effects. In the upper end of the therapeutic range (>70 μg/mL), some patients begin to have the concentration-dependent adverse effects of ethosuximide treatment—drowsiness, fatigue, lethargy, dizziness, ataxia, hiccups, euphoria, and headaches. Idiosyncratic side effects that are independent of concentration include rash, systemic lupus-like syndromes, and blood dyscrasia (leukopenia, pancytopenia).

TABLE 14-1 International Classification of Epileptic Seizures

MAJOR CLASS	SUBSET OF CLASS	DRUG THERAPY FOR SELECTED SEIZURE TYPE
Partial seizures (beginning locally)	1. Simple partial seizures (without impaired consciousness) a. With motor symptoms b. With somatosensory or special sensory symptoms c. With autonomic symptoms d. With psychological symptoms	Carbamazepine Phenytoin Valproic acid Phenobarbital Primidone
	2. Complex partial seizures (with impaired consciousness) a. Simple partial onset followed by impaired consciousness b. Impaired consciousness at onset	Carbamazepine Phenytoin Valproic acid Phenobarbital Primidone
	3. Partial seizures evolving into secondary generalized seizures	Carbamazepine Phenytoin Valproic acid Phenobarbital Primidone
Generalized seizures (convulsive or nonconvulsive)	1. Absence seizures (typical or atypical; also known as petit mal seizures)	Valproic acid Ethosuximide
	2. Tonic-clonic seizures (also known as grand mal seizures)	Phenytoin Carbamazepine Valproic acid Phenobarbital Primidone

Adapted from Brodie MJ, Dichter MA. Antiepileptic drugs. N Engl J Med 1996;334:168–75.

CLINICAL MONITORING PARAMETERS

The goals of therapy with anticonvulsants are to reduce seizure frequency and maximize quality of life with a minimum of adverse drug effects. Although it is desirable to abolish all seizure episodes, it may not be possible to accomplish this for many patients. Patients should be observed for concentration-related side effects (drowsiness, fatigue, lethargy, dizziness, ataxia, hiccups, euphoria, headaches) and for gastrointestinal upset associated with local irritation of the gastric mucosa (gastric distress, nausea, vomiting, anorexia). Serious but rare idiosyncratic side effects include systemic lupus-like syndromes, leukopenia, and pancytopenia.

Serum concentration of ethosuximide should be measured for most patients. Because epilepsy is an episodic disease, patients do not have seizures on a continuous basis. During dosage titration, it is difficult to determine whether the patient is responding to drug therapy or simply is not having abnormal central nervous system discharges at the time. Measurement of serum concentration of ethosuximide also is valuable to avoid adverse drug effects. Patients are more likely to accept drug therapy if adverse reactions are held to the absolute minimum.

BASIC CLINICAL PHARMACOKINETIC PARAMETERS

Most ethosuximide (70% to 80%) is eliminated from the body through hepatic metabolism by means of hydroxylation and then conjugated to inactive metabolites.[5] About 20% to 30% of an ethosuximide dose is recovered as unchanged drug in the urine.[6] Ethosuximide is not substantially bound to plasma proteins. At concentrations exceeding 100 μg/mL, the drug may follow nonlinear pharmacokinetics, presumably owing to Michaelis-Menten (concentration-dependent or saturable) metabolism.[7] Because an intravenous form of the drug is not commercially available, the absolute bioavailability in humans is not known. However, based on animal studies, the oral bioavailability of ethosuximide capsules (250 mg) and syrup (250 mg/5 mL) is assumed to be 100%.[4] The typical maintenance dose of ethosuximide is 20 mg/kg per day for patients younger than 12 years and 15 mg/kg per day for older patients.[4]

EFFECTS OF DISEASES AND CONDITIONS ON PHARMACOKINETICS AND DOSING

The oral clearance rate (Cl/F) of ethosuximide among children 12 years and older and among adults is 12 mL/h per kilogram. For children it is 16 mL/h per kilogram.[4] The volume of distribution (V/F) of ethosuximide is 0.7 L/kg. Half-life averages 30 hours in children and 60 hours in adults.[4] Although results of studies involving patients with hepatic disease are not available, 70% to 80% of the drug is eliminated through hepatic metabolism. Because of this, patients with cirrhosis of the liver or acute hepatitis may have low ethosuximide clearance because of destruction of the liver parenchyma. This loss of functional hepatic cells decreases the amount of enzymes available to metabolize the drug and decreases clearance. An index of liver dysfunction can be gained by applying the Child-Pugh clinical classification system (Table 14-2).[8] Child-Pugh scores are discussed in detail in Chapter 3, but are briefly discussed here.

The Child-Pugh score consists of five laboratory tests or clinical symptoms: serum albumin, total bilirubin, prothrombin time, ascites, and hepatic encephalopathy. Each of these areas is given a score of 1 (normal) to 3 (severely abnormal; see Table 14-2), and the scores for the five areas are summed. The Child-Pugh score for a patient with normal liver function is 5. The score for a patient with grossly abnormal serum albumin, total bilirubin, and prothrombin time values in addition to severe ascites and hepatic encephalopathy is 15. A Child-Pugh score greater than 8 is grounds for a decrease of 25%

TABLE 14-2 Child-Pugh Scores for Patients with Liver Disease

TEST/SYMPTOM	SCORE 1 POINT	SCORE 2 POINTS	SCORE 3 POINTS
Total bilirubin (mg/dL)	<2.0	2.0–3.0	>3.0
Serum albumin (g/dL)	>3.5	2.8–3.5	<2.8
Prothrombin time (seconds prolonged over control)	<4	4–6	>6
Ascites	Absent	Slight	Moderate
Hepatic encephalopathy	None	Moderate	Severe

Adapted from Pugh RN, Murray-Lyon IM, Dawson JL, Pietroni MC, Williams R. Transection of the oesophagus for bleeding oesophageal varices. Br J Surg 1973;60:646–9.

to 50% in the initial daily dose of ethosuximide. As in the case of any patient with or without liver dysfunction, initial doses are meant as starting points for dosage titration based on patient response and avoidance of adverse effects. Serum concentration of ethosuximide and the presence of adverse drug effects should be monitored frequently for patients with cirrhosis of the liver.

A small amount (20% to 30%) of ethosuximide usually is eliminated unchanged by the kidneys, so patients with renal dysfunction (creatinine clearance, <30 mL/min) receiving ethosuximide should be closely observed.[6] A large amount of ethosuximide is removed during hemodialysis, and supplemental doses may be needed after a dialysis session.[9] The drug crosses into the placenta and enters breast milk, achieving concentrations at both sites similar to concurrent maternal serum concentrations.[10–12]

DRUG INTERACTIONS

Unlike other antiepileptic drugs, ethosuximide is not a hepatic enzyme inducer or inhibitor, and it appears to cause no clinically important drug interactions.[13] Valproic acid can inhibit ethosuximide metabolism and increase steady-state concentration, especially when ethosuximide serum concentrations are in the upper end of the therapeutic range.[7]

INITIAL DOSAGE DETERMINATION METHODS

Pharmacokinetic Dosing Method

The goal of initial dosing of ethosuximide is to compute the best dose possible for the patient given the diseases and conditions that influence ethosuximide pharmacokinetics and the epileptic disorder for which the patient is being treated. To do this, pharmacokinetic parameters for the patient are estimated with average parameters measured for other patients with similar disease and condition profiles.

ESTIMATE OF CLEARANCE

Ethosuximide is metabolized predominately by liver. There is no good way to estimate the elimination characteristics of liver-metabolized drugs using an endogenous marker of liver function in the same manner that serum creatinine and estimated creatinine clearance are used to estimate the elimination of agents that are eliminated by the kidney. Because of this, a patient is categorized according to the diseases and conditions known to change ethosuximide clearance, and the published clearance is used as an estimate of the current patient's clearance. For example, for a 20-kg pediatric patient, ethosuximide clearance is assumed to be 16 mL/h per kilogram: 20 kg · 16 mL/h/kg = 320 mL/h, or 0.32 L/h. To produce the most conservative ethosuximide doses for patients with several diseases or conditions that affect ethosuximide pharmacokinetics, the disease state or condition with the smallest clearance is used to compute doses. This approach avoids accidental overdosage as much as currently possible.

ESTIMATE OF VOLUME OF DISTRIBUTION

The volume of distribution of ethosuximide is assumed to be 0.7 L/kg for adults and children. For a 20-kg pediatric patient, the estimated ethosuximide volume of distribution is 14 L: V = 0.7 L/kg · 20 kg = 14 L.

ESTIMATE OF HALF-LIFE AND ELIMINATION RATE CONSTANT

Once the correct clearance and volume of distribution estimates are identified for the patient, they can be converted into ethosuximide half-life ($t_{1/2}$) and elimination rate constant (k) estimates with the following equations: $t_{1/2} = (0.693 \cdot V)/Cl$; $k = 0.693/t_{1/2} = Cl/V$.

SELECTION OF APPROPRIATE PHARMACOKINETIC MODEL AND EQUATIONS

Ethosuximide follows a one-compartment pharmacokinetic model. Oral ethosuximide has good bioavailability (F = 1), and dosing once or twice a day provides a relatively smooth serum concentration–time curve that emulates intravenous infusion. Because of this, a very simple pharmacokinetic equation for computing the average steady-state serum concentration of ethosuximide (Css in μg/mL = mg/L) is widely used and allows calculation of the maintenance dosage: $Css = [F(D/\tau)]/Cl$, or $D = (Css \cdot Cl \cdot \tau)/F$, where F is the bioavailability fraction of the oral dosage form (F = 1 for oral ethosuximide products), D is the dose of ethosuximide in milligrams, Cl is ethosuximide clearance in liters per hour, and τ is the dosage interval in hours.

Example 1 LK is a 13-year-old, 47-kg (height, 155 cm) girl who has absence seizures. She needs therapy with oral ethosuximide. She has normal liver and renal function. Suggest an initial ethosuximide dosage regimen designed to achieve a steady-state ethosuximide concentration of 50 μg/mL.

1. *Estimate clearance and volume of distribution according to disease states and conditions present in the patient.*

The clearance rate for an older patient is 12 mL/h per kilogram. At this value, estimated clearance is 0.564 L/h: Cl = 47 kg · 12 mL/h/kg = 564 mL/h, or 0.564 L/h. The estimated volume of distribution is 33 L: 47 kg · 0.7 L/kg = 33 L.

2. *Estimate half-life and elimination rate constant.*

Once the correct clearance and volume of distribution estimates are identified for the patient, they can be converted into ethosuximide half-life ($t_{1/2}$) and elimination rate constant (k) estimates with the following equations: $t_{1/2} = (0.693 \cdot V)/Cl = (0.693 \cdot 33\ L)/(0.564\ L/h) = 41\ h$; $k = Cl/V = (0.564\ L/h)/33\ L = 0.017\ h^{-1}$.

3. *Compute the dosage regimen.*

Oral ethosuximide capsules are prescribed to this patient (F = 1). (Note: μg/mL = mg/L, and this concentration unit was substituted for Css in the calculations to avoid unit conversion.) The dosage equation for oral ethosuximide is $D = (Css \cdot Cl \cdot \tau)/F = (50\ mg/L \cdot 0.564\ L/h \cdot 12\ h)/1 = 338\ mg$, rounded to 250 every 12 hours.

Steady-state minimum serum concentration of ethosuximide should be measured after steady state is attained in 3 to 5 half-lives. Because the drug is expected to have a half-life of 41 hours in this patient, steady-state concentration of ethosuximide can be measured any time after the ninth day of dosing (5 half-lives = $5 \cdot 41\ h = 205\ h$, or 9 d). Serum concentration of ethosuximide should be measured if the patient has an exacerbation of epilepsy or if the patient has signs or symptoms of ethosuximide toxicity.

Example 2 CT is a 10-year-old, 40-kg (height, 127 cm) boy who has absence seizures. He needs therapy with oral ethosuximide. He has normal liver and renal function. Suggest an initial ethosuximide dosage regimen designed to achieve a steady-state ethosuximide concentration of 50 μg/mL.

1. *Estimate clearance and volume of distribution according to disease states and conditions present in the patient.*

The clearance rate for a child is 16 mL/h per kilogram. At this value, estimated clearance is 0.640 L/h: $Cl = 40\ kg \cdot 16\ mL/h/kg = 640\ mL/h$, or 0.640 L/h. At 0.7 L/kg, the estimated volume of distribution is 28 L: $40\ kg \cdot 0.7\ L/kg = 28\ L$.

2. *Estimate half-life and elimination rate constant.*

Once the correct clearance and volume of distribution estimates are identified for the patient, they can be converted into ethosuximide half-life ($t_{1/2}$) and elimination rate constant (k) estimates with the following equations: $t_{1/2} = (0.693 \cdot V)/Cl = (0.693 \cdot 28\ L)/(0.640\ L/h) = 30\ h$; $k = Cl/V = (0.640\ L/h)/28\ L = 0.023\ h^{-1}$.

3. *Compute the dosage regimen.*

Oral ethosuximide syrup is prescribed to this patient (F = 1). (Note: μg/mL = mg/L, and this concentration unit was substituted for Css in the calculations to avoid unit conversion.) The dosage equation for oral ethosuximide is $D = (Css \cdot Cl \cdot \tau)/F = (50\ mg/L \cdot 0.640\ L/h \cdot 12\ h)/1 = 384\ mg$, rounded to 400 mg every 12 hours.

Steady-state minimum serum concentration of ethosuximide should be measured after steady state is attained in 3 to 5 half-lives. Because the drug is expected to have a half-life of 30 hours in this patient, steady-state concentration of ethosuximide can be measured any time after the sixth day of dosing (5 half-lives = $5 \cdot 30\ h = 150\ h$, or 6 d). Serum concentration of ethosuximide should be measured if the patient has an exacerbation of epilepsy or if the patient has signs or symptoms of ethosuximide toxicity.

Literature-Based Recommended Dosing

Because of the large variability in the pharmacokinetics of ethosuximide, even when concurrent diseases and conditions are identified, most clinicians believe that use of standard ethosuximide doses in various situations is warranted. The original computation of these doses was based on pharmacokinetic dosing methods and modified according to clinical experience. In general, the expected steady-state serum concentration of ethosuximide used to compute these doses was 40 to 50 μg/mL. The usual initial maintenance dose for patients younger than 12 years is 20 mg/kg per day. For older patients, the initial maintenance dose is 15 mg/kg per day. One or two divided daily doses are initially used for these total doses. To avoid gastrointestinal side effects, doses greater than 1500 mg at one time should be avoided. Dosage increases of 3 to 7 mg/kg per day are made every 1 to 2 weeks depending on response and adverse effects. Although maximal doses are 40 mg/kg per day for children younger than 12 years and 30 mg/kg per day for older patients, serum concentration of ethosuximide and the presence of adverse effects should be used to judge optimal response to the drug. If the patient has marked hepatic dysfunction (Child-Pugh score, ≥8), maintenance doses prescribed with this method should be decreased 25% to 50% depending on the aggressiveness of therapy. To illustrate the similarities and differences between this method of dosage calculation and the pharmacokinetic dosing method, the previous examples are used.

Example 3 LK is a 13-year-old, 47-kg (height, 155 cm) girl who has absence seizures. She needs therapy with oral ethosuximide. She has normal liver and renal function. Suggest an initial ethosuximide dosage regimen designed to achieve a steady-state ethosuximide concentration of 50 μg/mL.

1. *Estimate the ethosuximide dose according to disease states and conditions present in the patient.*

Oral ethosuximide capsules are prescribed to this patient. The suggested initial maintenance dose of ethosuximide for an older patient is 15 mg/kg per day: 47 kg · 15 mg/kg/d = 705 mg/d, rounded to 750 mg/d. The dose can be given as 250 mg in the morning and 500 mg in the evening. The dose is titrated upward in increments of 3 to 7 mg/kg per day every 1 to 2 weeks while the patient is observed for adverse and therapeutic effects. The goals of therapy are maximal suppression of seizures and avoidance of side effects.

Steady-state minimum total serum concentration of ethosuximide should be measured after steady state is attained in 1 to 2 weeks. Serum concentration of ethosuximide also should be measured if the patient has an exacerbation of epilepsy or if the patient has signs or symptoms of ethosuximide toxicity.

Example 4 CT is a 10-year-old, 40-kg (height, 127 cm) boy who has absence seizures. He needs therapy with oral ethosuximide. He has normal liver and renal function. Suggest an initial ethosuximide dosage regimen designed to achieve a steady-state ethosuximide concentration of 50 μg/mL.

1. *Estimate the ethosuximide dose according to disease states and conditions present in the patient.*

Oral ethosuximide syrup is prescribed to this patient. The suggested initial maintenance dose of ethosuximide for a child is 20 mg/kg per day: 40 kg · 20 mg/kg/d = 800 mg/d, or 400 mg every 12 hours. This dose is titrated upward in increments of 3 to 7 mg/kg per day every 1 to 2 weeks while the patient is observed for adverse and therapeutic effects. The goals of therapy are maximal suppression of seizures and avoidance of side effects.

Steady-state minimum total serum concentration of ethosuximide should be measured after steady state is attained in 1 to 2 weeks. Serum concentration of ethosuximide also should be measured if the patient has an exacerbation of epilepsy or if the patient has signs or symptoms of ethosuximide toxicity.

USE OF ETHOSUXIMIDE SERUM CONCENTRATIONS TO ALTER DOSES

Because of the large pharmacokinetic variability among patients, it is likely that doses computed with patient population characteristics will not always produce ethosuximide serum concentrations that are expected or desirable. Because of pharmacokinetic variability, the possible nonlinear pharmacokinetics followed by the drug at high concentrations, the narrow therapeutic index of ethosuximide, and the desire to avoid adverse side effects of ethosuximide, measurement of ethosuximide serum concentration is conducted for most patients to ensure that therapeutic, nontoxic levels are present. In addition to serum concentration of ethosuximide, important patient parameters such as seizure frequency and risk of side effects should be followed to confirm that the patient is responding to treatment and not having adverse drug reactions. When serum concentration of ethosuximide is measured and a dosage change is necessary, clinicians should use the simplest, most straightforward method available to determine a dose that will provide safe and effective treatment.

Linear Pharmacokinetics Method

Because ethosuximide follows linear, dose-proportional pharmacokinetics in most patients with concentrations within and below the therapeutic range, steady-state serum concentrations change in proportion to dose according to the following equation: $D_{new}/Css_{new} = D_{old}/Css_{old}$ or $D_{new} = (Css_{new}/Css_{old})D_{old}$, where D is the dose, Css is the steady-state concentration, old indicates the dose that produced the steady-state concentration that the patient is currently receiving, and new denotes the dose necessary to produce the desired steady-state concentration. The advantages of this method are that it is quick and simple. The disadvantages are steady-state concentrations are required, and the assumption of linear pharmacokinetics may not be valid for all patients. When steady-state serum concentrations increase more than expected after a dosage increase or decrease less than expected after a dosage decrease, nonlinear ethosuximide pharmacokinetics is a possible explanation for the observation. Because of this, suggested dosage increases greater than 75% with this method should be scrutinized by the prescribing clinician, and the risk versus benefit for the patient assessed before large dosage increases (>75% over current dose) are initiated.

Example 5 LK is a 13-year-old, 47-kg (height, 155 cm) girl who has absence seizures. She needs therapy with oral ethosuximide. After dosage titration, the patient is given a prescription for 500 mg every 12 hours of ethosuximide capsules (1000 mg/d) for 1 month. Steady-state total concentration of ethosuximide is 38 μg/mL. The patient is found to be compliant with the dosage regimen. Suggest an ethosuximide dosage regimen designed to achieve a steady-state ethosuximide concentration of 80 μg/mL.

1. *Compute a new dose to achieve the desired serum concentration.*

According to linear pharmacokinetics, the resulting total steady-state serum concentration of ethosuximide is $D_{new} = (Css_{new}/Css_{old})D_{old}$ = [(80 μg/mL)/(38 μg/mL)] 1000 mg/d = 2105 mg/d, rounded to 2000 mg/d, or 1000 mg every 12 hours.

Steady-state minimum total serum concentration of ethosuximide should be measured after steady state is attained in 1 to 2 weeks. Serum concentration of ethosuximide also should be measured if the patient has an exacerbation of epilepsy or if the patient has signs or symptoms of ethosuximide toxicity.

Example 6 CT is a 10-year-old, 40-kg (height, 127 cm) boy who has absence seizures. He needs therapy with oral ethosuximide. After dosage titration, the patient is given a prescription for 500 mg twice a day (1000 mg/d) of ethosuximide syrup for 1 month. Steady-state total concentration of ethosuximide is 130 μg/mL. The patient is found to be compliant with the dosage regimen. Suggest an ethosuximide dosage regimen designed to achieve a steady-state ethosuximide concentration of 75 μg/mL.

1. *Compute a new dose to achieve the desired serum concentration.*

According to linear pharmacokinetics, the resulting total steady-state serum concentration of ethosuximide is $D_{new} = (Css_{new}/Css_{old})D_{old}$ = [(75 μg/mL)/(130 μg/mL)] 1000 mg/d = 577 mg/d, rounded to 500 mg/d, or 250 mg every 12 hours.

Steady-state minimum total serum concentration of ethosuximide should be measured after steady state is attained in 1 to 2 weeks. Serum concentration of ethosuximide also should be measured if the patient has an exacerbation of epilepsy or if the patient has signs or symptoms of ethosuximide toxicity.

Pharmacokinetic Parameter Method

The pharmacokinetic parameter method of adjusting drug doses was among the first techniques for changing doses with serum concentrations. It allows computation of a patient's unique pharmacokinetic constants and uses those to calculate a dose that achieves desired ethosuximide concentrations. The pharmacokinetic parameter method requires that steady state has been achieved, and only steady-state concentration of ethosuximide (Css) is used. Ethosuximide clearance (Cl) can be calculated with the following formula: $Cl = [F(D/\tau)]/Css$, where F is the bioavailability fraction for the oral dosage form (F = 1 for oral ethosuximide products), D is the dose of ethosuximide in milligrams, Css is the steady-state ethosuximide concentration in milligrams per liter, and τ is the dosage interval in hours. To illustrate the similarities and differences between this method of dosage calculation and the pharmacokinetic parameter method, the previous examples are used.

Example 7 LK is a 13-year-old, 47-kg (height, 155 cm) girl who has absence seizures. She needs therapy with oral ethosuximide. After dosage titration, the patient is given a prescription for 500 mg every 12 hours of ethosuximide capsules (1000 mg/d) for 1 month. Steady-state total concentration of ethosuximide is 38 μg/mL. The patient is found to be compliant with the dosage regimen. Suggest an ethosuximide dosage regimen designed to achieve a steady-state ethosuximide concentration of 80 μg/mL.

1. *Compute pharmacokinetic parameters.*

The patient is expected to achieve steady-state conditions after 1 to 2 weeks of therapy. Ethosuximide clearance can be computed with steady-state ethosuximide concentration: $Cl = [F(D/\tau)]/Css = [1(500\ mg/12\ h)]/(38\ mg/L) = 1.1\ L/h$. (Note: μg/mL = mg/L, and this concentration unit was substituted for Css in the calculations to avoid unit conversion.)

2. *Compute the ethosuximide dose.*

Ethosuximide clearance is used to compute the new dose: $D = (Css \cdot Cl \cdot \tau)/F = (80\ mg/L \cdot 1.1\ L/h \cdot 12\ h)/1 = 1056\ mg$, rounded to 1000 mg every 12 hours.

Steady-state trough minimum serum concentration of ethosuximide should be measured after steady state is attained in 1 to 2 weeks. Serum concentration of ethosuximide also should be measured if the patient has an exacerbation of epilepsy or if the patient has signs or symptoms of ethosuximide toxicity.

Example 8 CT is a 10-year-old, 40-kg (height, 127 cm) boy who has absence seizures. He needs therapy with oral ethosuximide. After dosage titration, the patient is given a prescription for 500 mg twice a day (1000 mg/d) of ethosuximide syrup for 1 month. Steady-state total concentration of ethosuximide is 130 μg/mL. The patient is found to be compliant with the dosage regimen. Suggest an ethosuximide dosage regimen designed to achieve a steady-state ethosuximide concentration of 75 μg/mL.

1. *Compute pharmacokinetic parameters.*

The patient is expected to achieve steady-state conditions after 1 to 2 weeks of therapy. Ethosuximide clearance can be computed with steady-state ethosuximide concentration: $Cl = [F(D/\tau)]/Css = [1(500\ mg/12\ h)]/(130\ mg/L) = 0.32\ L/h$. (Note: μg/mL = mg/L, and this concentration unit was substituted for Css in the calculations to avoid unit conversion.)

2. *Compute the ethosuximide dose.*

Ethosuximide clearance is used to compute the new dose: $D = (Css \cdot Cl \cdot \tau)/F = (75\ mg/L \cdot 0.32\ L/h \cdot 12\ h)/1 = 288\ mg$, rounded to 250 mg every 12 hours.

Steady-state minimum total serum concentration of ethosuximide should be measured after steady state is attained in 1 to 2 weeks. Serum concentration of ethosuximide also should be measured if the patient has an exacerbation of epilepsy or if the patient has signs or symptoms of ethosuximide toxicity.

BAYESIAN PHARMACOKINETICS COMPUTER PROGRAMS

Computer programs can assist in the computation of pharmacokinetic parameters for patients. In the most reliable computer programs, a nonlinear regression algorithm incorporates components of Bayes' theorem.[14] Nonlinear regression is a statistical technique in which an iterative process is used to compute the best pharmacokinetic parameters for a concentration–time data set. The patient's drug dosage schedule and serum concentrations are entered into the computer. The computer program has a pharmacokinetic equation programmed for the drug and administration method, such as oral, intravenous bolus, or intravenous infusion. A one-compartment model typically is used, although some programs allow the user to choose among several different equations. With population estimates based on demographic information for the patient, such as age, weight, sex, liver function, cardiac status, supplied by the user, the program computes estimated serum concentration whenever the actual serum concentration is measured. Kinetic parameters are then changed by the computer program, and a new set of estimated serum concentrations are computed. The pharmacokinetic parameters that generate estimated serum concentrations closest to the actual values are stored in the computer memory, and the process is repeated until the set of pharmacokinetic parameters that give estimated serum concentrations statistically closest to the actual serum concentrations are generated. These pharmacokinetic parameters can be used to compute improved dosing schedules for patients. Bayes' theorem is used in the computer algorithm to balance the results of the computations between values based solely on the patient's serum drug concentrations and those based only on patient population parameters. Results of studies in which various methods of dosage adjustment have been compared have consistently shown that these types of computer dosing programs perform at least as well as experienced clinical pharmacokineticists and clinicians and better than inexperienced clinicians.

Some clinicians use Bayesian pharmacokinetics computer programs exclusively to alter drug doses based on serum concentrations. An advantage of this approach is that consistent dosage recommendations are made when several practitioners are involved in therapeutic drug monitoring programs. However, because simpler dosing methods work just as well for patients with stable pharmacokinetic parameters and steady-state drug concentrations, many clinicians reserve the use of computer programs for more difficult situations. Those situations include serum concentrations that are not at steady state, serum concentrations not obtained at the specific times needed to use simpler methods, and unstable pharmacokinetic parameters. Many Bayesian pharmacokinetics computer programs are available. Most should provide answers similar to the ones in the following examples. The program used to solve problems in this book is DrugCalc written by Dr. Dennis Mungall. It is available on his Internet web site (http://members.aol.com/thertch/index.htm).

Example 9 LK is a 13-year-old, 47-kg (height, 155 cm) girl who has absence seizures. She needs therapy with oral ethosuximide. The patient has normal liver and renal function (bilirubin, 0.5 mg/dL; albumin, 4.6 g/dL; serum creatinine, 0.5 mg/dL). After dosage titration, the patient is given a prescription for 500 mg every 12 hours of ethosuximide capsules (1000 mg/d) for 2 weeks. Steady-state total concentration of ethosuximide is 38 μg/mL. The patient is found to be compliant with the dosage regimen. Suggest an ethosuximide dosage regimen designed to achieve a steady-state ethosuximide concentration of 80 μg/mL.

1. *Enter the patient's demographic, drug dosing, and serum concentration–time data into the computer program.*

2. *Compute pharmacokinetic parameters for the patient with a Bayesian pharmacokinetics computer program.*

The pharmacokinetic parameters computed with the program are a volume of distribution of 46 L, a half-life of 26 hours, and a clearance of 1.24 L/h.

3. *Compute the dose required to achieve the desired ethosuximide serum concentrations.*

The one-compartment model, first-order absorption equations used in the program to compute doses indicate that a dose of 1000 mg every 12 hours produces a steady-state ethosuximide concentration of 68 μg/mL.

Example 10 JB is an 8-year-old, 35-kg (height, 127 cm) boy who has absence seizures. Ethosuximide syrup 350 mg every 12 hours has been started. The ethosuximide concentration is 25 μg/mL before the fifth maintenance dose. What ethosuximide dose is needed to achieve a steady-state concentration of 75 μg/mL?

1. *Enter the patient's demographic, drug dosing, and serum concentration–time data into the computer program.*

In this case, it is unlikely that the patient is at steady state, so the linear pharmacokinetics method cannot be used.

2. *Compute pharmacokinetic parameters for the patient with a Bayesian pharmacokinetics computer program.*

The pharmacokinetic parameters computed with the program are a volume of distribution of 30 L, a half-life of 18 hours, and clearance of 1.12 L/h.

3. *Compute the dose required to achieve the desired serum concentration of ethosuximide.*

The one-compartment model, oral equations used in the program to compute doses indicate that a dose of ethosuximide 1000 mg every 12 hours produces a steady-state concentration of 69 μg/mL.

PROBLEMS

The following problems are intended to emphasize the computation of initial and individualized doses with clinical pharmacokinetic techniques. Clinicians always should consult the patient's chart to confirm that current anticonvulsant therapy is appropriate. All other medications that the patient is taking, including prescription and nonprescription drugs, should be recorded and checked to ascertain the risk of drug interaction with ethosuximide.

1. YH is a 4-year-old, 16-kg (height, 102 cm) boy who has absence seizures. He needs therapy with oral ethosuximide. He has normal liver function. Suggest an initial etho-

suximide dosage regimen designed to achieve a steady-state ethosuximide concentration of 50 μg/mL.

2. Patient YH (see problem 1) is given a prescription for 300 mg/d of ethosuximide syrup for 1 month. Steady-state total concentration of ethosuximide is 40 μg/mL. The patient is found to be compliant with the dosage regimen. Suggest an ethosuximide dosage regimen designed to achieve a steady-state ethosuximide concentration of 75 μg/mL.

3. FD is a 9-year-old, 35-kg (height, 137 cm) girl who has absence seizures. She needs therapy with oral ethosuximide. She has normal liver function. Suggest an initial ethosuximide dosage regimen designed to achieve a steady-state ethosuximide concentration of 75 μg/mL.

4. Patient FD (see problem 3) is given a prescription for 350 mg every 12 hours (700 mg/d) of ethosuximide syrup for 2 weeks. Steady-state ethosuximide total concentration is 55 μg/mL. The patient is found to be compliant with the dosage regimen. Suggest an ethosuximide dosage regimen designed to achieve a steady-state ethosuximide concentration of 90 μg/mL.

5. LK is a 14-year-old, 60-kg (height, 168 cm) boy who has absence seizures. He needs therapy with ethosuximide capsules. He has normal liver and renal function. Suggest an initial ethosuximide dosage regimen designed to achieve a steady-state ethosuximide concentration of 50 μg/mL.

6. Patient LK (see problem 5) is given a prescription for 500 mg every 12 hours (1000 mg/d) of ethosuximide capsules for 2 weeks. Steady-state total concentration of ethosuximide is 40 μg/mL. The patient is found to be compliant with the dosage regimen. Suggest an ethosuximide dosage regimen designed to achieve a steady-state ethosuximide concentration of 60 μg/mL.

7. DG is a 15-year-old, 68-kg (height, 173 cm) boy who has absence seizures. He is receiving 1000 mg/d of ethosuximide capsules. He has normal liver and renal function. Total ethosuximide concentration is 22 μg/mL before the fourth dose. Compute an ethosuximide dose that will provide a steady-state concentration of 50 μg/mL.

8. YF is a 5-year-old, 20-kg (height, 107 cm) girl who has absence seizures. She is given a new prescription of 250 mg every 12 hours of oral ethosuximide syrup. She has normal liver and renal function. The minimum ethosuximide concentration before the fifth dose is 42 μg/mL. Compute an ethosuximide dose that will provide a total steady-state concentration of 75 μg/mL.

ANSWERS TO PROBLEMS

1. Solution to problem 1.

Pharmacokinetic Dosing Method

1. *Estimate clearance and volume of distribution according to disease states and conditions present in the patient.*

The clearance rate for a pediatric patient is 16 mL/h per kilogram. At this value, estimated clearance is 0.256 L/h: Cl = 16 kg · 16 mL/h/kg = 256 mL/h, or 0.256 L/h. At 0.7 L/kg, the estimated volume of distribution is 11 L: 16 kg · 0.7 L/kg = 11 L.

2. *Estimate half-life and elimination rate constant.*

Once the correct clearance and volume of distribution estimates are identified for the patient, they can be converted into ethosuximide half-life ($t_{1/2}$) and elimination rate constant (k) estimates with the following equations: $t_{1/2} = (0.693 \cdot V)/Cl = (0.693 \cdot 11\ L)/(0.256\ L/h) = 30\ h$; $k = Cl/V = (0.256\ L/h)/11\ L = 0.023\ h^{-1}$.

3. *Compute the dosage regimen.*

Oral ethosuximide syrup is prescribed to this patient (F = 1). (Note: µg/mL = mg/L, and this concentration unit was substituted for Css in the calculations to avoid unit conversion.) The dosage equation for oral ethosuximide is $D = (Css \cdot Cl \cdot \tau)/F = (50\ mg/L \cdot 0.256\ L/h \cdot 12\ h)/1 = 154\ mg$, rounded to 150 every 12 hours.

Steady-state minimum serum concentration of ethosuximide should be measured after steady state is attained in 3 to 5 half-lives. Because the drug is expected to have a half-life of 30 hours in this patient, steady-state concentration of ethosuximide can be measured any time after the sixth day of dosing (5 half-lives = 5 · 30 h = 150 h, or 6 d). Serum concentration of ethosuximide should be measured if the patient has an exacerbation of epilepsy or if the patient has signs or symptoms of ethosuximide toxicity.

Literature-Based Recommended Dosing

1. *Estimate the ethosuximide dose according to disease states and conditions present in the patient.*

Oral ethosuximide syrup is prescribed to this patient. The suggested initial maintenance dose of ethosuximide for a pediatric patient is 20 mg/kg per day: 16 kg · 20 mg/kg/d = 320 mg/d, rounded to 300 mg/d, or 150 mg every 12 hours. This dose is titrated upward in increments of 3 to 7 mg/kg per day every 1 to 2 weeks while the patient is observed for adverse and therapeutic effects. The goals of therapy are maximal suppression of seizures and avoidance of side effects.

Steady-state minimum total serum concentration of ethosuximide should be measured after steady state is attained in 1 to 2 weeks. Serum concentration of ethosuximide also should be measured if the patient has an exacerbation of epilepsy or if the patient has signs or symptoms of ethosuximide toxicity.

2. Solution to problem 2.

Linear Pharmacokinetics Method

1. *Compute a new dose to achieve the desired serum concentration.*

According to linear pharmacokinetics, the resulting total steady-state ethosuximide serum concentration is $D_{new} = (Css_{new}/Css_{old})D_{old} = [(75\ \mu g/mL)/(40\ \mu g/mL)]\ 300\ mg/d = 563\ mg/d$, rounded to 600 mg/d.

Steady-state minimum total serum concentration of ethosuximide should be measured after steady state is attained in 1 to 2 weeks. Serum concentration of ethosuximide also should be measured if the patient has an exacerbation of epilepsy or if the patient has signs or symptoms of ethosuximide toxicity.

Pharmacokinetic Parameter Method

1. *Compute pharmacokinetic parameters.*

The patient is expected to achieve steady-state conditions after 1 to 2 weeks of therapy. Ethosuximide clearance can be computed with steady-state ethosuximide concentration: $Cl = [F(D/\tau)]/Css = [1(300\ mg/24\ h)]/(40\ mg/L) = 0.31\ L/h$. (Note: μg/mL = mg/L, and this concentration unit was substituted for Css in the calculations to avoid unit conversion.)

2. *Compute the ethosuximide dose.*

Ethosuximide clearance is used to compute the new dose: $D = (Css \cdot Cl \cdot \tau)/F = (75\ mg/L \cdot 0.31\ L/h \cdot 24\ h)/1 = 558\ mg$, rounded to 600 mg every 24 hours.

Steady-state minimum total serum concentration of ethosuximide should be measured after steady state is attained in 1 to 2 weeks. Serum concentration of ethosuximide also should be measured if the patient has an exacerbation of epilepsy or if the patient has signs or symptoms of ethosuximide toxicity.

Bayesian Pharmacokinetics Computer Program Method

1. *Enter the patient's demographic, drug dosing, and serum concentration–time data into the computer program.*

2. *Compute pharmacokinetic parameters for the patient with a Bayesian pharmacokinetics computer program.*

The pharmacokinetic parameters computed with the program are a volume of distribution of 11.3 L, a half-life of 32 hours, and a clearance of 0.24 L/h.

3. *Compute the dose required to achieve the desired serum concentration of ethosuximide.*

The one-compartment model, first-order absorption equations used in the program to compute doses indicate that a dose of 500 mg/d produces a steady-state ethosuximide concentration of 68 μg/mL.

3. Solution to problem 3.

Pharmacokinetic Dosing Method

1. *Estimate clearance and volume of distribution according to disease states and conditions present in the patient.*

The clearance rate for a pediatric patient is 16 mL/h per kilogram. At this value, estimated clearance is 560 L/h: $Cl = 35\ kg \cdot 16\ mL/h/kg = 560\ mL/h$, or 0.560 L/h. At 0.7 L/kg, the estimated volume of distribution is 25 L: $35\ kg \cdot 0.7\ L/kg = 25\ L$.

2. *Estimate half-life and elimination rate constant.*

Once the correct clearance and volume of distribution estimates are identified for the patient, they can be converted into ethosuximide half-life ($t_{1/2}$) and elimination rate constant (k) estimates with the following equations: $t_{1/2} = (0.693 \cdot V)/Cl = (0.693 \cdot 25\ L)/(0.560\ L/h) = 31\ h$; $k = Cl/V = (0.560\ L/h)/25\ L = 0.022\ h^{-1}$.

3. *Compute the dosage regimen.*

Oral ethosuximide syrup is prescribed to this patient (F = 1). (Note: μg/mL = mg/L, and this concentration unit was substituted for Css in the calculations to avoid unit conversion.) The dosage equation for oral ethosuximide is $D = (Css \cdot Cl \cdot \tau)/F = (75\ mg/L \cdot 0.560\ L/h \cdot 12\ h)/1 = 504\ mg$, rounded to 500 mg every 12 hours.

Steady-state minimum serum concentration of ethosuximide should be measured after steady state is attained in 3 to 5 half-lives. Because the drug is expected to have a half-life of 31 hours in this patient, steady-state concentration of ethosuximide can be measured any time after the sixth day of dosing (5 half-lives = 5 · 31 h = 155 h, or 6 d). Serum concentration of ethosuximide should be measured if the patient has an exacerbation of epilepsy or if the patient has signs or symptoms of ethosuximide toxicity.

Literature-Based Recommended Dosing

1. *Estimate the ethosuximide dose according to disease states and conditions present in the patient.*

Oral ethosuximide syrup is prescribed to this patient. The suggested initial maintenance dose of ethosuximide for a pediatric patient is 20 mg/kg per day: 35 kg · 20 mg/kg/d = 700 mg/d, or 350 mg every 12 hours. This dose is titrated upward in increments of 3 to 7 mg/kg per day every 1 to 2 weeks while the patient is observed for adverse and therapeutic effects. The goals of therapy are maximal suppression of seizures and avoidance of side effects.

Steady-state minimum total serum concentration of ethosuximide should be measured after steady state is attained in 1 to 2 weeks. Serum concentration of ethosuximide also should be measured if the patient has an exacerbation of their epilepsy or if the patient has signs or symptoms of ethosuximide toxicity.

4. Solution to problem 4.

Linear Pharmacokinetics Method

1. *Compute a new dose to achieve the desired serum concentration.*

According to linear pharmacokinetics, the resulting total steady-state ethosuximide serum concentration is $D_{new} = (Css_{new}/Css_{old})D_{old} = [(90\ \mu g/mL)/(55\ \mu g/mL)]\ 700\ mg/d = 1145\ mg/d$, rounded to 1100 mg/d, or 550 mg every 12 hours.

Steady-state minimum total serum concentration of ethosuximide should be measured after steady state is attained in 1 to 2 weeks. Serum concentration of ethosuximide also should be measured if the patient has an exacerbation of epilepsy or if the patient has signs or symptoms of ethosuximide toxicity.

Pharmacokinetic Parameter Method

1. *Compute pharmacokinetic parameters.*

The patient is expected to achieve steady-state conditions after 1 to 2 weeks of therapy. Ethosuximide clearance can be computed with steady-state ethosuximide concentration: Cl = [F(D/τ)]/Css = [1(350 mg/12 h)]/(55 mg/L) = 0.53 L/h. (Note: μg/mL = mg/L, and this concentration unit was substituted for Css in the calculations to avoid unit conversion.)

2. *Compute the ethosuximide dose.*

Ethosuximide clearance is used to compute the new dose: D = (Css · Cl · τ)/F = (90 mg/L · 0.53 L/h · 12 h)/1 = 572 mg, rounded to 600 mg every 12 hours.

Steady-state minimum total serum concentration of ethosuximide should be measured after steady state is attained in 1 to 2 weeks. Serum concentration of ethosuximide also should be measured if the patient has an exacerbation of epilepsy or if the patient has signs or symptoms of ethosuximide toxicity.

Bayesian Pharmacokinetics Computer Program Method

1. *Enter the patient's demographic, drug dosing, and serum concentration–time data into the computer program.*

2. *Compute pharmacokinetic parameters for the patient with a Bayesian pharmacokinetics computer program.*

The pharmacokinetic parameters computed with the program are a volume of distribution of 25 L, a half-life of 36 hours, and a clearance of 0.48 L/h.

3. *Compute the dose required to achieve the desired ethosuximide serum concentrations.*

The one-compartment model, first-order absorption equations used in the program to compute doses indicate that a dose of 600 mg every 12 hours produces a steady-state ethosuximide concentration of 95 μg/mL.

5. Solution to problem 5.

Pharmacokinetic Dosing Method

1. *Estimate clearance and volume of distribution according to disease states and conditions present in the patient.*

The clearance rate for an older patient is 12 mL/h per kilogram. At this value, estimated clearance is 0.720 L/h: Cl = 60 kg · 12 mL/h/kg = 720 mL/h, or 0.720 L/h. At 0.7 L/kg, the estimated volume of distribution is 42 L: 60 kg · 0.7 L/kg = 42 L.

2. *Estimate half-life and elimination rate constant.*

Once the correct clearance and volume of distribution estimates are identified for the patient, they can be converted into ethosuximide half-life ($t_{1/2}$) and elimination rate constant (k) estimates with the following equations: $t_{1/2} = (0.693 \cdot V)/Cl = (0.693 \cdot 42\ L)/(0.720\ L/h) = 40\ h$; $k = Cl/V = (0.720\ L/h)/42\ L = 0.017\ h^{-1}$.

3. *Compute the dosage regimen.*

Oral ethosuximide capsules are prescribed to this patient (F = 1). (Note: μg/mL = mg/L, and this concentration unit was substituted for Css in the calculations to avoid unit conversion.) The dosage equation for oral ethosuximide is $D = (Css \cdot Cl \cdot \tau)/F = (50\ mg/L \cdot 0.720\ L/h \cdot 24\ h)/1 = 864\ mg$, rounded to 750 mg/d.

Steady-state minimum serum concentration of ethosuximide should be measured after steady state is attained in 3 to 5 half-lives. Because the drug is expected to have a half-life of 40 hours in this patient, steady-state concentration of ethosuximide can be measured any time after the sixth day of dosing (5 half-lives = 5 · 40 h = 200 h, or 8 d). Serum concentration of ethosuximide should be measured if the patient has an exacerbation of epilepsy or if the patient has signs or symptoms of ethosuximide toxicity.

Literature-Based Recommended Dosing

1. *Estimate the ethosuximide dose according to disease states and conditions present in the patient.*

Oral ethosuximide capsules are prescribed to this patient. The suggested initial maintenance dose of ethosuximide for an older patient is 15 mg/kg per day: 60 kg · 15 mg/kg/d = 900 mg/d, rounded to 1000 mg/d. This dose is titrated upward in increments of 3 to 7 mg/kg per day every 1 to 2 weeks while the patient is observed for adverse and therapeutic effects. The goals of therapy are maximal suppression of seizures and avoidance of side effects.

Steady-state minimum total serum concentration of ethosuximide should be measured after steady state is attained in 1 to 2 weeks. Serum concentration of ethosuximide also should be measured if the patient has an exacerbation of epilepsy or if the patient has signs or symptoms of ethosuximide toxicity.

6. Solution to problem 6.

Linear Pharmacokinetics Method

1. *Compute a new dose to achieve the desired serum concentration.*

According to linear pharmacokinetics, the resulting total steady-state ethosuximide serum concentration is $D_{new} = (Css_{new}/Css_{old})D_{old} = [(60\ \mu g/mL)/(40\ \mu g/mL)]\ 1000\ mg/d = 1500\ mg/d$, or 750 mg every 12 hours.

Steady-state minimum total serum concentration of ethosuximide should be measured after steady state is attained in 1 to 2 weeks. Serum concentration of ethosuximide also should be measured if the patient has an exacerbation of epilepsy or if the patient has signs or symptoms of ethosuximide toxicity.

Pharmacokinetic Parameter Method

1. *Compute pharmacokinetic parameters.*

The patient is expected to achieve steady-state conditions after 1 to 2 weeks of therapy. Ethosuximide clearance can be computed with a steady-state ethosuximide concentration: $Cl = [F(D/\tau)]/Css = [1(500\ mg/12\ h)]/(40\ mg/L) = 1.0\ L/h$. (Note: μg/mL = mg/L, and this concentration unit was substituted for Css in the calculations to avoid unit conversion.)

2. *Compute the ethosuximide dose.*

Ethosuximide clearance is used to compute the new dose: $D = (Css \cdot Cl \cdot \tau)/F = (60\ mg/L \cdot 1.0\ L/h \cdot 12\ h)/1 = 720\ mg$, rounded to 750 mg every 12 hours.

Steady-state minimum total serum concentration of ethosuximide should be measured after steady state is attained in 1 to 2 weeks. Serum concentration of ethosuximide also should be measured if the patient has an exacerbation of epilepsy or if the patient has signs or symptoms of ethosuximide toxicity.

Bayesian Pharmacokinetics Computer Program Method

1. *Enter the patient's demographic, drug dosing, and serum concentration–time data into the computer program.*

2. *Compute pharmacokinetic parameters for the patient with a Bayesian pharmacokinetics computer program.*

The pharmacokinetic parameters computed with the program are a volume of distribution of 42 L, a half-life of 32 hours, and a clearance of 0.93 L/h.

3. *Compute the dose required to achieve the desired serum concentration of ethosuximide.*

The one-compartment model, first-order absorption equations used in the program to compute doses indicate that a dose of 750 mg every 12 hours produces a steady-state ethosuximide concentration of 61 μg/mL.

7. Solution to problem 7.

Bayesian Pharmacokinetics Computer Program Method

1. *Enter the patient's demographic, drug dosing, and serum concentration–time data into the computer program.*

This patient is not at steady state, so linear pharmacokinetics cannot be used.

2. *Compute pharmacokinetic parameters for the patient with a Bayesian pharmacokinetics computer program.*

The pharmacokinetic parameters computed with the program are a volume of distribution of 48 L, a half-life of 29 hours, and a clearance of 1.2 L/h.

3. *Compute the dose required to achieve the desired serum concentration of ethosuximide.*

The one-compartment model, first-order absorption equations used in the program to compute doses indicate that a dose of 1750 mg every 24 hours produces a steady-state ethosuximide concentration of 48 μg/mL. To avoid possible gastrointestinal side effects, this daily dose should be given as a divided dose of 750 mg in the morning and 1000 mg in the evening.

8. Solution to problem 8.

Bayesian Pharmacokinetics Computer Program Method

1. *Enter the patient's demographic, drug dosing, and serum concentration–time data into the computer program.*

2. *Compute pharmacokinetic parameters for the patient with a Bayesian pharmacokinetics computer program.*

The pharmacokinetic parameters computed with the program are a volume of distribution of 13 L, a half-life of 31 hours, and a clearance of 0.30 L/h.

3. *Compute the dose required to achieve the desired serum concentration of ethosuximide.*

The one-compartment model, first-order absorption equations used in the program to compute doses indicate that a dose of 300 mg every 12 hours produces a steady-state ethosuximide concentration of 76 μg/mL.

REFERENCES

1. Brodie MJ, Dichter MA. Antiepileptic drugs. N Engl J Med 1996;334:168–75.
2. McNamara JO. Drugs effective in the therapy of the epilepsies. In: Hardman JG, Limbird LE, Molinoff PB, Ruddon RW, Gilman AG, eds. The pharmacological basis of therapeutics. New York: McGraw-Hill, 1996:461–86.
3. Graves NM, Garnett WR. Epilepsy. In: DiPiro JT, Talbert RL, Yee GC, Matzke GR, Wells BG, Posey LM, eds. Pharmacotherapy: a pathophysiologic approach. Stamford, CT: Appleton & Lange, 1999:952–75.
4. Garnett WR. Antiepileptics. In: Schumacher GE, ed. Therapeutic drug monitoring. Stamford, CT: Appleton & Lange, 1995:345–95.
5. Chang T. Ethosuximide: biotransformation. In: Levy RH, Mattson R, Meldrum B, eds. Antiepileptic drugs. New York: Raven Press, 1989:679–83.
6. Glazko AJ. Antiepileptic drugs: biotransformation, metabolism, and serum half-life. Epilepsia 1975;16:367–91.
7. Bauer LA, Harris C, Wilensky AJ, Raisys VA, Levy RH. Ethosuximide kinetics: possible interaction with valproic acid. Clin Pharmacol Ther 1982;31:741–5.
8. Pugh RN, Murray-Lyon IM, Dawson JL, Pietroni MC, Williams R. Transection of the oesophagus for bleeding oesophageal varices. Br J Surg 1973;60:646–9.
9. Marbury TC, Lee CS, Perchalski RJ, Wilder BJ. Hemodialysis clearance of ethosuximide in patients with chronic renal disease. Am J Hosp Pharm 1981;38:1757–60.

10. Chang T. Ethosuximide: absorption, distribution, and excretion. In: Levy RH, Mattson R, Meldrum B, eds. Antiepileptic drugs. New York: Raven Press, 1989:679–83.
11. Rane A, Tunell R. Ethosuximide in human milk and in plasma of a mother and her nursed infant. Br J Clin Pharmacol 1981;12:855–8.
12. Koup JR, Rose JQ, Cohen ME. Ethosuximide pharmacokinetics in a pregnant patient and her newborn. Epilepsia 1978;19:535–9.
13. Hansten PD, Horn JR. Drug interactions analysis and management. Vancouver, WA: Applied Therapeutics, 1999:480.
14. Wandell M, Mungall D. Computer assisted drug interpretation and drug regimen optimization. Am Assoc Clin Chem 1984;6:1–11.

Part V

IMMUNOSUPPRESSANTS

15

CYCLOSPORINE

INTRODUCTION

Cyclosporine is a cyclic polypeptide with immunosuppressant properties that is used for the prevention of graft-versus-host disease in the care of recipients of bone marrow transplant, for the prevention of graft rejection among recipients of solid-organ transplants, and for the management of psoriasis, rheumatoid arthritis, and a variety of other autoimmune diseases.[1–5] The immunomodulating properties of cyclosporine are caused by its ability to block the production of interleukin-2 and other cytokines secreted by T lymphocytes.[6] Cyclosporine binds to cyclophilin, an intracellular cytoplasmic protein in T cells. The cyclosporine-cyclophilin complex interacts with calcineurin, inhibits the catalytic activity of calcineurin, and prevents production of intermediaries involved in the expression of genes that regulate the production of cytokines.

THERAPEUTIC AND TOXIC CONCENTRATIONS

The therapeutic range of cyclosporine used by clinicians varies greatly according to the type of assay used to measure cyclosporine and whether blood or serum concentrations are measured by the clinical laboratory (Table 15-1).[1–5,7,8] Because cyclosporine is bound to erythrocytes, blood concentration is higher than simultaneously measured serum or plasma concentrations. High-pressure liquid chromatography (HPLC) assay techniques are specific for measurement of cyclosporine in blood, serum, or plasma. However, older immunoassays conducted with fluorescence polarization (polyclonal TDx® assay; Abbott Diagonostics) or radioimmunoassay (polyclonal RIA; various manufacturers) are nonspe-

TABLE 15-1 Therapeutic Concentrations of Cyclosporine for Different Assay Techniques and Biologic Fluids

ASSAY	BIOLOGIC FLUID	THERAPEUTIC CONCENTRATION (ng/mL)
High-pressure liquid chromatography (HPLC), monoclonal fluorescence polarization immunoassay (monoclonal TDx® assay; Abbott Diagnostics), or monocolonal radioimmunoassay (various manufacturers)	Blood	100–400
High-pressure liquid chromatography (HPLC), monoclonal fluorescence polarization immunoassay (monoclonal TDx® assay; Abbott Diagnostics), or monoclonal radioimmunoassay (various manufacturers)	Plasma	50–150
Polyclonal fluorescence polarization immunoassay (polyclonal TDx® assay; Abbott Diagnostics), or polyclonal radioimmunoassay (various manufacturers)	Blood	200–800
Polyclonal fluorescence polarization immunoassay (polyclonal TDx® assay; Abbott Diagnostics), or polyclonal radioimmunoassay (various manufacturers)	Plasma	100–400

cific and measure both cyclosporine and its metabolites. Newer monoclonal fluorescence polarization (monoclonal TDx® assay) and radioimmunoassays (various) are now available that are relatively specific for cyclosporine and produce results similar to those of HPLC. Cyclosporine concentration measured simultaneously with a specific HPLC technique or a specific immunoassay will be lower than that measured at the same time with a nonspecific immunoassay.

Because cyclosporine metabolites are excreted in the bile, recipients of liver transplants can have extremely high concentrations of cyclosporine metabolites in the blood, serum, and plasma immediately after transplantation because bile production has not begun in the newly transplanted organ. If nonspecific immunoassays are used to measure cyclosporine concentration immediately after transplantation before the graft has begun to produce bile, the predominate species measured with this assay may be cyclosporine metabolites and not cyclosporine. One reason some laboratories favor the use of immunoassays for the measurement of cyclosporine concentration, although they are less specific for the parent compound, is that it takes less time to perform the procedure and cyclosporine concentrations can be returned to clinicians more rapidly. For the purposes of the pharmacokinetic calculations and problems in this book, cyclosporine concentration in the blood measured with cyclosporine-specific HPLC is used.

Desired cyclosporine concentrations often differ among the various types of organ transplantation, change during the posttransplantation phase, and are determined with protocols specific to the transplantation service and institution.[1–5,7,8] It is especially important for clinicians to be aware of these factors, because acceptable cyclosporine concentrations under these different circumstances may be different from those listed by the clinical laboratory or those given in this text.

For patients receiving cyclosporine after bone marrow transplantation, the goals of therapy are to prevent graft-versus-host disease and avoid adverse effects of immunosuppressant therapy.[4,7,8] Graft-versus-host disease occurs when donor T lymphocytes detect antigens on host tissues and produce an immunologic response against these antigens and host tissues. Acute graft-versus-host disease usually occurs within the first 60 days of transplantation of donor marrow and causes epithelial tissue damage in organs. The most common tissues attacked are skin, gastrointestinal tract, and liver. To prevent acute graft-versus-host disease among recipients of allogeneic bone marrow transplants who have HLA-antigen–identical sibling donors, cyclosporine therapy usually is instituted on the day of transplantation (day 0). Doses are adjusted to provide therapeutic minimum concentrations. Methotrexate or glucocorticoids usually are given in conjunction with cyclosporine. If prophylaxis of acute graft-versus-host disease is successful, cyclosporine doses can be tapered starting on approximately posttransplantation day 50. The goal is to discontinue the drug by about posttransplantation day 180. For recipients of allogeneic bone marrow transplants who have HLA-mismatched or HLA-identical unrelated donors, the risk of acute graft-versus-host disease is higher, so cyclosporine therapy may be more prolonged for these patients. After posttransplantation day 100, chronic graft-versus-host disease may occur and can be managed with cyclosporine.

For patients receiving solid-organ transplants, such as kidney, liver, heart, lung, or heart and lung, the goals of cyclosporine therapy are to prevent acute or chronic rejection of the transplanted organ and to minimize the side effects of the drug.[1–3,5,7,8] The immune system of a recipient of a solid-organ transplant detects foreign antigens on the donor organ that produce an immunologic response to the graft. This response causes inflammatory and cytotoxic effects on the transplanted tissue and produces the risk of tissue damage and organ failure. In the case of a rejected kidney transplant, it is possible to remove the graft and begin dialysis to sustain their life. However, for recipients of other solid organs, graft rejection can cause death. Because cyclosporine can cause nephrotoxicity, many centers delay cyclosporine treatment of recipients of renal transplants for a few days or until the kidney begins functioning to avoid untoward effects on the newly transplanted organ. Desired cyclosporine concentration generally is lower among renal transplant recipients than among recipients of other organs (typically 100 to 200 ng/mL versus 150 to 300 ng/mL in whole blood with specific HPLC) to avoid toxicity in the renal graft. For recipients of other solid-organ transplants, cyclosporine therapy may be started several hours before the operation. During the immediately postoperative phase, intravenous cyclosporine may be given to these patients. For long-term immunosuppression of recipients of solid-organ transplants, cyclosporine doses are gradually tapered to the lowest concentration and dose possible over a 6- to 12-month period as long as rejection episodes do not occur.

Hypertension, nephrotoxicity, hyperlipidemia, tremor, hirsutism, and gingival hyperplasia are typical adverse effects of cyclosporine treatment.[1–8] Hypertension is the most common side effect. It is controlled with traditional antihypertensive drug therapy. Nephrotoxicity is separated into acute and chronic varieties. *Acute nephrotoxicity* is concentration- or dose-dependent and reverses with a dosage decrease. Renal damage in this situation is thought to be due to renal vasoconstriction, which increases renal vascular resistance, decreases renal blood flow, and decreases glomerular filtration rate. *Chronic nephrotoxicity* is accompanied by renal tissue damage, including interstitial fibrosis, nonspecific tubular vacuolization, and structural changes in the arteries, arterioles, and proximal tubular epithelium. Increased serum creatinine and blood urea nitrogen values, hyperkalemia, hyperuricemia, proteinuria, and increased renal sodium excretion occur with cyclosporine-induced nephrotoxicity. The clinical features of cyclosporine nephrotoxicity and *acute* graft rejection are similar among renal transplant patients. Renal biopsy may be performed to differentiate these possibilities.[1] Because biopsy findings are similar for cyclosporine-induced nephrotoxicity and *chronic* rejection of renal transplants, this technique is less helpful in this situation. Hyperlipidemia is managed with dietary counseling and antilipid drug therapy. Decreases in cyclosporine dosage may be necessary to decrease tremors associated with drug therapy. Hirsutism usually is addressed with counseling. Gingival hyperplasia can be minimized with dental hygiene and care.

CLINICAL MONITORING PARAMETERS

Recipients of bone marrow transplants should be observed for the signs and symptoms of graft-versus-host disease.[4] These include generalized maculopapular skin rash, diarrhea, abdominal pain, ileus, hyperbilirubinemia, and increased levels of serum alanine aminotransferase (ALT), aspartate aminotransferase (AST), and alkaline phosphatase, which indicate abnormal liver function. Patients with severe chronic graft-versus-host disease may have involvement of the skin, liver, eyes, mouth, esophagus, or other organs that resembles that of systemic autoimmune disease.

Recipients of solid-organ transplants should be observed for graft rejection. Among renal transplant patients, increased serum creatinine level, azotemia, hypertension, edema, weight gain due to fluid retention, graft tenderness, fever, and malaise may be caused by acute rejection.[1] Hypertension, proteinuria, a continuous decline in renal function (increases in serum creatinine and blood urea nitrogen levels), and uremia indicate chronic rejection of renal transplants. Among recipients of hepatic transplants, signs and symptoms of acute rejection include fever, lethargy, graft tenderness, increased leukocyte count, change in color or amount of bile, hyperbilirubinemia, and increased levels of liver enzymes.[5] Chronic rejection of a liver transplant may be accompanied only by increased levels of liver enzymes and jaundice. For recipients of heart transplants, acute rejection is accompanied by low-grade fever, malaise, heart failure (presence of S_3 heart sound), or atrial arrhythmia.[2] Chronic rejection in heart transplant patients, also known as *cardiac allograft vasculopathy*, is characterized by accelerated coronary artery atherosclerosis. The symptoms include arrhythmia, decreased left ventricular function, heart failure, myocardial infarction, and sudden cardiac death. For all recipients of solid-organ transplants, results of tissue biopsy of the transplanted tissue confirm the diagnosis of organ rejection.[1–5]

Typical adverse effects of cyclosporine include hypertension, nephrotoxicity, hyperlipidemia, tremor, hirsutism, and gingival hyperplasia.[1–8] The management of these more common drug side effects are discussed earlier. Adverse reactions that occur less frequently include gastrointestinal side effects (nausea, vomiting, diarrhea), headache, hepatotoxicity, hyperglycemia, acne, leukopenia, hyperkalemia, and hypomagnesemia.

Because of the pivotal role of cyclosporine as an immunosuppressant in the care of transplant recipients and because of the severity of the concentration- and dose-dependent side effects, concentration of cyclosporine should be measured for every patient receiving the drug. If a patient has signs or symptoms of graft-versus-host disease or organ rejection, cyclosporine concentration should be measured to ensure that levels have not fallen below the therapeutic range. If a patient has a clinical problem that may be an adverse effect of cyclosporine therapy, cyclosporine concentration should be measured to determine whether levels are in the toxic range. Immediately after transplantation, cyclosporine concentration is measured daily for most patients even though steady state may not yet have been achieved. The aim is to prevent acute rejection among recipients of solid-organ transplants or acute graft-versus-host disease among recipients of bone marrow transplants. After discharge from the hospital, cyclosporine concentrations are measured at most clinic visits. For patients receiving allogeneic bone marrow transplants from HLA-identical sibling donors, it usually is possible to decrease cyclosporine doses and concentrations about 2 months after transplantation and to stop cyclosporine therapy altogether about 6 months after transplantation if no or mild acute rejection episodes have taken place. However, patients who have undergone allogeneic transplantation of marrow from HLA-mismatched related or HLA-identical unrelated donors and all solid-organ transplant patients need long-term cyclosporine therapy. To decrease the risk of adverse effects, cyclosporine doses and concentration are decreased to the minimum required to prevent graft-versus-host reactions or rejection. Methods to adjust cyclosporine doses with cyclosporine concentration are discussed later. Although some newer data are available that suggest determination of cyclosporine area under the concentration–time curve using multiple concentrations[9,10] or 2-hour postdose cyclosporine concentrations[11] may be useful in the future, most transplant centers continue to use predose minimum cyclosporine concentration determinations to adjust drug doses.

BASIC CLINICAL PHARMACOKINETIC PARAMETERS

Cyclosporine is almost completely (>99%) eliminated through hepatic metabolism.[12] Hepatic metabolism is mainly through the CYP3A4 enzyme system, and the drug is a substrate for P-glycoprotein. There are more than 25 identified cyclosporine metabolites.[7,8] None of these metabolites appear to have appreciable immunosuppressive effects on humans. Most of the metabolites are eliminated in the bile. Less than 1% of a cyclosporine dose is recovered as unchanged drug in the urine. Within the therapeutic range, cyclosporine follows linear pharmacokinetics.[13]

A great deal of intrasubject variability in cyclosporine concentration occurs on a day-to-day basis, even when the patient should be at steady state. There are many reasons for this variability. Cyclosporine has low water solubility, and gastrointestinal absorption can be influenced by many variables.[7,8,14,15] To improve the consistency of absorption rate and bioavailability of the original dosage form (Sandimmune®; Novartis), a microemulsion version of the drug (Neoral®; Novartis) was marketed. Although use of microemulsion cyclosporine does decrease the variability in steady-state concentration (10% to 30% for Neoral® versus 16% to 38% for Sandimmune® for minimum concentration), there are still substantial day-to-day changes in cyclosporine concentration regardless of the dosage form used.[16] The fat content of meals has an influence on the absorption of oral cyclosporine.[17] Food containing a large amount of fat enhances the absorption of cyclosporine.

Oral cyclosporine solution is prepared with olive oil and alcohol to enhance the solubility of the drug. Immediately before it is swallowed, the solution is mixed in milk, chocolate milk, or orange juice in a glass container. When the entire dose has been given, the glass container should be rinsed with the diluting liquid and the contents of the container should be immediately consumed. If microemulsion cyclosporine solution is administered, it should be mixed in a similar manner with apple or orange juice. In either case, grapefruit juice should not be used because this vehicle inhibits CYP3A4 and/or P-glycoprotein in the gastrointestinal tract and markedly increases bioavailability. Variation in the absorption of cyclosporine solution depends on the accuracy of reproduction of the administration technique for each dose.

After liver transplantation, bile production and flow may not begin immediately, or bile flow may be diverted from the gastrointestinal tract with a T tube.[18,19] In the absence of bile salts, absorption of cyclosporine can be greatly decreased. Bile appears to assist in the dissolution of cyclosporine, which increases absorption of the drug. Diarrhea also impairs absorption of cyclosporine,[20,21] and patients who have undergone bone marrow transplantation may have diarrhea as a part of graph-versus-host disease.[4] Other drug therapy also can increase or decrease the intestinal first-pass clearance of cyclosporine.[22]

Cyclosporine is a low-to-moderate hepatic extraction ratio drug with an average liver extraction ratio of ~30%.[23] Because of this, hepatic clearance is influenced by unbound fraction in the blood (f_B), intrinsic clearance (Cl'_{int}), and liver blood flow. Cyclosporine binds primarily to erythrocytes and lipoproteins, yielding unbound fractions in the blood that are highly variable (1.4% to 12%).[24–29] Erythrocyte concentrations vary among transplant patients, especially those who have received bone marrow or kidney transplants. Lipoprotein concentrations also vary among patients, and hyperlipidemia is an adverse effect of cyclosporine. Hepatic intrinsic clearance is different among individuals, and there is a large amount of variability in this value within individual liver transplant patients that changes according to the viability of the graft and time after transplantation. Other drug therapy also can increase or decrease the hepatic intrinsic clearance of cyclosporine.[22] Liver blood flow exhibits a great deal of day-to-day intrasubject variability, which also changes hepatic clearance of cyclosporine. Of course, changing the unbound fraction in the blood, hepatic intrinsic clearance, or liver blood flow also changes the hepatic first-pass metabolism of cyclosporine. Taking into consideration all possible factors that alter absorption and clearance allows one to gain a better appreciation of why cyclosporine concentrations change on a day-to-day basis.

Cyclosporine capsules and solution are available in regular (25-, 50-, and 100-mg capsules; 100-mg/mL solution) and microemulsion (25- and 100-mg capsules; 100-mg/mL solution) form. Although the oral absorption characteristics are more consistent and bioavailability is higher for microemulsion forms of cyclosporine, it is recommended that when treatment is switched from intravenous cyclosporine to microemulsion cyclosporine doses be converted on a 1:1 basis. Subsequent dosage adjustments of microemulsion cyclosporine are based on concentration monitoring. Cyclosporine for intravenous administration is available at a concentration of 50 mg/mL. Before administration, it should be diluted in 20 to 100 mL of normal saline solution or 5% dextrose, and the drug should be infused over 2 to 6 hours. Anaphylactic reactions have occurred with this dosage form, possibly owing to the castor oil diluent used to enhance dissolution of the drug. The initial dose of cyclosporine varies greatly among transplantation centers. Cyclosporine therapy is commonly started 4 to 12 hours before the transplantation procedure. According to a survey of transplantation centers in the United States, the average initial oral doses, ± standard deviation, for renal, liver, and heart transplant recipients were 9 ± 3 mg/kg per day, 8 ± 4 mg/kg per day, and 7 ± 3 mg/kg per day.[16] For both rheumatoid arthritis and psoriasis, the recommended initial dose is 2.5 mg/kg per day with a maximal recommended dosage of 4 mg/kg per day.

EFFECTS OF DISEASES AND CONDITIONS ON CYCLOSPORINE PHARMACOKINETICS AND DOSING

Transplantation type does not appear to have a substantial effect on cyclosporine pharmacokinetics. The overall mean for all transplantation groups is a clearance of 6 mL/min per kilogram, a volume of distribution of 5 L/kg, and a half-life of 10 hours for adults.[7,8,14,15] Average clearance is higher (10 mL/min per kilogram) and mean half-life is shorter (6 hours) among children 16 years and younger.[7,8,14,15] Determination of the half-life of cyclosporine is difficult for patients receiving the drug twice a day because only a few concentrations can be measured in the postabsorption, postdistribution phase. Because of this, half-life measurements are obtained from studies in which at least 24 hours was allowed between doses. These results, as with the other pharmacokinetic parameters discussed in this chapter, are based on a specific HPLC assay conducted with samples of whole blood. As discussed earlier, nonspecific cyclosporine assays measure metabolite concentrations in addition to parent drug, and concurrently measured plasma or serum concentrations are lower than whole blood concentrations.

Because the drug is eliminated primarily through hepatic metabolism, clearance is lower (3 mL/min per kilogram) and half-life longer (20 hours) among patients with liver failure.[7,8,30] Immediately after liver transplantation, cyclosporine metabolism is depressed until the graft begins functioning in a stable manner. Patients with transient liver dysfunction, regardless of transplantation type, have decreased cyclosporine clearance and increased half-life values. Immediately after transplantation, oral absorption of cyclosporine, especially among recipients of liver transplants who have T tubes, is highly variable.[18,19] Obesity does not influence the pharmacokinetics of cyclosporine, so doses should be based on ideal body weight for these patients.[31–35] Renal failure also does not change the pharmacokinetics of cyclosporine, and the drug is not significantly removed in hemodialysis or peritoneal dialysis.[36–38]

DRUG INTERACTIONS

Drugs that interact with cyclosporine fall into two basic categories. The first are agents known to cause nephrotoxicity when administered by themselves.[22] The fear is that administration of a known nephrotoxin with cyclosporine will increase the incidence of renal damage over that which occurs when cyclosporine or the other agent is given separately. Compounds in this category of drug interaction include aminoglycoside antibiotics, vancomycin, cotrimoxazole (trimethoprim-sulfamethoxazole), amphotericin B, and anti-inflammatory drugs (diclofenac, naproxen, and other nonsteroidal antiinflammatory drugs). Other agents are melphalan, ketoconazole, cimetidine, ranitidine, and tacrolimus.

The second category of drug interaction involves inhibition or induction of cyclosporine metabolism. Cyclosporine is metabolized by CYP3A4 and is a substrate for P-glycoprotein, so the potential for many pharmacokinetic drug interactions exists with agents that inhibit these pathways or are cleared by these mechanisms.[22] Because both of these drug elimination systems also exist in the gastrointestinal tract, inhibition of drug interaction may enhance the oral bioavailability of cyclosporine by diminishing the intestinal and hepatic first-pass effects. Drugs that inhibit cyclosporine clearance include calcium channel blockers (verapamil, diltiazem, nicardipine), azole antifungals (fluconazole, itraconazole, ketoconazole), macrolide antibiotics (erythromycin, clarithromycin, troleandomycin), antivirals (indinavir, nelfinavir, ritonavir, saquinavir), steroids (methylprednisolone, oral contraceptives, androgens), and psychotropic agents (fluvoxamine, nefazodone) as well as other agents (amiodarone, chloroquine, allopurinol, bromocriptine, metoclopramide, cimetidine, grapefruit juice). Inducing agents include other antibiotics (nafcillin, rifampin, rifabutin), anticonvulsants (phenytoin, carbamazepine, phenobarbital, primidone), barbiturates, aminoglutethimide, troglitazone, octreotide, and ticlopidine. Because of the large number of interacting agents and the critical nature of the drugs involved in the treatment of transplant recipients, complete avoidance of drug interactions with cyclosporine is not possible. Most drug interactions with cyclosporine are managed with modification of cyclosporine dosage in which monitoring of cyclosporine concentration is a guide.

Cyclosporine can change the clearance of other drugs by means of competitive inhibition of CYP3A4 or P-glycoprotein.[22] Drugs that may decrease in clearance and increase in serum concentration when given with cyclosporine include prednisolone, digoxin, calcium channel blockers (verapamil, diltiazem, bepridil, nifedipine and most other dihydropyridine analogues, sildenafil), ergot alkaloids, vinca alkaloids, simvastatin, and lovastatin.

INITIAL DOSAGE DETERMINATION METHODS

Pharmacokinetic Dosing Method

The goals of initial dosing of cyclosporine are to compute the best dose possible for the patient to prevent graft rejection or graft-versus-host disease given the diseases and conditions that influence cyclosporine pharmacokinetics and to avoid adverse drug reactions. To do this, pharmacokinetic parameters for the patient are estimated with average parameters measured for other patients with similar diseases and conditions.

ESTIMATE OF CLEARANCE

Cyclosporine is almost completely metabolized by the liver. There is no good way to estimate the elimination characteristics of liver-metabolized drugs with an endogenous marker of liver function in the same manner that serum creatinine level and estimated creatinine clearance are used to estimate the elimination of agents elimated by the kidney. Because of this, a patient is categorized according to the diseases and conditions known to change cyclosporine clearance, and the clearance previously published is used as an estimate of the current patient's clearance rate. For example, an adult transplant recipient with normal liver function is assigned a cyclosporine clearance rate of 6 mL/min per kilogram, whereas a pediatric patient with the same profile is assumed to have a cyclosporine clearance of 10 mL/min per kilogram.

SELECTION OF APPROPRIATE PHARMACOKINETIC MODEL AND EQUATIONS

When given by means of intravenous infusion or orally, cyclosporine follows a two-compartment model.[38] When oral therapy is chosen, the drug is often erratically absorbed with variable absorption rates, and some patients may have a double-peak phenomenon whereby a maximum concentration is achieved 2 to 3 hours after administration and a second maximum concentration occurs 2 to 4 hours after that.[17,39] Because of the complex absorption profile and the fact that the drug is usually administered twice a day, a simple pharmacokinetic equation is used in which average steady-state concentration of cyclosporine is calculated (Css in ng/mL = μg/L). This equation is widely used and allows computation of a maintenance dose: $Css = [F(D/\tau)]/Cl$, or $D = (Css \cdot Cl \cdot \tau)/F$, where F is the bioavailability fraction for the oral dosage form (F averages 0.3, or 30% for most patient populations and oral dosage forms), D is the dose of cyclosporine in milligrams, Cl is cyclosporine clearance in liters per hour, and τ is the dosage interval in hours. If the drug is to be given intravenously as an intermittent infusion, the equivalent equation for that route of administration is $Css = (D/\tau)/Cl$, or $D = Css \cdot Cl \cdot \tau$. If the drug is to be given as a continuous intravenous infusion, the equation for that method of administration is $Css = k_0/Cl$, or $k_0 = Css \cdot Cl$, where k_0 is the infusion rate.

SELECTION OF STEADY-STATE CONCENTRATION

The generally accepted therapeutic ranges for cyclosporine in blood, serum, or plasma obtained with various specific and nonspecific (parent drug plus metabolite) assays are given in Table 15-1. More important than these general guidelines are the specific requirements for each graft type as defined by the transplantation center where the operation was performed. Clinicians should become familiar with the cyclosporine protocols used at the institutions at which they practice. Although it is unlikely that steady state has been achieved, cyclosporine concentration usually is measured daily, even when dosage changes are made the previous day, because of the critical nature of the therapeutic effect of the drug.

Example 1 HO is a 50-year-old, 75-kg (height, 178 cm) man who has undergone renal transplantation. Two days after transplantation, liver function test results are normal. Suggest an initial oral cyclosporine dose designed to achieve a steady-state minimum blood concentration of cyclosporine of 250 ng/mL.

1. *Estimate clearance according to disease states and conditions present in the patient.*

The mean cyclosporine clearance for adult patients is 6 mL/min per kilogram. The blood clearance of cyclosporine for this patient is expected to be 27 L/h: Cl = 6 mL/min/kg · 75 kg · [(60 min/h)/(1000 mL/L)] = 27 L/h.

2. *Compute dosage regimen.*

A 12-hour dosage interval is used for this patient. (Note: ng/mL = μg/L, and this concentration was substituted for Css in the calculations to avoid unit conversion. A conversion constant of 1000 μg/mg is used to change the dose amount to milligrams.) The dosage equation for oral cyclosporine is D = (Css · Cl · τ)/F = (250 μg/L · 27 L/h · 12 h)/(0.3 · 1000 μg/mg) = 270 mg, rounded to 300 mg every 12 hours. Cyclosporine concentrations are obtained daily, and steady state is expected to occur in about 2 days (5 half-lives = 5 · 10 h = 50 h, or ~2 d).

Example 2 For the patient in example 1, compute an initial dosage of intravenous cyclosporine.

1. *Estimate clearance according to disease states and conditions present in the patient.*

The mean cyclosporine clearance for adult patients is 6 mL/min per kilogram. The blood clearance of cyclosporine for this patient is expected to be 27 L/h: Cl = 6 mL/min/kg · 75 kg · [(60 min/h)/(1000 mL/L)] = 27 L/h.

2. *Compute the dosage regimen.*

A 12-hour dosage interval is used for this patient. (Note: ng/mL = μg/L, and this concentration was substituted for Css in the calculations to avoid unit conversion. A conversion constant of 1000 μg/mg is used to change the dose amount to milligrams.) The dosage equation for intravenous cyclosporine is D = Css · Cl · τ = (250 μg/L · 27 L/h · 12 h)/(1000 μg/mg) = 81 mg, rounded to 75 mg every 12 hours. If the cyclosporine dose is given as a continuous infusion instead of intermittent infusions, the dosage equation is k_0 = Css · Cl = (250 μg/L · 27 L/h)/(1000 μg/mg) = 6.8 mg/h, rounded to 7 mg/h. Cyclosporine concentration is measured daily, and steady state is expected to occur in about 2 days (5 half-lives = 5 · 10 h = 50 h, or ~2 d).

Literature-Based Recommended Dosing

Because of the large variability in pharmacokinetics of cyclosporine, even when concurrent diseases and conditions are identified, many clinicians believe that the use of standard cyclosporine doses for various situations is warranted. Most transplant centers use doses that are determined with a cyclosporine dosage protocol. The original computation of these doses was based on the pharmacokinetic dosing method described earlier and modified according to clinical experience. In general, the expected steady-state concentration of cyclosporine used to compute these doses depends on the type of tissue transplanted and the posttransplantation time line. In general, initial oral doses of 8 to 18 mg/kg per day or intravenous doses of 3 to 6 mg/kg per day (one-third the oral dose to account for ~30% oral bioavailability) are used and vary greatly from institution to institution.[1–5,7,8,15] For obese patients (>30% over ideal body weight), ideal body weight is used to compute initial doses.[31–35] To illustrate how this technique is used, the previous patient examples are repeated for this dosage approach.

Example 3 HO is a 50-year-old, 75-kg (height, 178 cm) man who received a renal transplant. Two days after transplantation, the results of liver function tests are normal. Suggest an initial oral cyclosporine dosage designed to achieve a steady-state minimum blood concentration of cyclosporine within the therapeutic range.

1. *Choose the cyclosporine dose based on disease states and conditions present in the patient and transplantation type.*

The oral dosage range of cyclosporine for adult patients is 8 to 18 mg/kg per day. Because this patient underwent renal transplantation, a dose in the lower end of the range (8 mg/kg per day) is used to avoid nephrotoxicity. The initial cyclosporine dose for this patient is 600 mg/d given as 300 mg every 12 hours: Dose = 8 mg/kg/d · 75 kg = 600 mg/d, or 300 mg every 12 hours. Cyclosporine concentration is measured daily, and steady state is expected to occur after 2 days (5 half-lives = 5 · 10 h = 50 h, or ~2 d) of treatment.

Example 4 For the patient in example 3, compute an initial dosage of intravenous cyclosporine.

1. *Choose the cyclosporine dose based on disease states and conditions present in the patient and transplantation type.*

The intravenous dosage range of cyclosporine for adult patients is 3 to 6 mg/kg per day. Because this patient underwent renal transplantation, a dose in the lower end of the range (3 mg/kg per day) is used to avoid nephrotoxicity. The initial cyclosporine dose for this patient is 200 mg/d given as 100 mg every 12 hours: Dose = 3 mg/kg/d · 75 kg = 225 mg/d, rounded to 200 mg/d, or 100 mg every 12 hours. If the cyclosporine dose is given as a continuous infusion instead of intermittent infusions, the infusion rate is k_0 = (3 mg/kg/d · 75 kg)/(24 h/d) = 9.4 mg/h, rounded to 9 mg/h. Cyclosporine concentration is measured daily. Steady state is expected to occur after 2 days (5 half-lives = 5 · 10 h = 50 h, or ~2 d) of treatment.

USE OF CYCLOSPORINE CONCENTRATIONS TO ALTER DOSES

Because of the large pharmacokinetic variability among patients, it is likely that doses computed with patient population characteristics will not always produce cyclosporine concentrations that are expected or desirable. Because of pharmacokinetic variability, the narrow therapeutic index of cyclosporine, and the severity of adverse side effects of cyclosporine, measurement of cyclosporine concentration is mandatory to ensure that therapeutic, nontoxic levels are present. In addition to cyclosporine concentration, important patient parameters, such as function tests or biopsy of the transplanted organ, clinical signs and symptoms of graft rejection or graft-versus-host disease, and risk of side effects of cyclosporine, should be followed to confirm that the patient is responding to treatment and not having adverse drug reactions.

When cyclosporine concentration is measured, and a dosage change is necessary, clinicians should use the simplest, most straightforward method available to determine a dose that will provide safe and effective treatment. In most cases, a simple dosage ratio can be used to change cyclosporine doses if the drug follows linear pharmacokinetics. Sometimes it is useful to compute cyclosporine pharmacokinetic constants for a patient and base dosage adjustments on these constants. In this case, it may be possible to calculate and use pharmacokinetic parameters to alter the cyclosporine dose. Finally, computerized methods that incorporate expected population pharmacokinetic characteristics (Bayesian pharmacokinetics computer programs) can be used when concentrations are obtained at suboptimal times or the patient is not at steady state when concentration is measured.

Linear Pharmacokinetics Method

Because cyclosporine follows linear, dose-proportional pharmacokinetics,[13] steady-state concentrations change in proportion to dose according to the following equation: $D_{new}/Css_{new} = D_{old}/Css_{old}$, or $D_{new} = (Css_{new}/Css_{old})D_{old}$, where D is the dose, Css is the steady-state concentration, old indicates the dose that produced the steady-state concentration that the patient is currently receiving, and new denotes the dose necessary to produce the desired steady-state concentration. The advantages of this method are that it is quick and simple. The disadvantage is that a steady-state concentration is required.

Example 5 LK is a 50-year-old, 75-kg (height, 178 cm) man who has undergone renal transplantation. He is receiving 400 mg every 12 hours of oral cyclosporine capsules. He has normal liver function. The current steady-state blood concentration of cyclosporine is 375 ng/mL. Compute a cyclosporine dose that will provide a steady-state concentration of 200 ng/mL.

1. *Compute the new dose to achieve the desired concentration.*

The patient is expected to achieve steady-state conditions after the second day (5 half-lives = 5 · 10 h = 50 h) of therapy. According to linear pharmacokinetics, the new dose to attain the desired concentration should be proportional to the old dose that produced the measured concentration (total daily dose = 400 mg/dose · 2 doses/d = 800 mg/d):

$$D_{new} = (Css_{new}/Css_{old})D_{old} = [(200 \text{ ng/mL})/(375 \text{ ng/mL})]\ 800 \text{ mg/d}$$
$$= 427 \text{ mg/d, rounded to } 400 \text{ mg/d}$$

The new suggested dose is 400 mg/d, or 200 mg every 12 hours of cyclosporine capsules to be started at the next scheduled dosing time.

Steady-state minimum cyclosporine concentration should be measured after steady state is attained in 3 to 5 half-lives. Because the drug is expected to have a half-life of 10 hours in this patient, steady-state concentration of cyclosporine can be measured any time after the second day of dosing (5 half-lives = 5 · 10 h = 50 h). Cyclosporine concentration should be measured if the patient has signs or symptoms of graft rejection or if the patient has signs or symptoms of cyclosporine toxicity.

Example 6 FD is a 60-year-old, 85-kg (height, 185 cm) man who has undergone liver transplantation. He is receiving 75 mg every 12 hours of intravenous cyclosporine. The current steady-state cyclosporine concentration is 215 ng/mL. Compute a cyclosporine dose that will provide a steady-state concentration of 350 ng/mL.

1. *Compute the new dose to achieve the desired concentration.*

The patient recently received a liver transplant and is expected to have a longer cyclosporine half-life if the organ is not yet functioning at an optimal level ($t_{1/2}$ = 20 h). Because of this, it can take as long as 4 days of consistent cyclosporine therapy to achieve steady-state conditions (5 half-lives = 5 · 20 h = 100 h, or ~4 d). According to linear pharmacokinetics, the new dose to attain the desired concentration should be proportional to the old dose that produced the measured concentration (total daily dose = 75 mg/dose · 2 doses/d = 150 mg/d):

$$D_{new} = (Css_{new}/Css_{old})D_{old} = [(350 \text{ ng/mL})/(215 \text{ ng/mL})]\ 150 \text{ mg/d}$$
$$= 244 \text{ mg/d, rounded to } 250 \text{ mg/d, or } 125 \text{ mg every } 12 \text{ hours}$$

Steady-state trough cyclosporine concentration should be measured after steady state is attained in 3 to 5 half-lives. Because the drug is expected to have a half-life up to 20 hours in this patient, steady-state concentration of cyclosporine can be measured any time after the fourth day of dosing (5 half-lives = 5 · 20 h = 100 h, or 4 d). Cyclosporine concentration should be measured if the patient has signs or symptoms of graft rejection or if the patient has signs or symptoms of cyclosporine toxicity.

If the patient in example 6 received cyclosporine as a continuous infusion at a rate of 6 mg/h, the equivalent dosage adjustment computation would be:

$$D_{new} = (Css_{new}/Css_{old})D_{old} = [(350 \text{ ng/mL})/(215 \text{ ng/mL})]\ 6 \text{ mg/h}$$
$$= 9.8 \text{ mg/h, rounded to } 10 \text{ mg/h}$$

Pharmacokinetic Parameter Method

The pharmacokinetic parameter method of adjusting drug doses was among the first techniques for changing doses with drug concentration. It allows computation of a patient's unique pharmacokinetic constants and use of those constants to calculate a dose that achieves the desired cyclosporine concentration. The pharmacokinetic parameter method requires that steady-state has been achieved, and uses only a steady-state cyclosporine concentration. Cyclosporine clearance can be measured with a single steady-state cyclosporine concentration and the following formula for orally administered drug: $Cl = [F(D/\tau)]/Css$, where Cl is cyclosporine clearance in liters per hour, F is the bioavailability factor for cyclosporine (F = 0.3), τ is the dosage interval in hours, and Css is the steady-state concentration of cyclosporine in nanograms per milliliter, or micrograms per liter. If cyclosporine is administered intravenously, bioavailability does not have to be taken into account: $Cl = (D/\tau)/Css$, where Cl is cyclosporine clearance in liters per hour, τ is the dosage interval in hours, and Css is the steady-state concentration of cyclosporine in nanograms per milliliter, or micrograms per liter. Although this method allows computation of cyclosporine clearance, it yields the same cyclosporine dose supplied with linear pharmacokinetics. Most clinicians prefer to directly calculate the new dosage with the simpler linear pharmacokinetics method. To demonstrate this point, the patient cases used to illustrate the linear pharmacokinetics method are used as examples of the pharmacokinetic parameter method.

Example 7 LK is a 50-year-old, 75-kg (height, 178 cm) man who has received a renal transplant. He is receiving 400 mg every 12 hours of oral cyclosporine capsules. He has normal liver function. The current steady-state blood concentration of cyclosporine is 375 ng/mL. Compute a cyclosporine dose that will provide a steady-state concentration of 200 ng/mL.

1. *Compute pharmacokinetic parameters.*

The patient is expected to achieve steady-state conditions after the second day (5 half-lives = 5 · 10 h = 50 h, or 2 d) of therapy. Cyclosporine clearance can be computed with steady-state cyclosporine concentration: Cl = [F(D/τ)]/Css = [0.3 · (400 mg/12 h) · 1000 μg/mg]/(375 μg/L) = 26.7 L/h. (Note: μg/L = ng/mL, and this concentration unit was substituted for Css in the calculations to avoid unit conversion.)

2. *Compute the cyclosporine dose.*

Cyclosporine clearance is used to compute the new dose: D = (Css · Cl · τ)/F = (200 μg/L · 26.7 L/h · 12 h)/(0.3 · 1000 μg/mg) = 214 mg, rounded to 200 mg every 12 hours.

Steady-state minimum concentration of cyclosporine should be measured after steady state is attained in 3 to 5 half-lives. Because the drug is expected to have a half-life of 10 hours in this patient, steady-state concentration of cyclosporine can be measured any time after the second day of dosing (5 half-lives = 5 · 10 h = 50 h). Cyclosporine concentration also should be measured if the patient has signs or symptoms of graft rejection or if the patient has signs or symptoms of cyclosporine toxicity.

Example 8 FD is a 60-year-old, 85-kg (height, 185 cm) man who has undergone liver transplantation. He is receiving 75 mg every 12 hours of intravenous cyclosporine. The current steady-state cyclosporine concentration is 215 ng/mL. Compute a cyclosporine dose that will provide a steady-state concentration of 350 ng/mL.

1. *Compute pharmacokinetic parameters.*

The patient recently received a liver transplant and is expected to have a longer cyclosporine half-life if the organ is not yet functioning at an optimal level ($t_{1/2}$ = 20 h). Because of this, it can take as long as 4 days of consistent cyclosporine therapy to achieve steady-state conditions (5 half-lives = 5 · 20 h = 100 h, or ~4 d). Cyclosporine clearance can be computed with steady-state cyclosporine concentration: Cl = (D/τ)/Css = [(75 mg/12 h) · 1000 μg/mg]/(215 μg/L) = 29.1 L/h. (Note: μg/L = ng/mL, and this concentration unit was substituted for Css in the calculations to avoid unit conversion.)

2. *Compute the cyclosporine dose.*

Cyclosporine clearance is used to compute the new dose: D = Css · Cl · τ = (350 μg/L · 29.1 L/h · 12 h)/1000 μg/mg = 122 mg, rounded to 125 mg every 12 hours.

Steady-state minimum concentration of cyclosporine should be measured after steady state is attained in 3 to 5 half-lives. Because the drug is expected to have a half-life up to 20 hours in this patient, steady-state concentration of cyclosporine can be measured any time after the fourth day of dosing (5 half-lives = 5 · 20 h = 100 h, or 4 d). Cyclosporine concentration should be measured if the patient has signs or symptoms of graft rejection or if the patient has signs or symptoms of cyclosporine toxicity.

If the patient in example 8 received cyclosporine as a continuous infusion at a rate of 6 mg/h, the equivalent clearance and dosage adjustment computations would be:

Cl = k_0/Css = (6 mg/h · 1000 μg/mg)/(215 μg/L)] = 27.9 L/h

k_0 = Css · Cl = (350 μg/L · 27.9 L/h)/(1000 μg/mg) = 9.8 mg/h, rounded to 10 mg/h

BAYESIAN PHARMACOKINETICS COMPUTER PROGRAMS

Computer programs can be used for computation of pharmacokinetic parameters for patients.[40–42] In the most reliable computer programs, a nonlinear regression algorithm incorporates components of Bayes' theorem. Nonlinear regression is a statistical technique in which an iterative process is used to compute the best pharmacokinetic parameters for a concentration–time data set. The patient's drug dosage schedule and drug concentrations are entered into the computer. The computer program has a pharmacokinetic equation programmed for the drug and administration method, such as oral, intravenous bolus, or intravenous infusion. A one-compartment model typically is used, although some programs allow the user to choose among several different equations. With population estimates based on demographic information for the patient, such as age, weight, sex, liver function, and cardiac status, supplied by the user, the program computes estimated drug concentrations for each actual drug concentration. Kinetic parameters are changed by the computer program, and a new set of estimated drug concentrations are computed. The pharmacokinetic parameters that generated the estimated drug concentrations closest to the actual values are stored in the computer memory, and the process is repeated until the set of pharmacokinetic parameters that provides the estimated drug concentrations statistically closest to the actual drug concentrations is generated. These pharmacokinetic parameters can be used to compute improved dosing schedules for patients. Bayes' theorem is used in the computer algorithm to balance the results of the computations between values based solely on the patient's drug concentrations and those based only on patient population parameters. Results of studies in which various methods of dosage adjustment have been compared have consistently shown that these types of computer dosing programs perform at least as well as experienced clinical pharmacokineticists and clinicians and better than inexperienced clinicians.

Some clinicians use Bayesian pharmacokinetics computer programs exclusively to alter doses based on drug concentrations. An advantage of this approach is that consistent dosage recommendations are made when several practitioners are involved in therapeutic drug-monitoring programs. However, because simpler dosing methods work just as well for patients with stable pharmacokinetic parameters and steady-state drug concentrations, many clinicians reserve the use of computer programs for more difficult situations. Those situations include drug concentrations that are not at steady state, drug concentrations not obtained at the specific times needed to use simpler methods, and unstable pharmacokinetic parameters. Many Bayesian pharmacokinetics computer programs are available, and most should provide answers similar to the one used in the following examples. The program used to solve problems in this book is DrugCalc written by Dr. Dennis Mungall. It is available at his Internet web site (http://members.aol.com/thertch/index.htm).[43]

Example 9 LK is a 50-year-old, 75-kg (height, 178 cm) man who has received a renal transplant. He is receiving 400 mg every 12 hours of oral cyclosporine capsules. He has normal liver (bilirubin, 0.7 mg/dL; albumin, 4.0 g/dL). The current steady-state blood concentration of cyclosporine is 375 ng/mL. Compute a cyclosporine dose that will provide a steady-state concentration of 200 ng/mL.

1. *Enter the patient's demographic, drug dosing, and concentration–time data into the computer program.*

2. *Compute pharmacokinetic parameters for the patient with a Bayesian pharmacokinetics computer program.*

The pharmacokinetic parameters computed with the program are a volume of distribution of 403 L, a half-life of 17.6 hours, and a clearance of 15.9 L/h.

3. *Compute the dose required to achieve the desired cyclosporine concentration.*

The one-compartment model, first-order absorption equations used in the program to compute doses indicate that a dose of 200 mg every 12 hours produces a steady-state cyclosporine concentration of 210 ng/mL. Using the linear pharmacokinetics and pharmacokinetic parameter methods described earlier produces the same answer for this patient.

Example 10 FD is a 60-year-old, 85-kg (height, 185 cm) man who has undergone liver transplantation. He is receiving 75 mg every 12 hours of intravenous cyclosporine. He has elevated liver function results (bilirubin, 3.2 mg/dL; albumin, 2.5 g/dL). The current steady-state cyclosporine concentration is 215 ng/mL. Compute a cyclosporine dose that will provide a steady-state concentration of 350 ng/mL.

1. *Enter the patient's demographic, drug dosing, and concentration–time data into the computer program.*

2. *Compute pharmacokinetic parameters for the patient with a Bayesian pharmacokinetics computer program.*

The pharmacokinetic parameters computed with the program are a volume of distribution of 403 L, a half-life of 13.8 hours, and a clearance of 20.3 L/h.

3. *Compute the dose required to achieve the desired cyclosporine concentration.*

The one-compartment model, first-order absorption equations used in the program to compute doses indicate that a dose of 125 mg every 12 hours produces a steady-state cyclosporine concentration of 380 ng/mL. Using the linear pharmacokinetics and pharmacokinetic parameter methods described earlier produces the same answer for this patient.

Example 11 YT is a 25-year-old, 55-kg (height, 157 cm) woman who has received a bone marrow transplant. She received 300 mg every 12 hours of oral cyclosporine capsules for two doses after transplantation, but because her renal function decreased, the dosage was empirically changed to 200 mg every 12 hours. The patient has normal liver function (bilirubin, 0.9 mg/dL; albumin, 3.9 g/dL). The blood concentration of cyclosporine obtained 12 hours after the first dose of the lower dosage regimen is 280 ng/mL. Compute a cyclosporine dose that will provide a steady-state concentration of 250 ng/mL.

1. *Enter the patient's demographic, drug dosing, and concentration–time data into the computer program.*

2. *Compute pharmacokinetic parameters for the patient with a Bayesian pharmacokinetics computer program.*

The pharmacokinetic parameters computed with the program are a volume of distribution of 401 L, a half-life of 35 hours, and a clearance of 8 L/h.

3. *Compute the dose required to achieve the desired cyclosporine concentration.*

The one-compartment model, first-order absorption equations used in the program to compute doses indicate that a dose of 100 mg every 12 hours produces a steady-state cyclosporine concentration of 250 ng/mL.

PROBLEMS

The following problems are intended to emphasize the computation of initial and individualized doses with clinical pharmacokinetic techniques. Clinicians always should consult the patient's chart to confirm that current immunosuppressive therapy is appropriate. All other medications that the patient is taking, including prescription and nonprescription drugs, should be recorded and checked to ascertain the risk of interaction with cyclosporine.

1. VI is a 37-year-old, 85-kg (height, 185 cm) man who has received a heart transplant. He needs therapy with oral cyclosporine. He has normal liver function. Suggest an initial dosage regimen designed to achieve a steady-state cyclosporine concentration of 300 ng/mL.
2. Patient VI (see problem 1) is given a prescription for 400 mg every 12 hours of cyclosporine capsules for 4 days. Steady-state cyclosporine concentration is 426 ng/mL. The patient is found to be compliant with the dosage regimen. Suggest a cyclosporine dosage regimen designed to achieve a steady-state cyclosporine concentration of 300 ng/mL.
3. AS is a 9-year-old, 35-kg (height, 137 cm) girl who has undergone bone marrow transplantation. She needs therapy with oral cyclosporine. She has normal liver function. Suggest an initial cyclosporine dosage regimen designed to achieve a steady-state cyclosporine concentration of 250 ng/mL.
4. Patient AS (see problem 3) is given a prescription for 150 mg every 12 hours of cyclosporine solution for 3 days. Steady-state cyclosporine concentration is 173 ng/mL. The patient is found to be compliant with the dosage regimen. Suggest an oral cyclosporine dosage regimen designed to achieve a steady-state cyclosporine concentration of 250 ng/mL.
5. FL is a 29-year-old, 78-kg (height, 180 cm) man who has received a liver transplant. He needs therapy with oral cyclosporine. He has poor liver function because of liver disease. Suggest an initial cyclosporine dosage regimen to be started 24 hours before transplantation to achieve a steady-state cyclosporine concentration of 300 ng/mL.
6. Patient FL (see problem 5) has been receiving 400 mg every 12 hours of cyclosporine capsules since transplantation. Ten days after transplantation, steady-state cyclosporine concentration is 531 ng/mL. The patient is found to be compliant with the dosage regimen. Suggest a cyclosporine dosage regimen designed to achieve a steady-state cyclosporine concentration of 250 ng/mL.
7. PH is a 22-year-old, 67-kg (height, 165 cm) woman who has received a renal transplant. She needs therapy with oral cyclosporine. Thirty-six hours after transplanta-

tion, the new kidney is beginning to function normally. Liver function is normal. Suggest an initial cyclosporine dosage regimen designed to achieve a steady-state cyclosporine concentration of 200 ng/mL.

8. Patient PH (see problem 7) is given a prescription for 200 mg every 12 hours of cyclosporine capsules for 3 days. Steady-state cyclosporine concentration is 125 ng/mL. The patient is found to be compliant with the dosage regimen. Suggest a cyclosporine dosage regimen designed to achieve a steady-state cyclosporine concentration of 200 ng/mL.

9. PU is a 55-year-old, 68-kg (height, 173 cm) man who has received a heart transplant. He has received two intravenous cyclosporine doses (125 mg every 12 hours), and therapy is switched to oral cyclosporine capsules 300 mg every 12 hours. The patient has normal liver function (bilirubin, 0.7 mg/dL; albumin, 4.0 g/dL). Cyclosporine concentration is 190 ng/mL 12 hours after the first oral dose of the drug. Compute a cyclosporine dose that will provide a steady-state concentration of 325 ng/mL.

10. LH is a 25-year-old, 60-kg (height, 160 cm) woman who has received a renal transplant. She is given a new prescription for cyclosporine capsules 200 mg every 12 hours 2 days after transplantation. The patient has normal liver function (bilirubin, 0.4 mg/dL; albumin, 3.7 g/dL) and also is being treated with phenytoin. The minimum cyclosporine concentration before the third dose is 90 ng/mL. Compute a cyclosporine dose that will provide a steady-state concentration of 200 ng/mL.

ANSWERS TO PROBLEMS

1. Answer to problem 1.

Pharmacokinetic Dosing Method

1. *Estimate clearance according to disease states and conditions present in the patient.*

The mean cyclosporine clearance for adult patients is 6 mL/min per kilogram. The blood clearance of cyclosporine for this patient is expected to be 30.6 L/h: Cl = 6 mL/min/kg · 85 kg · [(60 min/h)/(1000 mL/L)] = 30.6 L/h.

2. *Compute the dosage regimen.*

A 12-hour dosage interval is used for this patient. (Note: ng/mL = μg/L, and this concentration was substituted for Css in the calculations to avoid unit conversion. A conversion constant of 1000 μg/mg is used to change the dose amount to milligrams.) The dosage equation for oral cyclosporine is D = (Css · Cl · τ)/F = (300 μg/L · 30.6 L/h · 12 h)/(0.3 · 1000 μg/mg) = 367 mg, rounded to 400 mg every 12 hours. Cyclosporine concentration is measured daily, and steady state is expected to occur in about 2 days (5 half-lives = 5 · 10 h = 50 h, or ~2 d).

Literature-Based Recommended Dosing

1. *Choose the cyclosporine dose based on disease states and conditions present in the patient and transplantation type.*

The oral dosage range of cyclosporine for adult patients is 8 to 18 mg/kg per day. Because this patient underwent heart transplantation, a dose in the middle of the range (10 mg/kg per day) is used to avoid graft rejection. The initial cyclosporine dose for this patient is 800 mg/d given as 400 mg every 12 hours: Dose = 10 mg/kg/d · 85 kg = 850 mg/d, rounded to 800 mg/d, or 400 mg every 12 hours. Cyclosporine concentration is measured daily, and steady state is expected to occur after 2 days (5 half-lives = 5 · 10 h = 50 h, or ~2 d) of treatment.

2. Answer to problem 2.

Linear Pharmacokinetics Method

1. *Compute the new dose to achieve the desired concentration.*

The patient is expected to achieve steady-state conditions after the second day (5 half-lives = 5 · 10 h = 50 h) of therapy. According to linear pharmacokinetics, the new dose to attain the desired concentration should be proportional to the old dose that produced the measured concentration (total daily dose = 400 mg/dose · 2 doses/d = 800 mg/d):

$$D_{new} = (Css_{new}/Css_{old})D_{old} = [(300\ \text{ng/mL})/(426\ \text{ng/mL})]\ 800\ \text{mg/d}$$
$$= 563\ \text{mg/d, rounded to } 600\ \text{mg/d}$$

The new suggested dose is 600 mg/d, or 300 mg every 12 hours, of cyclosporine capsules to be started at the next scheduled dosing time.

Steady-state minimum concentration of cyclosporine should be measured after steady state is attained in 3 to 5 half-lives. Because the drug is expected to have a half-life of 10 hours in this patient, steady-state concentration of cyclosporine can be measured any time after the second day of dosing (5 half-lives = 5 · 10 h = 50 h). Cyclosporine concentration should be measured if the patient has signs or symptoms of graft rejection or if the patient has signs or symptoms of cyclosporine toxicity.

Pharmacokinetic Parameter Method

1. *Compute pharmacokinetic parameters.*

The patient is expected to achieve steady-state conditions after the second day (5 half-lives = 5 · 10 h = 50 h, or 2 d) of therapy. Cyclosporine clearance can be computed with steady-state cyclosporine concentration: $Cl = [F(D/\tau)]/Css = [0.3 \cdot (400\ \text{mg}/12\ \text{h}) \cdot 1000\ \mu\text{g/mg}]/(426\ \mu\text{g/L}) = 23.5\ \text{L/h}$. (Note: μg/L = ng/mL, and this concentration unit was substituted for Css in the calculations to avoid unit conversion.)

2. *Compute the cyclosporine dose.*

Cyclosporine clearance is used to compute the new dose: $D = (Css \cdot Cl \cdot \tau)/F = (300\ \mu\text{g/L} \cdot 23.5\ \text{L/h} \cdot 12\ \text{h})/(0.3 \cdot 1000\ \mu\text{g/mg}) = 282\ \text{mg}$, rounded to 300 mg every 12 hours.

Steady-state minimum concentration of cyclosporine should be measured after steady state is attained in 3 to 5 half-lives. Because the drug is expected to have a half-life of 10 hours in this patient, steady-state concentration of cyclosporine can be measured any time after the second day of dosing (5 half-lives = 5 · 10 h = 50 h). Cyclosporine concentration should be measured if the patient has signs or symptoms of graft rejection or if the patient has signs or symptoms of cyclosporine toxicity.

3. Answer to problem 3.

Pharmacokinetic Dosing Method

1. *Estimate clearance according to disease states and conditions present in the patient.*

The mean cyclosporine clearance for pediatric patients is 10 mL/min per kilogram. The blood clearance of cyclosporine for this patient is expected to be 21 L/h: Cl = 10 mL/min/kg · 35 kg · [(60 min/h)/(1000 mL/L)] = 21 L/h.

2. *Compute the dosage regimen.*

A 12-hour dosage interval is used for this patient. (Note: ng/mL = μg/L, and this concentration was substituted for Css in the calculations to avoid unit conversion. A conversion constant of 1000 μg/mg is used to change the dose amount to milligrams.) The dosage equation for oral cyclosporine is D = (Css · Cl · τ)/F = (250 μg/L · 21 L/h · 12 h)/(0.3 · 1000 μg/mg) = 210 mg, rounded to 200 mg every 12 hours of cyclosporine solution. Cyclosporine concentration is measured daily, and steady state is expected to occur in about 1 to 2 days (5 half-lives = 5 · 6 h = 30 h).

Literature-Based Recommended Dosing

1. *Choose the cyclosporine dose based on disease states and conditions present in the patient and transplantation type.*

The oral dosage range of cyclosporine is 8 to 18 mg/kg per day. Because the patient is a child, a dose in the middle of the range (12 mg/kg per day) is used to avoid graft-versus-host disease. The initial cyclosporine dose for this patient is 400 mg/d given as 200 mg every 12 hours: Dose = 12 mg/kg/d · 35 kg = 420 mg/d, rounded to 400 mg/d, or 200 mg every 12 hours of cyclosporine solution. Cyclosporine concentration is measured daily, and steady state is expected to occur in about 1 to 2 days (5 half-lives = 5 · 6 h = 30 h) of treatment.

4. Answer to problem 4.

Linear Pharmacokinetics Method

1. *Compute the new dose to achieve the desired concentration.*

The patient is expected to achieve steady-state conditions by the second day (5 half-lives = 5 · 6 h = 30 h) of therapy. According to linear pharmacokinetics, the new dose to attain the desired concentration should be proportional to the old dose that produced the measured concentration (total daily dose = 150 mg/dose · 2 doses/d = 300 mg/d):

$$D_{new} = (Css_{new}/Css_{old})D_{old} = [(250 \text{ ng/mL})/(173 \text{ ng/mL})]\ 300 \text{ mg/d}$$
$$= 434 \text{ mg/d, rounded to } 400 \text{ mg/d}$$

The new suggested dose is 400 mg/d, or 200 mg every 12 hours, of cyclosporine solution to be started at the next scheduled dosing time.

Steady-state minimum concentration of cyclosporine should be measured after steady state is attained in 3 to 5 half-lives. Because the drug is expected to have a half-life of 6 hours in this patient, steady-state concentration of cyclosporine can be measured any time after the first day of dosing (5 half-lives = 5 · 6 h = 30 h). Cyclosporine concentration should be measured if the patient has signs or symptoms of graft rejection or if the patient has signs or symptoms of cyclosporine toxicity.

Pharmacokinetic Parameter Method

1. *Compute pharmacokinetic parameters.*

The patient is expected to achieve steady-state conditions after the second day (5 half-lives = 5 · 6 h = 30 h) of therapy. Cyclosporine clearance can be computed with steady-state cyclosporine concentration: Cl = [F(D/τ)]/Css = [0.3 · (150 mg/12 h) · 1000 μg/mg]/(173 μg/L) = 21.7 L/h. (Note: μg/L = ng/mL, and this concentration unit was substituted for Css in the calculations to avoid unit conversion.)

2. *Compute the cyclosporine dose.*

Cyclosporine clearance is used to compute the new dose: D = (Css · Cl · τ)/F = (250 μg/L · 21.7 L/h · 12 h)/(0.3 · 1000 μg/mg) = 217 mg, rounded to 200 mg every 12 hours, of cyclosporine solution.

Steady-state minimum concentration of cyclosporine should be measured after steady state is attained in 3 to 5 half-lives. Because the drug is expected to have a half-life of 6 hours in this patient, steady-state concentration of cyclosporine can be measured any time after the first day of dosing (5 half-lives = 5 · 6 h = 30 h). Cyclosporine concentration should be measured if the patient has signs or symptoms of graft rejection or if the patient has signs or symptoms of cyclosporine toxicity.

5. Answer to problem 5.

Pharmacokinetic Dosing Method

1. *Estimate clearance according to disease states and conditions present in the patient.*

The mean cyclosporine clearance for adult patients is 6 mL/min per kilogram. The blood clearance of cyclosporine for this patient is expected to be 28.1 L/h: Cl = 6 mL/min/kg · 78 kg · [(60 min/h)/(1000 mL/L)] = 28.1 L/h.

2. *Compute the dosage regimen.*

A 12-hour dosage interval is used for this patient. (Note: ng/mL = μg/L, and this concentration was substituted for Css in the calculations to avoid unit conversion. A conversion constant of 1000 μg/mg is used to change the dose amount to milligrams.) The dosage equation for oral cyclosporine is D = (Css · Cl · τ)/F = (300 μg/L · 28.1 L/h · 12 h)/(0.3 · 1000 μg/mg) = 337 mg, rounded to 300 mg every 12 hours. Cyclosporine concentration is measured daily, and steady state is expected to occur in about 2 days (5 half-lives = 5 · 10 h = 50 h, or ~2 d).

Literature-Based Recommended Dosing

1. *Choose the cyclosporine dose based on disease states and conditions present in the patient and transplantation type.*

The oral dosage range of cyclosporine for adult patients is 8 to 18 mg/kg per day. Because the patient has received a liver transplant, a dose in the middle of the range (10 mg/kg per day) is used to avoid graft rejection. The initial cyclosporine dose for this patient is 800 mg/d given as 400 mg every 12 hours: Dose = 10 mg/kg/d · 78 kg = 780 mg/d, rounded to 800 mg/d, or 400 mg every 12 hours. Cyclosporine concentration is measured daily, and steady state is expected to occur after 2 days (5 half-lives = 5 · 10 h = 50 h, or ~2 d) of treatment.

6. Answer to problem 6.

Linear Pharmacokinetics Method

1. *Compute the new dose to achieve the desired concentration.*

The patient is expected to achieve steady-state conditions after the second day (5 half-lives = 5 · 10 h = 50 h) of therapy. According to linear pharmacokinetics, the new dose to attain the desired concentration should be proportional to the old dose that produced the measured concentration (total daily dose = 400 mg/dose · 2 doses/d = 800 mg/d):

$$D_{new} = (Css_{new}/Css_{old})D_{old} = [(250 \text{ ng/mL})/(531 \text{ ng/mL})]\ 800 \text{ mg/d}$$
$$= 377 \text{ mg/d, rounded to } 400 \text{ mg/d}$$

The new suggested dose is 400 mg/d, or 200 mg every 12 hours, of cyclosporine capsules to be started at the next scheduled dosing time.

Steady-state minimum concentration of cyclosporine should be measured after steady state is attained in 3 to 5 half-lives. Because the drug is expected to have a half-life of 10 hours in this patient, steady-state concentration of cyclosporine can be measured any time after the second day of dosing (5 half-lives = 5 · 10 h = 50 h). Cyclosporine concentration should be measured if the patient has signs or symptoms of graft rejection or if the patient has signs or symptoms of cyclosporine toxicity.

Pharmacokinetic Parameter Method

1. *Compute pharmacokinetic parameters.*

The patient is expected to achieve steady-state conditions after the second day (5 half-lives = 5 · 10 h = 50 h, or 2 d) of therapy. Cyclosporine clearance can be computed with steady-state cyclosporine concentration: $Cl = [F(D/\tau)]/Css = [0.3 \cdot (400 \text{ mg}/12 \text{ h}) \cdot 1000\ \mu\text{g/mg}]/(531\ \mu\text{g/L}) = 18.8$ L/h. (Note: μg/L = ng/mL, and this concentration unit was substituted for Css in the calculations to avoid unit conversion.)

2. *Compute the cyclosporine dose.*

Cyclosporine clearance is used to compute the new dose: $D = (Css \cdot Cl \cdot \tau)/F = (250\ \mu\text{g/L} \cdot 18.8 \text{ L/h} \cdot 12 \text{ h})/(0.3 \cdot 1000\ \mu\text{g/mg}) = 188$ mg, rounded to 200 mg every 12 hours.

Steady-state minimum concentration of cyclosporine should be measured after steady state is attained in 3 to 5 half-lives. Because the drug is expected to have a half-life of 10 hours in this patient, steady-state concentration of cyclosporine can be measured any time after the second day of dosing (5 half-lives = 5 · 10 h = 50 h). Cyclosporine concentrations should be measured if the patient has signs or symptoms of graft rejection or if the patient has signs or symptoms of cyclosporine toxicity.

7. Answer to problem 7.

Pharmacokinetic Dosing Method

1. *Estimate clearance according to disease states and conditions present in the patient.*

The mean cyclosporine clearance for adult patients is 6 mL/min per kilogram. The blood clearance of cyclosporine for this patient is expected to be 24.1 L/h: Cl = 6 mL/min/kg · 67 kg · [(60 min/h)/(1000 mL/L)] = 24.1 L/h.

2. *Compute the dosage regimen.*

A 12-hour dosage interval is used for this patient. (Note: ng/mL = μg/L, and this concentration was substituted for Css in the calculations to avoid unit conversion. A conversion constant of 1000 μg/mg is used to change the dose amount to milligrams.) The dosage equation for oral cyclosporine is D = (Css · Cl · τ)/F = (200 μg/L · 24.1 L/h · 12 h)/(0.3 · 1000 μg/mg) = 193 mg, rounded to 200 mg every 12 hours. Cyclosporine concentration is measured daily, and steady state is expected to occur in about 2 days (5 half-lives = 5 · 10 h = 50 h, or ~2 d).

Literature-Based Recommended Dosing

1. *Choose the cyclosporine dose based on disease states and conditions present in the patient and transplantation type.*

The oral dosage range of cyclosporine for adult patients is 8 to 18 mg/kg per day. Because the patient has received a kidney transplant, a dose in the lower end of the range (8 mg/kg per day) is used to avoid nephrotoxicity. The initial cyclosporine dose for this patient is 500 mg/d: Dose = 8 mg/kg/d · 67 kg = 536 mg/d, rounded to 500 mg/d, or 200 mg every morning and 300 mg every evening. Cyclosporine concentration is measured daily, and steady state is expected to occur after 2 days (5 half-lives = 5 · 10 h = 50 h, or ~2 d) of treatment.

8. Answer to problem 8.

Linear Pharmacokinetics Method

1. *Compute the new dose to achieve the desired concentration.*

The patient is expected to achieve steady-state conditions after the second day (5 half-lives = 5 · 10 h = 50 h) of therapy. According to linear pharmacokinetics, the new dose to attain the desired concentration should be proportional to the old dose that produced the measured concentration (total daily dose = 200 mg/dose · 2 doses/d = 400 mg/d):

$$D_{new} = (Css_{new}/Css_{old})D_{old} = [(200\ \text{ng/mL})/(125\ \text{ng/mL})]\ 400\ \text{mg/d}$$
$$= 640\ \text{mg/d, rounded to } 600\ \text{mg/d}$$

The new suggested dose is 600 mg/d, or 300 mg every 12 hours, of cyclosporine capsules to be started at the next scheduled dosing time.

Steady-state minimum concentration of cyclosporine should be measured after steady state is attained in 3 to 5 half-lives. Because the drug is expected to have a half-life of 10 hours in this patient, steady-state concentration of cyclosporine can be measured any time after the second day of dosing (5 half-lives = 5 · 10 h = 50 h). Cyclosporine concentration should be measured if the patient has signs or symptoms of graft rejection or if the patient has signs or symptoms of cyclosporine toxicity.

Pharmacokinetic Parameter Method

1. *Compute pharmacokinetic parameters.*

The patient is expected to achieve steady-state conditions after the second day (5 half-lives = 5 · 10 h = 50 h, or 2 d) of therapy. Cyclosporine clearance can be computed with steady-state cyclosporine concentration: $Cl = [F(D/\tau)]/Css = [0.3 \cdot (200\ mg/12\ h) \cdot 1000\ \mu g/mg]/(125\ \mu g/L) = 40\ L/h$. (Note: μg/L = ng/mL, and this concentration unit was substituted for Css in the calculations to avoid unit conversion.)

2. *Compute the cyclosporine dose.*

Cyclosporine clearance is used to compute the new dose: $D = (Css \cdot Cl \cdot \tau)/F = (200\ \mu g/L \cdot 40\ L/h \cdot 12\ h)/(0.3 \cdot 1000\ \mu g/mg) = 320\ mg$, rounded to 300 mg every 12 hours.

Steady-state minimum concentration of cyclosporine should be measured after steady state is attained in 3 to 5 half-lives. Because the drug is expected to have a half-life of 10 hours in this patient, steady-state concentration of cyclosporine can be measured any time after the second day of dosing (5 half-lives = 5 · 10 h = 50 h). Cyclosporine concentration should be measured if the patient has signs or symptoms of graft rejection or if the patient has signs or symptoms of cyclosporine toxicity.

9. Solution to problem 9.

Bayesian Pharmacokinetics Computer Program Method

1. *Enter the patient's demographic, drug dosing, and concentration–time data into the computer program.*

2. *Compute pharmacokinetic parameters for the patient with a Bayesian pharmacokinetics computer program.*

The pharmacokinetic parameters computed with the program are a volume of distribution of 401 L, a half-life of 35 hours, and a clearance of 8 L/h.

3. *Compute the dose required to achieve the desired cyclosporine concentration.*

The one-compartment model, first-order absorption equations used in the program to compute doses indicate that a dose of 100 mg every 12 hours produces a steady-state cyclosporine concentration of 250 μg/mL.

10. Solution to problem 10.

Bayesian Pharmacokinetics Computer Program Method

1. *Enter the patient's demographic, drug dosing, and concentration–time data into the computer program.*

Because the patient is also being treated with phenytoin, an enzyme-induction drug interaction for cyclosporine should be entered into the program at the appropriate place.

2. *Compute pharmacokinetic parameters for the patient with a Bayesian pharmacokinetics computer program.*

The pharmacokinetic parameters computed with the program are a volume of distribution of 240 L, a half-life of 7 hours, and a clearance of 23.7 L/h.

3. *Compute the dose required to achieve the desired cyclosporine concentration.*

The one-compartment model, first-order absorption equations used in the program to compute doses indicate that a dose of 400 mg every 12 hours produces a steady-state cyclosporine concentration of 200 μg/mL.

REFERENCES

1. Johnson HJ, Heim-Duthoy KL, Ptachcinski RJ. Renal transplantation. In: DiPiro JT, Talbert RL, Yee GC, Matzke GR, Wells BG, Posey LM, eds. Pharmacotherapy: a pathophysiologic approach. Stamford, CT: Appleton & Lange, 1999:771–94.
2. Lake KD, Olivari MT. Cardiac transplantation. In: DiPiro JT, Talbert RL, Yee GC, Matzke GR, Wells BG, Posey LM, eds. Pharmacotherapy: a pathophysiologic approach. Stamford, CT: Appleton & Lange, 1999:280–94.
3. Maurer JR. Lung transplantation. In: Fauci AS, Braunwald E, Isselbacher KJ, et al, eds. Principles of internal medicine. New York: McGraw-Hill, 1998:1491–3.
4. Perkins JB, Yee GC. Bone marrow transplantation. In: DiPiro JT, Talbert RL, Yee GC, Matzke GR, Wells BG, Posey LM, eds. Pharmacotherapy: a pathophysiologic approach. Stamford, CT: Appleton & Lange, 1999:2195–220.
5. Somani AZ, Burckart GJ. Liver transplantation. In: DiPiro JT, Talbert RL, Yee GC, Matzke GR, Wells BG, Posey LM, eds. Pharmacotherapy: a pathophysiologic approach. Stamford, CT: Appleton & Lange, 1999:676–85.
6. Diasio RB, LoBuglio AF. Immunomodulators: immunosuppressive agents and immunostimulants. In: Hardman JG, Limbird LE, Molinoff PB, Ruddon RW, Gilman AG, eds. The pharmacological basis of therapeutics. New York: McGraw-Hill, 1996:1291–1308.
7. Yee GC, Salomon DR. Cyclosporine. In: Evans WE, Schentag JJ, Jusko WJ, Relling MV, eds. Applied pharmacokinetics. Vancouver, WA: Applied Therapeutics, 1992:28-1–28-40.
8. Min DI. Cyclosporine. In: Schumacher GE, ed. Therapeutic drug monitoring. Stamford, CT: Appleton & Lange, 1995:449–68.
9. Wacke R, Rohde B, Engel G, et al. Comparison of several approaches of therapeutic drug monitoring of cyclosporine A based on individual pharmacokinetics. Eur J Clin Pharmacol 2000;56:43–8.
10. Grevel J. Area-under-the-curve versus trough level monitoring of cyclosporine concentration: critical assessment of dosage adjustment practices and measurement of clinical outcome. Ther Drug Monit 1993;15:488–91.
11. Grant D, Kneteman N, Tchervenkov J, et al. Peak cyclosporine levels (C_{max}) correlate with freedom from liver graft rejection: results of a prospective, randomized comparison of Neoral and Sandimmune for liver transplantation (NOF-8). Transplantation 1999;67:1133–7.
12. Kronbach T, Fischer V, Meyer UA. Cyclosporine metabolism in human liver: identification of a cytochrome P-450III gene family as the major cyclosporine-metabolizing enzyme explains interactions of cyclosporine with other drugs. Clin Pharmacol Ther 1988;43:630–5.

13. Grevel J, Welsh MS, Kahan BD. Linear cyclosporine phamacokinetics. Clin Pharmacol Ther 1988;43:175.
14. Lindholm A. Factors influencing the pharmacokinetics of cyclosporine in man. Ther Drug Monit 1991;13:465–77.
15. Fahr A. Cyclosporine clinical pharmacokinetics. Clin Pharmacokinet 1993;24:472–95.
16. Neoral [package insert]. East Hanover, NJ: Novartis Pharmaceuticals, 1999.
17. Gupta SK, Manfro RC, Tomlanovich SJ, Gambertoglio JG, Garovoy MR, Benet LZ. Effect of food on the pharmacokinetics of cyclosporine in healthy subjects following oral and intravenous administration. J Clin Pharmacol 1990;30:643–53.
18. Naoumov NV, Tredger JM, Steward CM, et al. Cyclosporin A pharmacokinetics in liver transplant recipients in relation to biliary T-tube clamping and liver dysfunction. Gut 1989; 30:391–6.
19. Tredger JM, Naoumov NV, Steward CM, et al. Influence of biliary T tube clamping on cyclosporine pharmacokinetics in liver transplant recipients. Transplant Proc 1988;20:512–5.
20. Burckart GJ, Starzl T, Williams L. Cyclosporine monitoring and pharmacokinetics in pediatric liver transplant patients. Transplant Proc 1985;17:1172.
21. Atkinson K, Britton K, Paull P. Detrimental effect of intestinal disease on absorption of orally administered cyclosporine. Transplant Proc 1983;15:2446.
22. Hansten PD, Horn JR. Drug interactions analysis and management. Vancouver, WA: Applied Therapeutics, 1999:480.
23. Wu CY, Benet LZ, Hebert MF, et al. Differentiation of absorption and first-pass gut and hepatic metabolism in humans: studies with cyclosporine. Clin Pharmacol Ther 1995;58:492–7.
24. Legg B, Rowland M. Cyclosporin: measurement of fraction unbound in plasma. J Pharm Pharmacol 1987;39:599–603.
25. Legg B, Gupta SK, Rowland M, Johnson RW, Solomon LR. Cyclosporin: pharmacokinetics and detailed studies of plasma and erythrocyte binding during intravenous and oral administration. Eur J Clin Pharmacol 1988;34:451–60.
26. Lemaire M, Tillement JP. Role of lipoproteins and erythrocytes in the in vitro binding and distribution of cyclosporin A in the blood. J Pharm Pharmacol 1982;34:715–8.
27. Rosano TG. Effect of hematocrit on cyclosporine (cyclosporin A) in whole blood and plasma of renal-transplant patients. Clin Chem 1985;31:410–12.
28. Sgoutas D, MacMahon W, Love A, Jerkunica I. Interaction of cyclosporin A with human lipoproteins. J Pharm Pharmacol 1986;38:583–8.
29. Henricsson S. A new method for measuring the free fraction of cyclosporin in plasma by equilibrium dialysis. J Pharm Pharmacol 1987;39:384–5.
30. Ptachcinski RJ, Venkataramanan R, Burckart GJ. Clinical pharmacokinetics of cyclosporin. Clin Pharmacokinet 1986;11:107–32.
31. Flechner SM, Kolbeinsson M, Lum B, Tam J, Moran T. The effect of obesity on cyclosporine pharmacokinetics in uremic patients. Transplant Proc 1989;21:1446–8.
32. Flechner SM, Kolbeinsson M, Tam J, Lum B. The impact of body weight on cyclosporine pharmacokinetics in renal transplant recipients. Transplantation 1989;47:806–10.
33. Flechner SM, Haug M, Fisher RK, Modlin CS. Cyclosporine disposition and long-term renal function in a 500-pound kidney transplant recipient. Am J Kidney Dis 1998;32:E4.
34. Yee GC, McGuire TR, Gmur DJ, Lennon TP, Deeg HJ. Blood cyclosporine pharmacokinetics in patients undergoing marrow transplantation: influence of age, obesity, and hematocrit. Transplantation 1988;46:399–402.
35. Yee GC, Lennon TP, Gmur DJ, Cheney CL, Oeser D, Deeg HJ. Effect of obesity on cyclosporine disposition. Transplantation 1988;45:649–51.
36. Swan SK, Bennett WM. Drug dosing guidelines in patients with renal failure. West J Med 1992;156:633–8.

37. Bennett WM. Guide to drug dosage in renal failure. Clin Pharmacokinet 1988;15:326–54.
38. Follath F, Wenk M, Vozeh S, et al. Intravenous cyclosporine kinetics in renal failure. Clin Pharmacol Ther 1983;34:638–43.
39. Lindholm A, Henricsson S, Lind M, Dahlqvist R. Intraindividual variability in the relative systemic availability of cyclosporin after oral dosing. Eur J Clin Pharmacol 1988;34:461–4.
40. Anderson JE, Munday AS, Kelman AW, et al. Evaluation of a Bayesian approach to the pharmacokinetic interpretation of cyclosporin concentrations in renal allograft recipients. Ther Drug Monit 1994;16:160–5.
41. Kahan BD, Kramer WG, Williams C, Wideman CA. Application of Bayesian forecasting to predict appropriate cyclosporine dosing regimens for renal allograft recipients. Transplant Proc 1986;18:200–3.
42. Ruggeri A, Martinelli M. A program for the optimization of cyclosporine therapy using population kinetics modeling. Comput Methods Programs Biomed 2000;61:61–9.
43. Wandell M, Mungall D. Computer assisted drug interpretation and drug regimen optimization. Am Assoc Clin Chem 1984;6:1–11.

16

TACROLIMUS (FK506)

INTRODUCTION

Tacrolimus, also known as FK506, is a macrolide compound with immunosuppressant actions. It is used to prevent rejection of solid-organ transplants.[1–5] Currently, it is approved for use in liver and renal transplantation.[1,5] It is also used for heart, heart–lung, and other types of solid-organ transplantation and is under investigation for the management of graft-versus-host disease in bone marrow transplantation.[2–4] The immunomodulating effects of tacrolimus are caused by its ability to block production of interleukin-2 and other cytokines produced by T lymphocytes.[6] Tacrolimus binds to FK-binding protein (FKBP), an intracellular cytoplasmic protein in T cells. The tacrolimus–FKBP complex interacts with calcineurin, inhibits the catalytic activity of calcineurin, and blocks production of intermediaries involved with the expression of genes that regulate production of cytokines.

THERAPEUTIC AND TOXIC CONCENTRATIONS

The therapeutic range of tacrolimus used at most transplantation centers is 5 to 20 ng/mL in blood.[5,7,8] Although plasma tacrolimus concentrations have been measured and an equivalent therapeutic range in this matrix suggested (0.5 to 2 ng/mL), the two most widely used assays for the drug are performed with blood samples.[7,8] Because tacrolimus is extensively bound to erythrocytes, blood concentration averages about 15 times greater than concurrently measured serum or plasma concentration.[7] Two assay systems are in widespread use. The enzyme-linked immunosorbent assay (ELISA, Pro-Trac®; IncStar) and microparticulate enzyme immunoassay (MEIA, IMx®; Abbott Diagnostics) incorporate the same monoclonal antibody. With blood as the assay matrix, these two assay systems produce similar results.[9–11] For the purposes of the pharmacokinetic computations and problems in this book, tacrolimus concentrations in the blood determined with ELISA or MEIA are used. Because predose minimum steady-state concentration correlates well with steady-state area under the concentration–time curve, minimum concentration of tacrolimus is used for monitoring.[7,12,13]

Desired tacrolimus concentrations differ among the various types of organ transplantation, change during the posttransplantation phase, and are determined with protocols specific to the transplantation service and institution.[1–5,7] It is important for clinicians to be aware of these factors because acceptable tacrolimus concentrations may be different than those given by the clinical laboratory or those suggested in this textbook.

For patients receiving solid-organ transplants such as kidney, liver, heart, lung, or heart and lung, the goals of tacrolimus therapy are to prevent acute or chronic rejection of the transplanted organ and to minimize side effects of the drug.[1–3,5,7] The recipient's immune system detects foreign antigens on the donor organ and produces an immunologic response to the graft. This leads to inflammatory and cytotoxic effects on the transplanted tissue and produces risk of organ damage and failure. In the case of a rejected kidney transplant, it is possible to remove the graft and perform dialysis to sustain life. However, for patients undergoing other types of solid-organ transplantation, graft rejection can cause death. Because tacrolimus can cause nephrotoxicity, some centers delay tacrolimus treatment of renal transplant recipients for a few days or until the kidney begins functioning to avoid untoward effects on the newly transplanted organ. Desired tacrolimus concentration among recipients of renal transplants generally is lower than for other transplant patients (typically 5 to 15 ng/mL versus 5 to 20 ng/mL in whole blood) to avoid toxicity in the new renal graft. For recipients of other solid-organ transplants, tacrolimus therapy may be started several hours before the operation. During the immediately postoperative phase, intravenous tacrolimus may be given to these patients. For long-term immunosuppression among recipients of solid-organ transplants, tacrolimus doses are tapered over a 6- to 12-month period to the lowest concentration and dose possible as long as rejection does not occur.

Although not currently approved for use in the care of recipients of bone marrow transplants, tacrolimus is being investigated as an immunosuppressant for this patient population.[4] For patients receiving tacrolimus after bone marrow transplantation, the goals of therapy are to prevent graft-versus-host disease and to avoid adverse effects of immunosuppressant therapy. Graft-versus-host disease occurs when donor T lymphocytes detect antigens on host tissues and produce an immunologic response to these antigens and host tissues. Acute graft-versus-host disease usually occurs within the first 60 days of transplantation of donor marrow and causes epithelial tissue damage in organs. The most common tissues attacked are skin, gastrointestinal tract, and liver. To prevent acute graft-versus-host disease among recipients of allogeneic bone marrow transplants with HLA-identical sibling donors, tacrolimus therapy usually is instituted on the day of marrow transplantation (day 0). Doses are adjusted to provide therapeutic minimum concentration. Methotrexate and/or glucocorticoids usually are given in conjunction with tacrolimus to recipients of bone marrow transplants. If prophylaxis of acute graft-versus-host disease is successful, tapering of tacrolimus dosage begins approximately 50 days after transplantation. The goal is discontinuation by about posttransplantation day 180.

For recipients of allogeneic bone marrow transplants from HLA-mismatched or HLA-identical unrelated donors, the risk of acute graft-versus-host disease is higher, so tacrolimus therapy may be longer among these patients. After posttransplantation day 100, chronic graft-versus-host disease may occur. Tacrolimus is being investigated as an agent to manage this type of immunologic response.

Neurotoxicity (coma, delirium, psychosis, encephalopathy, seizures, tremor, confusion, headaches, paresthesia, insomnia, nightmares, photophobia, anxiety), nephrotoxicity, hypertension, electrolyte imbalances (hyperkalemia, hypomagnesemia), glucose intolerance, gastrointestinal upset (diarrhea, nausea, vomiting, anorexia), hepatotoxicity, pruritus, alopecia, and leukocytosis are typical adverse effects of tacrolimus.[1–7] Neurologic side effects tend to be associated with a high (≥25 ng/mL) blood concentration of tacrolimus and usually respond to dosage decreases. Hypertension is a common side effect of tacrolimus therapy and is managed with traditional antihypertensive drug therapy. Nephrotoxicity is similar to that which occurs with cyclosporine and is separated into acute and chronic varieties. *Acute nephrotoxicity* is concentration- or dose-dependent and reverses with a dosage decrease. *Chronic nephrotoxicity* is accompanied by kidney tissue damage, including interstitial fibrosis, nonspecific tubular vacuolization, and structural changes in arteries, arterioles, and proximal tubular epithelium. Increased serum creatinine and blood urea nitrogen values and hyperkalemia occur with tacrolimus-induced nephrotoxicity. The clinical features of tacrolimus nephrotoxicity and acute graft rejection among renal transplant patients are similar, so renal biopsy may be performed to differentiate these possibilities. Because biopsy findings are similar for tacrolimus-induced nephrotoxicity and chronic rejection of renal transplants, this technique is not helpful in this situation.[1] Dosage decreases may be necessary to limit adverse drug effects of tacrolimus therapy.

CLINICAL MONITORING PARAMETERS

Recipients of solid-organ transplants should be observed for graft rejection.[1–3,5] For renal transplant patients, increased serum creatinine level, azotemia, hypertension, edema, weight gain due to fluid retention, graft tenderness, fever, and malaise may be caused by acute rejection.[1] Hypertension, proteinuria, continuous decline in renal function (increases in serum creatinine and blood urea nitrogen levels), and uremia indicate chronic rejection among renal transplant patients. For recipients of hepatic transplants, signs and symptoms of acute rejection include fever, lethargy, graft tenderness, increased leukocyte count, change in color or amount of bile, hyperbilirubinemia, and abnormal results of liver function tests.[5] Chronic rejection of a liver transplant may be accompanied only by abnormal results of liver function tests and jaundice. For heart transplant patients, acute rejection is accompanied by low-grade fever, malaise, heart failure (presence of S_3 heart sound), or atrial arrhythmia.[2] Chronic rejection among heart transplant patients, also known as *cardiac allograft vasculopathy* is characterized by accelerated coronary artery atherosclerosis. The symptoms include arrhythmia, decreased left ventricular function, heart failure, myocardial infarction, and sudden cardiac death. For all recipients of solid-organ transplants, biopsy of the transplanted tissue may be performed to confirm the diagnosis of organ rejection.[1–3,5]

Recipients of bone marrow transplants should be observed for signs and symptoms of graft-versus-host disease.[4] These include a generalized maculopapular skin rash, diarrhea, abdominal pain, ileus, hyperbilirubinemia, and abnormal results of liver function tests—including increased serum levels of aspartate aminotransferase (AST), alanine aminotransferase (ALT), and alkaline phosphatase. Patients with severe chronic graft-versus-host disease may have involvement of the skin, liver, eyes, mouth, esophagus, or other organs that resembles systemic autoimmune disease.

Typical adverse effects of tacrolimus include neurotoxicity, nephrotoxicity, hypertension, hyperkalemia, hypomagnesemia, glucose intolerance, gastrointestinal upset, hepatotoxicity, pruritus, alopecia, and leukocytosis.[1–6] Management of these more common side effects is discussed earlier. Less frequent adverse reactions to tacrolimus include hyperlipidemia and thrombocytopenia.

Because of the pivotal role of tacrolimus as an immunosuppressant and the severity of the concentration- and dose-dependent side effects, tacrolimus concentration should be measured for every patient receiving the drug. If a patient has signs or symptoms of organ rejection or graft-versus-host disease, tacrolimus concentration should be measured to ensure that levels have not fallen below the therapeutic range. If a patient has a clinical problem that may be an adverse effect of tacrolimus therapy, tacrolimus concentration should be measured to determine whether levels are in the toxic range.

During the immediately posttransplantation phase, tacrolimus concentration is measured daily for most patients even though steady state may not have been achieved. The aim is to prevent acute rejection of solid-organ transplants or acute graft-versus-host disease associated with bone marrow transplantation. After discharge from the hospital, tacrolimus concentration is measured at most clinic visits. For patients receiving allogeneic bone marrow transplants from HLA-identical sibling donors, it is usually possible to decrease tacrolimus doses and concentrations about 2 months after transplantation and stop tacrolimus therapy altogether about 6 months after transplantation if no or mild acute rejection has occurred. However, recipients of allogeneic bone marrow transplants from HLA-mismatched related or HLA-identical unrelated donors and all recipients of solid-organ transplants need long-term tacrolimus therapy. To decrease risk of drug adverse effects, doses and concentrations of tacrolimus are decreased to the minimum required to prevent graft-versus-host reactions or rejection. Methods to adjust tacrolimus dosage with tacrolimus concentration are discussed later. Because of a good correlation with the steady-state area under the concentration–time curve for tacrolimus, predose steady-state minimum concentration of tacrolimus is used to adjust doses.[7,12,13]

BASIC CLINICAL PHARMACOKINETIC PARAMETERS

Tacrolimus is almost completely (>99%) eliminated through hepatic metabolism. Hepatic metabolism is mainly through the CYP3A4 enzyme system, and the drug is a substrate for P-glycoprotein.[14–17] There are more than 15 identified metabolites of tacrolimus.[7] None of these metabolites appear to have an appreciable immunosuppressive effect on humans. Most of the metabolites are eliminated in the bile.[18] Less than 1% of a tacrolimus dose is recovered as unchanged drug in the urine.[19]

There is large intrasubject variability in tacrolimus concentration from day to day, even when the patient should be at steady state.[7] There are many causes of this variability. Tacrolimus has low water solubility, and its gastrointestinal absorption can be influenced by many variables. Although oral absorption rate is generally fast for most patients (time to maximum concentration of 0.5 to 1 hour), some patients absorb tacrolimus very slowly, which yields a flat concentration–time profile.[12,19–21] Absorption lag times as long as 2 hours have been reported among recipients of liver transplants.[12] Although average oral bioavailability is 25%, there is a large amount of variation in this parameter among patients (4% to 89%).[7] Renal transplant recipients may have decreased oral bioavailability of tacrolimus. When tacrolimus is given with meals, especially with foods that have a high fat content, oral bioavailability decreases.[7] To avoid the possible effect of food on the bioavailability of tacrolimus, the drug should be given at a constant time in relation to meals. Oral tacrolimus should not be taken with grapefruit juice because this vehicle inhibits CYP3A4 and P-glycoprotein contained in the gastrointestinal tract and markedly increases bioavailability.[22] After liver transplantation, bile production and flow may not begin immediately, or bile flow may be diverted from the gastrointestinal tract with a T tube. Unlike that of cyclosporine, gastrointestinal absorption of tacrolimus does not seem to be influenced by the presence or absence of bile.[19,23] Other drug therapy can increase or decrease the intestinal first-pass clearance of tacrolimus.[22]

Tacrolimus is a low hepatic extraction ratio drug.[7] Because of this, hepatic clearance is influenced by unbound fraction in the blood (f_B) and intrinsic clearance (Cl'_{int}). Tacrolimus binds primarily to erythrocytes, α_1-acid glycoprotein, and albumin.[24–27] The exact value for protein binding (72% to 99%) depends on the technique used and matrix tested, and these factors have resulted in a large range of reported values for unbound fractions in the blood.[7] Erythrocyte concentrations vary among patients, especially those who have received bone marrow or kidney transplants. α_1-Acid glycoprotein concentrations also vary greatly among patients. Hepatic intrinsic clearance is different among individuals, and there is great variability in this value among individual liver transplant patients that changes according to the viability of the graft and time after transplantation. Other drug therapy can increase or decrease the hepatic intrinsic clearance of tacrolimus.[22] Taking into consideration all of these factors that alter absorption and clearance allows one to gain a better appreciation of why tacrolimus concentrations change day to day.

Tacrolimus capsules are available in 0.5-, 1-, and 5-mg strengths. Tacrolimus injection for intravenous administration is available at a concentration of 5 mg/mL. The drug should be diluted in normal saline solution or 5% dextrose before administration, and it should be given as a continuous infusion. Anaphylactic reactions have occurred with this dosage form, possibly owing to the castor oil diluent used to enhance dissolution of the drug. The initial dose of tacrolimus varies greatly among various transplantation centers. The range is 0.1 to 0.3 mg/kg per day for orally administered drug and 0.03 to 0.1 mg/kg per day for intravenously administered drug.[5,7] For patients with liver dysfunction, these doses may be reduced 25% to 50%.[23,28,29] Tacrolimus therapy may be started before transplantation.[1–5] Recommended initial oral doses of tacrolimus are 0.2 mg/kg per day for adults receiving kidney transplants, 0.10 to 0.15 mg/kg per day for adults receiving liver transplants, and 0.15 to 0.2 mg/kg per day for children receiving hepatic transplants. Oral tacrolimus is usually given in two divided daily doses, one every 12 hours.

EFFECTS OF DISEASES AND CONDITIONS ON TACROLIMUS PHARMACOKINETICS AND DOSING

Transplantation type does not appear to have a substantial effect on the pharmacokinetics of tacrolimus.[7] The overall mean for all transplantation groups is a clearance of 0.06 L/h per kilogram, a volume of distribution of 1 L/kg, and a half-life of 12 hours for adults.[7] For children 16 years or younger, average clearance and volume of distribution are higher than in adults (0.138 L/h per kilogram and 2.6 L/kg, respectively), but the mean half-life is about the same as that of adults (12 hours).[7] Determination of the half-life of tacrolimus is difficult for patients receiving the drug twice a day because only a few concentrations can be measured in the postabsorption, postdistribution phase. These results, as are the other pharmacokinetic parameters discussed in this chapter, are based on an enzyme-linked immunosorbent assay (ELISA, Pro-Trac®; IncStar) or a microparticulate enzyme immunoassay (MEIA, IMx®; Abbott Diagnostics) performed with samples of whole blood. As discussed earlier, concurrently measured plasma or serum concentrations are lower than are whole-blood concentrations.

Because the drug is eliminated primarily through hepatic metabolism, average clearance is lower (0.04 L/h per kilogram) among adult patients with liver dysfunction than it is among other patients.[23,28,29] Mean volume of distribution is larger (3 L/kg) and half-life prolonged and variable (mean, 60 hours; range, 28 to 141 hours) in this patient population. Immediately after liver transplantation, tacrolimus metabolism is depressed until the graft begins functioning in a stable manner. Patients with transient liver dysfunction, regardless of transplantation type, have decreased tacrolimus clearance and increased half-life values. Renal failure does not markedly change the pharmacokinetics of tacrolimus, and tacrolimus dosage adjustments are not necessary for patients receiving hemodialysis or peritoneal dialysis.[30,31]

DRUG INTERACTIONS

Drug interactions with tacrolimus are not as well documented as those with cyclosporine. Many drug interactions that are reported with cyclosporine are assumed also to occur with tacrolimus.[22] Drugs that interact with tacrolimus fall into two basic categories. The first are agents known to cause nephrotoxicity when administered by themselves. The fear is that administration of a known nephrotoxin with tacrolimus will increase the incidence of renal damage over that which occurs when tacrolimus or the other agent is given separately. Compounds in this category of drug interactions include aminoglycoside antibiotics, vancomycin, cotrimoxazole (trimethoprim-sulfamethoxazole), amphotericin B, and nonsteroidal antiinflammatory drugs. Coadministration of tacrolimus with cyclosporine can augment nephrotoxic side effects.

The second category of drug interaction involves inhibition or induction of tacrolimus metabolism.[22] Tacrolimus is metabolized by CYP3A4 and is a substrate for P-glycoprotein, so the risk for many pharmacokinetic drug interactions exists when an agent is used that inhibits these pathways or is cleared by these mechanisms. Because both of these drug elimination systems exist in the gastrointestinal tract, inhibition drug interactions can enhance the oral bioavailability of tacrolimus by means of diminishing the intestinal and hepatic first-pass effects. Drugs that can inhibit tacrolimus clearance include the calcium channel blockers (verapamil, diltiazem, nicardipine), azole antifungals (fluconazole, itraconazole, ketoconazole), macrolide antibiotics (erythromycin, clarithromycin, troleandomycin), antivirals (indinavir, nelfinavir, ritonavir, saquinavir), steroids, (methylprednisolone, oral contraceptives, androgens), psychotropic agents (fluvoxamine, nefazodone), and other compounds (cimetidine, grapefruit juice). Inducing agents include other antibiotics (nafcillin, rifampin, rifabutin), anticonvulsants (phenytoin, carbamazepine, phenobarbital, primidone), barbiturates, aminoglutethimide, and troglitazone. Because of the large number of potentially interacting agents, and the critical nature of the drugs involved in the treatment of transplant recipients, complete avoidance of drug interactions with tacrolimus is not possible. Most drug interactions with tacrolimus are managed with dosage modification of tacrolimus, and concentration of tacrolimus is used as a guide.

If the drug is given with antacids, tacrolimus concentration may decrease.[22] The mechanisms of action of this drug interaction appears to be pH-mediated destruction of tacrolimus by sodium bicarbonate or magnesium oxide and physical adsorption of tacrolimus to the antacid for aluminum hydroxide gel. Gastrointestinal prokinetic agents (cisapride, metoclopramide) may increase tacrolimus concentration by means of an unknown mechanism. Tacrolimus has the potential to change the clearance of other drugs by means of competitive inhibition of CYP3A4 or P-glycoprotein.[22]

INITIAL DOSAGE DETERMINATION METHODS

Pharmacokinetic Dosing Method

The goals of initial dosing of tacrolimus are to compute the best dose possible for the patient to prevent graft rejection or graft-versus-host disease, given the diseases and conditions that influence the pharmacokinetics of tacrolimus, and to avoid adverse drug reactions. To do this, pharmacokinetic parameters for the patient are estimated with average parameters measured for other patients with similar diseases and conditions.

ESTIMATE OF CLEARANCE

Tacrolimus is almost completely metabolized by the liver. There is no good way to estimate the elimination characteristics of liver-metabolized drugs with an endogenous marker of liver function in the same manner that serum creatinine and estimated creatinine clearance are used to estimate the elimination of agents that are removed by the kidney. Because of this, patients are categorized according to the diseases and conditions known to change the clearance of tacrolimus. Published clearance rate is used as an estimate of the current patient's clearance rate. For example, an adult transplant patient with normal liver function is assigned a tacrolimus clearance rate of 0.06 L/h per kilogram. A pediatric transplant patient with the same profile is assumed to have a tacrolimus clearance rate of 0.138 L/h per kilogram.

SELECTION OF APPROPRIATE PHARMACOKINETIC MODEL AND EQUATIONS

Given by intravenous infusion or orally, tacrolimus follows a two-compartment model. When oral therapy is chosen, the drug often is erratically absorbed and has variable absorption rates. Because of the complex absorption profile and the fact that the drug is usually administered twice a day, a simple pharmacokinetic equation for calculating average steady-state concentration of tacrolimus (Css in ng/mL = μg/L) is widely used and allows computation of a maintenance dose: Css = [F(D/τ)]/Cl, or D = (Css · Cl · τ)/F, where F is the bioavailability fraction for the oral dosage form (F averages 0.25, or 25% for most patient populations), D is the dose of tacrolimus in milligrams, Cl is tacrolimus clearance in liters per hour, and τ is the dosage interval in hours. If the drug is to be given as a continuous intravenous infusion, the equivalent equation for that route of administration is Css = k_0/Cl, or k_0 = Css · Cl, where k_0 is the infusion rate in milligrams per hour.

SELECTION OF STEADY-STATE CONCENTRATION

The generally accepted therapeutic range of tacrolimus in the blood is 5 to 20 ng/mL. More important than this general guideline are the specific requirements for each graft type at the transplantation center where the operation was performed. Clinicians should become familiar with the tacrolimus protocols used at the various institutions at which they practice. Although it is unlikely that steady state has been achieved, tacrolimus concentration usually is measured daily, even when dosage changes are made the previous day, because of the critical nature of the therapeutic effect provided by the drug.

Example 1 HO is a 50-year-old, 75-kg (height, 178 cm) man who has received a renal transplant. Two days after transplantation, results of liver function tests are normal. Suggest an initial oral tacrolimus dose designed to achieve a steady-state minimum blood concentration of tacrolimus of 15 ng/mL.

1. *Estimate clearance according to disease states and conditions present in the patient.*

The mean tacrolimus clearance for adult patients is 0.06 L/h per kilogram. The blood clearance of tacrolimus for this patient is expected to be 4.5 L/h: Cl = 0.06 L/h/kg · 75 kg = 4.5 L/h.

2. *Compute the dosage regimen.*

A 12-hour dosage interval is used for this patient. (Note: ng/mL = μg/L, and this concentration was substituted for Css in the calculations to avoid unit conversion. A conversion constant of 1000 μg/mg is used to change the dose amount to milligrams.) The dosage equation for oral tacrolimus is D = (Css · Cl · τ)/F = (15 μg/L · 4.5 L/h · 12 h)/(0.25 · 1000 μg/mg) = 3.2 mg, rounded to 3 mg every 12 hours. Tacrolimus concentration is measured daily, and steady state is expected to occur in about 3 days (5 half-lives = 5 · 12 h = 60 h).

Example 2 For the patient in example 1, compute an initial dose of intravenous tacrolimus.

1. *Estimate clearance according to disease states and conditions present in the patient.*

The mean tacrolimus clearance for adult patients is 0.06 L/h per kilogram. The blood clearance of tacrolimus for this patient is expected to be 4.5 L/h: Cl = 0.06 L/h/kg · 75 kg = 4.5 L/h.

2. *Compute the dosage regimen.*

A continuous infusion is used for this patient. (Note: ng/mL = μg/L, and this concentration was substituted for Css in the calculations to avoid unit conversion. A conversion constant of 1000 μg/mg is used to change the dose amount to milligrams.) The dosage equation for intravenous tacrolimus is $k_0 = Css \cdot Cl = (15\ \mu g/L \cdot 4.5\ L/h)/(1000\ \mu g/mg) = 0.07\ mg/h$. Tacrolimus concentration is measured daily, and steady state is expected to occur in about 3 days (5 half-lives = 5 · 12 h = 60 h).

Literature-Based Recommended Dosing

Because of the large variability in pharmacokinetics of tacrolimus, even when concurrent diseases and conditions are identified, many clinicians believe that the use of standard tacrolimus doses for various situations is warranted. Most transplantation centers use doses determined with a tacrolimus dosage protocol. The original computation of these doses was based on the pharmacokinetic dosing method described earlier and modified according to clinical experience. In general, the expected steady-state concentration of tacrolimus used to compute these doses depends on the type of tissue transplanted and the posttransplantation time line. In general, initial oral doses of 0.1 to 0.3 mg/kg per day are needed to achieve a therapeutic steady-state concentration of tacrolimus.[5,7] The usual initial dose for continuous intravenous infusion is 0.03 to 0.1 mg/kg per day.[5,7] For patients with liver dysfunction, this dosage can be reduced 25% to 50%.[23,28,29] To illustrate how this technique is used, the previous patient examples are repeated.

Example 3 HO is a 50-year-old, 75-kg (height, 178 cm) man who has received a renal transplant. Two days after transplantation, results of liver function tests are normal. Suggest an initial oral tacrolimus dose designed to achieve a steady-state tacrolimus minimum blood concentration within the therapeutic range.

1. *Choose the tacrolimus dose based on disease states and conditions present in the patient and transplantation type.*

The oral dosage range of tacrolimus for adult patients is 0.1 to 0.3 mg/kg per day. Because the patient has received a renal transplant, a dose in the lower end of the range (0.1 mg/kg per day) is used to avoid nephrotoxicity. The initial tacrolimus dose for this patient is 8 mg/d given as 4 mg every 12 hours: Dose = 0.1 mg/kg/d · 75 kg = 7.5 mg/d, rounded to 8 mg/d, or 4 mg every 12 hours. Tacrolimus concentration is measured daily, and steady state is expected to occur after 3 days (5 half-lives = 5 · 12 h = 60 h) of treatment.

Example 4 For the patient in example 3, compute an initial dose of intravenous tacrolimus.

1. *Choose the tacrolimus dose based on disease states and conditions present in the patient and transplantation type.*

The intravenous dosage range of tacrolimus for adult patients is 0.03 to 0.1 mg/kg per day. Because the patient has received a renal transplant, a dose in the lower end of the range (0.03 mg/kg per day) is used to avoid nephrotoxicity. The initial intravenous infusion dose of tacrolimus for this patient is 0.09 mg/h: Dose = (0.03 mg/kg/d · 75 kg)/

24 h/d = 0.09 mg/h. Tacrolimus concentration is measured daily, and steady state is expected to occur after 3 days (5 half-lives = 5 · 12 h = 60 h) of treatment.

USE OF TACROLIMUS CONCENTRATIONS TO ALTER DOSES

Because of the large pharmacokinetic variability among patients, it is likely that doses computed with patient population characteristics will not always produce tacrolimus concentrations that are expected or desirable. Because of pharmacokinetic variability, the narrow therapeutic index of tacrolimus, and the severity of the adverse side effects of tacrolimus, measurement of tacrolimus concentration is mandatory to ensure that therapeutic, nontoxic levels are present. In addition to tacrolimus concentration, important patient parameters, such as results of function tests or biopsy of the transplanted organ, clinical signs and symptoms of graft rejection or graft-versus-host disease, or risk of side effects, should be followed to confirm that the patient is responding to treatment and not having adverse drug reactions.

When tacrolimus concentration is measured, and a dosage change is necessary, clinicians should use the simplest, most straightforward method available to determine a dose that will provide safe and effective treatment. In most cases, a simple dosage ratio can be used to change tacrolimus doses, assuming the drug follows linear pharmacokinetics. Sometimes it is useful to compute tacrolimus pharmacokinetic constants for a patient and base dosage adjustments on them. In this case, it may be possible to calculate and use pharmacokinetic parameters to alter the tacrolimus dose. Computerized methods that incorporate expected population pharmacokinetic characteristics (Bayesian pharmacokinetics computer programs) can be used in difficult cases when concentrations are obtained at suboptimal times or the patient was not at steady state when concentration was measured.

Linear Pharmacokinetics Method

Assuming tacrolimus follows linear, dose-proportional pharmacokinetics,[32] steady-state concentration changes in proportion to dose according to the following equation: $D_{new}/Css_{new} = D_{old}/Css_{old}$, or $D_{new} = (Css_{new}/Css_{old})D_{old}$, where D is the dose, Css is steady-state concentration, old indicates the dose that produced the steady-state concentration that the patient is currently receiving, and new denotes the dose necessary to produce the desired steady-state concentration. The advantages of this method are that it is quick and simple. The disadvantage is that steady-state concentration is required.

Example 5 LK is a 50-year-old, 75-kg (height, 178 cm) man who has received a renal transplant. He is receiving 5 mg every 12 hours of oral tacrolimus capsules. He has normal liver function. The current steady-state blood concentration of tacrolimus is 24 ng/mL. Compute a tacrolimus dose that will provide a steady-state concentration of 15 ng/mL.

1. *Compute the new dose to achieve the desired concentration.*

The patient is expected to achieve steady-state conditions after the third day (5 half-lives = 5 · 12 h = 60 h) of therapy. According to linear pharmacokinetics, the new dose to attain the desired concentration should be proportional to the old dose that produced the measured concentration (total daily dose = 5 mg/dose · 2 doses/d = 10 mg/d):

$$D_{new} = (Css_{new}/Css_{old})D_{old} = [(15\ ng/mL)/(24\ ng/mL)]\ 10\ mg/d$$
$$= 6.3\ mg/d,\ \text{rounded to}\ 6\ mg/d$$

The new suggested dose is 6 mg/d, or 3 mg every 12 hours, of tacrolimus capsules to be started at the next scheduled dosing time.

Steady-state minimum concentration of tacrolimus should be measured after steady state is attained in 3 to 5 half-lives. Because the drug is expected to have a half-life of 12 hours in this patient, steady-state concentration of tacrolimus can be measured any time after the third day of dosing (5 half-lives = 5 · 12 h = 60 h). Tacrolimus concentration should be measured if the patient has signs or symptoms of graft rejection or if the patient has signs or symptoms of tacrolimus toxicity.

Example 6 FD is a 60-year-old, 85-kg (height, 185 cm) man who has received a liver transplant. He is receiving 0.15 mg/h of intravenous tacrolimus as a continuous infusion. The current steady-state concentration of tacrolimus is 9 ng/mL. Compute a tacrolimus dose that will provide a steady-state concentration of 15 ng/mL.

1. *Compute the new dose to achieve the desired concentration.*

The patient is expected to achieve steady-state conditions after the third day (5 half-lives = 5 · 12 h = 60 h) of therapy. According to linear pharmacokinetics, the new dose to attain the desired concentration should be proportional to the old dose that produced the measured concentration:

$$D_{new} = (Css_{new}/Css_{old})D_{old} = [(15\ ng/mL)/(9\ ng/mL)]\ 0.15\ mg/h = 0.25\ mg/h$$

Tacrolimus concentration should be measured after steady state is attained in 3 to 5 half-lives. Because the drug is expected to have a half-life of 12 hours in this patient, steady-state concentration of tacrolimus can be measured any time after the third day of dosing (5 half-lives = 5 · 12 h = 60 h). Tacrolimus concentration should be measured if the patient has signs or symptoms of graft rejection or if the patient has signs or symptoms of tacrolimus toxicity.

Pharmacokinetic Parameter Method

The pharmacokinetic parameter method of adjusting drug doses was among the first techniques for changing doses with drug concentration. It allows computation of a patient's unique pharmacokinetic constants, which are used to calculate a dose that achieves the desired concentration of tacrolimus. The pharmacokinetic parameter method requires that steady state has been achieved, and only steady-state tacrolimus concentration is used. Tacrolimus clearance can be measured with a single steady-state tacrolimus concentration and the following formula for orally administered drug: $Cl = [F(D/\tau)]/Css$, where Cl is tacrolimus clearance in liters per hour, F is the bioavailability factor for tacrolimus (F = 0.25), τ is the dosage interval in hours, and Css is steady-state concentration of tacrolimus in nanograms per milliliter, which convert to micrograms per liter. If tacrolimus is administered intravenously, it is not necessary to take bioavailability into account: $Cl = k_0/Css$, where Cl is tacrolimus clearance in liters per hour, k_0 is tacrolimus infusion rate in milligrams per hour, and Css is steady-state concentration of tacrolimus in nanograms per milliliter, which convert to micrograms per liter. Although this method does allow computation of tacrolimus clearance, it yields exactly the same tacrolimus dose as that supplied with linear pharmacokinetics. As a result, most clinicians prefer to calculate directly the new dose with the simpler linear pharmacokinetics method. To demonstrate this point, the patient cases used to illustrate the linear pharmacokinetics method are repeated for the pharmacokinetic parameter method.

Example 7 LK is a 50-year-old, 75-kg (height, 178 cm) man who has received a renal transplant. He is receiving 5 mg every 12 hours of oral tacrolimus capsules. He has normal liver function. The current steady-state blood concentration of tacrolimus is 24 ng/mL. Compute a tacrolimus dose that will provide a steady-state concentration of 15 ng/mL.

1. *Compute pharmacokinetic parameters.*

The patient is expected to achieve steady-state conditions after the third day (5 half-lives = 5 · 12 h = 60 h) of therapy. Tacrolimus clearance can be computed with steady-state concentration of tacrolimus: $Cl = [F(D/\tau)]/Css = [0.25 \cdot (5\ mg/12\ h) \cdot 1000\ \mu g/mg]/(24\ \mu g/L) = 4.3\ L/h$. (Note: μg/L = ng/mL, and this concentration unit was substituted for Css in the calculations to avoid unit conversion.)

2. *Compute the tacrolimus dose.*

Tacrolimus clearance is used to compute the new dose: $D = (Css \cdot Cl \cdot \tau)/F = (15\ \mu g/L \cdot 4.3\ L/h \cdot 12\ h)/(0.25 \cdot 1000\ \mu g/mg) = 3.1\ mg$, rounded to 3 mg every 12 hours.

Steady-state minimum tacrolimus concentration should be measured after steady state is attained in 3 to 5 half-lives. Because the drug is expected to have a half-life of 12 hours in this patient, steady-state concentration of tacrolimus can be measured any time after the third day of dosing (5 half-lives = 5 · 12 h = 60 h). Tacrolimus concentration should be measured if the patient has signs or symptoms of graft rejection or if the patient has signs or symptoms of tacrolimus toxicity.

Example 8 FD is a 60-year-old, 85-kg (height, 185 cm) man who has received a liver transplant. He is receiving 0.15 mg/h of intravenous tacrolimus as a continuous infusion. The current steady-state concentration of tacrolimus is 9 ng/mL. Compute a tacrolimus dose that will provide a steady-state concentration of 15 ng/mL.

1. *Compute pharmacokinetic parameters.*

The patient is expected to achieve steady-state conditions after the third day (5 half-lives = 5 · 12 h = 60 h) of therapy. Tacrolimus clearance can be computed with steady-state tacrolimus concentration: $Cl = k_0/Css = (0.15\ mg/h \cdot 1000\ \mu g/mg)/(9\ \mu g/L) = 16.7\ L/h$. (Note: μg/L = ng/mL, and this concentration unit was substituted for Css in the calculations to avoid unit conversion.)

2. *Compute the tacrolimus dose.*

Tacrolimus clearance is used to compute the new dose: $k_0 = Css \cdot Cl = (15\ \mu g/L \cdot 16.7\ L/h)/(1000\ \mu g/mg) = 0.25\ mg/h$.

Steady-state minimum tacrolimus concentration should be measured after steady state is attained in 3 to 5 half-lives. Because the drug is expected to have a half-life of 12 hours in this patient, steady-state concentration of tacrolimus can be measured any time after the third day of dosing (5 half-lives = 5 · 12 h = 60 h). Tacrolimus concentration should be measured if the patient has signs or symptoms of graft rejection or if the patient has signs or symptoms of tacrolimus toxicity.

BAYESIAN PHARMACOKINETICS COMPUTER PROGRAMS

Computer programs can assist in computation of pharmacokinetic parameters for patients. In the most reliable computer programs, a nonlinear regression algorithm incorporates components of Bayes' theorem. Nonlinear regression is a statistical technique in which an iterative process is used to compute the best pharmacokinetic parameters for a concentration–time data set. The patient's drug dosage schedule and drug concentrations are entered into the computer. The computer program has a pharmacokinetic equation programmed for the drug and administration method, such as oral, intravenous bolus, or intravenous infusion. A one-compartment model typically is used, although some programs allow the user to choose among several different equations. With population estimates based on demographic information for the patient, such as age, weight, sex, liver function, and cardiac status, supplied by the user, the program is used to compute estimated drug concentrations for each actual drug concentration. Kinetic parameters are changed by the computer program, and a new set of estimated drug concentrations are computed. The pharmacokinetic parameters that generated the estimated drug concentrations closest to the actual values are stored in the computer memory, and the process is repeated until the set of pharmacokinetic parameters that provides estimated drug concentrations statistically closest to the actual drug concentrations is generated. These pharmacokinetic parameters can be used to compute improved dosing schedules for patients. Bayes' theorem is used in the computer algorithm to balance the results of the computations between values based solely on the patient's drug concentrations and those based only on patient population parameters. Results of studies in which various methods of dosage adjustment have been compared have consistently shown that these types of computer dosing programs perform at least as well as experienced clinical pharmacokineticists and clinicians and better than inexperienced clinicians.

Some clinicians use Bayesian pharmacokinetics computer programs exclusively to alter drug doses based on drug concentrations. An advantage of this approach is that consistent dosage recommendations are made when several practitioners are involved in therapeutic drug monitoring programs. However, because simpler dosing methods work just as well for patients with stable pharmacokinetic parameters and steady-state drug concentrations, many clinicians reserve the use of computer programs for more difficult situations. Those situations include drug concentrations that are not at steady state, drug concentrations not obtained at the specific times needed to use simpler methods, and unstable pharmacokinetic parameters. Many Bayesian pharmacokinetics computer programs are available, and most should provide answers similar to the ones used in the examples. The program used to solve problems in this book is DrugCalc written by Dr. Dennis Mungall. It is available on his Internet web site (http://members.aol.com/thertch/index.htm).[33]

Example 9 LK is a 50-year-old, 75-kg (height, 178 cm) man who has received a renal transplant. He is receiving 5 mg every 12 hours of oral tacrolimus capsules. He has normal liver function (bilirubin, 0.7 mg/dL; albumin, 4.0 g/dL). The current steady-state blood concentration of tacrolimus is 24 ng/mL. Compute a tacrolimus dose that will provide a steady-state concentration of 15 ng/mL.

1. *Enter the patient's demographic, drug dosing, and concentration–time data into the computer program.*

2. *Compute pharmacokinetic parameters for the patient with a Bayesian pharmacokinetics computer program.*

The pharmacokinetic parameters computed with the program are a volume of distribution of 76 L, a half-life of 15.8 hours, and a clearance of 3.3 L/h.

3. *Compute the dose required to achieve the desired concentration of tacrolimus.*

The one-compartment model, first-order absorption equations used in the program to compute doses indicate that a dose of 2 mg every 12 hours produces a steady-state tacrolimus concentration of 15 ng/mL. Use of the linear pharmacokinetics and pharmacokinetic parameter methods described earlier produces a similar answer for this patient.

Example 10 FD is a 60-year-old, 85-kg (height, 185 cm) man who has received a liver transplant. He is receiving 0.15 mg/h of intravenous tacrolimus as a continuous infusion. He has normal liver function (bilirubin, 1.1 mg/dL; albumin, 3.5 g/dL). The current steady-state tacrolimus concentration is 9 ng/mL. Compute a tacrolimus dose that will provide a steady-state concentration of 15 ng/mL.

1. *Enter the patient's demographic, drug dosing, and concentration–time data into the computer program.*

2. *Compute pharmacokinetic parameters for the patient with a Bayesian pharmacokinetics computer program.*

The pharmacokinetic parameters computed with the program are a volume of distribution of 85 L, a half-life of 3.6 hours, and a clearance of 16.3 L/h.

3. *Compute the dose required to achieve the desired concentration of tacrolimus.*

The one-compartment model, continuous infusion equations used in the program to compute doses indicate that a dose of 0.24 mg/h produces a steady-state tacrolimus concentration of 15 ng/mL. Use of the linear pharmacokinetics and pharmacokinetic parameter methods described earlier produces a similar answer for this patient.

Example 11 YT is a 25-year-old, 55-kg (height, 157 cm) woman who has received a renal transplant. She received 4 mg every 12 hours of oral tacrolimus capsules for two doses after transplantation, but because renal function decreased, the dose was empirically changed to 2 mg every 12 hours. The patient has normal liver function (bilirubin, 0.9 mg/dL; albumin, 3.9 g/dL). The blood concentration of tacrolimus measured 12 hours after the first dose at the lower dosage is 22 ng/mL. Compute a tacrolimus dose that will provide a steady-state concentration of 15 ng/mL.

1. *Enter the patient's demographic, drug dosing, and concentration–time data into the computer program.*

2. *Compute pharmacokinetic parameters for the patient with a Bayesian pharmacokinetics computer program.*

The pharmacokinetic parameters computed with the program are a volume of distribution of 54 L, a half-life of 1.8 hours, and a clearance of 21 L/h.

3. *Compute the dose required to achieve the desired concentration of tacrolimus.*

The one-compartment model, first-order absorption equations used in the program to compute doses indicate that a dose of 1 mg every 12 hours produces a steady-state tacrolimus concentration of 15 ng/mL.

PROBLEMS

The following problems are intended to emphasize the computation of initial and individualized doses with clinical pharmacokinetic techniques. Clinicians always should consult the patient's chart to confirm that current immunosuppressive therapy is appropriate. All other medications that the patient is taking, including prescription and nonprescription drugs, should be recorded and checked to ascertain the risk of drug interaction with tacrolimus.

1. VI is a 37-year-old, 85-kg (height, 185 cm) man who has received a heart transplant. He needs therapy with oral tacrolimus. He has normal liver function. Suggest an initial dosage regimen designed to achieve a steady-state tacrolimus concentration of 15 ng/mL.

2. Patient VI (see problem 1) is given a prescription for 5 mg every 12 hours of tacrolimus capsules for 4 days. Steady-state tacrolimus concentration is 28 ng/mL. The patient is found to be compliant with the dosage regimen. Suggest a tacrolimus dosage regimen designed to achieve a steady-state tacrolimus concentration of 15 ng/mL.

3. AS is a 9-year-old, 35-kg (height, 137 cm) girl who has undergone bone marrow transplantation. She needs therapy with oral tacrolimus. She has normal liver function. Suggest an initial tacrolimus dosage regimen designed to achieve a steady-state tacrolimus concentration of 12 ng/mL.

4. Patient AS (see problem 3) is given a prescription for 3 mg every 12 hours of tacrolimus capsules for 3 days. Steady-state tacrolimus concentration is 9 ng/mL. The patient is found to be compliant with the dosage regimen. Suggest an oral tacrolimus dosage regimen designed to achieve a steady-state tacrolimus concentration of 12 ng/mL.

5. FL is a 29-year-old, 78-kg (height, 180 cm) man who is scheduled to receive a liver transplant. He needs therapy with oral tacrolimus before the surgery is conducted. He has poor liver function because of liver disease. Suggest an initial tacrolimus dosage regimen to be started 24 hours before transplantation that is designed to achieve a steady-state tacrolimus concentration of 15 ng/mL.

6. For the 10 days since liver transplantation, patient FL (see problem 5) has been receiving 4 mg every 12 hours of tacrolimus capsules. Steady-state tacrolimus concentration is 33 ng/mL. The patient is found to be compliant with the dosage regimen. Suggest a tacrolimus dosage regimen designed to achieve a steady-state tacrolimus concentration of 15 ng/mL.

7. PH is a 22-year-old, 67-kg (height, 165 cm) woman who has received a renal transplant. She needs therapy with oral tacrolimus. Thirty-six hours after transplantation, the new kidney is beginning to function normally. Liver function is normal. Suggest an initial tacrolimus dosage regimen designed to achieve a steady-state tacrolimus concentration of 15 ng/mL.

8. Patient PH (see problem 7) is given a prescription for 3 mg every 12 hours of tacrolimus capsules for 3 days. Steady-state tacrolimus concentration is 11 ng/mL. The patient is found to be compliant with the dosage regimen. Suggest a tacrolimus dosage regimen designed to achieve a steady-state tacrolimus concentration of 15 ng/mL.

9. PU is a 55-year-old, 68-kg (height, 173 cm) man who has received a heart transplant. He was given a continuous intravenous infusion of tacrolimus (0.25 mg/h for 24 hours), and therapy was switched to oral tacrolimus capsules 3 mg every 12 hours. The patient has normal liver function (bilirubin, 0.7 mg/dL; albumin, 4.0 g/dL). Tacrolimus concentration is 25 ng/mL 12 hours after the first oral dose of the drug. Compute a tacrolimus dose that will provide a steady-state concentration of 20 ng/mL.

10. LH is a 25-year-old, 60-kg (height, 160 cm) woman who has received a renal transplant. She is given a new prescription for tacrolimus capsules 4 mg every 12 hours 2 days after transplantation. She has normal liver function (bilirubin, 0.4 mg/dL; albumin, 3.7 g/dL) and is being treated with phenytoin. The minimum tacrolimus concentration before the fourth dose is 10 ng/mL. Compute a tacrolimus dose that will provide a steady-state concentration of 20 ng/mL.

ANSWERS TO PROBLEMS

1. Answer to problem 1.

Pharmacokinetic Dosing Method

1. *Estimate clearance according to disease states and conditions present in the patient.*

The mean tacrolimus clearance for adult patients is 0.06 L/h per kilogram. The blood clearance of tacrolimus for this patient is expected to be Cl = 0.06 L/h/kg · 85 kg = 5.1 L/h.

2. *Compute the dosage regimen.*

A 12-hour dosage interval is used for this patient. (Note: ng/mL = μg/L, and this concentration was substituted for Css in the calculations to avoid unit conversion. A conversion constant of 1000 μg/mg is used to change the dose amount to milligrams.) The dosage equation for oral tacrolimus is D = (Css · Cl · τ)/F = (15 μg/L · 5.1 L/h · 12 h)/(0.25 · 1000 μg/mg) = 3.7 mg, rounded to 4 mg every 12 hours. Tacrolimus concentration is measured daily, and steady state is expected to occur after about 3 days of therapy (5 half-lives = 5 · 12 h = 60 h).

Literature-Based Recommended Dosing

1. *Choose the tacrolimus dose based on disease states and conditions present in the patient and transplantation type.*

The oral dosage range of tacrolimus for adult patients is 0.1 to 0.3 mg/kg per day. Because the patient has received a heart transplant, a dose in the middle of the range (0.15 mg/kg per day) is used to avoid graft rejection. The initial tacrolimus dose for this patient is: Dose = 0.15 mg/kg/d · 85 kg = 12.8 mg/d, rounded to 12 mg/d, or 6 mg every 12 hours. Tacrolimus concentration is measured daily, and steady state is expected to occur after 3 days (5 half-lives = 5 · 12 h = 60 h) of treatment.

2. Answer to problem 2.

Linear Pharmacokinetics Method

1. *Compute the new dose to achieve the desired concentration.*

The patient is expected to achieve steady-state conditions after the third day (5 half-lives = 5 · 12 h = 60 h) of therapy. According to linear pharmacokinetics, the new dose to attain the desired concentration should be proportional to the old dose that produced the measured concentration (total daily dose = 5 mg/dose · 2 doses/d = 10 mg/d):

$$D_{new} = (Css_{new}/Css_{old})D_{old} = [(15 \text{ ng/mL})/(28 \text{ ng/mL})]\ 10 \text{ mg/d}$$
$$= 5.4 \text{ mg/d, rounded to } 6 \text{ mg/d}$$

The new suggested dose is 6 mg/d, or 3 mg every 12 hours, of tacrolimus capsules to be started at the next scheduled dosing time.

Steady-state minimum tacrolimus concentration should be measured after steady state is attained in 3 to 5 half-lives. Because the drug is expected to have a half-life of 12 hours in this patient, steady-state concentration of tacrolimus can be measured any time after the third day of dosing (5 half-lives = 5 · 12 h = 60 h). Tacrolimus concentration should be measured if the patient has signs or symptoms of graft rejection or if the patient has signs or symptoms of tacrolimus toxicity.

Pharmacokinetic Parameter Method

1. *Compute pharmacokinetic parameters.*

The patient is expected to achieve steady-state conditions after the third day (5 half-lives = 5 · 12 h = 60 h) of therapy. Tacrolimus clearance can be computed with a steady-state tacrolimus concentration: Cl = [F(D/τ)]/Css = [0.25 · (5 mg/12 h) · 1000 μg/mg]/ (28 μg/L) = 3.7 L/h. (Note: μg/L = ng/mL, and this concentration unit was substituted for Css in the calculations to avoid unit conversion.)

2. *Compute the tacrolimus dose.*

Tacrolimus clearance is used to compute the new dose: D = (Css · Cl · τ)/F = (15 μg/L · 3.7 L/h · 12 h)/(0.25 · 1000 μg/mg) = 2.7 mg, rounded to 3 mg every 12 hours.

Steady-state minimum tacrolimus concentration should be measured after steady state is attained in 3 to 5 half-lives. Because the drug is expected to have a half-life of 12 hours in this patient, steady-state concentration of tacrolimus can be measured any time after the third day of dosing (5 half-lives = 5 · 12 h = 60 h). Tacrolimus concentration should be measured if the patient has signs or symptoms of graft rejection or if the patient has signs or symptoms of tacrolimus toxicity.

3. Answer to problem 3.

Pharmacokinetic Dosing Method

1. *Estimate clearance according to disease states and conditions present in the patient.*

The mean tacrolimus clearance for pediatric patients is 0.138 L/h per kilogram. The blood clearance of tacrolimus for this patient is expected to be Cl = 0.138 L/h/kg · 35 kg = 4.8 L/h.

2. *Compute the dosage regimen.*

A 12-hour dosage interval is used for this patient. (Note: ng/mL = μg/L, and this concentration was substituted for Css in the calculations to avoid unit conversion. A conversion constant of 1000 μg/mg is used to change the dose amount to milligrams.) The dosage equation for oral tacrolimus is D = (Css · Cl · τ)/F = (12 μg/L · 4.8 L/h · 12 h)/(0.25 · 1000 μg/mg) = 2.8 mg, rounded to 3 mg every 12 hours, of tacrolimus capsules. Tacrolimus concentration is measured daily, and steady state is expected to occur after about 3 days (5 half-lives = 5 · 12 h = 60 h).

Literature-Based Recommended Dosing

1. *Choose the tacrolimus dose based on disease states and conditions present in the patient and transplantation type.*

The oral dosage range of tacrolimus is 0.1 to 0.3 mg/kg per day. Because this is a pediatric patient, a dose in the middle of the range (0.15 mg/kg per day) is used to avoid graft-versus-host disease. The initial tacrolimus dose for this patient is: Dose = 0.15 mg/kg/d · 35 kg = 5.3 mg/d, rounded to 6 mg/d, or 3 mg every 12 hours, of tacrolimus capsules. Tacrolimus concentration is measured daily, and steady state is expected to occur after about 3 days (5 half-lives = 5 · 12 h = 60 h) of treatment.

4. Answer to problem 4.

Linear Pharmacokinetics Method

1. *Compute the new dose to achieve the desired concentration.*

The patient is expected to achieve steady-state conditions by the third day (5 half-lives = 5 · 12 h = 60 h) of therapy. According to linear pharmacokinetics, the new dose to attain the desired concentration should be proportional to the old dose that produced the measured concentration (total daily dose = 3 mg/dose · 2 doses/d = 6 mg/d):

$$D_{new} = (Css_{new}/Css_{old})D_{old} = [(12\ ng/mL)/(9\ ng/mL)]\ 6\ mg/d = 8\ mg/d$$

The new suggested dose is 8 mg/d, or 4 mg every 12 hours, of tacrolimus capsules to be started at the next scheduled dosing time.

Steady-state minimum tacrolimus concentration should be measured after steady state is attained in 3 to 5 half-lives. Because the drug is expected to have a half-life of 12 hours in this patient, steady-state concentration of tacrolimus can be measured any time after the third day of dosing (5 half-lives = 5 · 12 h = 60 h). Tacrolimus concentration should be measured if the patient has signs or symptoms of graft rejection or if the patient has signs or symptoms of tacrolimus toxicity.

Pharmacokinetic Parameter Method

1. *Compute pharmacokinetic parameters.*

The patient is expected to achieve steady-state conditions after the third day (5 half-lives = 5 · 12 h = 60 h) of therapy. Tacrolimus clearance can be computed with steady-state tacrolimus concentration: $Cl = [F(D/\tau)]/Css = [0.25 \cdot (3\ mg/12\ h) \cdot 1000\ \mu g/mg]/(9\ \mu g/L) = 6.9\ L/h$. (Note: μg/L = ng/mL, and this concentration unit was substituted for Css in the calculations to avoid unit conversion.)

2. *Compute the tacrolimus dose.*

Tacrolimus clearance is used to compute the new dose: $D = (Css \cdot Cl \cdot \tau)/F = (12\ \mu g/L \cdot 6.9\ L/h \cdot 12\ h)/(0.25 \cdot 1000\ \mu g/mg) = 4\ mg$, given as 4 mg every 12 hours, of tacrolimus capsules.

Steady-state minimum tacrolimus concentration should be measured after steady state is attained in 3 to 5 half-lives. Because the drug is expected to have a half-life of 12 hours in this patient, steady-state concentration of tacrolimus can be measured any time after the third day of dosing (5 half-lives = 5 · 12 h = 60 h). Tacrolimus concentration should be measured if the patient has signs or symptoms of graft rejection or if the patient has signs or symptoms of tacrolimus toxicity.

5. Answer to problem 5.

Pharmacokinetic Dosing Method

1. *Estimate clearance according to disease states and conditions present in the patient.*

The mean tacrolimus clearance for adult patients with liver dysfunction is 0.04 L/h per kilogram. The blood clearance of tacrolimus for this patient is expected to be $Cl = 0.04\ L/h/kg \cdot 78\ kg = 3.1\ L/h$.

2. *Compute the dosage regimen.*

A 12-hour dosage interval is used for this patient. (Note: ng/mL = μg/L, and this concentration was substituted for Css in the calculations to avoid unit conversion. A conversion constant of 1000 μg/mg is used to change the dose amount to milligrams.)

The dosage equation for oral tacrolimus is D = (Css · Cl · τ)/F = (15 μg/L · 3.1 L/h · 12 h)/(0.25 · 1000 μg/mg) = 2.2 mg, rounded to 2 mg every 12 hours. Tacrolimus concentration is measured daily, and steady state is expected to occur after about 12 days of therapy (5 half-lives = 5 · 60 h = 300 h, or 12.5 d). However, this patient is scheduled to undergo transplantation the next day.

Literature-Based Recommended Dosing

1. *Choose the tacrolimus dose based on disease states and conditions present in the patient and transplantation type.*

The oral dosage range of tacrolimus for adult patients is 0.1 to 0.3 mg/kg per day. Because this patient has liver dysfunction, a dose in the lower end of the range (0.1 mg/kg per day) is used to avoid graft rejection. The initial tacrolimus dose for this patient is: Dose = 0.1 mg/kg/d · 78 kg = 7.8 mg/d, rounded to 8 mg/d. Because this patient has liver dysfunction, this dose should be empirically reduced 50%; 8 mg/d · 0.5 = 4 mg/d, or 2 mg every 12 hours. Tacrolimus concentration is measured daily, and steady state is expected to occur after about 12 days of therapy (5 half-lives = 5 · 60 h = 300 h, or 12.5 d). However, this patient is scheduled to undergo transplantation the next day.

6. Answer to problem 6.

Linear Pharmacokinetics Method

1. *Compute the new dose to achieve the desired concentration.*

The patient is expected to achieve steady-state conditions after the third day (5 half-lives = 5 · 12 h = 60 h) of therapy. According to linear pharmacokinetics, the new dose to attain the desired concentration should be proportional to the old dose that produced the measured concentration (total daily dose = 4 mg/dose · 2 doses/d = 8 mg/d):

$$D_{new} = (Css_{new}/Css_{old})D_{old} = [(15\ \text{ng/mL})/(33\ \text{ng/mL})]\ 8\ \text{mg/d}$$
$$= 3.6\ \text{mg/d, rounded to } 4\ \text{mg/d}$$

The new suggested dose is 4 mg/d, or 2 mg every 12 hours, of tacrolimus capsules to be started at the next scheduled dosing time.

Steady-state minimum tacrolimus concentration should be measured after steady state is attained in 3 to 5 half-lives. Because the drug is expected to have a half-life of 12 hours in this patient, steady-state concentration of tacrolimus can be measured any time after the third day of dosing (5 half-lives = 5 · 12 h = 60 h). Tacrolimus concentration should be measured if the patient has signs or symptoms of graft rejection or if the patient has signs or symptoms of tacrolimus toxicity.

Pharmacokinetic Parameter Method

1. *Compute pharmacokinetic parameters.*

The patient is expected to achieve steady-state conditions after the third day (5 half-lives = 5 · 12 h = 60 h) of therapy. Tacrolimus clearance can be computed with steady-state tacrolimus concentration: Cl = [F(D/τ)]/Css = [0.25 · (4 mg/12 h) ·

1000 μg/mg]/(33 μg/L) = 2.5 L/h. (Note: μg/L = ng/mL, and this concentration unit was substituted for Css in the calculations to avoid unit conversion.)

2. *Compute the tacrolimus dose.*

Tacrolimus clearance is used to compute the new dose: D = (Css · Cl · τ)/F = (15 μg/L · 2.5 L/h · 12 h)/(0.25 · 1000 μg/mg) = 1.8 mg, rounded to 2 mg every 12 hours.

Steady-state minimum tacrolimus concentration should be measured after steady state is attained in 3 to 5 half-lives. Because the drug is expected to have a half-life of 12 hours in this patient, steady-state concentration of tacrolimus can be measured any time after the third day of dosing (5 half-lives = 5 · 12 h = 60 h). Tacrolimus concentration should be measured if the patient has signs or symptoms of graft rejection or if the patient has signs or symptoms of tacrolimus toxicity.

7. Answer to problem 7.

Pharmacokinetic Dosing Method

1. *Estimate clearance according to disease states and conditions present in the patient.*

The mean tacrolimus clearance for adult patients is 0.06 L/h per kilogram. The blood clearance of tacrolimus for this patient is expected to be Cl = 0.06 L/h/kg · 67 kg = 4.0 L/h.

2. *Compute the dosage regimen.*

A 12-hour dosage interval is used for this patient. (Note: ng/mL = μg/L, and this concentration was substituted for Css in the calculations to avoid unit conversion. A conversion constant of 1000 μg/mg is used to change the dose amount to milligrams.) The dosage equation for oral tacrolimus is D = (Css · Cl · τ)/F = 15 μg/L · 4.0 L/h · 12 h)/(0.25 · 1000 μg/mg) = 2.9 mg, rounded to 3 mg every 12 hours. Tacrolimus concentration is measured daily, and steady state is expected to occur after about 3 days of therapy (5 half-lives = 5 · 12 h = 60 h).

Literature-Based Recommended Dosing

1. *Choose the tacrolimus dose based on disease states and conditions present in the patient and transplantation type.*

The oral dosage range of tacrolimus for adult patients is 0.1 to 0.3 mg/kg per day. Because the patient has received a kidney transplant, a dose in the lower end of the range (0.1 mg/kg per day) is used to avoid nephrotoxicity. The initial tacrolimus dose for this patient is: Dose = 0.1 mg/kg/d · 67 kg = 6.7 mg/d, rounded to 6 mg/d, or 3 mg every 12 hours. Tacrolimus concentration is measured daily, and steady state is expected to occur after 3 days (5 half-lives = 5 · 12 h = 60 h) of treatment.

8. Answer to problem 8.

Linear Pharmacokinetics Method

1. *Compute the new dose to achieve the desired concentration.*

The patient is expected to achieve steady-state conditions after the third day (5 half-lives = 5 · 12 h = 60 h) of therapy. According to linear pharmacokinetics, the new dose to attain the desired concentration should be proportional to the old dose that produced the measured concentration (total daily dose = 3 mg/dose · 2 doses/d = 6 mg/d):

$$D_{new} = (Css_{new}/Css_{old})D_{old} = [(15\ ng/mL)/(11\ ng/mL)]\ 6\ mg/d = 8.2\ mg/d, \text{ rounded to } 8\ mg/d$$

The new suggested dose is 8 mg/d, or 4 mg every 12 hours, of tacrolimus capsules to be started at the next scheduled dosing time.

Steady-state minimum tacrolimus concentration should be measured after steady state is attained in 3 to 5 half-lives. Because the drug is expected to have a half-life of 12 hours, steady-state concentration of tacrolimus can be measured any time after the third day of dosing (5 half-lives = 5 · 12 h = 60 h). Tacrolimus concentration should be measured if the patient has signs or symptoms of graft rejection or if the patient has signs or symptoms of tacrolimus toxicity.

Pharmacokinetic Parameter Method

1. *Compute pharmacokinetic parameters.*

The patient is expected to achieve steady-state conditions after the third day (5 half-lives = 5 · 12 h = 60 h) of therapy. Tacrolimus clearance can be computed with steady-state tacrolimus concentration: $Cl = [F(D/\tau)]/Css = [0.25 \cdot (3\ mg/12\ h) \cdot 1000\ \mu g/mg]/(11\ \mu g/L) = 5.7\ L/h$. (Note: μg/L = ng/mL, and this concentration unit was substituted for Css in the calculations to avoid unit conversion.)

2. *Compute the tacrolimus dose.*

Tacrolimus clearance is used to compute the new dose: $D = (Css \cdot Cl \cdot \tau)/F = (15\ \mu g/L \cdot 5.7\ L/h \cdot 12\ h)/(0.25 \cdot 1000\ \mu g/mg) = 4.1\ mg$, rounded to 4 mg every 12 hours.

Steady-state minimum tacrolimus concentration should be measured after steady state is attained in 3 to 5 half-lives. Because the drug is expected to have a half-life of 12 hours, steady-state concentration of tacrolimus can be measured any time after the third day of dosing (5 half-lives = 5 · 12 h = 60 h). Tacrolimus concentration should be measured if the patient has signs or symptoms of graft rejection or if the patient has signs or symptoms of tacrolimus toxicity.

9. Solution to problem 9.

Bayesian Pharmacokinetics Computer Program Method

1. *Enter the patient's demographic, drug dosing, and concentration–time data into the computer program.*

2. *Compute pharmacokinetic parameters for the patient with a Bayesian pharmacokinetics computer program.*

The pharmacokinetic parameters computed with the program are a volume of distribution of 69 L, a half-life of 14 hours, and a clearance of 3.4 L/h.

3. *Compute the dose required to achieve the desired concentration of tacrolimus.*

The one-compartment model infusion and first-order absorption equations used in the program to compute doses indicate that a dose of 4 mg every 12 hours produces a steady-state tacrolimus concentration of 20 μg/mL.

10. Solution to problem 10.

Bayesian Pharmacokinetics Computer Program Method

1. *Enter the patient's demographic, drug dosing, and concentration–time data into the computer program.*

Because the patient is also being treated with phenytoin, an enzyme-induction drug interaction for tacrolimus should be entered into the program at the appropriate place.

2. *Compute pharmacokinetic parameters for the patient with a Bayesian pharmacokinetics computer program.*

The pharmacokinetic parameters computed with the program are a volume of distribution of 60 L, a half-life of 9 hours, and a clearance of 4.5 L/h.

3. *Compute the dose required to achieve the desired tacrolimus concentration.*

The one-compartment model, first-order absorption equations used in the program to compute doses indicate that a dose of 6 mg every 12 hours produces a steady-state tacrolimus concentration of 20 μg/mL.

REFERENCES

1. Johnson HJ, Heim-Duthoy KL, Ptachcinski RJ. Renal transplantation. In: DiPiro JT, Talbert RL, Yee GC, Matzke GR, Wells BG, Posey LM, eds. Pharmacotherapy: a pathophysiologic approach. Stamford, CT: Appleton & Lange, 1999:771–94.
2. Lake KD, Olivari MT. Cardiac transplantation. In: DiPiro JT, Talbert RL, Yee GC, Matzke GR, Wells BG, Posey LM, eds. Pharmacotherapy: a pathophysiologic approach. Stamford, CT: Appleton & Lange, 1999:280–94.
3. Maurer JR. Lung transplantation. In: Fauci AS, Braunwald E, Isselbacher KJ, et al, eds. Principles of internal medicine. New York: McGraw-Hill, 1998:1491–3.
4. Perkins JB, Yee GC. Bone marrow transplantation. In: DiPiro JT, Talbert RL, Yee GC, Matzke GR, Wells BG, Posey LM, eds. Pharmacotherapy: a pathophysiologic approach. Stamford, CT: Appleton & Lange, 1999:2195–220.
5. Somani AZ, Burckart GJ. Liver transplantation. In: DiPiro JT, Talbert RL, Yee GC, Matzke GR, Wells BG, Posey LM, eds. Pharmacotherapy: a pathophysiologic approach. Stamford, CT: Appleton & Lange, 1999:676–85.
6. Diasio RB, LoBuglio AF. Immunomodulators: immunosuppressive agents and immunostimulants. In: Hardman JG, Limbird LE, Molinoff PB, Ruddon RW, Gilman AG, eds. The pharmacological basis of therapeutics. New York: McGraw-Hill, 1996:1291–308.
7. Venkataramanan R, Swaminathan A, Prasad T, et al. Clinical pharmacokinetics of tacrolimus. Clin Pharmacokinet 1995;29:404–30.
8. Jusko WJ, Thomson AW, Fung J, et al. Consensus document: therapeutic monitoring of tacrolimus (FK-506). Ther Drug Monit 1995;17:606–14.

9. D'Ambrosio R, Girzaitis N, Jusko WJ. Multicenter comparison of tacrolimus (FK 506) whole blood concentrations as measured by the Abbott IMX analyzer and enzyme immunoassay with methylene chloride extraction. Ther Drug Monit 1994;16:287–92.
10. Matsunami H, Tada A, Makuuchi M, Lynch SV, Strong RW. New technique for measuring tacrolimus concentrations in blood [letter]. Am J Hosp Pharm 1994;51:123.
11. Winkler M, Christians U, Stoll K, Baumann J, Pichlmayr R. Comparison of different assays for the quantitation of FK 506 levels in blood or plasma. Ther Drug Monit 1994;16:281–6.
12. Jusko WJ, Piekoszewski W, Klintmalm GB, et al. Pharmacokinetics of tacrolimus in liver transplant patients. Clin Pharmacol Ther 1995;57:281–90.
13. Regazzi MB, Rinaldi M, Molinaro M, et al. Clinical pharmacokinetics of tacrolimus in heart transplant recipients. Ther Drug Monit 1999;21:2–7.
14. Floren LC, Bekersky I, Benet LZ, et al. Tacrolimus oral bioavailability doubles with coadministration of ketoconazole. Clin Pharmacol Ther 1997;62:41–9.
15. Hebert MF, Fisher RM, Marsh CL, Dressler D, Bekersky I. Effects of rifampin on tacrolimus pharmacokinetics in healthy volunteers. J Clin Pharmacol 1999;39:91–6.
16. Sattler M, Guengerich FP, Yun CH, Christians U, Sewing KF. Cytochrome P-450 3A enzymes are responsible for biotransformation of FK506 and rapamycin in man and rat. Drug Metab Dispos 1992;20:753–61.
17. Karanam BV, Vincent SH, Newton DJ, Wang RW, Chiu SH. FK 506 metabolism in human liver microsomes: investigation of the involvement of cytochrome P450 isozymes other than CYP3A4 [published correction appears in Drug Metab Dispos 1994;22:979]. Drug Metab Dispos 1994;22:811–4.
18. Iwasaki K, Shiraga T, Nagase K, Hirano K, Nozaki K, Noda K. Pharmacokinetic study of FK 506 in the rat. Transplant Proc 1991;23:2757–9.
19 Venkataramanan R, Jain A, Warty VS, et al. Pharmacokinetics of FK 506 in transplant patients. Transplant Proc 1991;23:2736–40.
20. Gruber SA, Hewitt JM, Sorenson AL, et al. Pharmacokinetics of FK506 after intravenous and oral administration in patients awaiting renal transplantation. J Clin Pharmacol 1994;34: 859–64.
21. Venkataramanan R, Jain A, Warty VW, et al. Pharmacokinetics of FK 506 following oral administration: a comparison of FK 506 and cyclosporine. Transplant Proc 1991;23:931–3.
22. Hansten PD, Horn JR. Drug interactions analysis and management. Vancouver, WA: Applied Therapeutics, 1999:480.
23. Jain AB, Venkataramanan R, Cadoff E, et al. Effect of hepatic dysfunction and T tube clamping on FK 506 pharmacokinetics and trough concentrations. Transplant Proc 1990;22:57–9.
24. Kobayashi M, Tamura K, Katayama N, et al. FK 506 assay past and present: characteristics of FK 506 ELISA. Transplant Proc 1991;23:2725–9.
25. Kay JE, Sampare-Kwateng E, Geraghty F, Morgan GY. Uptake of FK 506 by lymphocytes and erythrocytes. Transplant Proc 1991;23:2760–2.
26. Piekoszewski W, Jusko WJ. Plasma protein binding of tacrolimus in humans. J Pharm Sci 1993;82:340–1.
27. Nagase K, Iwasaki K, Nozaki K, Noda K. Distribution and protein binding of FK506, a potent immunosuppressive macrolide lactone, in human blood and its uptake by erythrocytes. J Pharm Pharmacol 1994;46:113–7.
28. Winkler M, Ringe B, Rodeck B, et al. The use of plasma levels for FK 506 dosing in liver-grafted patients. Transpl Int 1994;7:329–33.
29. Jain AB, Abu-Elmagd K, Abdallah H, et al. Pharmacokinetics of FK506 in liver transplant recipients after continuous intravenous infusion [see comments]. J Clin Pharmacol 1993;33: 606–11.

30. Bennett WM. Guide to drug dosage in renal failure. Clin Pharmacokinet 1988;15:326–54.
31. Swan SK, Bennett WM. Drug dosing guidelines in patients with renal failure. West J Med 1992;156:633–8.
32. Bekersky I, Dressler D, Mekki QA. Dose linearity after oral administration of tacrolimus 1-mg capsules at doses of 3, 7, and 10 mg. Clin Ther 1999;21:2058–64.
33. Wandell M, Mungall D. Computer assisted drug interpretation and drug regimen optimization. Am Assoc Clin Chem 1984;6:1–11.

Part VI

OTHER DRUGS

17

LITHIUM

INTRODUCTION

Lithium is an alkali metal administered as a monovalent cation (Li^+) in the management of bipolar disorder. In the United States, orally administered carbonate and citrate salts of lithium are available. Although lithium is still used as primary therapy for bipolar disorder, its use as the primary agent is being challenged by valproic acid and carbamazepine for some forms of the disease.[1] Although this drug has been used in psychiatric medicine since the 1940s, the mechanism of action of lithium is largely unknown. Among the current theories are competition with other cations at receptor and tissue sites, dopamine-receptor supersensitivity blockage, decreased stimulation of β-receptor–induced adenylate cyclase, and enhanced sensitivity to serotonin (5-HT), acetylcholine, and γ-aminobutyric acid (GABA).[1,2]

THERAPEUTIC AND TOXIC CONCENTRATIONS

The general therapeutic range of lithium is 0.6 to 1.5 mmol/L. Because lithium is a monovalent cation, the therapeutic range expressed in milliequivalents per liter is identical to these values (i.e., 0.6 to 1.5 mEq/L). However, most clinicians apply different therapeutic concentration ranges depending on the clinical situation.[3] For patients with acute mania, a minimum lithium concentration of 0.8 mmol/L usually is recommended. The usual desired range for these patients is 0.8 to 1 mmol/L. If patients with acute mania do not respond to these levels, it occasionally is necessary to use a lithium concentration of 1 to 1.2 mmol/L. In some instances, a concentration as high as 1.2 to 1.5 mmol/L is needed. For long-term maintenance, the usual desired range is 0.6 to 0.8 mmol/L. If patients do not respond to these levels during maintenance treatment, occasional use of a lithium concentration of 0.9 to 1 mmol/L is required. In some cases, a concentration as high as 1 to 1.2 mmol/L is necessary for an adequate outcome.

The therapeutic ranges are based on steady-state lithium serum concentration measured 12 hours after a dose. Adoption of a standardized 12-hour postdose lithium concentration to assess dose and response has been paramount in establishing the aforementioned therapeutic ranges of the agent.[4] After oral administration, lithium concentration follows a complex concentration–time curve that is best described with a multicompartment model (Figure 17-1).[4–8] The time needed for distribution between serum and tissues varies greatly among patients, so using a uniform time to determine steady-state serum concentration is important. When monitoring of serum concentration of lithium is anticipated, the patient needs to understand that it is important to take the medication as instructed for 2 to 3 days before the blood sample is obtained, to have the blood sample withdrawn 12 ± 0.5 hours after the last dose, and to report any discrepancies in compliance and blood sampling time to the care provider.

Short-term side effects that occur when lithium therapy is begun or after a dosage increase include muscle weakness, lethargy, polydipsia, polyuria, nocturia, headache, impairment of memory or concentration, confusion, impaired fine motor performance, and hand tremors.[1,2,9] Many of these adverse effects diminish with continued dosing of lithium. However, intervention may be needed for the tremor, including a shorter dosage interval with the same total daily dose to decrease peak lithium concentration, a decreased lithium dose, or concurrent treatment with a β-blocker. Long-term adverse effects include drug-induced diabetes insipidus, renal toxicity (glomerulosclerosis, renal tubular atrophy, interstitial nephritis, urinary casts), hypothyroidism with or without goiter formation, electrocardiographic abnormalities, leukocytosis, weight gain, and dermatologic changes.[1,2,9]

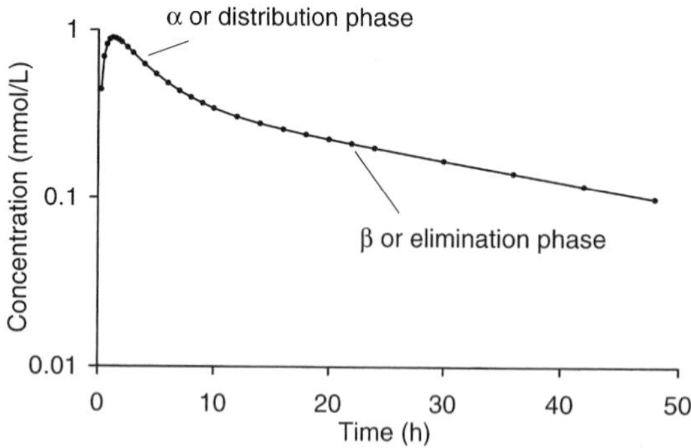

FIGURE 17-1 Lithium ion serum concentration–time curve after a single 900-mg oral dose of lithium carbonate (24.4 mmol or mEq of lithium ion) rapid-release capsules. Maximum serum concentration occurs 2 to 3 hours after the dose is given. After peak concentration is achieved, the distribution phase lasts 6 to 10 hours and is followed by the elimination phase. Among patients with good renal function (creatinine clearance, >80 mL/min), the average elimination half-life of lithium is 24 hours. Because of the long distribution phase, the serum concentration of lithium used for dosage adjustment should be measured no sooner than 12 hours after administration.

At lithium serum concentrations within the upper end of the therapeutic range (1.2 to 1.5 mmol/L), the following adverse effects can occur: decreased memory and concentration, drowsiness, fine hand tremor, weakness, lack of coordination, nausea, diarrhea, vomiting, or fatigue.[1,2,9] At concentrations slightly above the therapeutic range (1.5 to 3 mmol/L), confusion, giddiness, agitation, slurred speech, lethargy, blackouts, ataxia, nystagmus, blurred vision, tinnitus, vertigo, hyperreflexia, hypertonia, dysarthia, coarse hand tremors, and muscle fasciculations can occur. If concentrations exceed 3 mmol/L, severe toxicity occurs with choreoathetosis, seizures, irreversible brain damage, arrhythmia, hypotension, respiratory and cardiovascular complications, stupor, coma, and death. At toxic concentrations, lithium can cause a nonspecific decrease in glomerular filtration, which decreases lithium clearance. The decrease in lithium clearance further increases lithium serum concentration. This phenomenon can cause a viscious circle of decreased clearance leading to increased lithium serum concentration, which leads to additional decreases in lithium clearance. Because of this and the severe toxic side effects, lithium concentrations above 3.5 to 4 mmol/L may necessitate hemodialysis to remove the drug as quickly as possible.[1,9]

CLINICAL MONITORING PARAMETERS

The signs and symptoms of bipolar disease include those of depression (depressed affect, sad mood, decreased interest and pleasure in normal activities, decreased appetite and weight loss, insomnia or hypersomnia, psychomotor retardation or agitation, decreased energy or fatigue, feelings of worthlessness or guilt, impaired decision making and concentration, and suicidal ideation or attempts) and of mania (abnormal and persistently elevated mood, grandiosity, decreased need for sleep, pressure of speech, flight of ideas, distractibility with poor attention span, increased activity or agitation, and excessive involvement in high-risk activities).[1] Generally, onset of action for lithium is 1 to 2 weeks, and a 4- to 6-week treatment period is required to assess complete therapeutic response to the drug.[1,9]

Before beginning lithium therapy, patients should undergo a complete physical examination, general serum chemistry panel (including serum electrolytes and serum creatinine), complete blood cell count with differential, thyroid function tests, urinalysis (including osmolality and specific gravity), and urine toxicologic screen for substances of abuse. For patients with renal dysfunction or baseline cardiac disease, additional testing (measured 24-hour creatinine clearance or electrocardiogram, respectively) is recommended. Clinicians should consider ordering a pregnancy test for women of child-bearing age. Follow-up testing in the following areas should be conducted every 6 to 12 months: serum electrolytes, serum creatinine (measured 24-hour creatinine clearance in patients with renal dysfunction), thyroid function tests, and complete blood cell count with differential. If urine output exceeds 3 L/d, urinalysis with osmolality and specific gravity should be measured.

Serum concentration of lithium should be measured for every patient receiving the drug. Dosage schedules should be arranged so that serum samples for lithium measurement are obtained 12 ± 0.5 hours after a dose.[4] This usually necessitates administration of the drug every 12 hours for dosing twice a day. For dosing three times a day, it is necessary to administer the drug so that there is a 12-hour period overnight. Examples of two common dosage schemes are 0900 H, 1500 H, and 2100 H and 0800 H, 1400 H, and 2000 H. The choice should be individualized according to the patient's lifestyle. At initiation of therapy, serum concentration can be measured every 2 to 3 days for safety reasons for patients who are predisposed to lithium toxicity, even though steady state has not been achieved. Once the desired steady-state lithium concentration has been achieved, lithium concentration should be measured every 1 to 2 weeks for approximately 2 months or until the concentration has stabilized. Because patients with acute mania can have increased lithium clearance, lithium concentration should be measured again for these patients once the manic episode is over and clearance returns to normal. Otherwise, lithium concentrations can accumulate to toxic levels owing to the decrease in lithium clearance. During lithium maintenance therapy, steady-state serum concentration of lithium should be repeated every 3 to 6 months. This period should be altered to every 6 to 12 months for patients whose mood is stable or every 1 to 2 months for patients with frequent mood alterations. If alterations of lithium dosage are needed or if therapy with another drug known to interact with lithium is added, serum concentration of lithium should be measured within 1 to 2 weeks after the change.

BASIC CLINICAL PHARMACOKINETIC PARAMETERS

Lithium is eliminated almost completely (>95%) unchanged in the urine.[8] The ion is filtered freely at the glomerulus, and 60% to 80% of the amount filtered is reabsorbed by the proximal tubule of the nephron. Lithium eliminated in the saliva, sweat, and feces accounts for less than 5% of the administered dose.[9] On average, lithium clearance is approximately 20% of the patient's creatinine clearance.[9–11] Lithium is administered orally as carbonate or citrate salts. Lithium carbonate capsules (150, 300, 600 mg) and tablets (rapid-release, 300 mg; sustained-release, 300 and 450 mg) are available. There are 8.12 mmol (8.12 mEq) of lithium in 300 mg of lithium carbonate. Lithium citrate syrup (8 mmol or mEq/5 mL) is another oral dosage form. Oral bioavailability is good for all lithium salts and dosage forms and is 100%.[12,13] The peak lithium concentration occurs 15 to 30 minutes after a dose of lithium citrate syrup, 1 to 3 hours after a dose of rapid-release lithium carbonate tablets or capsules, and 4 to 8 hours after a dose of sustained-release lithium carbonate tablets. Lithium ion is not plasma protein bound. The typical dose of lithium carbonate is 900 to 2400 mg/d for adults with normal renal function.

EFFECTS OF DISEASES AND CONDITIONS ON LITHIUM PHARMACOKINETICS

Adults with normal renal function (creatinine clearance >80 mL/min) have an average elimination half-life of lithium of 24 hours, volume of distribution of 0.9 L/kg, and clearance of 20 mL/min for lithium.[4–8] During an acute manic phase, lithium clearance can increase as much as 50%, which produces a half-life about half the normal value.[14] Among children 9 to 12 years of age, average elimination half-life of the ion is 18 hours, volume of distribution is 0.9 L/kg, and clearance is 40 mL/min.[15] Because glomerular filtration and creatinine clearance decrease with age, lithium clearance can decrease among elderly patients; the half-life can be as long as 36 hours.[10,11] Because of the circadian rhythm of glomerular filtration, lithium clearance is about 30% higher during the day.[16]

Because lithium is eliminated almost exclusively by the kidney, renal dysfunction is the most important disorder that affects lithium pharmacokinetics. The clearance rate of lithium decreases in proportion to creatinine clearance. In adults, the ratio of lithium clearance to creatinine clearance is 20%, but during a manic phase it increases to about 30%.[10,11,14] This relation between renal function and lithium clearance forms the basis for initial dosage computation. Because of the decrease in clearance, the average half-life of lithium is 40 to 50 hours among patients with renal failure.

Renal clearance of lithium is influenced by the state of sodium balance and fluid hydration. Lithium is reabsorbed in the proximal tubule of the nephron through the same mechanisms that maintain sodium balance.[4] When a patient is in negative sodium balance, the kidney increases sodium reabsorption as a compensatory maneuver, and lithium reabsorption increases. The kidney also increases sodium reabsorption when a patient becomes dehydrated, and lithium reabsorption increases secondary to this alteration. In both cases, increased lithium reabsorption leads to decreased lithium clearance. Common causes of sodium depletion and/or dehydration include sodium-restricted diets for the management of other conditions; vomiting, diarrhea, or fever that might be due to viral or other illnesses; heavy or intense exercise; excessive sweating; use of saunas or hot tubs; and hot weather. Overuse of coffee, tea, soft drinks, or other caffeine-containing liquids and ethanol should be avoided by patients taking lithium. Patients should be advised to maintain adequate fluid intake at all times (2.5 to 3 L/d) and to increase fluid intake as needed.[1]

During periods of acute mania, lithium clearance can be increased as much as 50%.[14] Lithium is generally not used in the first trimester of pregnancy because of the risk of teratogenic effects on the fetus.[1,9] Because of increased glomerular filtration, lithium clearance may be higher in pregnant women, especially during the third trimester. Lithium crosses the placenta, and the concentration in human milk is 30% to 100% that of concurrent serum concentration.[17] Lithium is removed from the body during hemodialysis, peritoneal dialysis, and arteriovenous hemodiafiltration; the clearance values are 30 to 50 mL/min, 13 to 15 mL/min, and 21 mL/min, respectively.[9,18,19]

DRUG INTERACTIONS

Many diuretics have drug interactions with lithium.[20] Thiazide diuretics cause sodium and water depletion, which leads to increased sodium reabsorption in the proximal tubule of the kidney as a compensatory mechanism. Because lithium is reabsorbed by the same mechanisms as sodium, lithium reabsorption increases and lithium clearance decreases 40% to 50% during treatment with thiazide diuretics. Other diuretics, such as chlorthalidone and metolazone, that work at the site of the distal tubule of the kidney may cause a similar interaction with lithium. Although there are case reports of loop diuretics causing a similar interaction, there are also reports of no drug interaction between lithium and these agents. Because of this, many clinicians who treat patients taking lithium favor use of a loop diuretic with careful monitoring of adverse effects and lithium serum concentrations. Amiloride has also been reported to have minimal effects on lithium clearance.

Nonsteroidal antiinflammatory agents (NSAIDs) decrease lithium clearance and increase lithium concentration. The probable mechanism is an NSAID-induced decrease in renal blood flow due to inhibition of prostaglandins. Of these agents, sulindac and aspirin appear to have little or no drug interaction with lithium. Angiotensin-converting enzyme (ACE) inhibitors and angiotensin receptor blockers have been reported to inhibit elimination of lithium by an undefined mechanism. Of the two classes of drugs, more documentation exists for ACE inhibitors, in the presence of which serum concentration of lithium can increase as much as 200% to 300% from pretreatment level.

Some serotonin-specific reuptake inhibitors (SSRIs) have been reported to cause serotonergic hyperarousal syndrome when taken in conjunction with lithium. Case reports of this problem are available for fluoxetine, sertraline, and fluvoxamine. In addition to elevated lithium concentration, patients can have stiffness of the arms and legs, coarse tremors, dizziness, ataxia, dysarthria, and seizures when taking these SSRIs with lithium. Although there are also literature reports of these combinations used safely, caution should be exercised when concurrent treatment with SSRIs and lithium is indicated.

Theophylline increases the ratio of lithium clearance to creatinine clearance as much as 58%, resulting in an average decrease of 21% in steady-state lithium concentration. A rare but severe drug interaction between lithium and antipsychotic drugs has been reported in which patients are more susceptible to the development of extrapyramidal symptoms or irreversible brain damage. Although there are reports of the successful use of antipsychotic agents and lithium together, patients who need this combination therapy should be closely observed for adverse drug reactions.

INITIAL DOSAGE DETERMINATION METHODS

Pharmacokinetic Dosing Method

The goal of initial dosing of lithium is to compute the best dose possible for the patient, given the diseases and conditions that influence lithium pharmacokinetics and the type and severity of the bipolar disease. To do this, pharmacokinetic parameters for the patient are estimated with average parameters measured for other patients with similar diseases and conditions.

ESTIMATE OF CLEARANCE

Lithium ion is almost totally eliminated unchanged in the urine, and there is a consistent relation between lithium clearance and creatinine clearance with a ratio of 20% between the two (lithium clearance to creatinine clearance).[9–11] This relation allows estimation of lithium clearance for a patient, and the estimate can be used to compute an initial dose of the drug. The equation for the straight line shown in Figure 17-2 is Cl = 0.2(CrCl), where Cl is lithium clearance in milliliters per minute and CrCl is creatinine clearance in milliliters per minute. For dosing purposes, it is more useful to have lithium clearance expressed in liters per day. The equation converted to this unit is Cl = 0.288(CrCl), where Cl is lithium clearance in liters per day and CrCl is creatinine clearance in milliliters per minute. If a patient has acute mania, lithium clearance increases about 50%. The corresponding equation is Cl = 0.432(CrCl), where Cl is lithium clearance in liters per day and CrCl is creatinine clearance in millilters per minute.[14]

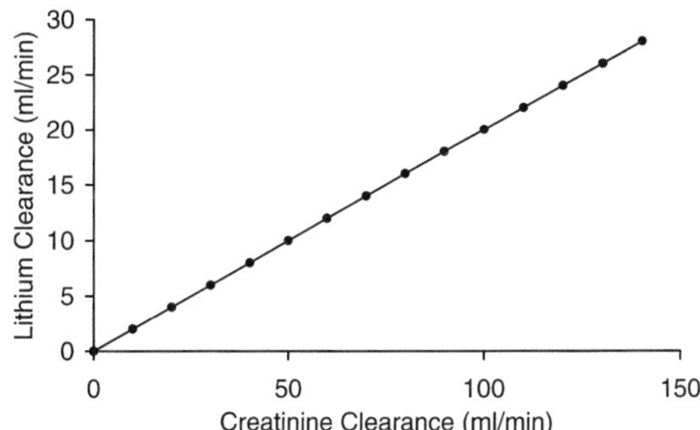

FIGURE 17-2 The ratio between lithium clearance and creatinine clearance is 0.2 for patients who need maintenance therapy with lithium. This relation is used to estimate lithium clearance for patients who need initial dosing with the drug.

SELECTION OF APPROPRIATE PHARMACOKINETIC MODEL AND EQUATION

When given orally, lithium follows a two-compartment model (see Figure 17-1).[4–8] After peak concentration is achieved, serum concentration decreases rapidly because of distribution of drug from blood to tissues (α or distribution phase). Six to 10 hours after administration, lithium concentration declines more slowly. The elimination rate constant for this segment of the concentration–time curve is the one that varies with renal function (β or elimination phase). Although this model is the most correct from a strict pharmacokinetic viewpoint, it cannot easily be used clinically because of the mathematical complexity. During the elimination phase of the concentration-time curve, lithium serum concentration decreases slowly because of the long elimination half-life (24 hours with normal renal function, as long as 50 hours with end-stage renal disease). A simple pharmacokinetic equation for computing average steady-state serum concentration of lithium (Css in mmol/L = mEq/L) is widely used and allows calculation of a maintenance dose: $Css = [F(D/\tau)]/Cl$, or $D/\tau = (Css \cdot Cl)/F$, where F is the bioavailability fraction for the oral dosage form (F = 1 for oral lithium), D is the lithium dose in millimoles, τ is the dosage interval in days, and Cl is lithium clearance in liters per day. Because this equation is used to compute lithium ion requirement and because lithium carbonate doses are prescribed in milligrams, the ratio of lithium ion content to lithium carbonate salt (8.12 mmol Li^+ per 300 mg lithium carbonate) is used to convert the result from this equation into a lithium carbonate dose. Total daily amounts of lithium usually are given as almost equally divided doses twice or three times a day. Single doses greater than 1200 mg/d of lithium carbonate usually are not given to avoid gastrointestinal upset.

SELECTION OF STEADY-STATE CONCENTRATION

Serum concentration of lithium is based on the presence or absence of acute mania, and the drug is titrated to response.[3] For persons with acute mania, a minimum lithium concentration of 0.8 mmol/L usually is recommended. The usual desired range for these patients is 0.8 to 1 mmol/L. If patients with acute mania do not respond to these levels, it may be necessary to use lithium concentrations of 1 to 1.2 mmol/L and in some instances concentrations as high as 1.2 to 1.5 mmol/L. For long-term maintenance, the usual desired range is 0.6 to 0.8 mmol/L. If patients do not respond to these levels during maintenance treatment, occasional use of a lithium concentration of 0.9 to 1 mmol/L is needed. In some cases, a concentration as high as 1 to 1.2 mmol/L is necessary to gain an adequate outcome.

Example 1 MJ is a 50-year-old, 70-kg (height, 178 cm) man who has bipolar disease. He is not currently experiencing acute mania. Serum creatinine level is 0.9 mg/dL. Compute an oral lithium dose for maintenance therapy.

1. *Estimate creatinine clearance.*

This patient has a stable serum creatinine level and is not obese. The Cockcroft-Gault equation can be used to estimate creatinine clearance, where BW is body weight and S_{Cr} is serum creatinine level:

$$CrCl_{est} = [(140 - age)BW]/(72 \cdot S_{Cr}) = [(140 - 50\ y)70\ kg]/(72 \cdot 0.9\ mg/dL)$$

$$CrCl_{est} = 97\ mL/min$$

2. *Estimate clearance.*

The drug clearance versus creatinine clearance relation is used to estimate lithium clearance for this patient:

$$Cl = 0.288(CrCl) = 0.288(97\ mL/min) = 27.9\ L/d$$

3. *Use the average steady-state concentration equation to compute a maintenance dose of lithium.*

For a patient who needs maintenance therapy for bipolar disease, the desired lithium concentration is 0.6 to 0.8 mmol/L. A serum concentration of 0.6 mmol/L is chosen for this patient, and oral lithium carbonate is used ($F = 1$, 8.12 mmol Li^+ per 300 mg of lithium carbonate).

$$D/\tau = (Css \cdot Cl)/F = [(0.6\ mmol/L) \cdot (27.9\ L/d)]/1 = 16.7\ mmol/d$$

D/τ = (300 mg lithium carbonate/8.12 mmol Li^+) 16.7 mmol/d = 617 mg/d, rounded to 600 mg/d of lithium carbonate. This dose is given as 300 mg of lithium carbonate every 12 hours. Upon initiation of therapy, serum concentration can be measured every 2 to 3 days for safety in the care of patients predisposed to lithium toxicity, even though steady state has not yet been achieved. Once the desired steady-state lithium concentration has been achieved, lithium concentration should be measured every 1 to 2 weeks for approximately 2 months or until concentration has stabilized.

Example 2 The patient in example 1 has a serum creatinine level of 3.5 mg/dL, which indicates renal impairment.

1. *Estimate creatinine clearance.*

This patient has a stable serum creatinine level and is not obese. The Cockcroft-Gault equation can be used to estimate creatinine clearance:

$$CrCl_{est} = [(140 - age)BW]/(72 \cdot S_{Cr}) = [(140 - 50\ y)70\ kg]/(72 \cdot 3.5\ mg/dL)$$

$$CrCl_{est} = 25\ mL/min$$

2. *Estimate clearance.*

The drug clearance versus creatinine clearance relation is used to estimate lithium clearance for this patient:

$$Cl = 0.288(CrCl) = 0.288(25\ mL/min) = 7.2\ L/d$$

3. *Use the average steady-state concentration equation to compute a maintenance dose of lithium.*

For a patient who needs maintenance therapy for bipolar disease, the desired lithium concentration is 0.6 to 0.8 mmol/L. A serum concentration of 0.6 mmol/L is chosen for this patient, and oral lithium carbonate is used (F = 1, 8.12 mmol/Li^+ per 300 mg of lithium carbonate).

$$D/\tau = (Css \cdot Cl)/F = [(0.6\ mmol/L) \cdot (7.2\ L/d)]/1 = 4.3\ mmol/d$$

D/τ = (300 mg lithium carbonate/8.12 mmol Li^+) 4.3 mmol/d = 159 mg/d, rounded to 150 mg/d of lithium carbonate. This dose is given as 150 mg of lithium carbonate daily.

Upon initiation of therapy, serum concentration can be measured every 2 to 3 days for safety in the care of patients predisposed to lithium toxicity, even though steady state has not yet been achieved. Once the desired steady-state lithium concentration has been achieved, lithium concentration should be measured every 1 to 2 weeks for approximately 2 months or until concentration has stabilized.

Example 3 The patient in example 1 has a serum creatinine level of 0.9 mg/dL and is being treated for acute mania. Compute an oral lithium carbonate dose for this patient.

1. *Estimate creatinine clearance.*

This patient has a stable serum creatinine level and is not obese. The Cockcroft-Gault equation can be used to estimate creatinine clearance:

$$CrCl_{est} = [(140 - age)BW]/(72 \cdot S_{Cr}) = [(140 - 50\ y)70\ kg]/(72 \cdot 0.9\ mg/dL)$$

$$CrCl_{est} = 97\ mL/min$$

2. *Estimate clearance.*

The drug clearance versus creatinine clearance relation is used to estimate lithium clearance for this patient:

$$Cl = 0.432\ (CrCl) = 0.432\ (97\ mL/min) = 41.9\ L/d$$

3. *Use the average steady-state concentration equation to compute a maintenance dose of lithium.*

For a patient who needs therapy for the acute manic phase of bipolar disease, the desired lithium concentration is 0.8 mmol/L. Oral lithium carbonate is used (F = 1, 8.12 mmol Li^+ per 300 mg of lithium carbonate).

$$D/\tau = (Css \cdot Cl)/F = [(0.8\ mmol/L) \cdot (41.9\ L/d)]/1 = 33.5\ mmol/d$$

D/τ = (300 mg lithium carbonate/8.12 mmol Li^+) 33.5 mmol/d = 1238 mg/d, rounded to 1200 mg/d of lithium carbonate. This dose is given as 600 mg of lithium carbonate every 12 hours.

Upon initiation of therapy, serum concentration can be measured every 2 to 3 days for safety in the care of patients predisposed to lithium toxicity, even though steady state has not yet been achieved. Once the desired steady-state lithium concentration has been achieved, lithium concentration should be measured every 1 to 2 weeks for approximately 2 months or until concentration has stabilized. Because patients with acute mania can have increased lithium clearance, lithium concentration should be measured when the manic episode is over and clearance returns to normal.

Literature-Based Recommended Dosing

Because of the large variability in the pharmacokinetics of lithium, even when concurrent diseases and conditions are identified, many clinicians believe that use of standard lithium doses for varied situations is warranted. The original computation of these doses was based on the pharmacokinetic dosing method described earlier and modified according to clinical experience. For the management of acute mania, initial doses are usually 900 to 1200 mg/d of lithium carbonate.[1,9] If the drug is being used for prophylaxis of bipolar disease, an initial dose of 600 mg/d lithium carbonate is recommended.[1,9] In both cases, the total daily dose is given in two or three divided doses each day. To avoid adverse side effects, lithium doses are slowly increased 300 to 600 mg/d every 2 to 3 days according to clinical response and serum concentration of lithium. Renal dysfunction is the main condition that alters lithium pharmacokinetics and dosage.[21–24] If creatinine clearance is 10 to 50 mL/min, the prescribed initial dose is 50% to 75% of that recommended for patients with normal renal function. For creatinine clearance values less than 10 mL/min, the prescribed dose should be 25% to 50% of the usual dose in the treatment of patients with good renal function.

Zetin and associates[25,26] developed a multiple regression equation for computing lithium carbonate doses based on hospitalization status, age, sex, and weight of the patient as well as whether the patient is using a tricyclic antidepressant. However, because renal function was not assessed as an independent parameter in the studies, this dosage method is not presented herein.

To illustrate the similarities and differences between the literature-based method of initial dosage calculation and the pharmacokinetic dosing method, the previous examples are used.

Example 4 MJ is a 50-year-old, 70-kg (height, 178 cm) man who has bipolar disease. He is not currently experiencing acute mania. Serum creatinine is 0.9 mg/dL. Recommend an oral lithium dose for maintenance therapy.

1. *Estimate creatinine clearance.*

This patient has a stable serum creatinine level and is not obese. The Cockcroft-Gault equation can be used to estimate creatinine clearance:

$$CrCl_{est} = [(140 - \text{age})BW]/(72 \cdot S_{Cr}) = [(140 - 50\text{ y})70\text{ kg}]/(72 \cdot 0.9\text{ mg/dL})$$

$$CrCl_{est} = 97\text{ mL/min}$$

2. *Choose the lithium dose based on disease states and conditions present in the patient.*

The patient needs prophylactic lithium therapy for bipolar disease and has good renal function. A lithium carbonate dose of 600 mg/d, given as 300 mg every 12 hours, is recommended as the initial amount. The dosage rate is increased 300 to 600 mg/d every 2 to 3 days as needed to provide adequate therapeutic effect, avoid adverse effects, and produce therapeutic steady-state concentration of lithium.

Example 5 The patient in example 4 has a serum creatinine level of 3.5 mg/dL, which indicates renal impairment.

1. *Estimate creatinine clearance.*

This patient has a stable serum creatinine level and is not obese. The Cockcroft-Gault equation can be used to estimate creatinine clearance:

$$CrCl_{est} = [(140 - age)BW]/(72 \cdot S_{Cr}) = [(140 - 50\ y)70\ kg]/(72 \cdot 3.5\ mg/dL)$$

$$CrCl_{est} = 25\ mL/min$$

2. *Choose the lithium dose based on disease states and conditions present in the patient.*

The patient needs prophylactic lithium therapy for bipolar disease and has moderate renal function. With an estimated creatinine clearance of 25 mL/min, lithium carbonate doses should be 50% to 75% of the usual amount. A lithium carbonate dose of 300 mg/d, given as 150 mg every 12 hours, is recommended as the initial amount. The dose is increased 150 to 300 mg/d every 5 to 7 days as needed to provide adequate therapeutic effect, avoid adverse effects, and produce a therapeutic steady-state concentration of lithium.

Example 6 The patient in example 4 has a serum creatinine level of 0.9 mg/dL and is being treated for the acute mania phase of bipolar disease. Compute an oral lithium carbonate dose for this patient.

1. *Estimate creatinine clearance.*

This patient has a stable serum creatinine level and is not obese. The Cockcroft-Gault equation can be used to estimate creatinine clearance:

$$CrCl_{est} = [(140 - age)BW]/(72 \cdot S_{Cr}) = [(140 - 50\ y)70\ kg]/(72 \cdot 0.9\ mg/dL)$$

$$CrCl_{est} = 97\ mL/min$$

2. *Choose the lithium dose based on disease states and conditions present in the patient.*

The patient needs lithium therapy for acute mania and has good renal function. A lithium carbonate dose of 900 mg/d, given as 300 mg at 0800 H, 1400 H, and 2000 H, is recommended as the initial amount. The dosage rate is increased 300 to 600 mg/d every 2 to 3 days as needed to provide adequate therapeutic effect, avoid adverse effects, and produce a therapeutic steady-state concentration of lithium.

Test Dose Methods to Assess Initial Lithium Dosage Requirements

There are several methods for assessing an initial dosage of lithium with one or more test doses and one or more serum concentrations of lithium.

COOPER NOMOGRAM

Use of the Cooper nomogram for assessment of maintenance dose of lithium necessitates administration of a single test dose of 600 mg lithium carbonate and one measurement of serum concentration of lithium 24 hours later.[27,28] The 24-hour serum concentration of lithium is compared with a table that converts the observed concentration into the dose of lithium carbonate required to produce a steady-state lithium concentration of 0.6 to 1.2 mmol/L (Table 17-1). The theoretical basis for this dosage approach lies in the relation between serum concentration of a drug measured about one half-life after dosage and the elimination rate constant for the drug in a particular patient. This nomogram can be expressed as an equation for the total daily lithium dosage requirement (D in mmol/d): $D = e^{(4.80 - 7.5\,C_{test})}$, where C_{test} is the 24-hour postdose lithium concentration for a 600-mg lithium carbonate dose.[9] Perry and associates suggested a similar nomogram with a test dose of 1200 mg lithium carbonate.[29,30] An important requirement for these methods is an accurate lithium assay for measuring lithium concentration after a single dose of the drug. When the lithium carbonate test dose is given, serum concentration of lithium in the patient must be zero.

Example 7 LK is a 47-year-old, 65-kg (height, 165 cm) woman who has bipolar disease. She is not currently experiencing acute mania. Serum creatinine level is 0.9 mg/dL. Use the Cooper nomogram to compute an oral lithium dose for maintenance therapy.

1. *Administer test dose of 600 mg lithium carbonate and measure 24-hour postdose lithium concentration. Use nomogram to recommend a maintenance dose of lithium carbonate.*

TABLE 17-1 Cooper Nomogram for Dosage of Lithium: Lithium Carbonate Dosage Required to Produce Steady-State Lithium Serum Concentration of 0.6 to 1.2 mmol/L*

LITHIUM SERUM CONCENTRATION 24 HOURS AFTER THE TEST DOSE (mmol/L)	LITHIUM CARBONATE DOSAGE REQUIREMENT†
<0.05	1200 mg three times a day (3600 mg/d)‡
0.05–0.09	900 mg three times a day (2700 mg/d)
0.10–0.14	600 mg three times a day (1800 mg/d)
0.15–0.19	300 mg four times a day (1200 mg/d)
0.20–0.23	300 mg three times a day (900 mg/d)
0.24–0.30	300 mg twice a day (600 mg/d)
>0.30	300 mg twice a day (600 mg/d)§

* Lithium dosage requirements should be reassessed with changes in clinical status (mania versus maintenance treatment), renal function, or other factors that alter lithium pharmacokinetics.

† Dosage schedule determined to provide minimum fluctuation in lithium serum concentration and maximum patient compliance. A change in dosage interval can be made by the prescribing clinician, but the total daily dose should remain the same.

‡ Use extreme caution. Patient appears to have an increased clearance and short half-life for lithium, which would require large maintenance doses of lithium carbonate. However, this large of a maintenance dose requires careful patient monitoring for response and adverse side effects.

§ Use extreme caution. Patient appears to have a reduced clearance and long half-life of lithium and may accumulate steady-state lithium concentrations above the therapeutic range.

Adapted from Cooper TB, Bergner PE, Simpson GM. The 24-hour lithium level as a prognosticator of dosage requirements. Am J Psychiatry 1973;130:601–63 and Cooper TB, Simpson GM. The 24-hour lithium level as a prognosticator of dosage requirements: a 2-year follow-up study. Am J Psychiatry 1976;133:440–3.

After the test dose is given, 24-hour lithium concentration is 0.12 mmol/L. The recommended maintenance dose of lithium carbonate is 600 mg three times a day. The doses are given at 0900 H, 1500 H, and 2100 H to allow a 12-hour window after the evening dose for measurement of serum concentration of lithium.

Upon initiation of therapy, serum concentration can be measured every 2 to 3 days for safety in the care of patients predisposed to lithium toxicity, even though steady state has not yet been achieved. Once the desired steady-state lithium concentration has been achieved, lithium concentration should be measured every 1 to 2 weeks for approximately 2 months or until concentration has stabilized. Because patients with acute mania can have increased lithium clearance, lithium concentration should be measured when the manic episode is over and clearance returns to normal.

PERRY METHOD

In this technique, a small pharmacokinetic experiment is conducted after administration of a test dose of lithium carbonate.[31] Twelve and 36 hours after the test dose (600 to 1500 mg) of lithium carbonate is administered, serum concentration of lithium is measured. The two lithium concentrations are used to compute the elimination rate constant for the patient: $k = [(\ln C_{12\text{ h}}) - (\ln C_{36\text{ h}})]/\Delta t$, where k is the elimination rate constant in h^{-1} for lithium, $C_{12\text{ h}}$ and $C_{36\text{ h}}$ are the lithium concentrations in mmol/L (or mEq/L) 12 hours and 36 hours after the test dose is given, and Δt is the difference between times (24 h) that the two serum concentrations were measured. When the elimination rate constant (k) is known, the accumulation ratio (R) can be computed for any dosage interval: $R = 1/(1 - e^{-k\tau})$, where τ is the dosage interval in hours. The accumulation ratio (R) also is the ratio of concentration at any time, *t,* after a single dose ($C_{SD,t}$ in mmol/L) and the steady-state concentration at that same time after the dose during multiple dosing (Css_t in mmol/L): $R = Css_t/C_{SD,t}$, or $Css_t = R \cdot C_{SD,t}$. Once a steady-state concentration can be computed for a dosage regimen, linear pharmacokinetic principles can be used to compute the dose required to achieve a target steady-state serum concentration of lithium: $D_{new} = (Css_{new}/Css_{old})D_{old}$, where D is the dose, Css is the steady-state concentration, old indicates the dose that produced the steady-state concentration that the patient is currently receiving, and new denotes the dose necessary to produce the desired steady-state concentration. As with the Cooper nomogram, the serum concentration of lithium must be zero before the test dose is administered.

Example 8 HG is a 32-year-old, 58-kg (height, 155 cm) woman who has bipolar disease. She is not currently experiencing acute mania. Serum creatinine level is 0.9 mg/dL. A single test dose of lithium (1200 mg) is given to the patient. Lithium concentration is 0.6 mmol/L 12 hours and 0.3 mmol/L 36 hours after the drug is given. Use the Perry method to compute an oral lithium dose for this patient to produce a steady-state serum concentration of 0.8 mmol/L.

1. *Administer test dose of lithium carbonate and measure 12- and 36-hour postdose lithium concentrations. Compute the lithium elimination rate constant and accumulation ratio for the patient.*

The lithium elimination rate constant is computed with the two serum concentrations: $k = [(\ln C_{12\text{ h}}) - (\ln C_{36\text{ h}})]/\Delta t = [\ln (0.6\text{ mmol/L}) - \ln (0.3\text{ mmol/L})]/24\text{ h} = 0.0289\text{ h}^{-1}$.

The lithium accumulation ratio is computed with the elimination rate constant and desired lithium dosage interval of 12 hours: $R = 1/(1 - e^{-k\tau}) = 1/(1 - e^{-(0.0289\ h^{-1})(12\ h)}) = 3.4$.

2. *Compute the estimated lithium concentration at steady state for the test dose. Use this relation to compute the dosage regimen for the patient.*

With the lithium concentration obtained at 12 hours, the steady-state concentration of lithium for 1200 mg every 12 hours can be computed: $Css_t = R \cdot C_{SD,t} = 3.4 \cdot 0.6$ mmol/L = 2.0 mmol/L. Linear pharmacokinetic principles can be used to compute the dose required to achieve the target steady-state serum concentration of lithium: D_{new} = [(0.8 mmol/L)/(2 mmol/L)] 1200 mg = 480 mg, rounded to 450 mg every 12 hours, of lithium carbonate.

Upon initiation of therapy, serum concentration can be measured every 2 to 3 days for safety in the care of patients predisposed to lithium toxicity, even though steady state has not yet been achieved. Once the desired steady-state lithium concentration has been achieved, lithium concentration should be measured every 1 to 2 weeks for approximately 2 months or until concentration has stabilized. Because patients with acute mania can have increased lithium clearance, lithium concentration should be measured when the manic episode is over and clearance returns to normal.

REPEATED ONE-POINT OR RITSCHEL METHOD

The method to individualize lithium dose proposed by Ritschel and associates is another way to compute the elimination rate constant for a patient.[32,33] In this case, two equal lithium doses are administered apart from each other by the desired dosage interval (usually 12 hours). Serum concentration is measured before the second test dose is given and again after the second dose is given at a time equaling the anticipated dosage interval. These values are used to compute the elimination rate constant (k in h^{-1}) for the patient: $k = \{\ln [C_1/(C_2 - C_1)]\}/\tau$, where C_1 is the lithium concentration in millimoles per liter obtained after the first test dose, C_2 is the lithium concentration in millimoles per liter obtained after the second test dose, and τ is the expected dosage interval in hours for lithium dosing and also is the postdose time at which the lithium concentrations are obtained.

With knowledge of the elimination rate constant (k), the accumulation ratio (R) can be computed for the dosage interval: $R = 1/(1 - e^{-k\tau})$, where τ is the dosage interval in hours. The accumulation ratio (R) also is the ratio of the concentration at any time, *t*, after a single dose ($C_{SD,t}$ in mmol/L) and the steady-state concentration at that same time after the dose is administered as multiple doses (Css_t in mmol/L): $R = Css_t/C_{SD,t}$, or $Css_t = R \cdot C_{SD,t}$. Once a steady-state concentration can be computed for a dosage regimen, linear pharmacokinetic principles can be used to compute the dose required to achieve a target steady-state serum concentration of lithium: $D_{new} = (Css_{new}/Css_{old})D_{old}$, where D is the dose, Css is the steady-state concentration, old indicates the dose that produced the steady-state concentration that the patient is currently receiving, and new denotes the dose necessary to produce the desired steady-state concentration. As with the Cooper and Perry methods, serum concentration of lithium must be zero before the test dose is administered.

Example 9 CB is a 27-year-old, 75-kg (height, 188 cm) man who has bipolar disease. He is currently experiencing acute mania. Serum creatinine is 1.0 mg/dL. Two test doses of lithium (600 mg each, 12 hours apart) are given to the patient. Lithium concentration is 0.3 mmol/L 12 hours after the first dose and 0.5 mmol/L 12 hours after the second dose. Use the Ritschel repeated one-point method to compute an oral lithium dose for this patient to produce a steady-state serum concentration of 1.2 mmol/L.

1. *Administer test dose of lithium carbonate and measure lithium concentration. Compute the lithium elimination rate constant and accumulation ratio for the patient.*

The lithium elimination rate constant is computed with the two serum concentrations: $k = \{\ln [C_1/(C_2 - C_1)]\}/\tau = \ln [(0.3 \text{ mmol/L})/(0.5 \text{ mmol/L} - 0.3 \text{ mmol/L})]/12 \text{ h} = 0.0338 \text{ h}^{-1}$. The lithium accumulation ratio is computed with the elimination rate constant and desired lithium dosage interval of 12 hours: $R = 1/(1 - e^{-k\tau}) = 1/(1 - e^{-(0.0338 \text{ h}^{-1})(12 \text{ h})}) = 3.0$.

2. *Compute the estimated lithium concentration at steady state for the test dose. Use this relation to compute the dosage regimen for the patient.*

With the lithium concentration obtained at 12 hours, the steady-state lithium concentration for 600 mg every 12 hours can be computed: $Css_t = R \cdot C_{SD,t} = 3.0 \cdot 0.3 \text{ mmol/L} = 0.9 \text{ mmol/L}$. Linear pharmacokinetic principles can be used to compute the dose required to achieve the target steady-state serum concentration of lithium: $D_{new} = [(1.2 \text{ mmol/L})/(0.9 \text{ mmol/L})]\ 600 \text{ mg} = 800 \text{ mg}$, rounded to 900 mg every 12 hours, of lithium carbonate.

Upon initiation of therapy, serum concentration can be measured every 2 to 3 days for safety in the care of patients predisposed to lithium toxicity, even though steady state has not yet been achieved. Once the desired steady-state lithium concentration has been achieved, lithium concentration should be measured every 1 to 2 weeks for approximately 2 months or until concentration has stabilized. Because patients with acute mania can have increased lithium clearance, lithium concentration should be measured when the manic episode is over and clearance returns to normal.

USE OF LITHIUM SERUM CONCENTRATIONS TO ALTER DOSES

Because of pharmacokinetic variability among patients, it is likely that doses computed with patient population characteristics do not always produce lithium serum concentrations that are expected. Because of this, serum concentration of lithium is measured for all patients to ensure that therapeutic, nontoxic levels are present. Important patient parameters should be followed to confirm that the patient is responding to treatment and not having adverse drug reactions.

When serum concentration of lithium is measured and a dosage change is necessary, clinicians should use the simplest, most straightforward method available to determine a dose that will provide safe and effective treatment. In most cases, a simple dosage ratio can be used to change lithium doses because this drug follows linear pharmacokinetics. Computerized methods that incorporate expected population pharmacokinetic characteristics (Bayesian pharmacokinetics computer programs) can be used when renal function is changing, serum concentration is measured at suboptimal times, or the patient is not at steady state when serum concentration is measured.

Linear Pharmacokinetics Method

Because lithium follows linear, dose-proportional pharmacokinetics, steady-state serum concentration changes in proportion to dose according to the following equation: $D_{new}/Css_{new} = D_{old}/Css_{old}$, or $D_{new} = (Css_{new}/Css_{old})D_{old}$, where D is the dose, Css is the steady-state concentration, old indicates the dose that produced the steady-state concentration that the patient is currently receiving, and new denotes the dose necessary to produce the desired steady-state concentration. The advantages of this method are that it is quick and simple. The principal disadvantage is that steady-state concentration is required.

Example 10 YC is a 37-year-old, 55-kg (height, 155 cm) woman who has bipolar disease. She is currently not experiencing acute mania and needs prophylactic treatment with lithium. Serum creatinine level is 0.6 mg/dL. The patient is receiving 900 mg of lithium carbonate at 0800 H, 1400 H, and 2000 H. Steady-state serum concentration of lithium is 1.1 mmol/L 12 hours after administration of the drug. Compute a new lithium dose to achieve a steady-state concentration of 0.6 mmol/L.

1. *Compute the new dose to achieve the desired serum concentration.*

According to linear pharmacokinetics, the new dose to attain the desired concentration should be proportional to the old dose (2700 mg/d) that produced the measured concentration:

$$D_{new} = (Css_{new}/Css_{old})D_{old} = [(0.6 \text{ mmol/L})/(1.1 \text{ mmol/L})]\ 2700 \text{ mg/d}$$
$$= 1473 \text{ mg/d, rounded to } 1500 \text{ mg/d}$$

The patient is given 600 mg of lithium carbonate at 0800 H and 2000 H and 300 mg of lithium carbonate at 1400 H. When lithium dosage alterations are needed, serum concentration of lithium should be measured within 1 to 2 weeks after the change. During lithium maintenance therapy, steady-state serum concentration of lithium should be measured every 3 to 6 months. This period should be altered to every 6 to 12 months for patients whose mood is stable or every 1 to 2 months for patients with frequent mood alterations.

BAYESIAN PHARMACOKINETICS COMPUTER PROGRAMS

Computer programs can assist in the computation of pharmacokinetic parameters for patients.[14] In the most reliable computer programs, a nonlinear regression algorithm incorporates components of Bayes' theorem. Nonlinear regression is a statistical technique in which an iterative process is used to compute the best pharmacokinetic parameters for a concentration–time data set. The patient's drug dosage schedule and serum concentration values are entered into the computer. The computer program has a pharmacokinetic equation programmed for the drug and administration method, such as oral, intravenous bolus, or intravenous infusion. A one-compartment model typically is used, although some programs allow the user to choose among several different equations. With population estimates based on demographic information for the patient, such as age, weight, sex, and renal function, supplied by the user, the program computes estimated serum concentrations for each time there is an actual serum concentration. Kinetic parameters are changed by the computer program, and a new set of estimated serum concentrations are computed. The pharmacokinetic parameters that generated the estimated serum concentrations closest to the actual values are stored in the computer memory, and the process is repeated until the set of pharmacokinetic parameters that produced estimated serum concentrations statistically closest to the actual serum concentrations is generated. These pharmacokinetic parameters can then be used to compute improved dosing schedules for patients. Bayes' theorem is used in the computer algorithm to balance the results of the computations between values based solely on the patient's serum drug concentrations and those based only on patient population parameters. Results of studies in which various methods of dosage adjustment have been compared have consistently shown that these types of computer dosing programs perform at least as well as experienced clinical pharmacokineticists and clinicians and better than inexperienced clinicians.

Some clinicians use Bayesian pharmacokinetics computer programs exclusively to alter drug doses based on serum concentrations. An advantage of this approach is that consistent dosage recommendations are made when several practitioners are involved in therapeutic drug monitoring programs. However, because simpler dosing methods work just as well for patients with stable pharmacokinetic parameters and steady-state drug concentrations, many clinicians reserve the use of computer programs for more difficult situations. Those situations include serum concentrations that are not at steady state, serum concentrations not obtained at the specific times needed to use simpler methods, and unstable pharmacokinetic parameters. Many Bayesian pharmacokinetics computer programs are available, and most should provide answers similar to the ones used in the examples. The program used to solve problems in this book is DrugCalc, written by Dr. Dennis Mungall, and is available on his Internet web site (http://members.aol.com/thertch/index.htm). For comparison, three cases for other dosage methods are presented as examples of use of a Bayesian pharmacokinetics computer program.

Example 11 YC is a 37-year-old, 55-kg (height, 155 cm) woman who has bipolar disease. She is currently not experiencing acute mania and needs prophylactic treatment with lithium. Serum creatinine level is 0.6 mg/dL. The patient is receiving 900 mg of lithium carbonate at 0800 H, 1400 H, and 2000 H. Steady-state serum concentration of lithium is 1.1 mmol/L. Compute a new lithium dose to achieve a steady-state concentration of 0.6 mmol/L.

1. *Enter the patient's demographic, drug dosing, and serum concentration–time data into the computer program.*

Lithium doses must be entered into DrugCalc as millimoles of lithium ion. 900 mg of lithium carbonate provides 24.4 mmol of lithium ion: 900 mg (8.12 mmol Li^+/300 mg lithium carbonate) = 24.4 mmol Li^+.

2. *Compute pharmacokinetic parameters for the patient with a Bayesian pharmacokinetics computer program.*

The pharmacokinetic parameters computed with the program are a volume of distribution of 38 L, a half-life of 17.9 hours, and a clearance of 1.48 L/h.

3. *Compute the dose required to achieve the desired serum concentration of lithium.*

The one-compartment, first-order absorption equations used in the program to compute doses indicate that a dose of 13 mmol Li^+ every 12 hours produces a steady-state concentration of 0.6 mmol/L. This dose is equivalent to 480 mg of lithium carbonate (13 mmol [300 mg lithium carbonate/8.12 mmol Li^+] = 480 mg lithium carbonate). This amount is rounded to an amount available as an oral dosage form, and 450 mg of lithium carbonate is given every 12 hours.

Example 12 LK is a 47-year-old, 65-kg (height, 165 cm) woman who has bipolar disease. She is not currently experiencing acute mania. Serum creatinine level is 0.9 mg/dL. After the test dose of 600 mg lithium carbonate, 24-hour lithium concentration is 0.12 mmol/L. Compute an oral lithium dose for maintenance therapy that would achieve a steady-state concentration of 0.6 mmol/L.

1. *Enter the patient's demographic, drug dosing, and serum concentration–time data into the computer program.*

Lithium doses must be entered into DrugCalc as millimoles of lithium ion. Six hundred milligrams of lithium carbonate provides 16.2 mmol of lithium ion: 600 mg (8.12 mmol Li^+/300 mg lithium carbonate) = 16.2 mmol Li^+.

2. *Compute pharmacokinetic parameters for the patient with a Bayesian pharmacokinetics computer program.*

The pharmacokinetic parameters computed with the program are a volume of distribution of 77 L, a half-life of 38 hours, and a clearance of 1.42 L/h.

3. *Compute the dose required to achieve the desired serum concentration of lithium.*

The one-compartment, first-order absorption equations used in the program to compute doses indicate that a dose of 10 mmol Li^+ every 8 hours produces a steady-state concentration of 0.8 mmol/L. This dose is equivalent to 369 mg of lithium carbonate (10 mmol [300 mg lithium carbonate/8.12 mmol Li^+] = 369 mg lithium carbonate). This amount is rounded to an amount available as an oral dosage form, and 300 mg of lithium carbonate is given three times a day at 0800 H, 1400 H, and 2000 H to provide a 12-hour window for monitoring of serum concentration after the evening dose.

Example 13 CB is a 27-year-old, 75-kg (height, 188 cm) man who has bipolar disease. He is currently experiencing acute mania. Serum creatinine level is 1.0 mg/dL. Two test doses of lithium (600 mg each) are administered at 0800 H and 2000 H. Lithium concentration is 0.3 mmol/L 12 hours after the first dose and 0.5 mmol/L after the second dose. Compute an oral lithium dose for this patient to produce a steady-state serum concentration of 1.2 mmol/L.

1. *Enter the patient's demographic, drug dosing, and serum concentration–time data into the computer program.*

Lithium doses must be entered into DrugCalc as millimoles of lithium ion. Six hundred milligrams of lithium carbonate provides 16.2 mmol of lithium ion: 600 mg (8.12 mmol Li^+/300 mg lithium carbonate) = 16.2 mmol Li^+.

2. *Compute pharmacokinetic parameters for the patient with a Bayesian pharmacokinetics computer program.*

The pharmacokinetic parameters computed with the program are a volume of distribution of 38 L, a half-life of 19.2 hours, and a clearance of 1.37 L/h.

3. *Compute the dose required to achieve the desired serum concentration of lithium.*

The one-compartment, first-order absorption equations used in the program to compute doses indicate that a dose of 22 mmol Li^+ every 12 hours produces a steady-state concentration of 1.2 mmol/L. This dose is equivalent to 813 mg of lithium carbonate (22 mmol [300 mg lithium carbonate/8.12 mmol Li^+] = 813 mg lithium carbonate). This amount is rounded to an amount available as an oral dosage form, and 900 mg of lithium carbonate is given every 12 hours.

When lithium dosage alterations are needed, serum concentration of lithium should be measured within 1 to 2 weeks after the change. During lithium maintenance therapy, steady-state lithium serum concentration should be repeated every 3 to 6 months. This period should be altered to every 6 to 12 months for patients whose mood is stable or every 1 to 2 months for patients with frequent mood alterations.

PROBLEMS

The following problems are intended to emphasize the computation of initial and individualized doses with clinical pharmacokinetic techniques. Clinicians always should consult the patient's chart to confirm that current therapy is appropriate. All other medications that the patient is taking, including prescription and nonprescription drugs, should be recorded and checked to ascertain the risk of drug interaction with lithium.

1. PG is a 67-year-old, 72-kg (height, 185 cm) man who has bipolar disease. He needs maintenance therapy with oral lithium. Serum creatinine level is 1.2 mg/dL. Suggest an initial lithium carbonate dosage regimen designed to achieve a steady-state lithium concentration of 0.6 mmol/L.

2. Patient PG (see problem 1) is given a prescription for lithium carbonate 900 mg orally every 12 hours. The current 12-hour postdose steady-state concentration of lithium is 1.0 mmol/L. Compute a new lithium carbonate dose that will provide a steady-state concentration of 0.6 mmol/L.

3. DU is a 21-year-old, 70-kg (height, 175 cm) woman who has bipolar disease. She needs therapy with lithium. Serum creatinine level is 0.8 mg/dL. The patient is currently experiencing acute mania. Suggest an initial lithium carbonate dosage regimen designed to achieve a steady-state lithium concentration of 0.8 mmol/L.

4. Patient DU (see problem 3) is given a prescription for lithium carbonate 600 mg orally at 0800 H, 1400 H, and 2000 H. The current 12-hour postdose steady-state concentration of lithium is 0.6 mmol/L. Compute a new oral lithium dose that will provide a steady-state concentration of 1 mmol/L.

5. JH is a 35-year-old, 60-kg (height, 157 cm) woman who has bipolar disease. She needs maintenance treatment with lithium. Serum creatinine level is 0.8 mg/dL. The patient is given a test dose of 600 mg lithium carbonate, and the 24-hour postdose lithium concentration is 0.07 mmol/L. Suggest an initial lithium dosage regimen designed to achieve a steady-state concentration of 0.8 mmol/L.

6. Patient JH (see problem 5) is given a prescription for lithium carbonate 600 mg orally every 12 hours starting 12 hours after the concentration for the test dose is measured. Serum concentration of lithium immediately before the tenth dose of this regimen is 0.4 mmol/L. Compute a new oral lithium carbonate dose that will provide a steady-state concentration of 0.6 mmol/L.

7. PZ is a 24-year-old, 80-kg (height, 180 cm) man in the acute manic phase of bipolar disease. He needs therapy with oral lithium. Serum creatinine level is 1.1 mg/dL. He is administered a test dose of lithium carbonate 600 mg at 0800 H, and 24-hour postdose lithium concentration is 0.21 mmol/L. Suggest an initial lithium dosage regimen designed to achieve a steady-state concentration of 0.8 mmol/L.

8. Patient PZ (see problem 7) is given a prescription for lithium carbonate 600 mg orally at 0800 H, 1400 H, and 2000 H (first dose at 1400 H on the same day the lithium test dose concentration is obtained). Serum concentration of lithium just before the 12th dose of this regimen is 1.5 mmol/L. Compute a new lithium carbonate dose that will provide a steady-state concentration of 1 mmol/L.

9. WG is a 41-year-old, 130-kg (height, 180 cm) man in the acute phase of bipolar disease. He needs treatment with lithium carbonate. Serum creatinine level is 1.2 mg/dL. He is given a test dose of lithium carbonate 1200 mg at 0800 H, and lithium concentration is measured 12 and 36 hours after dosing. Lithium concentration is 0.42 mmol/L 12 hours after and 0.28 mmol/L 36 hours after administration of the drug. Suggest an initial lithium carbonate dosage regimen designed to achieve a steady-state concentration of 1 mmol/L.

10. FY is a 32-year-old, 68-kg (height, 162 cm) woman who has bipolar disease. She needs treatment with lithium carbonate. Serum creatinine level is 0.9 mg/dL. The patient is given a test dose of 900 mg lithium carbonate at 0800 H, and lithium concentration is measured 12 and 36 hours after dosing. Lithium concentration is 0.3 mmol/L 12 hours after and 0.11 mmol/L 36 hours after administration of the drug. Suggest an initial lithium carbonate dosage regimen designed to achieve a steady-state concentration of 1.0 mmol/L.

11. MW is a 22-year-old, 81-kg (height, 188 cm) man who has bipolar disease. He is currently experiencing acute mania. Serum creatinine level is 0.9 mg/dL. Two test doses of lithium (900 mg each, 12 hours apart) are given to the patient. Lithium concentration is 0.19 mmol/L 12 hours after the first dose and 0.31 mmol/L 12 hours after the second dose. Compute an oral lithium dose for this patient to produce a steady-state serum concentration of 1 mmol/L.

12. YT is a 42-year-old, 66-kg (height, 152 cm) woman who has bipolar disease. She needs prophylactic therapy for bipolar disease. Serum creatinine level is 1.4 mg/dL.

Two test doses of lithium (300 mg each, 12 hours apart) are given to the patient. Lithium concentration is 0.11 mmol/L 12 hours after the first dose and 0.2 mmol/L 12 hours after the second dose. Compute an oral lithium dose for this patient to produce a steady-state serum concentration of 0.6 mmol/L.

ANSWERS TO PROBLEMS

1. Answer to problem 1.

Pharmacokinetic Dosing Method

1. *Estimate creatinine clearance.*

This patient has a stable serum creatinine level and is not obese. The Cockcroft-Gault equation can be used to estimate creatinine clearance:

$$CrCl_{est} = [(140 - age)BW]/(72 \cdot S_{Cr}) = [(140 - 67\ y)72\ kg]/(72 \cdot 1.2\ mg/dL)$$

$$CrCl_{est} = 61\ mL/min$$

2. *Estimate clearance.*

The drug clearance versus creatinine clearance relation is used to estimate lithium clearance for this patient:

$$Cl = 0.288(CrCl) = 0.288\ (61\ mL/min) = 17.6\ L/d$$

3. *Use the average steady-state concentration equation to compute a maintenance dose of lithium.*

For a patient who needs maintenance therapy for bipolar disease, the desired lithium concentration is 0.6 to 0.8 mmol/L. A serum concentration of 0.6 mmol/L is chosen for this patient, and oral lithium carbonate is used (F = 1, 8.12 mmol Li^+ per 300 mg of lithium carbonate).

$$D/\tau = (Css \cdot Cl)/F = [(0.6\ mmol/L) \cdot (17.6\ L/d)]/1 = 10.6\ mmol/d$$

D/τ = (300 mg lithium carbonate/8.12 mmol Li^+) 10.6 mmol/d = 392 mg/d, rounded to 450 mg/d of lithium carbonate. This dose is given as 150 mg of lithium carbonate in the morning and 300 mg of lithium carbonate in the evening.

Upon initiation of therapy, serum concentration can be measured every 2 to 3 days for safety in the care of patients predisposed to lithium toxicity, even though steady state has not yet been achieved. Once the desired steady-state lithium concentration has been achieved, lithium concentration should be measured every 1 to 2 weeks for approximately 2 months or until concentration has stabilized.

Literature-Based Recommended Dosing

1. *Estimate creatinine clearance.*

This patient has a stable serum creatinine level and is not obese. The Cockcroft-Gault equation can be used to estimate creatinine clearance:

$$CrCl_{est} = [(140 - age)BW]/(72 \cdot S_{Cr}) = [(140 - 67\ y)72\ kg]/(72 \cdot 1.2\ mg/dL)$$

$$CrCl_{est} = 61\ mL/min$$

2. *Choose the lithium dose based on disease states and conditions present in the patient.*

The patient needs prophylactic lithium therapy for bipolar disease and has good renal function. A lithium carbonate dose of 600 mg/d, given as 300 mg every 12 hours, is recommended as the initial amount. The dosage rate is increased 300 to 600 mg/d every 2 to 3 days as needed to provide adequate therapeutic effect, avoid adverse effects, and produce a therapeutic steady-state concentration of lithium.

2. Answer to problem 2.

Linear Pharmacokinetics Method

1. *Compute the new dose to achieve the desired serum concentration.*

According to linear pharmacokinetics, the new dose to attain the desired concentration should be proportional to the old dose (1800 mg/d) that produced the measured concentration:

$$D_{new} = (Css_{new}/Css_{old})D_{old} = [(0.6\ mmol/L)/(1.0\ mmol/L)]\ 1800\ mg/d$$
$$= 1080\ mg/d,\ \text{rounded to}\ 900\ mg/d$$

The patient is given 450 mg of lithium carbonate every 12 hours. When lithium dosage alterations are needed, serum concentration of lithium should be measured within 1 to 2 weeks after the change. During lithium maintenance therapy, steady-state lithium serum concentration should be measured every 3 to 6 months. This period should be altered to every 6 to 12 months for patients whose mood is stable or every 1 to 2 months for patients with frequent mood alterations.

3. Answer to problem 3.

Pharmacokinetic Dosing Method

1. *Estimate creatinine clearance.*

This patient has a stable serum creatinine level and is not obese. The Cockcroft-Gault equation can be used to estimate creatinine clearance:

$$CrCl_{est} = \{[(140 - age)BW]/(72 \cdot S_{Cr})\} \cdot 0.85$$
$$= \{[(140 - 21\ y)70\ kg]/(72 \cdot 0.8\ mg/dL)\} \cdot 0.85$$

$$CrCl_{est} = 123\ mL/min$$

2. *Estimate clearance.*

The drug clearance versus creatinine clearance relation for a patient with acute mania is used to estimate lithium clearance for this patient:

$$Cl = 0.432(CrCl) = 0.432(123\ mL/min) = 53.1\ L/d$$

3. *Use the average steady-state concentration equation to compute a maintenance dose of lithium.*

For a patient who needs therapy for the acute mania phase of bipolar disease, the desired lithium concentration is 0.8 to 1 mmol/L. A serum concentration of 0.8 mmol/L was chosen for this patient, and oral lithium carbonate is used (F = 1, 8.12 mmol Li^+ per 300 mg of lithium carbonate).

$$D/\tau = (Css \cdot Cl)/F = (0.8 \text{ mmol/L} \cdot 53.1 \text{ L/d})/1 = 42.5 \text{ mmol/d}$$

D/τ = (300 mg lithium carbonate/8.12 mmol Li^+) 42.5 mmol/d = 1570 mg/d, rounded to 1500 mg/d of lithium carbonate. This dose is given as 600 mg of lithium carbonate at 0800 H and 2000 H and 300 mg of lithium carbonate at 1400 H.

Upon initiation of therapy, serum concentration can be measured every 2 to 3 days for safety in the care of patients predisposed to lithium toxicity, even though steady state has not yet been achieved. Once the desired steady-state concentration of lithium has been achieved, lithium concentrations should be measured every 1 to 2 weeks for approximately 2 months or until concentration has stabilized.

Literature-Based Recommended Dosing

1. *Estimate creatinine clearance.*

This patient has a stable serum creatinine level and is not obese. The Cockcroft-Gault equation can be used to estimate creatinine clearance:

$$CrCl_{est} = \{[(140 - age)BW]/(72 \cdot S_{Cr})\} \cdot 0.85$$
$$= \{[(140 - 21 \text{ y})70 \text{ kg}]/(72 \cdot 0.8 \text{ mg/dL})\} \cdot 0.85$$

$$CrCl_{est} = 123 \text{ mL/min}$$

2. *Choose the lithium dose based on disease states and conditions present in the patient.*

The patient needs immediate lithium therapy to manage the acute manic phase of bipolar disease. She has good renal function. A lithium carbonate dose of 1200 mg/d, given as 600 mg every 12 hours, is recommended as the initial amount. The dosage is increased 300 to 600 mg/d every 2 to 3 days as needed to provide adequate therapeutic effect, avoid adverse effects, and produce a therapeutic steady-state concentration of lithium.

4. Answer to problem 4.

Linear Pharmacokinetics Method

1. *Compute the new dose to achieve the desired serum concentration.*

According to linear pharmacokinetics, the new dose to attain the desired concentration should be proportional to the old dose (1800 mg/d) that produced the measured concentration:

$$D_{new} = (Css_{new}/Css_{old})D_{old} = [(1 \text{ mmol/L})/(0.6 \text{ mmol/L})]\ 1800 \text{ mg/d}$$
$$= 3000 \text{ mg/d, rounded to 2700 mg/d}$$

The patient is given 900 mg of lithium carbonate at 0800 H, 1400 H, and 2000 H.

When lithium dosage alterations are needed, serum concentration of lithium should be measured within 1 to 2 weeks after the change. During lithium maintenance therapy, steady-state serum concentration of lithium should be measured every 3 to 6 months. This period should be altered to every 6 to 12 months for patients whose mood is stable or every 1 to 2 months for patients with frequent mood alterations.

5. Answer to problem 5.

Cooper Nomogram

1. *Administer a test dose of 600 mg lithium carbonate and measure 24-hour postdose lithium concentration. Use Cooper nomogram to recommend a maintenance dose of lithium carbonate.*

After the test dose is given, 24-hour postdose lithium concentration is 0.07 mmol/L. The recommended maintenance dose of lithium carbonate is 900 mg three times a day. The doses are given at 0900 H, 1500 H, and 2100 H to allow a 12-hour window after the evening dose for measurement of serum concentration of lithium.

Upon initiation of therapy, serum concentration can be measured every 2 to 3 days for safety in the care of patients predisposed to lithium toxicity, even though steady state has not yet been achieved. Once the desired steady-state concentration of lithium has been achieved, lithium concentration should be measured every 1 to 2 weeks for approximately 2 months or until concentration has stabilized.

Bayesian Pharmacokinetics Computer Program Method

1. *Enter the patient's demographic, drug dosing, and serum concentration–time data into the computer program.*

Lithium doses must be entered into DrugCalc as millimoles of lithium ion. Six hundred milligrams of lithium carbonate provides 16.2 mmol of lithium ion: 600 mg (8.12 mmol Li^+/300 mg lithium carbonate) = 16.2 mmol Li^+.

2. *Compute pharmacokinetic parameters for the patient with a Bayesian pharmacokinetics computer program.*

The pharmacokinetic parameters computed with the program are a volume of distribution of 99 L, a half-life of 27 hours, and a clearance of 2.53 L/h.

3. *Compute the dose required to achieve the desired serum concentration of lithium.*

The one-compartment, first-order absorption equations used in the program to compute doses indicate that a dose of 34 mmol Li^+ every 12 hours produces a steady-state concentration of 0.8 mmol/L. This dose is equivalent to 1256 mg of lithium carbonate (34 mmol [300 mg lithium carbonate/8.12 mmol Li^+] = 1256 mg lithium carbonate). This amount is rounded to an amount available as an oral dosage form, and 1200 mg of lithium carbonate is given every 12 hours.

Upon initiation of therapy, serum concentration can be measured every 2 to 3 days for safety in the care of patients predisposed to lithium toxicity, even though steady state has not yet been achieved. Once the desired steady-state concentration of lithium has been achieved, lithium concentration should be measured every 1 to 2 weeks for approximately 2 months or until concentration has stabilized.

6. Solution to problem 6.

Linear Pharmacokinetics Method

1. *Compute the new dose to achieve the desired serum concentration.*

According to linear pharmacokinetics, the new dose to attain the desired concentration should be proportional to the old dose (1200 mg/d) that produced the measured concentration:

$$D_{new} = (Css_{new}/Css_{old})D_{old} = [(0.6\ \text{mmol/L})/(0.4\ \text{mmol/L})]\ 1200\ \text{mg/d} = 1800\ \text{mg/d}$$

The patient is administered 900 mg of lithium carbonate every 12 hours.

When lithium dosage alterations are needed, serum concentration of lithium should be measured within 1 to 2 weeks after the change. During lithium maintenance therapy, steady-state serum concentration of lithium should be measured every 3 to 6 months. This period should be altered to every 6 to 12 months for patients whose mood is stable or every 1 to 2 months for patients with frequent mood alterations.

Bayesian Pharmacokinetics Computer Program Method

1. *Enter the patient's demographic, drug dosing, and serum concentration–time data into the computer program.*

Lithium doses must be entered into DrugCalc as millimoles of lithium ion. Six hundred milligrams of lithium carbonate provides 16.2 mmol of lithium ion: 600 mg (8.12 mmol Li^+/300 mg lithium carbonate) = 16.2 mmol Li^+. In this case, the concentration after the test dose (see problem 5) and the concentration just before the tenth dose can be used in the program.

2. *Compute pharmacokinetic parameters for the patient with a Bayesian pharmacokinetics computer program.*

The pharmacokinetic parameters computed with the program are a volume of distribution of 112 L, a half-life of 35 hours, and a clearance of 2.22 L/h.

3. *Compute the dose required to achieve desired serum concentration of lithium.*

The one-compartment, first-order absorption equations used in the program to compute doses indicate that a dose of 21 mmol Li^+ every 12 hours produces a steady-state concentration of 0.8 mmol/L. This dose is equivalent to 776 mg of lithium carbonate (21 mmol [300 mg lithium carbonate/8.12 mmol Li^+] = 776 mg lithium carbonate). This amount is rounded to an amount available as an oral dosage form, and 750 mg of lithium carbonate is given every 12 hours.

When lithium dosage alterations are needed, serum concentration of lithium should be measured within 1 to 2 weeks after the change. During lithium maintenance therapy, steady-state serum concentration of lithium should be repeated every 3 to 6 months. This period should be altered to every 6 to 12 months for patients whose mood is stable or every 1 to 2 months for patients with frequent mood alterations.

7. Answer to problem 7.

Cooper Nomogram

1. *Administer a test dose of 600 mg lithium carbonate and measure 24-hour postdose lithium concentration. Use Cooper nomogram to recommend a maintenance dose of lithium carbonate.*

After the test dose is given, the 24-hour lithium concentration is 0.21 mmol/L. The recommended maintenance dose of lithium carbonate is 300 mg three times a day. The doses are given at 0900 H, 1500 H, and 2100 H to allow a 12-hour window after the evening dose for measurement of serum concentration of lithium.

Upon initiation of therapy, serum concentration can be measured every 2 to 3 days for safety in the care of patients predisposed to lithium toxicity, even though steady state has not yet been achieved. Once the desired steady-state concentration of lithium has been achieved, lithium concentration should be measured every 1 to 2 weeks for approximately 2 months or until concentration has stabilized.

Bayesian Pharmacokinetics Computer Program Method

1. *Enter the patient's demographic, drug dosing, and serum concentration–time data into the computer program.*

Lithium doses must be entered into DrugCalc as millimoles of lithium ion. Six hundred milligrams of lithium carbonate provides 16.2 mmol of lithium ion: 600 mg (8.12 mmol Li^+/300 mg lithium carbonate) = 16.2 mmol Li^+.

2. *Compute pharmacokinetic parameters for the patient with a Bayesian pharmacokinetics computer program.*

The pharmacokinetic parameters computed with the program are a volume of distribution of 44 L, a half-life of 25 hours, and a clearance of 1.2 L/h.

3. *Compute the dose required to achieve the desired serum concentration of lithium.*

The one-compartment, first-order absorption equations used in the program to compute doses indicate that a dose of 8 mmol Li^+ every 8 hours produces a steady-state concentration of 0.8 mmol/L. This dose is equivalent to 296 mg of lithium carbonate (8 mmol [300 mg lithium carbonate/8.12 mmol Li^+] = 296 mg lithium carbonate). This amount is rounded to an amount available as an oral dosage form, and 300 mg of lithium carbonate is given at 0900 H, 1500 H, and 2100 H to allow a 12-hour window after the evening dose for measurement of serum concentration of lithium.

Upon initiation of therapy, serum concentration can be measured every 2 to 3 days for safety in the care of patients predisposed to lithium toxicity, even though steady state has not yet been achieved. Once the desired steady-state concentration of lithium has been achieved, lithium concentration should be measured every 1 to 2 weeks for approximately 2 months or until concentration has stabilized.

8. Solution to problem 8.

Linear Pharmacokinetics Method

1. *Compute the new dose to achieve the desired serum concentration.*

According to linear pharmacokinetics, the new dose to attain the desired concentration should be proportional to the old dose (1800 mg/d) that produced the measured concentration:

$$D_{new} = (Css_{new}/Css_{old})D_{old} = [(1 \text{ mmol/L})/(1.5 \text{ mmol/L})]\ 1800 \text{ mg/d} = 1200 \text{ mg/d}$$

The patient is given 600 mg of lithium carbonate every 12 hours.

When lithium dosage alterations are needed, serum concentration of lithium should be measured within 1 to 2 weeks after the change. During lithium maintenance therapy, steady-state serum concentration of lithium should be repeated every 3 to 6 months. This period should be altered to every 6 to 12 months for patients whose mood is stable or every 1 to 2 months for patients with frequent mood alterations.

Bayesian Pharmacokinetics Computer Program Method

1. *Enter the patient's demographic, drug dosing, and serum concentration–time data into the computer program.*

Lithium doses must be entered into DrugCalc as millimoles of lithium ion. Six hundred milligrams of lithium carbonate provides 16.2 mmol of lithium ion: 600 mg (8.12 mmol Li^+/300 mg lithium carbonate) = 16.2 mmol Li^+. In this case, the concentration after the test dose (see problem 7) and the concentration just before the twelfth dose can be used in the program.

2. *Compute pharmacokinetic parameters for the patient with a Bayesian pharmacokinetics computer program.*

The pharmacokinetic parameters computed with the program are a volume of distribution of 44 L, a half-life of 25 hours, and a clearance of 1.2 L/h.

3. *Compute the dose required to achieve the desired serum concentration of lithium.*

The one-compartment, first-order absorption equations used in the program to compute doses indicate that a dose of 16 mmol Li^+ every 12 hours produces a steady-state concentration of 1 mmol/L. This dose is equivalent to 591 mg of lithium carbonate (16 mmol [300 mg lithium carbonate/8.12 mmol Li^+] = 591 mg lithium carbonate). This amount is rounded to an amount available as an oral dosage form, and 600 mg of lithium carbonate is given every 12 hours.

When lithium dosage alterations are needed, serum concentration of lithium should be measured within 1 to 2 weeks after the change. During lithium maintenance therapy, steady-state serum concentration of lithium should be repeated every

3 to 6 months. This period should be altered to every 6 to 12 months for patients whose mood is stable or every 1 to 2 months for patients with frequent mood alterations.

9. Answer to problem 9.

Perry Method

1. *Administer a test dose of lithium carbonate and measure 12- and 36-hour postdose lithium concentrations. Compute the lithium elimination rate constant and accumulation ratio for the patient.*

The lithium elimination rate constant is computed with the two serum concentrations: $k = (\ln C_{12\,h} - \ln C_{36\,h})/\Delta t = [\ln (0.42\ \text{mmol/L}) - \ln (0.28\ \text{mmol/L})]/24\ h = 0.0169\ h^{-1}$. The lithium accumulation ratio is computed with the elimination rate constant and desired lithium dosage interval of 12 hours: $R = 1/(1 - e^{-k\tau}) = 1/(1 - e^{-(0.0169\ h^{-1})(12\ h)}) = 5.4$.

2. *Compute the estimated lithium concentration at steady state for the test dose given. Use this relation to compute the dosage regimen for the patient.*

Using the lithium concentration at 12 hours, the steady-state lithium concentration for 1200 mg every 12 hours can be computed: $Css_t = R \cdot C_{SD,t} = 5.4 \cdot 0.42$ mmol/L = 2.3 mmol/L. Linear pharmacokinetic principles can be used to compute the dose required to achieve the target lithium steady-state serum concentration: D_{new} = [(1 mmol/L)/(2.3 mmol/L)] 1200 mg = 522 mg, rounded to 600 mg every 12 hours, of lithium carbonate.

Upon initiation of therapy, serum concentration can be measured every 2 to 3 days for safety in the care of patients predisposed to lithium toxicity, even though steady state has not yet been achieved. Once the desired steady-state concentration of lithium has been achieved, lithium concentration should be measured every 1 to 2 weeks for approximately 2 months or until concentration has stabilized. Because patients with acute mania can have increased lithium clearance, lithium concentration should be measured once the manic episode is over and clearance returns to normal.

Bayesian Pharmacokinetics Computer Program Method

1. *Enter the patient's demographic, drug dosing, and serum concentration–time data into the computer program.*

Lithium doses must be entered into DrugCalc as millimoles of lithium ion. Twelve hundred milligrams of lithium carbonate provides 32.5 mmol of lithium ion: 1200 mg (8.12 mmol Li^+/300 mg lithium carbonate) = 32.5 mmol Li^+.

2. *Compute pharmacokinetic parameters for the patient with a Bayesian pharmacokinetics computer program.*

The pharmacokinetic parameters computed with the program are a volume of distribution of 67 L, a half-life of 41 hours, and a clearance of 1.13 L/h.

3. *Compute the dose required to achieve the desired serum concentration of lithium.*

The one-compartment, first-order absorption equations used in the program to compute doses indicate that a dose of 14 mmol Li^+ every 12 hours produces a steady-state concentration of 1 mmol/L. This dose is equivalent to 517 mg of lithium carbonate (14 mmol [300 mg lithium carbonate/8.12 mmol Li^+] = 517 mg lithium carbonate). This amount is rounded to an amount available as an oral dosage form, and 600 mg of lithium carbonate is given every 12 hours.

Upon initiation of therapy, serum concentration can be measured every 2 to 3 days for safety in the care of patients predisposed to lithium toxicity, even though steady state has not yet been achieved. Once the desired steady-state concentration of lithium has been achieved, lithium concentration should be measured every 1 to 2 weeks for approximately 2 months or until concentration has stabilized.

10. Answer to problem 10.

Perry Method

1. *Administer a test dose of lithium carbonate and measure 12- and 36-hour postdose lithium concentrations. Compute the lithium elimination rate constant and accumulation ratio for the patient.*

The lithium elimination rate constant is computed with the two serum concentrations: $k = (\ln C_{12\text{ h}} - \ln C_{36\text{ h}})/\Delta t$ = [ln (0.3 mmol/L) – ln (0.11 mmol/L)]/24 h = 0.0418 h^{-1}. The lithium accumulation ratio is computed with the elimination rate constant and desired lithium dosage interval of 12 hours: $R = 1/(1 - e^{-k\tau}) = 1/(1 - e^{-(0.0418\text{ h}^{-1})(12\text{ h})}) = 2.5$.

2. *Compute the estimated lithium concentration at steady state for the test dose given. Use this relation to compute the dosage regimen for the patient.*

With the lithium concentration obtained at 12 hours, steady-state concentration of lithium for 900 mg every 12 hours can be computed: $Css_t = R \cdot C_{SD,t} = 2.5 \cdot$ 0.3 mmol/L = 0.75 mmol/L. Linear pharmacokinetic principles can be used to compute the dose required to achieve the target steady-state serum concentration of lithium: D_{new} = [(1 mmol/L)/(0.75 mmol/L)] 900 mg = 1200 mg every 12 hours of lithium carbonate.

Upon initiation of therapy, serum concentration can be measured every 2 to 3 days for safety in the care of patients predisposed to lithium toxicity, even though steady state has not yet been achieved. Once the desired steady-state concentration of lithium has been achieved, lithium concentrations should be measured every 1 to 2 weeks for approximately 2 months or until concentration has stabilized. Because patients with acute mania can have increased lithium clearance, lithium concentration should be measured once the manic episode is over and clearance returns to normal.

Bayesian Pharmacokinetics Computer Program Method

1. *Enter the patient's demographic, drug dosing, and serum concentration–time data into the computer program.*

Lithium doses must be entered into DrugCalc as millimoles of lithium ion. Nine hundred milligrams of lithium carbonate provides 24.4 mmol of lithium ion: 900 mg (8.12 mmol Li^+/300 mg lithium carbonate) = 24.4 mmol Li^+.

2. *Compute pharmacokinetic parameters for the patient with a Bayesian pharmacokinetics computer program.*

The pharmacokinetic parameters computed with the program are a volume of distribution of 47 L, a half-life of 17 hours, and a clearance of 1.94 L/h.

3. *Compute the dose required to achieve the desired serum concentration of lithium.*

The one-compartment, first-order absorption equations used in the program to compute doses indicate that a dose of 31 mmol Li^+ every 12 hours produces a steady-state concentration of 1 mmol/L. This dose is equivalent to 1145 mg of lithium carbonate (31 mmol [300 mg lithium carbonate/8.12 mmol Li^+] = 1145 mg lithium carbonate). This amount is rounded to an amount available as an oral dosage form, and 1200 mg of lithium carbonate is given every 12 hours.

Upon initiation of therapy, serum concentration can be measured every 2 to 3 days for safety in the care of patients predisposed to lithium toxicity, even though steady state has not yet been achieved. Once the desired steady-state concentration of lithium has been achieved, lithium concentration should be measured every 1 to 2 weeks for approximately 2 months or until concentration has stabilized.

11. Solution to problem 11.

Ritschel Method

1. *Administer test dose of lithium carbonate and measure lithium concentration. Compute the lithium elimination rate constant and accumulation ratio for the patient.*

The lithium elimination rate constant is computed with the two serum concentrations: $k = \{\ln [C_1/(C_2 - C_1)]\}/\tau = \ln [(0.19 \text{ mmol/L})/(0.31 \text{ mmol/L} - 0.19 \text{ mmol/L})]/12 \text{ h} = 0.0383 \text{ h}^{-1}$. The lithium accumulation ratio is computed with the elimination rate constant and desired lithium dosage interval of 12 hours: $R = 1/(1 - e^{-k\tau}) = 1/(1 - e^{-(0.0383 \text{ h}^{-1})(12 \text{ h})}) = 2.7$.

2. *Compute the estimated lithium concentration at steady state for the test dose given. Use this relation to compute the dosage regimen for the patient.*

With the lithium concentration obtained at 12 hours, steady-state concentration of lithium for 900 mg every 12 hours can be computed: $Css_t = R \cdot C_{SD,t} = 2.7 \cdot 0.19$ mmol/L = 0.5 mmol/L. Linear pharmacokinetic principles can be used to compute the dose required to achieve the target steady-state serum concentration of lithium: D_{new} = [(1 mmol/L)/(0.5 mmol/L)] 900 mg = 1800 mg every 12 hours of lithium carbonate. Because the dose exceeds 1200 mg per administration time, the total daily dose of 3600 mg/d is split into three equal doses of 1200 mg and is given at 0900 H, 1500 H, and 2100 H.

Upon initiation of therapy, serum concentration can be measured every 2 to 3 days for safety in the care of patients predisposed to lithium toxicity, even though steady state has not yet been achieved. Once the desired steady-state concentration of lithium has been achieved, lithium concentration should be measured every 1 to 2 weeks for approximately 2 months or until concentration has stabilized. Because patients with acute mania can have increased lithium clearance, lithium concentration should be measured once the manic episode is over and clearance returns to normal.

Bayesian Pharmacokinetics Computer Program Method

1. *Enter the patient's demographic, drug dosing, and serum concentration–time data into the computer program.*

Lithium doses must be entered into DrugCalc as millimoles of lithium ion. Nine hundred milligrams of lithium carbonate provides 24.4 mmol of lithium ion: 900 mg (8.12 mmol Li^+/300 mg lithium carbonate) = 24.4 mmol Li^+.

2. *Compute pharmacokinetic parameters for the patient with a Bayesian pharmacokinetics computer program.*

The pharmacokinetic parameters computed with the program are a volume of distribution of 79 L, a half-life of 19 hours, and a clearance of 2.89 L/h.

3. *Compute the dose required to achieve the desired serum concentration of lithium.*

The one-compartment, first-order absorption equations used in the program to compute doses indicate that a dose of 27 mmol Li^+ every 8 hours produces a steady-state concentration of 1 mmol/L. This dose is equivalent to 998 mg of lithium carbonate (27 mmol [300 mg lithium carbonate/8.12 mmol Li^+] = 998 mg lithium carbonate). This amount is rounded to an amount available as an oral dosage form, and 900 mg of lithium carbonate is given at 0900 H, 1500 H, and 2100 H.

Upon initiation of therapy, serum concentration can be measured every 2 to 3 days for safety in the care of patients predisposed to lithium toxicity, even though steady state has not yet been achieved. Once the desired steady-state concentration of lithium has been achieved, lithium concentration should be measured every 1 to 2 weeks for approximately 2 months or until concentration has stabilized.

12. Solution to problem 12.

Ritschel Method

1. *Administer test dose of lithium carbonate and measure lithium concentration. Compute the lithium elimination rate constant and accumulation ratio for the patient.*

The lithium elimination rate constant is computed with the two serum concentrations: $k = \{\ln [C_1/(C_2 - C_1)]\}/\tau = \ln [(0.11 \text{ mmol/L})/(0.2 \text{ mmol/L} - 0.11 \text{ mmol/L})]/12 \text{ h} = 0.0167 \text{ h}^{-1}$. The lithium accumulation ratio is computed with the elimination rate constant and desired lithium dosage interval of 12 hours: $R = 1/(1 - e^{-k\tau}) = 1/(1 - e^{-(0.0167 \text{ h}^{-1})(12 \text{ h})}) = 5.5$.

2. *Compute the estimated lithium concentration at steady state for the test dose given. Use this relation to compute the dosage regimen for the patient.*

With the lithium concentration obtained at 12 hours, steady-state concentration of lithium for 300 mg every 12 hours can be computed: $Css_t = R \cdot C_{SD,t} = 5.5 \cdot 0.11$ mmol/L =

0.6 mmol/L. This is the desired steady-state concentration, so 300 mg every 12 hours of lithium carbonate is prescribed.

Upon initiation of therapy, serum concentration can be measured every 2 to 3 days for safety in the care of patients predisposed to lithium toxicity, even though steady state has not yet been achieved. Once the desired steady-state concentration of lithium has been achieved, lithium concentration should be measured every 1 to 2 weeks for approximately 2 months or until concentration has stabilized. Because patients with acute mania can have increased lithium clearance, lithium concentration should be measured once the manic episode is over and clearance returns to normal.

Bayesian Pharmacokinetics Computer Program Method

1. *Enter the patient's demographic, drug dosing, and serum concentration–time data into the computer program.*

Lithium doses must be entered into DrugCalc as millimoles of lithium ion. Three hundred milligrams of lithium carbonate provides 8.12 mmol of lithium ion: 300 mg (8.12 mmol Li^+/300 mg lithium carbonate) = 8.12 mmol Li^+.

2. *Compute pharmacokinetic parameters for the patient with a Bayesian pharmacokinetics computer program.*

The pharmacokinetic parameters computed with the program are a volume of distribution of 61 L, a half-life of 65 hours, and a clearance of 0.65 L/h.

3. *Compute the dose required to achieve the desired serum concentration of lithium.*

The one-compartment, first-order absorption equations used in the program to compute doses indicate that a dose of 5 mmol Li^+ every 12 hours produces a steady-state concentration of 0.6 mmol/L. This dose is equivalent to 185 mg of lithium carbonate (5 mmol [300 mg lithium carbonate/8.12 mmol Li^+] = 185 mg lithium carbonate). This amount is rounded to an amount available as an oral dosage form, and 150 mg of lithium carbonate is given every 12 hours. Because of the long half-life of lithium in this patient, a dose of 300 mg/d can be prescribed.

Upon initiation of therapy, serum concentration can be measured every 2 to 3 days for safety in the care of patients predisposed to lithium toxicity, even though steady state has not yet been achieved. Once the desired steady-state concentration of lithium has been achieved, lithium concentration should be measured every 1 to 2 weeks for approximately 2 months or until concentration has stabilized.

REFERENCES

1. Fankhauser MP, Benefield WH. Bipolar disorder. In: DiPiro JT, Talbert RL, Yee GC, Matzke GR, Wells BG, Posey LM, eds. Pharmacotherapy: a pathophysiologic approach. Stamford, CT: Appleton & Lange, 1999:1161–81.
2. Baldessarini RJ. Drugs and the treatment of psychiatric disorders: depression and mania. In: Hardman JG, Limbird LE, Molinoff PB, Ruddon RW, Gilman AG, eds. The pharmacological basis of therapeutics. New York: McGraw-Hill, 1996:431–59.

3. Weber SS, Saklad SR, Kastenholz KV. Bipolar affective disorders. In: Koda-Kimble MA, Young LY, Kradjan WA, Guglielmo BJ, eds. Applied therapeutics. Vancouver, WA: Applied Therapeutics, 1992:58-1–58-17.
4. Amdisen A. Serum level monitoring and clinical pharmacokinetics of lithium. Clin Pharmacokinet 1977;2:73–92.
5. Thornhill DP, Field SP. Distribution of lithium elimination rates in a selected population of psychiatric patients. Eur J Clin Pharmacol 1982;21:351–4.
6. Nielsen-Kudsk F, Amdisen A. Analysis of the pharmacokinetics of lithium in man. Eur J Clin Pharmacol 1979;16:271–7.
7. Goodnick PJ, Meltzer HL, Fieve RR, Dunner DL. Differences in lithium kinetics between bipolar and unipolar patients. J Clin Psychopharmacol 1982;2:48–50.
8. Mason RW, McQueen EG, Keary PJ, James NM. Pharmacokinetics of lithium: elimination half-time, renal clearance and apparent volume of distribution in schizophrenia. Clin Pharmacokinet 1978;3:241–6.
9. Vertrees JE, Ereshefsky L. Lithium. In: Schumacher GE, ed. Therapeutic drug monitoring. Stamford, CT: Appleton & Lange, 1995:493–526.
10. Hardy BG, Shulman KI, Mackenzie SE, Kutcher SP, Silverberg JD. Pharmacokinetics of lithium in the elderly. J Clin Psychopharmacol 1987;7:153–8.
11. Chapron DJ, Cameron IR, White LB, Merrall P. Observations on lithium disposition in the elderly. J Am Geriatr Soc 1982;30:651–5.
12. Caldwell HC, Westlake WJ, Schriver RC, Bumbier EE. Steady-state lithium blood level fluctuations in man following administration of a lithium carbonate conventional and controlled-release dosage form. J Clin Pharmacol 1981;21:106–9.
13. Meinhold JM, Spunt AL, Trirath C. Bioavailability of lithium carbonate: in vivo comparison of two products. J Clin Pharmacol 1979;19:701–3.
14. Williams PJ, Browne JL, Patel RA. Bayesian forecasting of serum lithium concentrations: comparison with traditional methods. Clin Pharmacokinet 1989;17:45–52.
15. Vitiello B, Behar D, Malone R, Delaney MA, Ryan PJ, Simpson GM. Pharmacokinetics of lithium carbonate in children. J Clin Psychopharmacol 1988;8:355–9.
16. Lauritsen BJ, Mellerup ET, Plenge P, Rasmussen S, Vestergaard P, Schou M. Serum lithium concentrations around the clock with different treatment regimens and the diurnal variation of the renal lithium clearance. Acta Psychiatr Scand 1981;64:314–9.
17. Schou M. Lithium treatment during pregnancy, delivery, and lactation: an update. J Clin Psychiatry 1990;51:410–3.
18. Pringuey D, Yzombard G, Charbit JJ, et al. Lithium kinetics during hemodialysis in a patient with lithium poisoning. Am J Psychiatry 1981;138:249–51.
19. Zetin M, Plon L, Vaziri N, Cramer M, Greco D. Lithium carbonate dose and serum level relationships in chronic hemodialysis patients. Am J Psychiatry 1981;138:1387–8.
20. Hansten PD, Horn JR. Drug interactions analysis and management. Vancouver, WA: Applied Therapeutics, 1998:527.
21. Bennett WM, Aronoff GR, Morrison G, et al. Drug prescribing in renal failure: dosing guidelines for adults. Am J Kidney Dis 1983;3:155–93.
22. Swan SK, Bennett WM. Drug dosing guidelines in patients with renal failure. West J Med 1992;156:633–8.
23. Bennett WM, Muther RS, Parker RA, et al. Drug therapy in renal failure: dosing guidelines for adults: II. Sedatives, hypnotics, and tranquilizers; cardiovascular, antihypertensive, and diuretic agents; miscellaneous agents. Ann Intern Med 1980;93:286–325.
24. Bennett WM, Muther RS, Parker RA, et al. Drug therapy in renal failure: dosing guidelines for adults: I. Antimicrobial agents, analgesics. Ann Intern Med 1980;93:62–89.
25. Zetin M, Garber D, Cramer M. A simple mathematical model for predicting lithium dose requirement. J Clin Psychiatry 1983;44:144–5.

26. Zetin M, Garber D, De Antonio M, et al. Prediction of lithium dose: a mathematical alternative to the test-dose method. J Clin Psychiatry 1986;47:175–8.
27. Cooper TB, Bergner PE, Simpson GM. The 24-hour serum lithium level as a prognosticator of dosage requirements. Am J Psychiatry 1973;130:601–3.
28. Cooper TB, Simpson GM. The 24-hour lithium level as a prognosticator of dosage requirements: a 2-year follow-up study. Am J Psychiatry 1976;133:440–3.
29. Perry PJ, Prince RA, Alexander B, Dunner FJ. Prediction of lithium maintenance doses using a single point prediction protocol. J Clin Psychopharmacol 1983;3:13–27.
30. Perry PJ, Alexander B, Prince RA, Dunner FJ. The utility of a single-point dosing protocol for predicting steady-state lithium levels. Br J Psychiatry 1986;148:401–5.
31. Perry PJ, Alexander B, Dunner FJ, Schoenwald RD, Pfohl B, Miller D. Pharmacokinetic protocol for predicting serum lithium levels. J Clin Psychopharmacol 1982;2:114–8.
32. Ritschel WA, Banarer M. Lithium dosage regimen designed by the repeated one-point method. Arzneimittelforschung 1982;32:98–102.
33. Marr MA, Djuric PE, Ritschel WA, Garver DL. Prediction of lithium carbonate dosage in psychiatric inpatients using the repeated one-point method. Clin Pharm 1983;2:243–8.

18

THEOPHYLLINE

INTRODUCTION

Theophylline is a methylxanthine compound used to manage asthma, chronic obstructive pulmonary disease (COPD; chronic bronchitis and emphysema), and premature apnea. The bronchodilatory effects of theophylline are useful primarily to patients with asthma because bronchospasm is a key component of that disease.[1] The use of theophylline to treat patients with COPD is controversial because chronic bronchitis and emphysema have different pathophysiologic profiles, although some patients do have a mixed disease profile with a limited reversible airway component. Even patients with COPD who do not have significant bronchospasm have clinical improvement when they take theophylline.[2–4] Theophylline is a central nervous system stimulant, so it is useful for the treatment of premature apnea.

In the long-term management of asthma or COPD, theophylline is considered to be a third-line agent.[5,6] Asthma is now recognized as an inflammatory disease, and inhaled glucocorticoids are considered the mainstay of therapy.[6] Inhaled selective β_2-agonists are used as bronchodilators in the care of patients with asthma. Other useful drugs for patients with asthma are cromolyn, nedocromil, inhaled anticholinergics, and the leukotriene modifiers zafirlukast and zileuton. Inhaled bronchodilators are preferred therapy for COPD. Many clinicians favor the use of ipratropium for initial therapy followed by an inhaled selective β_2-agonist as a second-line agent.[5] Theophylline is considered for use in the care of patients with asthma and of patients with COPD after other treatment has been started. Theophylline also is useful in the care of patients who are unable or unwilling to use a multiple-metered dose inhaler (MDI) or if an intravenous drug is needed. To manage premature apnea, most clinicians prefer to use caffeine, a related methylxanthine agent, rather than theophylline because caffeine provides smoother apnea control and causes fewer adverse effects.

The bronchodilatory response to theophylline by means of smooth muscle relaxation in the lung is postulated to be caused by several mechanisms.[7] Of these, the two predominant mechanisms of action are antagonism of adenosine receptors and inhibition of phosphodiesterases, which increases the amount of cyclic adenosine monophosphate (cAMP) in the cells. In addition to bronchodilation, theophylline increases diaphragmatic contractility, increases mucociliary clearance, and exerts some antiinflammatory effects. Theophylline is a general central nervous system stimulant and specifically stimulates the medullary respiratory center. For these reasons, it is a useful agent in the management of premature apnea.

THERAPEUTIC AND TOXIC CONCENTRATIONS

The accepted therapeutic ranges of theophylline are 10 to 20 μg/mL for the management of asthma or COPD and 6 to 13 μg/mL for the management of premature apnea. Recent guidelines suggest that for initial management of pulmonary disease, clinical response to theophylline concentrations of 5 to 15 μg/mL be assessed before higher concentrations are used.[8] Many patients who need long-term theophylline therapy derive sufficient bronchodilatory response with a low likelihood of adverse effects at concentrations of 8 to 12 μg/mL. However, theophylline therapy must be individualized for each patient to achieve optimal responses and minimal side effects.

Some patients receiving theophylline in the upper end of the therapeutic range (>15 μg/mL) have minor side effects similar to those of caffeine.[1] These adverse effects include nausea, vomiting, dyspepsia, insomnia, nervousness, and headache. Theophylline concentration exceeding 20 to 30 μg/mL can cause various forms of tachyarrhythmia, including sinus tachycardia. At theophylline concentrations greater than 40 μg/mL, serious life-threatening adverse effects, including ventricular arrhythmia (premature ventricular contractions, ventricular tachycardia or fibrillation) or seizures, can occur. Theophylline-induced seizures are an ominous sign because they respond poorly to antiepileptic therapy and can result in postseizure neurologic sequelae or death. Unfortunately, minor side effects do not always occur before severe, life-threatening adverse effects. Seizures due to theophylline therapy have been reported to occur among patients with theophylline concentrations as low as 25 μg/mL. Monitoring of serum concentration is mandatory for patients receiving theophylline. Clinicians should understand that not all patients with "toxic" theophylline serum concentrations in the listed ranges have signs or symptoms of theophylline toxicity. Rather, theophylline concentrations in the ranges given increase the likelihood that an adverse effect will occur.

CLINICAL MONITORING PARAMETERS

Pulmonary function testing is an important component of bronchodilator therapy among patients with asthma or COPD.[5,6] Forced expiratory volume in 1 second (FEV_1) should be measured on a regular basis for patients with asthma, and peak-flow monitoring can be routinely performed by these patients at home. Successful bronchodilator therapy increases both FEV_1 and peak flow. In addition to the use of FEV_1 to monitor bronchodilator effects, spirometric tests useful to patients with COPD include measurement of vital capacity (VC), total lung capacity (TLC), forced vital capacity (FVC), and forced expiratory flow over the middle 50% of the expiratory curve ($FEF_{25\%-75\%}$ or $FEF_{50\%}$). Patients should be observed for clinical signs and symptoms, such as frequency and severity of dyspnea, coughing, wheezing, and impairment of normal activity. During acute exacerbations or in severe cases of COPD or asthma, arterial blood gases can be measured and used as a monitoring parameter. When theophylline is used to treat premature infants with apnea, the frequency of apneic events is monitored as a measure of therapeutic effect.

Monitoring of serum concentration of theophylline is mandatory in the care of patients receiving the drug. If a patient has clinical signs or symptoms that could be due to an adverse effect of theophylline, a serum theophylline concentration should be measured to rule out drug-induced toxicity. For dosage adjustment, serum concentration of theophylline should be measured at steady state after the patient has received a consistent dose for 3 to 5 half-lives of the drug. The half-life of theophylline varies from 3 to 5 hours in children and persons who smoke tobacco to 50 hours or more in patients with severe heart or liver failure. If the theophylline is given as a continuous intravenous infusion, it can take a long time for some patients to achieve effective concentrations, so an intravenous loading dose is commonly administered (Figure 18-1). The ideal situation is to administer an intravenous loading dose that will achieve the desired concentration immediately, then start an intravenous continuous infusion that will maintain that concentration (see Figure 18-1). To derive this perfect situation, the theophylline volume of distribution (V, in liters) would have to be known to compute the loading dose (LD, in milligrams): $LD = Css \cdot V$, where Css is the desired theophylline concentration in milligrams per liter. However, this pharmacokinetic parameter is rarely, if ever, known for a patient, so a loading dose based on a population average volume of distribution is used to calculate the amount of theophylline needed.

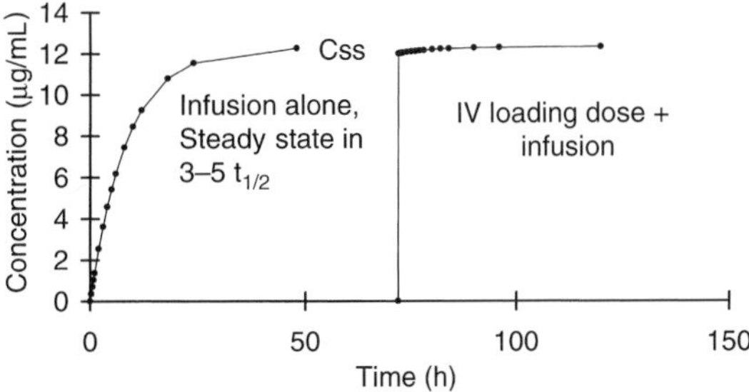

FIGURE 18-1 When intravenous theophylline or aminophylline is administered to a patient as a continuous infusion, it takes 3 to 5 half-lives for serum theophylline concentration to reach steady-state level. Because of this, a considerable amount of time elapses before maximal drug response is achieved. To hasten the onset of drug action, loading doses are given to attain effective theophylline concentration immediately.

Because the patient's unique volume of distribution most likely is greater (resulting in too low a loading dose) or less (resulting in too large a loading dose) than the population average volume of distribution used to compute the loading dose, the desired steady-state theophylline concentration is not achieved. Because of this, it still takes 3 to 5 half-lives for the patient to reach steady-state conditions while receiving an intravenous infusion at a constant rate (Figure 18-2). Thus, intravenous loading doses of theophylline do not usually achieve steady-state serum concentrations immediately. They should, however, produce a therapeutic concentration and response sooner than simply starting an intravenous infusion alone. If oral theophylline-containing products are used, steady-state predose, or "trough" minimum, concentrations should be used to monitor therapy after the patient has received a stable dosage regimen for 3 to 5 half-lives.

After an efficacious theophylline dosage regimen has been established for a patient, serum concentration of theophylline remains fairly stable among patients receiving long-term therapy. In these cases, dosage requirements and steady-state serum concentration of theophylline should be reassessed on a yearly basis. For patients with congestive heart failure or cirrhosis of the liver, dosage requirements of theophylline can vary greatly according to the status of the patient. For example, if a patient with compensated heart failure is receiving a stable dose of theophylline but has an exacerbation of heart disease, it is likely he or she will need to have the theophylline dosage reassessed to avoid theophylline toxicity. Acute viral diseases, especially in children, also have been associated with adverse effects of theophylline among patients whose condition had been stablized with effective, nontoxic theophylline dosage regimens.[9,10] Methods to adjust theophylline doses with serum concentration are discussed later.

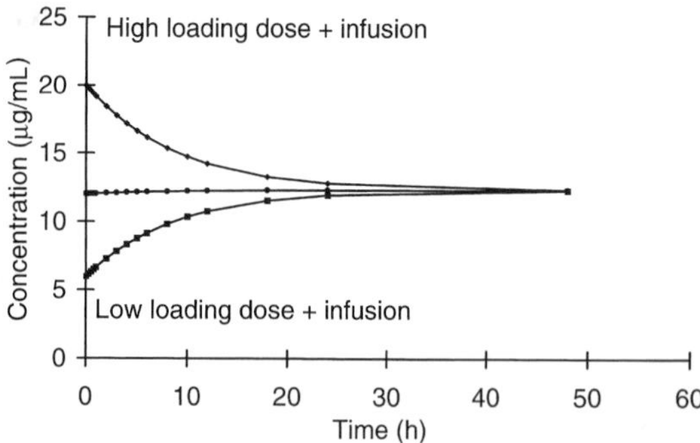

FIGURE 18-2 If the patient's unique volume of distribution (V) of theophylline is known, the exact loading dose (LD) of intravenous theophylline or aminophylline to immediately achieve steady-state theophylline concentration (Css) can be calculated (LD = Css · V). However, the volume of distribution for the patient is rarely known when loading doses have to be administered. For practical purposes, an average population volume of distribution for theophylline is used to estimate the parameter for the patient (V = 0.5 L/kg; ideal body weight is used if the patient is >30% overweight). Because of this, the computed loading dose almost always is too large or too small to reach the desired steady-state theophylline concentration, and it still takes 3 to 5 half-lives to attain steady-state conditions.

BASIC CLINICAL PHARMACOKINETIC PARAMETERS

Theophylline is primarily (>90%) eliminated through hepatic metabolism. Hepatic metabolism is mainly through the CYP1A2 enzyme system, with a smaller amount metabolized by CYP2E1 and CYP3A. About 10% of a theophylline dose is recovered in the urine as unchanged drug.[11,12] Theophylline follows nonlinear pharmacokinetics.[13–15] However, for clinical drug dosing, linear pharmacokinetic concepts and equations can be used to compute doses and estimate serum concentration. Serum concentration of theophylline can increase occasionally more than expected after a dosage increase; nonlinear pharmacokinetics may explain the observation.[13–15.]

Three different forms of theophylline are available. Aminophylline is the ethylenediamine salt of theophylline. Anhydrous aminophylline contains about 85% theophylline, and aminophylline dihydrate contains about 80% theophylline. Oxtriphylline is the choline salt of theophylline and contains about 65% theophylline. Theophylline and aminophylline are available for intravenous injection and oral use. Oxtriphylline is available only for oral use. The oral bioavailability of all three theophylline-based drugs is good and generally is 100%. However, some older sustained-release oral dosage forms have been reported to have incomplete bioavailability and loss of slow-release characteristics under certain circumstances because of tablet or capsule design. Plasma protein binding of theophylline is only 40%.[16,17]

The recommended dose of theophylline or one of its salt forms is based on the concurrent diseases and conditions present in the patient that can influence the pharmacokinetics of theophylline. Pharmacokinetic parameters used to compute doses of theophylline are presented for specific patient profiles.

EFFECTS OF DISEASES AND CONDITIONS ON THEOPHYLLINE PHARMACOKINETICS AND DOSING

In healthy adults without the diseases and conditions described later and who have normal liver function, the average half-life of theophylline is 8 hours (range, 6 to 12 hours) and the volume of distribution is 0.5 L/kg (range, 0.4 to 0.6 L/kg; Table 18-1).[18–20] Most diseases and conditions that change the pharmacokinetics and dosage requirements of theophylline alter clearance, but volume of distribution remains stable at ~0.5 L/kg in these situations. Tobacco and marijuana smoke causes induction of hepatic CYP1A2, which accelerates clearance of theophylline.[18–23] In patients who smoke these substances, the average half-life of theophylline is 5 hours. When patients stop smoking these compounds, theophylline clearance slowly approaches baseline level for the patient over 6 to 12 months if the patient does not encounter secondhand smoke produced by other users.[24] If the patient inhales a sufficient amount of secondhand smoke, theophylline clearance for the ex-smoker can remain in the fully induced state or at an intermediate state.[25]

Patients with cirrhosis of the liver or acute hepatitis have low theophylline clearance, which prolongs the average half-life of theophylline, which is 24 hours.[19,26–28] However, the effect of liver disease on theophylline pharmacokinetics is highly variable and difficult to predict. It is possible for a patient with liver disease to have relatively normal or grossly abnormal clearance and half-life of theophylline. For example, a patient with liver

TABLE 18-1 Diseases and Conditions That Alter the Pharmacokinetics of Theophylline

DISEASE/ CONDITION	HALF-LIFE (h)	VOLUME OF DISTRIBUTION (L/kg)	COMMENT
Adult, normal liver function	8 (range, 6–12)	0.5 (range, 0.4–0.6)	—
Adult, tobacco or marijuana smoker	5	0.5	Tobacco and marijuana smoke induces CYP1A2 enzyme system and accelerates theophylline clearance
Adult, hepatic disease (cirrhosis or acute hepatitis)	24	0.5	Theophylline is metabolized >90% by hepatic microsomal enzymes (primary, CYP1A2; secondary, CYP2E1, CYP3A), so loss of functional liver tissue decreases theophylline clearance. Pharmacokinetic parameters highly variable among patients with liver disease.
Adult, mild heart failure (NYHA CHF class I or II)	12	0.5	Decrease in liver blood flow secondary to decrease in cardiac output due to heart failure decreases theophylline clearance.
Adult, moderate to severe heart failure (NYHA CHF class III or IV) or cor pulmonale	24	0.5	Moderate to severe heart failure reduces cardiac output even more than mild heart failure. The result is large and variable decreases in theophylline clearance. Cardiac status must be monitored closely for patients with heart failure receiving theophylline, because theophylline clearance changes with acute changes in cardiac output.
Adult, obese (>30% over IBW)	According to other diseases or conditions that affect theophylline pharmacokinetics	0.5 (IBW)	Theophylline doses should be based on ideal body weight (IBW) for patients more than 30% above IBW.

TABLE 18-1 *(continued)*

DISEASE/ CONDITION	HALF-LIFE (h)	VOLUME OF DISTRIBUTION (L/kg)	COMMENT
Children, 1–9 years, normal cardiac and hepatic function	3.5	0.5	Children have increased theophylline clearance. When puberty is reached, adult doses can be used to account for diseases and conditions that alter theophylline pharmacokinetics.
Older than 65 years	12	0.5	For elderly persons with concurrent diseases or conditions known to alter theophylline clearance, the drug should be administered according to the specific recommendations.

NYHA, New York Heart Association; CHF, congestive heart failure; IBW, ideal body weight.

disease who smokes cigarettes can have a half-life of theophylline of 5 hours if some liver parenchyma is present and tobacco-induced enyzme induction has occurred or of 50 hours if little or no functional liver tissue remains. An index of liver dysfunction can be gained by applying the Child-Pugh clinical classification system (Table 18-2). Child-Pugh scores are discussed in detail in Chapter 3, but are briefly discussed here. The Child-Pugh score consists of five laboratory tests or clinical symtpoms: serum albumin, total bilirubin, prothrombin time, ascites, and hepatic encephalopathy. Each of these areas is given a score of 1 (normal) to 3 (severely abnormal; see Table 18-2), and the scores for the five

TABLE 18-2 Child-Pugh Scores for Patients with Liver Disease

TEST/SYMPTOM	SCORE 1 POINT	SCORE 2 POINTS	SCORE 3 POINTS
Total bilirubin (mg/dL)	<2.0	2.0–3.0	>3.0
Serum albumin (g/dL)	>3.5	2.8–3.5	<2.8
Prothrombin time (seconds prolonged over control)	<4	4–6	>6
Ascites	Absent	Slight	Moderate
Hepatic encephalopathy	None	Moderate	Severe

Adapted from Pugh RN, Murray-Lyon IM, Dawson JL, Pietroni MC, Williams R. Transection of the oesophagus for bleeding oesophageal varices. Br J Surg 1973;60:646–9.

areas are summed. The Child-Pugh score for a patient with normal liver function is 5. The score for a patient with grossly abnormal serum albumin, total bilirubin, and prothrombin time values in addition to severe ascites and hepatic encephalopathy is 15. A Child-Pugh score greater than 8 is grounds for a decrease in the initial daily dose of theophylline ($t_{1/2}$ = 24 hours). As in the care of any patient with or without liver dysfunction, initial doses are meant as starting points for dosage titration based on patient response and avoidance of adverse effects. Serum theophylline concentration and the presence of adverse drug effects should be monitored frequently in the care of patients with cirrhosis of the liver.

Heart failure reduces theophylline clearance because of a decrease in hepatic blood flow due to compromise of cardiac output.[19,29–32] Venous stasis of blood within the liver also may contribute to the decrease in theophylline clearance among patients with heart failure. Patients with mild heart failure (New York Heart Association [NYHA] class I or II; Table 18-3) have an average theophylline half-life of 12 hours (range, 5 to 24 hours). Those with moderate to severe heart failure (NYHA class III or IV) or cor pulmonale have an average theophylline half-life of 24 hours (5 to 50 hours). The effect of heart failure on the pharmacokinetics of theophylline is highly variable and difficult to predict. It is possible for a patient with heart failure to have a relatively normal or grossly abnormal clearance and half-life of theophylline. In the care of patients with heart failure, initial doses are meant as starting points for dosage titration based on patient response and avoidance of adverse effects. Serum theophylline concentration and the presence of adverse drug effects should be monitored frequently for patients with heart failure.

For obese patients (>30% above ideal body weight [IBW]), volume of distribution estimates should be based on ideal body weight.[33–36] The half-life of theophylline should be based on the concurrent diseases and conditions present in the patient. If weight-based dosage recommendations (mg/kg per day or mg/kg per hour) are to be used, IBW should be used to compute doses for obese patients.

Patient age has an effect on theophylline clearance and half-life. Newborns have decreased theophylline clearance because hepatic drug-metabolizing enzymes are not yet

TABLE 18-3 New York Heart Association Functional Classification of Heart Failure

CLASS	DESCRIPTION
I	Cardiac disease but no limitation of physical activity. Ordinary physical activity does not cause undue fatigue, dyspnea, or palpitation.
II	Cardiac disease that causes slight limitation of physical activity. Ordinary physical activity causes fatigue, palpitation, dyspnea, or angina.
III	Cardiac disease that causes marked limitation of physical activity. Although patients are comfortable at rest, less than ordinary activity causes symptoms.
IV	Cardiac disease that causes an inability to perform physical activity without discomfort. Symptoms of congestive heart failure are present even at rest. With any physical activity, discomfort increases.

Adapted from Johnson JA, Parker RB, Geraci SA. Heart failure. In: DiPiro JT, Talbert RL, Yee GC, Matzke GR, Wells BG, Posey LM, eds. Pharmacotherapy: a pathophysiologic approach. Stamford, CT: Appleton & Lange, 1999:153–81.

fully developed at birth. Premature neonates have an average theophylline half-life of 30 hours 3 to 15 days after birth and 20 hours 25 to 57 days after birth.[37–39] Term infants have an average theophylline half-life of 25 hours 1 to 2 days after birth and 11 hours 3 to 30 weeks after birth.[40–42] Children 1 to 9 years of age have accelerated theophylline clearance, and the average half-life is 3.5 hours (range, 1.5 to 5 hours).[43–45] As children reach puberty, theophylline clearance and half-life approach the values for adults. For persons older than 65 years, results of some studies indicate that theophylline clearance and half-life are the same as for younger adults. Other investigators have found that theophylline clearance is slower and half-life is longer among elderly patients (average half-life, 12 hours; range, 8 to 16 hours).[46–50] A confounding factor in pharmacokinetic studies of theophylline conducted with older adults is the possible accidental inclusion of subjects with subclinical or mild cases of the diseases associated with reduced theophylline clearance, such as heart failure and liver disease. Thus, the pharmacokinetics of theophylline in elderly persons is controversial.

Febrile illnesses can temporarily decrease the clearance of theophylline and necessitate an immediate dosage decrease to avoid toxicity.[9,10] The mechanism of this acute change in theophylline disposition is unclear, but it probably involves decreased clearance due to production of interleukins. Children seem to be at especially high risk of adverse reactions to theophylline because febrile illnesses are prevalent among this population, and high theophylline doses are prescribed on a mg/kg per day basis. Patients with hypothyroidism have decreased basal metabolic rates and need smaller theophylline doses until a euthyroid condition is established.[51] Because only a small amount of theophylline is eliminated unchanged in urine (<10% of a dose), dosage adjustments are not necessary for patients with renal impairment.[11,12] Theophylline is removed by hemodialysis; if possible, doses should be held until after the dialysis procedure is complete.[52–57] If a pulmonary exacerbation occurs because theophylline concentration is decreased, individualized supplemental doses of theophylline may be needed during or after the dialysis session. Theophylline is not appreciably removed by peritoneal dialysis.[55]

DRUG INTERACTIONS

Drug interactions with theophylline are common and occur with a variety of medications.[58] Serious inhibition drug interactions are those that decrease theophylline clearance more than 30%. Clinicians should consider an arbitrary decrease in theophylline dose of 30% to 50% for patients receiving these agents until the actual degree of hepatic enzyme inhibition can be assessed by means of monitoring of serum theophylline concentration. Patients should also be actively observed for the signs and symptoms of theophylline toxicity. The magnitude of drug interactions due to inhibition of hepatic enzymes is highly variable. Some patients may need even larger theophylline dosage decreases, and others have no drug interactions at all. Cimetidine given at higher doses three or more times a day (≥1000 mg/d) decreases theophylline clearance 30% to 50%. Other cimetidine doses given once or twice a day (≤800 mg/d) decrease theophylline clearance 20% or less.[59,60] Ciprofloxacin and enoxacin, both quinolone antibiotics, and troleandomycin, a macrolide antibiotic, also decrease theophylline clearance 30% to 50%. Estrogen and estrogen-containing oral contraceptives, propranolol, metoprolol, mexiletine, propafenone, pentoxifyline, ticlopidine, tacrine, thiabendazole, disulfiram, and fluvoxamine also can decrease theophylline clearance 30% to 50%.

Moderate inhibition drug interactions are those that decrease theophylline clearance 10% to 30%. For this magnitude drug interaction, many clinicians believe that a routine decrease in theophylline dose is unnecessary for patients with steady-state theophylline concentrations less than 15 μg/mL but should be considered on a case-by-case basis for those with concentrations greater than this level. If a decrease is warranted, theophylline doses can be cut 20% to avoid adverse effects. Patients should be actively observed for the signs and symptoms of theophylline toxicity. The calcium channel blockers verapamil and diltiazem have been reported to cause decreases in theophylline clearance of 15% to 25%. Clarithromycin and erythromycin, both macrolide antibiotics, and norfloxacin, a quinolone antibiotic, also can decrease theophylline clearance 15% to 25%. At doses of 600 mg/d or greater, allopurinol has been reported to decrease theophylline clearance 25%.

Theophylline elimination is subject to induction of hepatic microsomal enzymes, which increases theophylline clearance. Because hepatic microsomal enzyme induction is variable, some patients may need theophylline dosage increases whereas others need no alteration in dosage requirements. Hepatic microsomal enzyme induction takes time, and maximal effects may not be seen for 2 to 4 weeks of treatment with enzyme inducers. Patients treated with a drug that increases theophylline clearance need to be carefully observed for signs and symptoms of the disease for which they are taking the drug, and steady-state theophylline concentration should be measured. Disease exacerbations may be caused by a decrease in theophylline concentration, and a dosage increase may be warranted for some patients. Phenytoin, carbamazepine, phenobarbital, rifampin, and moricizine all increase theophylline clearance.

INITIAL DOSAGE DETERMINATION METHODS

Pharmacokinetic Dosing Method

The goal of initial dosing of theophylline is to compute the best dose possible for the patient, given the diseases and conditions that influence theophylline pharmacokinetics and the pulmonary disorder for which the patient is being treated. To do this, pharmacokinetic parameters for the patient are estimated with average parameters measured for other patients with similar diseases and conditions.

ESTIMATE OF HALF-LIFE AND ELIMINATION RATE CONSTANT

Theophylline is predominately metabolized by the liver. There is no good way to estimate the elimination characteristics of liver-metabolized drugs with an endogenous marker of liver function in the same manner that serum creatinine and estimated creatinine clearance are used to estimate the elimination of agents removed by the kidney. Because of this, a patient is categorized according to the diseases and conditions known to change the half-life of theophylline. The previously published half-life is used as an estimate of the half-life in the current patient. For example, for a patient with COPD who currently smokes tobacco-containing cigarettes, the half-life of theophylline is assumed to be 5 hours. For a patient with moderate heart failure (NYHA class III), theophylline half-life is assumed to be 24 hours. A patient with severe liver disease (Child-Pugh score, 12) is assigned an estimated half-life of 24 hours. To produce the most conservative theophylline doses for patients with several concurrent diseases or conditions that affect the pharmacokinetics of theophylline, the disease or condition that causes the longest half-life should be used to compute doses. This approach avoids accidental overdosage as much as currently possible. For instance, for a patient with asthma who currently smokes tobacco-containing cigarettes and has severe liver disease, an estimated theophylline half-life of 24 hours is used to compute initial dosage requirements. Once the current half-life is identified for the patient, it can be converted into the theophylline elimination rate constant (k) with the following equation: $k = 0.693/t_{1/2}$.

ESTIMATE OF VOLUME OF DISTRIBUTION

The volume of distribution of theophylline is relatively stable in patients regardless of the diseases and conditions present. Volume of distribution is assumed to be 0.5 L/kg for nonobese patients. For obese patients (>30% above ideal body weight or IBW), IBW is used to compute the volume of distribution of theophylline. For an 80-kg patient, the estimated volume of distribution of theophylline is 40 L: $V = 0.5 \text{ L/kg} \cdot 80 \text{ kg} = 40 \text{ L}$. For a 150-kg obese patient with an IBW of 60 kg, the estimated theophylline volume of distribution is 30 L: $V = 0.5 \text{ L/kg} \cdot 60 \text{ kg} = 30 \text{ L}$.

SELECTION OF APPROPRIATE PHARMACOKINETIC MODEL AND EQUATIONS

When given by means of continuous intravenous infusion or orally, theophylline follows a one-compartment pharmacokinetic model (Figures 18-1, 18-3, 18-4). When oral therapy is needed, most clinicians use a sustained-release dosage form that has good bioavailability (F = 1), supplies a continuous release of theophylline into the gastrointestinal tract, and provides a smooth theophylline serum concentration–time curve that emulates an intravenous infusion after once- or twice-daily dosing. Because of this, a simple pharmacokinetic equation for computing average steady-state serum concentration of theophylline (Css in μg/mL = mg/L) is widely used and allows calculation of a mainte-

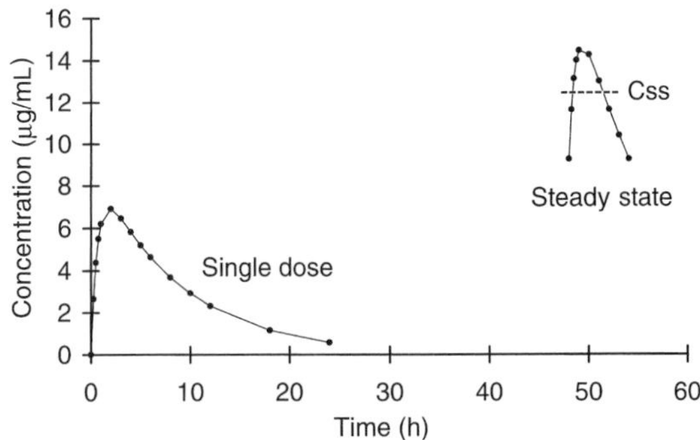

FIGURE 18-3 Serum concentration–time profile for rapid-release theophylline or aminophylline oral dosage forms after a single dose and at steady state (given every 6 hours). The curves shown are typical for an adult cigarette smoker receiving 300 mg theophylline. The steady-state serum concentration (*Css*) expected from an equivalent continuous infusion of theophylline or aminophylline is shown by the *dashed line* in the steady-state concentrations.

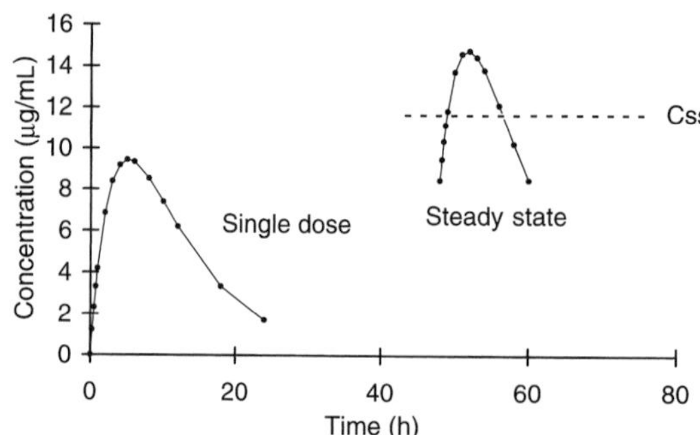

FIGURE 18-4 Serum concentration–time profile for sustained-release theophylline or aminophylline oral dosage forms after a single dose and at steady state (given every 12 hours). The curves shown are typical for an adult cigarette smoker receiving 600 mg theophylline. The steady-state serum concentration (*Css*) expected from an equivalent continuous infusion of theophylline or aminophylline is shown by the *dashed line* in the steady-state concentrations.

nance dosage: Css = [F · S(D/τ)]/Cl, or D = (Css · Cl · τ)/(F · S), where *F* is the bioavailability fraction for the oral dosage form (F = 1 for most oral theophylline sustained-release products), S is the fraction of the theophylline salt form that is active theophylline (S = 1 for theophylline, S = 0.85 for anhydrous aminophylline, S = 0.80 for aminophylline dihydrate, S = 0.65 for oxtriphylline), D is the dose of theophylline salt in milligrams, and τ is the dosage interval in hours. Cl is theophylline clearance in liters per hour and is computed with estimates of theophylline elimination rate constant (k) and volume of distribution: Cl = kV. For example, for a patient with an estimated elimination rate constant of 0.139 h^{-1} and an estimated volume of distribution of 35 L, estimated clearance is 4.87 L/h: Cl = 0.139 h^{-1} · 35 L = 4.87 L/h.

When intravenous therapy is needed, a similar pharmacokinetic equation for computing steady-state serum concentration of theophylline (Css in μg/mL = mg/L) is widely used and allows dosage calculation for a continuous infusion: Css = [S · k_0]/Cl or k_0 = (Css · Cl)/S, where S is the fraction of the theophylline salt form that is active theophylline (S = 1 for theophylline, S = 0.85 for anhydrous aminophylline, S = 0.80 for aminophylline dihydrate), k_0 is the dose of theophylline salt in milligrams per hour, and Cl is theophylline clearance in liters per hour and is computed with estimates of theophylline elimination rate constant (k) and volume of distribution: Cl = kV.

The equation used to calculate an intravenous loading dose (LD, in milligrams) is based on a simple one-compartment model: LD = (Css · V)/S, where Css is the desired steady-state concentration of theophylline in micrograms per milliliter, which is equivalent to milligrams per liter; V is the volume of distribution of theophylline in liters; and S is the fraction of the theophylline salt form that is active theophylline (S = 1 for theophylline, S = 0.85 for anhydrous aminophylline, S = 0.80 for aminophylline dihydrate). Intravenous loading doses of theophylline should be infusions over at least 20 to 30 minutes.

SELECTION OF STEADY-STATE CONCENTRATION

The accepted therapeutic ranges of theophylline are 10 to 20 μg/mL for the management of asthma or COPD and 6 to 13 μg/mL for the management of premature apnea. Recent guidelines suggest that for initial management of pulmonary disease, clinical response to theophylline concentrations of 5 to 15 μg/mL be assessed before higher concentrations are used.[8] Many patients who need long-term theophylline therapy derive sufficient bronchodilatory response with a low likelihood of adverse effects at concentrations of 8 to 12 μg/mL. However, theophylline therapy must be individualized to achieve optimal responses and minimal side effects.

Example 1 LK is a 50-year-old, 75-kg (height, 178 cm) man who has chronic bronchitis. He needs therapy with oral theophylline. He smokes 2 packs of cigarettes a day and has normal liver and heart function. Suggest an initial theophylline dosage regimen designed to achieve a steady-state theophylline concentration of 8 μg/mL. (Note: μg/mL = mg/L, and this concentration unit was substituted for Css in the calculations to avoid unit conversion.)

1. *Estimate half-life and elimination rate constant according to disease states and conditions present in the patient.*

Cigarette smoke induces the enzyme systems responsible for theophylline metabolism, and the expected theophylline half-life ($t_{1/2}$) is 5 hours. The elimination rate constant is computed with the following formula: $k = 0.693/t_{1/2} = 0.693/5\ h = 0.139\ h^{-1}$.

2. *Estimate volume of distribution and clearance.*

The patient is not obese, so the estimated volume of distribution of theophylline is based on actual body weight: $V = 0.5\ L/kg \cdot 75\ kg = 38\ L$. Estimated theophylline clearance is computed by multiplying volume of distribution by elimination rate constant: $Cl = kV = 0.139\ h^{-1} \cdot 38\ L = 5.28\ L/h$.

3. *Compute the dosage regimen.*

Oral sustained-release theophylline tablets are prescribed to this pateint (F = 1, S = 1). Because theophylline has a rapid clearance and short half-life in this patient, the initial dosage interval (τ) is set to 8 hours. (Note: μg/mL = mg/L, and this concentration unit was substituted for Css in the calculations to avoid unit conversion.) The dosage equation for oral theophylline is $D = (Css \cdot Cl \cdot \tau)/(F \cdot S) = (8\ mg/L \cdot 5.28\ L/h \cdot 8\ h)/(1 \cdot 1) = 338\ mg$, rounded to 300 mg every 8 hours.

Steady-state minimum theophylline serum concentration should be measured after steady state is attained in 3 to 5 half-lives. Because the drug is expected to have a half-life of 5 hours in this patient, steady-state concentration of theophylline can be measured any time after the first day of dosing (5 half-lives = 5 · 5 h = 25 h). Serum concentration of theophylline should be measured if the patient has an exacerbation of lung disease or if the patient has signs or symptoms of theophylline toxicity.

Example 2 OI is a 60-year-old, 85-kg (height, 185 cm) man who has emphysema. He needs therapy with oral theophylline. He has cirrhosis of the liver (Child-Pugh score, 11) and normal cardiac function. Suggest an initial theophylline dosage regimen designed to achieve a steady-state theophylline concentration of 10 μg/mL.

1. *Estimate half-life and elimination rate constant according to disease states and conditions present in the patient.*

Patients with severe liver disease have highly variable theophylline pharmacokinetics and dosage requirements. Hepatic disease destroys liver parenchyma, where hepatic drug-metabolizing enzymes are contained. The expected half-life ($t_{1/2}$) of theophylline is 24 hours. The elimination rate constant is computed with the following formula: $k = 0.693/t_{1/2} = 0.693/24\ h = 0.029\ h^{-1}$.

2. *Estimate volume of distribution and clearance.*

The patient is not obese, so the estimated volume of distribution of theophylline is based on actual body weight: $V = 0.5\ L/kg \cdot 85\ kg = 43\ L$. Estimated theophylline clearance is computed by multiplying volume of distribution by elimination rate constant: $Cl = kV = 0.029\ h^{-1} \cdot 43\ L = 1.25\ L/h$.

3. *Compute the dosage regimen.*

Oral sustained-release theophylline tablets are prescribed to this patient ($F = 1$, $S = 1$). The initial dosage interval (τ) is set to 12 hours. (Note: μg/mL = mg/L, and this concentration unit was substituted for Css in the calculations to avoid unit conversion.) The dosage equation for oral theophylline is $D = (Css \cdot Cl \cdot \tau)/(F \cdot S) = (10\ mg/L \cdot 1.25\ L/h \cdot 12\ h)/(1 \cdot 1) = 150$ mg every 12 hours.

Steady-state minimum theophylline serum concentration should be measured after steady state is attained in 3 to 5 half-lives. Because the drug is expected to have a half-life of 24 hours in this patient, steady-state concentration of theophylline can be measured any time after the fifth day of dosing (5 half-lives = $5 \cdot 24\ h = 120\ h$, or 5 d). Serum concentrations of theophylline should be measured if the patient has an exacerbation of lung disease or if the patient has signs or symptoms of theophylline toxicity.

To illustrate the differences and similarities between oral and intravenous theophylline dosage regimen design, the previous cases are used to compute intravenous loading doses and continuous infusions of theophylline.

Example 3 LK is a 50-year-old, 75-kg (height, 178 cm) man who has chronic bronchitis. He needs therapy with intravenous theophylline. He smokes 2 packs of cigarettes a day and has normal liver and heart function. Suggest an initial intravenous dose of aminophylline designed to achieve a steady-state theophylline concentration of 8 μg/mL.

1. *Estimate half-life and elimination rate constant according to disease states and conditions present in the patient.*

Cigarette smoke induces the enzyme systems responsible for theophylline metabolism, and the expected half-life ($t_{1/2}$) of theophylline is 5 hours. The elimination rate constant is computed with the following formula: $k = 0.693/t_{1/2} = 0.693/5\ h = 0.139\ h^{-1}$.

2. *Estimate volume of distribution and clearance.*

The patient is not obese, so the estimated volume of distribution of theophylline is based on actual body weight: $V = 0.5\ L/kg \cdot 75\ kg = 38\ L$. Estimated theophylline clearance is computed by multiplying volume of distribution by elimination rate constant: $Cl = kV = 0.139\ h^{-1} \cdot 38\ L = 5.28\ L/h$.

3. *Compute the dosage regimen.*

Theophylline is administered as the aminophylline dihydrate salt form (S = 0.8). (Note: μg/mL = mg/L, and this concentration unit was substituted for Css in the calculations to avoid unit conversion.) Therapy is started with administration of an intravenous loading dose of aminophylline: LD = (Css · V)/S = (8 mg/L · 38 L)/0.8 = 380 mg, rounded to 400 mg intravenously over 20 to 30 minutes. Continuous intravenous infusion of aminophylline is started immediately after the loading dose has been administered. The dosage equation for intravenous aminophylline is k_0 = (Css · Cl)/S = (8 mg/L · 5.28 L/h)/0.8 = 53 mg/h, rounded to 55 mg/h.

Steady-state serum concentration of theophylline should be measured after steady state is attained in 3 to 5 half-lives. Because the drug is expected to have a half-life of 5 hours, steady-state concentration of theophylline can be measured any time after the first day of dosing (5 half-lives = 5 · 5 h = 25 h). Serum concentration of theophylline should be measured if the patient has an exacerbation of lung disease or if the pateint has signs or symptoms of theophylline toxicity.

Example 4 OI is a 60-year-old, 85-kg (height, 185 cm) man who has emphysema. He needs therapy with intravenous aminophylline. He has cirrhosis of the liver (Child-Pugh score, 11) and normal cardiac function. Suggest an initial intravenous aminophylline dosage regimen designed to achieve a steady-state theophylline concentration of 10 μg/mL.

1. *Estimate half-life and elimination rate constant according to disease states and conditions present in the patient.*

Patients with severe liver disease have highly variable theophylline pharmacokinetics and dosage requirements. Hepatic disease destroys liver parenchyma, where hepatic drug-metabolizing enzymes are contained. The expected half-life ($t_{1/2}$) of theophylline is 24 hours. The elimination rate constant is computed with the following formula: k = $0.693/t_{1/2}$ = 0.693/24 h = 0.029 h^{-1}.

2. *Estimate volume of distribution and clearance.*

The patient is not obese, so the estimated volume of distribution of theophylline is based on actual body weight: V = 0.5 L/kg · 85 kg = 43 L. Estimated theophylline clearance is computed by multiplying volume of distribution by elimination rate constant: Cl = kV = 0.029 h^{-1} · 43 L = 1.25 L/h.

3. *Compute the dosage regimen.*

Theophylline is administered as the aminophylline dihydrate salt form (S = 0.8). (Note: μg/mL = mg/L, and this concentration unit was substituted for Css in the calculations to avoid unit conversion.) Therapy is started with administration of an intravenous loading dose of aminophylline: LD = (Css · V)/S = (10 mg/L · 43 L)/0.8 = 538 mg, rounded to 500 mg intravenously over 20 to 30 minutes. Continuous intravenous infusion of aminophylline is started immediately after the loading dose has been administered. The dosage equation for intravenous aminophylline is k_0 = (Css · Cl)/S = (10 mg/L · 1.25 L/h)/0.8 = 16 mg/h, rounded to 15 mg/h.

Steady-state serum concentration of theophylline should be measured after steady state is attained in 3 to 5 half-lives. Because the drug is expected to have a half-life of 24 hours in this patient, steady-state concentration of theophylline can be measured any time after the fifth day of dosing (5 half-lives = 5 · 24 h = 120 h, or 5 d). Serum concentration of theophylline should be measured if the patient has an exacerbation of lung disease or if the patient has signs or symptoms of theophylline toxicity.

Literature-Based Recommended Dosing

Because of the large variability in theophylline pharmacokinetics, even when concurrent diseases and conditions are identified, many clinicians believe that the use of standard theophylline doses for various situations is warranted.[19,61,62] The original computation of these doses was based on the pharmacokinetic dosing method described earlier and modified according to clinical experience. In general, the expected steady-state serum concentration of theophylline used to compute these doses was 10 μg/mL. Suggested theophylline maintenance doses stratified by diseases and conditions known to alter theophylline pharmacokinetics are given in Table 18-4.[62] For obese persons (>30% over IBW), IBW should be used to compute doses.[33–36] Because the doses are given in terms of theophylline, doses for other theophylline salt forms must be adjusted accordingly (S = 0.85 for anhydrous aminophylline, S = 0.8 for aminophylline dihydrate, S = 0.65 for oxtriphylline). If theophylline is to be given orally, the dose given in Table 18-4 (in mg/kg per hour) must be multiplied by the appropriate dosage interval for the dosage form being used: D = (theophylline dose · Wt · τ)/S, where Wt is patient weight in kilograms, τ is the dosage interval in hours, and S is the appropriate salt form correction factor for aminophylline or oxtriphylline. If theophylline is to be given in a continuous intravenous infusion, the following equation is used to compute the infusion rate: k_0 = (theophylline dose · Wt)/S, where Wt is patient weight in kilograms, and S is the appropriate salt form correction factor for aminophylline. When a patient has more than one disease or condition, choosing the lowest dose suggested in Table 18-4 gives the safest, most conservative dosage recommendation. If an intravenous loading dose is necessary, theophylline

TABLE 18-4 Theophylline Clearance and Dosage Rates for Patients with Various Diseases and Conditions

DISEASE/CONDITION	MEAN DOSE (mg/kg per hour)
Child 1–9 y of age	0.8
Child 9–12 y of age or adult smokers	0.7
Adolescent 12–16 y of age	0.5
Adult nonsmoker	0.4
Nonsmoker older than 65 y	0.3
Decompensated congestive heart failure, cor pulmonale, cirrhosis	0.2

From Edwards DJ, Zarowitz BJ, Slaughter RL. Theophylline. In: Evans WE, Schentag JJ, Jusko WJ, Relling MV, eds. Applied pharmacokinetics. Vancouver, WA: Applied Therapeutics, 1992.

5 mg/kg or aminophylline 6 mg/kg is used. IBW is used to compute loading doses for obese patients (>30% over IBW).

To illustrate the similarities and differences between this method of dosage calculation and the pharmacokinetic dosing method, the previous examples are used.

Example 5 LK is a 50-year-old, 75-kg (height, 178 cm) man who has chronic bronchitis. He needs therapy with oral theophylline. He smokes 2 packs of cigarettes a day and has normal liver and heart function. Suggest an initial theophylline dosage regimen for this patient.

1. *Choose the theophylline dose based on disease states and conditions present in the patient.*

A theophylline dose of 0.7 mg/kg per hour is suggested in Table 18-4 for an adult cigarette smoker.

2. *Compute the dosage regimen.*

Oral sustained-release theophylline tablets are prescribed to this patient (F = 1, S = 1). Because theophylline has a rapid clearance and half-life in this patient, the initial dosage interval (τ) is set to 8 hours: D = (theophylline dose · weight · τ)/S = (0.7 mg/kg/h · 75 kg · 8 h)/1 = 420 mg, rounded to 400 mg every 8 hours. This dose is similar to that established with the pharmacokinetic dosing method, 300 mg every 8 hours.

Steady-state minimum serum concentration of theophylline should be measured after steady state is attained in 3 to 5 half-lives. Because the drug is expected to have a half-life of 5 hours in this patient, steady-state concentration of theophylline can be measured any time after the first day of dosing (5 half-lives = 5 · 5 h = 25 h). Serum concentration of theophylline should be measured if the patient has an exacerbation of lung disease or if the patient has signs or symptoms of theophylline toxicity.

Example 6 OI is a 60-year-old, 85-kg (height, 185 cm) man who has emphysema. He needs therapy with oral theophylline. He has cirrhosis of the liver (Child-Pugh score, 11) and normal cardiac function. Suggest an initial theophylline dosage regimen for this patient.

1. *Choose the theophylline dose based on disease states and conditions present in the patient.*

A theophylline dose of 0.2 mg/kg per hour is suggested by the table for an adult with cirrhosis.

2. *Compute the dosage regimen.*

Oral sustained-release theophylline tablets are prescribed to this patient (F = 1, S = 1). The initial dosage interval (τ) is set to 12 hours: D = (theophylline dose · weight · τ)/S = (0.2 mg/kg/h · 85 kg · 12 h)/1 = 204 mg, rounded to 200 mg every 12 hours. This dose is similar to that established with the pharmacokinetic dosing method, 150 mg every 12 hours.

Steady-state minimum serum concentration of theophylline should be measured after steady state is attained in 3 to 5 half-lives. Because the drug is expected to have a half-life of 24 hours in this patient, steady-state concentration of theophylline can be measured any time after the fifth day of dosing (5 half-lives = 5 · 24 h · 120 h, or 5 days). Serum concentration of theophylline should be measured if the patient has an exacerbation of lung disease or if the patient has signs or symptoms of theophylline toxicity.

To illustrate the differences and similarities between designs of oral and intravenous theophylline dosage regimens, the previous cases are used to compute intravenous loading doses and continuous infusions of theophylline.

Example 7 LK is a 50-year-old, 75-kg (height, 178 cm) man who has chronic bronchitis. He needs therapy with intravenous theophylline. He smokes 2 packs of cigarettes a day and has normal liver and heart function. Suggest an initial theophylline dosage regimen for this patient.

1. *Choose the theophylline dose based on disease states and conditions present in the patient.*

A theophylline dose of 0.7 mg/kg per hour is suggested in the Table 18-4 for an adult smoker.

2. *Compute the dosage regimen.*

Theophylline is administered intravenously (S = 1): k_0 = (theophylline dose · weight)/S = 0.7 mg/kg/h · 75 kg)/1 = 53 mg/h, rounded to 55 mg/h. A loading dose of theophylline 5 mg/kg also is prescribed: LD = 5 mg/kg · 75 kg = 375 mg, rounded to 400 mg of theophylline infused over 20 to 30 minutes. These are similar to the doses established with the pharmacokinetic dosing method.

Serum concentration of theophylline should be measured after steady state is attained in 3 to 5 half-lives. Because the drug is expected to have a half-life of 5 hours in this patient, steady-state concentration of theophylline can be measured any time after the first day of dosing (5 half-lives = 5 · 5 h = 25 h). Serum concentration of theophylline should be measured if the patient has an exacerbation of lung disease or if the patient has signs or symptoms of theophylline toxicity.

Example 8 OI is a 60-year-old, 85-kg (height, 185 cm) man who has emphysema. He needs therapy with intravenous theophylline. He has cirrhosis of the liver (Child-Pugh score, 11) and normal cardiac function. Suggest an initial intravenous aminophylline dosage regimen for this patient.

1. *Choose the theophylline dose based on disease states and conditions present in the patient.*

A theophylline dose of 0.2 mg/kg per hour is suggested in Table 18-4 for an adult with cirrhosis.

2. *Compute the dosage regimen.*

Theophylline is administered as the aminophylline dihydrate salt form (S = 0.8): D = (theophylline dose · weight)/S = (0.2 mg/kg/h · 85 kg)/0.8 = 21 mg/h, rounded to 20 mg/h. A loading dose of 6 mg/kg aminophylline also is prescribed: LD = 6 mg/kg · 85 kg = 510 mg, rounded to 500 mg of aminophylline infused over 20 to 30 minutes. These doses are similar to those established with the pharmacokinetic dosing method, a 500-mg loading dose followed by a 15-mg/h continuous infusion.

Steady-state serum concentration of theophylline should be measured after steady state is attained in 3 to 5 half-lives. Because the drug is expected to have a half-life of 24 hours in this patient, steady-state concentration of theophylline can be measured any time after the fifth day of dosing (5 half-lives = 5 · 24 h = 120 h, or 5 d). Serum concentration of theophylline should be measured if the patient has an exacerbation of lung disease or if the patient has signs or symptoms of theophylline toxicity.

USE OF THEOPHYLLINE SERUM CONCENTRATIONS TO ALTER DOSES

Because of the large pharmacokinetic variability among patients, it is likely that doses computed with patient population characteristics do not always produce serum theophylline concentrations that are expected or desirable. Because of pharmacokinetic variability, the narrow therapeutic index of theophylline, and the severity of side effects of theophylline, measurement of serum theophylline concentration is mandatory to ensure that therapeutic, nontoxic levels are present. In addition to serum theophylline concentrations, important patient parameters, such as results of pulmonary function tests, clinical signs and symptoms of the pulmonary disease, and presence of side effects of theophylline, should be followed to confirm that the patient is responding to treatment and not having adverse drug reactions.

When serum theophylline concentration is measured and a dosage change is necessary, clinicians should use the simplest, most straightforward method available to determine a dose that will provide safe and effective treatment. In most cases, a simple dosage ratio can be used to change theophylline doses if the drug follows linear pharmacokinetics. Although it has been clearly demonstrated in research studies that theophylline follows nonlinear pharmacokinetics,[13–15] in the clinical setting most patients' steady-state serum concentrations change proportionally to theophylline doses less than and within the therapeutic range, and assuming linear pharmacokinetics is adequate for dosage adjustments in most patients.

Sometimes it is useful to compute theophylline pharmacokinetic constants for a patient and base dosage adjustments on these. In this case, it may be possible to calculate and use pharmacokinetic parameters to alter theophylline dose. In some situations, it may be necessary to compute theophylline clearance for the patient during a continuous infusion before steady-state conditions occur using the Chiou method. This pharmacokinetic parameter can be used to calculate the best drug dose. Computerized methods that incorporate expected population pharmacokinetic characteristics (Bayesian pharmacokinetics computer programs) can be used when serum concentration is measured at suboptimal times or the patient is not at steady state when serum concentration is measured.

Linear Pharmacokinetics Method

Because theophylline follows linear, dose-proportional pharmacokinetics in most patients with concentrations within or below the therapeutic range, steady-state serum concentration changes in proportion to dose according to the following equation: $D_{new}/Css_{new} = D_{old}/Css_{old}$, or $D_{new} = (Css_{new}/Css_{old})D_{old}$, where D is the dose, Css is the steady-state concentration, old indicates the dose that produced the steady-state concentration that the patient is currently receiving, and new denotes the dose necessary to produce the desired steady-state concentration. The advantages of this method are that it is quick and simple. The disadvantages are that steady-state concentrations are required and that the assumption of linear pharmacokinetics may not be valid for all patients. When steady-state serum concentration increases more than expected after a dosage increase or decreases less than expected after a dosage decrease, nonlinear theophylline pharmacokinetics is a possible explanation. Because of this, suggested dosage increases greater than 75% with this method should be scrutinized by the prescribing clinician. The risk versus benefit for the patient should be assessed before large dosage increases (>75% over current dose) are made.

Example 9 LK is a 50-year-old, 75-kg (height, 178 cm) man who has chronic bronchitis. He is receiving 300 mg every 8 hours of oral theophylline sustained-release tablets. He smokes 2 packs of cigarettes a day and has normal liver and heart function. Current steady-state theophylline concentration is 8 μg/mL. Compute a theophylline dose to provide a steady-state concentration of 12 μg/mL.

1. *Compute the new dose to achieve the desired serum concentration.*

The patient smokes tobacco-containing cigarettes and is expected to achieve steady-state conditions after the first day (5 half-lives = 5 · 5 h = 25 h) of therapy. According to linear pharmacokinetics, the new dose to attain the desired concentration should be proportional to the old dose that produced the measured concentration (total daily dose = 300 mg/dose · 3 doses/d = 900 mg/d):

$$D_{new} = (Css_{new}/Css_{old})D_{old} = [(12\ \mu g/mL)/(8\ \mu g/mL)]\ 900\ mg/d = 1350\ mg/d$$

The new suggested dose is 1350 mg/d, or 450 mg every 8 hours, of theophylline sustained-release tablets to be started at the next scheduled dosing time.

Steady-state minimum serum concentration of theophylline should be measured after steady state is attained in 3 to 5 half-lives. Because the drug is expected to have a half-life of 5 hours in this patient, the steady-state concentration of theophylline can be obtained any time after the first day of dosing (5 half-lives = 5 · 5 h = 25 h). Serum concentration of theophylline should be measured if the patient has an exacerbation of lung disease or if the patient has signs or symptoms of theophylline toxicity.

Example 10 OI is a 60-year-old, 85-kg (height, 185 cm) man who has emphysema. He is receiving 200 mg every 12 hours of oral theophylline sustained-release tablets. He has cirrhosis of the liver (Child-Pugh score, 11) and normal cardiac function. Current steady-state theophylline concentration is 15 μg/mL. The patient has minor caffeine-type adverse effects (insomnia, jitteriness, nausea). Compute a theophylline dose to provide a steady-state concentration of 10 μg/mL.

1. *Compute the new dose to achieve the desired serum concentration.*

The patient has severe liver disease and is expected to achieve steady-state conditions after 5 days (5 half-lives = 5 · 24 h = 120 h, or 5 d) of therapy. According to linear pharmacokinetics, the new dose to attain the desired concentration should be proportional to the old dose that produced the measured concentration (total daily dose = 200 mg/dose · 2 doses/d = 400 mg/d):

$$D_{new} = (Css_{new}/Css_{old})D_{old} = [(10\ \mu g/mL)/(15\ \mu g/mL)]\ 400\ mg/d = 267\ mg/d$$

The new suggested dose is 267 mg/d, or 134 mg every 12 hours, rounded to 150 mg every 12 hours, of theophylline sustained-release tablets to be started after one or two doses are held and adverse effects have subsided.

Steady-state minimum serum concentration of theophylline should be measured after steady state is attained in 3 to 5 half-lives. Because the drug is expected to have a half-life of 24 hours in this patient, steady-state concentration of theophylline can be measured any time after the fifth day of dosing (5 half-lives = 5 · 24 h = 120 h, or 5 d). Serum concentration of theophylline should be measured if the patient has an exacerbation of lung disease or if the patient has signs or symptoms of theophylline toxicity.

To illustrate the differences and similarities between oral and intravenous designs of theophylline dosage regimens, the previous cases are used to compute altered intravenous continuous infusions of theophylline with steady-state serum concentration.

Example 11 LK is a 50-year-old, 75-kg (height, 178 cm) man who has chronic bronchitis. He is receiving a constant intravenous infusion of aminophylline at a rate of 50 mg/h. He smokes 2 packs of cigarettes a day and has normal liver and heart function. Current steady-state theophylline concentration is 8 μg/mL. Compute an aminophylline infusion rate to provide a steady-state concentration of 12 μg/mL.

1. *Compute the new dose to achieve the desired serum concentration.*

The patient smokes tobacco-containing cigarettes and is expected to achieve steady-state conditions after the first day (5 half-lives = 5 · 5 h = 25 h) of therapy. According to linear pharmacokinetics, the new infusion rate to attain the desired concentration should be proportional to the old infusion rate that produced the measured concentration:

$$D_{new} = (Css_{new}/Css_{old})D_{old} = [(12\ \mu g/mL)/(8\ \mu g/mL)]\ 50\ mg/h = 75\ mg/h$$

The new suggested infusion rate is 75 mg/h of aminophylline.

Steady-state serum concentration of theophylline should be measured after steady state is attained in 3 to 5 half-lives. Because the drug is expected to have a half-life of 5 hours in this patient, steady-state concentration of theophylline can be measured any time after the first day of dosing (5 half-lives = 5 · 5 h = 25 h). Serum concentrations of theophylline should be measured if the patient has an exacerbation of lung disease or if the patient has signs or symptoms of theophylline toxicity.

Example 12 OI is a 60-year-old, 85-kg (height, 185 cm) man who has emphysema. He is receiving a 20-mg/h continuous infusion of theophylline. He has cirrhosis of the liver (Child-Pugh score, 11) and normal cardiac function. Current steady-state theophylline concentration is 15 μg/mL. The patient has minor caffeine-type adverse effects (insomnia, jitteriness, nausea). Compute a theophylline dose to provide a steady-state concentration of 10 μg/mL.

1. *Compute the new dose to achieve the desired serum concentration.*

The patient has severe liver disease and is expected to achieve steady-state conditions after 5 days (5 half-lives = 5 · 24 h = 120 h, or 5 d) of therapy. According to linear pharmacokinetics, the new infusion rate to attain the desired concentration should be proportional to the old infusion rate that produced the measured concentration:

$$D_{new} = (Css_{new}/Css_{old})D_{old} = [(10\ \mu g/mL)/(15\ \mu g/mL)]\ 20\ mg/h$$
$$= 13\ mg/h,\ \text{rounded to}\ 15\ mg/h$$

The new suggested dose is 15 mg/h of theophylline in a continuous infusion. If necessary, the infusion can be stopped for 12 to 24 hours until adverse effects of theophylline have subsided.

Steady-state minimum serum concentration of theophylline should be measured after steady state is attained in 3 to 5 half-lives. Because the drug is expected to have a half-life of 24 hours in this patient, steady-state concentration of theophylline can be measured any time after the fifth day of dosing (5 half-lives = 5 · 24 h = 120 h, or 5 d). Serum concentration of theophylline should be measured if the patient has an exacerbation of lung disease or if the patient has signs or symptoms of theophylline toxicity.

Pharmacokinetic Parameter Method

The pharmacokinetic parameter method of adjusting drug dosages was among the first techniques whereby doses were changed according to serum concentration. It allows computation of a patient's unique pharmacokinetic constants and uses those to calculate a dose that achieves the desired theophylline concentration. The pharmacokinetic parameter method requires that steady state has been achieved, and only steady-state concentration (Css) of theophylline is used. During a continuous intravenous infusion, the following equation is used to compute theophylline clearance (Cl): $Cl = [S \cdot k_0]/Css$, where S is the fraction of the theophylline salt form that is active theophylline (S = 1 for theophylline, S = 0.85 for anhydrous aminophylline, S = 0.80 for aminophylline dihydrate) and k_0 is the dose of theophylline salt in milligrams per hour. If the patient is receiving oral theophylline therapy, theophylline clearance (Cl) can be calculated with the following formula: $Cl = [F \cdot S\ (D/\tau)]/Css$, where F is the bioavailability fraction for the oral dosage form (F = 1 for most oral theophylline sustained-release products), S is the fraction of the theophylline salt form that is active theophylline (S = 1 for theophylline, S = 0.85 for anhydrous aminophylline, S = 0.80 for aminophylline dihydrate, S = 0.65 for oxtriphylline), D is the dose of theophylline salt in milligrams, Css is steady-state theophylline concentration, and τ is the dosage interval in hours.

Theophylline serum concentration occasionally is measured before and after an intravenous loading dose. In a one-compartment model, the volume of distribution (V) is calculated with the following equation: $V = (S \cdot D)/(C_{postdose} - C_{predose})$, where S is the fraction of the theophylline salt form that is active theophylline (S = 1 for theophylline, S = 0.85 for anhydrous aminophylline, S = 0.80 for aminophylline dihydrate), D is the dose of theophylline salt in milligrams, $C_{postdose}$ is the concentration in milligrams per liter after the loading dose is administered, and $C_{predose}$ is the concentration in milligrams per liter before the loading dose is administered (both concentrations should be obtained within 30 to 60 minutes of administration). If the predose concentration is also a steady-state concentration, theophylline clearance can be computed. If both clearance (Cl) and volume of distribution (V) have been measured with these techniques, half-life [$t_{1/2} = (0.693 \cdot V)/Cl$] and elimination rate constant ($k = 0.693/t_{1/2} = Cl/V$) can be calculated. The clearance, volume of distribution, elimination rate constant, and half-life measured with these techniques are the patient's unique theophylline pharmacokinetic constants and can be used in one-compartment model equations to compute the required dose to achieve any desired serum concentration. Because linear pharmacokinetics are assumed in this method, theophylline doses computed with the pharmacokinetic parameter method and the linear pharmacokinetic method should be identical.

Example 13 LK is a 50-year-old, 75-kg (height, 178 cm) man who has chronic bronchitis. He is receiving 300 mg every 8 hours of oral theophylline sustained-release tablets. He smokes 2 packs of cigarettes a day and has normal liver and heart function. Current steady-state theophylline concentration is 8 μg/mL. Compute a theophylline dose to provide a steady-state concentration of 12 μg/mL.

1. *Compute pharmacokinetic parameters.*

The patient smokes tobacco-containing cigarettes and is expected to achieve steady-state conditions after the first day (5 half-lives = $5 \cdot 5$ h = 25 h) of therapy. Theophylline clearance can be computed with steady-state theophylline concentration: $Cl = [F \cdot S\ (D/\tau)]/Css = [1 \cdot 1\ (300\ mg/8\ h)]/(8\ mg/L) = 4.69\ L/h$. (Note: μg/mL = mg/L, and this concentration unit was substituted for Css in the calculations to avoid unit conversion.)

2. *Compute the theophylline dose.*

Theophylline clearance is used to compute the new dose: $D = (Css \cdot Cl \cdot \tau)/(F \cdot S) = (12\ mg/L \cdot 4.69\ L/h \cdot 8\ h)/(1 \cdot 1) = 450$ mg every 8 hours. The new theophylline dosage regimen is instituted at the next dosage time.

Steady-state minimum serum concentration of theophylline should be measured after steady state is attained in 3 to 5 half-lives. Because the drug is expected to have a half-life of 5 hours in this patient, steady-state concentration of theophylline can be measured any time after the first day of dosing (5 half-lives = $5 \cdot 5$ h = 25 h). Serum concentration of theophylline should be measured if the patient has an exacerbation of lung disease or if the patient has signs or symptoms of theophylline toxicity.

Example 14 OI is a 60-year-old, 85-kg (height, 185 cm) man who has emphysema. He is receiving 200 mg every 12 hours of oral theophylline sustained-release tablets. He has cirrhosis of the liver (Child-Pugh score, 11) and normal cardiac function. Current steady-state theophylline concentration is 15 μg/mL. The patient has minor caffeine-type adverse effects (insomnia, jitteriness, nausea). Compute a theophylline dose to provide a steady-state concentration of 10 μg/mL.

1. *Compute pharmacokinetic parameters.*

The patient has severe liver disease and is expected to achieve steady-state conditions after 5 days (5 half-lives = $5 \cdot 24$ h = 120 h, or 5 d) of therapy. Theophylline clearance can be computed with steady-state theophylline concentration: $Cl = [F \cdot S\ (D/\tau)]/Css = [1 \cdot 1$

(200 mg/12 h)]/(15 mg/L) = 1.11 L/h. (Note: μg/mL = mg/L, and this concentration unit was substituted for Css in the calculations to avoid unit conversion.)

2. *Compute the theophylline dose.*

Theophylline clearance is used to compute the new dose: D = (Css · Cl · τ)/(F · S) = (10 mg/L · 1.11 L/h · 12 h)/(1 · 1) = 133 mg, rounded to 150 mg every 12 hours. The new dose is started after one or two doses are held and adverse effects have subsided.

Steady-state minimum serum concentration of theophylline should be measured after steady state is attained in 3 to 5 half-lives. Because the drug is expected to have a half-life of 24 hours in this patient, steady-state concentration of theophylline can be measured any time after the fifth day of dosing (5 half-lives = 5 · 24 h = 120 h, or 5 d). Serum concentration of theophylline should be measured if the patient has an exacerbation of lung disease or if the patient has signs or symptoms of theophylline toxicity.

To illustrate the differences and similarities between designs of oral and intravenous theophylline dosage regimens, the previous cases are used to compute altered intravenous continuous infusions of theophylline with steady-state serum concentration.

Example 15 LK is a 50-year-old, 75-kg (height, 178 cm) man who has chronic bronchitis. He is receiving a constant intravenous infusion of aminophylline at a rate of 50 mg/h. He smokes 2 packs of cigarettes a day and has normal liver and heart function. Current steady-state theophylline concentration is 8 μg/mL. Compute an aminophylline infusion rate to provide a steady-state concentration of 12 μg/mL.

1. *Compute pharmacokinetic parameters.*

The patient smokes tobacco-containing cigarettes and is expected to achieve steady-state conditions after the first day (5 half-lives = 5 · 5 h = 25 h) of therapy. Theophylline clearance can be computed with steady-state theophylline concentration: Cl = [S · k_0]/Css = [0.8 · 50 mg/h]/(8 mg/L) = 5 L/h. (Note: μg/mL = mg/L, and this concentration unit was substituted for Css in the calculations to avoid unit conversion.)

2. *Compute the theophylline dose.*

Theophylline clearance is used to compute the new aminophylline infusion rate: k_0 = (Css · Cl)/S = (12 mg/L · 5 L/h)/(0.8) = 75 mg/h. The new aminophylline infusion rate is instituted immediately.

Steady-state serum concentration of theophylline should be measured after steady state is attained in 3 to 5 half-lives. Because the drug is expected to have a half-life of 5 hours in this patient, steady-state concentration of theophylline can be measured any time after the first day of dosing (5 half-lives = 5 · 5 h = 25 h). Serum concentration of theophylline should be measured if the patient has an exacerbation of lung disease or if the patient has signs or symptoms of theophylline toxicity.

Example 16 OI is a 60-year-old, 85-kg (height, 185 cm) man who has emphysema. He is receiving a 20-mg/h continuous infusion of theophylline. He has cirrhosis of the liver (Child-Pugh score, 11) and normal cardiac function. Current steady-state theophylline concentration is 15 μg/mL. The patient has minor caffeine-type adverse effects (insomnia, jitteriness, nausea). Compute a theophylline dose to provide a steady-state concentration of 10 μg/mL.

1. *Compute pharmacokinetic parameters.*

The patient has severe liver disease and is expected to achieve steady-state conditions after 5 days (5 half-lives = 5 · 24 h = 120 h, or 5 d) of therapy. Theophylline clearance can be computed with steady-state theophylline concentration: Cl = [S · k_0]/Css = [1 · 20 mg/h]/(15 mg/L) = 1.33 L/h. (Note: μg/mL = mg/L, and this concentration unit was substituted for Css in the calculations to avoid unit conversion.)

2. *Compute the theophylline dose.*

Theophylline clearance is used to compute the new theophylline infusion rate: k_0 = (Css · Cl)/S = (10 mg/L · 1.33 L/h)/(1) = 13 mg/h, rounded to 15 mg/h. The new suggested dose is 15 mg/h of theophylline in a continuous infusion. If necessary, the infusion can be stopped for 12 to 24 hours until adverse effects of theophylline have subsided.

Steady-state serum concentration of theophylline should be measured after steady state is attained in 3 to 5 half-lives. Because the drug is expected to have a half-life of 24 hours in this patient, steady-state concentration of theophylline can be measured any time after the fifth day of dosing (5 half-lives = 5 · 24 h = 120 h, or 5 d). Serum concentration of theophylline should be measured if the patient has an exacerbation of lung disease or if the patient has signs or symptoms of theophylline toxicity.

Example 17 PP is a 59-year-old, 65-kg (height, 173 cm) man who has emphysema. He is receiving a constant intravenous infusion of aminophylline at a rate of 15 mg/h. He smokes 2 packs of cigarettes a day and has normal liver function. He has heart failure (NYHA class IV). Steady-state theophylline concentration is 6 μg/mL. Compute an infusion rate of aminophylline that will provide a steady-state concentration of 10 μg/mL. In an attempt to boost theophylline concentration as soon as possible, an intravenous bolus of 300 mg aminophylline is given over 30 minutes before the infusion rate is increased. Serum concentration of theophylline after the additional bolus dose is 12 μg/mL.

1. *Compute pharmacokinetic parameters.*

The patient has severe heart failure and is expected to achieve steady-state conditions after 5 days (5 half-lives = 5 · 24 h = 120 h, or 5 d) of therapy. Theophylline clearance can be computed with steady-state theophylline concentration: Cl = [S · k_0]/Css = [0.8 · 15 mg/h]/(6 mg/L) = 2 L/h. (Note: μg/mL = mg/L, and this concentration unit was substituted for Css in the calculations to avoid unit conversion.)

The volume of distribution of theophylline can be computed with the concentrations before the bolus dose (Css = 6 μg/mL) and after the bolus dose: V = (S · D)/($C_{postdose}$ − $C_{predose}$) = (0.8 · 300 mg)/(12 mg/L − 6 mg/L) = 40 L. (Note: μg/mL = mg/L, and this concentration unit was substituted for Css in the calculations to avoid unit conversion.) Theophylline half-life ($t_{1/2}$) and elimination rate constant (k) can be computed: $t_{1/2}$ = (0.693 · V)/Cl = (0.693 · 40 L)/(2 L/h) = 14 h; k = Cl/V = (2 L/h)/(40 L) = 0.05 h^{-1}.

2. *Compute the theophylline dose.*

Theophylline clearance is used to compute the new aminophylline infusion rate: $k_0 = (Css \cdot Cl)/S = (10 \text{ mg/L} \cdot 2 \text{ L/h})/(0.8) = 25 \text{ mg/h}$. The new aminophylline infusion rate is instituted immediately after the additional loading dose is given.

Serum concentration of theophylline should be measured after steady state is attained in 3 to 5 half-lives. Because the drug has a half-life of 14 hours in this patient, steady-state concentration of theophylline can be measured after 3 days of continuous dosing (5 half-lives = 5 · 14 h = 70 h). Serum concentration of theophylline should be measured if the patient has an exacerbation of lung disease or if the patient has signs or symptoms of theophylline toxicity.

CHIOU METHOD

For some patients, it is desirable to individualize theophylline infusion rates as rapidly as possible before steady state is achieved. Examples are patients with heart failure or hepatic cirrhosis who have variable theophylline pharmacokinetic parameters and long half-lives of theophylline. In this situation, two theophylline serum concentrations measured at least 4 to 6 hours apart during continuous infusion can be used to compute theophylline clearance and dosing rates.[63–65] In addition to this requirement, the only way theophylline can be entering the patient's body must be through intravenous infusion. Thus, the last dose of sustained-release theophylline must have been administered no less than 12 to 16 hours before this technique is used, or some residual oral theophylline will still be absorbed from the gastrointestinal tract and cause computation errors.

The following equation is used to compute theophylline clearance (Cl) using theophylline concentrations:

$$Cl = \frac{2 \cdot S \cdot k_0}{C_1 + C_2} + \frac{2V(C_1 - C_2)}{(C_1 + C_2)\,(t_2 - t_1)}$$

where S is the fraction of the theophylline salt form that is active theophylline (S = 1 for theophylline, S = 0.85 for anhydrous aminophylline, S = 0.80 for aminophylline dihydrate), k_0 is the infusion rate of the theophylline salt, V is volume of distribution of theophylline (assumed to be 0.5 L/kg; IBW is used for patients >30% overweight), C_1 and C_2 are the first and second theophylline serum concentrations, and t_1 and t_2 are the times that C_1 and C_2 were obtained. Once theophylline clearance (Cl) is determined, it can be used to adjust the infusion rate (k_0) of theophylline salt with the following relation: $k_0 = (Css \cdot Cl)/S$, where S is the fraction of the theophylline salt form that is active theophylline (S = 1 for theophylline, S = 0.85 for anhydrous aminophylline, S = 0.80 for aminophylline dihydrate).

Example 18 JB is a 50-year-old, 60-kg (height, 170 cm) man who has heart failure (NYHA class III). A 50-mg/h aminophylline infusion is started after administration of an intravenous loading dose. Theophylline concentration is 15.6 μg/mL at 1000 H and 18.3 μg/mL at 1400 H. What aminophylline infusion rate is needed to achieve a steady-state concentration of 15 μg/mL?

1. *Compute theophylline clearance and dose.*

$$Cl = \frac{2 \cdot S \cdot k_0}{C_1 + C_2} + \frac{2V(C_1 - C_2)}{(C_1 + C_2)(t_2 - t_1)}$$

$$Cl = \frac{2[0.8(50 \text{ mg/h})]}{15.6 \text{ mg/L} + 18.3 \text{ mg/L}} + \frac{2(0.5 \text{ L/kg} \cdot 60 \text{ kg})(15.6 \text{ mg/L} - 18.3 \text{ mg/L})}{(15.6 \text{ mg/L} + 18.3 \text{ mg/L})\ 4 \text{ h}} = 1.17 \text{ L/h}$$

(Note: μg/mL = mg/L, and this concentration unit was substituted for concentrations to avoid unit conversion. The difference between t_2 and t_1 is determined and placed directly in the calculation.)

$$k_0 = (Css \cdot Cl)/S = (15 \text{ mg/L} \cdot 1.17 \text{ L/h})/0.8$$
$$= 22 \text{ mg/h, rounded to 20 mg/h of aminophylline}$$

Example 19 YU is a 64-year-old, 80-kg (height, 175 cm) man who has COPD. He smokes 1½ packs of cigarettes per day. A 40-mg/h theophylline infusion is started after administration of an intravenous loading dose at 0900 H. Theophylline concentration is 11.6 μg/mL at 1000 H and 8.1 μg/mL at 1600 H. What theophylline infusion rate is needed to achieve a steady-state concentration of 10 μg/mL?

1. *Compute theophylline clearance and dose.*

$$Cl = \frac{2 \cdot S \cdot k_0}{C_1 + C_2} + \frac{2V(C_1 - C_2)}{(C_1 + C_2)(t_2 - t_1)}$$

$$Cl = \frac{2[1(40 \text{ mg/h})]}{11.6 \text{ mg/L} + 8.1 \text{ mg/L}} + \frac{2(0.5 \text{ L/kg} \cdot 80 \text{ kg})(11.6 \text{ mg/L} - 8.1 \text{ mg/L})}{(11.6 \text{ mg/L} + 8.1 \text{ mg/L})\ 6 \text{ h}} = 6.43 \text{ L/h}$$

(Note: μg/mL = mg/L, and this concentration unit was substituted for concentrations to avoid unit conversion. The difference between t_2 and t_1 is determined and placed directly in the calculation.)

$$k_0 = (Css \cdot Cl)/S = (10 \text{ mg/L} \cdot 6.43 \text{ L/h})/1 = 64 \text{ mg/h, rounded to 65 mg/h of theophylline}$$

BAYESIAN PHARMACOKINETICS COMPUTER PROGRAMS

Computer programs are available to assist in computation of pharmacokinetic parameters for patients. In the most reliable computer programs, a nonlinear regression algorithm incorporates components of Bayes' theorem. Nonlinear regression is a statistical technique in which an iterative process is used to compute the best pharmacokinetic parameters for a concentration–time data set. The patient's drug dosage schedule and serum concentrations are entered into the computer. The computer program has a pharmacokinetic equation programmed for the drug and administration method, such as oral, intravenous bolus, or intravenous infusion. A one-compartment model typically is used, although some programs allow the user to choose among several different equations. With population estimates based on demographic information for the patient, such as age, weight, sex, liver function, and cardiac status, supplied by the user, the computer program estimates serum concentrations for each time at which there are actual serum concentrations. Kinetic parameters are changed by the program, and a new set of estimated serum concentrations are computed. The pharmacokinetic parameters that generate the estimated serum concentrations closest to the actual values are stored in the computer memory, and the process is repeated until the set of pharmacokinetic parameters that produces estimated serum concentrations statistically closest to the actual serum concentrations is generated. These pharmacokinetic parameters can be used to compute improved dosing schedules for patients. Bayes' theorem is used in the computer algorithm to balance the results of the computations between values based solely on the patient's serum drug concentrations and those based only on patient population parameters. Results of studies in which various methods of dosage adjustment have been compared have shown consistently that these types of computer dosing programs perform at least as well as experienced clinical pharmacokineticists and clinicians and better than inexperienced clinicians.

Some clinicians use Bayesian pharmacokinetics computer programs exclusively to alter drug doses based on serum concentrations. An advantage of this approach is that consistent dosage recommendations are made when several practitioners are involved in therapeutic drug monitoring programs. However, because simpler dosing methods work just as well for patients with stable pharmacokinetic parameters and steady-state drug concentrations, many clinicians reserve the use of computer programs for more difficult situations. Those situations include serum concentrations that are not at steady state, serum concentrations not obtained at the specific times needed to use simpler methods, and unstable pharmacokinetic parameters. Many Bayesian pharmacokinetics computer programs are available, and most should provide answers similar to the ones used in the following examples. The program used to solve problems in this book is DrugCalc written by Dr. Dennis Mungall. It is available at his Internet web site (http://members.aol.com/thertch/index.htm).[66]

Example 20 LK is a 50-year-old, 75-kg (height, 178 cm) man who has chronic bronchitis. He is receiving 300 mg every 8 hours of oral theophylline sustained-release tablets. He smokes 2 packs of cigarettes a day and has normal liver (bilirubin, 0.7 mg/dL; albumin, 4.0 g/dL) and heart function. The current steady-state theophylline concentration is 8 μg/mL. Compute a theophylline dose to provide a steady-state concentration of 12 μg/mL.

1. *Enter the patient's demographic, drug dosing, and serum concentration–time data into the computer program.*

2. *Compute pharmacokinetic parameters for the patient with a Bayesian pharmacokinetics computer program.*

The pharmacokinetic parameters computed with the program are a volume of distribution of 37 L, a half-life of 5.9 hours, and a clearance of 4.33 L/h.

3. *Compute the dose required to achieve the desired serum concentration of theophylline.*

The one-compartment model, first-order absorption equations used in the program to compute doses indicate that a dose of 450 mg every 8 hours produces a steady-state theophylline concentration of 12 μg/mL. Use of the linear pharmacokinetics and pharmacokinetic parameter methods described earlier produces the same answer for this patient.

Example 21 HJ is a 62-year-old, 87-kg (height, 185 cm) man who has emphysema. He is given a new prescription for 300 mg every 12 hours of oral theophylline sustained-release tablets. He has cirrhosis of the liver (Child-Pugh score, 12; bilirubin, 3.2 mg/dL; albumin, 2.5 g/dL) and normal cardiac function. The theophylline concentration after the sixth dose is 15 μg/mL. The patient has minor caffeine-type adverse effects (insomnia, jitteriness, nausea). Compute a theophylline dose that will provide a steady-state concentration of 10 μg/mL.

1. *Enter the patient's demographic, drug dosing, and serum concentration–time data into the computer program.*

In this case, it is unlikely that the patient is at steady state, so the linear pharmacokinetics method cannot be used.

2. *Compute pharmacokinetic parameters for the patient with a Bayesian pharmacokinetics computer program.*

The pharmacokinetic parameters computed with the program are a volume of distribution of 38 L, a half-life of 19 hours, and a clearance of 1.41 L/h.

3. *Compute the dose required to achieve the desired serum concentration of theophylline.*

The one-compartment, first-order absorption equations used in the program to compute doses indicate that a dose of 200 mg every 12 hours produces a steady-state concentration of 11 μg/mL.

Example 22 JB is a 50-year-old, 60-kg (height, 170 cm) man who has heart failure (NYHA class III). A 50-mg/h aminophylline infusion is started after administration at 0800 H of an intravenous loading dose of 500 mg aminophylline over 20 minutes. Theophylline concentration is 15.6 μg/mL at 1000 H and 18.3 μg/mL at 1400 H. What aminophylline infusion rate is needed to achieve a steady-state concentration of 15 μg/mL?

1. *Enter the patient's demographic, drug dosing, and serum concentration–time data into the computer program.*

In this case, it is unlikely that the patient is at steady state, so the linear pharmacokinetics method cannot be used. DrugCalc requires that doses be entered in terms of theophylline, so aminophylline doses must be converted to theophylline doses (LD = 500 mg aminophylline · 0.8 = 400 mg theophylline; k_0 = 50 mg/h aminophylline · 0.8 = 40 mg/h theophylline).

2. *Compute pharmacokinetic parameters for the patient with a Bayesian pharmacokinetics computer program.*

The pharmacokinetic parameters computed with the program are a volume of distribution of 29 L, a half-life of 21 hours, and clearance of 0.98 L/h.

3. *Compute the dose required to achieve the desired serum concentration of theophylline.*

The one-compartment model, intravenous infusion equations used in the program to compute doses indicate that a dose of aminophylline 20 mg/h produces a steady-state concentration of 16 μg/mL. Use of the Chiou method described earlier produces a comparable answer for this patient (20 mg/h to produce a steady-state concentration of 15 μg/mL).

USE OF THEOPHYLLINE BOOSTER DOSES FOR IMMEDIATE INCREASES IN SERUM CONCENTRATIONS

If a patient has a subtherapeutic theophylline serum concentration in an acute situation, it may be desirable to increase theophylline concentration as quickly as possible. In this setting, it is not acceptable simply to increase the maintenance dose and wait 3 to 5 half-lives for therapeutic serum concentrations to be established. A rational way to increase serum concentrations rapidly is to administer a booster dose of theophylline (a process also known as "re-loading" the patient with theophylline) computed with pharmacokinetic techniques. A modified loading dose equation is used to compute the booster dose (BD). The equation takes into account current theophylline concentration: $BD = [(C_{desired} - C_{actual})V]/S$, where $C_{desired}$ is the desired theophylline concentration, C_{actual} is the actual current theophylline concentration for the patient, S is the fraction of the theophylline salt form that is active theophylline (S = 1 for theophylline, S = 0.85 for anhydrous aminophylline, S = 0.80 for aminophylline dihydrate), and V is the volume of distribution of theophylline. If the volume of distribution of theophylline is known for the patient, it can be used in the calculation. However, this value usually is not known and is assumed to be the population average of 0.5 L/kg (IBW is used for patients >30% overweight).

Concurrent with administration of the booster dose, the maintenance dose of theophylline usually is increased. Clinicians need to recognize that administration of a booster dose does not alter the time required to achieve steady-state conditions when a new theophylline dosage rate is prescribed. It still takes 3 to 5 half-lives to attain steady state when the dosage rate is changed. However, the difference between theophylline concentration after the booster dose and the ultimate steady-state concentration usually is reduced when the extra dose of drug is given.

Example 23 BN is a 22-year-old, 50-kg (height, 157 cm) woman who has asthma. She is receiving therapy with intravenous theophylline. She does not smoke cigarettes and has normal liver and heart function. After an initial loading dose of aminophylline (300 mg) and a maintenance infusion of 20 mg/h aminophylline for 16 hours, theophylline concentration is 5.6 μg/mL. The pulmonary function test results are worsening. Compute a booster dose of aminophylline to achieve a theophylline concentration of 10 μg/mL.

1. *Estimate volume of distribution according to disease states and conditions present in the patient.*

In the case of theophylline, the population average volume of distribution is 0.5 L/kg. This value is used to estimate the parameter for the patient. The patient is not obese, so actual body weight is used in the computation: $V = 0.5\ L/kg \cdot 50\ kg = 25\ L$.

2. *Compute the booster dose.*

The booster dose is computed with the following equation: $BD = [(C_{desired} - C_{actual})V]/S = [(10\ mg/L - 5.6\ mg/L)25\ L]/0.8 = 138\ mg$, rounded to 150 mg of aminophylline infused over 20 to 30 minutes. (Note: μg/mL = mg/L, and this concentration unit was substituted for concentration variables in the calculations to avoid unit conversion.) If the maintenance dose is increased, an additional 3 to 5 estimated half-lives elapse before new steady-state conditions are achieved. Theophylline serum concentration should be measured at that time.

CONVERSION OF THEOPHYLLINE DOSES FROM INTRAVENOUS TO ORAL ROUTE OF ADMINISTRATION

Patients whose condition is stablized with theophylline therapy sometimes need a change from the oral route of administration to an equivalent continuous infusion or vice versa.[67] In general, oral theophylline dosage forms, including most sustained-release tablets and capsules, have a bioavailability of 1. If equal serum theophylline concentrations are desired, conversion between the intravenous [$k_0 = (Css \cdot Cl)/S$] and oral [$D = (Css \cdot Cl \cdot \tau)/(F \cdot S)$] routes of administration is simple because equivalent doses of drug (corrected for theophylline salt form) are prescribed: $k_0 = D_{po}/(24\ h/d \cdot S_{iv})$, or $D_{po} = S_{iv} \cdot k_0 \cdot 24\ h/d$, where k_0 is the equivalent rate of intravenous infusion of theophylline salt in milligrams per hour, D_{po} is the equivalent dose of oral theophylline in milligrams per day, and S_{iv} is the fraction of the intravenously administered theophylline salt form that is active theophylline.

Example 24 JH is receiving oral sustained-release theophylline 600 mg every 12 hours. She is responding well to therapy, has no adverse drug effects, and has a steady-state theophylline concentration of 14.7 μg/mL. Suggest an equivalent dose of aminophylline given as an intravenous infusion.

1. *Calculate the equivalent intravenous dose of aminophylline.*

The patient is receiving 600 mg every 12 hours, or 1200 mg/d (600 mg/dose · 2 doses/d = 1200 mg/d) of theophylline. The equivalent intravenous aminophylline dose is $k_0 = D_{po}/(24\ h/d \cdot S_{iv}) = (1200\ mg/d)/(24\ h/d \cdot 0.8) = 62.5\ mg/h$, rounded to 65 mg/h of aminophylline as a continuous intravenous infusion.

Example 25 LK is receiving a continuous infusion of aminophylline at the rate of 40 mg/h. He is responding well to therapy, has no adverse drug effects, and has a steady-state theophylline concentration of 11.3 μg/mL. Suggest an equivalent dose of sustained-release oral theophylline.

1. *Calculate the equivalent oral dose of theophylline.*

The patient is receiving 40 mg/h of intravenous aminophylline as a constant infusion. The equivalent oral sustained-release theophylline dose is $D_{po} = S_{iv} \cdot k_0 \cdot 24\ h/d = 0.8 \cdot 40\ mg/h \cdot 24\ h/d = 768\ mg/d$, rounded to 800 mg/d. The patient is given a prescription for theophylline sustained-release tablets 400 mg orally every 12 hours.

REMOVAL OF THEOPHYLLINE BODY STORES IN MANAGEMENT OF THEOPHYLLINE OVERDOSE

In addition to supportive care, management of seizures with anticonvulsant agents, and management of cardiac arrhythmia with antiarrhythmic agents, removal of theophylline from the body should be considered in cases of acute and chronic overdosage.[61] Extracorporeal methods to remove theophylline in emergencies include hemodialysis[52–57] and charcoal hemoperfusion.[68,69] Hemoperfusion is a technique similar to hemodialysis except the blood is passed through a column of activated charcoal instead of through an artificial kidney. Charcoal hemoperfusion is effective in removing theophylline from the blood. The extraction ratio across the column is greater than 90%, but theophylline serum concentration can rebound 5 to 10 μg/mL on discontinuation of the procedure as theophylline in the tissues comes into equilibrium with the blood.[68,69] Serum theophylline concentration should be closely monitored when charcoal hemoperfusion is instituted. Other complications of charcoal hemoperfusion include hypotension, hypocalcemia, platelet consumption, and bleeding.

Theophylline can be removed from the body with oral doses of activated charcoal.[70,71] This method to reduce theophylline body stores is about as effective as hemodialysis removal. Activated charcoal adsorbs theophylline, rendering it nonabsorbable from the gastrointestinal tract. If the patient is vomiting, appropriate antiemetic therapy must be instituted so that the charcoal is retained in the stomach. Phenothiazine antiemetics should be avoided because they can decrease the seizure threshold. For an acute theophylline overdose, oral activated charcoal (0.5 g/kg up to 20 g, repeated at least once in 1 to 2 hours) binds theophylline that has not yet been absorbed and holds it in the gastrointestinal tract. Oral activated charcoal also enhances the clearance of theophylline by binding theophylline secreted in gastrointestinal juices and eliminating the drug in the stool. Used this way, oral activated charcoal (0.5 g/kg up to 20 g) is given every 2 hours. For both methods of administration, a dose of oral sorbitol should be given to hasten removal of charcoal-bound theophylline from the intestine.

After acute and chronic theophylline overdoses, a single dose of oral activated charcoal is recommended if serum theophylline concentration is 20 to 30 μg/mL. For serum theophylline concentrations >30 μg/mL, multiple doses of oral activated charcoal should be used. Patients should be observed for signs and symptoms of theophylline toxicity and treated appropriately. Theophylline serum concentration should be measured every 2 to 4 hours to guide further therapy.

PROBLEMS

The following problems are intended to emphasize the computation of initial and individualized doses with clinical pharmacokinetic techniques. Clinicians always should consult the patient's chart to confirm that current pulmonary therapy, including inhaled bronchodilators and steroids, is appropriate. All other medications that the patient is taking, including prescription and nonprescription drugs, should be recorded and checked to ascertain the risk of drug interaction with theophylline.

1. NJ is a 67-year-old, 72-kg (height, 185 cm) man who has chronic bronchitis. He needs therapy with oral theophylline. He smokes 3 packs of cigarettes a day and has normal liver and heart function. Suggest an initial oral theophylline dosage regimen designed to achieve a steady-state theophylline concentration of 10 μg/mL.

2. Patient NJ (see problem 1) is given a prescription for theophylline sustained-release tablets 500 mg orally every 8 hours. Current steady-state theophylline concentration is 18 μg/mL. Compute a new oral theophylline dose to provide a steady-state concentration of 12 μg/mL.

3. GF is a 56-year-old, 81-kg (height, 175 cm) man who has emphysema. He needs therapy with oral theophylline. He has cirrhosis of the liver (Child-Pugh score, 12) and normal cardiac function. Suggest an initial theophylline dosage regimen designed to achieve a steady-state theophylline concentration of 8 μg/mL.

4. Patient GF (see problem 3) is given a prescription for theophylline sustained-release tablets 100 mg orally every 12 hours. Current steady-state theophylline concentration is 8 μg/mL. Compute a new oral theophylline dose to provide a steady-state concentration of 12 μg/mL.

5. YU is a 71-year-old, 60-kg (height, 157 cm) woman who has COPD. She needs therapy with oral theophylline. She has severe heart failure (NYHA class IV) and normal liver function. Suggest an initial theophylline dosage regimen designed to achieve a steady-state theophylline concentration of 8 μg/mL.

6. Patient YU (see problem 5) is given a prescription for theophylline sustained-release tablets 200 mg orally every 12 hours. Serum concentration of theophylline just before the sixth dose of this regimen is 19.5 μg/mL. Assuming the theophylline concentration was zero before the first dose, compute a new oral theophylline dose to provide a steady-state concentration of 12 μg/mL.

7. WE is a 24-year-old, 55-kg (height, 165 cm) woman who has asthma. She needs therapy with oral theophylline. She does not smoke cigarettes and has normal liver and heart function. Suggest an initial oral theophylline dosage regimen designed to achieve a steady-state theophylline concentration of 12 μg/mL.

8. Patient WE (see problem 7) is given a prescription for theophylline sustained-release tablets 400 mg orally every 12 hours. Serum concentration of theophylline just before the third dose of this regimen is 13.5 μg/mL. Assuming theophylline concentration was zero before the first dose, compute a new oral theophylline dose to provide a steady-state concentration of 10 μg/mL.

9. IO is a 62-year-old, 130-kg (height, 180 cm) man who has COPD. He needs therapy with oral theophylline. He has mild heart failure (NYHA class I) and normal liver function. Suggest an initial theophylline dosage regimen designed to achieve a steady-state theophylline concentration of 8 μg/mL.

10. Patient IO (see problem 9) is given a prescription for theophylline sustained-release tablets 200 mg orally every 12 hours. Serum concentration of theophylline just before the sixth dose of this regimen is 6.2 μg/mL. Assuming the theophylline concentration was zero before the first dose, compute a new oral theophylline dose to provide a steady-state concentration of 10 μg/mL.

11. LG is a 53-year-old, 69-kg (height, 178 cm) man who has chronic bronchitis. He needs therapy with intravenous theophylline. He smokes 2 packs of cigarettes a day and has normal liver and heart function. Suggest an initial aminophylline dosage regimen designed to achieve a steady-state theophylline concentration of 8 μg/mL.

12. Patient LG (see problem 11) is given a prescription for intravenous aminophylline 50 mg/h. Serum concentration of theophylline after 24 hours of this regimen is

7.4 μg/mL. Compute a new intravenous aminophylline infusion and an aminophylline booster dose that will provide a steady-state concentration of 11 μg/mL.

13. CV is a 69-year-old, 90-kg (height, 185 cm) man who has emphysema. He needs therapy with intravenous theophylline. He has cirrhosis of the liver (Child-Pugh score, 11) and normal cardiac function. Suggest an initial intravenous aminophylline dosage regimen designed to achieve a steady-state theophylline concentration of 10 μg/mL.

14. Patient CV (see problem 13) is given a prescription for intravenous aminophylline 25 mg/h. A loading dose of 400 mg aminophylline is administered over 30 minutes before the continuous infusion is begun. Theophylline serum concentration after 72 hours of infusion is 25.2 μg/mL. Compute a new intravenous aminophylline infusion to provide a steady-state concentration of 15 μg/mL.

15. PE is a 61-year-old, 67-kg (height, 168 cm) woman who has COPD. She needs therapy with intravenous theophylline. She has severe heart failure (NYHA class IV) and normal liver function. Suggest an initial intravenous aminophylline dosage regimen designed to achieve a steady-state theophylline concentration of 8 μg/mL.

16. Patient PE (see problem 15) is given a prescription for 20 mg/h intravenous aminophylline. A loading dose of 350 mg aminophylline is administered over 20 minutes before the continuous infusion is begun. Serum theophylline concentrations 12 hours and 24 hours after the start of infusion are 14.2 μg/mL and 18.6 μg/mL. Compute a new intravenous aminophylline infusion to provide a steady-state concentration of 18 μg/mL.

ANSWERS TO PROBLEMS

1. The initial theophylline dose for patient NJ is calculated as follows.

Pharmacokinetic Dosing Method

1. *Estimate half-life and elimination rate constant according to disease states and conditions present in the patient.*

Cigarette smoke induces the enzyme systems responsible for theophylline metabolism. The expected half-life ($t_{1/2}$) of theophylline is 5 hours. The elimination rate constant is computed with the following formula: $k = 0.693/t_{1/2} = 0.693/5\ h = 0.139\ h^{-1}$.

2. *Estimate volume of distribution and clearance.*

The patient is not obese, so the estimated volume of distribution of theophylline is based on actual body weight: $V = 0.5\ L/kg \cdot 72\ kg = 36\ L$. Estimated theophylline clearance is computed by multiplying volume of distribution by elimination rate constant: $Cl = kV = 0.139\ h^{-1} \cdot 36\ L = 5.0\ L/h$.

3. *Compute the dosage regimen.*

Oral sustained-release theophylline tablets are prescribed to this patient ($F = 1$, $S = 1$). Because the patient has a rapid clearance and half-life of theophylline, the initial dosage interval (τ) is set to 8 hours. (Note: μg/mL = mg/L, and this concentration unit was substituted for Css in the calculations to avoid unit conversion.) The dosage equation for oral theophylline is D = (Css · Cl · τ)/(F · S) = (10 mg/L · 5.0 L/h · 8 h)/(1 · 1) = 400 mg every 8 hours.

Steady-state minimum serum concentration of theophylline should be measured after steady state is attained in 3 to 5 half-lives. Because the drug is expected to have a half-life of 5 hours in this patient, steady-state concentration of theophylline can be measured any time after the first day of dosing (5 half-lives = 5 · 5 h = 25 h). Serum concentration of theophylline should be measured if the patient has an exacerbation of lung disease or if the patient has signs or symptoms of theophylline toxicity.

Literature-Based Recommended Dosing

1. *Choose the theophylline dose based on disease states and conditions present in the patient.*

A theophylline dose of 0.7 mg/kg per hour is suggested in Table 18-4 for an adult smoker.

2. *Compute the dosage regimen.*

Oral sustained-release theophylline tablets are prescribed to this patient (F = 1, S = 1). Because the patient has a rapid clearance and half-life of theophylline, the initial dosage interval (τ) is set to 8 hours: D = (theophylline dose · weight · τ)/S = (0.7 mg/kg/h · 72 kg · 8 h)/1 = 403 mg, rounded to 400 mg every 8 hours. This dose is identical to that established with the pharmacokinetic dosing method.

Steady-state minimum serum concentration of theophylline should be measured after steady state is attained in 3 to 5 half-lives. Because the drug is expected to have a half-life of 5 hours in this patient, steady-state concentration of theophylline can be measured any time after the first day of dosing (5 half-lives = 5 · 5 h = 25 h). Serum concentration of theophylline should be measured if the patient has an exacerbation of lung disease or if the patient has signs or symptoms of theophylline toxicity.

2. The revised theophylline dose for patient NJ is calculated as follows.

Linear Pharmacokinetics Method

1. *Compute the new dose to achieve the desired serum concentration.*

The patient smokes tobacco-containing cigarettes and is expected to achieve steady-state conditions after the first day (5 half-lives = 5 · 5 h = 25 h) of therapy. According to linear pharmacokinetics, the new dose to attain the desired concentration should be proportional to the old dose that produced the measured concentration (total daily dose = 500 mg/dose · 3 doses/d = 1500 mg/d):

$$D_{new} = (Css_{new}/Css_{old})D_{old} = [(12\ \mu g/mL)/(18\ \mu g/mL)]\ 1500\ mg/d = 1000\ mg/d$$

The new suggested dose is rounded to 900 mg/d, or 300 mg every 8 hours, of theophylline sustained-release tablets to be started at the next scheduled dosing time.

Steady-state minimum serum concentration of theophylline should be measured after steady state is attained in 3 to 5 half-lives. Because the drug is expected to have a half-life of 5 hours in this patient, steady-state concentration of theophylline can be measured any time after the first day of dosing (5 half-lives = 5 · 5 h = 25 h). Serum concentration of theophylline should be measured if the patient has an exacerbation of lung disease or if the patient has signs or symptoms of theophylline toxicity.

Pharmacokinetic Parameter Method

1. *Compute pharmacokinetic parameters.*

The patient smokes tobacco-containing cigarettes and is expected to achieve steady-state conditions after the first day (5 half-lives = 5 · 5 h = 25 h) of therapy. Theophylline clearance can be computed with steady-state theophylline concentration: Cl = [F · S (D/τ)]/Css = [1 · 1 (500 mg/8 h)]/(18 mg/L) = 3.47 L/h. (Note: μg/mL = mg/L, and this concentration unit was substituted for Css in the calculations to avoid unit conversion.)

2. *Compute the theophylline dose.*

Theophylline clearance is used to compute the new dose: D = (Css · Cl · τ)/(F · S) = (12 mg/L · 3.47 L/h · 8 h)/(1 · 1) = 333 mg, rounded to 300 mg every 8 hours. The new theophylline dosage regimen is instituted at the next dosage time.

Steady-state minimum serum concentration of theophylline should be measured after steady state is attained in 3 to 5 half-lives. Because the drug is expected to have a half-life of 5 hours in this patient, steady-state concentration of theophylline can be measured any time after the first day of dosing (5 half-lives = 5 · 5 h = 25 h). Serum concentration of theophylline should be measured if the patient has an exacerbation of lung disease or if the patient has signs or symptoms of theophylline toxicity.

3. The initial theophylline dose for patient GF is calculated as follows.

Pharmacokinetic Dosing Method

1. *Estimate half-life and elimination rate constant according to disease states and conditions present in the patient.*

Patients with severe liver disease have highly variable theophylline pharmacokinetics and dosage requirements. Hepatic disease destroys liver parenchyma, where hepatic drug-metabolizing enzymes are contained. The expected half-life ($t_{1/2}$) of theophylline is 24 hours. The elimination rate constant is computed with the following formula: $k = 0.693/t_{1/2} = 0.693/24\ h = 0.029\ h^{-1}$.

2. *Estimate volume of distribution and clearance.*

The patient is not obese, so the estimated volume of distribution of theophylline is based on actual body weight: V = 0.5 L/kg · 81 kg = 41 L. Estimated theophylline clearance is computed by multiplying volume of distribution by elimination rate constant: $Cl = kV = 0.029\ h^{-1} \cdot 41\ L = 1.19\ L/h$.

3. *Compute the dosage regimen.*

Oral sustained-release theophylline tablets are prescribed to this patient (F = 1, S = 1). The initial dosage interval (τ) is set to 12 hours. (Note: μg/mL = mg/L, and this concentration unit was substituted for Css in the calculations to avoid unit conversion.) The dosage equation for oral theophylline is D = (Css · Cl · τ)/(F · S) = (8 mg/L · 1.19 L/h · 12 h)/(1 · 1) = 114 mg, rounded to 100 mg every 12 hours.

Steady-state minimum serum concentration of theophylline should be measured after steady state is attained in 3 to 5 half-lives. Because the drug is expected to have a half-life of 24 hours in this patient, steady-state concentration of theophylline can be measured any time after the fifth day of dosing (5 half-lives = 5 · 24 h = 120 h, or 5 d). Serum concentration of theophylline should be measured if the patient has an exacerbation of lung disease or if the patient has signs or symptoms of theophylline toxicity.

Literature-Based Recommended Dosing

1. *Choose the theophylline dose based on disease states and conditions present in the patient.*

A theophylline dose of 0.2 mg/kg per hour is suggested in Table 18-4 for an adult with cirrhosis.

2. *Compute the dosage regimen.*

Oral sustained-release theophylline tablets are prescribed to this patient (F = 1, S = 1). The initial dosage interval (τ) is set to 12 hours: D = (theophylline dose · weight · τ)/S = (0.2 mg/kg/h · 81 kg · 12 h)/1 = 194 mg, rounded to 200 mg every 12 hours. This dose is similar to that established with the pharmacokinetic dosing method, 100 mg every 12 hours.

Steady-state minimum serum concentration of theophylline should be measured after steady state is attained in 3 to 5 half-lives. Because the drug is expected to have a half-life of 24 hours in this patient, steady-state concentration of theophylline can be measured any time after the fifth day of dosing (5 half-lives = 5 · 24 h = 120 h, or 5 d). Serum concentration of theophylline should be measured if the patient has an exacerbation of lung disease or if the patient has signs or symptoms of theophylline toxicity.

4. The revised theophylline dose for patient GF is calculated as follows.

Linear Pharmacokinetics Method

1. *Compute the new dose to achieve the desired serum concentration.*

The patient has liver disease and is expected to achieve steady-state conditions after the fifth day (5 half-lives = 5 · 24 h = 120 h, or 5 d) of therapy. According to linear pharmacokinetics, the new dose to attain the desired concentration should be proportional to the old dose that produced the measured concentration (total daily dose = 100 mg/dose · 2 doses/d = 200 mg/d):

$$D_{new} = (Css_{new}/Css_{old})D_{old} = [(12\ \mu g/mL)/(8\ \mu g/mL)\ 200\ mg/d] = 300\ mg/d$$

The new suggested dose is 300 mg/d, or 150 mg every 12 hours, of theophylline sustained-release tablets to be started at the next scheduled dosing time.

Steady-state minimum serum concentration of theophylline should be measured after steady state is attained in 3 to 5 half-lives. Because the drug is expected to have a half-life of 24 hours in this patient, steady-state concentration of theophylline can be measured any time after the fifth day of dosing (5 half-lives = 5 · 24 h = 120 h, or 5 d). Serum concentration of theophylline should be measured if the patient has an exacerbation of lung disease or if the patient has signs or symptoms of theophylline toxicity.

Pharmacokinetic Parameter Method

1. *Compute pharmacokinetic parameters.*

The patient has liver disease and is expected to achieve steady-state conditions after the fifth day (5 half-lives = 5 · 24 h = 120 h, or 5 d) of therapy. Theophylline clearance can be computed with steady-state theophylline concentration: $Cl = [F \cdot S\ (D/\tau)]/Css = [1 \cdot 1\ (100\ mg/12\ h)]/(8\ mg/L) = 1.04\ L/h$. (Note: μg/mL = mg/L, and this concentration unit was substituted for Css in the calculations to avoid unit conversion.)

2. *Compute the theophylline dose.*

Theophylline clearance is used to compute the new dose: $D = (Css \cdot Cl \cdot \tau)/(F \cdot S) = (12\ mg/L \cdot 1.04\ L/h \cdot 12\ h)/(1 \cdot 1) = 150$ mg every 12 hours. The new theophylline dosage regimen is instituted at the next dosage time.

Steady-state minimum serum concentration of theophylline should be measured after steady state is attained in 3 to 5 half-lives. Because the drug is expected to have a half-life of 24 hours in this patient, steady-state concentration of theophylline can be measured any time after the fifth day of dosing (5 half-lives = 5 · 24 h = 120 h, or 5 d). Serum concentration of theophylline should be measured if the patient has an exacerbation of lung disease or if the patient has signs or symptoms of theophylline toxicity.

5. The initial theophylline dose for patient YU is calculated as follows.

Pharmacokinetic Dosing Method

1. *Estimate half-life and elimination rate constant according to disease states and conditions present in the patient.*

Patients with severe heart failure have highly variable theophylline pharmacokinetics and dosage requirements. Patients with heart failure have decreased cardiac output, which leads to decreased liver blood flow. The expected half-life ($t_{1/2}$) of theophylline is 24 hours. The elimination rate constant is computed with the following formula: $k = 0.693/t_{1/2} = 0.693/24\ h = 0.029\ h^{-1}$.

2. *Estimate volume of distribution and clearance.*

The patient is not obese, so the estimated volume of distribution of theophylline is based on actual body weight: $V = 0.5\ L/kg \cdot 60\ kg = 30\ L$. Estimated theophylline clearance is computed by multiplying volume of distribution by elimination rate constant: $Cl = kV = 0.029\ h^{-1} \cdot 30\ L = 0.87\ L/h$.

3. *Compute the dosage regimen.*

Oral sustained-release theophylline tablets are prescribed to this patient (F = 1, S = 1). The initial dosage interval (τ) is set to 12 hours. (Note: μg/mL = mg/L, and this concentration unit was substituted for Css in the calculations to avoid unit conversion.) The dosage equation for oral theophylline is D = (Css · Cl · τ)/(F · S) = (8 mg/L · 0.87 L/h · 12 h)/(1 · 1) = 84 mg, rounded to 100 mg every 12 hours.

Steady-state minimum serum concentration of theophylline should be measured after steady state is attained in 3 to 5 half-lives. Because the drug is expected to have a half-life of 24 hours in this patient, steady-state concentration of theophylline can be measured any time after the fifth day of dosing (5 half-lives = 5 · 24 h = 120 h, or 5 d). Serum concentration of theophylline should be measured if the patient has an exacerbation of lung disease or if the patient has signs or symptoms of theophylline toxicity. The pharmacokinetic parameters of theophylline can change as cardiac status changes. If heart failure improves, cardiac output increases. The increase in cardiac output increases liver blood flow and theophylline clearance. If heart failure worsens, cardiac output, liver blood flow, and theophylline clearance decrease. Patients with heart failure receiving theophylline must be observed carefully.

Literature-Based Recommended Dosing

1. *Choose the theophylline dose based on disease states and conditions present in the patient.*

A theophylline dose of 0.2 mg/kg per hour is suggested by Table 18-4 for an adult with severe heart failure.

2. *Compute the dosage regimen.*

Oral sustained-release theophylline tablets are prescribed to this patient (F = 1, S = 1). The initial dosage interval (τ) is set to 12 hours: D = (theophylline dose · weight · τ)/S = (0.2 mg/kg/h · 60 kg · 12 h)/1 = 144 mg, rounded to 150 mg every 12 hours. This dose is similar to that established with the pharmacokinetic dosing method, 100 mg every 12 hours.

Steady-state minimum serum concentration of theophylline should be measured after steady state is attained in 3 to 5 half-lives. Because the drug is expected to have a half-life of 24 hours in this patient, steady-state concentration of theophylline can be measured any time after the fifth day of dosing (5 half-lives = 5 · 24 h = 120 h, or 5 d). Serum concentration of theophylline should be measured if the patient has an exacerbation of lung disease or if the patient has signs or symptoms of theophylline toxicity. The pharmacokinetic parameters of theophylline can change as cardiac status changes. If heart failure improves, cardiac output increases. The increase in cardiac output increases liver blood flow and theophylline clearance. If heart failure worsens, cardiac output, liver blood flow, and theophylline clearance decrease. Patients with heart failure receiving theophylline must be observed carefully.

6. The revised theophylline dose for patient YU is calculated as follows.

The patient has severe heart failure and is expected to achieve steady-state conditions after the fifth day (5 half-lives = 5 · 24 h = 120 h, or 5 d) of therapy. Because serum theophylline concentration was measured on the third day of therapy, it is unlikely that steady state has been attained, so the linear pharmacokinetics and pharmacokinetic parameter methods cannot be used.

Bayesian Pharmacokinetics Computer Program Method

1. *Enter the patient's demographic, drug dosing, and serum concentration–time data into the computer program.*

2. *Compute pharmacokinetic parameters for the patient with a Bayesian pharmacokinetics computer program.*

The pharmacokinetic parameters computed with the program are a volume of distribution of 24.5 L, a half-life of 26.6 hours, and a clearance of 0.64 L/h.

3. *Compute the dose required to achieve the desired serum concentration of theophylline.*

The one-compartment model, first-order absorption equations used by the program to compute doses indicate that a dose of 100 mg every 12 hours will produce a steady-state theophylline concentration of 12.4 μg/mL.

7. The initial theophylline dose for patient WE is calculated as follows.

Pharmacokinetic Dosing Method

1. *Estimate half-life and elimination rate constant according to disease states and conditions present in the patient.*

The expected theophylline half-life ($t_{1/2}$) is 8 hours. The elimination rate constant is computed with the following formula: $k = 0.693/t_{1/2} = 0.693/8\ h = 0.087\ h^{-1}$.

2. *Estimate volume of distribution and clearance.*

The patient is not obese, so the estimated volume of distribution of theophylline is based on actual body weight: $V = 0.5\ L/kg \cdot 55\ kg = 28\ L$. Estimated theophylline clearance is computed by multiplying volume of distribution by elimination rate constant: $Cl = kV = 0.087\ h^{-1} \cdot 28\ L = 2.44\ L/h$.

3. *Compute the dosage regimen.*

Oral sustained-release theophylline tablets are prescribed to this patient (F = 1, S = 1), and the initial dosage interval (τ) is set to 12 hours. (Note: μg/mL = mg/L, and this concentration unit was substituted for Css in the calculations to avoid unit conversion.) The dosage equation for oral theophylline is $D = (Css \cdot Cl \cdot \tau)/(F \cdot S) = (12\ mg/L \cdot 2.44\ L/h \cdot 12\ h)/(1 \cdot 1) = 351\ mg$, rounded to 300 mg every 12 hours. (Note: dose is rounded down because of the narrow therapeutic index of theophylline.)

Steady-state minimum serum concentration of theophylline should be measured after steady state is attained in 3 to 5 half-lives. Because the drug is expected to have a half-life of 8 hours in this patient, steady-state concentration of theophylline can be measured any time after the second day of dosing (5 half-lives = 5 · 8 h = 40 h). Serum concentration of theophylline should be measured if the patient has an exacerbation of lung disease or if the patient has signs or symptoms of theophylline toxicity.

Literature-Based Recommended Dosing

1. *Choose the theophylline dose based on disease states and conditions present in the patient.*

A theophylline dose of 0.4 mg/kg per hour is suggested in Table 18-4 for an adult without other diseases or conditions that alter theophylline dosing.

2. *Compute the dosage regimen.*

Oral sustained-release theophylline tablets are prescribed to this patient (F = 1, S = 1), and the initial dosage interval (τ) is set to 12 hours: D = (theophylline dose · weight · τ)/S = (0.4 mg/kg/h · 55 kg · 12 h)/1 = 264 mg, rounded to 300 mg every 12 hours. This dose is identical to that established with the pharmacokinetic dosing method.

Steady-state minimum serum concentration of theophylline should be measured after steady state is attained in 3 to 5 half-lives. Because the drug is expected to have a half-life of 8 hours in this patient, steady-state concentration of theophylline can be measured any time after the second day of dosing (5 half-lives = 5 · 8 h = 40 h). Serum concentration of theophylline should be measured if the patient has an exacerbation of lung disease or if the patient has signs or symptoms of theophylline toxicity.

8. The revised theophylline dose for patient WE is calculated as follows.

The patient has normal cardiac and hepatic function and is expected to achieve steady-state conditions after the second day (5 half-lives = 5 · 8 h = 40 h) of therapy. Because serum theophylline concentration is measured before the third dose, it is unlikely that serum concentration is at steady state, so the linear pharmacokinetics and pharmacokinetic parameter methods cannot be used.

Bayesian Pharmacokinetics Computer Program Method

1. *Enter the patient's demographic, drug dosing, and serum concentration–time data into the computer program.*

2. *Compute pharmacokinetic parameters for the patient with a Bayesian pharmacokinetics computer program.*

The pharmacokinetic parameters computed with the program are a volume of distribution of 24.6 L, a half-life of 15 hours, and a clearance of 1.14 L/h.

3. *Compute the dose required to achieve the desired serum concentration of theophylline.*

The one-compartment model, first-order absorption equations used in the program to compute doses indicate that a dose of 150 mg every 12 hours produces a steady-state theophylline concentration of 10 μg/mL.

9. The initial theophylline dose for patient IO is calculated as follows.

Pharmacokinetic Dosing Method

1. *Estimate half-life and elimination rate constant according to disease states and conditions present in the patient.*

Patients with mild heart failure have highly variable theophylline pharmacokinetics and dosage requirements. Patients with heart failure have decreased cardiac output, which leads to decreased liver blood flow. The expected half-life ($t_{1/2}$) of theophylline is 12 hours. The elimination rate constant is computed with the following formula: $k = 0.693/t_{1/2} = 0.693/12\ h = 0.058\ h^{-1}$.

2. *Estimate volume of distribution and clearance.*

The patient is obese {IBW_{male} (in kg) = 50 kg + [2.3(Ht − 60)] = 50 kg + [2.3 (71″ − 60)] = 75 kg, where *Ht* is patient height in inches, patient >30% over IBW}, so the estimated theophylline volume of distribution is based on the ideal body weight: V = 0.5 L/kg · 75 kg = 38 L. (Note: height in inches is height in centimeters divided by 2.54.) Estimated theophylline clearance is computed by multiplying volume of distribution by elimination rate constant: $Cl = kV = 0.058\ h^{-1} \cdot 38\ L = 2.20\ L/h$.

3. *Compute dosage regimen.*

Oral sustained-release theophylline tablets are prescribed to this patient (F = 1, S = 1). The initial dosage interval (τ) is set to 12 hours. (Note: μg/mL = mg/L, and this concentration unit was substituted for Css in the calculations to avoid unit conversion.) The dosage equation for oral theophylline is D = (Css · Cl · τ)/(F · S) = (8 mg/L · 2.20 L/h · 12 h)/(1 · 1) = 211 mg, rounded to 200 mg every 12 hours.

Steady-state minimum serum concentration of theophylline should be measured after steady state is attained in 3 to 5 half-lives. Because the drug is expected to have a half-life of 12 hours in this patient, steady-state concentration of theophylline can be measured any time after the third day of dosing (5 half-lives = 5 · 12 h = 60 h). Serum concentration of theophylline should be measured if the patient has an exacerbation of lung disease or if the patient has signs or symptoms of theophylline toxicity. The pharmacokinetic parameters of theophylline can change as cardiac status changes. If heart failure improves, cardiac output increases. The increase in cardiac output increases liver blood flow and theophylline clearance. If heart failure worsens, cardiac output, liver blood flow, and theophylline clearance decrease. Patients with heart failure receiving theophylline must be observed carefully.

Literature-Based Recommended Dosing

1. *Choose the theophylline dose based on disease states and conditions present in the patient.*

A theophylline dose of 0.2 mg/kg per hour is suggested in Table 18-4 for an adult with heart failure. Because the patient is obese {IBW_{male} (in kg) = 50 kg + [2.3(Ht − 60)] = 50 kg + [2.3(71″ − 60)] = 75 kg, where *Ht* is patient height in inches, patient >30% over ideal body weight}, ideal body weight is used to compute doses. (Note: height in inches is height in centimeters divided by 2.54.)

2. *Compute the dosage regimen.*

Oral sustained-release theophylline tablets are prescribed to this patient (F = 1, S = 1). The initial dosage interval (τ) is set to 12 hours: D = (theophylline dose · weight · τ)/S = (0.2 mg/kg/h · 75 kg · 12 h)/1 = 180 mg, rounded to 200 mg every 12 hours. This dose is the same as that established with the pharmacokinetic dosing method.

Steady-state minimum serum concentration of theophylline should be measured after steady state is attained in 3 to 5 half-lives. Because the drug is expected to have a half-life of 12 hours in this patient, steady-state theophylline concentration can be measured any time after the third day of dosing (5 half-lives = 5 · 12 h = 60 h). Serum concentration of theophylline should be measured if the patient has an exacerbation of lung disease or if the patient has signs or symptoms of theophylline toxicity. The pharmacokinetic parameters of theophylline can change as cardiac status changes. If heart failure improves, cardiac output increases. The result is increased liver blood flow and theophylline clearance. If heart failure worsens, cardiac output, liver blood flow, and theophylline clearance decrease. Patients with heart failure receiving theophylline must be observed carefully.

10. The revised theophylline dose for patient IO is calculated as follows.

The patient has mild heart failure and is expected to achieve steady-state conditions after the third day (5 half-lives = 5 · 12 h = 60 h) of therapy. Because serum theophylline concentration is measured on the third day of therapy, it is unlikely that serum concentration is at steady state, so the linear pharmacokinetics and pharmacokinetic parameter methods cannot be used.

Bayesian Pharmacokinetics Computer Program Method

1. *Enter the patient's demographic, drug dosing, and serum concentration–time data into the computer program.*

2. *Compute pharmacokinetic parameters for the patient with a Bayesian pharmacokinetics computer program.*

The pharmacokinetic parameters computed with the program are a volume of distribution of 39.4 L, a half-life of 12.4 hours, and a clearance of 2.20 L/h.

3. *Compute the dose required to achieve the desired serum concentration of theophylline.*

The one-compartment model, first-order absorption equations used in the program to compute doses indicate that a dose of 300 mg every 12 hours produces a steady-state theophylline concentration of 10.2 μg/mL.

Steady-state minimum serum concentration of theophylline should be measured after steady state is attained in 3 to 5 half-lives. Because the drug is expected to have a half-life of 12 hours in this patient, steady-state concentration of theophylline can be obtained any time after the third day of dosing (5 half-lives = 5 · 12 h = 60 h). Serum concentration of theophylline should be measured if the patient has an exacerbation of lung disease or if the patient has signs or symptoms of theophylline toxicity. The pharmacokinetic parameters of theophylline can change as cardiac status changes. If heart failure improves, cardiac output increases. The result is increased liver blood flow and theophylline clearance. If heart failure worsens, cardiac output, liver blood flow, and theophylline clearance decrease. Patients with heart failure receiving theophylline must be observed carefully.

11. The initial theophylline dose for patient LG is calculated as follows.

Pharmacokinetic Dosing Method

1. *Estimate half-life and elimination rate constant according to disease states and conditions present in the patient.*

Cigarette smoke induces the enzyme systems responsible for theophylline metabolism, and the expected half-life ($t_{1/2}$) of theophylline is 5 hours. The elimination rate constant is computed with the following formula: $k = 0.693/t_{1/2} = 0.693/5\ h = 0.139\ h^{-1}$.

2. *Estimate volume of distribution and clearance.*

The patient is not obese, so estimated theophylline volume of distribution is based on actual body weight: $V = 0.5\ L/kg \cdot 69\ kg = 35\ L$. Estimated theophylline clearance is computed by multiplying volume of distribution by elimination rate constant: $Cl = kV = 0.139\ h^{-1} \cdot 35\ L = 4.87\ L/h$.

3. *Compute the dosage regimen.*

Theophylline is administered as the aminophylline dihydrate salt form (S = 0.8). (Note: μg/mL = mg/L, and this concentration unit was substituted for Css in the calculations to avoid unit conversion.) Therapy will be started by administering an intravenous loading dose of aminophylline to the patient: $LD = (Css \cdot V)/S = (8\ mg/L \cdot 35\ L)/0.8 = 350\ mg$ intravenously over 20 to 30 minutes.

Continuous intravenous infusion of aminophylline is started immediately after the loading dose is administered. (Note: μg/mL = mg/L, and this concentration unit was substituted for Css in the calculations to avoid unit conversion.) The dosage equation for intravenous aminophylline is $k_0 = (Css \cdot Cl)/S = (8\ mg/L \cdot 4.87\ L/h)/0.8 = 49\ mg/h$, rounded to 50 mg/h.

Steady-state serum concentration of theophylline should be measured after steady state is attained in 3 to 5 half-lives. Because the drug is expected to have a half-life of 5 hours in this patient, steady-state concentration of theophylline can be measured any time after the first day of dosing (5 half-lives = 5 · 5 h = 25 h). Serum concentration of theophylline should be measured if the patient has an exacerbation of lung disease or if the patient has signs or symptoms of theophylline toxicity.

Literature-Based Recommended Dosing

1. *Choose the theophylline dose based on disease states and conditions present in the patient.*

A theophylline dose of 0.7 mg/kg per hour is suggested in Table 18-4 for an adult cigarette smoker.

2. *Compute the dosage regimen.*

Theophylline is administered as the aminophylline dihydrate salt form (S = 0.8): k_0 = (theophylline dose · weight)/S = (0.7 mg/kg/h · 69 kg)/0.8 = 60 mg/h. A loading dose of aminophylline 6 mg/kg is prescribed: LD = 6 mg/kg · 69 kg = 414 mg, rounded to 400 mg of aminophylline infused over 20 to 30 minutes. Similar doses were established with the pharmacokinetic dosing method.

Serum concentration of theophylline should be measured after steady state is attained in 3 to 5 half-lives. Because the drug is expected to have a half-life of 5 hours in this patient, steady-state concentration of theophylline can be measured any time after the first day of dosing (5 half-lives = 5 · 5 h = 25 h). Serum concentration of theophylline should be measured if the patient has an exacerbation of lung disease or if the patient has signs or symptoms of theophylline toxicity.

12. The revised theophylline dose for patient LG is calculated as follows.

Linear Pharmacokinetics Method

1. *Compute the new dose to achieve the desired serum concentration.*

The patient smokes tobacco-containing cigarettes and is expected to achieve steady-state conditions after the first day (5 half-lives = 5 · 5 h = 25 h) of therapy. According to linear pharmacokinetics, the new infusion rate to attain the desired concentration should be proportional to the old infusion rate that produced the measured concentration:

$$D_{new} = (Css_{new}/Css_{old})D_{old} = [(11\ \mu g/mL)/(7.4\ \mu g/mL)]\ 50\ mg/h$$
$$= 74.3\ mg/h,\ \text{rounded to}\ 75\ mg/h$$

The new suggested infusion rate is 75 mg/h of aminophylline. A booster dose of aminophylline is computed using an estimated volume of distribution for the patient (0.5 L/kg · 69 kg = 35 L): BD = $[(C_{desired} - C_{actual})V]/S$ = [(11 mg/L − 7.4 mg/L) 35 L]/0.8 = 157 mg, rounded to 150 mg of aminophylline infused over 20 to 30 minutes. The booster dose is given before the infusion rate is increased to the new value.

Steady-state serum theophylline concentration should be measured after steady state is attained in 3 to 5 half-lives. Because the drug is expected to have a half-life of 5 hours in this patient, steady-state concentration of theophylline can be measured any time after the first day of dosing (5 half-lives = 5 · 5 h = 25 h). Serum concentration of theophylline should be measured if the patient has an exacerbation of lung disease or if the patient has signs or symptoms of theophylline toxicity.

Pharmacokinetic Parameter Method

1. *Compute pharmacokinetic parameters.*

The patient smokes tobacco-containing cigarettes and is expected to achieve steady-state conditions after the first day (5 half-lives = 5 · 5 h = 25 h) of therapy. Theophylline clearance can be computed with steady-state theophylline concentration: Cl = $[S \cdot k_0]/Css$ = [0.8 · 50 mg/h]/(7.4 mg/L) = 5.41 L/h. (Note: μg/mL = mg/L, and this concentration unit was substituted for Css in the calculations to avoid unit conversion.)

2. *Compute the theophylline dose.*

Theophylline clearance is used to compute the new aminophylline infusion rate: k_0 = (Css · Cl)/S = (11 mg/L · 5.41 L/h)/(0.8) = 74 mg/h, rounded to 75 mg/h. A booster dose of aminophylline is computed with the estimated volume of distribution for the patient (0.5 L/kg · 69 kg = 35 L): BD = [($C_{desired}$ − C_{actual})V]/S = [(11 mg/L − 7.4 mg/L)35 L]/0.8 = 157 mg, rounded to 150 mg of aminophylline infused over 20 to 30 minutes. The booster dose is given before the infusion rate is increased to the new value.

Steady-state serum theophylline concentration should be measured after steady state is attained in 3 to 5 half-lives. Because the drug is expected to have a half-life of 5 hours in this patient, steady-state concentration of theophylline can be measured any time after the first day of dosing (5 half-lives = 5 · 5 h = 25 h). Serum concentration of theophylline should be measured if the patient has an exacerbation of lung disease or if the patient has signs or symptoms of theophylline toxicity.

13. The initial theophylline dose for patient CV is calculated as follows.

Pharmacokinetic Dosing Method

1. *Estimate half-life and elimination rate constant according to disease states and conditions present in the patient.*

Patients with severe liver disease have highly variable theophylline pharmacokinetics and dosage requirements. Hepatic disease destroys liver parenchyma, where hepatic drug-metabolizing enzymes are contained. The expected half-life ($t_{1/2}$) of theophylline is 24 hours. The elimination rate constant is computed with the following formula: k = 0.693/$t_{1/2}$ = 0.693/24 h = 0.029 h^{-1}.

2. *Estimate volume of distribution and clearance.*

The patient is not obese, so estimated theophylline volume of distribution is based on actual body weight: V = 0.5 L/kg · 90 kg = 45 L. Estimated theophylline clearance is computed by multiplying volume of distribution by elimination rate constant: Cl = kV = 0.029 h^{-1} · 45 L = 1.31 L/h.

3. *Compute the dosage regimen.*

Theophylline is administered as the aminophylline dihydrate salt form (S = 0.8). (Note: μg/mL = mg/L, and this concentration unit was substituted for Css in the calculations to avoid unit conversion.) Therapy is started with administration of an intravenous loading dose of aminophylline: LD = (Css · V)/S = (10 mg/L · 45 L)/0.8 = 563 mg, rounded to 550 mg intravenously over 20 to 30 minutes.

Continuous intravenous infusion of aminophylline is started immediately after the loading dose is administered. (Note: μg/mL = mg/L, and this concentration unit was substituted for Css in the calculations to avoid unit conversion.) The dosage equation for oral theophylline is k_0 = (Css · Cl)/S = (10 mg/L · 1.31 L/h)/0.8 = 16 mg/h, rounded to 15 mg/h.

Steady-state serum theophylline concentration should be measured after steady state is attained in 3 to 5 half-lives. Because the drug is expected to have a half-life of 24 hours in this patient, steady-state concentration of theophylline can be measured any time after the fifth day of dosing (5 half-lives = 5 · 24 h = 120 h, or 5 d). Serum concentration of theophylline should be measured if the patient has an exacerbation of lung disease or if the patient has signs or symptoms of theophylline toxicity.

Literature-Based Recommended Dosing

1. *Choose the theophylline dose based on disease states and conditions present in the patient.*

A theophylline dose of 0.2 mg/kg per hour is suggested in Table 18-4 for an adult with cirrhosis.

2. *Compute the dosage regimen.*

Theophylline is administered as the aminophylline dihydrate salt form (S = 0.8): D = (theophylline dose · weight)/S = (0.2 mg/kg/h · 90 kg)/0.8 = 23 mg/h, rounded to 20 mg/h. A loading dose of aminophylline 6 mg/kg is prescribed: LD = 6 mg/kg · 90 kg = 540 mg, rounded to 550 mg of aminophylline infused over 20 to 30 minutes. These doses are similar to those established with the pharmacokinetic dosing method, a 550-mg loading dose followed by a 15-mg/h continuous infusion.

Steady-state serum theophylline concentration should be measured after steady state is attained in 3 to 5 half-lives. Because the drug is expected to have a half-life of 24 hours in this patient, steady-state concentration of theophylline can be measured any time after the fifth day of dosing (5 half-lives = 5 · 24 h = 120 h, or 5 d). Serum concentration of theophylline should be measured if the patient has an exacerbation of lung disease or if the patient has signs or symptoms of theophylline toxicity.

14. The revised theophylline dose for patient CV is calculated as follows.

The patient has cirrhosis of the liver and is expected to achieve steady-state conditions after the fifth day (5 half-lives = 5 · 24 h = 120 h, or 5 d) of therapy. Because serum theophylline concentration is measured after 72 hours of therapy, it is unlikely that serum concentration is at steady state, even though a loading dose is given, so the linear pharmacokinetics and pharmacokinetic parameter methods cannot be used.

Bayesian Pharmacokinetics Computer Program Method

1. *Enter the patient's demographic, drug dosing, and serum concentration–time data into the computer program.*

In this case, it is unlikely that the patient is at steady state, so the linear pharmacokinetics method cannot be used. DrugCalc requires that doses be entered in terms of theophylline, so aminophylline doses must be converted to theophylline doses (LD = 400 mg aminophylline · 0.8 = 320 mg theophylline; k_0 = 25 mg/h aminophylline · 0.8 = 20 mg/h theophylline).

2. *Compute pharmacokinetic parameters for the patient with a Bayesian pharmacokinetics computer program.*

The pharmacokinetic parameters computed with the program are a volume of distribution of 37 L, a half-life of 38 hours, and a clearance of 0.67 L/h.

3. *Compute the dose required to achieve the desired serum concentration of theophylline.*

The one-compartment model, infusion equations used in the program to compute doses indicate that an aminophylline infusion of 13 mg/h produces a steady-state theophylline concentration of 15 μg/mL. This dose is started after the infusion is held for 40 hours (~1 half-life) to allow serum theophylline concentration to decrease 50%.

15. The initial theophylline dose for patient PE is calculated as follows.

Pharmacokinetic Dosing Method

1. *Estimate half-life and elimination rate constant according to disease states and conditions present in the patient.*

Patients with severe heart failure have highly variable theophylline pharmacokinetics and dosage requirements. Patients with heart failure have decreased cardiac output, which leads to decreased liver blood flow. The expected half-life ($t_{1/2}$) of theophylline is 24 hours. The elimination rate constant is computed with the following formula: $k = 0.693/t_{1/2} = 0.693/24\ h = 0.029\ h^{-1}$.

2. *Estimate volume of distribution and clearance.*

The patient is not obese, so estimated theophylline volume of distribution is based on actual body weight: V = 0.5 L/kg · 67 kg = 34 L. Estimated theophylline clearance is computed by multiplying volume of distribution by elimination rate constant: $Cl = kV = 0.029\ h^{-1} \cdot 34\ L = 0.99\ L/h$.

3. *Compute the dosage regimen.*

Theophylline is administered as the aminophylline dihydrate salt form (S = 0.8). (Note: μg/mL = mg/L, and this concentration unit was substituted for Css in the calculations to avoid unit conversion.) Therapy is started with administration of an intravenous loading dose of aminophylline: LD = (Css · V)/S = (8 mg/L · 34 L)/0.8 = 340 mg, rounded to 350 mg intravenously over 20 to 30 minutes.

Continuous intravenous infusion of aminophylline is started immediately after the loading dose is administered. (Note: μg/mL = mg/L, and this concentration unit was substituted for Css in the calculations to avoid unit conversion.) The dosage equation for intravenous aminophylline is $k_0 = (Css \cdot Cl)/S = (8\ mg/L \cdot 0.99\ L/h)/0.8 = 9.9\ mg/h$, rounded to 10 mg/h.

Steady-state serum theophylline concentration should be measured after steady state is attained in 3 to 5 half-lives. Because the drug is expected to have a half-life of 24 hours in this patient, steady-state concentration of theophylline can be measured any time after the fifth day of dosing (5 half-lives = 5 · 24 h = 120 h, or 5 d). Serum concentration of theophylline should be measured if the patient has an exacerbation of lung disease or if the patient has signs or symptoms of theophylline toxicity. The pharmacokinetic parameters of theophylline can change as cardiac status changes. If heart failure improves, cardiac output increases. The result is increased liver blood flow and theophylline clearance. If heart failure worsens, cardiac output, liver blood flow, and theophylline clearance decrease. Patients with heart failure who receive theophylline must be observed carefully.

Literature-Based Recommended Dosing

1. *Choose the theophylline dose based on disease states and conditions present in the patient.*

A theophylline dose of 0.2 mg/kg per hour is suggested in Table 18-4 for an adult with severe heart failure.

2. *Compute the dosage regimen.*

Theophylline is administered as the aminophylline dihydrate salt form (S = 0.8): D = (theophylline dose · weight)/S = (0.2 mg/kg/h · 67 kg)/0.8 = 17 mg/h, rounded to 15 mg/h. A loading dose of aminophylline 6 mg/kg is prescribed: LD = 6 mg/kg · 67 kg = 402 mg, rounded to 400 mg of aminophylline infused over 20 to 30 minutes. These doses are similar to those established with the pharmacokinetic dosing method.

Steady-state serum theophylline concentration should be measured after steady state is attained in 3 to 5 half-lives. Because the drug is expected to have a half-life of 24 hours in this patient, steady-state concentration of theophylline can be measured any time after the fifth day of dosing (5 half-lives = 5 · 24 h = 120 h, or 5 d). Serum concentration of theophylline should be measured if the patient has an exacerbation of lung disease or if the patient has signs or symptoms of theophylline toxicity. The pharmacokinetic parameters of theophylline can change as cardiac status changes. If heart failure improves, cardiac output increases. The result is increased liver blood flow and theophylline clearance. If heart failure worsens, cardiac output, liver blood flow, and theophylline clearance decrease. Patients with heart failure who receive theophylline must be observed carefully.

16. The revised theophylline dose for patient PE is calculated as follows.

The patient has severe heart failure and is expected to achieve steady-state conditions after the fifth day (5 half-lives = 5 · 24 h = 120 h, or 5 d) of therapy. Because serum theophylline concentrations measured after 12 hours and 24 hours of therapy are not equal, it is unlikely that steady state has been attained, even though a loading dose was given, so the linear pharmacokinetics and pharmacokinetic parameter methods cannot be used.

Chiou Method

1. *Compute theophylline clearance.*

$$Cl = \frac{2 \cdot S \cdot k_0}{C_1 + C_2} + \frac{2V(C_1 - C_2)}{(C_1 + C_2)\,(t_2 - t_1)}$$

$$Cl = \frac{2[0.8(20\text{ mg/h})]}{14.2\text{ mg/L} + 18.6\text{ mg/L}} + \frac{2(0.5\text{ L/kg} \cdot 67\text{ kg})(14.2\text{ mg/L} - 18.6\text{ mg/L})}{(14.2\text{ mg/L} + 18.6\text{ mg/L})\ 12\text{ h}} = 0.23\text{ L/h}$$

(Note: μg/mL = mg/L, and this concentration unit was substituted for concentrations to avoid unit conversion. The difference between t_2 and t_1 was determined and placed directly in the calculation.)

$$k_0 = (Css \cdot Cl)/S = (18\ mg/L \cdot 0.23\ L/h)/0.8 = 5\ mg/h \text{ of aminophylline}$$

Bayesian Pharmacokinetics Computer Program Method

1. *Enter the patient's demographic, drug dosing, and serum concentration–time data into the computer program.*

In this case, the patient is not at steady state, so the linear pharmacokinetics method cannot be used. DrugCalc requires that doses be entered in terms of theophylline, so aminophylline doses must be converted to theophylline doses (LD = 350 mg aminophylline · 0.8 = 280 mg theophylline; k_0 = 20 mg/h aminophylline · 0.8 = 16 mg/h theophylline).

2. *Compute pharmacokinetic parameters for the patient with a Bayesian pharmacokinetics computer program.*

The pharmacokinetic parameters computed with the program are a volume of distribution of 26 L, a half-life of 31 hours, and a clearance of 0.59 L/h.

3. *Compute the dose required to achieve the desired serum concentration of theophylline.*

The one-compartment model, infusion equations used in the program to compute doses indicate that an aminophylline infusion of 14 mg/h produces a steady-state theophylline concentration of 18 μg/mL.

REFERENCES

1. Weinberger M, Hendeles L. Drug therapy: theophylline in asthma. N Engl J Med 1996;334: 1380–8.
2. COMBIVENT Inhalation Aerosol Study Group. In chronic obstructive pulmonary disease, a combination of ipratropium and albuterol is more effective than either agent alone: an 85-day multicenter trial. Chest 1994;105:1411–9.
3. Vaz Fragoso CA, Miller MA. Review of the clinical efficacy of theophylline in the treatment of chronic obstructive pulmonary disease. Am Rev Respir Dis 1993;147:S40–7.
4. Wesseling G, Mostert R, Wouters EF. A comparison of the effects of anticholinergic and beta 2-agonist and combination therapy on respiratory impedance in COPD. Chest 1992;101:166–73.
5. Konzem SL, Stratton MA. Chronic obstructive lung disease. In: DiPiro JT, Talbert RL, Yee GC, Matzke GR, Wells BG, Posey LM, eds. Pharmacotherapy: a pathophysiologic approach. New York: McGraw-Hill, 1999:460–77.
6. Kelly HW, Kamada AK. Asthma. In: DiPiro JT, Talbert RL, Yee GC, Matzke GR, Wells BG, Posey LM, eds. Pharmacotherapy: a pathophysiologic approach. New York: McGraw-Hill, 1999:430–59.
7. Serafin WE. Drugs used in the treatment of asthma. In: Hardman JG, Limbird LE, Molinoff PB, Ruddon RW, Gillman AG, eds. The pharmacologic basis of therapeutics. New York: McGraw-Hill, 1996:659–82.

8. Asthma Sepotmo. Guidelines for the diagnosis and management of asthma. NIH publication 97-4051. Bethesda, MD: National Institutes of Health, 1997:86.
9. Chang KC, Bell TD, Lauer BA, Chai H. Altered theophylline pharmacokinetics during acute respiratory viral illness. Lancet 1978;1:1132–3.
10. Koren G, Greenwald M. Decreased theophylline clearance causing toxicity in children during viral epidemics. J Asthma 1985;22:75–9.
11. Levy G, Koysooko R. Renal clearance of theophylline in man. J Clin Pharmacol 1976;16: 329–32.
12. Bauer LA, Bauer SP, Blouin RA. The effect of acute and chronic renal failure on theophylline clearance. J Clin Pharmacol 1982;22:65–8.
13. Sarrazin E, Hendeles L, Weinberger M, Muir K, Riegelman S. Dose-dependent kinetics for theophylline: observations among ambulatory asthmatic children. J Pediatr 1980;97:825–8.
14. Weinberger M, Ginchansky E. Dose-dependent kinetics of theophylline disposition in asthmatic children. J Pediatr 1977;91:820–4.
15. Tang-Liu DD, Williams RL, Riegelman S. Nonlinear theophylline elimination. Clin Pharmacol Ther 1982;31:358–69.
16. Vallner JJ, Speir WA Jr, Kolbeck RC, Harrison GN, Bransome ED Jr. Effect of pH on the binding of theophylline to serum proteins. Am Rev Respir Dis 1979;120:83–6.
17. Shaw LM, Fields L, Mayock R. Factors influencing theophylline serum protein binding. Clin Pharmacol Ther 1982;32:490–6.
18. Hunt SN, Jusko WJ, Yurchak AM. Effect of smoking on theophylline disposition. Clin Pharmacol Ther 1976;19:546–51.
19. Jusko WJ, Gardner MJ, Mangione A, Schentag JJ, Koup JR, Vance JW. Factors affecting theophylline clearances: age, tobacco, marijuana, cirrhosis, congestive heart failure, obesity, oral contraceptives, benzodiazepines, barbiturates, and ethanol. J Pharm Sci 1979;68:1358–66.
20. Jusko WJ, Schentag JJ, Clark JH, Gardner M, Yurchak AM. Enhanced biotransformation of theophylline in marijuana and tobacco smokers. Clin Pharmacol Ther 1978;24:405–10.
21. Jenne H, Nagasawa H, McHugh R, MacDonald F, Wyse E. Decreased theophylline half-life in cigarette smokers. Life Sci 1975;17:195–8.
22. Grygiel JJ, Birkett DJ. Cigarette smoking and theophylline clearance and metabolism. Clin Pharmacol Ther 1981;30:491–6.
23. Powell JR, Thiercelin JF, Vozeh S, Sansom L, Riegelman S. The influence of cigarette smoking and sex on theophylline disposition. Am Rev Respir Dis 1977;116:17–23.
24. Lee BL, Benowitz NL, Jacob PD. Cigarette abstinence, nicotine gum, and theophylline disposition. Ann Intern Med 1987;106:553–5.
25. Matsunga SK, Plezia PM, Karol MD, Katz MD, Camilli AE, Benowitz NL. Effects of passive smoking on theophylline clearance. Clin Pharmacol Ther 1989;46:399–407.
26. Mangione A, Imhoff TE, Lee RV, Shum LY, Jusko WJ. Pharmacokinetics of theophylline in hepatic disease. Chest 1978;73:616–22.
27. Staib AH, Schuppan D, Lissner R, Zilly W, von Bomhard G, Richter E. Pharmacokinetics and metabolism of theophylline in patients with liver diseases. Int J Clin Pharmacol Ther Toxicol 1980;18:500–2.
28. Piafsky KM, Sitar DS, Rangno RE, Ogilvie RI. Theophylline disposition in patients with hepatic cirrhosis. N Engl J Med 1977;296:1495–7.
29. Piafsky KM, Sitar DS, Rangno RE, Ogilvie RI. Theophylline kinetics in acute pulmonary edema. Clin Pharmacol Ther 1977;21:310–6.
30. Vicuna N, McNay JL, Ludden TM, Schwertner H. Impaired theophylline clearance in patients with cor pulmonale. Br J Clin Pharmacol 1979;7:33–7.
31. Jenne JW, Chick TW, Miller BA, Strickland RD. Apparent theophylline half-life fluctuations during treatment of acute left ventricular failure. Am J Hosp Pharm 1977;34:408–9.

32. Powell JR, Vozeh S, Hopewell P, Costello J, Sheiner LB, Riegelman S. Theophylline disposition in acutely ill hospitalized patients: the effect of smoking, heart failure, severe airway obstruction, and pneumonia. Am Rev Respir Dis 1978;118:229–38.
33. Gal P, Jusko WJ, Yurchak AM, Franklin BA. Theophylline disposition in obesity. Clin Pharmacol Ther 1978;23:438–44.
34. Blouin RA, Elgert JF, Bauer LA. Theophylline clearance: effect of marked obesity. Clin Pharmacol Ther 1980;28:619–23.
35. Slaughter RL, Lanc RA. Theophylline clearance in obese patients in relation to smoking and congestive heart failure. Drug Intell Clin Pharm 1983;17:274–6.
36. Rohrbaugh TM, Danish M, Ragni MC, Yaffe SJ. The effect of obesity on apparent volume of distribution of theophylline. Pediatr Pharmacol 1982;2:75–83.
37. Hilligoss DM, Jusko WJ, Koup JR, Giacoia G. Factors affecting theophylline pharmacokinetics in premature infants with apnea. Dev Pharmacol Ther 1980;1:6–15.
38. Giacoia G, Jusko WJ, Menke J, Koup JR. Theophylline pharmacokinetics in premature infants with apnea. J Pediatr 1976;89:829–32.
39. Aranda JV, Sitar DS, Parsons WD, Loughnan PM, Neims AH. Pharmacokinetic aspects of theophylline in premature newborns. N Engl J Med 1976;295:413–6.
40. Rosen JP, Danish M, Ragni MC, Saccar CL, Yaffe SJ, Lecks HI. Theophylline pharmacokinetics in the young infant. Pediatrics 1979;64:248–51.
41. Simons FE, Simons KJ. Pharmacokinetics of theophylline in infancy. J Clin Pharmacol 1978; 18:472–6.
42. Nassif EG, Weinberger MM, Shannon D, et al. Theophylline disposition in infancy. J Pediatr 1981;98:158–61.
43. Zaske DE, Miller KW, Strem EL, Austrian S, Johnson PB. Oral aminophylline therapy: increased dosage requirements in children. JAMA 1977;237:1453–5.
44. Loughnan PM, Sitar DS, Ogilvie RI, Eisen A, Fox Z, Neims AH. Pharmacokinetic analysis of the disposition of intravenous theophylline in young children. J Pediatr 1976;88:874–9.
45. Ginchansky E, Weinberger M. Relationship of theophylline clearance to oral dosage in children with chronic asthma. J Pediatr 1977;91:655–60.
46. Bauer LA, Blouin RA. Influence of age on theophylline clearance in patients with chronic obstructive pulmonary disease. Clin Pharmacokinet 1981;6:469–74.
47. Antal EJ, Kramer PA, Mercik SA, Chapron DJ, Lawson IR. Theophylline pharmacokinetics in advanced age. Br J Clin Pharmacol 1981;12:637–45.
48. Cusack B, Kelly JG, Lavan J, Noel J, O'Malley K. Theophylline kinetics in relation to age: the importance of smoking. Br J Clin Pharmacol 1980;10:109–14.
49. Crowley JJ, Cusack BJ, Jue SG, Koup JR, Park BK, Vestal RE. Aging and drug interactions: II. Effect of phenytoin and smoking on the oxidation of theophylline and cortisol in healthy men. J Pharmacol Exp Ther 1988;245:513–23.
50. Nielsen-Kudsk F, Magnussen I, Jakobsen P. Pharmacokinetics of theophylline in ten elderly patients. Acta Pharmacol Toxicol (Copenh) 1978;42:226–34.
51. Pokrajac M, Simic D, Varagic VM. Pharmacokinetics of theophylline in hyperthyroid and hypothyroid patients with chronic obstructive pulmonary disease. Eur J Clin Pharmacol 1987;33: 483–6.
52. Blouin RA, Bauer LA, Bustrack JA, Record KE, Bivins BA. Theophylline hemodialysis clearance. Ther Drug Monit 1980;2:221–3.
53. Slaughter RL, Green L, Kohli R. Hemodialysis clearance of theophylline. Ther Drug Monit 1982;4:191–3.
54. Levy G, Gibson TP, Whitman W, Procknal J. Hemodialysis clearance of theophylline. JAMA 1977;237:1466–7.

55. Lee CS, Peterson JC, Marbury TC. Comparative pharmacokinetics of theophylline in peritoneal dialysis and hemodialysis. J Clin Pharmacol 1983;23:274–80.
56. Lee CS, Marbury TC, Perrin JH, Fuller TJ. Hemodialysis of theophylline in uremic patients. J Clin Pharmacol 1979;19:219–26.
57. Kradjan WA, Martin TR, Delaney CJ, Blair AD, Cutler RE. Effect of hemodialysis on the pharmacokinetics of theophylline in chronic renal failure. Nephron 1982;32:40–4.
58. Hansten PD, Horn JR. Drug interactions analysis and management. Vancouver, WA: Applied Therapeutics, 1999:480.
59. Loi CM, Parker BM, Cusack BJ, Vestal RE. Aging and drug interactions: III. Individual and combined effects of cimetidine and cimetidine and ciprofloxacin on theophylline metabolism in healthy male and female nonsmokers. J Pharmacol Exp Ther 1997;280:627–37.
60. Nix DE, Di Cicco RA, Miller AK, et al. The effect of low-dose cimetidine (200 mg twice daily) on the pharmacokinetics of theophylline. J Clin Pharmacol 1999;39:855–65.
61. Hendeles L, Jenkins J, Temple R. Revised FDA labeling guideline for theophylline oral dosage forms [see comments]. Pharmacotherapy 1995;15:409–27.
62. Edwards DJ, Zarowitz BJ, Slaughter RL. Theophylline. In: Evans WE, Schentag JJ, Jusko WJ, Relling MV, eds. Applied pharmacokinetics. Vancouver, WA: Applied Therapeutics, 1992.
63. Anderson G, Koup J, Slaughter R, Edwards WD, Resman B, Hook E. Evaluation of two methods for estimating theophylline clearance prior to achieving steady state. Ther Drug Monit 1981;3:325–32.
64. Chiou WL, Gadalla MA, Peng GW. Method for the rapid estimation of the total body drug clearance and adjustment of dosage regimens in patients during a constant-rate intravenous infusion. J Pharmacokinet Biopharm 1978;6:135–51.
65. Pancorbo S, Davies S, Raymond JL. Use of a pharmacokinetic method for establishing doses of aminophylline to treat acute bronchospasm. Am J Hosp Pharm 1981;38:851–6.
66. Wandell M, Mungall D. Computer assisted drug interpretation and drug regimen optimization. Am Assoc Clin Chem 1984;6:1–11.
67. Stein GE, Haughey DB, Ross RJ, Vakoutis J. Conversion from intravenous to oral dosing using sustained-release theophylline tablets. Ann Pharmacother 1982;16:772–4.
68. Ehlers SM, Zaske DE, Sawchuk RJ. Massive theophylline overdose: rapid elimination by charcoal hemoperfusion. JAMA 1978;240:474–5.
69. Russo ME. Management of theophylline intoxication with charcoal-column hemoperfusion. N Engl J Med 1979;300:24–6.
70. Sintek C, Hendeles L, Weinberger M. Inhibition of theophylline absorption by activated charcoal. J Pediatr 1979;94:314–6.
71. Davis R, Ellsworth A, Justus RE, Bauer LA. Reversal of theophylline toxicity using oral activated charcoal. J Fam Pract 1985;20:73–4.

INDEX

B

F

G

H

NOTES

NOTES

NOTES

NOTES

NOTES

NOTES

NOTES

NOTES

NOTES

NOTES

NOTES

NOTES

NOTES

NOTES

NOTES

NOTES

NOTES

NOTES